Ferrets, Rabbits, and Rodents

Clinical Medicine and Surgery

Ferrets, Rabbits, and Rodents

Clinical Medicine and Surgery

SECOND EDITION

Includes Sugar Gliders and Hedgehogs

Katherine E. Quesenberry, DVM, Diplomate ABVP

Service Head
Avian and Exotic Pet Service
The Animal Medical Center
New York, New York

James W. Carpenter, MS, DVM, Diplomate ACZM

Professor
Zoological Medicine
Department of Clinical Sciences
College of Veterinary Medicine
Kansas State University
Manhattan, Kansas

SAUNDERS
An Imprint of Elsevier

SAUNDERS
An Imprint of Elsevier

11830 Westline Industrial Drive
St. Louis, Missouri 63146

FERRETS, RABBITS, AND RODENTS: CLINICAL MEDICINE AND SURGERY ISBN 0-7216-9377-6

Notice

Veterinary medicine is an ever-changing field. Standard safety precautions must be followed, but as new research and clinical experience broaden our knowledge, changes in treatment and drug therapy may become necessary or appropriate. Readers are advised to check the most current product information provided by the manufacturer of each drug to be administered to verify the recommended dose, the method and duration of administration, and contraindications. It is the responsibility of the licensed prescriber, relying on experience and knowledge of the patient, to determine dosages and the best treatment for each individual patient. Neither the publisher nor the author assumes any liability for any injury and/or damage to persons or property arising from this publication.

International Standard Book Number 0-7216-9377-6

Acquisitions Editor: Liz Fathman
Developmental Editor: Jolynn Gower
Publishing Services Manager: Linda McKinley
Project Manager: Judy Ahlers
Designer: Julia Dummitt

Printed in the United States of America

Last digit is the print number: 9 8 7 6 5 4 3 2

CONTRIBUTORS

Sean Aiken, DVM, MS, Diplomate ACVS
The Animal Medical Center
New York, New York

Natalie Antinoff, DVM, Diplomate ABVP
Gulf Coast Avian and Exotics
Gulf Coast Veterinary Specialists
Houston, Texas

Louise Bauck, DVM, MVSc
Alexandria Veterinary Clinic
Alexandria, Ontario, Canada

Judith A. Bell, DVM, MSc, PhD
Department of Population Medicine
Ontario Veterinary College
University of Guelph
Guelph, Ontario, Ontario

R. Avery Bennett, DVM, MS, Diplomate ACVS
Associate Professor of Surgery
Department of Small Animal Clinical Studies
School of Veterinary Medicine
University of Pennsylvania
Philadelphia, Pennsylvania

Craig Bihun, DVM, DVSc
NRC Senior Veterinarian
National Research Council
Ottawa, Ontario, Canada

Rosie Booth, BVSc
Brisbane
Queensland, Australia

Dale L. Brooks, DVM, PhD
School of Veterinary Medicine
University of California
Davis, California

Susan A. Brown, DVM
Midwest Bird & Exotic Animal Hospital
Westchester, Illinois

David A. Crossley, BVetMed, MRCVS, FAVD, Diplomate EVDC
Unit of Oral Pathology
University Dental Hospital of Manchester
Manchester, United Kingdom
Department of Surgery
Rutland House Referrals
St. Helens, United Kingdom
Department of Surgery
Animal Medical Centre Referral Services
Manchester, United Kingdom

Barbara J. Deeb, DVM, MS
All Pet Veterinary Clinic
Shoreline, Washington
Affiliate Clinical Assistant Professor
Department of Comparative Medicine
University of Washington
Seattle, Washington

Thomas M. Donnelly, BVSc, Diplomate ACLAM
Member, Warren Institute
Ossining, New York
Consultant in Laboratory Animal Medicine and Exotic Pets
New York, New York

Richard S. Funk, MA, DVM
Department of Exotic Pets
Mesa Veterinary Hospital
Mesa, Arizona

Darryl J. Heard, BVMS, PhD, Diplomate ACZM
Associate Professor of Zoological Medicine
Department of Small Animal Clinical Sciences
College of Veterinary Medicine
University of Florida
Gainesville, Florida

Stephen J. Hernandez-Divers, BVetMed, CBiol MIBiol, DZooMed, MRCVS, Diplomate RCVS Zoological Medicine, RCVS Recognised Specialist in Zoo and Wildlife Medicine
Assistant Professor of Exotic Animal, Wildlife and Zoological Medicine
Department of Small Animal Medicine and Surgery
College of Veterinary Medicine
University of Georgia
Athens, Georgia

Laurie Hess, DVM, Diplomate ABVP
The Animal Medical Center
New York, New York

Elizabeth V. Hillyer, DVM
Oldwick, New Jersey

Heidi L. Hoefer, DVM, Diplomate ABVP
West Hills Animal Hospital
Huntington Station, New York

Sharon M. Huston, DVM, Diplomate ACVIM (Cardiology)
Staff Cardiologist
Veterinary Internal Medicine and Allergy Specialists
New York, New York

Evelyn Ivey, DVM, Diplomate ABVP
Department of Clinical Studies
University of Pennsylvania
School of Veterinary Medicine
Philadelphia, Pennsylvania

Jeffrey R. Jenkins, DVM, Diplomate ABVP
Avian and Exotic Animal Hospital
San Diego, California

Amy Kapatkin, DVM, Diplomate ACVS
Assistant Professor of Orthopaedic Surgery
Department of Clinical Studies
School of Veterinary Medicine
University of Pennsylvania
Philadelphia, Pennsylvania

Andrew S. Loar, DVM, Diplomate ACVIM
Consultant, Department of Pathology
The Animal Medical Center
New York, New York

Lori Ludwig, VMD, MS, Diplomate ACVS
The Animal Medical Center
New York, New York

Douglas R. Mader, MS, DVM, Diplomate ABVP
Big Pine Key, Florida

Mark A. Mitchell, DVM, MS, PhD
Assistant Professor
Department of Veterinary Clinical Sciences
School of Veterinary Medicine
Louisiana State University
Baton Rouge, Louisiana

James K. Morrisey, DVM, Diplomate ABVP
Chief of Companion Exotic Animal Medicine Service
Department of Clinical Sciences
College of Veterinary Medicine
Cornell University
Ithaca, New York

Holly S. Mullen, DVM, Diplomate ACVS
Chief of Surgery, California Veterinary Surgical Practice
Emergency Animal Hospital and Referral Center of San Diego
San Diego, California

Michael J. Murray, DVM
Monterey, California

Robert D. Ness, DVM
Ness Exotic Wellness Center
Lisle, Illinois

Connie Orcutt, DVM, Diplomate ABVP
Angell Memorial Animal Hospital
Boston, Massachusetts

Dorcas P. O'Rourke, DVM, MS, Diplomate ACLAM
Associate Professor
Department of Comparative Medicine
College of Veterinary Medicine
University of Tennessee
Knoxville, Tennessee

Jean A. Paré, DMV, DVSc, Diplomate ACZM
Assistant Professor
Special Species Health
Department of Surgical Sciences
School of Veterinary Medicine
University of Wisconsin
Madison, Wisconsin

Joanne Paul-Murphy, DVM, Diplomate ACZM
Assistant Professor
Department of Surgical Sciences
School of Veterinary Medicine
University of Wisconsin
Madison, Wisconsin

Jean-Paul Petrie, DVM, Diplomate ACVIM (Cardiology)
Staff Cardiologist
Department of Medicine
Bobst Hospital of the Animal Medical Center
New York, New York

Christal G. Pollock, DVM, Diplomate ABVP
Clinical Assistant Professor
Zoological Medicine
Department of Clinical Sciences
College of Veterinary Medicine
Kansas State University
Manhattan, Kansas

Karen L. Rosenthal, DVM, MS, Diplomate ABVP
Clinical Assistant Professor
Director of Special Species Medicine
Matthew J. Ryan Veterinary Hospital
University of Pennsylvania
Philadelphia, Pennsylvania

Joseph D. Stefanacci, VMD, Diplomate ACVR
Radiology Department
Long Island Veterinary Specialists
Plainview, New York

Thomas N. Tully, Jr., DVM, MS, Diplomate ABVP
Professor
Department of Veterinary Clinical Sciences
School of Veterinary Medicine
Louisiana State University
Baton Rouge, Louisiana

James Walberg, DVM, Diplomate ACVP
Consultant, Department of Pathology
The Animal Medical Center
New York, New York

Charles A. Weiss, DVM
Bradley Hills Animal Hospital
Bethesda, Maryland

Bruce H. Williams, DVM, Diplomate ACVP
Department of Telemedicine
Armed Forces Institute of Pathology
Washington, District of Columbia

Alexandra van der Woerdt, DVM, MS, Diplomate ACVO, ECVO
Staff Ophthalmologist
Associate Director, Bobst Hospital of the Animal Medical Center
New York, New York

I dedicate this book with love to my husband, Robert, for his patience and support, and to my wonderful children, Zachary and Chelsea, who are the center of my world. I extend special and heartfelt thanks to my friend and colleague, Dr. Elizabeth Hillyer, who envisioned this project with me and was my co-editor on the first edition. I give a special dedication to the late Dr. Si-Kwang Liu, who was a pioneer in the field of exotic animal pathology. He never stopped teaching or learning, and he was a constant source of encouragement and inspiration during the 20 years that I was privileged to work with him at the Animal Medical Center.

KEQ

I dedicate this book to my associates in the Zoological Medicine Service at the College of Veterinary Medicine, Kansas State University, and to the 22 interns and 4 residents we have trained since 1990. Their understanding, support, and encouragement, which have allowed me to undertake projects such as this book, are greatly appreciated. In addition, I wish to thank veterinary students Gretchen Cole and Christopher J. Marion for assisting us in the preparation of this book.

Special thanks to my wife, Terry, and children, Erin and Michael, for their support during this $2^1/_2$-year project.

JWC

PREFACE

Since the first edition of this book was published, the specialty area of veterinary exotic pet practice has undergone tremendous growth. Whereas small mammal species were once considered novelty pets, many veterinarians have now incorporated these species into their general small animal practices. Increasing numbers of veterinarians now practice exclusively with exotic pets, including small mammals, birds, and reptiles. Many books, periodicals, and on-line sources pertaining to the veterinary care of these animals have become available. The information in many of these sources is excellent, whereas in others, it is anecdotal at best.

Parallel to this growth and perhaps a driving force in this change, the owners of these types of pets are no longer satisfied with simply finding a veterinarian who is willing to examine their pet. Because of the wealth of information now available at the touch of a computer keyboard, owners are much more informed and demand a higher level of care. Many will go to great lengths and travel long distances for access to the best that veterinary medicine has to offer their animals.

Just as advances in medicine and surgery have increased our capacity to help individual animals, recent outbreaks of infectious diseases such as monkeypox and SARS have re-emphasized the link between these types of animals and the broader concerns of public health. The potential of exotic and novelty pets to serve as carriers of diseases infectious to humans must be an ongoing concern to veterinarians on both an individual and a public health level.

In this second edition, we have again tried to provide a concise, reader-friendly source of information about small mammal species commonly kept as pets. In addition to ferrets, rabbits, and the more common small rodents, we have expanded the species list to include prairie dogs, sugar gliders, and African hedgehogs. Along with the more traditional small mammals kept as pets, these species are now commonly presented for veterinary care.

We have included chapters on cutting-edge topics that were just developing when the first edition was prepared. New chapters on small mammal dentistry, cardiovascular and lymphoproliferative diseases of rabbits, zoonotic diseases, endoscopy, and cytology and hematology provide much-needed information in one source that is difficult to find elsewhere. The chapters on cytology and hematology and on endoscopy include full-color plates with detailed descriptions, clearly illustrating important topics. Other chapters in the first edition have been completely updated, many written by new authors and including new and updated information.

As in the first edition, the authors reflect a broad background of expertise and interests. Included in the contributor list are practitioners, university faculty members, laboratory animal veterinarians, and board-certified specialists in such diverse fields as surgery, cardiology, ophthalmology, pathology, and zoo animal medicine. This varied group provides a wealth of information and perspectives, all tremendously instructive and helpful. We hope that you will find their viewpoints and experiences valuable.

In bringing this project together into its final form, we thank the authors for their hard work, the editors at Elsevier for their willingness and patience in working with us, and especially, Ray Kersey for supporting us so completely and in spearheading this second edition. It could not have happened without him.

KATHERINE E. QUESENBERRY
JAMES W. CARPENTER

CONTENTS

SECTION THREE
Guinea Pigs, Chinchillas, and Prairie Dogs

SECTION FOUR
Small Rodents

SECTION FIVE
Other Small Mammals

SECTION SIX
General Topics

SECTION SEVEN
Special Topics

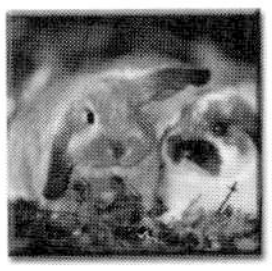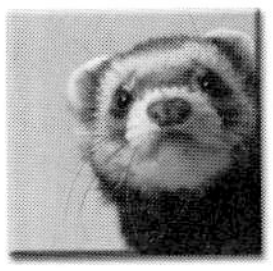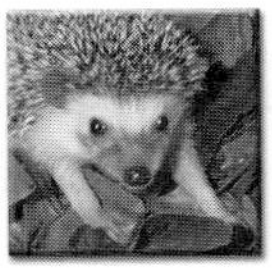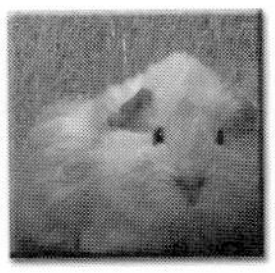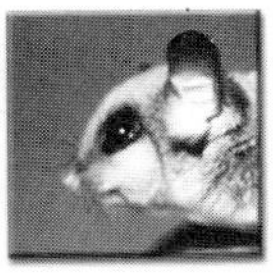

SECTION ONE

FERRETS

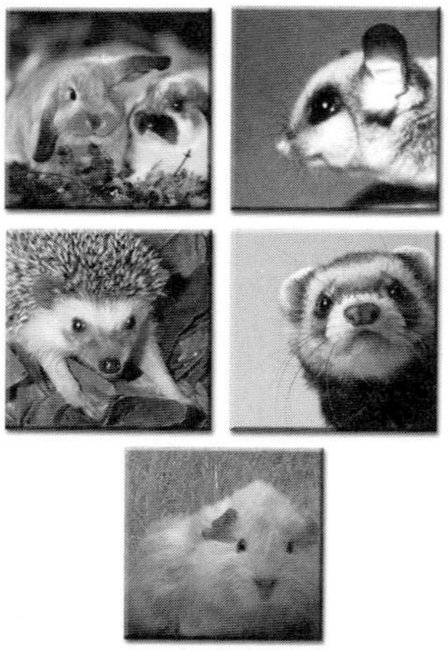

CHAPTER 1

Basic Anatomy, Physiology, and Husbandry

Susan A. Brown, DVM

"There is something about ferrets. Some people find them good working partners for a frosty morning's rabbiting. Some enjoy their individuality and admire their courage, or appreciate their affable companionship. Some react with a knowing laugh or shudder. The majority, perhaps, dismiss ferrets as smelly animals that bite and that spend much of their time down the trousers of foolhardy men. The majority are very wrong indeed."[19]

HISTORY

Ferrets belong to the family Mustelidae and are related to weasels, mink, otters, badgers, stoats, martens, and skunks. There are three species of ferrets (also known as polecats in Europe and Asia): the European polecat (*Mustela putorius*), the Steppe or Siberian polecat (*Mustela eversmanni*), and the black-footed ferret (*Mustela nigripes*). The European polecat is found in various areas from the Atlantic to the Ural mountains and dwells along the edges of woodlands and wetlands.[8] The Siberian polecat is found in Eurasia from the thirtieth to the sixtieth degree of latitude, may be larger than the European polecat, and lives primarily in open areas such as steppes, slopes of ravines, and semi-deserts.[8] The black-footed ferret is native to the prairies of North America. It almost became extinct in the wild because of habitat destruction and the decimation of its main food source, the prairie dog, from poisoning and hunting.[8] Currently, captive breeding and reintroduction programs are under way in an attempt to reestablish the black-footed ferret into its native range. It is illegal to own this endangered species.

The origin of the domestic ferret (*Mustela putorius furo*) is shrouded in mystery. The Latin name translates loosely as "mouse-eating (*mustela*) smelly (*putorius*) thief (*furo*)." This species may have originated from either the Siberian or the European polecat.[5,23] It is difficult to find archaelogic evidence of domestication, possibly because of the ferret's small skeleton, which may have deteriorated rapidly, or the lack of paraphernalia associated with the ferret. We know that European ferret kits, if taken into captivity before their eyes open, can imprint readily on human beings and become tame.[16] The first recorded reference that can be reasonably assumed to refer to a ferret is around 350 BC by Aristotole.[5,23] Ferrets were introduced into Europe possibly by the Romans or the Normans during their invasions.[10] Over the centuries, numerous references have been made to the use of ferrets in Europe, including for rodent control in homes, farms, and ships, and for hunting rabbits both for damage control and for human food.

The domestic ferret was introduced into Australia from Europe in the 1800s to control the populations of European rabbits that had been previously released.[10] Fortunately, enough other predators, such as foxes, dingoes, and hawks, preyed on the ferret so that feral populations never developed.[10] However, when they were introduced into New Zealand for the same reason in the late 1800s along with stoats and weasels, there were no predators to control their numbers.[10] Feral populations of domestic ferrets therefore developed and are still present today.[5,10] The impact of feral ferrets on native wildlife has been controversial.

The domestic ferret was probably introduced into the United States from Europe by the shipping industry in the 1700s. They may have come as pets or as hunting companions.[5,10,19]

USES

Early references to ferrets record their use for rodent or rabbit control.[5,10,19] Ferrets are efficient little predators that can bring down prey quite a bit larger than themselves and can maneuver in small spaces more effectively than cats. Ferrets were used on ships in colonial days to control the rat populations.[5] In the early 1900s, the U.S. Department of Agriculture encouraged the use of ferrets as a means of controlling rabbits, raccoons, gophers, mice, and rats around granaries and farms.[5,19] One needed only to call the local "ferret master" to bring out his ferrets, which were set loose to do their work and then recaptured to work another day. Large facilities kept their own ferrets on site. Ferrets are still used for rodent and rabbit control in some areas of Europe and Australia today. However, hunting with ferrets is prohibited in the United States.

Ferrets have long been used to hunt rabbits—not only for control, but as a food source for human beings (Fig. 1-1). "Ferreting" was a common sport in the United Kingdom and many other areas of Europe. It is still practiced today but to a much lesser degree. Ferrets are released in a rabbit warren area, where they investigate burrows and flush out rabbits. The rabbits are then caught in nets or by dogs or shot by the waiting hunter.

Domestic ferrets have been bred for their pelts. A coat made of ferret fur is referred to as *fitch*. Ferret fur never really took hold in the United States, but it still exists in a few areas of Northern Europe.

An entertainment peculiar to English pubs and still found in a few isolated areas of the United Kingdom is called *ferret-legging*. This is a sport in which a man securely ties his trouser legs closed at the ankles and then places two ferrets, each with a full set of teeth, into his trousers. He then securely ties the trousers closed at the waist. The contest is to see how long he can stand having the ferrets in his trousers. If a ferret bites, it can only be dislodged from the outside of the trousers. The record of 5 hours and 26 minutes was set by a 72-year-old Yorkshire man.[5]

Domestic ferrets have also been used to transport cables through long stretches of conduit. They have been used to string cable for oilmen of the North Sea, for camera crews, in jets, and for the telephone company.[5]

Ferrets have been used in biomedical research since the early 1900s, when they were used to study human influenza and other viral diseases.[5] Today ferrets are used in the fields of virology, reproductive physiology, anatomy, endocrinology, and toxicology.[5] Although the use of ferrets in research is very distasteful to some, much of the information gained has directly benefited the pet ferret as well.

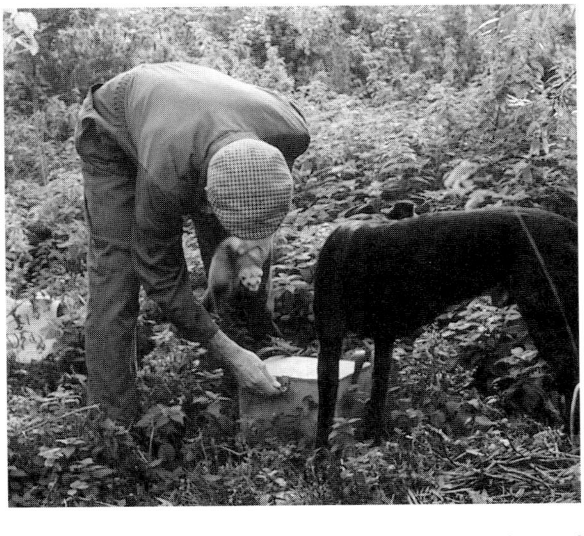

Figure 1-1 Ferreter in the United Kingdom hunting rabbits with his ferret.

The main use for ferrets today, however, particularly in the United States, is as a companion animal. Their popularity has increased dramatically over the past few decades. There has been a proliferation of ferret organizations dedicated to the well-being of this pet. It is difficult to say when the first ferret was kept strictly as a pet, but it is hard to imagine people in the distant past not feeling some attraction to the engaging personalities of this animal.

Ferrets make suitable pets for many people. They are small, clean, and very interactive with human beings and each other. However, as with all companion animals, the prospective owner should be educated on their husbandry requirements and behavior. For instance, ferrets (as with most pets) are not suitable for children younger than 6 years. Another consideration is that the majority of ferrets in the United States will likely be afflicted by one or more neoplastic diseases as they age. In addition, certain legal restrictions relate to the ownership of ferrets. Ferrets are still not considered domestic animals in most areas of the United States despite their long history. In some areas owning a ferret as a pet is illegal, and in other areas permits must be obtained for ownership.

With the advent of an approved rabies vaccine for the domestic ferret, restrictions on their use as pets have been lifted in many parts of the United States. However, in some localities, even if the ferret is appropriately vaccinated, it can be seized and destroyed if it bites a human being. Veterinarians should therefore be familiar with legislation in their localities regarding the keeping of ferrets before they engage in ferret veterinary care.

ANATOMY AND PHYSIOLOGY

The following is a brief overview of the important anatomic and physiologic features of domestic ferrets for the practitioner. The extensive literature on the anatomy and physiology of the ferret provides a more detailed discussion. The skeletal anatomy is depicted in Fig. 1-2, and the visceral anatomy is presented in Fig. 1-3, 1-4, and 1-5.

Body Morphology

Ferrets have a long tubular body with short legs; this body shape allows them to get in and out of small holes in the ground during hunting. The ferret's spine is very flexible, enabling the animal to easily turn 180 degrees in a narrow passageway. The ferret's neck is long and thick and of approximately the same diameter as the mandibular area; this anatomic feature makes it difficult for owners to use collars on their pets. Even though their legs are short and their claws are primarily used for traction and digging, ferrets can climb along surfaces such as screen or wire mesh and may reach dangerous heights.

If male ferrets are allowed to reach sexual maturity before they are neutered, their body size is normally twice that of female ferrets. This discrepancy in size is repeated throughout the mustelid family. One theory for the large size of males is that it facilitates defending their territories against other males and allows them to successfully overpower and mate with

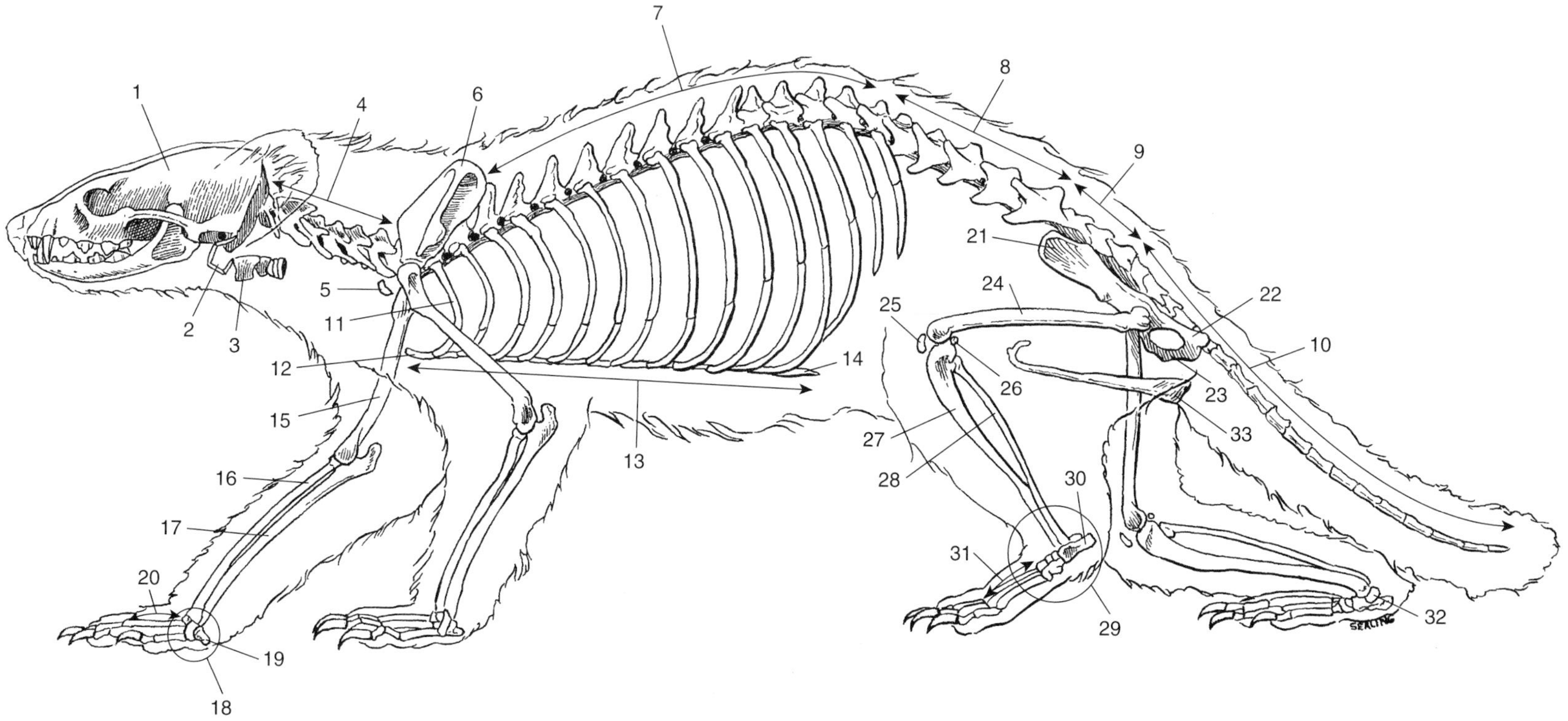

Figure 1-2 Skeletal anatomy of a ferret. *1,* Calvaria; *2,* hyoid apparatus; *3,* larynx; *4,* seven cervical vertebrae; *5,* clavicle; *6,* scapula; *7,* 15 thoracic vertebrae; *8,* five lumbar vertebrae; *9,* three sacral vertebrae; *10,* 18 caudal vertebrae; *11,* first rib; *12,* manubrium; *13,* sternum; *14,* xiphoid process; *15,* humerus; *16,* radius; *17,* ulna; *18,* carpal bones; *19,* accessory carpal bone; *20,* metacarpal bones; *21,* ilium; *22,* ischium; *23,* pubis; *24,* femur; *25,* patella; *26,* fabella; *27,* tibia; *28,* fibula; *29,* tarsal bones; *30,* calcaneus; *31,* metatarsal bones; *32,* talus; *33,* os penis. *(Adapted from An NQ, Evans HE: Anatomy of the ferret.* In *Fox JG, ed: Biology and Diseases of the Ferret. Philadelphia, Lea & Febiger, 1988, pp 14-65.)*

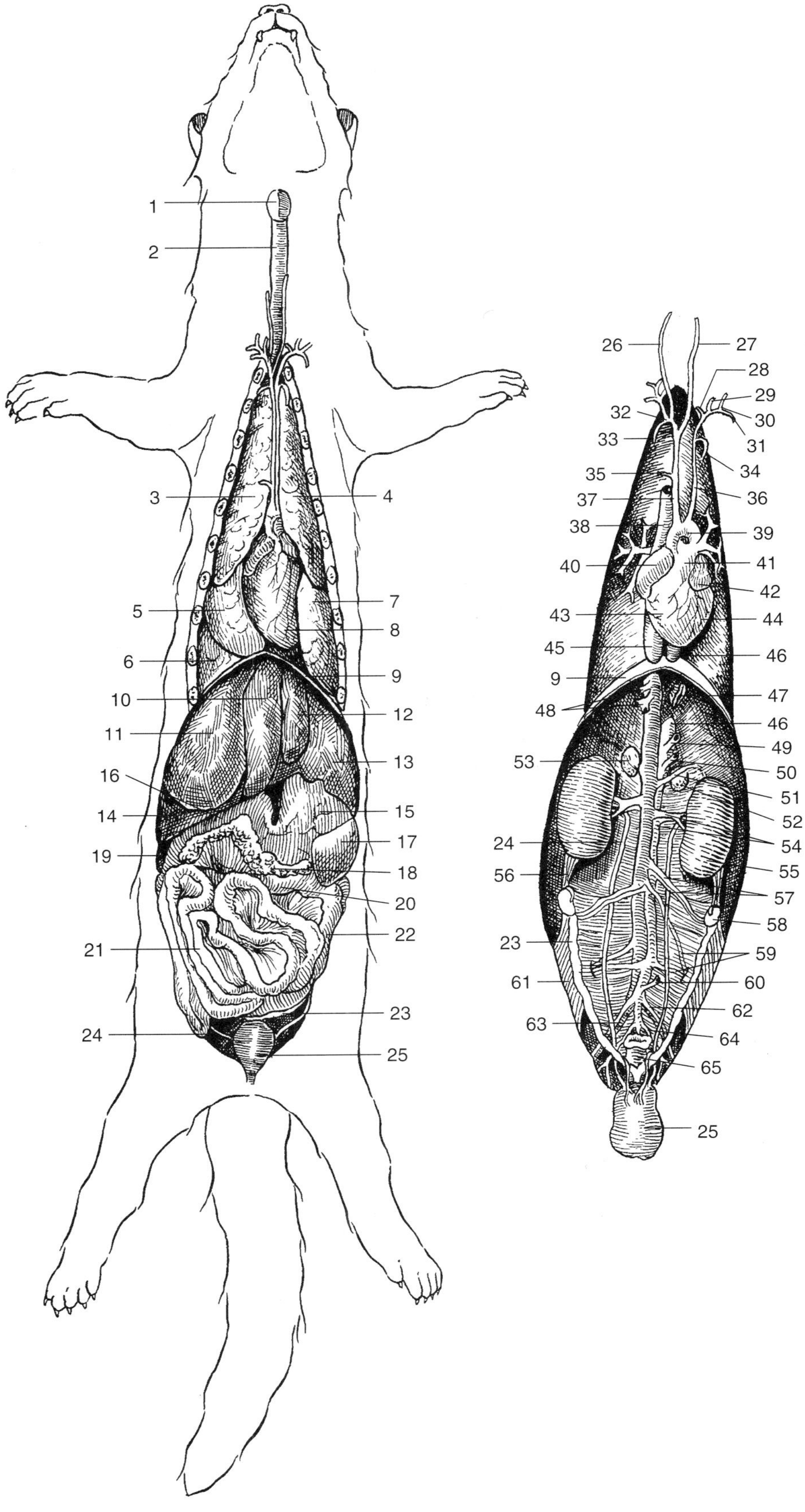

Figure 1-3 *A,* Ventral aspect of the viscera of a ferret in situ. *B,* Anatomy of the viscera and most important blood vessels as seen after removal of the lungs, liver, and gastrointestinal tract. *1,* Larynx; *2,* trachea; *3,* right cranial lobe of lung; *4,* left cranial lobe of lung; *5,* right middle lobe of lung; *6,* right caudal lobe of lung; *7,* left caudal lobe of lung; *8,* heart; *9,* diaphragm; *10,* quadrate lobe of liver; *11,* right medial lobe of liver; *12,* left medial lobe of liver; *13,* left lateral lobe of liver; *14,* right lateral lobe of liver; *15,* stomach; *16,* right kidney; *17,* spleen; *18,* pancreas; *19,* duodenum; *20,* transverse colon; *21,* jejunoileum; *22,* descending colon; *23,* uterus; *24,* ureter; *25,* urinary bladder; *26,* right common carotid artery; *27,* left common carotid artery; *28,* vertebral artery; *29,* costocervical artery; *30,* superficial cervical artery; *31,* axillary artery; *32,* right subclavian artery; *33,* right internal thoracic artery; *34,* left internal thoracic artery; *35,* branch to thymus; *36,* left subclavian artery; *37,* brachiocephalic (innominate) artery; *38,* cranial vena cava; *39,* aortic arch; *40,* right atrium; *41,* pulmonary trunk; *42,* left atrium; *43,* right ventricle; *44,* left ventricle; *45,* caudal vena cava; *46,* aorta; *47,* esophagus; *48,* hepatic veins; *49,* celiac artery; *50,* cranial mesenteric artery; *51,* left adrenolumbar vein; *52,* left adrenal gland; *53,* right adrenal gland; *54,* left renal artery and vein; *55,* left kidney; *56,* suspensory ligament of ovary; *57,* left ovarian artery and vein; *58,* left ovary; *59,* left deep circumflex iliac artery and vein; *60,* caudal mesenteric artery; *61,* broad ligament of uterus; *62,* left external iliac artery; *63,* right common iliac vein; *64,* left internal iliac artery; *65,* rectum. *(Adapted from An NQ, Evans HE: Anatomy of the ferret. In Fox JG, ed: Biology and Diseases of the Ferret. Philadelphia, Lea & Febiger, 1988, pp 14-65.)*

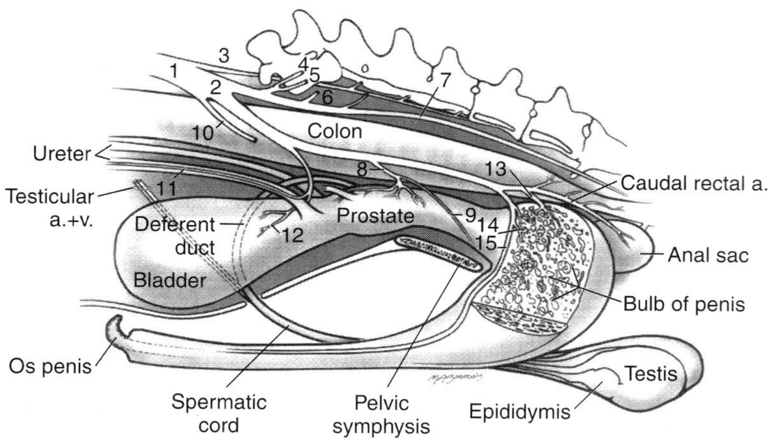

Figure 1-4 Pelvic arteries and structures of the male. *1,* Internal iliac artery; *2,* internal pudendal artery; *3,* medial sacral artery; *4,* iliolumbar artery; *5,* cranial gluteal artery; *6,* caudal gluteal artery; *7,* lateral caudal artery; *8,* prostatic artery; *9,* urethral branch; *10,* umbilical artery; *11,* ureteral branch; *12,* caudal vesicle artery; *13,* artery of the bulb; *14,* deep artery of penis; *15,* dorsal artery of penis. *(From Fox JG, ed: Biology and Diseases of the Ferret. 2nd ed. Baltimore, Williams & Wilkins, 1998, p 67.)*

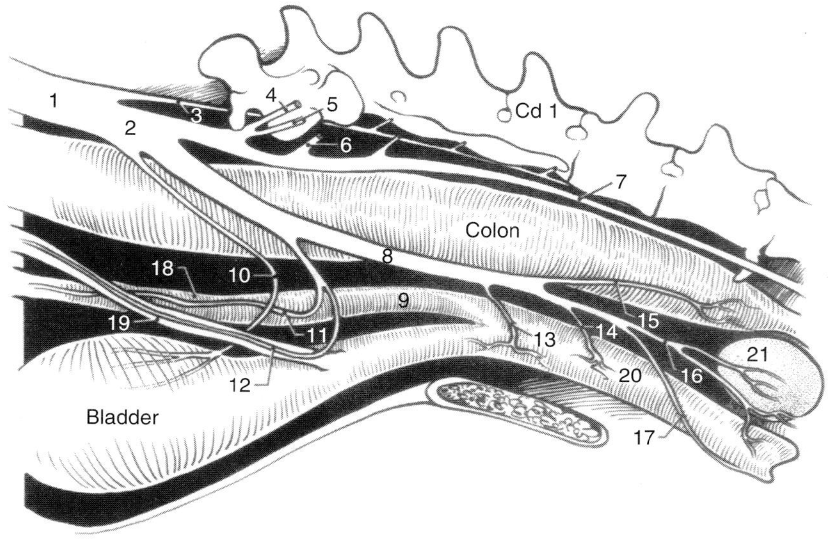

Figure 1-5 Pelvic viscera of the female (left lateral view). *1,* Internal iliac artery; *2,* internal pudendal artery; *3,* medial sacral artery; *4,* iliolumbar artery; *5,* cranial gluteal artery; *6,* caudal gluteal artery; *7,* lateral caudal artery; *8,* vaginal artery; *9,* uterine horn; *10,* umbilical artery; *11,* uterine artery; *12,* ureteral branch; *13,* urethral artery; *14,* artery to vestibular bulb; *15,* caudal rectal artery; *16,* perineal artery; *17,* artery of the clitoris; *18,* uterine horn; *19,* ureter; *20,* vagina; *21,* anal sac. *(From Fox JG, ed: Biology and Diseases of the Ferret. 2nd ed. Baltimore, Williams & Wilkins, 1998, p 64.)*

females.[13] A theory for the small size of the females suggests that because they are confined near a nest for the energy-intensive task of raising young, which they do entirely on their own, a small body size means the female needs less to feed herself and thus more of the food is available to the young.[13] In other words, the male's reproductive success may be determined by his ability to defend his territory and mate with many females, and the female's reproductive success may be determined by her ability to secure food.[13] The body weight of intact male ferrets ranges from 1 to 2 kg and that of females from 0.6 to 1 kg.[11] If neutered before weaning, female ferrets become larger and male ferrets stay smaller than intact individuals of the same sex. Ferrets neutered before sexual maturity weigh between 0.8 and 1.2 kg. Males that have been neutered early do not develop the heavy muscular neck and shoulder area that is characteristic of intact males.

Ferrets experience a normal seasonal change in body fat—that is, they lose weight in the summer and regain it in the winter. In intact animals, the weight change is most dramatic: the weight difference that occurs from season to season may be as great as 40%.

Hair Coat and Skin

The "wild" coat color of the domestic ferret most closely resembles that of the European ferret. This color is referred to as *fitch-ferret, polecat-ferret,* or *sable* and consists of black guard hair with a cream undercoat, black feet and tail, and a black mask on the face (Fig. 1-6). The other two naturally occurring colors are albino, which is denoted by yellow-white fur and unpigmented eyes, and cinnamon, which is also called *sandy.* Interestingly, the cinnamon coloring—with its beige guard hair, cream undercoat, and faint mask—closely resembles the natural coloring of the Siberian ferret. In the United States, more than 30 color variations are recognized by the American Ferret Association. Color variations include silver (dark gray guard hair with a cream undercoat and little or no mask), black-eyed white (white body hair but pigmented irises), chocolate (similar to sable but with

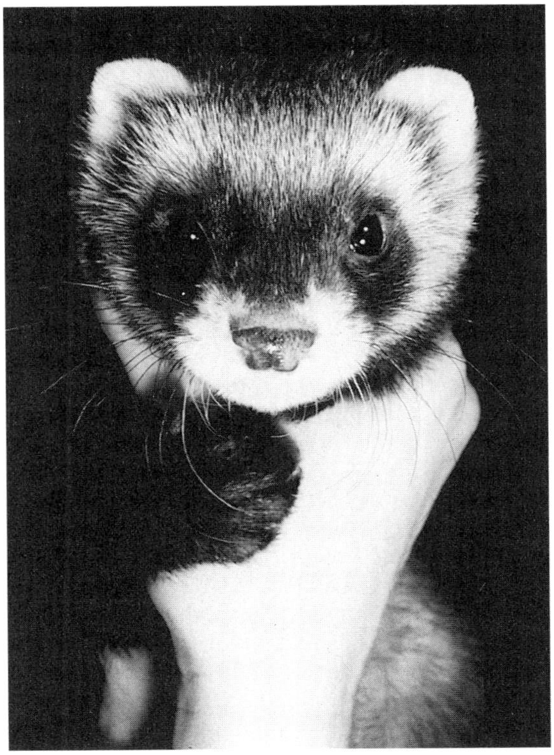

Figure 1-6 Sable coloring of a domestic ferret.

dark brown rather than black guard hair), Siamese (guard hairs that are a lighter brown than chocolate and a light-colored mask), panda (white hair on the head and shoulders and body hair of various colors), and shetland sable (sable body coloring but with a white stripe running vertically on the face from the nose to the top of the head).

Ferrets molt in the spring and the fall, concomitantly with their change in weight. The molting can be subtle or dramatic. The hair itself may vary in length from season to season, typically being shorter in the summer and longer in the fall. Hair color also may change, usually being lighter in the winter and darker in the fall. In intact females, hair loss will follow the first ovulation of the season followed by hair regrowth after successful mating.[6] The regrown hair usually is sleeker and darker then the original coat. This loss and regrowth can be repeated if more than one mating occurs during the season.[6] If a female molts the coat and does not successfully mate, areas of alopecia may result. If a ferret is in estrus when an ovariohysterectomy is performed, a new coat will grow in within a month after surgery. Neutered ferrets of either sex have a less dramatic molt and color change than intact ferrets. A large percentage of silver ferrets become black-eyed whites as they mature in years. Ferrets may lose or change their mask configuration from season to season and from year to year; for this reason, dependence on photographs alone for pet identification is unreliable. A more permanent form of identification, such as a microchip or tattoo, should be used.

The clinician should consider the hair coat cycles of the ferret when removing hair for surgery or diagnostic procedures. The hair may not grow back for weeks to months, which should be explained to the owner. In addition, the regrown hair can be a different texture or shade than the previous hair and it may suddenly appear under the skin, giving a bluish appearance that can be misinterpreted as a skin disease.

The skin of the ferret is thick, especially over the neck and shoulders where it protects the ferret during fights with other ferrets or during mating when vigorous biting of the back of the neck occurs. Healthy skin should have a smooth appearance without flakes or scales. Ferrets do not have sweat glands in their skin and thus quickly succumb to heat prostration.[14] Ferrets have very active sebaceous glands, which account for their body odor. During the breeding season, intact animals have increased sebaceous secretions; this increase results in a noticeable increase in body odor, yellow discoloration of the undercoat, and oily fur.

Ferrets have a pair of well-developed anal glands, as do all members of the mustelid family. These glands produce a serous yellow liquid with a powerful odor. Ferrets that are frightened or threatened can express their anal glands frequently but are unable to project the fluid over a long distance, as can skunks. The odor only lasts a few minutes, and as ferrets mature and become accustomed to their environment they rarely express these glands. Routine removal of the anal glands (a procedure known as *descenting;* see Chapter 12) is not necessary because the anal gland secretion is not responsible for the musky body odor of ferrets. Rather, the sebaceous secretions of the skin produce these animals' overall odor. Nevertheless, pet ferrets originating from large breeding farms in the United States are routinely descented when they are 5 to 6 weeks of age.

Special Senses

Ferrets have good binocular vision and they can see fairly well in low-light levels because their ancestors were twilight or night hunters.[21] The retina contains cones and ganglions, but it is unknown how well colors are distinguished.[21] An experiment with moving targets indicated that ferrets consistently followed and attacked the "prey" when it was moving at 25 to 45 cm/sec, which is the approximate escape speed of a mouse.[3]

Ferrets have an elaborate turbinate system like other carnivores and appear to develop their olfactory preferences for food items during the first 3 months of life. By the fourth month, when in the wild they would be leaving the nest, these preferences are set.[2] This may explain why it can be difficult to change a ferret's diet as an adult.

Skeletal System

The long narrow skull of the ferret has no suture lines in the adult.[1] The dental formula for the ferret is $2(I\frac{3}{3}\ C\frac{1}{1}\ P\frac{3}{3}\ M\frac{1}{2}) = 34$. The deciduous teeth erupt at 20 to 28 days of age, and the permanent teeth erupt at 50 to 74 days of age.[1] The upper incisors are slightly longer than the lower incisors and cover the lower ones when the mouth is closed. The canines are prominent as in other members of the order Carnivora. In some ferrets, the tips of the upper canines extend beyond the most ventral portion of the chin. The canine roots are longer than the crown; this fact must be considered when extraction is necessary. Upper premolars 1 and 2 and all three of the lower premolars have two roots. The third upper premolar, or carnassial tooth, and the first upper molar have three roots. The second lower molar is very tiny and has only one root.[1]

The ferret's long, flexible spine has a vertebral formula of C7, T15, L5 (6 or 7), S3, Cd18.[1] Ferrets normally have 15 pairs of ribs (occasionally 14), and some ferrets have 14 on one side and 15 on the other.[1] The first 10 ribs are attached to the sternum, and the remaining 4 to 5 become the costal arch. In ferrets, the thoracic inlet is bordered by the first pair of ribs and the sternum and is very small.[1] The presence of anterior thoracic masses or megaesophagus can result in dysphagia or dyspnea.

Each of the ferret's four feet has five clawed digits. The first digit on each foot has only two phalanges, whereas each of the other digits has three.[1] The claws are not retractable as in cats and thus must be trimmed periodically. Ferrets should not routinely be declawed, in part because this causes difficulty with traction.

Thoracic Cavity and Pharyngeal Anatomy

The heart lies approximately between the sixth and eighth ribs. It is cone shaped, and, on a ventrodorsal view of the chest, its apex is directed to the left of midline.[1] The ligament that connects the heart to the sternum can be surrounded by a varying amount of fat. On lateral radiographic views, this gives the impression that the heart shadow is raised above the sternum. Loss of this raised effect (i.e., the heart shadow is in direct contact with the sternum) is one of the early signs of cardiac enlargement.

The lungs of the ferret have six lobes. The left lung is composed of two lobes—the left cranial and the left caudal lobes; the right lung is composed of four lobes—the right cranial, the right middle, the right caudal, and the accessory lobes.[1]

The thymus can vary in size depending on the age of the ferret. It can be quite prominent in the young ferret and is found within the thoracic inlet in the cranial mediastinum.[1] In my experience, it can be a common site of neoplasia presenting with a prominent cranial mediastinal mass in ferrets younger than 1 year.

The anatomy of the major arteries exiting the aorta in the direction of the head is unusual. In place of bilateral carotid arteries, ferrets have a single central artery, the innominate artery or the brachiocephalic artery, that exits the aortic arch just proximal to the left subclavian artery. The brachiocephalic artery divides into the left carotid, the right carotid, and the right subclavian arteries at the level of the thoracic inlet. This central artery may be an anatomic adaptation that allows the ferret to maintain blood flow to the brain while it turns its head 180 degrees.[22]

Ferrets have five pairs of salivary glands: the parotid, the zygomatic, the molar, the sublingual, and the mandibular.[1] Mucoceles are uncommon in ferrets. The mandibular lymph node lies cranial to the mandibular salivary gland and closer to the angle of the jaw. This lymph node can become enlarged, particularly in some cases of lymphoma, and thus may be confused with the salivary gland. A fine-needle aspirate of the mass should be obtained and examined to cytologically differentiate the two.

Abdominal Viscera

The ferret spleen varies greatly in size, depending on the animal's age and state of health. The spleen is located along the greater curvature of the stomach and is attached to the stomach and liver by the gastrosplenic ligament.[1] The caudal splenic tip can be located anywhere from the cranial pole of the left kidney to the caudal pole of the right kidney, depending on its size. When enlarged, the spleen extends in a diagonal fashion from the upper left to the lower right of the abdominal cavity.

The ferret's relatively large liver is composed of six lobes. The pear-shaped gallbladder is located between the quadrate lobe and the right medial lobe.[1] The opening of the bile duct is located in the duodenum in common with the pancreatic duct[1] (see Fig. 12-6). The pancreas is V shaped with a right and left limb connected at the midline near the pylorus.[1] The right limb is longer than the left and extends along the descending part of the duodenum. The left limb extends along an area between the stomach and the spleen.[1] Ferrets have a simple stomach that can expand greatly to accommodate large amounts of food.[1] It fits into the curve of the liver in the cranial abdomen. The pylorus is well developed and is easily distinguished grossly. Ferrets have the ability to vomit but do not always do so in the presence of gastric foreign bodies. Before vomiting, a ferret will back up, hold its head low, squint its eyes, and salivate excessively.

The small intestine is short, approximately 182 to 198 cm in length.[1] This length results in a short gastrointestinal transit time of about 3 to 4 hours in the adult animal.[4] The gut flora is simple, and therefore gastrointestinal upset with use of antibiotics is rare.[4] The ileum and jejunum are indistinguishable on gross examination. Ferrets do not have a cecum or ileocolonic valve. The large intestine of the ferret is approximately 10 cm in length.[1]

The adrenal glands (Fig. 1-7) of ferrets older than 2 years are frequently affected by disease. The left adrenal gland lies in fatty tissue just medial to the cranial pole of the left kidney. It is approximately 6 to 8 mm in length and is usually crossed by the adrenolumbar vein on the ventral surface.[9] Two or more branches of the left adrenolumbar artery supply blood. The right adrenal gland lies more dorsal than the left and is covered by the caudate lobe of the liver. It is intimately attached to the

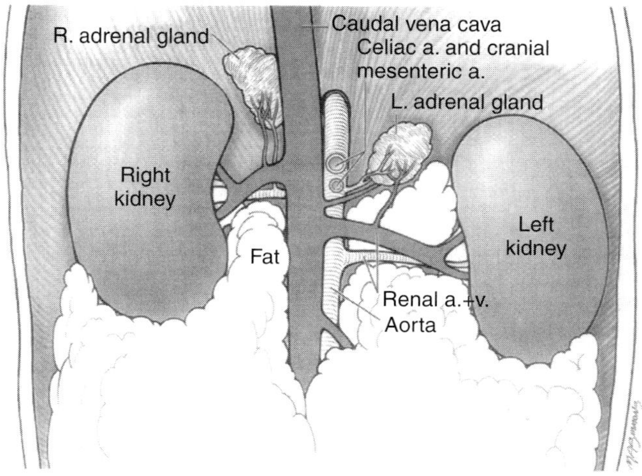

Figure 1-7 Ventral view of the abdominal cavity showing the arterial supply and venous drainage of the kidneys and adrenal glands. *(From Fox JG, ed: Biology and Diseases of the Ferret. 2nd ed. Baltimore, Williams & Wilkins, 1998, p 60.)*

caudal vena cava. The caudal vena cava may lie over part or all of the gland. The right adrenal gland is slightly larger than the left one and is longer, approximately 8 to 11 mm in length.[9] In another study, the adrenal gland length in females ranged from 5.0 to 10.0 mm for the left and 5.0 to 10.0 mm for the right; in males, it was 7.0 to 10.5 mm for the left and 7.5 to 13.5 for the right.[15] The right adrenal gland is supplied by three to five separate vessels that come from a combination of the right renal artery, the right adrenolumbar artery, and the aorta.[9] In two studies, accessory nodules of adrenal cortical tissue were found in 11 of 135 ferrets and 10 of 26 ferrets, respectively.[9,15] The accessory adrenal tissue was usually found either embedded in or adjacent to the adrenal gland.[15]

Urogenital Tract

The right kidney lies cranial to the left kidney in the retroperitoneal fat. The cranial end of the right kidney is covered by the caudate lobe of the liver. The bladder is small and easily holds 10 mL of urine at a low pressure.[21]

Male ferrets have a small prostate gland that is located at the base of the bladder and surrounds the urethra.[1] When the prostate is grossly enlarged, as in the presence of paraurethral or prostatic cysts, it appears on lateral radiographic views as a round mass just dorsal to the neck of the bladder. Male ferrets have a J-shaped os penis, which can complicate urethral catheterization.

Female ferrets have paired ovaries located just caudal to the kidneys and attached to the wall of the abdominal cavity by the broad ligament and by the suspensory ligament.[1] The uterus is bicornate with a short body and one cervix, similar to the cat uterus. The vulva becomes extremely enlarged during estrus.

Physiologic Values

Physiologic values for domestic ferrets are presented in Table 1-1.

TABLE 1-1
Selected Physiologic Values for Domestic Ferrets[7,11]

Parameter	Normal Values
Body weight, intact male	1-2 kg
Body weight, intact female	0.6-1.0 kg
Body weight, neutered; both sexes	0.8-1.2 kg
Life span	5-11 yr
Sexual maturity	6-12 mo of age
Gestation period	41-43 days
Litter size	1-18 kits, average 8
Normal weight at birth	6-12 g
Eyes and ears open	32-34 days
Weaning age	6-8 wk
Body temperature	37.8-40°C (100-104°F)
Average blood volume	Mature male, 60 mL; mature female, 40 mL
Heart rate	200-400 beats/min
Respirations	33-36 breaths/min
Urine volume	26-28 mL/24 hr
Urine pH	6.5-7.5

HUSBANDRY

The following discussion of husbandry is an overview of the keeping of ferrets as pets. A wealth of information is now available on all these topics, providing more details. The literature also contains ample information about maintaining ferrets as laboratory animals; thus this topic is not addressed here.

Behavior

The domestic ferret maintains the physiology and behavior of its predator ferret ancestors. Domestication has made ferrets unafraid of human beings and able to handle new environments without fear. The alertness for danger among feral relatives also is decreased.[16] In addition, their ancestors are solitary animals that do not interact with others except to mate. Ferrets, on the other hand, appear to be able to live in communal groups peacefully, particularly if neutered. Ferrets still maintain the instinctive behaviors for play, territory marking, and hunting.

Aggressive play behavior can serve as a tool to teach aggression and protection skills as well as hunting skills. Aggressive play begins at around 6 weeks of age and eventually merges into more serious adult aggressive behavior as ferrets mature.[17] Ferrets will still exhibit bouts of play behavior as adults, particularly during courtship or within their familiar group. Serious aggression occurs primarily when strangers are introduced or during periods when the animal feels fearful. Neck biting by both sexes is the most common aggressive and play behavior seen.[17] This behavior is also used by males to control females during mating. Ferrets have very thick skin over the back of the neck and they can sustain very aggressive biting without serious injury. In addition, the neck bite serves to quickly kill prey when used in hunting. Other offensive aggressive behaviors include lunging, sideways attack, dancing, and a staccato clucking sound.[18] Defensive threats include hissing, screaming, and snapping of the jaws.[18] A ferret scream can be quite loud, high-pitched, and alarming, but it is associated with fear and not pain.[18] To minimize biting among ferrets, a bitter-tasting product can be applied to the necks of ferrets. This type of product is also helpful when sprayed on an owner's hands, feet, or shoes to prevent nipping by a playful pet.

The polecat ancestors of the ferret lived in underground burrows. They usually took over other animals' burrows and then modified them by digging additional entryways and rooms.[20] In the home, the domestic ferret thoroughly enjoys digging in soft materials, including carpeting, furniture stuffing, and litter box material. Ferrets also appreciate being able to explore tunnel-like areas and having an enclosed sleeping area. Polecats are very fastidious about their dens and never defecate or urinate in or near the burrow. They use urine, stool, and anal gland secretions to mark their territory. Ferrets, like the polecats, prefer to back up to a vertical surface to defecate or urinate and then proceed to leave their scent with anal gland secretions by dragging their anus over the surrounding area.[20] In addition, an intact male ferret may mark his territory by rubbing his abdomen or side around the perimeter, leaving the scent of skin oils in the area.[18]

Ferrets appear to use olfactory clues rather then visual clues when searching for prey.[3] However, once the prey is located they are stimulated by a range of movement somewhere between 25 and 45 cm/sec, which is the escape speed of a small rodent.[3] In addition, ferrets learn to attack the neck area of the prey as they experience success with an efficient kill.[3] Ferrets in the home like to run after and sometimes grab moving targets such as feet, objects rolling across the floor, and other pets.

Because they are close to the ground, ferrets spend a great deal of time with their noses to the floor investigating their environment. This behavior results in the inhalation of dust and debris and subsequent sneezes. A ferret's sneeze, which is very loud and sounds like a combination of a cough and a sneeze, may be alarming to its owner. Unless sneezing is frequent or associated with other clinical signs, owners need not be concerned.

Reproduction

Ferrets are easily sexed. The preputial opening in the male ferret is located on the ventrum, as in male dogs, just caudal to the umbilical area. The os penis is readily palpable. In female ferrets, the urogenital opening is located in the perineal region ventral to the anus. The urogenital opening looks like a slit in nonestrous females; during estrus, the vulva becomes swollen and protuberant, appearing like a doughnut of tissue.

Both male and female reproductive cycles are controlled by the photoperiod; they become fertile as the days get longer.[6] The natural breeding season for ferrets in the northern hemisphere is from March to August. Under artificial lighting conditions, they can be induced to breed year-round.[6] Spermatogenic activity occurs in the seminiferous tubules from December to July, and the testicles enlarge during this time. In addition, both sexes have an increase in the intensity of the odor of the skin oils and urine during the fertile period. White ferret fur becomes yellow with these oily secretions.

Female ferrets are seasonally polyestrous and induced ovulators. Ovulation occurs 30 to 40 hours after copulation. Copulation is a noisy, violent affair in which the male ferret grasps the female by the neck and drags her around, repeatedly mating with her. If the female is receptive, she will become limp in his grasp. The normal gestation is 41 to 43 days, and the female raises the kits entirely on her own. Pregnancy can be determined at around 14 days with gentle palpation or ultrasound. If fertilization does not occur, pseudopregnancy lasting 41 to 43 days will result. If not bred, females can stay in estrus indefinitely unless the photoperiod changes, she is bred, she is treated with hormones, or she dies from hyperestrogenism. (See Chapter 4 for a discussion of this disease.)

The kits are born blind and deaf, with a thin coat of white hair. By about 3 days of age, the hair starts to change color unless the kit is an albino. Kits start moving around actively and can eat soft food by 21 days of age, even before their eyes are open. The eyes and ears open at 32 to 34 days of age and they are weaned at 6 to 8 weeks. It is very difficult to raise neonate orphaned kits.

Housing

Ferrets can be housed either indoors or outdoors depending on the climatic conditions of the area. Ferrets are intelligent, curious animals that should not be continuously confined in a small cage. Pets need a safe play area where they can investigate a variety of objects, such as boxes, bags, and plastic pipes. Ferrets should be allowed a minimum of 2 hours a day of exercise. Lewington[12] has an extensive description of an entire "ferretarium" and other outside enclosures for ferrets that are rich in environmental stimuli.

A play or living area for ferrets must first be "ferret proofed"—that is, all holes to the outside or to areas from which the ferrets cannot be retrieved must be blocked off. In addition, ferrets like to burrow into the soft foam rubber of furniture and mattresses. Owners should be advised to cover the bottom of all couches, chairs, and mattresses with a piece of thin wood or hardware cloth. The burrowing is not only destructive but also potentially life threatening because ferrets may swallow the foam rubber and develop gastrointestinal obstructive disease. Reclining chairs have been implicated in the deaths of many ferrets and should be removed from the environment. In addition, all access to any foam or latex rubber items, such as dog and cat toys, athletic shoes, rubber bands, stereo speakers and headphones, and pipe insulation, should be eliminated. Ferrets will often chew these substances, and ingestion of rubber foreign bodies is the most frequent cause of gastrointestinal obstruction, particularly in ferrets younger than 1 year.

Up to two ferrets can use a wire cage of 24 × 24 × 18 inches in height as a home base when it is necessary to confine them. The floor can be either solid or wire. Glass tanks are not suitable for caging ferrets because they provide poor ventilation. Custom-built wooden cages can also be used, but care must be taken to protect corners, the lower third of walls, and the floor from contamination with urine. If ferrets are kept outdoors, a portion of the cage should be shaded for protection from extremes of heat and cold and a well-insulated nest box should be provided. They do not tolerate temperatures above 90°F (32°C), especially in the presence of high humidity, and may need to be brought indoors. In climates where the temperature drops below 20°F (−7°C), a heated shelter is necessary. When caring for ferrets in a clinical setting, ensure that cages are escape proof. Ferrets have been known to squeeze between the bars of a standard dog or cat hospital cage.

Ferrets need a dark, enclosed sleeping area. This is essential in the clinical setting as well because the patient may become more anxious and stressed if denied access to such a "safe" area. Towels, old shirts, and cloth hats can be used in addition to specific products designed for ferrets to sleep in, such as cloth tubes and tents. For the occasional ferret that insists on eating its cloth sleeping material, use a small cardboard, plastic, or wooden box with an access hole cut into it. Some owners use slings, hammocks, or shelves that are built into the cage to provide additional sleep and play areas. In a multiple-ferret household, at least one sleep area should be provided per ferret.

Toys for ferrets should not include any latex rubber toys intended for dogs or cats. Instead, paper bags, cloth toys for cats or babies, or hard plastic or metal toys can be used. Ferrets love to run through cylindrical objects, such as polyvinyl chloride pipe, large mailing tubes, and dryer vent tubing; these items make good toys and promote exercise.

Ferrets can be trained to use a litter box relatively easily. Because ferrets like to back up in corners to defecate or urinate, the litter box sides should be high enough to contain the excreted material. Pelleted litter material is recommended instead of clay or clumping litter. Because of the ferret's short digestive transit time, the pet may not always reach the cage to use the litter box if it is not close by. Therefore owners should be advised to have several litter boxes available in various rooms of the house for use by the pet when it is uncaged.

Nutrition

Ferrets are strict carnivores that are designed to eat whole, small prey animals. Their polecat ancestors would bring their kill home and store the excess in the den and eat small frequent meals rather then gorging.[4] They have a very short gastrointestinal tract with minimal gut flora and few brush border enzymes, so they cannot use carbohydrates efficiently or digest fiber.[4] Ferrets in nature would only encounter carbohydrates as found in the partially digested stomach contents of their prey. Ferrets should therefore be fed a diet high in fat for energy, high in good-quality meat protein, and minimal carbohydrate and fiber. A whole prey diet or a balanced fresh or freeze-dried carnivore diet is the most appropriate for a ferret, and such diets are currently fed in some areas of the world. Disease-free sources of prey food such as chicks, mice, and rats are now available in many areas thanks to the reptile market, which uses these foods for carnivorous pets. The stools of a ferret on a whole prey diet are very firm and of low volume.

The most common diet fed to pet ferrets in the United States is dry kibble. Although there have been advancements in dry ferret food formulation, these diets still contains high levels of grain, which is necessary to hold the food in its solid shape. Very high levels of plant proteins in the diet can lead to urolithiasis.[4] Furthermore, excess dietary carbohydrates can affect the pancreas and may contribute to disease of the beta cells. Unfortunately, ferrets seem to enjoy sweet foods, and some commercial pet food companies have capitalized on this preference by producing ferret treats that are little more than sugar-coated grains. These treat foods are particularly dangerous to the health of the pet ferret. The stools of a ferret eating a dry kibble diet is formed but soft, voluminous, and may contain visible undigested grain.

If a dry diet is fed to the ferret, the owner should read the diet ingredients carefully. The crude protein should be 30% to 35% and composed primarily of high-quality meat sources, not grains; the fat content should be 15% to 20%.[4] Dry food ingredients are listed on the label in descending order of their amount in the product. The first three ingredients of a ferret diet should be meat products. Because the diet is dry, it can be left out at all times. However, the ferret may establish stashes of food around the house, mimicking the storage of extra prey in its ancestral den. Growing kits need 35% protein and 20% fat, and lactating females require 20% fat and twice the calories of the nonpregnant ferret.[4]

Acceptable supplemental foods to a dry diet include fresh raw organ or muscle meat and raw egg. It is not necessary to cook the meat or eggs if they are fresh and are suitable for human consumption. Omega-3 oils, fish oils, or meat fat can be added to increase the fat content of the diet provided these additions are not allowed to become rancid. Dairy products have also been used as a fat and protein supplement, but some ferrets develop soft stools when fed these products. Even though ferrets enjoy eating fruits, they should be avoided because owners often overfeed these items, leading to a reduction in the consumption of a healthier diet and the overfeeding of sugars and fiber. Ferrets develop their dietary preferences by 4 months of age; therefore changing an adult ferret's diet can be difficult without some innovation.

Because of the short gastrointestinal transit time, fasting a ferret for longer than 3 hours is not necessary to check the fasting blood glucose level. Six hours is more than sufficient to empty the gastrointestinal tract for surgery. Ferrets older than 2 years in the United States are prone to develop insulinoma, and a longer fast could result in a serious hypoglycemic condition.

Water should always be available in either a sipper bottle or a heavy crock-type bowl. Ferrets love to play in the water, so the bowl should not be easy to overturn. Supplements should not be added to the ferrets' water supply.

REFERENCES

1. An NQ, Evans HE: Anatomy of the ferret. *In* Fox JG, ed. Biology and Diseases of the Ferret, 2nd ed. Baltimore, Williams & Wilkins, 1998, pp 19-69.
2. Apfelbach R: Olfactory sign stimulus for prey selection in polecats. Zeitschrift fur Tierpsychol 1973; 33:270-273.
3. Apflebach R, Wester U: The quantitative effect of visual and tactile stimuli on the prey-catching behaviour of ferrets (*Putorius furo* L.). Behav Processes 1977; 2:187-200.
4. Bell JA: Ferret nutrition. Vet Clin North Am Exotic Anim Pract 1999; 2:169-192.
5. Fox JG: Taxonomy, history, and use. *In* Fox JG, ed. Biology and Diseases of the Ferret, 2nd ed. Baltimore, Williams & Wilkins, 1998, pp 3-18.
6. Fox JG, Bell JA: Growth, reproduction, and breeding. *In* Fox JG, ed. Biology and Diseases of the Ferret, 2nd ed. Baltimore, Williams & Wilkins, 1998, pp 211-227.
7. Fox JG: Normal clinical and biologic parameters. *In* Fox JG, ed. Biology and Diseases of the Ferret, 2nd ed. Baltimore, Williams & Wilkins, 1998, pp 183-210.
8. Grzimek B, ed: Grzimek's Encyclopedia of Mammals, Vol 3. New York, McGraw-Hill, 1990, pp 401-405.
9. Holmes RL: The adrenal glands of the ferret, *Mustela putorius*. J Anat 1961; 95:325-339.
10. Lewington JH: Classification, history and current status of ferrets. *In* Ferret Husbandry, Medicine & Surgery. Oxford, Butterworth-Heinemann, 2000, pp 3-9.
11. Lewington JH: External features and anatomy profile. *In* Ferret Husbandry, Medicine & Surgery. Oxford, Butterworth-Heinemann, 2000, pp 10-25.
12. Lewington JH: Accommodation. *In* Ferret Husbandry, Medicine & Surgery. Oxford, Butterworth-Heinemann, 2000, pp 26-53.
13. MacDonald D: The Velvet Claw: A Natural History of the Carnivores. London, BBC Books, 1992, pp 211-215.
14. Moody KD, Bowman TA, Lang CM: Laboratory management of the ferret for biomedical research. Lab Anim Sci 1985; 35:272-279.
15. Neuwirth L, Collins B, Calderwood-Mays M, et al: Adrenal ultrasonography correlated with histopathology in ferrets. Vet Radiol Ultrasound 1997; 38:69-74.
16. Poole TB: Some behavioral differences between the European polecat, *Mustela putorius*, the ferret, *Mustela furo*, and their hybrids. J Zool 1972; 166:25-35.

17. Poole TB: Aggressive play in polecats. Symp Zool Soc Lond 1966; 18:23-44.
18. Poole TB: Aspects of aggressive behavior in polecats. Zeitschrift fur Tierpsychol 1967; 24:351-364.
19. Porter V, Brown N: The Complete Book of Ferrets. London, Pelham Books, 1987.
20. Sleeman P: Stoats & Weasels, Polecats & Martens. London, Whittet Books, 1989, pp 67-70.
21. Whary MT, Andrews PLR: Physiology of the ferret. *In* Fox JG, ed. Biology and Diseases of the Ferret. 2nd ed. Baltimore, Williams & Wilkins, 1998, pp 103-148.
22. Willis LS, Barrow MV: The ferret *(Mustela putorius furo* L.*)* as a laboratory animal. Lab Anim Sci 1971; 21:712–716.
23. Zeuner FE: A History of Domesticated Animals. New York, Harper & Row, 1963, pp 401-403.

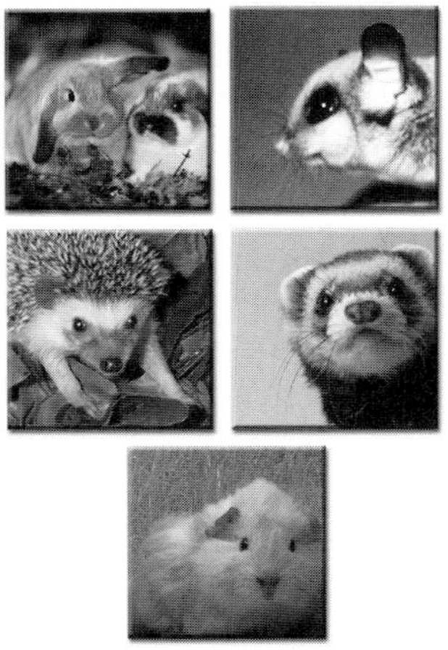

CHAPTER 2

Basic Approach to Veterinary Care

Katherine E. Quesenberry, DVM, Diplomate ABVP, and
Connie Orcutt, DVM, Diplomate ABVP

Ferrets can easily be accommodated in an existing small animal veterinary practice. Special equipment needs are minimal, and the approach to handling ferrets is similar in many ways to that for dogs and cats. Ferret owners regularly seek veterinary care for a variety of reasons: ferrets need preventive vaccinations for canine distemper and rabies; ferret owners generally are very attuned to their pets and are responsible pet owners; ferrets have a relatively short life span compared with that of cats and dogs; ferrets in the United States have a high incidence of endocrine, gastrointestinal, and neoplastic diseases, especially middle-aged and geriatric ferrets; and many of the diseases common to ferrets are not easily ignored by the pet owner (e.g., alopecia resulting from adrenal disease and hypoglycemic episodes caused by insulinoma).

RESTRAINT AND PHYSICAL EXAMINATION

Restraint

Most ferrets are docile and can be easily examined without assistance. However, an assistant is usually needed when taking the rectal temperature, when administering injections or oral medications, or if an animal has a tendency to bite. Young ferrets often nip, and nursing females and ferrets that are handled infrequently may bite. Unlike dogs and cats, which growl, ferrets will bite without warning. Therefore always ask the owner if the ferret will bite before handling it and take precautions accordingly. Also be aware of local laws pertaining to required procedures if an unvaccinated ferret bites an employee or other person in your clinic.

Depending on the ferret's disposition, one of two basic restraint methods can be used for physical examination. For a very active animal or one that bites, scruff the ferret at the back of its neck and suspend it with all four legs off the table (Fig. 2-1). Most ferrets become very relaxed with this hold, and the veterinarian is able to examine the oral cavity, head, and body, auscultate the chest, and palpate the abdomen easily.

For more tractable animals, lightly restrain the ferret on the examination table. Examine the mucous membranes, oral cavity, head, and integument. Then pick the ferret up and use one hand for support under its body while using the second hand to auscultate the thorax and palpate the abdomen. The ferret can be scruffed at any time for vaccination, ear cleaning, or other procedures that may elicit an attempt to escape or bite.

To restrain a ferret for procedures such as venipuncture or ultrasound, hold it firmly by the scruff of its neck and around the hips without pulling the legs back. Most ferrets struggle if their legs are extended by pulling on the feet. Many animals can be distracted during a procedure by feeding Nutri-Cal (Tomlyn, Buena, NJ) or a meat-based canned food (a/d Prescription Diet, Hill's Pet Nutrition, Topeka, KS; Eukanuba Maximum-Calorie, The Iams Company, Dayton, OH) by syringe. However, if a blood sample is to be collected subsequently to measure the blood glucose concentration, feeding Nutri-Cal or other products containing sugar, which will cause the blood glucose concentration to increase, should be avoided. Leather gloves are not recommended because they interfere with the handler's dexterity, they cannot be disinfected between animals, and a determined ferret can bite through them.

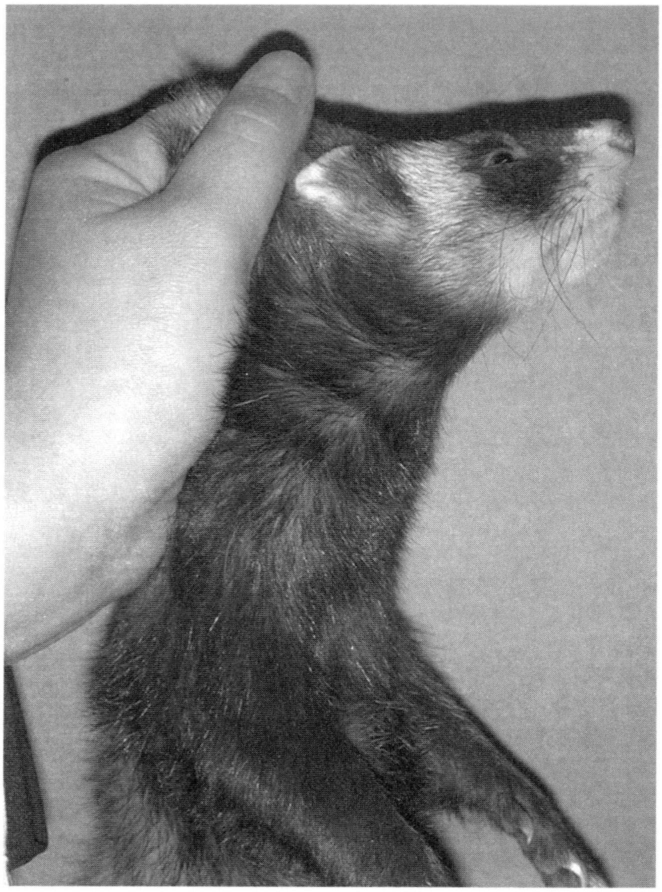

Figure 2-1 Restrain an active ferret by scruffing the loose skin on the back of the neck. The ferret will relax and allow you to palpate the abdomen or administer a vaccine.

Physical Examination

Most ferrets strenuously object to having their temperature taken with a rectal thermometer. If a ferret struggles during the examination, the temperature taken at the end of the examination may be artificially high. Therefore measuring the rectal temperature early in the physical examination is the best approach. A flexible digital thermometer is preferred because it is unbreakable and the temperature can be rapidly recorded. If a glass rectal thermometer is used, the end of the thermometer should be held to prevent it from breaking if the ferret struggles. The reference range for body temperature of a ferret is reported as 100° to 104°F (37.8°-40°C), with an average of 101.9°F (38.8°C).[40] However, in clinical practice the rectal temperature of a healthy ferret is usually not above 103°F unless the ferret is excited or the ambient temperature is high.

The physical examination of a ferret is basically the same as that of any small mammal and can be performed quickly and efficiently if a few simple guidelines are followed. Observe the attitude and alertness of the animal. Ferrets may sleep in the carrier in the veterinary office; however, once awakened for the examination, a ferret should be alert and responsive. Assess hydration by observing the skin turgor of the eyelids, the tenting of the skin at the back of the neck, and the moistness of the oral mucous membranes. However, skin turgor can be difficult to evaluate in a cachectic animal. Estimate the capillary refill time by digitally pressing on the gingiva above the teeth.

Examine the eyes, nose, ears, and facial symmetry. Cataracts can develop in both juvenile and adult animals. Retinal degeneration is another ophthalmic disorder seen in ferrets and may be indicated by abnormal pupil dilation. Inspect for nasal discharge and ask the owner about any history of sneezing or coughing. The ears may have a brown waxy discharge, but the presence of excessive brown exudate may indicate infestation with ear mites *(Otodectes cynotis)*. Bruxism often indicates gastrointestinal discomfort.

The teeth of ferrets should be clean and the gums pink. Dental tartar is commonly present and is exacerbated by the feeding of soft foods or sugary treats such as raisins. Tartar most commonly accumulates on the first and second premolars of the maxilla. Excessive dental tartar should be removed by dental techniques used in dogs and cats, and measures to prevent tartar buildup should be implemented. As a preventative, a pet dentifrice or tartar control toothpaste[18] can be applied to the teeth to decrease formation of calculi. Gingival disease, which is manifest by erythematous gums that sometimes bleed, is a common sequela of excessive dental tartar.

Ferrets often break off the tip of one or both canine teeth; however, they rarely exhibit clinical signs of sensitivity or pain associated with a broken canine (see Chapter 34). If the tooth turns dark or the ferret exhibits sensitivity when eating, recommend a root canal or extraction, depending on the degree of damage to the tooth. Rarely, an infected root of a broken canine can cause swelling of the submandibular lymph node on the corresponding side. If swelling is present, dental radiographs, canine tooth extraction, and possibly lymph node biopsy are indicated.

Observe the symmetry of the face. Although uncommon, salivary mucoceles do occur in ferrets and are noticeable as a unilateral swelling on the side of the face, usually in the cheek or temporal area (see Chapter 3).

Palpate the regional lymph nodes of the neck, axillary, popliteal, and inguinal areas. Nodes should be soft and may sometimes feel enlarged in large or overweight animals because of surrounding fat. Any degree of firmness or asymmetry in one or more nodes is suspicious and warrants a fine needle aspirate or a biopsy. If two or more nodes are enlarged and firm, a full diagnostic workup is indicated.

Auscultate the heart and the lungs in a quiet room. Ferrets have a rapid heart rate (180-250 beats/min) and often a very pronounced sinus arrhythmia. If a ferret is excited and has a very rapid heart rate, subtle murmurs may be missed. Cardiomyopathies are seen in ferrets, and any murmur or abnormal heart rhythm should be investigated further (see Chapter 6).

Palpate the abdomen while holding the ferret off the table, either by scruffing the neck or supporting the ferret with one hand. This allows the abdominal organs to displace downward, making palpation easier. If the history is consistent with an intestinal foreign body or urinary blockage, palpate gently to avoid causing iatrogenic injury, such as a ruptured stomach or bladder. Palpate the cranial abdomen, paying particular attention to the presence of gas or any irregularly shaped mass in the stomach area, especially in ferrets with a history of vomiting, melena, or chronic weight loss. The spleen is commonly enlarged in ferrets; this may or may not be significant, depending on other clinical findings (see Chapter 6). Palpate a large spleen gently to avoid iatrogenic damage. A very enlarged spleen may indicate systemic disease or, very rarely, idiopathic hypersplenism, and further diagnostic workup is warranted. Always note any degree of splenic enlargement in the medical record so that this finding can be rechecked at future examinations.

Examine the genital area, observing the size of the vulva in females. Vulvar enlargement in a spayed female is consistent with either adrenal disease or an ovarian remnant; the former is much more common. If the vulva is of normal size, point this out to the owner so that any vulvar enlargement in the future will be noticed. Examine the size of the testicles of male ferrets; testicular tumors are sometimes seen.

Check the fur coat for evidence of alopecia. Alopecia of the tail tip is common in ferrets and may be incidental and transient or an early sign of adrenal disease. Symmetric, bilateral alopecia or thinning of the hair coat that begins at the tail base and progresses cranially is a common clinical finding in ferrets with adrenal disease. Examine the skin on the back and neck for evidence of scratching or alopecia. Pruritus may be present with adrenal disease (common) or with ectoparasites (fleas, *Sarcoptes scabiei*). Check closely visually and by searching through the hair coat with your fingers for evidence of skin masses. Mast cell tumors are very common and can range in size from a small pimple to the size of a nickel. Often, the fur around a mast cell tumor is parted and matted with dark blood from the animal's scratching. Other types of skin tumors, such as sebaceous adenomas and basal cell tumors, are also common (see Chapter 10). Do an excisional biopsy of any bump or lump found on the skin.

PREVENTIVE MEDICINE

Young, recently purchased ferrets need serial distemper vaccinations until they are 13 to 14 weeks of age.[1] Rabies vaccines should be given annually beginning at 3 months of age.[7] Ferrets should be examined annually until they are 4 to 5 years of age; middle-aged and older animals should be examined twice yearly because of the high incidence of metabolic disease and neoplasia. Annual blood tests (consisting of a complete blood count and plasma [or serum] biochemical analysis) are recommended for older animals. Measure the blood glucose concentration twice yearly in healthy ferrets middle-aged and older; more frequent monitoring is needed in ferrets with insulinomas. An endocrine panel is indicated in ferrets with hair loss on the tail or other clinical signs suggestive of early adrenal disease (see Chapter 8). A screening test for the virus causing Aleutian disease is also advised, especially in new ferrets that will be introduced into a multiferret household or those that are taken to ferret shows (see Chapter 6). Currently ferrets can be tested for Aleutian disease virus by a counterimmunoelectrophoresis test (United Vaccines, Inc, Madison, WI, [608]-277-2030) or an enzyme-linked immunosorbent assay (Avecon Diagnostics Inc., Bath, PA; www.avecon.com).

Vaccinations

Canine Distemper

Ferrets must be vaccinated against canine distemper virus. Currently two vaccines are approved by the U.S. Department of Agriculture for use in ferrets: Fervac-D (United Vaccines, Inc, Madison, WI) and PureVax (Merial, Athens, GA). Fervac-D is a modified-live virus vaccine of chick cell origin. Vaccine reactions are seen with this product, but the true incidence of reactions is not known (see below). PureVax is a canarypox vectored recombinant vaccine. Because this recombinant vaccine does not contain adjuvants or the complete distemper virus, many of the postvaccination risks have been reduced or eliminated. This product has a wide safety margin and has proved effective in protecting ferrets against canine distemper infection.[37] Another modified live canine distemper vaccine (Galaxy D, Schering-Plough Animal Health Co, Omaha, NE) has been studied for safety and efficacy in ferrets. This product, attenuated in a primate cell line, has proved effective in preventing canine distemper in young ferrets challenged after serial vaccination.[41] However, duration of immunity with this product is not known and its use in clinical animals is extralabel, requiring informed owner consent. Although no vaccine reactions were reported in the study, the incidence of vaccine reactions with Galaxy D is unknown because experience with repeated long-term use in ferrets has been limited.[41] Because of the possibility of vaccine-induced disease, especially in immunosuppressed or sick ferrets, do not use combination canine vaccines or vaccines of ferret cell or low-passage canine cell origin.

In young ferrets, the half-life of maternal antibody to canine distemper virus is 9.43 days.[1] Vaccinate young ferrets for distemper at 8 weeks of age, then give 2 additional boosters at 3-week intervals for a total of 3 vaccinations. Give booster vaccines annually.

Rabies

Vaccination against rabies is recommended and is mandatory in some states.[7] A killed rabies vaccine is approved for use in ferrets (Imrab-3, Merial) and is effective in producing immunity for at least 1 year.[36] Reactions occur occasionally with this vaccine. Current recommendations are to vaccinate healthy ferrets at 3 months of age at a dose of 1 mL administered subcutaneously; give booster vaccinations annually. Titers develop within 30 days of rabies vaccination.[36]

In ferrets that were experimentally inoculated intramuscularly with skunk-origin rabies virus, the mean incubation period was 33 days and the mean morbidity period was 4 to 5 days.[26] Clinical signs were ascending paralysis, ataxia, cachexia, bladder atony, fever, hyperactivity, tremors, and paresthesia. Virus antigen was present in the brain tissue of all ferrets with clinical signs of rabies, and virus was isolated from the salivary gland of one ferret. In a similar study of ferrets inoculated with a raccoon rabies isolate, the mean incubation period was 28 days. Virus was isolated from the salivary glands of 63% of rabid ferrets, and 47% shed virus in saliva. Virus excretion began from 2 days before until 6 days after onset of illness.[27] In an earlier study of ferrets with experimentally induced rabies, only mild clinical signs were observed before death.[5] Infected ferrets exhibited restlessness and apathy, and some showed leg paresis. Sick animals did not attempt to bite when threatened, and virus was not excreted in the submaxillary salivary glands of animals that died. In this study, the authors concluded that ferrets are 50,000 times less susceptible to rabies than fox and 300 times less susceptible than hares. In another study, ferrets that were fed up to 25 carcasses of mice infected with rabies did not develop the disease; in contrast, skunks become fatally infected after the consumption of only one carcass.[3]

Local city and state regulations vary regarding rabies vaccination in ferrets, and veterinarians should contact their local governmental agencies regarding this issue. Ferrets are considered currently immunized 30 days after the initial rabies vaccination and immediately after a booster vaccination. If a healthy pet ferret bites a human being, current recommendations of the Compendium of Animal Rabies Prevention and Control are to confine and observe the animal for 10 days.[7] If signs of illness develop, the animal should be evaluated by a veterinarian. If signs suggest rabies, the ferret should be euthanatized and protocols for rabies evaluation should be followed. For a vaccinated ferret exposed to a possible rabid animal, recommendations are to revaccinate the ferret and quarantine for 45 days. An unvaccinated animal that is exposed to a rabid animal should be euthanatized.

Vaccine Reactions

In ferrets, adverse events associated with vaccination are primarily type I hypersensitivity reactions or anaphylaxis.[22] Type I hypersensitivity reactions involve lymphoid tissue associated with mucosal surfaces (skin, intestines, and lungs) and result from the interaction of antigen and immunoglobulin E in mast cells or basophils. Ferrets with mild reactions may exhibit pruritus and skin erythema. More severe reactions are typified by vomiting, diarrhea, piloerection, hyperthermia, cardiovascular collapse, or death.

Vaccine reactions are most common after distemper vaccination but also occur after rabies vaccination. Of vaccine reactions in ferrets reported to the United States Pharmacopeia Veterinary Practitioners' Reporting Program, 65% (54 of 83) of reports involved administration of FerVac D; 24% (20 of 83) involved concomitant administration of FerVac D and Imrab; and 11% (9 of 83) involved administration of Imrab alone (PureVax was not approved for use at the time data were collected).[22] According to the manufacturer's product information, the incidence of vaccine reactions with PureVax is 0.3%. No data are available for products not licensed for use in ferrets. Veterinarians are not required to report vaccine-associated adverse events, and surveillance of these events is passive, relying on voluntary reporting by practitioners.[22] Therefore the true incidence of adverse events for any of these products is not known. Currently, adverse vaccine reactions can be reported to the Center for Biologics, U.S. Department of Agriculture (1-800-752-6255; www.aphis.usda.gov/vs/cvb/adverseeventreport.htm).

Always follow the manufacturer's instructions for vaccine administration and inform the owner of the possibility of a reaction before vaccinating. Also have the owner monitor the ferret in the waiting area for 30 minutes or more after vaccination with any product. Although most reactions occur soon after vaccination, some reactions can be delayed for 24 to 48 hours.

If a ferret has an adverse reaction, administer an antihistamine (e.g., diphenhydramine hydrochloride [Benadryl, Parke-Davis, Morris Plains, NJ] (0.5-2.0 mg/kg IV or IM), epinephrine (20 µg/kg IV, IM, SC, or intratracheally), or a short-acting corticosteroid (e.g., dexamethasone sodium phosphate,1-2 mg/kg IV or IM), and give supportive care.

For any biologic product, veterinarians must assess risk versus benefit of vaccination. The treatment options for ferrets that have had a vaccine reaction include not vaccinating if risk of exposure is minimal; administering diphenhydramine (2 mg/kg PO or SC) at least 15 minutes before vaccination; or, for distemper, administering a different product.

Vaccine injection-site sarcoma has been described in ferrets.[24,25] In one report, 7 of 10 fibrosarcomas in ferrets were from locations used for vaccination.[24] Fibrosarcomas from injection sites had a higher degree of cellular pleomorphism and had similar histologic, immunohistochemical, and ultrastructural features as those reported for feline vaccine-associated sarcomas. In the reported cases in ferrets, no definitive association could be made between the fibrosarcoma and the type of vaccine. In cats, adjuvented vaccines are most likely to be involved in tumor development. However, ferrets appear less prone than cats to vaccine-associated sarcoma. In a study of early vaccine reactions in ferrets, mink, and cats, cats had more lymphocytes at the injection site than either ferrets or mink after vaccination with three different rabies vaccines.[10] Results of this study suggest a species susceptibility to vaccine-associated sarcomas in cats that is not present in ferrets or mink.

Parasites

Endoparasites

Gastrointestinal parasitism is uncommon in ferrets. There are no reports of natural hookworm or roundworm infections in ferrets or mink.[2] Rarely, ferrets may become infected with nematodes from other natural hosts through intermediate hosts or vectors. Protozoan parasites are occasionally seen. Therefore perform routine fecal flotations and direct fecal smears for all young ferrets at the initial examination.

Coccidiosis (*Isospora* species) is seen infrequently, usually in young ferrets, which shed oocysts between 6 and 16 weeks of age.[2] The infection is usually subclinical; occasionally, however, ferrets may have loose stool or bloody diarrhea. Treatment of ferrets with coccidiosis is similar to that of other small animals and should be continued for at least 2 weeks. Coccidiostats such as sulfadimethoxine and amprolium are effective and safe. The *Isospora* species that infect ferrets may cross-infect dogs and cats; therefore other pets in the household should be checked for coccidia and treated as needed.

Giardiasis is occasionally seen in ferrets and probably results from exposure to infected dogs or cats in pet stores.[2] *Giardia* species can be detected by identifying cysts or trophozoites in a fresh fecal smear or by zinc sulfate flotation. A fecal antigen enzyme-linked immunosorbent assay for giardia is available; however, results should be interpreted with results of fecal examination. Treat ferrets with giardiasis with metronidazole (20 mg/kg q12h PO) for 5 to 10 days. Fenbendazole (50 mg/kg q24h PO for 3 days) is used in dogs, but safety and efficacy in ferrets are unknown.

Cryptosporidiosis can occur in a high percentage of young ferrets.[35] Infection is usually subclinical in both immunocompetent and immunosuppressed animals. Although most immunocompetent animals recover from infection within 2 to 3 weeks, infection can persist for months in immunosuppressed animals. Oocysts of *Cryptosporidium* are small (3-5 µm) and difficult to detect but can be found in samples of fresh feces examined immediately after acid-fast staining.[2,35] No treatments exist for *Cryptosporidium* infection. Because of the zoonotic potential, ferrets may be a source of infection for human beings, especially immunocompromised individuals with AIDS.[35]

Heartworms *(Dirofilaria immitis)* can cause disease in ferrets. Ferrets that are housed outdoors in heartworm-endemic areas are most susceptible to infection; however, all ferrets in endemic areas should be given preventive medicine. Oral administration of ivermectin is currently the most practical preventive measure because it is administered once per month (see Chapters 6 and 41).

Ectoparasites

Ear mites *(Otodectes cynotis)* are very common in ferrets, but affected animals rarely exhibit pruritus or irritation. This mite species also infects dogs and cats, and animals in households with multiple pets can transmit mites to other animals. A red-brown, thick, waxy discharge in the ear canal and pinna characterizes infection. A direct smear of the exudate reveals adult mites or eggs. Because ferrets normally have brown ear wax, the color or appearance of debris in the ear canal is not pathognomonic for mites. At the initial examination, check all ferrets for ear mites and do follow-up checks at the annual examination in ferrets kept in multipet households (see Chapter 10).

Flea infestation (*Ctenocephalides* species) is most common in ferrets kept in households with dogs or cats. Ferrets with chronic infestation can become severely anemic. Check all ferrets during the physical examination for signs of fleas or flea dirt. Treat infested animals with products safe for use in cats, and institute flea control measures (see Chapter 10).

HOSPITALIZATION

Ferrets can be hospitalized in standard stainless steel hospital cages with some adaptations. Ferrets are agile escape artists and can squeeze through even very small openings. In many cages designed for dogs and cats, the bar spacing is too wide, allowing an easy avenue of escape. For housing ferrets, use only cages with very small spacing between vertical bars or use cages with small crossbars. If this type of caging is not available, adapt standard cages for use by attaching a Plexiglas plate to the front of the cage at least half the height of the cage door or higher. The plate will prevent escape through the bars yet can be easily detached and cleaned.

Special hospital cages with Plexiglas fronts and circular access ports made for birds can be used for ferrets. There is no avenue of escape, and ferrets are visible at all times. Acrylic or laminate animal intensive care cages (Lyon Electric Company, Inc., Chula Vista, CA; Snyder Mfg. Co., Englewood, CO) also can be used to house ferrets and are especially useful for animals that need supplemental heat or oxygen. The cage should be large enough to accommodate a sleeping area or box and an area for defecation and urination. Ferrets are very careful about not soiling their sleeping area, even when very sick.

All ferrets like to burrow and should be given opportunity to do so while hospitalized. Clean towels make excellent burrowing material. Alternatively, a mound of shredded paper provides much satisfaction to hospitalized animals. If not provided with burrowing material, many ferrets will burrow underneath the cage paper. Extra-small padded pet beds and fleece pet "pockets" work well as sleeping areas.

An oxygen cage should be available for use with dyspneic animals. Monitor the temperature in commercial oxygen cages closely, because ferrets can become hypothermic quickly at cool cage temperatures that are used for dogs and cats. Conversely, ferrets can overheat at temperatures used for avian patients.

Provide water for hospitalized ferrets in either water bottles or small weighted bowls. Ask the owner which type of watering system the ferret is accustomed to before hospitalization. Ferrets can be finicky eaters and should be fed their regular diet while hospitalized, if possible. Otherwise, feed a very palatable ferret food or a premium-quality, high-protein cat or kitten chow. If dietary changes are needed in the regular diet, recommend that changes be made gradually after the ferret has been released from the hospital. For animals that are anorexic, force-feed a high-calorie semisolid food or supplement until the animal is eating on its own (see below).

CLINICAL AND TREATMENT TECHNIQUES

Venipuncture

Obtaining a blood sample from a ferret is relatively easy and usually does not require anesthesia. Several venipuncture sites are readily accessible; the technique and site chosen depend on how much blood is needed and the availability of assistants for restraint. Anesthesia can be used if assistants are unavailable, but anesthesia may affect hematologic values.[21] Ferrets often can be distracted during restraint for venipuncture by offering food or Nutri-Cal (Tomlyn) by syringe. However, draw blood for glucose determination or other fasting samples before offering food.

Most veterinary laboratories offer small mammal hematologic and biochemical panels that can be done with 1.5 mL or less of blood. The blood volume of healthy ferrets is approximately 40 mL in average-sized females weighing 750 g and 60 mL in males weighing 1 kg.[13] Up to 10% of the blood volume can be safely withdrawn at one time in a normal ferret, but collect only the minimum needed for analysis. Repeated blood drawing can contribute to anemia in sick animals hospitalized for long periods.

Two techniques, jugular and anterior vena cava venipuncture, are commonly used to obtain large blood samples in ferrets. For jugular venipuncture, the technique is similar to that used in cats, with the forelegs extended over the edge of a table and the neck extended up (Fig. 2-2). Use a 25-gauge needle with a 1- to 3-mL syringe for venipuncture in most ferrets; a 22-gauge needle can be used in big males. Shave the neck at the venipuncture site to enhance visibility of the jugular vein. The vein is located more lateral in the neck than it is in dogs or cats, and it is sometimes difficult to locate in big males. Once the needle is inserted, the blood should flow easily into the syringe; if the neck is overextended and the head is arched back, the blood may not flow readily from the vein. Relax the hold on the head or gently "pump" the vein by moving the head slowly up and down to enhance blood flow into the syringe.

The second technique is venipuncture of the anterior vena cava (or a branch that drains into it, such as the subclavian vein). Restrain the ferret on its back with the forelegs pulled caudally and the head and neck extended (Fig. 2-3). In an unanesthetized ferret, two assistants are usually needed, one for restraint of the forelegs and head and the other for restraint of the rear just cranial to the pelvis. Insert a 25-gauge needle with an attached 3-mL syringe into the thoracic cavity between the first rib and the manubrium at a 45-degree angle to the body. Direct the needle toward the opposite rear leg or most caudal rib and insert it almost to the hub. Pull back on the plunger as the needle is slowly withdrawn until blood begins to fill the syringe. If the ferret struggles, quickly withdraw the needle and wait until the ferret is quiet before making a second attempt.

The lateral saphenous or the cephalic vein can be used if only a small amount of blood is needed for a packed cell volume or

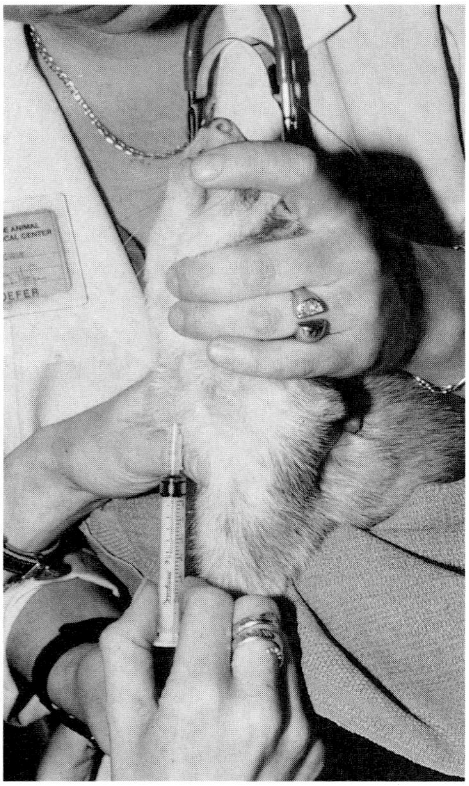

Figure 2-2 Jugular venipuncture in a ferret. Restrain the ferret similar to a cat, with the legs pulled down and the head back. After the vein is punctured, the head can be "pumped" up and down slowly to facilitate blood flow.

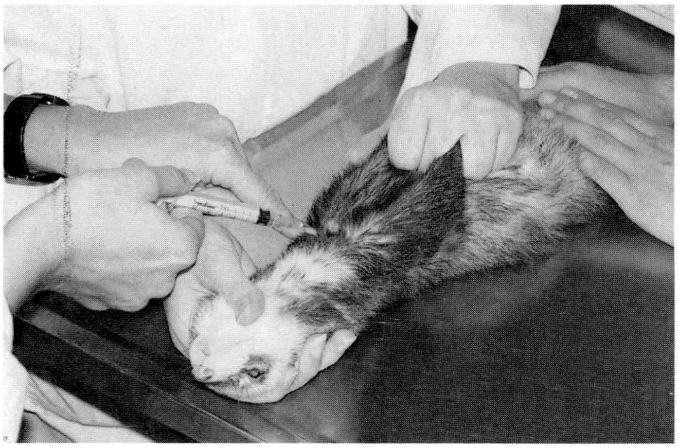

Figure 2-3 A ferret is restrained for venipuncture of the anterior vena cava. Both forelegs are pulled back, hindlegs are restrained, and the neck is extended.

blood glucose analysis. To prevent collapse of the vein during venipuncture, use an insulin syringe with an attached 27- or 28-gauge needle. The saphenous vein lies just above the hock joint on the lateral surface of the leg (Fig. 2-4); the cephalic vein is in the same anatomic location as in a dog. Before venipuncture, shave the fur from the area to enhance visibility of the vein.

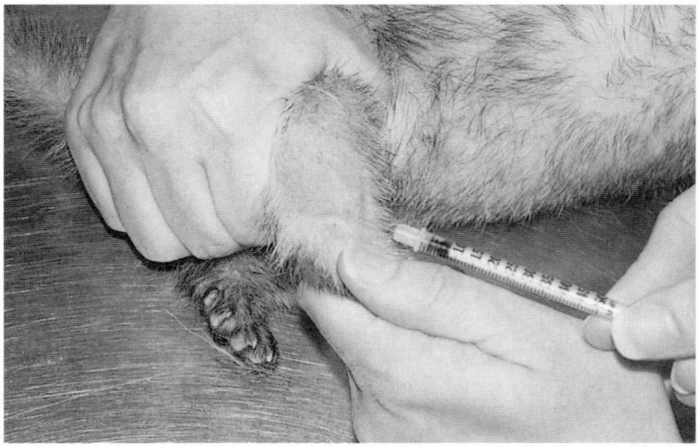

Figure 2-4 The lateral saphenous vein is visible just above the hock. Shaving the leg enhances visibility of the vein.

Although rarely used in pet ferrets, venipuncture of the tail artery can be performed to obtain blood samples in nonanesthetized animals.[6] For this technique, place the ferret in a heated environment for several minutes or apply moist heat to promote vasodilation and facilitate blood flow. Then restrain the ferret on its back. Because venipuncture at this site can be painful, apply topical lidocaine or prilocaine (EMLA cream, Astra Pharmaceuticals, Wayne, PA). Insert a syringe with a 21- or 20-gauge needle directed toward the body into the ventral side of the tail, in the groove along the midline. The artery is located 2 to 3 mm deep to the skin. Once the artery is entered, slowly withdraw the plunger until blood fills the syringe. Approximately 3 to 5 mL of blood can be withdrawn with this technique. Apply pressure to the venipuncture site for 2 to 3 minutes after the needle has been withdrawn.

Reference Ranges

Published reference ranges for hematologic and serum biochemical values in ferrets are listed in Tables 2-1 and 2-2. Most of these values were reported in studies of laboratory ferrets. Other sources of reference ranges for ferrets are available.[13,14] Additionally, most clinical veterinary laboratories routinely provide reference ranges for ferret hematologic and biochemical values.

Published reference values for white blood cell counts in ferrets range from 2.5 to 19.1 × 10^3 cells/μL[13,16,38]; however, white blood cell counts generally tend to be low in ferrets. In one study, mean white blood cell values were 5.7 and 5.6 × 10^3 cells/μL in male and female ferrets, respectively.[14] High white blood cell counts are not seen as commonly in ferrets as in dogs and cats, perhaps in part because infectious bacterial diseases are relatively uncommon in ferrets.

Isoflurane anesthesia can cause decreases in all hematologic values that begin at induction of anesthesia and reach maximal levels at 15 minutes after induction.[21] Therefore the complete blood count (CBC) values of blood samples collected while a ferret is anesthetized must be carefully interpreted.

Few sources have published reference ranges for blood coagulation times in ferrets. In male ferrets, the mean prothrombin time (PT) was 15.7 seconds with a range of 14.4 to 16.5 seconds.[38] In a study of 6 ferrets, values of clotting time of whole blood were 2 ± 0.5 minutes in glass tubes and 3 ± 0.9 minutes in siliconized tubes; PT was 10.3 ± 0.1 seconds; activated partial

TABLE **2-1**
Reference Ranges for Hematologic Values in Ferrets

		FITCH FARRETS[16]*		ALBINO FERRETS[38]†	
Value	**Sex**	**Range**	**Mean**	**Range**	**Mean**
Hematocrit (%)	♂	46-57	49.1	44-61	55.4
	♀	47-51	48.4	42-55	49.2
Hemoglobin (g/dL)	♂	15.2-17.7	16.1	16.3-18.2	17.8
	♀	15.2-17.4	15.9	14.8-17.4	16.2
Red blood cells ($\times 10^6/\mu L$)	♂			7.30-12.18	10.23
	♀			6.77-9.76	8.11
Reticulocytes (%)	♂			1-12	4.0
	♀			2-14	5.3
White blood cells ($\times 10^3/\mu L$)	♂	5.6-10.8	7.3	4.4-19.1	9.7
	♀	2.5-8.6	5.9	4.0-18.2	10.5
Neutrophils	♂	616-7020/μL	2659/μL	11-82%	57.0%
	♀	725-2409/μL	1825/μL	43-84%	59.5%
Lymphocytes	♂	1728-4704/μL	3791/μL	12-54%	35.6%
	♀	1475-5590/μL	3426/μL	12-50%	33.4%
Monocytes	♂	0-432/μL	176/μL	0-9%	4.4%
	♀	100-372/μL	263/μL	2-8%	4.4%
Eosinophils	♂	112-768/μL	378/μL	0-7%	2.4%
	♀	50-516/μL	214/μL	0-5%	2.6%
Basophils	♂	0-112/μL	50/μL	0-2%	0.1%
	♀	0-172/μL	48/μL	0-1%	0.2%
Bands	♂	0-972/μL	233/μL		
	♀	0-248/μL	99/μL		
Platelets ($\times 10^3/\mu L$)	♂			297-730	453
	♀			310-910	545
Mean corpuscular volume (μm^3)	♂				54
	♀				61
Mean corpuscular hemogiobin (pg)	♂				17.6
	♀				19.9
Mean corpuscular hemoglobin concentration (%)	♂				–32.2
	♀				32.8

Adapted with permission from Leo EJ, Moore WE, Fryer HC, et al: Hematological and serum chemistry profiles of ferrets (*Mustela putorius furo*). Lab Anim 1982; 16:133-137; and Thomton PC, Wright PA, Sacra PJ, et al: The ferret, *Mustela putorius furo*, as a new species in toxicology. Lab Anim 1979; 13:119-124. Copyright 1979 and 1982, Macmillan Magazines Limited.
*Males all castrated.
†Males all intact.

thromboplastin time (APPT) was 18.4 ± 1.4 seconds; and thrombin time was 28.8 ± 8.7 seconds.[17] In the same study, mean values for individual coagulation factors were also determined[17] and have also been reported elsewhere.[9] In a study of 30 intact ferrets (15 male, 15 female), mean bleeding time was less than 2 minutes; PT was 8 to 11 seconds for females and 9 to 10.6 seconds for males; and APPT was 16 to 21 seconds for females and 17 to 25 seconds for males (E. Ivey, DVM, unpublished data, 2000). In this study, PT and APPT were measured with the ACT II (Medtronic, Parker, CO).

Intravenous Catheters

Indwelling intravenous catheters are routinely used in ferrets. Catheters can be placed in the lateral saphenous or cephalic vein (Fig. 2-5). Jugular vein catheters are more difficult to place and are not commonly used. Except in very depressed animals, catheters are placed with the ferret anesthetized. First, puncture the skin over the vein with a 20- or 22-gauge needle, taking care to avoid the vein; then introduce a short 22-, 24-, or 26-gauge over-the-needle catheter into the vein. After placing the catheter, attach a T-connector and wrap the leg securely with a soft padded bandage. Closely monitor ferrets with indwelling catheters to prevent the fluid line from entangling. Most ferrets do not chew a catheter once it is placed and do not require an Elizabethan collar.

In ferrets that are collapsed with poor blood pressure or in young or very small ferrets, attempts to place an intravenous catheter may be unsuccessful. An intraosseous catheter can be placed in these animals and maintained for several days. The

TABLE 2-2
Reference Ranges for Serum Biochemical Values in Ferrets

Value	Albino*	Fitch†
Total protein (g/dL)	5.1-7.4	5.3-7.2
Albumin (g/dL)	2.6-3.8	3.3-4.1
Glucose (mg/dL)	94-207	62.5-134
Fasting glucose (mg/dL)		90-125‡
Blood urea nitrogen (mg/dL)	10-45	12-43
Creatinine (mg/dL)	0.4-0.9	0.2-0.6
Sodium (mmol/L)	137-162	146-160
Polasslum (mmol/L)	4.5-7.7	4.3-5.3
Choride (mmol/L)	106-125	102-121
Calcium (mg/dL)	8.0-11.8	8.6-10.5
Phosphorus (mg/dL)	4.0-9.1	5.6-8.7
Alanine aminotransferase (U/L)		82-289 78-149§
Aspartate aminotransferase (U/L)	28-120	57-248§
Alkaline phosphatase (U/L)	9-84	30-120 31-66§
Bilirubin (mg/dL)	<1.0	0-0.1§
Cholesterol (mg/dL)	64-296	119-209§
Carbon dioxide (mmol/L)	16.5-28	16-28§

*Combined values of male (n = 40) and female (n = 24) ferrets.[38]
†Combined values of intact male, female, and castrated male ferrets (total n = 13, aged 4-8 mo)[36] except where noted.
‡From Brown S: Personal communication, 1995.
§Combined values from cardiac and orbital venipuncture of male ferrets (n = 16).[13]

proximal femur is the most common site used. Unless the ferret is very depressed, anesthetize the animal to place the catheter. Insert a 20- or 22-gauge, 1.5-inch spinal needle into the marrow cavity. Alternatively, use a 20- or 22-gauge hypodermic needle with a surgical steel wire inserted into the lumen to prevent the needle from occluding during insertion.[29] If possible, change to an intravenous catheter as soon as the animal is rehydrated or blood pressure improves.

Vascular access ports, consisting of an indwelling intravenous catheter attached to an injection port placed in subcutaneous tissue, have been used in ferrets for repeated administration of chemotherapeutic medications. These ports can be used when repeated vascular access is required for any reason.[34] The technique used to place the catheter and port has been described and illustrated.[30]

Fluid Therapy

Hospitalized ferrets usually require fluid therapy to maintain hydration and correct dehydration. Daily fluid requirements of ferrets have not been determined; however, calculating fluid requirements based on rates used in cats (60-70 mL/kg per day) appears adequate for maintenance. One source estimates daily water consumption of adult ferrets as 75 to 100 mL/day.[23] Provide additional fluids to compensate for ongoing fluid loss and to correct dehydration calculated as a percentage of the body weight.

Give fluids subcutaneously or intravenously; intravenous fluids are preferred in ill animals. Administer subcutaneous fluids in the loose skin along the back and dorsal cervical area, dividing the calculated daily fluid volume into doses given 2 or 3 times daily. Ferrets often react painfully to subcutaneous fluid administration, and good restraint is needed to prevent a ferret from biting its handler.

If possible, administer intravenous fluids by continuous rate infusion. Alternatively, administer fluids by dividing the

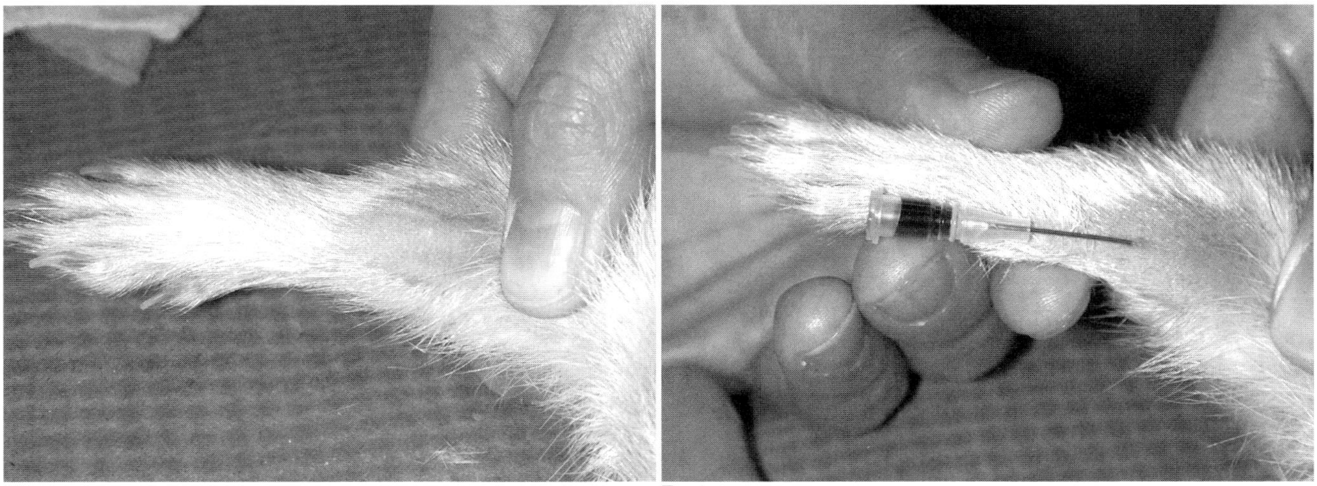

A B

Figure 2-5 Placing an indwelling catheter in the cephalic vein of a ferret. **A**, The hair over the vein is shaved and the vein held off. **B**, A 24-gauge, three-quarter–inch intravenous catheter is introduced into the cephalic vein and taped in place.

calculated daily fluid volume into 2 or 3 doses administered by a Buretrol (Baxter Healthcare, Glendale, CA) or a syringe pump. Depending on the clinical condition of the ferret, add dextrose (2.5%-5%), B vitamins, or potassium to maintenance fluids by using the same criteria and calculations as for dogs and cats.

Colloids are effective in improving intravascular fluid volume and oncotic pressure in ferrets that are hypoproteinemic or in shock. Dosage and administration are similar to those in small animals. Most commonly, hydroxyethyl starch (hetastarch) is given at a dose of 10 to 20 mL/kg per day. When hetastarch is coadministered with crystalloids, reduce the crystalloid fluid volume by 33% to 50%. In ferrets in shock, hetastarch can be given as a bolus at 5 mL/kg over a 15-minute period; this can be repeated to a total dose not exceeding 20 mL/kg per day.

Antibiotic and Drug Therapy

Ferrets are given antibiotics and other drugs at dosages similar to those used in cats (see Chapter 41). Intravenous antibiotics are preferred in sick animals if an indwelling catheter is in place. Intramuscular antibiotics can be given, but subcutaneous administration is preferred because of the limited muscle mass in cachectic animals if therapy continues over several days. Because pills are very difficult to administer, oral medications are most easily given in a liquid form. Many compounding pharmacists can prepare suspensions of drugs that are not commercially available as liquids. Avoid fish flavors in compounded formulas; ferrets do not generally like this taste.

Pain Management

Pain management is important in the postoperative period and for traumatic injuries (see Chapter 33). Both buprenorphine and torbugesic can be used in ferrets. However, ferrets given torbugesic after surgery can become very lethargic and immobile for long periods. If a heating lamp is used in the postoperative period, closely monitor the body temperature of any ferret given pain medication to prevent overheating.

Like cats, ferrets are sensitive to acetaminophen toxicity.[8] The activity of UDP-glucuronosyltransferase in their livers is similar to that of cats. Therefore, acetaminophen glucuronidation is slower in ferrets than in other non-felid species. Unlike cats, however, no genetic mutations are associated with this slow metabolism, and the exact cause is not known. When dosed inappropriately, ibuprofen can also be toxic in ferrets (see Chapter 6). Therefore use any nonsteroidal anti-inflammatory drugs with caution. The cyclooxygenase 2 (COX-2) inhibitors may prove a better choice for pain management; however, as yet little is known about their use in ferrets.

Nutritional Support

Many sick ferrets are either cachectic or have minimal body fat and require nutritional support. Force-feeding is also important to prevent hypoglycemia in anorexic ferrets with insulinomas. Ferrets can be syringe fed meat-based soft foods marketed for hospitalized dogs and cats such as Maximum-Calorie (The Iams Company) or Canine a/d (Hill's Pet Nutrition). Animals that refuse regular or semisolid food will often accept high-energy paste supplements such as Nutri-Cal (Tomlyn) or Furo-Vite (Marshall Pet Products, Wolcott, NY), chicken or beef broth, meat baby foods, liquid soy-based formulas (Deliver 2.0, Mead Johnson Nutritionals, Evansville, IN), or mixtures of any of these. However, these supplements are not nutritionally complete and should only be used for a few days until the ferret accepts a more complete diet. Some supplements have a high carbohydrate content and should be avoided in ferrets with insulinoma.

Force-feed anorectic ferrets as much as they will accept comfortably, usually 5 to 10 mL fed 3 to 4 times daily. Use a syringe to administer food. Once a ferret develops a taste for the food, it may eat it directly from a bowl.

Esophagostomy feeding tubes can be placed in ferrets to manage debilitated animals over the long term. The technique is similar to that used in cats.[12] Gastric feeding tubes have been placed in ferrets experimentally.[4] In a study of 14 ferrets, gastrostomy tubes were placed percutaneously by a nonendoscopic technique. However, the practicality of maintaining gastrostomy tubes in clinical patients has yet to be determined.

Total nutrient admixtures have been formulated to provide partial parenteral nutrition to ferrets.[29] Parenteral nutrition should be considered if an esophageal, gastric, or intestinal disorder precludes the use of enteral formulations, for example, in cases of malabsorptive diarrhea. The total nutrient mixture is formulated from a mixture of lipid and dextrose supplemented with amino acids, electrolytes, water-soluble vitamins, minerals, and enough fluids to meet daily fluid volume requirements. The solution should be administered by infusion pump through a silicone elastomer or polyurethane jugular catheter.

Ferret owners often prepare homemade diets of "duck soup" or "chicken gravy" to nurse their pets at home. Recipes for these preparations are readily available on various Internet sites. These recipes are usually based on canned dog food, kibble, or whole chicken with additives ranging from beef fat, Nutri-Cal, or brewers yeast to *Echinacea* capsules. Although many of these recipes appear acceptable, some are very high in fat and carbohydrates. Discuss any particular recipe that a ferret owner is using before endorsing it for long-term use.

Urine Collection and Urinalysis

Urine samples can be collected by cystocentesis or by free catch after natural voiding or gentle manual expression of the bladder. The techniques for manually expressing the bladder and cystocentesis are the same as those used in dogs and cats. Anesthetize fractious ferrets to avoid trauma to the thin bladder wall. Use a 25-gauge needle for cystocentesis.

Reference values for urinalysis are listed in Table 2-3. In one study, the reference range for urine pH in ferrets was reported as 6.5 to 7.5[40]; however urine pH can vary according to the diet, and the normal urine pH in ferrets fed a high-quality, meat-based diet is approximately 6.0 (see Chapter 4).

Urinary Catheterization

Urinary catheterization is commonly indicated in male ferrets, but the procedure can be difficult. Although techniques have been described for both sexes,[20] clinical indications to place a urinary catheter in females are rare. For females, tranquilize or anesthetize the ferret, then position it in ventral recumbency with the rear quarters elevated with a rolled towel. With a vaginal speculum, locate the urethral opening in the floor of the urethral vestibule, approximately 1 cm cranial to the clitoral fossa. Intro-

TABLE 2-3
Reference Ranges for Urinalysis in Ferrets

Value	Mean ± SD*	Range
24-hour urine volume (mL)	24.93 ± 14.31[11]	
	26 ♂[38]	8-48 ♂[38]
	28 ♀[38]	8-140 ♀[38]
pH		6.5-7.5[40]
Urine protein (mg/dL)		7-33 ♂[38]
		0-32 ♀[38]
Exogenous creatinine clearance (mL/min per kg)	3.32 ± 2.16 ♀[11]	
Insulin clearance (mL/min per kg)	3.02 ± 1.78 ♀[11]	
Endogenous creatinine clearance (mL/min per kg)	2.50 ± 0.93[11]	

*Mean 11-hour urine volume and endogenous creatinine clearance from reference 11 are based on values from 25 female and 2 male ferrets.

duce a 3.5-Fr, red rubber urethral catheter fitted with a wire stylet into the urethral orifice.

In male ferrets, urethral blockage is a common sequelae of adrenal disease. Hormonal influence causes the prostate gland to enlarge, which subsequently constricts the urethra. Placing a urinary catheter is difficult because the urethral opening is very small and located on the ventral surface of the penis, below the hook in the end of the os penis. If needed, use a surgical magnifying loupe to help see the orifice. Also, in ferrets with urethral blockage, the tip of the penis and the preputial area are often very swollen, and introducing a catheter can be challenging. If needed, a small incision can be made in the prepuce to facilitate exteriorizing the penis.

To place a catheter, use a 3.5-Fr rubber feeding catheter or a 3.0-Fr ferret urinary catheter (Slippery Sam, Global Veterinary Products, New Buffalo, MI; www.globalveterinaryproducts.com). If using a long rubber catheter, estimate the length of the catheter that must be inserted to reach the bladder before placing it. Use a stylet or sterile metal guitar string to stiffen the catheter while passing. Another option is to use a 20- or 22-gauge, 8-inch jugular catheter with the stylet removed.[29] If needed, the stylet can be retracted to provide stiffness, but be very careful when rounding the pelvic flexure to avoid perforating the urethra. Dilate the urethral opening by passing a 24-gauge intravenous catheter just inside the tip of the urethra and flushing gently with saline. Then slip the tip of the lubricated urinary catheter gently into the dilated opening alongside the intravenous catheter and, while gently flushing with saline solution, pass the catheter into the bladder. Often resistance is met at the pelvic flexure; if this occurs, try repeated gentle flushing and relubricating the catheter until it passes. Once in place, secure the catheter by placing butterfly tape strips around the catheter just as it enters the urethra and at another point 3 to 5 cm distal and suturing these to the skin. Tape the catheter to the tail to further prevent tension, and attach a urinary collection device. If needed, bandage the ferret's abdomen to minimize rotation of the catheter and to restrict the ferret from traumatizing it. Elizabethan collars are occasionally needed in some ferrets to prevent chewing at the catheter.

Temporary tube cystostomy has been used successfully to manage male ferrets with urinary obstruction caused by adrenal disease.[28] In these ferrets, a 5-Fr or 8-Fr Foley catheter was placed in the bladder at the time of adrenalectomy and left in place for 5 to 14 days. This technique was especially useful for ferrets in which a urinary catheter could not be placed before surgery; immediate treatment of urinary blockage was by cystocentesis.

Splenic Aspiration

Splenic aspiration is a common diagnostic technique that is used in ferrets with enlarged spleens (see Chapters 6 and 38). The technique is simple and usually can be done in unanesthetized ferrets. However, if a ferret is fractious, use inhalant anesthesia administered by face mask. Restrain the ferret on its back or in lateral recumbency and shave and prepare the abdominal skin in the area over the spleen. Palpate and immobilize the spleen directly under the prepped area with one hand while directing a 3-mL syringe with an attached 25-gauge needle into the spleen with the other hand. Quickly aspirate the syringe and withdraw the needle; a positive aspirate appears bloody. More preferably, "stab" the needle several times into the spleen without applying negative pressure. Then detach the needle, and reattach an air-filled syringe to express the contents of the needle onto slides. This technique will minimize blood contamination. Obtain aspirates from two sites and prepare several slides for cytologic staining. If an abnormal mass is found on ultrasound examination, perform an ultrasound-guided aspirate to improve chances of a positive result. The two most common findings on cytologic examination of a splenic aspirate are extramedullary hematopoiesis and lymphoma.

Bone Marrow Collection

Evaluating a bone marrow sample is a valuable diagnostic tool for many disease conditions, including anemia, thrombocytopenia, pancytopenia, proliferative abnormalities, and suspected hematopoietic malignancies. Anesthesia is necessary to aspirate the bone marrow or perform a core biopsy.

Although the proximal femur is usually the most readily accessible site, the iliac crest and humerus (Fig. 2-6) can also be used to collect bone marrow samples. After the ferret is anesthetized, place it in lateral recumbency and shave and aseptically prepare the area around the collection site. For the proximal femur,[33] make a small incision through the skin over the greater trochanter with a No. 15 scalpel blade. Hold and stabilize the femur with one hand while inserting a 20-gauge, 1.5-inch spinal needle into the bone medial to the greater trochanter. Use steady pressure and an alternating rotating motion to advance the needle into the marrow cavity. Withdraw the stylet, and attach a 6- to 12-mL syringe to the needle. Aspirate the marrow sample into the syringe, stopping suction as soon as the sample is visible (to prevent blood contamination). To collect a core biopsy sample, use the same technique, but use a 1.5-inch, 18-gauge needle in place of the spinal needle.[39] Collect samples from alternate sites by using the same basic technique.

Try to prepare at least 4 to 8 slides for cytologic evaluation. To do this, forcibly expel the bone marrow sample from the syringe onto glass slides. The slide can be held vertically to allow contaminating blood to drain, leaving only bony spicules. Place a clean slide on top of the slide with the sample and allow the

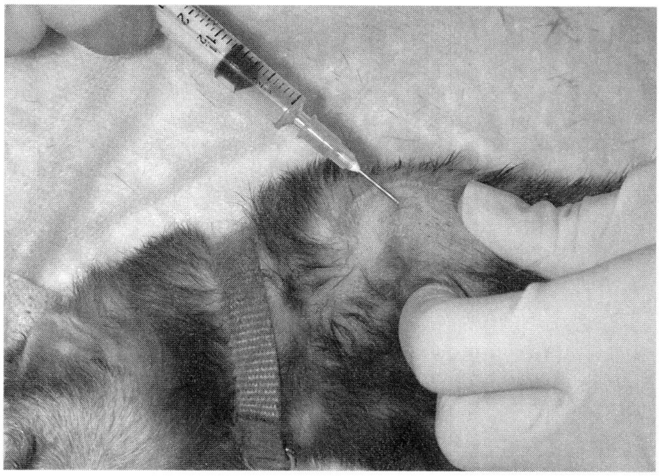

Figure 2-6 Collection of a bone marrow sample from the proximal humerus in a ferret.

marrow to spread between the slides, then draw the two slides apart in a horizontal plane.[39]

Tracheal Wash

Ferrets will occasionally present with clinical and radiographic evidence of respiratory disease. In these animals, a tracheal wash may be indicated to obtain samples for cytologic examination and bacterial culture and sensitivity testing. The procedure is similar to that in a cat. Anesthetize the ferret and intubate with a sterile endotracheal tube. Pass an open-end urinary catheter through the endotracheal tube, preferably to the level of tracheal bifurcation. Inject 2 to 3 mL of warm, sterile saline solution, then induce coughing by tapping on the rib cage. Aspirate the fluid, and prepare samples for submission for diagnostic testing.

Blood Transfusion

Blood transfusions may be needed in ferrets that are anemic from chronic disease, blood loss, or estrogen toxicosis or in ferrets that are thrombocytopenic. As in other species, evaluate the need for a transfusion based on the packed cell volume or platelet count and clinical status of the ferret. Consider a transfusion if the packed cell volume is 25% or less in a ferret that exhibits clinical signs of anemia or requires surgery (see Chapter 6) or if a ferret is thrombocytopenic and exhibits ecchymosis, petechiation, or bleeding.

Ferrets lack detectable blood groups and there is little risk of transfusion reaction, even without cross-matching.[19] Because they have a larger blood volume, large male ferrets are preferred over females as blood donors. Depending on the size of the donor ferret, 6 to 12 mL of blood can be safely collected for transfusion. Collect blood into an anticoagulant such as acid-citrate-dextrose at a ratio of 1 mL of anticoagulant to 6 mL of donor blood.[15] Intraosseous blood transfusions can be given to ferrets if an intravenous catheter cannot be placed.

Hemoglobin solutions can also be used safely in ferrets (see Chapter 6). A hemoglobin-based oxygen-carrying solution (Oxyglobin, Biopure Corp., Cambridge, MA) has been used in anemic ferrets at a dose of 11 to 15 mg/kg infused over a 4-hour period and administered once to twice during a 24-hour period.[31,32] Use of a hemoglobin-based oxygen-carrying solution obviates the need for a donor ferret and a filter for administration, and the solution can be administered through a catheter of any size.

REFERENCES

1. Appel MJ, Harris WV: Antibody titers in domestic ferret jills and their kits to canine distemper virus vaccine. J Am Vet Med Assoc 1988; 193:332-333.
2. Bell JA: Parasites of domesticated pet ferrets. Compend Cont Educ Pract Vet 1994; 16:617-620.
3. Bell JF, Moore GJ: Susceptibility of carnivore to rabies virus administered orally. Am J Epidemiol 1971; 93:176-182.
4. Benson KG, Paul-Murphy J, Carr A: Percutaneous placement of a gastric feeding tube in the ferret. Lab Anim 2000; 29:44-46.
5. Blancou J, Aubert MFA, Artois M: Experimental rabies in the ferret *(Mustela [putorius] furo)*: susceptibility—symptoms—excretion of the virus. Rev Med Vet 1982; 133:553–557.
6. Bleakley SP: Simple technique for bleeding ferrets (*Mustela putorius furo*). Lab Anim 1980; 14:59-60.
7. Compendium of Animal Rabies Prevention and Control, 2003. National Association of State Public Health Veterinarians. Available at: http://www.avma.org/pubhlth/rabcont.asp. Accessed April 1, 2003.
8. Court MH: Acetaminophen UDP-glucuronosyltransferase in ferrets: species and gender differences, and sequence analysis of ferret UGT1A6. J Vet Pharmacol Ther 2001; 24:415-422.
9. Dodds WJ: Rabbit and ferret hemostasis. *In* Fudge AM, ed. Laboratory Medicine: Avian and Exotic Pets. Philadelphia, WB Saunders, 2000, pp 285-290.
10. Eggers Carroll E, Dubielzig RR, Schultz RD: Cats differ from mink and ferrets in their response to commercial vaccines: a histologic comparison of early vaccine reactions. Vet Pathol 2002; 39:216-227.
11. Esteves MI, Marini RP, Ryden EB, et al: Estimation of glomerular filtration rate and evaluation of renal function in ferrets (*Mustela putorius furo*). Am J Vet Res 1994; 55:166-172.
12. Fisher PG: Esophagotomy feeding tube placement in the ferret. Exotic DVM 2001; 2:23-25.
13. Fox JG: Normal clinical and biologic parameters. *In* Fox JG, ed. Biology and Diseases of the Ferret, 2nd ed. Baltimore, Williams & Wilkins, 1998, pp 183-210.
14. Fudge AM: Ferret hematology. *In* Fudge AM, ed. Laboratory Medicine: Avian and Exotic Pets. Philadelphia, WB Saunders, 2000, pp 269-272.
15. Hoefer HL: Transfusions in exotic species. *In* Hohenhaus AE, ed. Transfusion Medicine. Philadelphia, JB Lippincott, 1992, pp 625-635.
16. Lee EJ, Moore WE, Fryer HC, et al: Haematological and serum chemistry profiles of ferrets (*Mustela putorius furo*). Lab Anim 1982; 16:133-137.
17. Lewis JH: Comparative Hemostasis in Vertebrates. New York, Plenum Press, 1996, pp 224-240.
18. Mann PH, Harper DS, Regnier S: Reduction of calculus accumulation in domestic ferrets with two dentifrices containing pyrophosphate. J Dent Res 1990; 69:451-453.
19. Manning DD, Bell JA: Lack of detectable blood groups in domestic ferrets: implications for transfusion. J Am Vet Med Assoc 1990; 197:84-86.
20. Marini RP, Esteves MI, Fox JG: A technique for catheterization of the urinary bladder in the ferret. Lab Anim 1994; 28:155-157.
21. Marini RP, Jackson LR, Esteves MI, et al: Effect of isoflurane on hematologic variables in ferrets. Am J Vet Res 1994; 55:1479-1483.

22. Meyer EK: Vaccine-associated adverse events. Vet Clin North Am Small Anim Pract 2001; 31:493-514.
23. Moody KD, Bowman TA, Lang CM: Laboratory management of the ferret for biomedical research. Lab Anim Sci 1985; 35:272-279.
24. Munday JS, Stedman NL, Richey LJ: Histology and immunochemistry of seven ferret vaccination-site fibrosarcomas. Vet Pathol 2003; 40:288-293.
25. Murray J: Vaccine injection-site sarcoma in a ferret [letter]. J Am Vet Med Assoc 1998; 213:955.
26. Niezgoda M, Briggs DJ, Shaddock J, et al: Pathogenesis of experimentally induced rabies in domestic ferrets. Am J Vet Res 1997; 58:1327-1331.
27. Niezgoda M, Briggs DJ, Shaddock J, et al: Viral excretion in domestic ferrets (*Mustela putorius furo*) inoculated with a raccoon rabies isolate. Am J Vet Res 1998; 59:1629-1632.
28. Nolte DM, Carberry CA, Gannon KM, et al: Temporary tube cystostomy as a treatment for urinary obstruction secondary to adrenal disease in four ferrets. J Am Anim Hosp Assoc 2002; 38:527-532.
29. Orcutt C: Emergency and critical care of ferrets. Vet Clin North Am Exotic Anim Pract 1998; 1:99-126.
30. Orcutt C: Use of vascular access ports in exotic animals. Exotic DVM 2000; 2.3:34-38.
31. Orcutt C: Oxyglobin administration for the treatment of anemia in ferrets. Exotic DVM 2000; 2.3:44-46.
32. Orcutt C: Update on oxyglobin use in ferrets. Exotic DVM 2001; 3.3:29-30.
33. Palley LS, Marini RP, Rosenblad WD, et al: A technique for femoral bone marrow collection in the ferret. Lab Anim Sci 1990; 40:654-655.
34. Rassnick KM, Gould WJ, Flanders JA: Use of a vascular access system for administration of chemotherapeutic agents to a ferret with lymphoma. J Am Vet Med Assoc 1995; 206:500-504.
35. Rehg JE, Gigliotti F, Stokes DC: Cryptosporidiosis in ferrets. Lab Anim Sci 1988; 38:155-158.
36. Rupprecht CE, Gilbert J, Pitts R, et al: Evaluation of an inactivated rabies vaccine in domestic ferrets. J Am Vet Med Assoc 1990; 196:1614-1616.
37. Tanner PA, Tseggai T, Rice Conlon JA, et al: Minimum protective dose (MPD) and efficacy determination of a recombinant canine distemper virus vaccine for ferrets. *In* Proceedings of 81st Annual Meeting of the Conference of Research Workers in Animal Diseases; Nov. 12-14, 2000; Chicago, IL. Abstract 156.
38. Thornton PC, Wright PA, Sacra PJ, et al: The ferret, *Mustela putorius furo*, as a new species in toxicology. Lab Anim 1979; 119-124.
39. Williams BH: Disorders of rabbit and ferret bone marrow. *In* Fudge AM, ed. Laboratory Medicine: Avian and Exotic Pets. Philadelphia, WB Saunders, 2000, pp 276-284.
40. Williams CSF: Practical Guide to Laboratory Animals. St Louis, Mosby, 1976, p 207.
41. Wimsatt J, Jay MT, Innes KE, et al: Serologic evaluation, efficacy, and safety of a commercial modified-live canine distemper vaccine in domestic ferrets. Am J Vet Res 2001; 62:736-740.

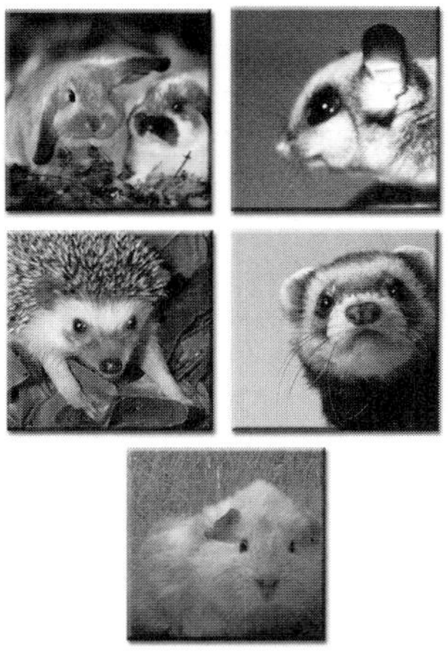

CHAPTER 3

Gastrointestinal Diseases

Part I: Heidi L. Hoefer, DVM, Diplomate ABVP
Part II: Judith A. Bell, DVM, MSc, PhD

PART I **GENERAL GASTROINTESTINAL DISORDERS**

Heidi L. Hoefer, DVM, Diplomate ABVP

Disease of the gastrointestinal (GI) tract is common in ferrets. Clinicians should be familiar with the more common GI disorders, able to recognize clinical signs, and able to differentiate among potential diagnoses.

DENTAL DISEASE

Dental tartar, gingivitis, and periodontal disease are common in middle-aged and older ferrets (see Chapter 34). Moist or semimoist diets may predispose these animals to dental calculi and periodontal disease.[30] Most ferrets, even on a dry diet, develop tartar that progresses with age. Tartar tends to accumulate most heavily on the second and third upper premolars. Biting and gnawing habits often result in discoloration, wearing, and breaking of the tips of the canine teeth (Fig. 3-1). Broken canine teeth do not usually result in obvious discomfort or pain unless the dental pulp is exposed. Root canal restoration or surgical removal of the affected teeth may be necessary in some ferrets.[33] Tooth root abscesses are not common but can occur at any age.

Although dysphagia and drooling are sometimes seen, dental disease is often an incidental finding during physical examination. Dental extractions and scaling can be performed with the animal under anesthesia. Follow the basic principles for dental disease management that apply in the care of the dog or cat.

SALIVARY MUCOCELE

Ferrets have five major pairs of salivary glands: the parotid, submandibular, sublingual, molar, and zygomatic.[44] Trauma to a gland can result in extravasation of saliva and salivary muco-

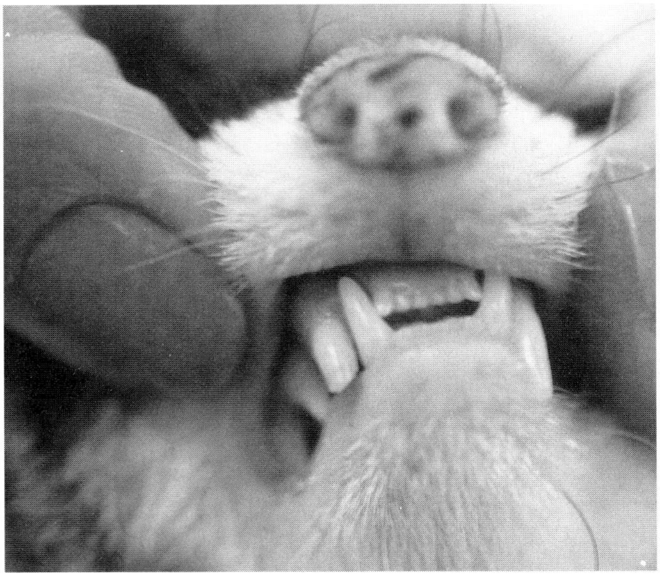

Figure 3-1 Broken canine teeth are common in ferrets.

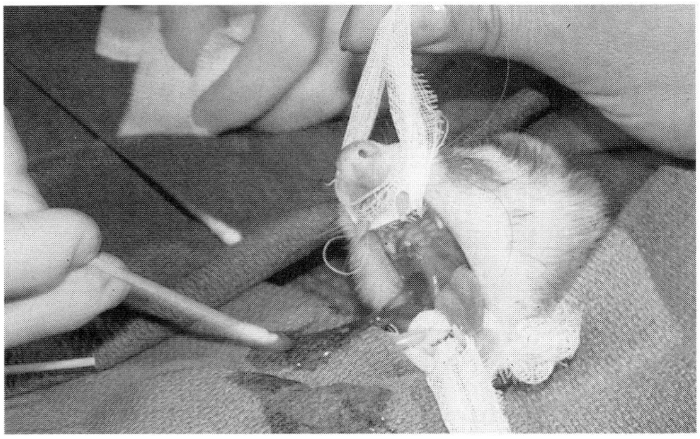

Figure 3-2 Surgical correction of a salivary mucocele. The medial aspect of the mucocele is marsupialized into the mouth.

cele formation. Although this lesion is uncommon in ferrets, mucocele diagnosis and treatment have been described.[3,39]

Diagnosis of a mucocele is relatively straightforward. Facial swellings are often seen in the commissures of the mouth or in the orbital area in the case of a zygomatic mucocele. Other locations also are possible. Aspirate the mass to obtain samples for cytologic analysis. The fluid is viscous or mucinous and clear or blood-tinged. Cytologic examination reveals amorphous debris and occasional red blood cells.

Treatment for salivary mucoceles is usually surgery. In one reported case, scalpel blade lancing of the medial wall of the mucocele resulted in drainage and no recurrence.[3] Marsupialization into the mouth with the use of a wide circular incision in the medial wall of the mucocele may be effective for mucoceles that bulge into the oral cavity (Fig. 3-2). Surgical excision of the affected salivary gland is ideal for avoiding recurrence (see Chapter 12). It may be possible to inject contrast medium into the mucocele in an effort to trace the origin of the saliva. Review the superficial anatomy of the head and neck region of the ferret before attempting surgical excision of a salivary gland.[44] Recurrence is possible.

ESOPHAGEAL DISEASE

Diseases of the esophagus are rare in ferrets. Acquired megaesophagus has been reported in ferrets, and I have seen the condition several times in my practice.[6,31] *Megaesophagus* describes an esophagus that is enlarged (dilated) on radiographic examination and that lacks normal motility. Recognizing this disease is important because the prognosis in ferrets with megaesophagus is poor. Clinical signs include lethargy, inappetence or anorexia, dysphagia, and weight loss. Regurgitation is common. Coughing or choking motions are sometimes described, and some ferrets have labored breathing. Differential diagnosis includes the presence of an esophageal or GI foreign body, gastritis, influenza, and respiratory diseases.

Diagnosis is based on clinical signs and radiographic evidence. On radiographs, the esophagus is often dilated in both the cervical and thoracic segments (Fig. 3-3). Food may be visualized in the esophagus. Aspiration pneumonia and gastric gas are sometimes evident in addition to esophageal dilation. Always take radiographs of the abdomen to exclude lower GI disease. Administer barium (10 mL/kg PO) to delineate the esophagus and to evaluate mural lesions, strictures, or obstructions (Fig. 3-4). An endoscope can also be used to evaluate the esophagus. Use fluoroscopy, if available, to determine the motility of the esophagus after a barium swallow.

The cause of megaesophagus in ferrets is unknown. Consider possibilities in the differential diagnosis as for dogs, and tailor the diagnostic workup accordingly. The management of ferrets with megaesophagus is similar to that of canine patients but is usually less successful. Supportive care and antibiotics are palliative at best. Administration of a GI motility enhancer such as metoclopramide (0.2-1 mg/kg q6-8h PO or SC) (Reglan, AH Robins Company, Inc., Richmond, VA) may be helpful. Cisapride, which until recently was marketed for gastroesophageal reflux and gastroparesis in humans, reduces the frequency of regurgitation in dogs with megaesophagus when it is given at 0.5 mg/kg q8-24h PO.[55] However, this drug is no longer available commercially in the United States because of adverse cardiac effects in humans. Its use in ferrets has not been evaluated. If esophagitis is suspected, add an H_2-receptor blocker, such as cimetidine, ranitidine (Zantac, Glaxo Pharmaceuticals, Research Triangle Park, NC), or famotidine (Pepcid AC, Johnson and Johnson, Fort Washington, PA).

The prognosis for ferrets with megaesophagus is poor; generally, they die or are euthanatized within days of diagnosis. Affected ferrets are debilitated and suffer from malnutrition, hepatic lipidosis, and aspiration pneumonia.

Other causes of esophageal disease in the ferret are rare. Esophageal foreign body has been reported in a ferret and was successfully managed surgically.[10]

GASTRITIS AND ULCERATION

Gastric and duodenal ulceration has been reported in laboratory ferrets and is seen sporadically in pet ferrets. Causes of GI

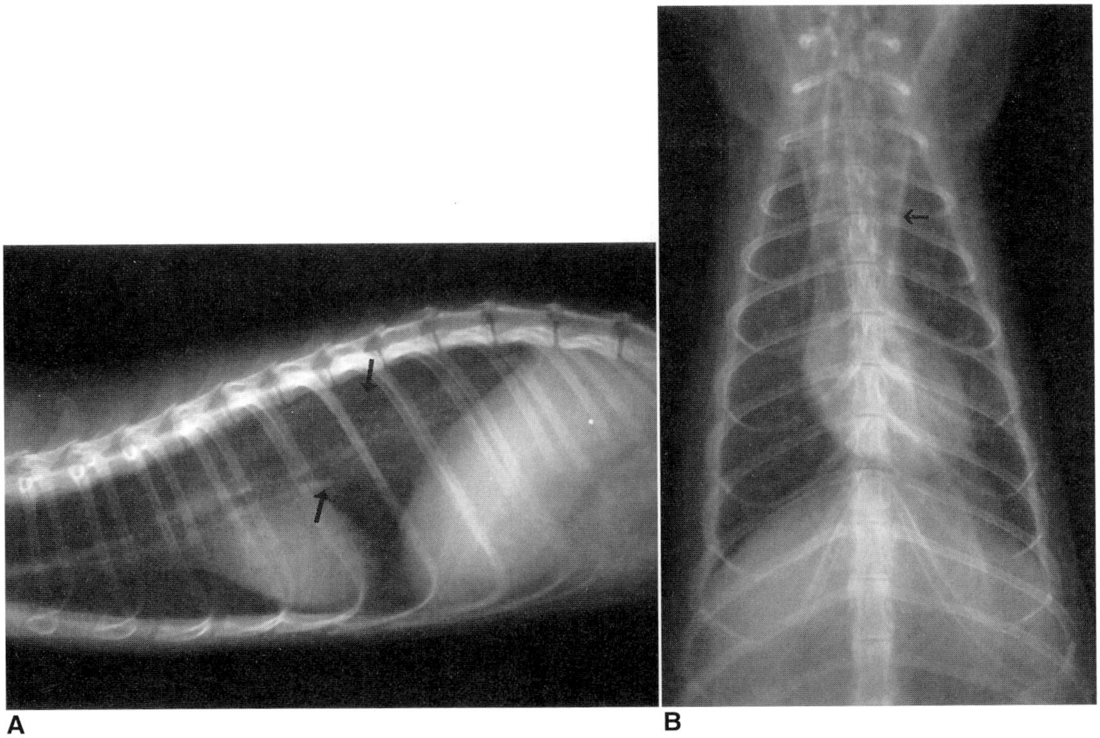

Figure 3-3 A, Lateral thoracic radiograph of a ferret with megaesophagus. Note the subtle dilation of the thoracic esophagus (*arrows*). B, Ventrodorsal radiograph of the same ferret in A. The cranial thoracic esophagus is dilated (*arrow*) and is much easier to visualize in this view than in the lateral view.

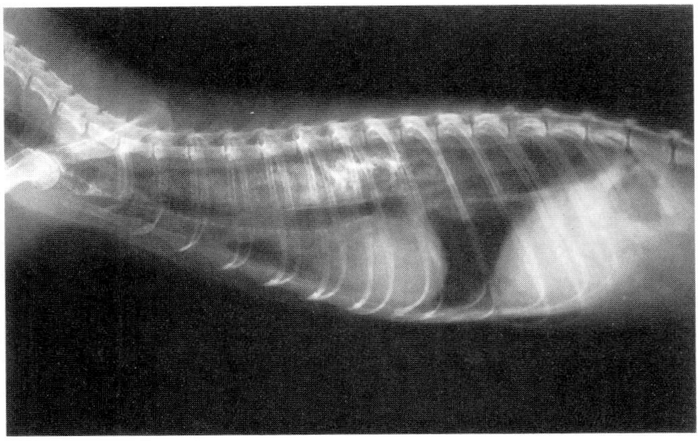

Figure 3-4 Lateral radiograph of a ferret with megaesophagus. Orally administered barium sulfate delineates the esophagus.

ulceration include foreign body or toxin ingestion, *Helicobacter mustelae* infection, treatment with ulcerogenic drugs, GI neoplasia, and azotemia caused by renal disease.

The laboratory ferret is used as an animal model for the study of *H. pylori* infection in humans. *H. mustelae* isolated from the gastric mucosa of ferrets shares many molecular and biochemical features of *H. pylori*. *H. mustelae* infection in ferrets is associated with varying degrees of gastritis, with or without duodenitis, and it can result in ulcer formation.[21] (See Part II for a discussion of *H. mustelae* infection.)

Ulcerogenic drugs such as nonsteroidal and steroidal anti-inflammatory agents can be associated with ulcer formation. It is rare for ferrets to have GI bleeding when they are treated with corticosteroids at appropriate dosages; however, ulceration is possible with the prolonged use or overdose of other anti-inflammatory agents such as ibuprofen (see Chapter 6). Severe uremia and associated melena can occur in ferrets with primary renal disease, but this is uncommon.

Gastritis in ferrets may be acute or chronic. Clinical signs may include weight loss and vomiting. Affected ferrets may hypersalivate and display tooth-grinding, which are indicative of nausea and abdominal pain. Clinical signs of gastric or duodenal ulceration include melena, anorexia, lethargy, and weight loss.

Basic diagnostic testing includes whole-body radiography and screening blood tests. Fast the ferret for a short time (6-8 hours) to facilitate visualization of a gastric foreign body or hairball. The diagnosis of *H. mustelae* gastritis may be a diagnosis of exclusion of other common disorders, such as the presence of a GI foreign body; treatment for *H. mustelae* gastritis is often based on a presumptive diagnosis. Establish definitive diagnosis of *Helicobacter* infection by histopathologic study of a gastric mucosal sample obtained by endoscopic or surgical biopsy. Specialized techniques are necessary for culturing the organism, which is not shed consistently in feces of infected ferrets.[26]

Treat gastritis and gastric ulceration with both specific therapy (according to the diagnosis) and supportive care. Hospitalize sick and anorexic ferrets for fluid therapy and parenteral treatment. A broad-spectrum antibiotic, administered parenterally, is indicated for sick ferrets. For ferrets that are not vomiting, offer multiple small feedings of a bland, moist diet; avoid dry, high-fiber foods. For vomiting animals, withhold food for 6 to 12 hours while closely monitoring for any sign of hypoglycemia (older ferrets often have subclinical insulinomas); then, if vomiting has resolved, introduce small, frequent feedings.

Bismuth compounds have action against pepsin, a proteolytic enzyme believed to be an important factor in the development of peptic ulcers. Administer bismuth subsalicylate at a dose of 1 mL/kg q8h PO. Sucralfate (Carafate, Marion Merrell Dow, Inc., Kansas City, MO) is a cytoprotective agent that binds to the erosion site and helps to form a protective barrier. It is a safe and useful adjunct to ulcer treatment and can be given orally in tablet ($^1/_8$–$^1/_{10}$ of a 1-g tablet) or suspension (100 mg/kg) form every 6 hours.

Systemic H_2-receptor antagonists, such as cimetidine and famotidine, are often used to treat gastric ulcers because they block the histamine receptor on the gastric parietal cell and reduce gastric acid secretion. The proton pump inhibitors, such as omeprazole (Prilosec, Astra Merck, Inc., Wayne, PA), are occasionally used in ferrets. One quarter of the contents of a 10-mg capsule can be mixed with soft food and given orally.

Antacid therapy may not be helpful in the early treatment of *Helicobacter* infection because affected ferrets usually develop hypochlorhydria.[26] A standard treatment for *Helicobacter* infection in humans is "triple therapy" with amoxicillin, metronidazole, and bismuth (see Part II). Bismuth interferes with the colonization of *H. pylori* in humans and suppresses colonization of *H. mustelae* in ferrets.[52]

Surgical removal is the treatment of choice for GI foreign bodies.

GASTROINTESTINAL POLYPS

Two ferrets with GI polyps have been seen at the Animal Medical Center (New York, NY). Both ferrets showed lethargy, inappetence, melena, and weakness from anemia. Abdominal radiographs suggested GI abnormalities. On surgical abdominal exploration, one ferret had a gastric polyp and the other had a small intestinal polyp. Both ferrets did well after surgical resection of the polyps, which were histologically benign.

GASTRIC BLOAT

Gastric bloat is rarely seen in pet ferrets, but it has been reported on domestic ferret farms and in black-footed ferrets (*Mustela nigripes*).[16,48] Clinical signs are usually observed in weanling ferrets and include acute gastric distention, dyspnea, and cyanosis. Sudden death can occur.

The cause of gastric bloat is unknown but is thought to be related to an overgrowth of *Clostridium perfringens* (previously called *C. welchii*). Certain conditions may predispose to clostridial overgrowth, including increased concentration of carbohydrates in the GI tract from overeating, dietary changes, and intestinal hypomotility. *C. perfringens* multiplies rapidly, producing enterotoxins that attack the villous epithelial cells of the gut. Gas production by the bacteria results in abdominal distention.

Prevention and treatment of the disease are difficult because of the ubiquitous nature of the organism and the short course

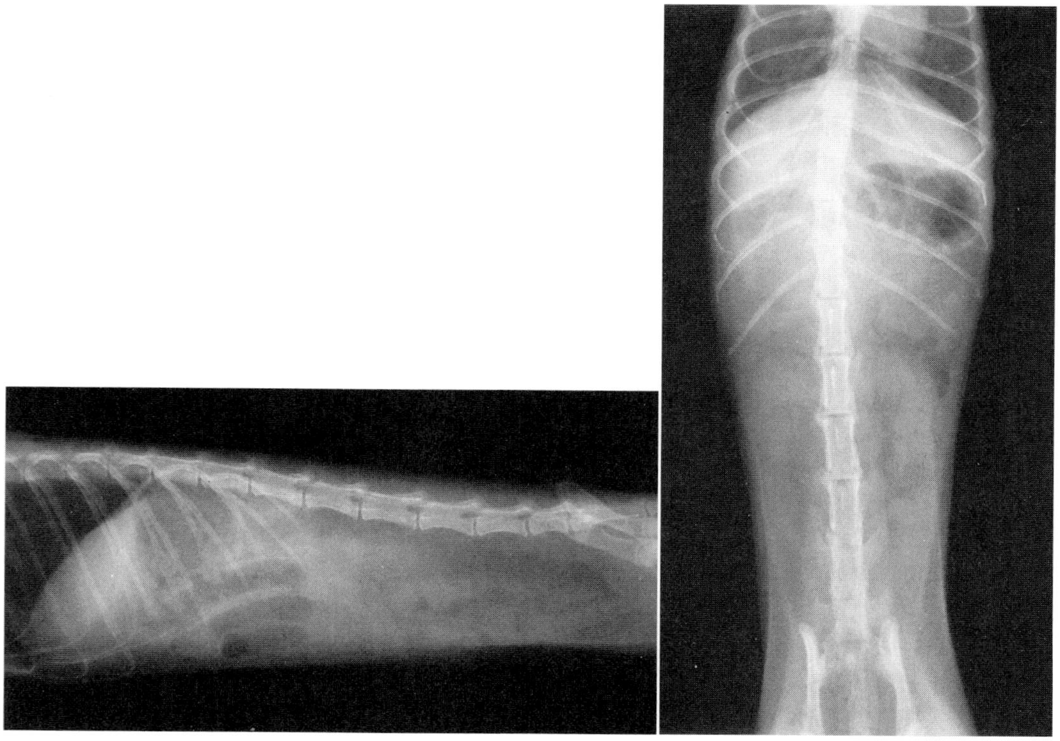

Figure 3-5 Lateral and ventrodorsal radiographic views of a ferret with a GI foreign body. There is a moderate amount of gastric gas present, and the proximal small intestine is markedly dilated. The foreign body is not visualized.

of disease. These animals are in shock and need immediate aggressive therapy. Relieve gastric pressure by trocharization or placement of an orogastric tube. Follow therapeutic protocols as for bloat in canine patients.

GASTROINTESTINAL FOREIGN BODIES

GI foreign bodies are very common in ferrets.[40] Ferrets are naturally very inquisitive and like to chew on miscellaneous environmental objects, particularly rubber or sponge products. Rubber foreign bodies are most commonly ingested by young ferrets (younger than 2 years of age); in contrast, trichobezoars (hair balls) are more common in older ferrets. Linear foreign bodies, commonly ingested by cats, are rare in ferrets.

The most common clinical signs of a GI foreign body in ferrets are lethargy, inappetence or anorexia, and diarrhea. Vomiting is often *not* reported by the owner. However, if vomiting is observed, consider a GI foreign body (Table 3-1). Some ferrets display signs of nausea, including bruxism, ptyalism, and face rubbing. Weakness can be profound in acutely obstructed animals; some of these ferrets are recumbent and reluctant to ambulate. If a GI foreign body is suspected, palpate the abdomen carefully. Foreign bodies in the small intestine often are associated with very localized discomfort or pain. Gastric foreign bodies are more difficult to palpate. Take whole-body survey radiographs in these cases. Although uncommon, esophageal disease is an important differential diagnosis in the anorexic, "vomiting" ferret. Abnormal abdominal radiographic findings include segmental ileus, gaseous distention of the stomach, and, occasionally, a visible foreign object or trichobezoar (Fig. 3-5). Contrast (barium) studies can be done but are rarely needed. Base the diagnosis on history, clinical signs, palpation, and the results of radiography. At a minimum, submit a blood sample for a complete blood count (CBC) and plasma biochemical analysis in ferrets that are sick for longer than 2 or 3 days.

Ferrets rarely pass GI foreign bodies unassisted. Occasionally, a small, partially obstructing object may pass with the administration of intestinal lubricants (cat laxatives) q8h and replacement fluids. However, most GI foreign bodies must be removed surgically. Stabilize debilitated ferrets before surgery. Parenteral fluids are usually essential because these ferrets often have varying degrees of dehydration. Perform an exploratory laparotomy as soon as possible. Collect biopsy specimens from the liver, the spleen (if enlarged), and the stomach or intestines (if ulcerated or abnormal in appearance). Some of these ferrets may also have *H. mustelae*–associated gastritis or GI lymphoma. Check the adrenal glands and the pancreas in older ferrets; discovery of concurrent abdominal disease is not unusual during surgery. (See Chapter 12 for a description of the surgical procedure.) In most instances, recovery is rapid after GI foreign body removal, and ferrets are able

TABLE 3-1
Differentiation of Common Gastrointestinal Diseases that Cause Weight Loss and Diarrhea in Ferrets by Typical History, Clinical Findings, and Laboratory and Radiographic Results*

Disease	Typical Diarrhea	Vomiting/ Bruxism	Prolapsed Rectum/ Tenesmus	Associated Physical Findings	Laboratory/ Radiographic Results	Comments/Pertinent History
Helicobacter mustelae gastritis	Black, tarry; mucoid, green	Yes	No	Enlarged mesenteric lymph nodes	± Reactive hepatitis ± Anemia Gas in stomach	Recent stress (i.e., surgery) Can increase in severity with age
Epizootic catarrhal enteritis	Acute—profuse mucoid, green Chronic—grainy ("bird seed")	Possible	No	± Thickened or fluid-filled intestinal loops	± Reactive hepatitis	Acute onset, can become chronic Recent exposure to new or young ferrets
Proliferative bowel disease	Mucoid, green	Rare	Yes	Palpably thickened large bowel	± High globulins	Affects young ferrets primarily
Eosinophilic gastroenteritis	Mucoid, green	Possible	No	± Thickened intestinal loops	Eosinophilia ± Reactive hepatitis	Rare occurrence Multiple tissue involvement (visceral lymph nodes, spleen)
Inflammatory bowel disease	Mucoid, green	Possible	No	± Enlarged mesenteric lymph nodes	Reactive hepatitis ± High globulins ± High lipase	May develop secondary to other GI diseases
Foreign body	Black, tarry or mucoid, green	Yes	No	Palpable gastric or intestinal gas Painful abdominal palpation	± Reactive hepatitis Anemia (chronic) Gas in stomach or intestinal loops	Acute or chronic Young ferrets—toys, etc; Adult ferrets—hairballs more common

*Although typical findings are listed, clinical signs and physical findings are variable in any of the described diseases.

to eat soft foods 24 hours after surgery. Most ferrets can be discharged within 36 to 48 hours after surgery.

Prevention of foreign body obstructions includes recommending the regular use of a cat laxative preparation during active shedding seasons and "ferret-proofing" the household. Ferrets should not be left uncaged or unsupervised. Advise owners to avoid giving small rubber "squeak" toys to pet ferrets.

GASTROINTESTINAL PARASITISM

GI parasites are uncommon in ferrets. However, any ferret with diarrhea should have a complete fecal parasite check, including a direct fresh wet mount and fecal flotation. In juvenile ferrets, nematodiasis is rare, but coccidiosis and giardiasis are occasionally seen. Coccidiosis can be subclinical in ferrets or it may be associated with diarrhea, lethargy, and dehydration.[7] Rectal prolapse is possible. Base the diagnosis of coccidiosis on fecal testing, either by direct wet mount and microscopic examination or by fecal flotation. Follow the same treatment protocols as for canine and feline patients with coccidiosis.

Cryptosporidiosis is described in ferrets but may not result in clinical disease.[4,46] Young ferrets can have a subclinical infection that can persist for several weeks. The oocysts can be shed in the feces of clinically normal ferrets. Histologically, the organism may be associated with an eosinophilic infiltrate in the lamina propria of the small intestine. It is not known whether zoonotic transmission of ferret cryptosporidia is possible; however, warn immunocompromised owners if the oocysts are detected in their ferrets.

ENTERITIS AND DIARRHEA

Salmonellosis

Salmonellosis is a contagious disease characterized by fever, bloody diarrhea, and lethargy. Conjunctivitis and anemia also may be present. *Salmonella newport*, *S. typhimurium*, and *S. choleraesuis* may be involved.[35] The incidence of salmonellosis in pet ferrets is very low and the infection may be associated with the feeding of uncooked meat, poultry, and meat by-products. Isolation of *Salmonella* organisms usually requires the collection of multiple fecal samples and the use of selective media. Treatment consists of aggressive supportive care, use of antimicrobials, and shock therapy as needed.

Mycobacteriosis

Ferrets may be naturally or experimentally infected by the bovine, avian, and human tubercle bacilli.[8,15,49] *Mycobacterium bovis* and *M. avium* infections have been recognized in research and farm ferrets in England, Europe, and New Zealand. These infections may have been associated with the feeding of raw meat and poultry and unpasteurized dairy products. More recently, a pet ferret was reported to have a visceral infection caused by *M. avium.*[49] The ferret had a long-term history of weight loss, diarrhea, and vomiting that was unresponsive to treatment. Intestinal biopsy results revealed granulomatous inflammation and acid-fast bacteria.

Base the diagnosis of mycobacteriosis on the findings of tissue biopsy, including histopathologic examination with acid-fast staining, polymerase chain reaction (PCR) testing, and culture. *M. avium* can be detected in the small intestine, liver, spleen, and lymph nodes of affected ferrets. Because of the zoonotic potential, treatment is not recommended.

Campylobacteriosis

Campylobacter jejuni is a bacterial enteric pathogen that is associated with diarrhea and enterocolitis in human beings and several animal species, including dogs, cats, calves, and sheep. *C. jejuni* can be isolated from the feces of normal ferrets. During the 1980s, it was suspected to be the cause of proliferative colitis, which has since been renamed "proliferative bowel disease (PBD)" in ferrets.[19,20] However, inoculation of *C. jejuni* in 54 conventionally reared and two gnotobiotic ferrets caused diarrhea but not the full spectrum of clinical signs and histopathologic lesions seen in PBD (see Part II).[4] The agent of porcine proliferative enteropathy, which is identical to that causing PBD in ferrets,[15] has now been assigned the new genus and species name *Lawsonia intracellularis*. The importance of *C. jejuni* as a primary pathogen in pet ferrets is not known.

Viral Diarrhea

Infection with rotavirus causes diarrhea in young ferrets. Farm outbreaks of diarrhea are associated with high morbidity and mortality rates in neonatal kits from 2 to 6 weeks of age.[5,56] The morbidity is low in adult ferrets, but infection may result in a transient green mucoid diarrhea. No antemortem testing is available for the diagnosis of rotaviral infection in ferrets. Treatment is supportive; administer fluids and antibiotics to affected ferrets.

Canine distemper virus is a highly contagious paramyxovirus that causes fatal disease in unvaccinated ferrets. Clinical signs are variable but often include diarrhea in conjunction with nasal and ocular discharges and a generalized orange-tinged dermatitis (see Chapter 7). Diarrhea may be acute or intermittent. Fortunately, the widespread practice of vaccinating ferrets against canine distemper virus has greatly limited the occurrence of distemper and it has now has become an uncommon disease in ferrets. Coldlike symptoms and diarrhea in newly purchased, unvaccinated ferrets should arouse suspicion. There is no treatment for distemper.

Ferrets affected with human influenza virus (an orthomyxovirus) sometimes have transient diarrhea. The virus also causes upper respiratory disease associated with coughing, sneezing, inappetence, and lethargy. Affected ferrets are often febrile (see Chapter 7).

Epizootic catarrhal enteritis (ECE) is a highly transmissible diarrheal disease of ferrets that first appeared in 1993 in several rescue and breeder operations in the eastern United States. The causative agent is thought to be a coronavirus.[57] In intestinal biopsy samples from affected ferrets, histologic findings include lymphocytic enteritis, villous atrophy, and blunting or degeneration of apical epithelium. Ferrets with ECE initially develop a profuse, green mucoid diarrhea that may progress to a loose, grainy stool resembling birdseed.

Adult ferrets are most susceptible to ECE, and the typical history includes recent exposure to a new, young ferret that acts as an asymptomatic carrier. The incubation period is 48 to 72 hours, and affected ferrets are anorexic and lethargic. Treat sick ferrets with signs of ECE with aggressive fluid therapy, antibiotics, and supportive care, and isolate these ferrets from asymptomatic or unexposed ferrets. Although the morbidity rate can be high, the mortality rate is low in ferrets that are treated appropriately. After recovering from ECE, some adult ferrets develop persistent, intermittent malabsorption with diarrhea. The clinical course can be prolonged in these ferrets, lasting weeks to months. Treatment with a short course of steroids (prednisone 1 mg/kg q12h for 14 days) and changing the diet to an easily absorbed food may speed recovery.

Inflammatory Bowel Disease

Inflammatory bowel disease is a relatively common cause of gastroenteritis in ferrets.[9] The cause is unknown but may be related to dietary intolerance, hypersensitivity reaction, or another aberrant immune response. The inflammation typically is lymphoplasmacytic and should be distinguished from eosinophilic gastroenteritis, which often involves multiple tissues. This condition is easily overlooked in ferrets because it resembles viral diarrhea (ECE), eosinophilic gastroenteritis, and *Helicobacter*-associated gastroenteritis.

Affected ferrets can have loose stools, intermittent nausea, occasional vomiting, and weight loss. Clinical signs can be subtle or, in rare cases, can resemble those of a GI foreign body in severity. These ferrets are usually young or middle-aged adults and in multiple-ferret households; typically only one ferret in the household is affected. Results of blood tests may reveal an increase in concentrations of liver enzymes and serum globulins, and lymphocytosis is occasionally present. In some ferrets, laboratory results are unremarkable.

Diagnosis is based on clinical signs, a detailed clinical history that eliminates the possibility of exposure to ECE, and results of diagnostic tests such as radiographs and routine blood tests. Diseases such as *Helicobacter* gastroenteritis and Aleutian mink disease should be ruled out. Definitive diagnosis can only be made by histologic examination of full-thickness gastric and intestinal biopsy samples.

Treatment is aimed at suppressing the immune response and dietary management. Corticosteroids such as prednisone (1 mg/kg PO q12-24h) can be used, but some ferrets with inflammatory bowel disease respond poorly to long-term treatment with steroids. Azathioprine (Imuran, Prometheus Laboratories, San Diego, CA) (0.9 mg/kg PO q24-72h) is another treatment option and seems to be well tolerated in ferrets.[3] Hypoallergenic diets made for cats (z/d feline; Hill's Pet Nutrition, Topeka, KS) can be tried.

LIVER DISEASE

Lymphoma is the most common hepatic neoplasm seen in ferrets. Other reported hepatic neoplasms include hemangiosarcoma, adenocarcinoma, and hepatocellular adenoma.[29] Pancreatic islet cell tumors can eventually metastasize to the liver. Prognosis is guarded regardless of tumor type.

Other than neoplastic diseases, primary hepatopathies are uncommon in ferrets. Vascular shunts have not been reported. Hepatic lipidosis can be found in association with long-term anorexia. Chronic GI diseases (e.g., trichobezoar formation) can lead to hepatic lipidosis. Steroid hepatopathy is rare in ferrets, even with long-term steroid administration or hyperadrenocorticism. Chronic-lymphocytic portal hepatitis has been found on histologic examination of hepatic biopsy samples. The cause of these entities is unknown but may be related to chronic visceral inflammation such as inflammatory bowel disease. Chronic cholangiohepatitis with biliary hyperplasia of variable intensity was reported in 8 of 34 cohabitating ferrets.[28] Three ferrets had neoplastic lesions in the liver. Spiral-shaped bacteria were identified in the livers of three ferrets, and bacteria with 97% similarity to *Helicobacter* species were identified by PCR in the feces of one ferret. Because of the clustering of cases and the pathologic findings, a possible infectious cause was suggested.

Copper toxicosis was diagnosed in two sibling ferrets on the basis of high hepatic copper concentrations and histologic changes in hepatic tissue.[27] Clinical signs in these two ferrets were mostly nonspecific and included severe central nervous system depression with hypothermia and hyperthermia, respectively. One ferret was icteric. Both ferrets died within a few days of clinical evaluation despite supportive care. A genetic predisposition to copper toxicosis in these two ferrets was proposed because they were siblings with the same phenotypic coat color and because no environmental source of copper could be identified.

A high concentration of alanine aminotransferase (>275 IU/L) is present on biochemical analysis in most ferrets with liver disease. Alkaline phosphatase concentration is sometimes elevated. High total bilirubin levels are uncommon, and ferrets are rarely icteric. Base the diagnosis of liver disease on observation of persistently high concentrations of liver enzymes, radiographic and ultrasound findings, and for definitive diagnosis, analysis of liver biopsy samples. Ultrasound-guided needle biopsy of the liver is possible, but full abdominal exploration is often recommended because of the likelihood of concomitant disease in ferrets.

NEOPLASIA

The GI tract is not a common site of primary neoplasia in ferrets. The oral cavity is a rare location for neoplastic lesions. Pyloric adenocarcinoma has been reported,[47] and I have seen intestinal adenocarcinoma in one ferret. Lymphoma frequently affects the GI tract of ferrets (see also Part II). Visceral and mesenteric lymph nodes and the liver are common sites for lymphoma; intestinal lymphoma is uncommon. Treatment involves surgical resection and debulking whenever possible. Chemotherapy for lymphoma is described in Chapter 9.

RECTAL DISEASE

Rectal prolapse can occur in ferrets. It is most often associated with diarrhea and is usually a disease of young ferrets. Possible causes include coccidiosis, PBD, colitis, campylobacteriosis, and neoplasia (see Part II).

Diagnostic tests should include a fecal wet mount and flotation to check for parasites. GI parasitism other than coccidiosis is uncommon. Treat with antibiotics and antiparasitics, as indicated. Prolapses often resolve with treatment of the causative condition. Although rarely needed, rectal purse-string sutures can be placed if the prolapse is extensive; these sutures can be left in place for 2 to 3 days.

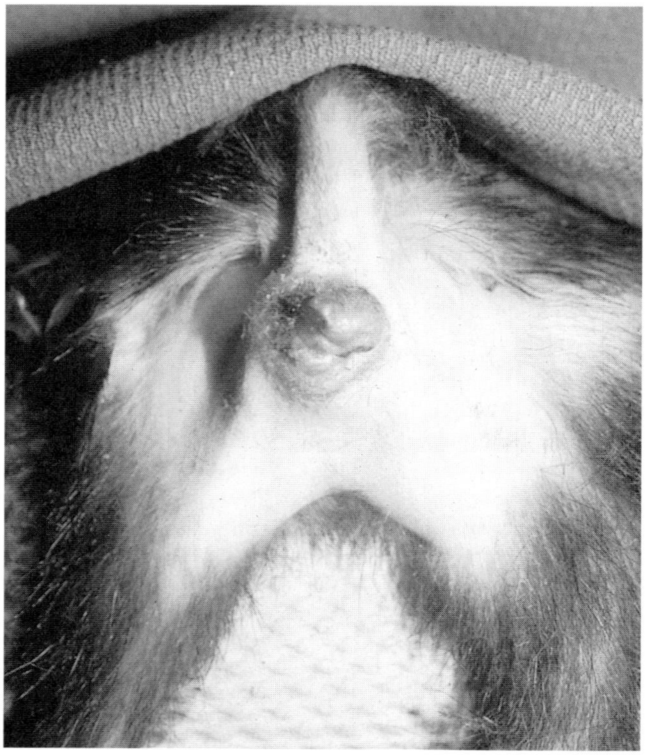

Figure 3-6 Rectal leiomyosarcoma in a ferret that presented for a recurrent rectal prolapse.

Include a careful rectal examination (visualization and palpation) in all ferret examinations. Undescented ferrets may develop anal gland disease, including impactions and abscessation. Palpation of the anal area may reveal either unilateral or 360-degree perianal swelling. Manage anal gland disease as in the dog. Be forewarned: anal gland odor is quite noxious. Anal gland removal is described in Chapter 12.

Neoplasia is rare in the rectal area, although I have seen one descented ferret with leiomyosarcoma that surrounded the rectal opening (Fig. 3-6). The ferret presented for a rectal prolapse, and a tumor was found on palpation. Treatment involves surgical debulking and, possibly, a rectoplasty. Prognosis is poor.

APPROACH TO VOMITING

Owners may describe "vomiting" in their ferrets, but some of these animals may actually be regurgitating. In light of this, the differential diagnoses for emesis in ferrets include both esophageal diseases and gastroenteric disorders. In the clinical history, vomiting is not as frequently described in ferrets as it is in canine or feline patients. For example, ferrets rarely vomit hairballs, and often vomiting is not part of the history associated with foreign body ingestion. The reason for this is unclear. No anatomic feature prevents emesis in ferrets; in fact, ferrets have long been laboratory animal models for human emesis studies because vomiting can readily be induced in them in a laboratory setting.[14]

The major differential diagnoses for vomiting or regurgitation in ferrets include the presence of a GI foreign body, *H. mustelae* gastritis, gastroenteritis, and, rarely, megaesophagus. It is uncommon for ferrets with metabolic problems such as azotemia or hepatic disease to vomit. Although definitive diagnosis is not always possible, it is important to recognize whether medical or surgical treatment is required. For example, most obstructions caused by a foreign body require surgery, whereas gastroenteritis is a medical disease. However, differentiating these two diagnoses is often quite challenging (see Table 3-1).

Diagnosis begins with the history. Pointedly question an owner regarding the chewing habits of the ferret: Does the ferret have a squeak toy? Is it unsupervised in the household or usually caged? Has vomiting been observed? The description of any vomiting behavior is significant. Also question the owner regarding the animal's appetite and obtain a description of the feces.

On physical examination, some foreign bodies in the small intestine can be distinctly palpated. However, enlarged mesenteric lymph nodes can sometimes feel like foreign objects. Also remember that foreign bodies in the stomach are difficult to detect on palpation. PBD may result in palpably thickened intestines in the ferret; however, vomiting is not usually a feature of this disease.

Radiography is the most important diagnostic test in the workup of a vomiting ferret. Survey radiographs should include the whole body. Radiographic signs of megaesophagus can be subtle. The heart may appear small because of hypovolemia from dehydration. Varying amounts of gas can be seen with foreign body–related obstruction, and sometimes the incriminating object is visible. Segmental ileus or a dilated and gas- or fluid-filled stomach is a typical radiographic sign of obstruction (see Fig. 3-5). Not all cases of GI foreign body are radiographically obvious. If evidence of foreign body obstruction is not well defined, consider medical therapy and perform repeat radiography in 24 hours. Alternatively, give barium contrast for a series of contrast-enhanced films.

If there is a strong indication of the presence of a foreign body, perform abdominal exploratory surgery the same day, preferably after parenteral fluid therapy has been started (see Chapter 12). Obtain tissue for biopsy as needed (e.g., the liver or spleen), and save any foreign object to show to the owner. Always check the entire gut for lesions and examine the pancreas and adrenal glands, especially in older ferrets. If a foreign body is not found, collect gastric and duodenal biopsy samples and request special staining for *Helicobacter* species. *Helicobacter* infection is associated with gastritis, especially in the antral region and the proximal duodenum (see Part II). Although results of exploratory surgery may be negative for a foreign object, histologic examination of biopsy samples may or may not reveal a diagnosis. The possibility of negative findings should be discussed with the owner before surgery.

If surgery is not an option or is not recommended, consider treatment for *H. mustelae*–associated gastritis (see Part II). If obstruction is still a possibility, administer a cat hairball preparation (Laxatone [EVSCO Pharmaceuticals, Buena, NJ] or Petromalt [VRx Products, Harbor City, CA]) at 1 mL q8-12h. Carefully examine all feces passed in the hospital; foreign objects or matter may sometimes be found in the stool.

APPROACH TO DIARRHEA

Normal ferrets nibble on food all day. Their GI transit time is short (3 hours), so defecation is frequent in the healthy state.

The normal stool is slightly soft and formed. Diarrhea can range from mucoid and green to hemorrhagic. Some owners describe a "birdseed" type of diarrhea that may be caused by malabsorption. Anorexic ferrets may produce a very dark green (bile) stool that can resemble melena. Unlike canine patients, diarrhea in ferrets is difficult to classify as originating in the small intestine or the large intestine. More important are the onset, duration, and severity of the diarrhea as well as concurrent clinical signs.

Several causes of diarrhea in ferrets are recognized. These can be separated into diseases of young or older ferrets as well as infectious or noninfectious causes. The most common noninfectious causes of diarrhea include dietary indiscretion, foreign body ingestion, trichobezoar, and inflammatory bowel disease. Occasionally, severe metabolic disease can result in a green (bile-tinged) mucoid diarrhea. Eosinophilic gastroenteritis typically affects mature ferrets but is uncommon (see Table 3-1 and Part II).

Infectious agents are rare causes of diarrhea in closed groups or isolated ferrets, such as those kept as individual household pets. Ferrets do not usually have GI parasites, but coccidia can be present in young, newly purchased ferrets. Rotavirus can cause outbreaks of severe diarrhea, but most reports of this are in very young, unweaned ferrets. Ferrets that have been exposed to unfamiliar ferrets, such as show ferrets, may be susceptible to ECE. Newly acquired young ferrets can also act as asymptomatic carriers of ECE and expose naïve, older ferrets in a household group. In contrast, PBD usually affects young ferrets. Canine distemper virus in the epitheliotropic form causes diarrhea in conjunction with respiratory and integumentary disease in unvaccinated ferrets.

The clinical approach to the diagnosis of diarrhea depends on the severity and duration of clinical signs. Obtain a vaccination and dietary history and perform a direct fecal wet mount and flotation to check for GI parasites. Treat ferrets with mild diarrhea, without anorexia or vomiting, on an outpatient basis with an antibiotic such as chloramphenicol or sulfadimethoxine or with a cat hairball preparation if a trichobezoar is a possibility. Sick ferrets need a more comprehensive workup that includes radiographs to check for obstructive lesions and a CBC and a plasma biochemical analysis to assess metabolic conditions. If simple diagnostic tests do not reveal a cause and therapy is unsuccessful, consider exploratory surgery to evaluate the GI tract and obtain biopsy samples. Endoscopy can be difficult in ferrets because of their small size but may be an alternative to surgery. Perform colonoscopy in ferrets with chronic colitis. Culture the feces for *C. jejuni* or *Salmonella* species, especially if the ferret is febrile or the feces are hemorrhagic.

Hospitalize sick or dehydrated ferrets for supportive care and a diagnostic workup. Give fluids subcutaneously if a ferret is stable or intravenously if it is weak and dehydrated. Administer antibiotics parenterally if possible. Metronidazole, chloramphenicol, and amoxicillin are good choices for GI disease in the ferret. Oral chloramphenicol does not usually cause the nausea and anorexia that it produces in some cats. A short course of a kaolin/pectin suspension (1-2 mL/kg PO q2-6h prn) can be administered as a GI protectant until a more definitive diagnosis is established. Drugs that affect the motility of the GI tract should never be administered without an initial diagnosis. Motility-enhancing drugs such as metoclopramide and cisapride are contraindicated if a GI obstruction is present, and anticholinergic drugs can produce an ileus that may be difficult to interpret radiographically.

Part II *HELICOBACTER MUSTALAE* GASTRITIS, PROLIFERATIVE BOWEL DISEASE, AND EOSINOPHILIC GASTROENTERITIS

Judith A. Bell, DVM, MSc, PhD

H. mustelae gastritis, PBD, and eosinophilic gastroenteritis all cause diarrhea and wasting in ferrets. Eosinophilic gastroenteritis has been infrequently diagnosed, and no specific causative agent has been identified. Virtually all North American ferrets are likely to be exposed to *H. mustelae* as kits, becoming persistently infected at weaning and developing some degree of gastritis.[17] PBD, also known as proliferative colitis or ileitis, is caused by an intracellular bacterium and is associated with chronic diarrhea and marked weight loss in ferrets.[18] Clinical or subclinical gastritis may develop concurrently with PBD and other GI or systemic diseases. Other entities to be ruled out include partial GI obstruction by a foreign body, lymphosarcoma or other gastric neoplasia, Aleutian mink disease, and persistent ECE.

HELICOBACTER MUSTELAE GASTRITIS

H. mustelae is a gram-negative rod morphologically similar to *Campylobacter* species that requires a microaerophilic environment for growth on artificial media. It is antigenically related and biochemically similar to *H. pylori*, a human pathogen associated with gastritis and ulcers.[21] Colonization of the antral area of the stomach and pyloric area of the duodenum with *H. mustelae* is very common in domestic ferrets, unless they are specifically treated or hand reared in isolation.[12,17] Colonization is accompanied by a specific immune response, but infection persists despite high serum antibody titers.[17] Although infection is common, clinical gastritis and ulcers occur relatively infrequently. Severe gastritis may be evident in gastric biopsy samples from ferrets showing no signs of clinical disease.[17]

The histopathologic lesions of *H. mustelae*–associated gastritis in human beings and ferrets consist of mucus depletion, gland loss and regeneration, and leukocyte infiltration. The organism can be observed in silver-stained histologic sections of gastric mucosa.[21] Affected ferrets that die usually have a single large pyloric ulcer or many small ones (Fig. 3-7), and the stomach and intestinal tract contain digested blood and mucus, causing the ingesta to appear very dark. Cultures of *H. mustelae* from fecal samples are usually difficult to obtain, even when the organism is readily identified histologically in gastric biopsy samples.

In humans, chronic infection with *H. pylori* leads to different clinical and pathologic outcomes, including chronic gastritis, peptic ulcer disease, and gastric neoplasia.[42] The severity and distribution of the *H. pylori*–induced inflammation are key deter-

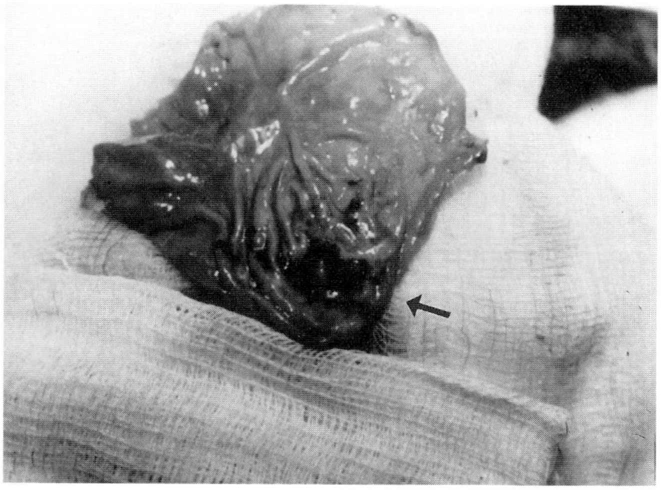

Figure 3-7 Single large ulcer (*arrow*) in the pyloric area of a ferret's stomach.

minants of these outcomes. Gastritis involving the antrum is associated with excessive acid secretion and a high risk of duodenal ulcer. Gastritis involving the acid-secreting corpus region of the stomach is associated with hypochlorhydria, gastric atrophy, and increased risk of gastric cancer.[41]

As in humans infected with *H. pylori*, transient hypochlorhydria develops in ferrets approximately 4 weeks after experimental infection.[36] This condition probably facilitates fecal-oral transmission as well as recovery of *H. mustelae* from feces.[37] Hypochlorhydria is associated with urease production, which is detectable in gastric biopsy samples. It also correlates with the degree of colonization and the occurrence of gastritis in biopsy results.[17] Urease production is associated with the ability of *H. mustelae* to colonize the stomach, with non-urease-producing strains being nonpathogenic.[17] A urease breath test is available for humans to aid in diagnosis, and a similar test has been used in ferrets under research conditions but is not practical for clinical use.[37] *H. mustelae* inhibits secretion of acid by parietal cells in vitro, and this mechanism may also contribute to hypochlorhydria.[21] In humans, chronic infection with *H. pylori* is associated with release of cytokines that impair function of enterochromaffin cells, which are neuroendocrine cells in the gastric mucosa that control acid secretion by releasing histamine. The impaired secretory function of these cells may predispose to hypochlorhydria and gastric carcinogenesis.[45]

Gastrin is a hormone that stimulates gastric acid secretion and is secreted by the G cells of the gastric antrum. In humans and probably in ferrets, high levels of gastrin may initiate GI mucosal damage and ulceration. Hypergastrinemia is probably a response to the presence of *H. mustelae* in the antrum or to its associated inflammation. Hypergastrinemia is abolished after antibiotic therapy eradicates the *Helicobacter* infection.[17]

In humans, *Helicobacter*-associated gastritis has been implicated as a risk factor for gastric adenocarcinoma and gastric lymphoma.[17] There is some evidence that this is also the case in ferrets. As *H. pylori* does in humans,[32] infection with *H. mustelae* in ferrets apparently stimulates cell proliferation in the gastric mucosa.[22] Under research conditions, gastric adenocarcinoma eventually developed in ferrets that were naturally infected with *H. mustelae* and treated with a known gastric carcinogen.[17] Spontaneously occurring gastric adenocarcinoma has been reported in pet ferrets. Although *H. mustelae* was neither cultured from the lesions nor identified histologically in some cases,[47,51,53] in others, silver-stained organisms that were morphologically compatible with *H. mustelae* were present in the neoplastic tissues.[22]

Lymphoid follicles (mucosa-associated lymphoid tissue [MALT]) are observed in the gastric mucosa of humans colonized with *H. pylori*[59] and in that of ferrets colonized with *H. mustelae*[21] but not in uninfected individuals. In humans this condition may progress to MALT lymphoma. Eradicating *H. pylori* usually causes early tumors to regress, implicating the infection as the cause of neoplasia.[58,59] Gastric MALT lymphoma associated with *H. mustelae* infection has also been reported in four ferrets 5 to 10 years of age.[12] None of the affected ferrets were treated with antibiotics to eradicate *H. mustelae* either before or during the illness associated with neoplasia.

Clinical Signs of *H. mustelae* Gastritis with Ulcers

Illness may develop in ferrets 12 to 20 weeks of age under conditions of stress caused by a combination of factors, such as rapid growth, dietary changes or inadequacy, and concurrent diseases. Infection is lifelong in untreated ferrets, and the severity of chronic gastritis increases with age.[24] In mature ferrets, the disease may become clinically apparent in animals that are stressed by concurrent disease or by surgery for other conditions such as adrenal disease or insulinoma. Ferrets with severe *H. mustelae* gastritis and ulcers are lethargic and anorexic, and they rapidly become emaciated. Chronic vomiting may occur. Excessive salivation and pawing at the mouth, which are signs of nausea in ferrets, may be evident. Affected ferrets are often moderately to severely dehydrated and may have mild anemia. Black, tarry fecal material often stains the fur of the tail and perineal region.

PROLIFERATIVE BOWEL DISEASE

PBD has been recognized for decades in pigs, hamsters, and ferrets. The cause in swine is a bacterium classified in a new genus and species, *Lawsonia intracellularis*.[38] The same agent causes PBD in hamsters and in ferrets[18] and has more recently been implicated in proliferative enteropathies of other species, including white-tailed deer, ratite birds, and domestic horse foals.[11] *L. intracellularis* is an obligate intracellular organism that cannot be propagated on artificial media. Two tests that detect this organism have been developed and are used in ferret tissues under research conditions: a PCR test specific for the swine isolate, and an indirect fluorescent antibody test that identifies the omega antigen common to organisms found in PBD lesions of swine, hamsters, and ferrets.[18] However, diagnosis of clinical cases usually depends on observing clinical signs and gross or histopathologic lesions.

Areas of intestine affected by PBD feel firm, appear grossly thickened, and are often discolored on the serosal surface. The colon, small intestine, or both may be involved. Ridges of proliferative tissue, distinct from adjacent normal tissue, are obvious on the mucosal surface (Fig. 3-8). Occasionally the affected

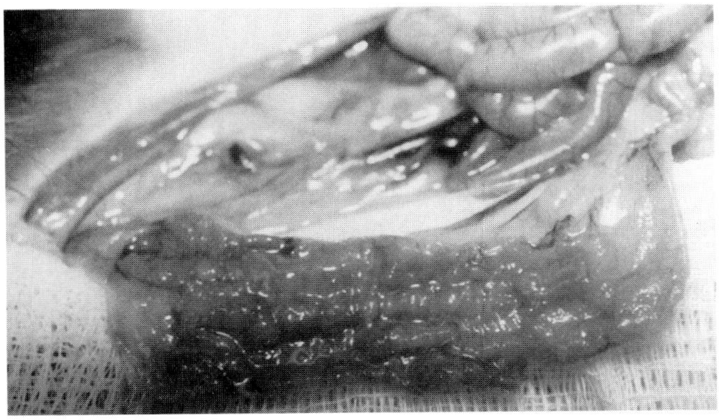

Figure 3-8 Ridges of proliferated tissue with adjacent areas of normal bowel mucosa in the colon of a ferret with proliferative colitis.

bowel perforates and causes fatal peritonitis. On histologic examination, epithelial proliferation with hypertrophy of the muscularis and infiltration of the bowel wall with either monocytic or granulocytic inflammatory cells, or both, are present.[25] In silver-stained sections, comma-shaped organisms can be found inside enterocytes lining crypts or glands. The normal architectural pattern of the mucosa is lost. Normally, straight tubular glands are covered evenly with enterocytes and numerous goblet cells. In PBD the irregular, branching, proliferative glands lack goblet cells, and necrotic debris accumulates in the crypts. Severe glandular hyperplasia resembles neoplasia and may metastasize to extraintestinal sites.[18]

Clinical Signs of Proliferative Bowel Disease

PBD occurs most frequently in rapidly growing juveniles, 10 to 16 weeks of age. Environmental and nutritional stress factors appear to play a role in resistance of infected animals to clinical disease. *L. intracellularis* is probably transmitted by the oral-fecal route,[18] and it may be assumed that all ferrets that are housed in groups will be equally exposed to the agent. However, clinical disease develops in only a small percentage (usually 1%-3%) of group-housed juvenile ferrets. Improvements in the quality of care and nutrition of pet ferrets may be responsible for the apparently decreasing incidence of PBD in recent years.

Affected ferrets have chronic diarrhea that may vary from dark, liquid feces streaked with bright red blood to scant, mucoid stool, often with bright green mucus. The fur of the tail and perineal area may be stained and wet with fecal material, and the preputial area of males is often wet with urine. Rectal tissue may continuously or intermittently prolapse (Fig. 3-9). Affected animals moan or cry while straining. Some continue to eat but lose weight at an alarming rate. If not appropriately treated, a ferret weighing 800 g may lose 400 g in less than 2 weeks. These animals are moderately to severely dehydrated and may be hypoalbuminemic. They are weak and sleep most of the time.

Because of their general debility, ferrets with PBD are more susceptible to other infectious diseases. They may have upper respiratory tract infections that do not affect other healthy ferrets housed with them and often develop clinical gastritis or ulcers. Severely affected animals will die if not treated appropriately,

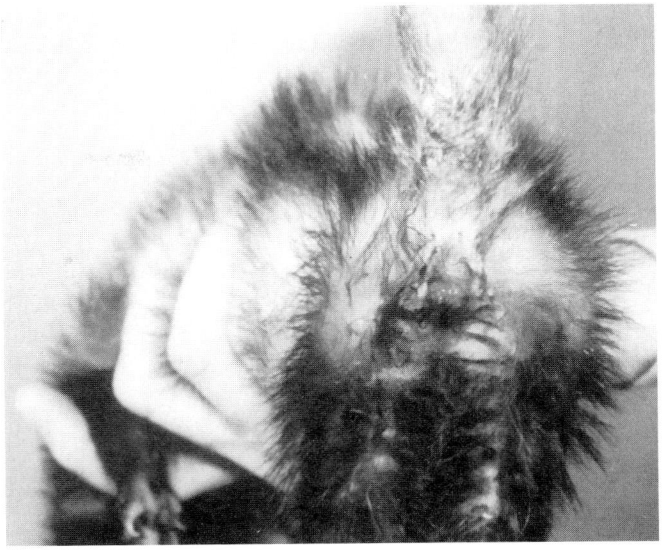

Figure 3-9 Prolapsed rectum and hair matted with fecal material in a wasted ferret with proliferative colitis.

and most of those that die despite treatment have proliferative ileitis alone or in combination with colitis.

EOSINOPHILIC GASTROENTERITIS

Eosinophilic gastroenteritis is a rare type of inflammatory bowel disease that occurs in ferrets as in other animals. In all reported cases, the ferrets were older than 6 months of age; however, because of the small number of reports available, finding this disease in a younger animal may be possible. No specific causative agent has been found in ferrets,[13,43] dogs,[50] or humans,[54] but food allergy is implicated in most humans and in some dogs. In specific cases in humans and in other species, clinical signs were relieved when appropriate treatment for food allergies or parasitism was instituted. Peripheral eosinophilia is a common but not a constant finding in affected dogs and humans[50] but has been reported in most of the relatively few ferrets diagnosed with this disease.[43] No reports of food elimination tests in affected ferrets have been published.

The lesion of eosinophilic gastritis in ferrets, as in other animals and humans, is a mild to extensive infiltration of the mucosa, submucosa, and muscularis of the stomach and small intestine with eosinophils. Focal eosinophilic granulomas may be found in the mesenteric lymph nodes of affected ferrets.[43] No pathogens have been observed in or isolated from the lesions of affected ferrets. In humans and other affected species, granulomas may cause partial bowel obstruction.

Clinical Signs of Eosinophilic Gastroenteritis

Affected animals typically have chronic diarrhea, with or without mucus and blood, and severe weight loss. Granulomas may be palpable. Vomiting, anorexia, and dehydration are variable signs. Signs may be clinically indistinguishable from those of gastritis, persistent ECE, or GI obstruction by a foreign body.

DIFFERENTIATION OF WASTING DISEASES

H. mustelae–associated gastritis and PBD may occur independently, sequentially, or concurrently in the same animal. PBD is a sufficient stressor to induce clinical gastritis in a ferret colonized with *H. mustelae*. Although these two diseases are most common in ferrets 12 to 16 weeks of age, sufficiently stressed mature ferrets may also be affected. However, clinical disease in adult animals is more often associated with *Helicobacter*-associated gastritis than with PBD. Although eosinophilic gastroenteritis has been confirmed only in adults, it also may be occurring undiagnosed in younger animals. Any of the wasting diseases can be diagnosed by gastric and intestinal biopsy. However, often a presumptive diagnosis may be based on clinical examination, an accurate history, and results of a CBC, without results from a complex or expensive laboratory workup. Diagnosis may be "confirmed" by the response to appropriate treatment. Characteristics of GI diseases that cause diarrhea and weight loss are summarized in Table 3-1. Other important differential diagnoses for diarrhea and weight loss in domestic ferrets include lymphoma and Aleutian disease.

Steps in Diagnosis

History Question the owner of a lethargic, anorexic ferret with diarrhea and sudden weight loss about changes in the ferret's diet, feeding schedule, and access to water. The stress factor most commonly associated with wasting diseases is restriction of food for any reason, including the following:

Self-denial of food Ferrets resist changing to a food that differs in flavor and texture from the one to which they are accustomed and may fast for several days rather than eat the new food. Fasting depletes fat stores, which should not be confused with the loss of muscle mass associated with wasting diseases.

Restriction of access to water Ferrets consume about three times as much water as dry food pellets and cannot meet their nutritional requirements if water is restricted.

Restriction of access to food Food hoppers used with some types of ferret cages may be easily blocked by large food pellets or pellets with unusual shapes, and the owner may not realize that the ferret is unable to get its food. Children caring for ferrets are less likely than adults to understand the significance of an unchanging level of food in the hopper for several days. In addition, some ferrets habitually dig their food out of the container and refuse to eat food that becomes wet or contaminated on the cage floor.

Inappropriate, nutritionally deficient diet Occasionally, new owners provide ferrets with inappropriate foods, such as dog food or poor-quality cat food, or offer them excessive amounts of treats, especially raisins, which are palatable but contain almost 100% sugar and no protein. Rapidly growing young animals with nutritional deficiencies are much more susceptible to all infectious diseases.

Environmental stress Exposure to extremes of temperature, particularly heat, is very stressful to ferrets. Animals may be stressed during inclement weather if they are housed outdoors without adequate protection from wind and rain, especially if their food is of poor quality or subject to wetting, caking, and molding. Ask the owner if the affected pet is their first ferret. You may identify stressors that the owner would not have taken into consideration.

Physical examination Palpate the abdomen of an emaciated ferret. Grossly thickened areas of gut in ferrets with PBD and eosinophilic gastroenteritis are usually palpable. A focal area of pain in the abdomen is more typical of the presence of a GI foreign body. Splenomegaly is common in ferrets in association with many diseases, and mesenteric lymph nodes are likely to be enlarged in ferrets with any of the wasting diseases. Projectile vomiting has been reported in one ferret with eosinophilic gastroenteritis.[13] Although rectal prolapse is not pathognomonic for PBD, it is safe to assume this diagnosis in a ferret with prolapse associated with diarrhea and weight loss. In young ferrets (younger than 16 weeks of age and usually younger than 10 weeks), coccidiosis may be associated with diarrhea and rectal prolapse, but coccidiosis is rarely associated with significant weight loss. Both Aleutian mink disease and lymphosarcoma are insidious; thin ferrets will have lost condition over a period of weeks or months and may not have diarrhea.

Radiography is the most useful tool for detecting a GI foreign body (see Part I). Contrast radiographs are sometimes helpful in identifying obstruction with a radiolucent foreign body, but radiographs may also suggest areas of gastric ulceration or intestinal mucosal proliferation in ferrets with either PBD or eosinophilic gastroenteritis.

Obtain a blood sample for a CBC to help eliminate the possibility of lymphosarcoma and eosinophilic gastroenteritis. Ferrets with eosinophilic gastroenteritis usually have dramatic eosinophilia (10%-35% eosinophils compared with 3%-5% in normal ferrets). Ferrets with lymphosarcoma may not be leukemic, and further tests, such as peripheral lymph node biopsy or a splenic aspirate, are necessary for diagnosis. Inflammation associated with PBD often causes leukocytosis with neutrophilia and a left shift. Ferrets with bleeding ulcers are usually anemic (normal hematocrit is 40%-55% in spayed or neutered pets, lower in jills in estrus). Dehydration may mask mild anemia and hypoproteinemia in emaciated animals; therefore repeat a CBC after rehydration. Aleutian disease may cause diarrhea, anemia, leukocytosis, and wasting. Serologic tests for Aleutian disease virus are available (see Chapter 6), but many ferrets with positive test results show no clinical signs of Aleutian mink disease. Clinicians should not assume that any illness in ferrets serologically positive for Aleutian disease virus is caused by the virus.

Treatment of Proliferative Bowel Disease

L. intracellularis is sensitive to chloramphenicol. No other antibiotic consistently resolves PBD in ferrets. Chloramphenicol is administered at a dose of 50 mg/kg q12h IM or SC (chloramphenicol sodium succinate) or orally (chloramphenicol palmitate oral suspension) for at least 10 days. A ferret with colitis of recent onset improves quickly with this treatment and gains 50 to 100 g/day within a few days of the first dose. *L. intracellularis* is also sensitive to tylosin, tetracyclines, tiamulin, and several other antimicrobials that are used to treat PBD in pigs[38] and to erythromycin, which is commonly used in affected foals,[34] but treatment of ferrets with any of these drugs is disappointing. Treatment of infected but clinically normal 6- to 9-week-old ferrets with oral tylosin (5 mg/kg mixed in soft food once daily) appears to reduce the incidence of clinical PBD in a colony, but only chloramphenicol produces a dramatic improvement in sick ferrets.

Repair of rectal prolapse with a purse-string suture is rarely necessary because, as the colon heals, the prolapse usually disappears spontaneously. It may appear intermittently for weeks but causes no apparent distress. If a purse-string suture is used, the owner must closely monitor the ferret to make sure that it can defecate, especially when the stool regains its normal consistency. Sutures should be removed in 2 to 3 days.

Treatment of *H. mustelae*–Associated Gastritis with Ulcers

Chloramphenicol has no effect on *H. mustelae*.[42] The original treatment for *Helicobacter* in humans and ferrets was "triple therapy," a combination of amoxicillin, metronidazole, and bismuth subsalicylate, administered q12h for at least 2 weeks (see Table 3-2 for dosages). Colloidal bismuth subcitrate (8 mg/kg PO q8h) may be substituted for bismuth subsalicylate. Although *H. mustelae* is sensitive to either amoxicillin or metronidazole, drug resistance quickly develops unless both are given simultaneously. Cimetidine (10 mg/kg PO q8h), other H_2-receptor blockers, or sucralfate suspension (25-100 mg/kg PO q8h) may be helpful in very sick animals that are bleeding from extensive gastric ulcers. Compounding pharmacists can prepare palatable suspensions of many drugs available in tablet form. Avoid fish-flavored suspensions when having drugs compounded because ferrets do not like this taste. When administering oral medications, scruff the ferret firmly and use a plastic dropper or dosing syringe. Oral veterinary or pediatric amoxicillin suspensions are palatable and well accepted by most ferrets.

Other drug combinations have been used in ferrets to eradicate *H. mustelae,* with advantages of improved palatability and convenience of dosing (see Table 3-2). A combination of ranitidine bismuth citrate and clarithromycin, recommended for treatment of *H. pylori* in humans, has been effective in treating ferrets under research conditions and has been used clinically.[36] Ranitidine bismuth citrate tablets may be crushed and mixed with a palatable liquid, and clarithromycin is available as a pediatric suspension (Biaxin, Abbott Laboratories, North Chicago, IL). Both drugs are administered for 14 days (dosages given in Table 3-2). A combination of clarithromycin, metronidazole, and omeprazole has proved more effective than the original "triple therapy" in eradicating *H. mustelae* in research ferrets.[1] Resistance to clarithromycin has not yet been reported in ferrets but does occur in humans.[36] To prevent development of macrolide-resistant strains, clarithromycin should be combined with a second antibiotic not in the macrolide class.[1]

Although eradication of *H. mustelae* is accompanied by decreasing antibody titers, lesions may take longer to resolve.[36] Ferrets from which the infection has been eradicated by antibiotic therapy may be reinfected with *H. mustelae* through contact with infected ferrets.[2] For treated ferrets to remain free of *H. mustelae,* they should not be exposed to ferrets of unknown *Helicobacter* status until the new ferrets have also been treated.

Table **3-2**
Summary of Treatment Regimens for *Helicobacter mustelae* Gastritis, Inflammatory Bowel Disease, Proliferative Bowel Disease, and Eosinophilic Gastroenteritis

Disease	Drug	Dosage
Helicobacter mustelae gastritis	Amoxicillin	10 mg/kg q12h PO
Original triple therapy*	Metronidazole	20 mg/kg q12h PO
	Bismuth subsalicylate	17 mg/kg (1 mL/kg) q12h PO
Alternative therapy*	Clarithromycin	12.5 mg/kg q8h PO[36]
	Ranitidine bismuth citrate	24 mg/kg q8h PO[36]
	or	
	Clarithromycin	50 mg/kg q24h PO[1]
	Omeprazole	4 mg/kg q24h PO[1]
	Metronidazole	75 mg/kg q24h PO[1]
Inflammatory bowel disease	Azathioprine	0.9 mg/kg PO q24-72h
	Prednisone	1 mg/kg PO q24h
	Sucralfate	100 mg/kg PO q6h
	Hypoallergenic diet	
Proliferative bowel disease	Chloramphenicol	50 mg/kg q12h PO, IM, SC
Eosinophilic gastroenteritis	Prednisone	1.25–2.5 mg/kg q24h PO
	Ivermectin	0.4 mg/kg SC, PO once; repeat in 14d

IM, Intramuscular; *PO,* per os; *SC,* subcutaneous.
Chloramphenicol, ranitidine bismuth citrate, azathioprine, and metronidazole can be prepared as suspensions by compounding pharmacists.
*Treat for a minimum of 14 days.

Treatment of Eosinophilic Gastroenteritis

Humans, dogs, and cats with eosinophilic gastroenteritis usually respond to steroid treatment. Because the disease in ferrets resembles that in other species, prednisone administration has been the treatment of choice.[43] Remission has occurred in ferrets treated with prednisone (1.25-2.5 mg/kg PO q24h for 7 days and q48h thereafter) until the ferret is clinically normal. Immediate recovery also followed removal of an enlarged mesenteric lymph node in one ferret and treatment with ivermectin (0.4 mg/kg SC) in another.[43] When eosinophilic gastroenteritis is a response to the presence of a parasite, eliminating the parasite is preferable to prolonged treatment with corticosteroids to relieve clinical signs.

Treatment of Emaciated Ferrets with Diarrhea

Rehydrate sick ferrets with either intravenously (preferred) or subcutaneously administered balanced electrolyte solutions. These animals are often very weak and may allow a saphenous or cephalic catheter to be inserted with little resistance. Among the advantages of giving intravenous fluids is that glucose can be administered by this route. However, if a catheter cannot be placed, fluids administered subcutaneously are well and rapidly absorbed. Hospitalize an emaciated, dehydrated ferret until fluid and electrolyte balances are reestablished. When the life-threatening episode is over, the owner will probably be willing and able to give the supportive care needed to restore the ferret to health.

While waiting for results of diagnostic tests, one can assume that most cachectic ferrets with diarrhea that do not have a GI foreign body or eosinophilia have both ileitis/colitis and *H. mustelae* gastritis with ulcers. If the ferret is treated for only one disease when it has both, the time required for recognizing treatment failure may be the factor that ultimately decides if the ferret will survive. Unfortunately, the effective drugs used for treatment of the two diseases are different, and therapy necessitates multiple daily doses of several drugs for at least 2 weeks. Because the gut flora of ferrets is very simple and plays no vital role in digestion, long-term administration of broad-spectrum antibiotics does not cause diarrhea in ferrets as it does in most animals. Emaciated animals that die despite proper treatment usually have either very extensive gastric ulcers or severe ileitis, each of which drastically reduces the absorption of essential nutrients. Age of the animal may help in the differential diagnosis; young ferrets are more likely to develop PBD, whereas older ferrets can develop severe, chronic gastritis associated with *H. mustelae* infection.[24] Also, *H. mustelae*–associated disease is more often associated with stress factors common in mature pet ferrets, such as concurrent disease or surgery (see Table 3-1).

Emaciated animals have no energy reserve and should receive intensive care. Offer a smorgasbord of premium cat foods and ferret diets. Some animals refuse to eat their regular diet of dry pellets but do accept the same food mixed with water and heated in a microwave until it develops a porridge-like consistency. Some ferrets eat meat baby foods, especially liver and chicken, and most drink milk. Milk causes loose stool in normal ferrets and in those with colitis, but it is very palatable. If milk fat is increased to 10% to 20% with cream, it appears to be absorbed well and contributes to weight gain even though diarrhea continues. Most sick ferrets accept Nutri-Cal (Tomlyn, Buena, NJ) at numerous times during the day. Many ferrets like the human food supplements such as Ensure Plus (Abbott Laboratories, Ross Products Division, Columbus, OH), Boost Plus (formerly Sustacal; Bristol Myers, Evansville, IN), or Isocal HN (Mead Johnston, Evansville, IN), and they sometimes eat softened pellets mixed with one of these products when they refuse pellets alone. Alternatively, offer nutritional recovery foods such as Maximum-Calorie (The Iams Company, Dayton, OH) or Canine a/d (Hill's Pet Nutrition); most sick ferrets accept these foods readily. Nutritional recovery diets such as Max-Cal can be used as the sole source of nutrition for weeks at a time if necessary. When using these diets, calculate a minimum daily intake of 400 kcal per kilogram of body weight. Sick ferrets may not make the effort to get up and drink from a water bottle but do usually drink from a dish. Offer fresh food and water by hand several times daily during hospitalization and home care; ferrets often take a few mouthfuls of every new offering but never go back for more. The first 2 days are critical for an animal that has lost 40% to 50% of its body weight, and intensive supportive care is essential.

When ferrets with PBD or ulcers regain their appetites, often within 48 hours of the first doses of medication, and diarrhea has resolved significantly, owners may be tempted to stop treatment. However, ferrets treated for less than 2 weeks often relapse, and some ferrets need antibiotic therapy for an additional 2 to 3 weeks if they are to recover completely. Ferrets with eosinophilic gastroenteritis that do not respond to ivermectin require longer periods of monitoring and prednisone therapy. Most ferrets with these wasting diseases can be saved with aggressive and persistent treatment.

REFERENCES

1. Alder JD, Ewing PJ, Mitten MJ, et al: Relevance of the ferret model of *Helicobacter*-induced gastritis to evaluation of antibacterial therapies. Am J Gastroenterol 1996; 91:2347-2354.
2. Batchelder M, Fox JG, Hayward A, et al: Natural and experimental *Helicobacter mustelae* reinfection following successful antimicrobial eradication ferrets. Helicobacter 1996; 1:34-42.
3. Bauck LS: Salivary mucocele in 2 ferrets. Mod Vet Pract 1985; 66:337-339.
4. Bell JA, Manning DD: Evaluation of *Campylobacter jejuni* colonization of the domestic ferret intestine as a model of proliferative colitis. Am J Vet Res 1991; 52:826-832.
5. Bernard S, Gorham JR, Ryland LM: Biology and diseases of ferrets. *In* Fox JG, Cohen BJ, Loew FM, eds. Laboratory Animal Medicine. New York, Academic Press, 1984, pp 385-397.
6. Blanco MC, Fox JG, Rosenthal K, et al: Megaesophagus in nine ferrets. J Am Vet Med Assoc 1994; 205:444-447.
7. Blankenship-Paris TL, Chang J, Bagnell CR: Enteric coccidiosis in a ferret. Lab Anim Sci 1993; 43:361-363.
8. Bryant JL, Hanner TL, Fultz DG, et al: A chronic granulomatous intestinal disease in ferrets caused by an acid-fast organism morphologically similar to *Mycobacterium paratuberculosis*. Lab Anim Sci 1988; 38:498-499.
9. Burgess M, Garner M: Clinical aspects of inflammatory bowel disease in ferrets. Exotic DVM 2002; 4.2:29-34.
10. Caliguiri R, Bellah JR, Collins BR, et al: Medical and surgical management of esophageal foreign body in a ferret. J Am Med Vet Assoc 1989; 195:969-971.
11. Cooper DM, Swanson DL, Gebhart CJ: Diagnosis of proliferative enteritis in frozen and formalin-fixed, paraffin-embedded

tissues from a hamster, horse, deer and ostrich using a *Lawsonia intracellularis*-specific multiplex PCR assay. Vet Microbiol 1997; 54:47-62.

12. Erdman SE, Correa P, Coleman LA, et al: *Helicobacter mustelae*-associated gastric MALT lymphoma in ferrets. Am J Pathol 1997; 151:273-280.
13. Fazakas S: Eosinophilic gastroenteritis in a domestic ferret. Can Vet J 2000; 41:707-709.
14. Florcyzk AP, Schurig JE, Bradner WT: Cisplatin-induced emesis in the ferret: a new animal model. Cancer Treat Rep 1982; 66:187-189.
15. Fox JG: Bacterial and mycoplasmal diseases. *In* Fox JG, ed. Biology and Diseases of the Ferret. Philadelphia, Lea & Febiger, 1988, pp 210-211.
16. Fox JG: Systemic diseases. *In* Fox JG, ed. Biology and Diseases of the Ferret. Philadelphia, Lea & Febiger, 1988, pp 258-259.
17. Fox JG: Bacterial and mycoplasmal diseases: *Helicobacter mustelae*. In Fox JG, ed. Biology and Diseases of the Ferret, 2nd ed. Baltimore, MD, Williams & Wilkins, 1998, pp 327-333.
18. Fox JG: Bacterial and mycoplasmal diseases: proliferative bowel disease—*Desulfovibrio* spp. (*Lawsonia intracellularis*). *In* Fox JG, ed. Biology and Diseases of the Ferret, 2nd ed. Baltimore, MD, Williams & Wilkins, 1998, pp 335-339.
19. Fox JG, Ackerman JI, Newcomer CE: Ferret as a potential reservoir for human campylobacteriosis. Am J Vet Res 1983; 44:1049-1052.
20. Fox JG, Ackerman JI, Taylor NS, et al: *Campylobacter jejuni* infection in the ferret: an animal model of human campylobacteriosis. Am J Vet Res 1987; 48:85-90.
21. Fox JG, Correa P, Taylor NS, et al: *Helicobacter mustelae*-associated gastritis in ferrets. An animal model of *Helicobacter pylori* gastritis in humans. Gastroenterology 1990; 99:352-361.
22. Fox JG, Dangler CA, Sager W, et al: *Helicobacter mustelae*-associated gastric adenocarcinoma in ferrets (*Mustela putorius furo*). Vet Path 1997; 34:225-229.
23. Fox JG, Dewhirst FE, Fraser GJ, et al: Intracellular *Campylobacter*-like organism from ferrets and hamsters with proliferative bowel disease is a *Desulfovibrio* sp. J Clin Microbiol 1994; 32:1229-1237.
24. Fox JG, Marini RP: *Helicobacter mustelae* infection in ferrets: pathogenesis, epizootiology, diagnosis, and treatment. Semin Avian Exotic Pet Med 2001; 10:36-44.
25. Fox JG, Murphy JC, Ackerman, JI, et al: Proliferative colitis in ferrets. Am J Vet Res 1982; 43:858-864.
26. Fox JG, Paster BJ, Dewhirst FE, et al: *Helicobacter mustelae* isolation from feces of ferrets: evidence to support fecal-oral transmission of a gastric *Helicobacter*. Infect Immun 1992; 60:606-611. (Published erratum appears in Infect Immun 1992; 60:4443.)
27. Fox JG, Zeman DH, Mortimer JD: Copper toxicosis in sibling ferrets. J Am Vet Med Assoc 1994; 205:1154-1156.
28. Garcia A, Erdman SE, Xu S, et al: Hepatobiliary inflammation, neoplasia, and argyrophilic bacteria in a ferret colony. Vet Pathol 2002; 39:173-179.
29. Goad ME, Fox JG: Neoplasia in ferrets. *In* Fox JG, ed. Biology and Diseases of the Ferret. Philadelphia, Lea & Febiger, 1988, pp 281-282.
30. Harper DS, Mann PH, Regner S: Measurement of dietary and dentifrice effects upon calculus accumulation rates in the domestic ferret. J Dent Res 1990; 69:447-450.
31. Harris CA, Andrews GA: Megaesophagus in a domestic ferret. Lab Anim Sci 1993; 43:506-508.
32. Havard TJ, Sarsfield P, Wotherspoon AC, et al: Increased gastric epithelial cell proliferation in *Helicobacter pylori* associated follicular gastritis. J Clin Pathol 1996; 49:68-71.
33. Johnson-Delaney CA, Nelson WB: A rapid procedure for filling fractured canine teeth of ferrets. J Sm Exotic Anim Med 1992; 1:100-102.
34. Lavoie JP, Drolet R, Parsons D, et al: Equine proliferative enteropathy: a cause of weight loss, colic, diarrhea and hypoproteinaemia in foals on three breeding farms in Canada. Eq Vet J 2000; 32:418-425.
35. Marini RP, Adkins JA, Fox JG: Proven or potential zoonotic diseases of ferrets. J Am Vet Med Assoc 1989; 195:990-993.
36. Marini RP, Fox JG, Taylor NS, et al: Ranitidine bismuth citrate and clarithromycin, alone or in combination, for eradication of *Helicobacter mustelae* in ferrets. Am J Vet Res 1999; 60:1280-1286.
37. McColm AA, Bagshaw JA, O'Malley CF: Development of a ^{14}C-urea breath test in ferrets colonised with *Helicobacter mustelae*: effects of treatment with bismuth, antibiotics, and urease inhibitors. Gut 1993; 34:181-186.
38. McOrist S, Mackie RA, Lawson GHK: Antimicrobial susceptibility of ileal symbiont intracellularis isolated from pigs with proliferative enteropathy. J Clin Microbiol 1995; 33:1314-1317.
39. Miller PE, Pickett JP: Zygomatic salivary gland mucocele in a ferret. J Am Vet Med Assoc 1989; 194:1437-1438.
40. Mullen HS, Scavelli TD, Quesenberry KE, et al: Gastrointestinal foreign body in ferrets: 25 cases (1986-1990). J Am Anim Hosp Assoc 1989; 28:13-19.
41. Naito Y, Yoshikawa T: Molecular and cellular mechanisms involved in *Helicobacter pylori*-induced inflammation and oxidative stress. Free Radic Biol Med 2002; 33:323-336.
42. Otto G, Fox JG, Wu P-Y, et al: Eradication of *Helicobacter mustelae* from the ferret stomach: an animal model of *Helicobacter (Campylobacter) pylori* chemotherapy. Antimicrob Agents Chemother 1990; 34:1232-1236.
43. Palley LS, Fox JG: Eosinophilic gastroenteritis in the ferret. *In* Kirk RW, Bonagura JD, eds. Kirk's Current Veterinary Therapy XI: Small Animal Practice. Philadelphia, WB Saunders, 1992, pp 1182-1184.
44. Poddar S, Jacob S: Gross and microscopic anatomy of the major salivary glands of the ferret. Acta Anat (Basel) 1977; 98:434-443.
45. Prinz C, Zanner R, Gratzl M: Physiology of gastric enterochromaffin-like cells. Annu Rev Physiol 2003; 65:371-382.
46. Rehg JE, Gigliotti F, Stokes DC: Cryptosporidiosis in ferrets. Lab Anim Sci 1988; 38:155-158.
47. Rice LE, Stahl SJ, McLeod C Jr: Pyloric adenocarcinoma in a ferret. J Am Vet Med Assoc 1992; 200:1117-1118.
48. Schulman FY, Montali RJ, Hauer PJ: Gastroenteritis associated with *Clostridium perfringens* type A in black-footed ferrets (*Mustela nigripes*). Vet Pathol 1993; 30:308-310.
49. Schultheiss PC, Dolginow SZ: Granulomatous enteritis caused by *Mycobacterium avium* in a ferret. J Am Vet Med Assoc 1994; 204:1217-1218.
50. Sherding RG, Johnston SE: Diseases of the intestines: eosinophilic gastroenteritis. *In* Sherding RG, ed. Saunders Manual of Small Animal Practice, 2nd ed, 2000, p 17.
51. Sleeman JM, Clyde VL, Jones MP, et al: Two cases of pyloric adenocarcinoma in the ferret (*Mustela putorius furo*). Vet Rec 1995; 17:272.
52. Stables R, Campbell C, Clayton N, et al: Gastric anti-secretory, mucosal protective, anti-pepsin and anti-*Helicobacter* properties of ranitidine bismuth citrate. Aliment Pharmacol Ther 1993; 7:237-246.
53. Stauber E, Kraft S, Roninette J, et al: Multiple tumors in a ferret. J Sm Exotic Anim Med 1991; 1:87-88.
54. Talley NJ, Shorter RG, Phillips SF, et al: Eosinophilic gastroenteritis: a clinicopathological study of patients with disease of the mucosa, muscle layer, and subserosal tissues. Gut 1990; 31:54-58.
55. Tams TR: Cisapride: clinical experience with the newest GI prokinetic drug. Proceedings of the Twelfth American College of

Veterinary Internal Medicine Forum, San Francisco, 1994, pp 100-101.
56. Torres-Medina A: Isolation of an atypical rotavirus causing diarrhea in neonatal ferrets. Lab Anim Sci 1987; 37:167-171.
57. Williams BH, Kiupel M, West KH, et al: Coronavirus-associated epizootic catarrhal enteritis in ferrets. J Am Vet Med Assoc 2000; 217:526-530.
58. Wotherspoon AC: A critical review of the effect of *Helicobacter pylori* eradication on gastric MALT lymphoma. Curr Gastroenterol Rep 2000; 2:494-498.
59. Wotherspoon AC: Gastric lymphoma of mucosa-associated lymphoid tissue and *Helicobacter pylori*. Ann Rev Med 1998; 49:289-299.

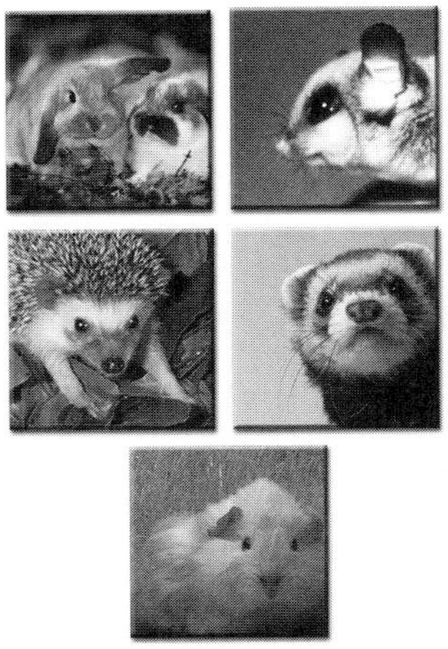

CHAPTER 4

Urogenital Diseases

Christal G. Pollock, DVM, Diplomate ABVP

Urogenital disease, such as renal failure, cystitis, and urolithiasis, is uncommon in pet ferrets. The incidence of prostatic cysts appears to be high, reflecting the high prevalence of adrenal disease in ferrets and our improved ability to diagnose this condition.

RENAL CYSTS

Renal cysts are a frequent finding in ferrets at necropsy.[20] At one institution, cysts were found in 10% to 15% of ferrets submitted for necropsy.[22] The cysts may be single or multiple and can be present on one or both kidneys.

The cause of renal cysts in ferrets is uncertain. There is no known hereditary basis for their formation, and the cysts are not associated with hepatic or biliary cysts.[25] Renal cysts in ferrets are usually an incidental finding during physical examination (as one or more smooth masses on the surface of the kidney) or during abdominal ultrasound examination (as a hypoechoic area with smooth walls). Cysts may be seen during surgery as translucent swellings that are visible through the renal capsule.

Polycystic disease is unusual in ferrets. Unlike the smooth masses palpable with renal cysts, polycystic kidneys are usually irregular. Cysts may be diffusely distributed throughout other organs, especially the liver. In rare instances, multiple cysts disrupt normal renal architecture and lead to renal failure (Fig. 4-1). Several renal cysts were found at necropsy in an adult ferret with seizure activity presumed to be caused by uremic encephalopathy.[13] Polycystic kidneys and bilateral perinephric pseudocysts were reported in an adult ferret.[39] In this ferret, pseudocyst formation led to marked abdominal distention and tachypnea (Fig. 4-2). Ultrasound-guided paracentesis was used initially as a palliative treatment. Plans were made to resect the renal capsule because of the rapid reaccumulation of fluid; however, the ferret rapidly declined and was euthanatized.

Diagnosis and Treatment

In ferrets with renal cysts, submit samples for a complete blood count (CBC), plasma biochemical analysis, and urinalysis. Ultrasonography is a noninvasive means of evaluating the architecture of the kidneys. Pyelography with intravenous contrast media or nuclear scintigraphy may be useful to evaluate renal function in some clinically affected ferrets.

There is no specific treatment for renal cysts. Monitor affected ferrets with periodic palpation and, if indicated, ultrasound examination, plasma biochemical analysis, and urinalysis. In humans, pain and hematuria are the most common clinical manifestations of renal cysts.[21] If a cyst becomes very large or painful, consider unilateral nephrectomy; however, be sure that the contralateral kidney is functioning adequately beforehand.

HYDRONEPHROSIS

Hydronephrosis has been reported in two young ferrets as a result of ligation of the ureter during ovariohysterectomy.[25,32] Both ferrets were seen for progressive abdominal distention, and abdominal radiographs showed a large fluid density. At exploratory laparotomy, a grossly enlarged, fluid-filled kidney was found (Fig. 4-3).

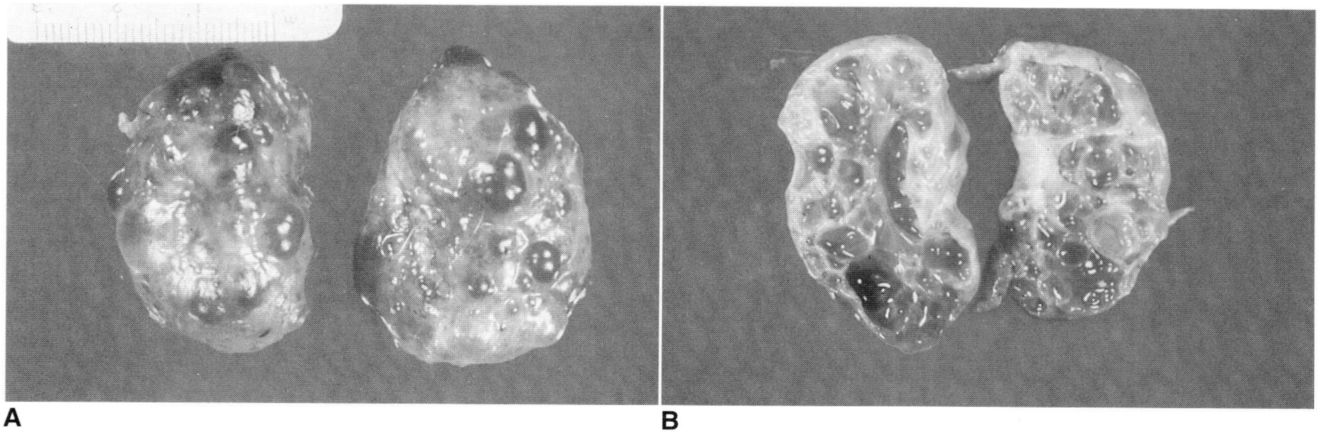

Figure 4-1 Polycystic kidney in a 3-year-old female ferret that presented with acute renal failure. **A,** Capsular aspect. **B,** Cut surface.

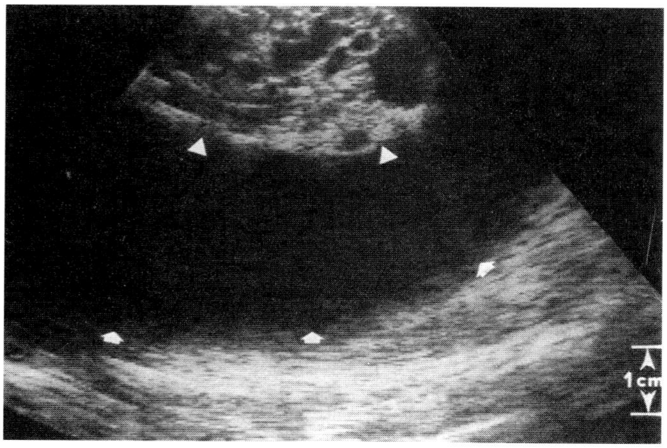

Figure 4-2 Sagittal ultrasound of the right polycystic kidney and perinephric pseudocyst in a 3-year-old male castrated ferret. The kidney (*arrowheads*) is surrounded by large amounts of pseudocyst fluid (*arrows*). *(From Puerto DA, Walker LM, Saunders M: Bilateral perinephric pseudocysts and polycystic kidneys in a ferret. Vet Radiol Ultrasound 1998; 39:309-312.)*

If hydronephrosis is suspected, submit samples for a CBC, serum biochemical analysis, and urinalysis. Abdominal ultrasound or intravenous pyelography may be used to further characterize the swelling. Fine-needle aspiration of the fluid-filled abdominal mass should reveal a transudate unless a secondary infection is present. The treatment is unilateral nephrectomy, and the prognosis is good if the function of the remaining kidney is normal.

RENAL DISEASE AND RENAL FAILURE

Although clinical renal disease is not common in ferrets, many ferrets older than 4 years submitted for necropsy at one institution had varying degrees of chronic interstitial nephritis.[27] Conditions uncommon to rare in pet ferrets include pyelonephritis, chronic interstitial nephritis, glomerulonephritis, bilirubinuric nephrosis (C. G. Pollock, personal observation, 2003), and immune complex–mediated glomerulonephropathy caused by Aleutian disease.[25,38] Renal failure has also been reported as a result of an epinephrine overdose administered to a ferret with a vaccine reaction.[14] Additionally, the use of nephrotoxic drugs may result in renal disease. Administration of amikacin (12 mg/kg SC q24h) appeared to induce renal disease in a 5-year old ferret despite concurrent administration of subcutaneous fluids (M. Loenser, personal communication, 2002). Although uncommon, renal tumors are another cause of renal failure in ferrets. Lymphoma, renal pelvic transitional cell carcinoma, renal adenocarcinoma, and papillary tubular cystadenoma have been reported.[4,49]

Diagnosis and Treatment

The approach to the diagnosis of renal disease in ferrets is the same as for other companion animal species. Clinical signs may include lethargy, anorexia, weight loss, oral ulcers, polyuria/polydipsia, and melena. Ill ferrets may also exhibit rear leg weakness or ataxia. Physical examination findings can include cachexia, dehydration, pallor, and irregularities in the size and shape of the kidneys.

In ferrets with clinical signs consistent with renal disease, perform a CBC, plasma biochemical analysis, and urinalysis. In ferrets with high concentrations of plasma proteins, submit a blood sample for Aleutian disease testing and serum protein electrophoresis. Isosthenuria in conjunction with dehydration and nonregenerative anemia may also be present; microscopic evaluation of urine sediment may therefore be helpful. Abdominal radiographs can reveal irregularities in kidney size or shape, and ultrasound examination can be used to evaluate renal architecture. Intravenous pyelography and nuclear scintigraphy are useful tests to evaluate renal function.

Abnormal results of plasma biochemical analysis in ferrets with renal disease may include hyperphosphatemia, hypocalcemia, reduced total carbon dioxide concentration, and high blood urea nitrogen concentration. Interestingly, increases in creatinine concentration are relatively moderate (generally less than 2 mg/dL). Kawasaki[27] described two ferrets with severe renal disease confirmed by histologic examination; both ferrets had a creatinine level of 1.1 mg/dL in conjunction with blood urea

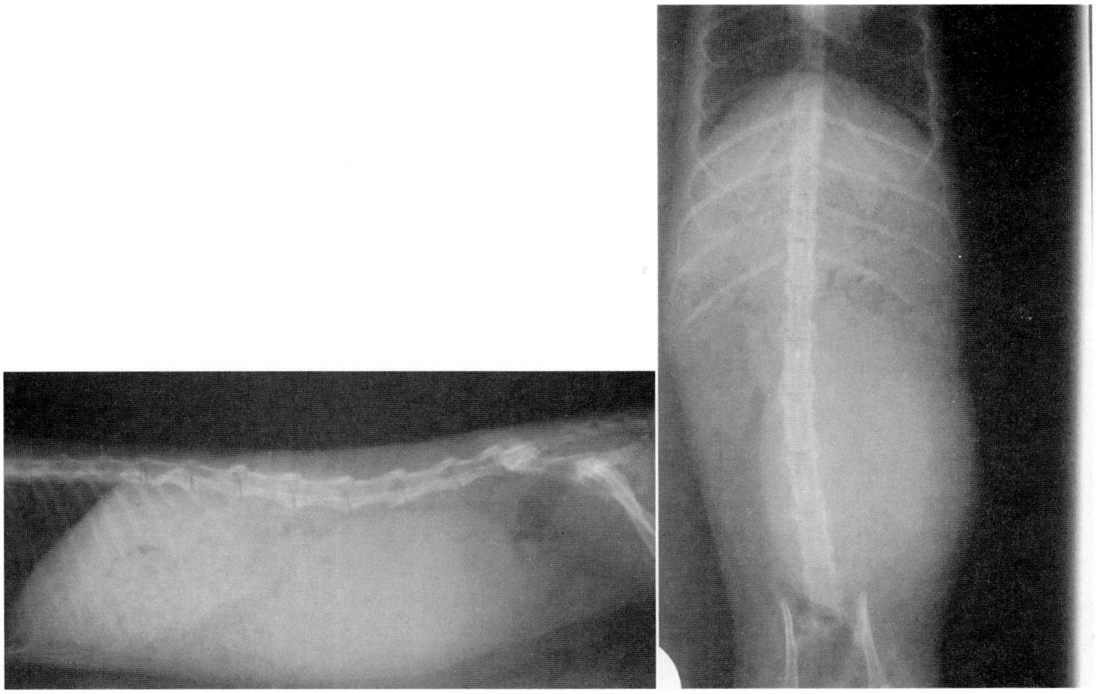

A B

Figure 4-3 Abdominal radiographs showing a hydronephrotic kidney (**A**, lateral view; **B**, ventrodorsal view). This 2-year-old spayed female ferret did well after unilateral nephrectomy. Hydronephrosis occurred as a result of inadvertent ligation of a ureter during ovariohysterectomy.

nitrogen values of 140 and 320 mg/dL. The reported normal mean creatinine level (0.4-0.6 mg/dL) is lower and the range for creatinine level (0.2-0.9 mg/dL) is narrower in ferrets than in dogs and cats.[17,19]

Reference values have been established for endogenous and exogenous creatinine and insulin clearance tests used to evaluate glomerular filtration in ferrets.[15,17] Although reference values for urine protein/creatinine ratios have not been established for ferrets, these ratios may also be an important tool for evaluating glomerular filtration. In dogs and cats, urine protein/creatinine ratios accurately reflect protein excretion over a 24-hour period regardless of sex, urine collection method, time of day, or whether the animal has been fasted or fed. Canine and feline reference values are generally less than 0.4.[12]

If renal disease is diagnosed in a ferret, try to identify the cause with ultrasound examination and, if necessary, ultrasound-guided renal biopsy (as for cats). Although treatment should be aimed at the primary cause, nonspecific therapy includes fluid therapy, supportive care, and antibiotic therapy if infection is suspected or documented. Select the antibiotic by using culture and sensitivity test results when available, and based on pharmacologic properties such as tissue distribution, route of excretion, and safety in renal failure. The prognosis for ferrets with renal failure depends on laboratory findings and response to therapy.

URETERAL RUPTURE

Traumatic avulsion of the ureter was reported in a ferret that had blunt trauma that also created a diaphragmatic hernia. No specific urinary tract signs or abnormal clinical pathologic findings were observed. Excretory urography was used to detect ureteral leakage, and treatment included ureteronephrectomy.[47]

UROLITHIASIS

Urinary calculi used to be a common cause of stranguria in ferrets; however, calculi are much less common today because of improvements in ferret diets.[9] Urolithiasis in ferrets may be characterized by solitary or multiple renal or cystic calculi or by the presence of sandy material in the bladder and urethra. Uroliths are seen most commonly in adult male ferrets, but they are also reported in pregnant jills fed a poor diet (see Chapter 5).

Although cystine urolithiasis was reported in an adult female ferret[15] and other types of stones are possible, magnesium ammonium phosphate (struvite) uroliths are most common. Dietary factors are believed to play an important role in the struvite urolith formation in ferrets. Struvite tends to precipitate in alkaline urine, and its solubility increases greatly when urine pH is 6.6 or less.[41] In turn, urine pH is greatly influenced by diet, specifically the source of dietary protein. Metabolism of animal protein tends to produce an acidic urine, whereas a plant protein–based diet produces an alkaline urine, which promotes struvite crystallization. The reported range for urine pH in normal ferrets can vary from 6.0 or 6.5 to 7.5.[25,48] Urine should be more acidic (approximately 6.0) in ferrets fed a high-quality, meat-based diet.[25]

Urolithiasis is rare in ferrets fed a high-quality feline or ferret food containing animal-based protein. The condition is much more common in ferrets fed dog food or a low-quality cat food.

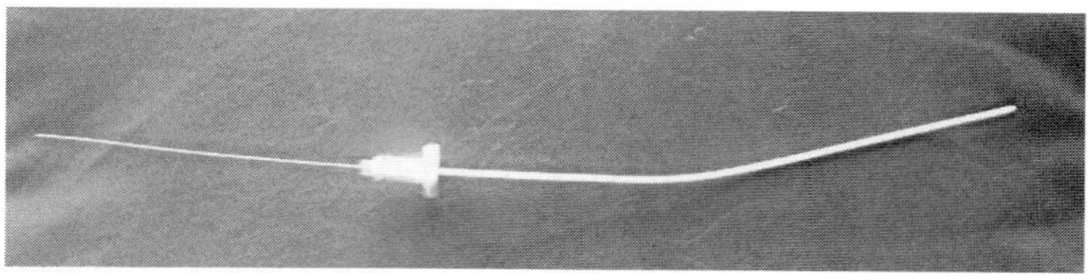

Figure 4-4 A 3.5-Fr II silicone Tomcat urethral catheter. This catheter has a closed endhole design. *(Courtesy Global Veterinary Products, New Buffalo, MI.)*

In one report, 6 (14%) of 43 ferrets fed a commercial pelleted dog food diet had renal or cystic calculi at necropsy.[33] Other factors that may predispose to the formation of struvite uroliths are infection with ascending urease-producing bacteria, particularly *Staphylococcus* and *Proteus* species, and metabolic or genetic factors.

Diagnosis

Obtain a complete history, including dietary history, from the owner. Clinical signs of urolithiasis in ferrets are dysuria, pollakiuria, wet fur in the perineal area, frequent licking of the perineum, urine dribbling, and hematuria. Ferrets with urethral obstruction may strain violently or cry when attempting to urinate. Occasionally, a ferret with blockage exhibits lethargy and inappetence without obvious signs of dysuria. If not corrected, urinary obstruction can result in severe metabolic disturbances, coma, and death. Although urethral obstruction is most common in male ferrets, females can also become obstructed.[25,36]

Cystic calculi and sand are often palpable in ferrets without obstruction, whereas a distended bladder is readily palpable in obstructed ferrets. Abdominal radiographs are a valuable diagnostic tool because the entire urinary tract can be evaluated for radiodense uroliths and other abnormalities. Unfortunately, calculi lodged at the os penis in male ferrets can be difficult to detect. Abdominal ultrasound examination is useful in identifying abnormal structures and other possible causes of urinary obstruction, such as prostatic enlargement (see below). In affected ferrets, submit samples for a full CBC, plasma biochemical analysis, and urinalysis.

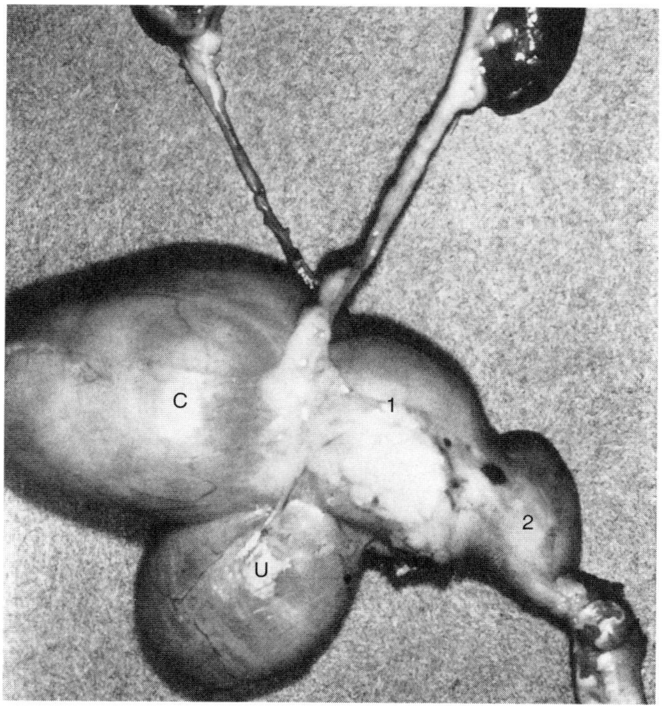

Figure 4-5 Urinary bladder and urethera in a 6-year-old male ferret. A thin-walled cyst (*C*) is on the dorsal surface of the urinary bladder (*U*) and two thick-walled cysts (*1, 2*) are on the dorsal aspect of the proximal urethra. *(From Li X, Fox JG, Erdman SE, et al: Cystic urogenital anomalies in ferrets. Vet Pathol 1996; 33:150-158.)*

Treatment

In ferrets with urolithiasis, provide supportive care, including parenteral fluids, and correct metabolic and acid-base disturbances. Begin antibiotic therapy after surgical removal of calculi or if you suspect infection, which is more common in females than in males. When possible, base the choice of antibiotic on the results of culture and sensitivity testing. Choose a broad-spectrum antibiotic that reaches high levels in the urinary tract, such as amoxicillin or cephalexin.

If the ferret is not obstructed, schedule surgical removal of calculi when the ferret is stable. Renal calculi may be managed by changing to an animal protein–based diet and antibiotic therapy, unless clinical signs warrant surgical removal.

Treatment of urinary obstruction in male ferrets is a challenge. Because of the small size of ferrets and their J-shaped os penis, urinary catheter placement may be difficult in males (see Chapter 2), particularly when they are obstructed. Use a 3.5-Fr silicone urethral catheter (Fig. 4-4), a 20- or 22-gauge 8-inch jugular catheter, or a 3.5-Fr red rubber catheter.[30,36] When placing a urinary catheter, use inhalant anesthesia to achieve adequate skeletal muscle relaxation (Fig. 4-5). Because it is excreted by the kidneys, avoid ketamine or use it with great caution.

If attempts at urinary catheterization are unsuccessful, two alternatives remain: cystocentesis followed by flushing of the urethra or emergency cystotomy. To decompress the bladder by cystocentesis, use a 22- to 25-gauge needle. Remove most, but not all, urine to protect against needle trauma. Even cystocentesis can be difficult in some ferrets with sludgy, turbid urine. Submit urine samples for urinalysis and bacterial culture and sensitivity testing. After removing the urine, place a catheter inside the prepuce and pinch the prepuce firmly closed as you flush. Ideally, the urethra will serve as the path of least resistance for the fluid, and it may be possible to flush calculi retrograde into the bladder. Alternatively, pass a feline metal urinary catheterization needle or other catheter as far as you can into the distal urethra and flush from there.[25]

An emergency cystotomy with anterograde flushing of the urethra is often the most expeditious and effective alternative to urinary catheterization (see Chapter 12). In rare instances, blockage is so severe that anterograde flushing of the urethra through the cystotomy is not possible; in such cases, an emergency perineal urethrostomy is necessary. Always submit a urolith sample for quantitative analysis and samples of crushed calculi and bladder mucosa for bacterial culture and sensitivity testing.

Long-term management of a ferret with urolithiasis involves antibiotic therapy for a minimum of 10 to 14 days and converting the ferret to an animal protein–based diet. Use the results of repeated urinalyses and urine culture and sensitivity tests to determine duration of antibiotic therapy.

Because the urine pH of a ferret on a high-quality, meat-based diet is approximately 6.0, urinary acidifiers are usually not necessary. In a study of six male ferrets, addition of phosphoric acid (H_3PO_4) to the diet at a level of 0.9% phosphorus and 0.6% calcium (dry matter basis) increased urine volume and maintained urine pH at a mean of 6.02-6.11; these conditions favor preventing as well as dissolving struvite caliculi.[16] However, this kind of dietary adjustment is impractical in the clinical setting.

Although a struvite-dissolving diet (Prescription Diet Feline s/d, Hill's Pet Nutrition, Topeka, KS) can be offered, it may not be palatable to some ferrets. This diet also contains insufficient protein for long-term use in ferrets. One ferret with a diagnosis of cystine urolithiasis was successfully managed on a prescription diet for advanced renal diseases (Prescription Diet Feline u/d, Hill's Pet Products). However, this ferret was also fed a protein supplement, and hemoglobin and albumin levels were monitored.[15] Consider a perineal urethrostomy for male ferrets with persistent problems (see Chapter 12). Fortunately, recurrence of urolithiasis is uncommon after successful therapy and management changes.

CYSTITIS

In ferrets, cystitis is generally associated with urolithiasis or prostatomegaly.[44] Prostatomegaly caused by adrenal disease reduces urine flow, thereby increasing urine stasis and the risk of bacterial overgrowth. Clinical signs of cystitis are pollakiuria, dysuria, crying with urination, urine staining of the perineum or inguinal region, and hematuria. The bladder wall may feel thickened on palpation. In a ferret with suspected cystitis, perform a cystocentesis to obtain a urine sample for urinalysis and culture and sensitivity testing. Consider a CBC and plasma biochemical analysis, particularly if the ferret is older than 3 years or if it shows signs of systemic illness. Abdominal radiographs and ultrasound examination may be indicated to rule out renal involvement and other causes of dysuria, such as urolithiasis, bladder neoplasia, the presence of an abdominal mass, or prostatomegaly.

Treat the ferret with a broad-spectrum antibiotic until the culture results are known. Then, adjust antibiotic therapy accordingly and continue treatment for a minimum of 2 weeks, as indicated by results of repeat urinalysis. Give fluid therapy and supportive care as needed and be sure that the ferret is fed a high-quality, meat-based diet (as for ferrets with urolithiasis).

BLADDER NEOPLASIA

Transitional cell carcinoma of the urinary bladder has been reported in ferrets. Presenting signs may include hematuria, dysuria, polyuria, or incontinence. The urinary bladder may also palpate abnormally. Excessive numbers of transitional cells, some abnormal in appearance, will be seen on urinalysis. Use contrast radiography or ultrasonography to visualize lesions in the bladder. Definitive diagnosis is based on biopsy results. The prognosis is poor.[40]

BLADDER ATONY

Although rabies is rarely reported in domestic ferrets, this disease should be considered a differential diagnosis in an animal with incontinence. Bladder atony and incontinence were reported in 65% of ferrets experimentally infected with rabies virus.[34]

NEOPLASIA OF THE REPRODUCTIVE TRACT

Tumors of the Female Reproductive Tract

Neoplasia of the reproductive tract is common in intact ferrets, with ovarian tumors being the most common tumor of the reproductive system. Leiomyoma is the most common ovarian tumor reported.[8,10,49] Other tumors that have been described are uterine leiomyoma, leiomyosarcoma, fibroleiomyoma, papillary adenocarcinoma, ovarian and uterine teratoma, luteoma, thecoma, uterine adenoma, fibromyoma, fibrosarcoma, granulosa cell tumor, arrhenoblastoma, dysgerminoma, and undifferentiated carcinoma of the uterine stump (see Chapter 9). Affected ferrets may be asymptomatic or show clinical signs of lethargy, depression, anorexia, persistent estrus (vulvar swelling and anemia), and dorsal alopecia that is bilaterally symmetrical. Ovariohysterectomy is the treatment of choice.[40,42]

Tumors of the Male Reproductive Tract

Interstitial cell tumors, Sertoli cell tumors, and seminomas have been reported in ferrets. These tumors cause the affected testicle to enlarge.[29,49] Total body alopecia and severe pruritus, presumably from hyperestrogenism, were described in a ferret with a Sertoli cell tumor. Although not reported in ferrets, feminization or androgenization can be seen with these tumors in other animal species.[31] The treatment of choice is castration.[1,25]

Preputial gland neoplasia has been reported in intact and neutered male ferrets (Fig. 4-6). Conflicting reports exist as to whether most of these tumors are malignant or benign. These tumors are located in the subcutis and appear either white or pink or are darkly pigmented. Careful surgical resection is the treatment of choice.[29,49]

PROSTATIC DISEASE

Prostatic disease is a potentially serious condition in middle-aged to geriatric castrated male ferrets. In fact, prostatomegaly with secondary urethral obstruction is now diagnosed more commonly than urolithiasis in male ferrets. Sterile or septic prostatic cysts can develop as a result of adrenal disease and, although the pathogenesis of prostatic cyst formation is unclear, androgens appear to stimulate prostatic tissue to proliferate.[9,44] Squamous metaplasia of glandular epithelium may lead to the development of multiple, thick-walled cysts that

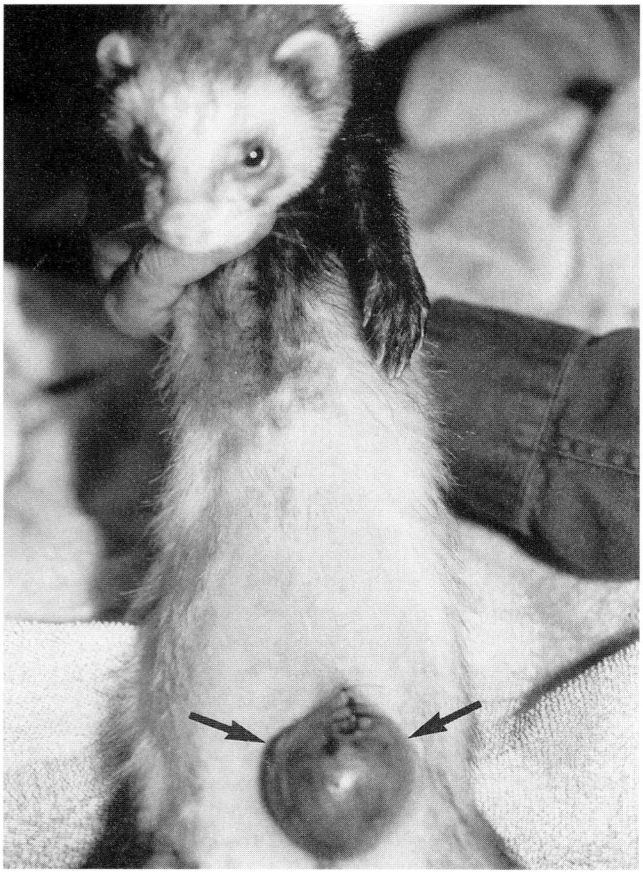

Figure 4-6 Preputial gland adenocarcinoma (*arrows*) in a 4-year-old male castrated ferret.

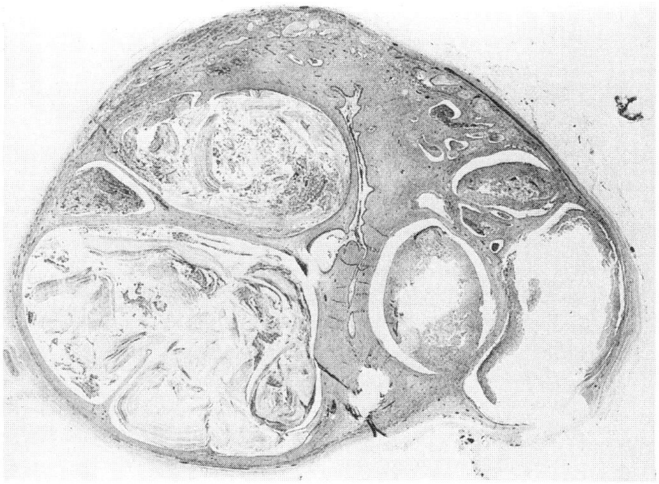

Figure 4-7 Prostate. The prostate is expanded by cysts of various sizes filled with keratin and proteinaceous debris. *(From Coleman GD, Chavez MA, Williams BH: Cystic prostatic disease associated with adrenocortical lesions in the ferret. Vet Pathol 1998; 35:547-549.)*

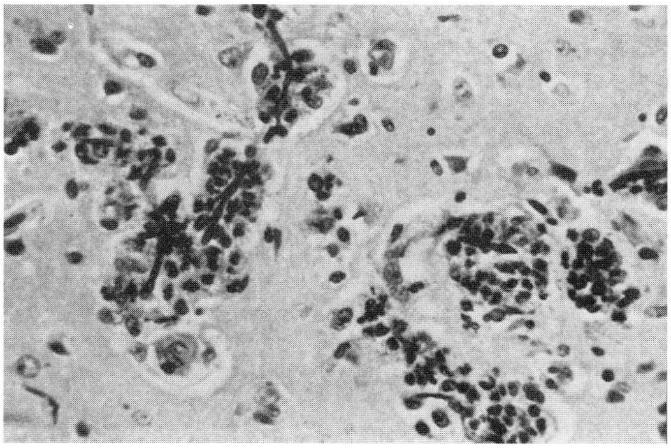

Figure 4-8 Prostate. Normal acini are separated widely by fibrous connective tissue and neutrophils, macrophages, lymphocytes, and plasma cells (hematoxylin and eosin stain, ×40). *(From Coleman GD, Chavez MA, Williams BH: Cystic prostatic disease associated with adrenocortical lesions in the ferret. Vet Pathol 1998; 35:547-549.)*

allow the prostate to potentially double in size. These cysts are filled with keratin and neutrophils and can measure up to 1 cm, and sometimes larger, in diameter (Fig. 4-7). Glandular tissue may be infiltrated with low to moderate numbers of neutrophils and fewer macrophages, lymphocytes, and plasma cells (Fig. 4-8).[9]

Prostatic disease unrelated to adrenal gland disease is rare.[44] Prostatic abscesses have been reported in association with transitional cell tumors of the bladder.[7] Prostatic seminoma and carcinoma have also been reported.[40]

Diagnosis and Treatment

Prostatomegaly can be associated with signs of a urinary tract infection, urethral obstruction, urinary incontinence, or preputial dermatitis. Most, but not all ferrets, have additional signs of adrenal disease. If the prostate is abscessed, a thick, yellow discharge may be associated with urination. An enlarged prostate may be palpable dorsal to the urinary bladder. The prostate may be even larger than the bladder (Fig. 4-9), although not all ferrets with prostatitis demonstrate prostatomegaly.[36]

Do a full medical workup in affected ferrets, remembering that adrenal disease is usually the underlying problem (see Chapter 8). On abdominal radiographs, prostatic enlargement may appear as a mass lesion dorsal to the urinary bladder, displacing the bladder ventrally. Abdominal ultrasonography to examine the architecture of the prostate is usually needed to confirm the diagnosis.[6] Ultrasound-guided fine-needle aspiration and culture of the cystic prostate may also be indicated but should be done cautiously.[36] If ultrasound is not available, contrast cystography may prove helpful.

Treatment involves managing the urethral obstruction (as with urolithiasis) and adrenalectomy if adrenal disease is present (see Chapter 12). To provide some relief for urethral obstruction, some clinicians treat ferrets with smooth muscle relaxants, such as diazepam (0.5 mg/kg IM, IV, PO q6-8h),[22] or alpha-adrenergic antagonists, such as phenoxybenzamine (Dibenzyline, SmithKline Beecham, Philadelphia, PA; 3.75-7.50 mg PO q24-72h)[44] (D. Mader, personal communication, 2003), or prazosin (Minipress, Pfizer, New York, NY; 0.05-0.10 mg/kg PO q8h) (C. G. Pollock, personal observation, 2003). Use phenoxybenza-

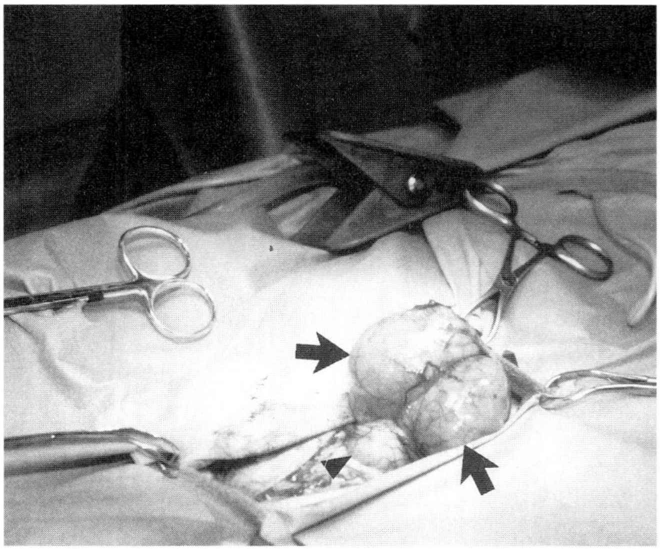

Figure 4-9 Enlarged prostate (*arrows*). The prostate may be identified dorsal to the urinary bladder (*arrowhead*). In some instances, the prostate may even be larger than the bladder in size.

mine and prazosin with caution because of the potential for adverse gastrointestinal and cardiovascular effects. A safer alternative than alpha-blockers is leuprolide acetate (Lupron Depot, Bristol-Myers-Squibb Oncology, Princeton, NJ) (see Chapter 8). In some individuals, use of high-dose leuprolide acetate (1-month form, 250 µg/kg IM) shrinks prostatic tissue within 12 to 48 hours, allowing better flow of urine through, and even voluntary micturition around, the catheter for several days. A dose of the monthly 3.75-mg formulation of leuprolide acetate has also been recommended for this purpose.[26]

Surgical management involves adrenalectomy and drainage of the cysts (see Chapter 12). With large cysts, surgical debulking is sometimes necessary. Within days after adrenalectomy, cystic hypertrophy of the prostate begins to resolve. The prevalence of infectious prostatitis associated with adrenal disease in the ferret is debatable. However, management of infectious prostatitis should include bacterial culture and sensitivity testing of cystic fluid.[7] One report describes an increased incidence of peritonitis caused by surgical debulking and drainage; instead, flushing and marsupializing the prostatic abscess to the abdominal wall are recommended. Once drainage of purulent discharge resolves, the stoma heals by secondary intention.[36] Although no complications were reported in five cases of marsupialization,[36] permanent cystotomy after marsupialization in one ferret has been described.[2]

PARAURETHRAL DISEASE

Urethral obstruction from adrenal disease is not always associated with prostatomegaly. Single or multiple, thin-walled cystic structures were reported on the dorsal aspect of the bladder and proximal urethra in six adult ferrets (four male, two female; see Fig. 4-9).[28] Clinical signs may include dysuria, hematuria, alopecia, or vulvar swelling. On physical examination, a caudal abdominal mass may be palpable. In the described cases, adrenal hyperplasia or neoplasia was detected in five ferrets; the adrenal gland was not evaluated in the sixth.[28] Although treatment was not attempted in these ferrets, initial therapy involves relief of the urethral obstruction, rehydration, and treatment of secondary bacterial infections.

Surgery is the definitive therapy for paraurethral disease. In one report, a paraurethral mass was diagnosed in a 3-year-old spayed female ferret with stranguria.[36] Physical findings included vulvar swelling and a fluctuant mass craniodorsal to the urinary bladder. On abdominal ultrasound examination, multiple cystic structures within the caudal abdomen, renal pelvic dilation, and unilateral adrenomegaly were identified. At exploratory surgery, a compartmentalized mass containing purulent material was found and marsupialized. Bacterial culture results were negative. Histologically, the cystic paraurethral tissue was described as reproductive in origin and was presumed to be a remnant of the cervix.

ESTROGEN TOXICOSIS

Ferrets are susceptible to estrogen-induced toxicosis of hematopoietic tissue.[46] Ferrets are induced ovulators, and approximately half of estrous females will remain in estrus until bred or artificially stimulated to ovulate. Short days (8 hours of light, 16 hours of dark) can also halt estrus.[45] Estrogen toxicosis has become uncommon since the large ferret breeding farms began to spay ferrets routinely before sale.[37,43] An estrogen-secreting ovarian remnant in spayed females or adrenal disease may also be associated with hyperestrogenism.[11] Clinical disease caused by an ovarian remnant is rarely observed before the ferret exceeds 1 year of age.[43] Adrenal disease rarely leads to estrogen toxicosis, and it does so only after long-standing disease has remained untreated.

Diagnosis and Treatment

Diagnosis of hyperestrogenism begins with a detailed history and careful physical examination. Clinical signs may include anorexia, lethargy, weakness, pallor, vulvar swelling, and vulvar discharge. Extended hyperestrogenism may cause melena, petechial or ecchymotic hemorrhages, and dorsally symmetric alopecia.[3,40,43]

High levels of estrogen in the ferret lead to bone marrow hypoplasia affecting all cell lines.[23,24,43] Results of a CBC will reveal a nonregenerative anemia (hematocrit less than 20%-25%), nucleated red blood cells, neutropenia, and thrombocytopenia (platelet count less than 50,000/mm^3).[40,43] Confirm nonregenerative anemia with a reticulocyte count. When results of the CBC or reticulocyte count are equivocal, submit samples of a bone marrow aspirate for cytologic evaluation.[43]

Necropsy findings may include vulvar swelling and vulvar discharge, melena, pale mucous membranes and bone marrow, endocrine alopecia, hematomyelia, hydrometra, pyometra, and petechial, ecchymotic, or subcutaneous hemorrhages.[3,40,43] Histologically, centrilobular hepatic degeneration, panmyelophthisis, and cystic endometrial hyperplasia may be detected.[3]

The primary goal of therapy is to reduce estrogen levels. Convert the estrous jill to anestrus by breeding her with a vasectomized male or mechanically induce ovulation with a vaginal probe such as a cotton-tipped applicator. The results of both procedures are unpredictable and often unsuccessful in the ill ferret.[40]

Medical manipulation of estrogen levels is most likely to be successful when estrogen levels have not been elevated for long (less than 4 weeks).[40] Administer gonadotropin-releasing hormone 20 μg/ferret SC or IM or human chorionic gonadotropin (100 IU/ferret IM).[40] Give human chorionic gonadotropin at least 10 days after the onset of estrus. Repeat in 7 days if vulvar swelling has not resolved.[37,40,43] Tamoxifen and clomiphene citrate are also contraindicated. Although both drugs demonstrate anti-estrogen effects in humans, they have been found to have estrogenic effects in the ferret. Do not use progestins because pyometra may result.[24,37,43]

Definitive therapy of hyperestrogenism is ovariohysterectomy or surgical removal of the ovarian remnant. Ovarian remnants, which are sometimes cystic, may be found near the ovarian pedicle or within mesenteric fat.[40]

Because these ferrets are often poor anesthetic and surgical risks, aggressive supportive care is often required before surgery. Give blood transfusions as needed; ferrets do not possess blood groups and multiple transfusions from multiple donors are possible.[40] The hemoglobin-based oxygen carrier Oxyglobin (Biopure Corporation, Cambridge, MA; 11-15 mL/kg IV over a 4-hour period) can be used in anemic ferrets.[35] Less commonly, bone marrow transfusions have also been described.[43]

Additional supportive care measures may include administration of anabolic steroids, corticosteroids, iron dextran, and erythropoietin (Epogen, Amgen Inc., Thousand Oaks, CA).[37,40] However, erythropoietin is reportedly not effective, possibly because of inhibition by estrogen.[40]

The prognosis for estrogen toxicosis has classically relied on the hematocrit value. A packed cell volume greater than 25% is associated with a fair to good prognosis, a packed cell volume between 15% and 25% is associated with a guarded prognosis, and a packed cell volume less than 15% is associated with a poor to grave prognosis.[40]

Estrogen toxicosis caused by persistent estrus is prevented by routine spaying of all female ferrets not intended for breeding by 6 months of age. At surgery, carefully identify all ovarian tissue that may be located within large fat deposits.[11] Do not allow breeding jills to remain in estrus for longer than 2 to 4 weeks.[40]

PYOMETRA

Because most female pet ferrets are spayed, pyometra is uncommon in clinical practice. Diagnosis and management are the same as in dogs and cats except that estrogen toxicosis must be ruled out in affected animals. Various bacteria have been cultured from infected uteri, including *Escherichia coli* and *Staphylococcus, Streptococcus,* and *Corynebacterium* species. Ovariohysterectomy is the treatment of choice (see section on metritis in Chapter 5). Occasionally, a ferret with adrenal disease develops stump pyometra. Treatment of this condition involves adrenalectomy and surgical excision of the infected stump, along with appropriate antibiotic therapy and supportive care.[25]

Stump pyometra was reported in a 4-year-old female spayed ferret. Clinical signs included dorsal alopecia, pollakiuria, and mild vulvar swelling. A turgid mass was palpable on physical examination. Peritonitis developed as a result of fine-needle aspiration of the mass.[18]

VAGINITIS

Vaginitis is sporadically seen in spayed female ferrets, most commonly caused by hyperestrogenism associated with an ovarian remnant or adrenal disease. Less commonly, vulvar swelling develops with cystitis or crystalluria. Irritation from foreign material within the vagina is common in breeding females kept on particulate bedding such as hay, straw, or shavings. Chronic vulvar swelling may lead to secondary overgrowth of bacteria such as *E. coli* and *Streptococcus* or *Klebsiella* species. Metritis and fever are occasionally present.[19] Treatment consists of systemic antibiotics and resolution of the underlying problem, such as reduction of estrogen levels medically with the use of human chorionic gonadotropin or leuprolide acetate or surgically by adrenalectomy or removal of the ovarian remnant.[40]

ACKNOWLEDGMENT

I thank Dr. Elizabeth V. Hillyer for authoring the chapter on urogenital diseases in the first edition of this book. Her work formed the basis for this chapter.

REFERENCES

1. Andrews PLR, Illman O, Mellersh A: Some observations of anatomical abnormalities and disease states in a population of 350 ferrets (*Mustela furo L.*). Z Versuchstierkd 1979; 21:346-353.
2. Antinoff N: Urinary disorders in ferrets. Semin Avian Exotic Pet Med 1998; 7:89-92.
3. Baumgartner W, Juchem R: Aplastic anemia in ferrets. Tierarztl Prax 1987; 15:333-335.
4. Bell RC, Moeller RB: Transitional cell carcinoma of the renal pelvis in a ferret. Lab Anim Sci 1990; 40:537-538.
5. Bernard SL, Leathers CW, Brobst DF, et al: Estrogen-induced bone marrow depression in ferrets. Am J Vet Res 1983; 44:657-661.
6. Besso JG, Tidwell AS, Gliatto JM: A retrospective review of the ultrasonographic features of adrenal lesions in 21 ferrets. Vet Radiol Ultrasound 1999; 40:549-550.
7. Brown SA: Ferrets. *In* Jenkins JR, Brown SA, eds. A Practitioner's Guide to Rabbits and Ferrets. Denver, The American Animal Hospital Association, 1993, pp 43-111.
8. Brown SA: Neoplasia. *In* Hillyer EV, Quesenberry KE, eds. Ferrets, Rabbits, and Rodents: Clinical Medicine and Surgery. Philadelphia, WB Saunders, 1997, p 111.
9. Coleman GD, Chavez MA, Williams BH: Cystic prostatic disease associated with adrenocortical lesions in the ferret. Vet Pathol 1998; 35:547-549.
10. Cotchin E: Smooth muscle hyperplasia and neoplasia in the ovaries of domestic ferrets and polecats. J Path Bacteriol 1980; 130:169-171.
11. de Wit M, Schoemaker NJ, van der Hage MH, et al: Signs of estrus in an ovariectomized ferret. Tijdschr Diergeneeskd 2001; 126:526-528.
12. DiBartola S: Clinical approach and laboratory evaluation of renal disease. *In* Ettinger SJ, Feldman EC, eds. Textbook of Veterinary Internal Medicine. Philadelphia, WB Saunders, 2000, pp 1600-1614.
13. Dillberger JE: Polycystic kidneys in a ferret. J Am Vet Med Assoc 1985; 186:74-75.
14. Donnelly TM, Orcutt CJ: Acute ataxia in a young ferret following canine distemper vaccination. Renal failure after epinephrine overdose. Lab Anim 2001; 30:25-27.

15. Dutton MA: Treatment of cystine bladder urolith in a ferret. Exotic Pet Pract 1996; 1:7.
16. Edfors CH, Ullrey DE, Aulerich RJ: Prevention of urolithiasis in the ferret (*Mustela putorius furo*) with phosphoric acid. J Zoo Wildl Med 1989; 20:12-19.
17. Esteves MI, Marini RP, Ryden EB, et al: Estimation of glomerular filtration rate and evaluation of renal function in ferrets (*Mustela putorius furo*). Am J Vet Res 1994; 55:166-172.
18. Fisher PG: Stump pyometra in a female ferret. Exotic Pet Pract 1996; 1:7.
19. Fox JG: Normal clinical and biologic parameters. *In* Fox JG, ed. Biology and Diseases of the Ferret, 2nd ed. Baltimore, Williams & Wilkins, 1998, pp 183-210.
20. Fox JG, Pearson RC, Bell JA: Diseases of the genitourinary system. *In* Fox JG, ed. Biology and Diseases of the Ferret, 2nd ed. Baltimore, Williams & Wilkins, 1998, pp 247-272.
21. Gabow PA: Cystic disease of the kidney. *In* Wyngaarden JB, Smith LH, Bennett JC, eds. Cecil Textbook of Medicine, 19th ed. Philadelphia, WB Saunders, 1992, pp 608-612.
22. Grauer GF: Disorders of micturition. *In* Nelson RW, Couto CG, eds. Small Animal Internal Medicine, 3rd ed, St Louis, Mosby, 2003, pp 650-659.
23. Hart JE: Endocrine factors in haematological changes seen in dogs and ferrets given oestrogens. Med Hypotheses 1985; 16:159-163.
24. Hart JE: Endocrine pathology of estrogens: species differences. Pharmacol Ther 1990; 47:203-218.
25. Hillyer EV: Urogenital diseases. *In* Hillyer EV, Quesenberry KE, eds. Ferrets, Rabbits, and Rodents: Clinical Medicine and Surgery. Philadelphia, WB Saunders, 1997, pp. 44-52.
26. Johnson-Delaney C: Ferret adrenal disease: alternatives to surgery. Exotic DVM 1999; 1:19-22.
27. Kawasaki TA: Normal parameters and laboratory interpretation of disease states in the domestic ferret. Semin Avian Exotic Pet Med 1994; 3:40-47.
28. Li X, Fox JG, Erdman SE, et al: Cystic urogenital anomalies in ferrets. Vet Pathol 1996; 33:150-158.
29. Li X, Fox J, Erdman S, et al: Spontaneous neoplasms in ferrets: a review of 204 cases. Vet Pathol 1996; 33:590.
30. Marini RP, Esteves MI, Fox JG: A technique for catheterization of the urinary bladder in the ferret. Lab Anim 1994; 28:155-157.
31. Meschter CL: Interstitial cell adenoma in a ferret. Lab Anim Sci 1989; 39:353-354.
32. Nelson WB: Hydronephrosis in a ferret. Vet Med 1984; April:516-521.
33. Nguyen HT, Moreland AF, Shields RP: Urolithiasis in ferrets (*Mustela putorius*). Lab Anim Sci 1979; 29:243-245.
34. Niezgoda M, Briggs DJ, Shaddock J, et al: Pathogenesis of experimentally induced rabies in domestic ferrets. Am J Vet Res 1997; 58:1327-1331.
35. Orcutt C: Oxyglobin administration for the treatment of anemia in ferrets. Exotic DVM 2000; 2:44-46.
36. Orcutt C: Treatment of urogenital disease in ferrets. Exotic DVM 2001; 3:31-37.
37. Orcutt CJ: Ferret urogenital diseases. Vet Clin North Am Exotic Anim Pract 2003; 6:113-138.
38. Palley LS, Corning BF, Fox JG, et al: Parvovirus-associated syndrome (Aleutian disease) in two ferrets. J Am Vet Med Assoc 1992; 201:100-106.
39. Puerto DA, Walker LM, Saunders M: Bilateral perinephric pseudocysts and polycystic kidneys in a ferret. Vet Radiol Ultrasound 1998; 39:309-312.
40. Purcell K, Brown SA: Essentials of Ferrets: A Guide for Practitioners. Philadelphia, American Animal Hospital Association Press, 1999, pp 41-43, 136-148, 186-187.
41. Rich LJ, Kirk RW: The relationship of struvite crystals to urethral obstruction in cats. J Am Vet Med Assoc 1969; 154:153-157.
42. Rodríguez JL, Martín de las Mulas J, Espinosa de los Monteros A, et al: Ovarian teratoma in a ferret: a morphological and immunohistochemical study. J Zoo Wildl Med 1994; 25:294-299.
43. Rosenthal KL: Ferrets. Vet Clin North Am Small Anim Pract 1994; 24:1-22.
44. Rosenthal KL, Peterson ME: Stranguria in a castrated male ferret. J Am Vet Med Assoc 1996; 209:62-64.
45. Ryan KD, Siegel SF, Robinson SL: Influence of day length and endocrine status on luteinizing hormone secretion in intact and ovariectomized adult ferrets. Biol Reprod 1985; 33:690-697.
46. Sherrill A, Gorham J: Bone marrow hypoplasia associated with estrus in ferrets. Lab Anim Sci 1985; 35:280-286.
47. Weiss C, Aronson LR, Drobatz K: Traumatic rupture of the ureter: 10 cases. J Am Anim Hosp Assoc 2002; 38:188-192.
48. Williams CF: Practical Guide to Laboratory Animals. St Louis, CV Mosby, 1976, pp 65-71.
49. Xiantang L, Fox JG: Neoplastic diseases. *In* Fox JG, ed. Biology and Diseases of the Ferret, 2nd ed. Baltimore, Williams & Wilkins, 1998, pp 405-447.

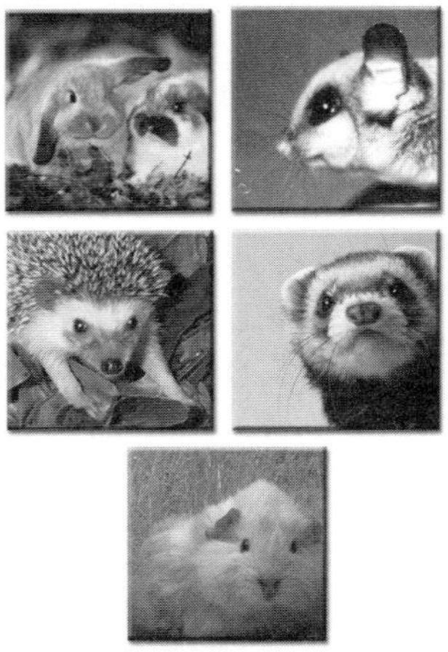

CHAPTER 5

Periparturient and Neonatal Diseases

Judith A. Bell, DVM, MSc, PhD

Well-fed and well-managed jills give birth to litters of 8 to 10 kits and lose about one kit per litter before weaning. Greater losses may stem from problems that begin before breeding and can be prevented with proper nutrition, housing, and management. Pregnancy toxemia, urolithiasis in pregnant jills, lactation failure, low conception rate, and small litter size result mainly from inadequate nutrition and management and can be virtually eliminated by improvements in diet, care, housing, and breeding techniques. The incidence of dystocia, mastitis, metritis, and neonatal kit diseases also can be reduced by improving management practices; however, because many variables are involved, a low frequency of these problems can be expected in any group of breeding ferrets.

GENERAL PRINCIPLES

Nutrition of Breeding Ferrets

The most important single factor in keeping any ferret healthy is nutrition. Feed male and female kits intended for breeding the highest-quality diet available at weaning and throughout their entire productive lives. Select a ration that contains 35% to 40% protein and 18% to 20% fat, with meat listed as the first ingredient.[2] Jills come in heat for the first time at 4 months of age if they are exposed to light for longer than 12 hours per day. If bred at this age, they must have an excellent diet that enables them to sustain both growth and pregnancy.

Feeding an inadequate diet to breeding ferrets leads to several serious sequelae. Multiparous jills fed poor-quality cat foods have small litters, and primiparous jills consuming such diets are susceptible to pregnancy toxemia. Failure to conceive or, more commonly, small litter size may be the result of several factors, including poor nutrition. Primiparous jills should have at least eight kits; smaller litters result from use of a hob of low fertility, breeding at the wrong time or only once during estrus, breeding of a jill and hob of an unusual color phase that carry lethal recessive genes, or feeding an inadequate diet. If the diet does not contain at least 35% protein and 15% fat, with most of the protein from meat products, suggest that the owner use a higher plane of nutrition for both the jill and hob as the first step in improving reproduction.

The first ingredient listed on the label of a diet suitable for ferrets should be meat or poultry meal. Food products vary in quality and may contain a high proportion of bone and undigestible tissue. The price of the food is a good indicator of its protein quality. Some older ferrets resist dietary changes; offer them a smorgasbord of premium cat and ferret foods so that they can make their own selections.[2] Some foods labeled as ferret diets were developed from commercial mink rations and contain poorly processed fish that is unpalatable to ferrets unaccustomed to the flavor of fish. Although fish is a natural diet for mink, it is not for ferrets. Ferrets prefer chicken or other meats, which are the usual ingredients in premium cat foods and diets formulated specifically for ferrets. Mink rations, premium cat foods, and high-quality ferret diets all can provide more than adequate nutrition for breeding ferrets; however, if a jill refuses to eat the diet, it obviously has no nutritional value for her.

Even if provided with a concentrated, meat-based diet, lactating jills become thin if they nurse litters of more than 10 kits. Jills bred on every estrous cycle must be fed very high-calorie diets between litters; the fat that they gain is not sufficient to cause obesity-related reproductive problems.

Management of Breeding Ferrets

Place a pregnant jill's cage in a quiet area well before parturition. This is particularly important for primiparous jills, which are more likely to settle down and care for their kits if they are not disturbed or distracted. A plastic dishpan with rolled edges makes a good nesting box. Place the dishpan in a corner of the cage and anchor it firmly or, ideally, drop it through an opening in the cage bottom so that the rolled edge of the pan is level with the cage floor. The jill must be able to easily enter and exit the nesting box without risking trauma to the mammary glands. The kits should not be able to climb out of the nesting box until they are close to weaning age. Shredded aspen or corn husks make good bedding for whelping nests. In small breeding operations, small terry cloth towels are a practical alternative for bedding material; do not use large towels, because kits can get lost in them. Discard old towels that begin to unravel to prevent kits' becoming entangled in loose threads. Avoid use of coarse wood shavings or shredded newspaper (which clumps in a solid mass when wet).

For the jill's comfort, the room temperature should not exceed 21.1°C (70°F). Place a heat lamp over part of the nesting box so that the jill and kits can select warmth as necessary. Be sure that food and water are readily accessible to the jill so that she can eat and drink without leaving the kits. Place a clip-on food dish and a water bottle near the edge of the nesting box so that the jill can eat and drink even while lying down.

Breeding Pet Ferrets

Discourage owners of single pet ferrets from trying to raise a litter unless they are prepared to devote most of their time for several weeks to observing and caring for the periparturient jill. Breeding ferrets and raising kits successfully requires constant supervision during gestation, parturition, and lactation; if not prevented or treated promptly, unattended problems can lead to death of the jill, kits, or both.

PROBLEMS OF PERIPARTURIENT JILLS

Pregnancy Toxemia

Pregnancy toxemia is a life-threatening disease caused by negative energy balance in late gestation.[1] Among primiparous jills carrying average litters and fed adequate diets, toxemia is most likely to develop when an accidental fast occurs during the last week of gestation. This sometimes happens when an owner tries to replace the normal ration with a higher-quality diet that the jill refuses to eat. Occasionally, pregnancy toxemia develops in well-fed primiparous jills that conceive 15 or more kits. With that many fetuses, nourishment of the dam and kits is compromised because the gravid uterus fills the abdomen and reduces the stomach capacity for a sufficient quantity of even a concentrated diet.

Warn owners to guard against accidental fasts during pregnancy. Pregnant jills must have palatable food and water available 24 hours a day. Provide both a bottle and a dish of water; most jills prefer to drink from a dish and use the bottle secondarily. Ferrets drink about three times the volume of water that they eat of dry pellets, and when deprived of water they soon stop eating. During the last week of gestation, even one overnight fast can induce toxemia in a jill with a large litter. Owners should place several small dishes of food in the cage so that accidental spillage or contamination does not restrict the jill's intake during this critical time. Although most owners take good care of their ferrets, the importance of providing constant access to an excellent diet during late gestation must be emphasized. Recommend that owners provide high-calorie foods or nutritional supplements such as Maximum-Calorie/Canine and Feline (Eukanuba, The Iams Company, Dayton, OH), Nutri-Cal (Tomlyn, Buena, NJ), or Ensure Plus (Abbott Laboratories, Ross Products Division, Columbus, OH) to jills that appear to be carrying very large litters.

Pregnancy toxemia should be suspected if a jill suddenly becomes lethargic just before her due date. Question the owner about the ration and its availability and about any recent changes in the food or feeding schedule. A toxemic jill is dehydrated, feels "doughy," and may have black, tarry stools. If the jill is severely dehydrated, the outline of the uterus, and sometimes the individual kits, can be seen in her abdomen. The hair easily epilates, the blood glucose concentration may be very low (less than 50 mg/dL), and the jill may be ketonuric and azotemic. A toxemic jill is cold but does not attempt to curl up or crawl into a warm spot. Instead, she lies flat on her abdomen with open, glazed eyes. The prognosis for such an animal is poor even with excellent care.

An immediate cesarean section is necessary to save the life of the jill, but the success of the procedure depends on the extent of liver damage. During surgery, use gas anesthesia and administer intravenous fluids containing dextrose. Insertion of an intravenous catheter can be very difficult in a jill that is severely dehydrated. If a catheter cannot be placed, give fluids subcutaneously; they are well absorbed if the jill is warm. If intravenous glucose is not given, offer or force-feed a dose of oral glucose or a high-calorie supplement before surgery. These jills must be kept warm, but, because ferrets are so susceptible to heat prostration, the use of a heating pad is risky. During and after surgery, place the jill on a circulating warm-water blanket, a forced warm-air pad, or a warmed terry cloth towel, and monitor the body temperature closely.

Perform the cesarean section as quickly as possible. A midline incision gives best access to both uterine horns. Remove all kits rapidly through an incision made midway along each horn.

Postsurgical care includes frequent force-feeding of small amounts of high-calorie supplements and maintaining hydration, as well as keeping the jill warm and comfortable. Position the heat source so that the jill can easily move away from the heat. Toxemic ferrets usually do not make the effort to climb over or out of anything, even when fully conscious. Continue intensive care as long as the jill is lethargic and until she begins to eat significant quantities on her own. Offer favorite foods (softened with warm water if she prefers it) at frequent intervals, and allow free access to drinking water at all times. The first 24 hours after surgery are critical, and ferrets that survive this period usually recover. Those that die have clay-colored, fatty livers and are anemic[1]; they may also have gastritis or gastric ulcers.

Jills that survive toxemia have no milk for at least several days after surgery. If a foster mother can be found, rotating the fostered kits so that some of them are always with their mother may induce sufficient lactation for her to raise at least part of the litter. If kits have no foster mother or if they are born before 40 days of gestation, they are best euthanatized, because hand-rearing of ferret kits from birth is extremely difficult.[4]

Struvite Urolithiasis in Pregnant Jills

In a large colony, 5% to 10% of pregnant jills consuming a diet containing mainly plant protein develop struvite bladder stones. Pregnant jills are particularly susceptible to urolithiasis because they constantly mobilize minerals; however, any ferret on a diet with ground yellow corn as its primary ingredient may develop this life-threatening problem. Magnesium ammonium phosphate (struvite) crystallizes when the urine pH is greater than 6.4. The mineral content of the food is not as important as the protein source in a diet chosen to prevent urolithiasis. Ferrets are obligate carnivores with a normal urine pH of about 6. Metabolism of cystine and methionine in animal proteins produces acid urine, whereas metabolism of the organic acids in plant protein produces alkaline urine that promotes struvite crystallization.[3] Moreover, when the urine pH is between 6 and 7, stones form to some extent in the pregnant ferret fed a corn-based diet, but not in one given a meat-based diet.

Jills are not as likely as hobs to develop complete urinary obstructions. However, straining eventually causes rectal or vaginal prolapse (or both), which may lead to self-mutilation and severe, possibly fatal, hemorrhage. If a jill in the last trimester of gestation or the first week of lactation presents with straining, carefully palpate for stones, which are often large and usually easy to feel (Fig. 5-1). If possible, take radiographs to confirm the diagnosis. If urolithiasis is diagnosed, perform a cystotomy as soon as possible (see also Chapter 12). Perform a cesarean section immediately before the cystotomy if the jill is due within 24 hours; this prevents the jill from putting strain on the fresh suture line while giving birth to the kits. Jills that receive good postoperative care nurse their kits normally.

Although gas anesthesia is ideal in uremic animals, ketamine (35 mg/kg) with xylazine (5 mg/kg) given intramuscularly, reversed with yohimbine (0.11 mg/kg IV or IM) after surgery, is also safe for both the jill and the unborn kits. Start intravenous or subcutaneous fluid administration before surgery.

The bladder is palpable and often visible in the lower abdomen after the jill is anesthetized. Carefully make an incision directly over the largest part of the bladder, allowing it to be pulled through the incision, folded back to expose its dorsal surface, and packed off. The bladder wall is often very thick and vascular. Make an incision in a relatively avascular area, and, after removing the stones from the bladder, search carefully for smaller stones. Palpate the urethra as far down as possible into the pelvic canal: stones in the distal urethra are usually responsible for tenesmus. After all stones are removed, swab the bladder mucosa to obtain a sample for culture and sensitivity testing, then flush the bladder with an acidifying solution (e.g., saline solution) to remove mucus, blood, and "sand" before closure. Close the bladder with two rows of 5-0 sutures placed as close as possible to the wound edges in a continuous Cushing pattern. Even very thick bladder walls can be closed well with this technique (see also Chapter 12).

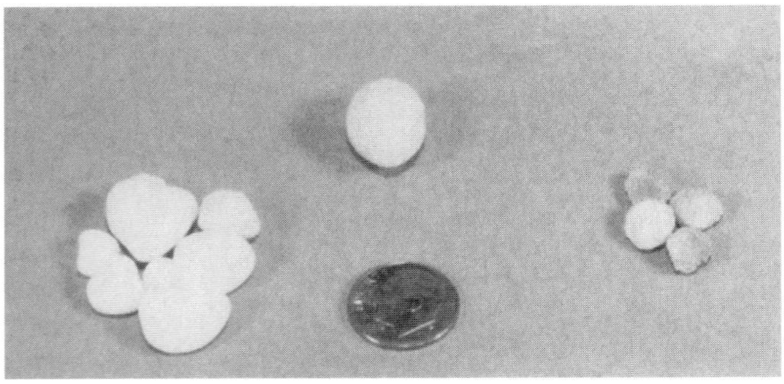

Figure 5-1 Struvite uroliths surgically removed from three pregnant ferrets that were fed a poor-quality diet.

Flunixin meglumine (Banamine, Schering-Plough Animal Health Corporation, Union, NJ) (2.5 mg per animal IM), administered before surgery and every 12 hours for 1 or 2 days thereafter reduces inflammation and pain and prevents straining. If possible, the ferret should continue to receive intravenous or subcutaneous fluids for 24 to 48 hours after surgery. Allow constant access to water in a dish. The use of urinary acidifiers slightly lowers the pH of urine but does not prevent the formation of more stones if the diet is poor. Trimethoprim-sulfa combinations (15-30 mg/kg PO q12h) are concentrated in urine and usually prevent postoperative bladder infection with urease producers such as *Staphylococcus* and *Proteus* species. These organisms raise urine pH rapidly, inducing struvite stone formation within hours. Perform antimicrobial sensitivity testing on any organisms cultured from bladder mucosal swabs obtained during surgery to confirm antibiotic efficacy in an individual animal.

The diet must be improved if recurrence of urolithiasis is to be prevented after surgery, but a drastic change in diet in late gestation can induce pregnancy toxemia. A safer approach is to mix several high-quality foods with the original diet, reducing the proportion of low-quality food until only premium food is available 1 week after surgery. Supplement the jill's diet with a high-calorie product that includes amino acids or with cow's milk with added cream or egg yolk to give a final fat concentration of 20%. Milk products can cause mild physiologic diarrhea, but they are excellent sources of animal protein and fat.

Problems Associated with Small Litter Size

The gestation period for ferrets is 41 to 42 days; this period is slightly shorter for primiparous jills. Litters of one or two kits often are overdue, probably because the hormonal stimulus from the fetuses is inadequate to induce parturition. After the 43rd day, the kits die, but until then they continue to grow and can cause dystocia if labor is induced.

If presented with a jill having only one palpable kit, induce labor on the 41st day of gestation. Give prostaglandin $F_{2\alpha}$ (Lutalyse, Pharmacia and Upjohn Company, Kalamazoo, MI) (0.5 mg per animal IM), then administer oxytocin (6 USP units) 1 to 4 hours later. Most jills deliver 2 to 12 hours after this treatment. If the kit is not delivered within 24 hours, repeat the treatment or perform a cesarean section. Waiting another day rarely harms the jill, but her milk will dry up, and the kits' chances of survival are greatly decreased by the 43rd day.

Some jills do not produce milk for fewer than five kits even after spontaneous delivery, and the smaller litters starve unless fostered within a few days after birth. The kits try to nurse from all of the mammary glands but do not stimulate any of the glands enough to induce lactation. Ideally, jills should be bred in pairs, so that if one has a very small litter the kits of both litters can be divided equally between the jills. Occasionally, kits in small litters nurse from only one or two glands, stimulating normal lactation in these glands, and the kits thrive.

Other Causes of Dystocia

Dystocia occurs at a rate of about 1% in a large group of ferrets, including those with small litters that are not delivered. Some jills repeatedly have whelping problems. Common causes of dystocia are kits of very large size (14-20 g; normal range, 8-10 g), deformed fetuses with bent necks, and anasarcous fetuses. Delayed parturition is associated with kits with congenital head deformities.

Cesarean Section

An average parturition in ferrets occurs over a period of 2 to 3 hours, with approximately five kits born per hour; however, some jills take longer than others to whelp. A good mother is attentive to the first-born kits before the births of subsequent kits, although she seldom settles down long enough to let them nurse. Progress should be steady and without distress on the part of the jill. Do not hesitate to perform a cesarean section if a jill has been in labor for longer than 24 hours or is in distress for a much shorter time. Jills recover well from surgery and usually nurse the litter uneventfully. The kits recover well even if the jill was given an injectable anesthetic; however, the best choice for cesarean section is a gas anesthetic. If injectable anesthetics must be used, a good combination is ketamine (35 mg/kg IM) plus xylazine (5 mg/kg IM), because it can be partially reversed with yohimbine (0.11 mg/kg IV or IM). Preanesthetic administration of atropine reduces the cardiovascular depressant effects of xylazine. Jills should be able to walk 10 minutes after the yohimbine is given; however, they may accidentally lie on and crush their kits if they are not fully recovered and should not be returned to the litter for at least 1 hour after yohimbine reversal.

Keep the kits warm by placing them on a heating pad or a circulating warm-water blanket after a cesarean delivery, but check often for overheating. Kits that are overdue by more than 2 days are inactive and may be very dehydrated. Kits that have a gray pallor at birth are not viable. Those that appear cyanotic usually are able to breathe with manual stimulation and benefit from a few minutes in an oxygen-rich environment.

Poor Mothering of Kits

Experienced jills rarely reject their kits, but primiparous jills often do. They may not mother their litter for several days, which is too late for many kits that are not aggressive enough to follow the jill and nurse. The more privacy these jills have, the more likely they are to bond with the litter. Although handling of the kits does not cause jills to reject their litter, unusual noise and confusion nearby may. Ferrets get very excited and may bury the kits in the bedding, or put them in a pile in a corner of the enclosure or in food or water containers. Some jills cannibalize the first few or all of their kits as they are born.

If a primiparous jill rejects but does not cannibalize her kits, place the jill and the litter inside a very small container, such as a dishpan, with a wire lid that allows air circulation but not exit by the jill. Offer moist food frequently, and attach a water bottle. Letting the jill out to eat her favorite snack and satisfy her appetite and then replacing her in the container with the kits sometimes helps her to concentrate, allowing her to accept the litter immediately. Once she accepts the kits, the jill can be allowed to move around more freely; however, some young jills seem to forget their young when they get out to play.

Even jills that are very excited by the birth of the first kits, or possibly by the pain of labor, may eventually make good mothers. If the jill is injuring or rejecting the kits, remove each one as it is born, and keep them in a warm place away from the jill until the whole litter is delivered. Provide clean bedding and feed the jill, and she may settle down and accept the kits when they are returned to her.

If the room temperature is too warm (greater than 21.1°C [70°F]), the jill may be reluctant to stay in the nest. To avoid accidental chilling of the kits, place a heat lamp near but not directly over the nest, so that the jill can move away from it when she becomes too warm.

Lactation Failure

Jills that fail to produce enough milk to feed kits in normal litters of eight or nine may be genetically incapable of doing so. However, before this conclusion is reached, examine at least four variables: management, nutrition, systemic diseases of the jill, and chronic mastitis.

Primiparous jills and older jills that are poorly managed at whelping time may never settle down with their newborn kits, and their milk quickly dries up if the stimulus from nursing is inadequate. Make sure the jill is housed away from unaccustomed noisy activity, and discourage visits by people unfamiliar to the jill until the litter is at least 5 days old. A good mother rarely leaves the nest for the first few days after whelping. Inadequate access to food and water limits the jill's ability to lactate. Place shallow dishes of food and water close to the nest so that the jill can reach them easily.

Nutrition determines the difference between adequate and outstanding milk production.[2] Jills fed a maintenance diet raise slow-growing kits with poor coats that are more susceptible to infectious diseases than are well-nourished kits. Three-week-old kits that are doing poorly benefit from milk and moist food supplements, but nothing ensures that kits will be healthy and robust as much as a steady and plentiful supply of ferret milk. Offer the best-quality diet available to lactating jills; at 2 to 3 weeks after parturition, the dietary fat level should be 25% to 30%. Jills need constant access to clean drinking water. Question owners whose jills consistently have small litters and poor kits about their ferrets' diet, and suggest upgrading to a premium food.

Postparturient jills with serious systemic diseases stop producing milk. Their kits are thin, and they cry and move around instead of nursing or lying quietly next to the jill. The common reasons for a sudden decrease in milk production are mastitis and metritis. Other diseases that may develop during the postparturient period include bacterial cystitis, urolithiasis, gastric ulcers, and lymphosarcoma.

If acute infections are promptly treated, the jill usually continues lactating; however, if she is very ill for a few days early in lactation, her milk will probably dry up. If a sick jill has little milk, feed the litter at least four times a day. However, leave the kits with the jill, so that as soon as she is able to produce milk the stimulus of nursing can induce lactation. Later in lactation, there is less tendency for the milk to dry up immediately if sickness or dehydration occurs. Whenever a lactating jill is ill, encourage her to take as much nourishment as possible by frequently offering high-calorie soft foods or supplements such as Maximum-Calorie, Nutri-Cal, or Ensure Plus, as well as her regular food mixed with warm water.

Acute Mastitis

Acute mastitis usually appears either soon after whelping or after the third week of lactation, when the kits begin to demand very great quantities of milk (stressing the dam) and have teeth that can damage the nipples. The affected glands are swollen, firm, red or purple, and painful, but the milk may not appear discolored. Common organisms isolated are *Staphylococcus* species and coliforms. Acute mastitis often becomes gangrenous within a few hours after clinical signs appear (Fig. 5-2, *A*). The skin turns black, and the jill becomes very ill and dehydrated.

Immediate aggressive treatment is needed to save a jill with acute mastitis. Debride necrotic tissue with a scalpel; this alone improves the jill's chances for survival. No anesthesia or sedation is necessary, because the gangrenous tissue is insensitive. Administer broad-spectrum antibiotics such as chloramphenicol, 50 mg/kg IM or SC q12h, or amoxicillin with clavulanate (Clavamox Drops, Pfizer Animal Health, Exton, PA), 18.75 mg PO q12h (combined dosage of amoxicillin and clavulanate; equal to 0.3 mL of the oral suspension). Avoid gentamicin in ferrets, because it causes renal damage, particularly in dehydrated animals, and can cause deafness in some ferrets. To confirm the sensitivity of the specific organism, culture a sample of the milk before beginning antibiotic therapy.

The toxins released by the necrotic tissue make the jills very ill, and jills with acute mastitis are reluctant to let their kits nurse because of pain. Flunixin meglumine (2.5 mg IM q12h PRN) relieves pain, reduces inflammation and toxemia, and is safe for use in ferrets. When flunixin is used in combination with antibiotics in jills with acute mastitis, the survival rate improves. Administer balanced electrolyte solutions subcutaneously as needed. Be sure that soft, palatable food is available, or give high-calorie supplements.

If treatment is instituted rapidly, the jill will continue to lactate, although the kits might need supplementation with a milk replacement formula for a few days. Avoid fostering the kits even temporarily, because they commonly infect the foster mother with the organism that caused mastitis in their dam. Persons handling the infected jill should wash their hands before handling another lactating ferret. Occasionally, the infected milk causes diarrhea in the kits. If this occurs, treat the kits twice daily (on a per kilogram basis) with the same antibiotic used for the mother.

Jills that have acute mastitis may heal completely but more often lose the gland (Fig. 5-2, *B*) or have recurrent mastitis. Loss of a single gland has little effect on the ability of a well-producing jill to raise an average litter, but if several glands are affected her kits will not do well. Breeding of a valuable jill can be synchronized with that of another dam that can take some extra kits when both whelp.

Chronic Mastitis

Chronic mastitis is so subtle that it can be missed by the owner. The glands are firm but not painful or discolored. They appear to be full of milk, but most of the milk-producing tissue has been replaced by scar tissue. The organism that is usually responsible, *Staphylococcus intermedius*, is commonly found on the skin of normal ferrets. Although this organism may be sensitive to several antibiotics in vitro, such agents are rarely effective in vivo. Jills with chronic mastitis are never able to nurse kits again. This type of mastitis is very contagious, and affected jills should be culled and kept separate from other breeders.

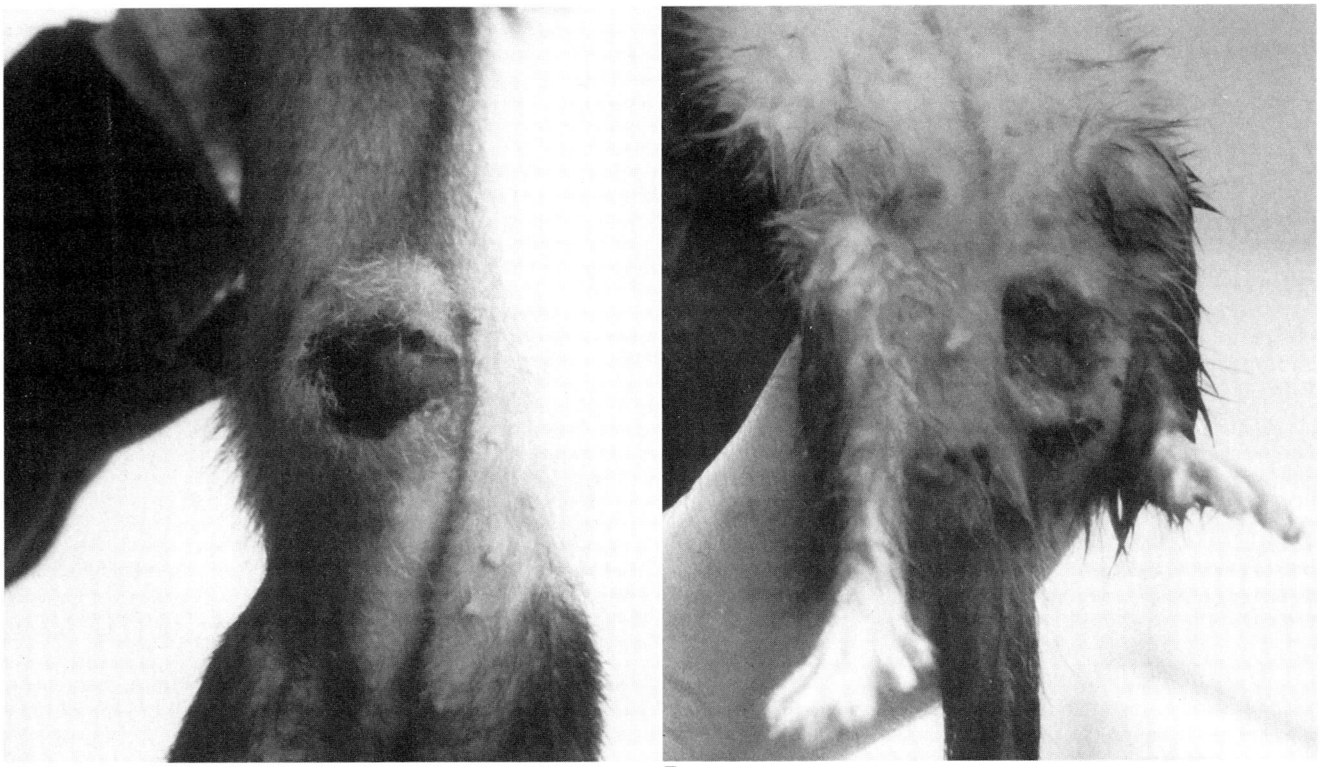

A B

Figure 5-2 A, Acute gangrenous mastitis in a jill, with a single gland affected. B, "Crater" resulting from necrosis caused by acute gangrenous mastitis.

Chronic mastitis may develop after acute mastitis, but it usually appears insidiously when the kits are 3 weeks of age. At this age, the jill ordinarily reaches peak milk production. If lactation regresses instead of peaking, the kits continue growing in stature but stop gaining weight. They look long and thin and have rough coats. To reduce the rate of infection to foster mothers, bathe the kits and keep them away from both jills for a few hours until their intestinal tracts empty of the infected milk. Treat them with an appropriate oral antibiotic. Neither this therapy nor treatment of the foster mother with antibiotics entirely prevents transmission of mastitis. Kits that are left with a jill with chronic mastitis need to be fed at least three times daily with as much warm milk replacer as they will take (see below).

Metritis

A jill with metritis may not have excessive vaginal discharge. Palpate the abdomen; if the uterus is distended, evacuate it with prostaglandin $F_{2\alpha}$ (0.5 mg IM) and initiate antibiotic therapy. A trimethoprim-sulfa combination drug is a good choice because it is concentrated in urine and helps prevent ascending bladder infection and subsequent urolithiasis. To reduce pain and toxemia, treat jills that have a red, sticky discharge without uterine distention with flunixin and trimethoprim-sulfa or another antibiotic. Because flunixin is a prostaglandin antagonist, it should not be given in conjunction with prostaglandin $F_{2\alpha}$.

The kits will appear more content and less gaunt within 24 hours after the appropriate treatment is given and the jill's milk production has improved. Continue treatment with antibiotics for at least 5 days, but stop flunixin therapy sooner because of the risk of gastritis or stomach ulcers.

PROBLEMS OF NEONATAL KITS

Ferret kits are altricial and have little ability to maintain their body temperature for the first 2 weeks of life. Normal kits weigh about 8 to 10 g at birth, 30 g at 1 week, 60 to 70 g at 2 weeks, and 100 g at 3 weeks of age. Their eyes usually open at 30 to 35 days of age but can open as early as 25 days of age.

Healthy, normal litters lie quietly and close to the jill and nurse or sleep except when the jill leaves the nest. By 3 weeks of age, even though their eyes are still closed, kits begin to explore and nibble on soft food, such as the jill's regular diet moistened with water. Ferrets are weaned at 6 to 8 weeks of age.

Fostering and Supplemental Feeding of Nursing Kits

Hand-rearing of ferret kits from birth is extremely difficult without a good supply of ferret milk and 24-hour-a-day attention.[4] If the jill is unable to care for her offspring, they should be fostered to another lactating jill if possible. Most jills accept kits of any size or age at any stage of lactation.

Providing supplemental nourishment for the kits is often the best alternative if the jill's milk production is reduced because of illness after parturition, but leave the kits with the jill so that the stimulus of nursing can induce lactation as she improves. Supplement neonatal kits with puppy or kitten milk replacer enriched with cream until the fat content is 20%. Kits drink much more if the milk is warm. Feed them at least four times a day with as much as they will take from a dropper or plastic pipette.

Kits that have reached 3 weeks of age can survive on enriched milk replacement formula alone, with no milk from the jill, until they are old enough to subsist on solid food. Use the same formula as for neonatal kits, and offer as much as the kits will take at least three times daily. Feed 3-week-old kits individually with a plastic pipette or dropper, because at this age, they might crawl into milk in a dish and get wet and cold. Older kits drink well from a dish after a few lessons. A low, flat dish is preferable to a saucer, because ferrets put their feet on the edge of the dish when they eat or drink. Kits cannot survive on solid food without milk until they are older than 4 weeks of age, and they do poorly on an adult diet before 5 weeks of age.

Medical Care of Neonatal Kits

If the jill is sick or is a poor mother and the nest area is not sufficiently warm, the kits may become chilled. They chill quickly and do not attempt to nurse when they are cold or hypoglycemic. Hold chilled kits in warm water or place them on a heating pad until they are active. If they are extremely cold, give them a few drops of glucose solution orally. Dehydrated neonatal kits rapidly absorb 0.5 to 1 mL of fluids warmed to body temperature and injected subcutaneously.

If antibiotic therapy is necessary for neonatal kits (see below), calculate the dose on a per kilogram basis. Amoxicillin with clavulanate must be diluted 4 : 1 with water so that a dose sufficiently low for a baby kit is obtained. Chloramphenicol formulated for intravenous use is effective orally in neonatal kits.

Entangled Umbilical Cords

Occasionally, kits in large litters are born so rapidly that the dam is unable to chew the attached placenta off each one and, as a result, a mass of kits is found bound together by their umbilical cords (Fig. 5-3). These kits cannot nurse, and they become

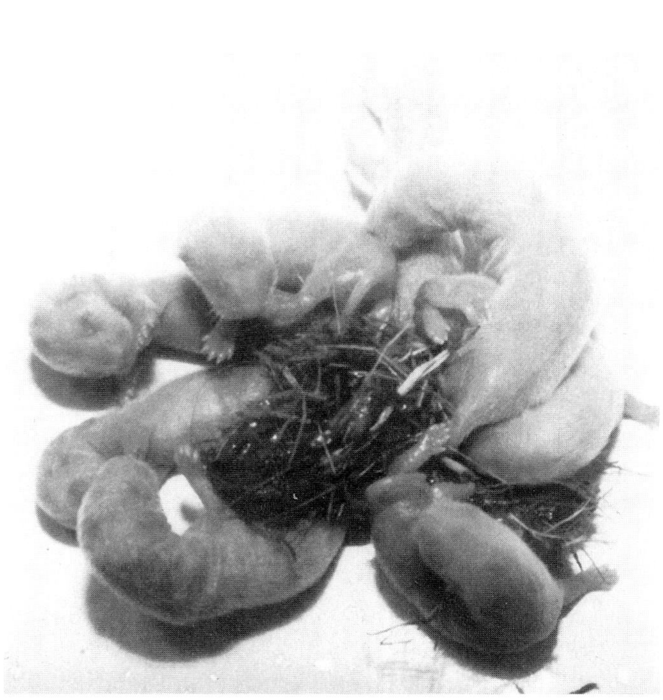

Figure 5-3 A ball of newborn kits bound together by tangled navel cords.

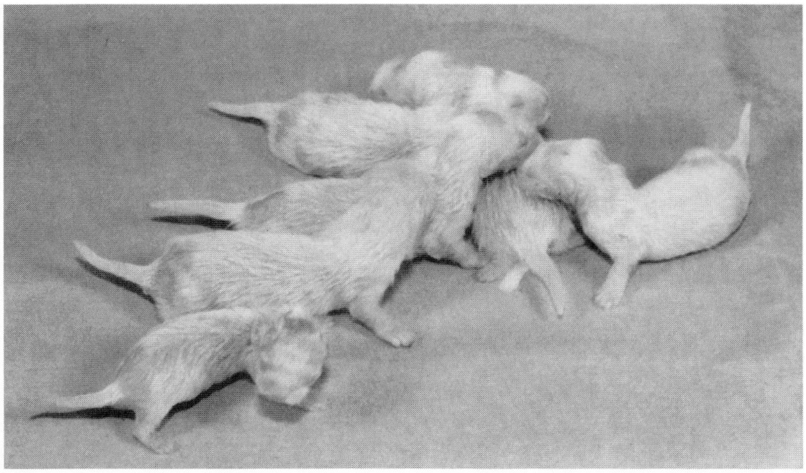

Figure 5-4 Litter of "sticky" kits with rotaviral diarrhea.

hypoglycemic and hypothermic because the jill cannot curl around them. Very coarse or sharp-edged shavings aggravate the problem of entangled placentas.

Separating the ball of kits without injuring any of them can be difficult. If the placentas have become dry, soften the tissue with warm water and remove as much of the shavings and debris as possible; then gently cut the umbilical cords with blunt scissors as far from the kits' abdomens as possible. If they have been tangled for more than a few hours, it may be necessary to sacrifice one kit to release the rest. To prevent umbilical cord tangling, owners should closely supervise births, picking up kits as they are born and shortening the umbilical cords.

Diarrhea of Neonatal Kits

Diarrhea of neonatal kits may be caused by rotavirus alone, rotavirus with secondary bacterial infection, or bacterial infection alone. Ferret rotavirus is similar but not identical to rotaviruses that infect human infants, pups, calves, and pigs.[5] The virus is carried by adult ferrets and may cause disease even in unstressed litters if they have no passive immunity. Rotaviral diarrhea is life threatening in kits 1 to 7 days of age. Older kits may not require treatment.

Kits with rotaviral diarrhea appear wet, and the hair on their heads and necks lies flat (Fig. 5-4). Because the jill grooms away all evidence of diarrhea, the owner may not notice it. Neonatal kits with severe enteritis dehydrate rapidly. Most survive if treated with fluids (0.5-1.0 mL SC q6-12h) and oral antibiotics for 4 to 5 days to prevent secondary bacterial enteritis. Useful antibiotics include spectinomycin, amoxicillin, amoxicillin with clavulanate, chloramphenicol, and trimethoprim-sulfa. The kits are anorectic early in the disease course, which allows pressure to build up in the jill's mammary glands, causing mastitis or inhibiting lactation.

Ophthalmia Neonatorum

Kits a few days to 3 weeks of age may develop infections in their unopened eyes. Purulent discharge accumulates in the conjunctival sac until it bulges and is noticed by the owner (Fig. 5-5). Usually these kits have empty stomachs, probably because nursing causes pain. A variety of skin flora are cultured from these eyes, but the route of infection is not known.

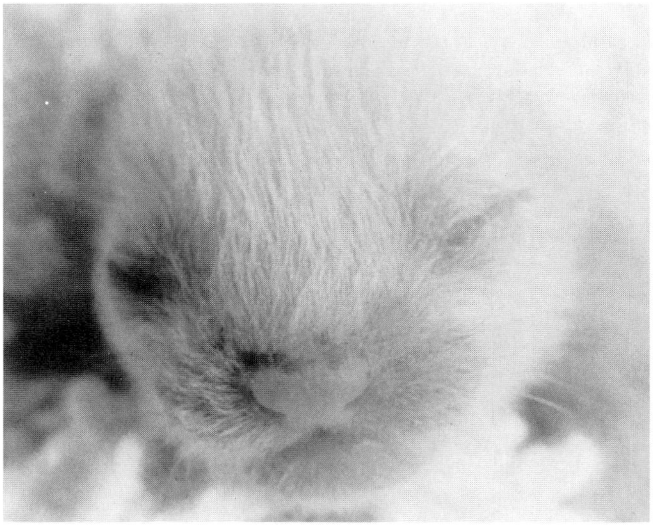

Figure 5-5 Kit with a swollen eye resulting from a bacterial infection. Note the encrusted material on the eyelid suture line.

To treat affected kits, cut along the natural suture line of the eyelids with a scalpel or 25-gauge needle bevel to allow the discharge to drain. One or two treatments with broad-spectrum ophthalmic ointment usually will clear the infection. The eye remains open if the kit is older than 3 weeks of age but will seal up if it is younger, and the infection may recur. Because several littermates usually are affected, carefully re-examine the litter twice daily.

REFERENCES

1. Batchelder MA, Bell JA, Erdman SE, et al: Pregnancy toxemia in the European ferret (*Mustela putorius furo*). Lab Anim Sci 1999; 49:372-379.

2. Bell JA: Ferret nutrition. *In* Jenkins JR, ed. Vet Clin North Am Exotic Anim Pract 1999; 2:169-192.
3. Buffington CAT: Nutritional diseases and nutritional therapy. *In* Sherding RG, ed. The Cat: Diseases and Clinical Management, 2nd ed, Vol. 1. New York, Churchill Livingstone, 1994, p 167.
4. Manning DD, Bell JA: Derivation of gnotobiotic ferrets: perinatal diet and hand-rearing requirements. Lab Anim Sci 1990; 40:51-55.
5. Torres-Medina A: Isolation of an atypical rotavirus causing diarrhea in neonatal ferrets. Lab Anim Sci 1987; 37:167-171.

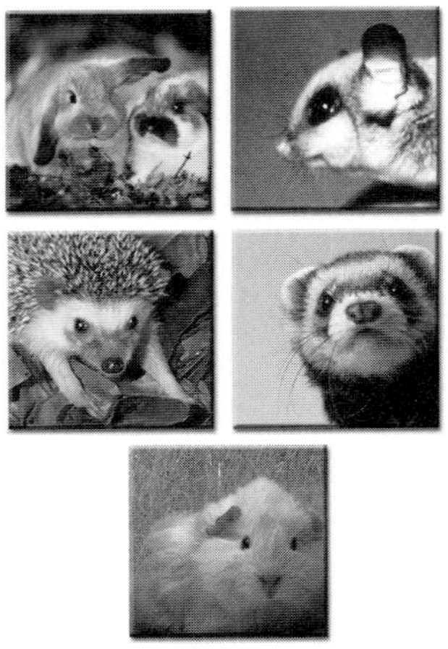

CHAPTER 6

Cardiovascular and Other Diseases

Part I: Jean-Paul Petrie, DVM, Diplomate ACVIM (Cardiology)
Part II: James K. Morrisey, DVM, Diplomate ABVP

PART I **CARDIAC DISEASE**

Jean-Paul Petrie, DVM, Diplomate ACVIM (Cardiology)

Cardiac disease is relatively common in pet ferrets and is suspected based on the presence of radiographic cardiomegaly, a heart murmur on auscultation, or clinical signs consistent with congestive heart failure (CHF). In addition, a thorough cardiac evaluation should be considered for any older ferret undergoing anesthesia. For these reasons, practitioners working with ferrets should be familiar with the clinical signs and diagnosis of heart disease as well as the treatment options available. Since the first edition of this book, reference data for common testing modalities, including echocardiography, electrocardiography (ECG), and radiography, have been published for ferrets. This section provides readers with this new information as well as my own accumulated clinical experience to facilitate the diagnosis and treatment of cardiovascular diseases in ferrets. To date, acquired heart disease is the only form of heart disease reported in ferrets. Congenital cardiac disease is not commonly recognized, and no case reports have been published. As echocardiography becomes more widely available, reports of congenital heart disease may be forthcoming.

GENERAL PRINCIPLES

History and Clinical Signs

Most ferrets that are presented because of cardiac disease are middle-aged to older (i.e., older than 3 years of age). Typical presenting clinical signs may be confused with those of other diseases, so a thorough history is important. The owner should be questioned about changes in the animal's appetite, activity level, sleep patterns, exposure to other ferrets, and exposure to the human influenza virus.

Ferrets with cardiac disease show a variety of clinical signs that are similar to those observed in other species, including lethargy, exercise intolerance, weight loss, anorexia, ascites, coughing, and dyspnea.[13,33,49] In addition, ferrets with cardiac disease may present with hind limb weakness. It is unclear why the hind limbs are preferentially affected compared with the front, but thromboembolic disease does not appear to be a cause. The diagnosis of cardiac disease may be an incidental finding in some ferrets; either these ferrets have compensated for mild cardiac disease or the owner has not noticed the often insidious signs.

Physical Examination

A thorough and systematic physical examination should be performed. Examine the oral mucus membranes for color and refill time (less than 2 seconds is normal). Pale or cyanotic mucus membranes with a prolonged capillary refill time may be related to CHF or reduced cardiac output. Jugular pulses may be visible in ferrets with right-sided CHF. Femoral pulses are palpated for quality, character, and the presence of any deficits. Pulses may be weak, irregular, or normal with cardiac disease. Bounding pulses are uncommon in my experience but could potentially be seen with a severe aortic insufficiency. Abdominal palpation of ferrets with heart disease may reveal ascites, hepatomegaly, and splenomegaly. Other physical examination findings may include hypothermia, lethargy, generalized weakness, and dehydration.

The ferret heart is auscultated between the sixth and eight ribs, much more caudally than in the dog or cat. The normal heart rate is between 180 and 250 beats/min. Ferrets may have a pronounced sinus arrhythmia that causes a dramatic decrease in heart rate or sinus pauses during auscultation. Relevant findings on auscultation include bradycardia, tachycardia, murmurs, gallop rhythms, and muffled heart sounds. Murmurs are usually associated with valvular insufficiency and increased outflow tract velocities. An S_3 gallop occurs secondary to dilation of the left ventricle, and an S_4 gallop occurs secondary to an accentuated atrial contraction filling a hypertrophied and noncompliant ventricle. Ferrets with cardiac disease may show signs of dyspnea and tachypnea. Auscultation of the lungs may reveal crackles, muffled lung sounds, or increased bronchovesicular sounds.

Diagnosis

A suspected diagnosis of heart disease can be made based on the historical and physical examination information previously discussed. A definitive diagnosis of cardiac disease requires objective data, such as an ECG, thoracic radiographs, and echocardiogram. These testing modalities are discussed in detail later. For all patients with documented or suspected heart disease, a minimum database, including a complete blood count (CBC), biochemical profile, and urinalysis, should be completed before therapy is instituted. Do heartworm testing for any ferrets with clinical signs suggestive of infection and for ferrets from heartworm-endemic areas. If thoracocentesis and abdominocentesis are done, cytologic and fluid analysis of the aspirated sample should be performed and may provide some insight into the cause of the effusion.

Radiography

Standard two-view thoracic radiographs can yield important information for the diagnosis of cardiac disease and CHF. Include the entire thorax in the radiographs, because problems in the anterior mediastinum are common. Physical restraint is usually adequate to obtain radiographs, although a short dose of inhalant anesthesia may be used safely. Until recently, the size of the normal ferret heart was described only qualitatively, because the typical landmarks used for dogs and cats are inaccurate in ferrets due to the shape of the thorax. The thoracic cavity of ferrets is elongated and flattened ventrodorsally. The normal ferret heart is more globoid in appearance than a dog or cat heart and it is located approximately between the sixth and eighth intercostal spaces. The right ventricle is slightly in contact with the sternum (Fig. 6-1). If heart disease is present, the cardiac silhouette may appear enlarged, resulting in tracheal elevation, rounding of the cardiac silhouette, and increased sternal contact on the lateral view. On the ventrodorsal view, the heart size may be elongated and widened, filling up a larger portion of the thorax.

The size of the cardiac silhouette can be quantified by the use of a modified vertebral heart score (VHS).[56] The technique involves measuring the length and the width of the heart on the right lateral radiograph and expressing this measurement in units of vertebral length (Fig. 6-2). This method corrects for differences in size between ferrets. Because the presence of pericardial fat on the ventrodorsal view makes the edges of the cardiac silhouette more difficult to discern, the lateral view is more accurate. On the lateral view, the long axis of the heart is the length

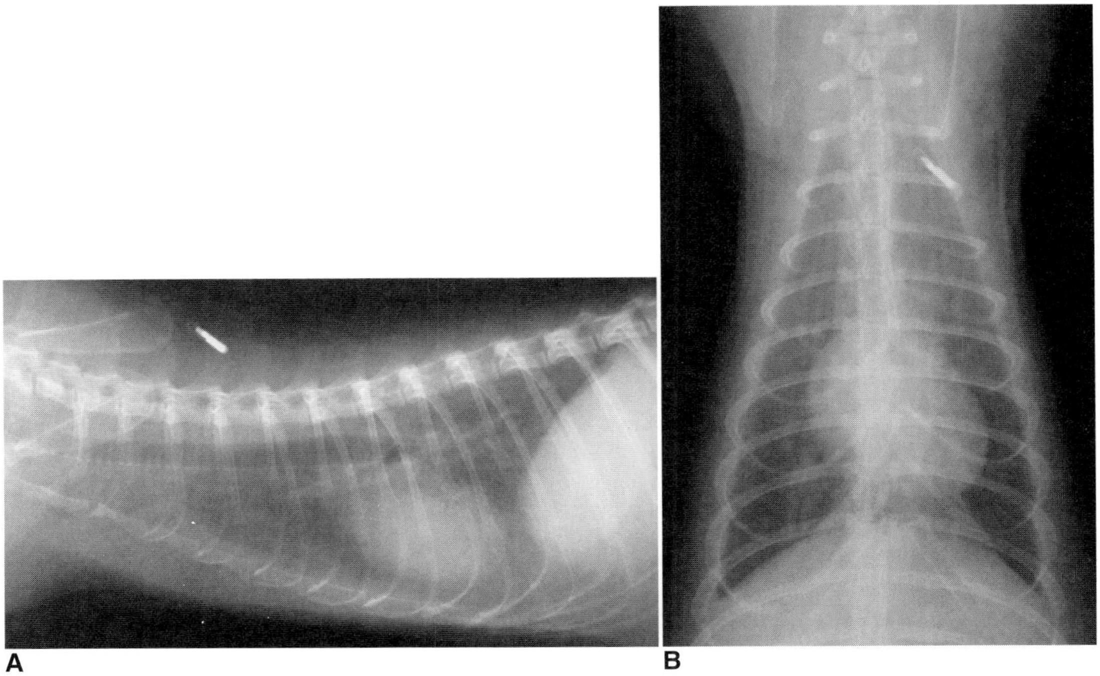

A B

Figure 6-1 Normal lateral (A) and ventrodorsal (B) thoracic radiographs of a 3-year-old, clinically normal ferret.

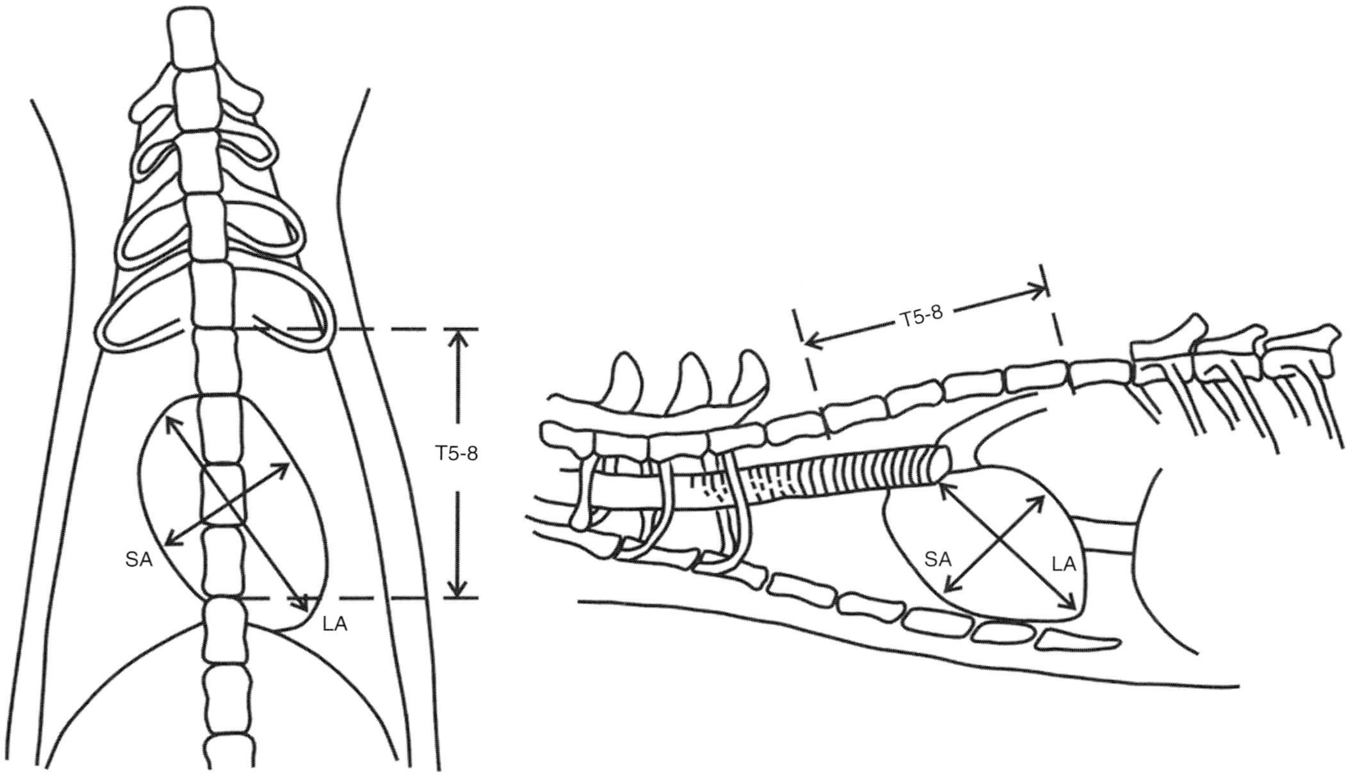

Figure 6-2 Drawings of lateral *(right)* and ventrodorsal *(left)* views of the thorax indicating measurements of the cardiac silhouette in both long axis *(LA)* and short axis *(SA)*. The sum of the LA and SA measurements is expressed in terms of vertebral length, beginning at the cranial edge of the fifth thoracic vertebra *(T5)* and estimated to the nearest 0.25 vertebra. The vertebral length and width measurements are then added to obtain a vertebral heart score. *(Adapted from Stepien RL, Benson KG, Forrest LJ: Radiographic measurement of cardiac size in normal ferrets. Vet Radiol Ultrasound 1999; 40:606-610).*

from the ventral border of the bifurcation of the trachea to the apex of the heart; the short axis is the maximum length from the cranial to the caudal edges. On the ventrodorsal view, the long axis is the length of the heart along midline from the cranial border of the heart to the apex. The short axis is the maximum width of the heart measured perpendicular to the long axis. These measurements are compared with the vertebral length, beginning with the cranial edge of the fifth thoracic vertebra (T5), and estimated to the nearest 0.25 vertebra. The length and width vertebral measurements from a single projection are then added to obtain a total score. Normal VHS values for the right lateral and ventrodorsal projections are 4.00 cm (95% confidence interval, 3.75-4.07 cm) and 4.08 cm (95% confidence interval, 3.85-4.15 cm), respectively.

CHF may be seen radiographically as pleural effusion, pulmonary edema, or pulmonary venous congestion. Pulmonary edema shows most typically a patchy interstitial and alveolar pattern. Abdominal radiographs may reveal hepatomegaly, splenomegaly, and ascites.

Electrocardiography

In ferrets, the ECG is used primarily to determine the presence of abnormal rhythms and conduction disturbances. Reference values for ECGs in ferrets have been published and are summarized in Table 6-1.[5,14,16,53] A variety of common arrhythmias have been seen in ferrets (Fig. 6-3). Sinus rhythm and sinus tachycardia are the most common rhythms seen on presentation with cardiac disease. Atrial and ventricular premature contractions may be recorded. Atrial fibrillation can occur in the presence of significant atrial enlargement. In one ferret I examined, short durations of nonsustained ventricular tachycardia were recorded. Sinus bradycardia can be associated with hypoglycemia, commonly seen in ferrets with insulinomas. Second-degree atrioventricular (AV) block can occur as a normal finding in healthy ferrets. High-grade second-degree AV block and complete (third-degree) AV block are rare. I have seen one case of complete AV block that was successfully treated by implantation of an epicardial transdiaphragmatic pacemaker. Other reported ECG changes include tall R waves, prolonged QRS complexes, and ST-segment depression.[54]

The ECG is ideally done without sedation with the animal in right lateral recumbency (Fig. 6-4). The ECG clips can be flattened to produce a smooth surface that does not result in pinching. Because most ferrets object to the use of alcohol, ECG coupling gel (or ultrasound gel) is recommended. The ferret can be distracted by offering Nutri-cal (EVSCO Pharmaceuticals, Buena, NJ) from a syringe while recording the ECG.

Echocardiography

The echocardiogram remains the test of choice for diagnosing structural and functional cardiac abnormalities.[36] In addition, the echocardiogram can be useful in identifying

TABLE 6-1
Electrocardiographic Variables for 52 Clinically Normal Ferrets*

Parameter	Mean Value ± SD (Range)† (N = 25)	Value‡ (N = 27)
Age (mo)	10–20	5.2
Male/female ratio	All male	1.25
Body weight (kg)	1.4 ± 0.2	Not available
Heart rate (beats/min)	196 ± 26.5 (140–240)	233 ± 22
Rhythm		
Normal sinus	Not available	67%
Sinus arrhythmia	Not available	33%
Mean electrical axis, frontal plane (degrees)	+86.13 ± 2.5 (79.6–90.0)	+77.22 ± 12
Lead II measurements		
P amplitude (mV)	Not available	0.122 ± 0.007
P duration (sec)	Not available	0.024 ± 0.004
PR interval (sec)	0.056 ± 0.0086 (0.04–0.08)	0.047 ± 0.003
QRS duration (sec)	0.044 ± 0.0079 (0.035–0.06)	0.043 ± 0.003
R amplitude (mV)	2.21 ± 0.42 (1.4–3.0)	1.46 ± 0.84
QT interval (sec)	0.109 ± 0.018 (0.08–0.14)	0.12 ± 0.04

*All ferrets were sedated with ketamine-xylazine.
†Data from Bone L, Battles AH, Goldfarb RD, et al: Electrocardiographic values from clinically normal, anesthetized ferrets (*Mustela putorius furo*). Am J Vet Res 1988; 49:1884-1887.
‡Data from Fox JG: Biology and Diseases of the Ferret. Philadelphia, Lea & Febiger, 1988, p 170.

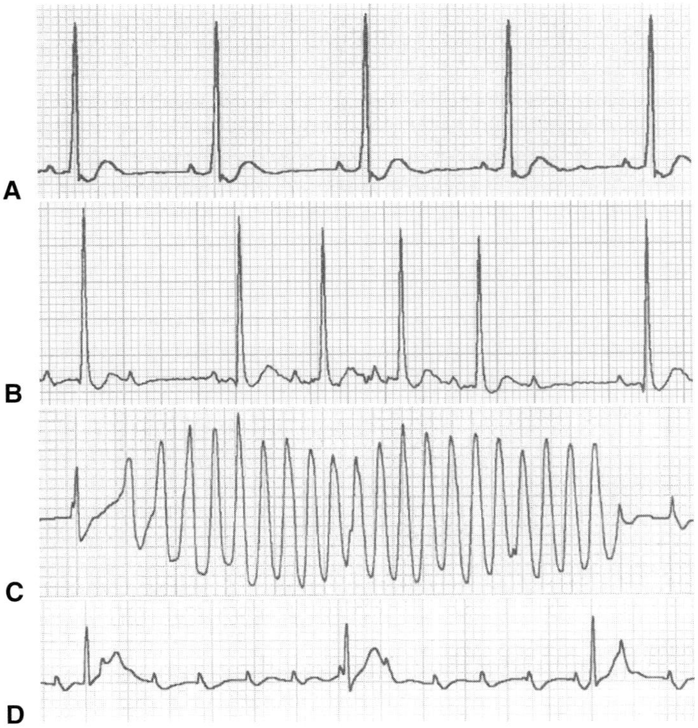

Figure 6-3 Electrocardiograms recorded from four ferrets, showing normal rhythm (**A**), second-degree atrioventricular (AV) block in an asymptomatic ferret (**B**), paroxysmal ventricular tachycardia (**C**), and complete AV block (**D**).

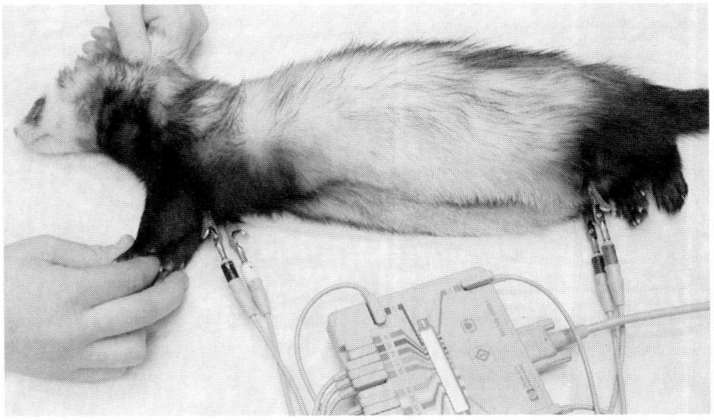

Figure 6-4 Technique for recording the electrocardiogram (ECG). The ferret is placed in right lateral recumbency, and the flattened ECG clips are placed distal on the limbs. Coupling gel is applied to the electrodes.

mediastinal masses and as an aid in detecting heartworm disease.[52] The echocardiogram can often be obtained without the use of sedation. If sedation is required, either a short-acting injectable anesthetic or an inhalant anesthetic may be used. The echocardiogram is done with the animal in both right and left lateral recumbency. Imaging planes similar to those obtained in other species are recorded.[63] Two-dimensional echocardiography provides an assessment of cardiac size and function. Standard M-mode measurements are obtained, including chamber dimensions, wall thickness, and indices of systolic function. Spectral Doppler imaging is used to quantitate the velocity of normal and abnormal blood flow. Color flow Doppler echocardiography provides a visual inspection of blood flow direction and detection of turbulent flow, including valvular regurgitation. Echocardiographic reference values in the sedated ferret have been published and are summarized in Table 6-2.[57] The echocardiogram is used in conjunction with good-quality thoracic radiographs to properly identify the severity of underlying cardiac disease and the presence of CHF.

Treatment

Basic therapeutic principles of CHF and cardiac disease are applied to ferrets. If a published ferret dose is not available, feline doses are often used as a starting point. Therapy for acute CHF focuses on improving oxygenation and reducing preload and afterload. Oxygen is provided by placing the animal in an oxygen-rich environment such as an incubator or closed cage. Diuretics reduce preload by reducing blood volume.[40] Furosemide is the most commonly used diuretic; it is most effective when given either intravenously or intramuscularly in the acute setting. Ferrets tolerate doses of 1 to 4 mg/kg every 8 to 12 hours. Nitroglycerin 2% ointment is a venous dilator applied to the skin in the axilla or inguinal area on a hairless body surface. Ferrets are sensitive to the hypotensive effects of nitroglycerin. Angiotensin-converting enzyme (ACE) inhibitors are given to reduce afterload by causing arterial vasodilation and to reduce preload by decreasing salt and water retention.[32] The dose is usually started at 0.5 mg/kg PO every 48 hours and then titrated up to every 24 hours if tolerated. In the first 24 to 48 hours of therapy, ACE inhibitors may result in hypotension or lethargy. The use of ACE inhibitors in ferrets with CHF and concurrent diuretic therapy can result in severe azotemia. Renal perfusion is reduced in CHF secondary to use of diuretics, decreased cardiac output, dehydration, and hypotension.[25] If significant pleural effusion is present, resulting in an increased inspiratory effort, perform pleurocentesis and submit the fluid for fluid analysis and cytologic examination. In acute disease, monitor ferrets closely for respiratory rate and effort, mucous membrane color, heart rate and rhythm, body weight, and hydration, as well as electrolyte, blood urea nitrogen (BUN), and creatinine values. Obtain serial radiographs to assess the response to therapy. Adjust medication dosages based on the listed monitoring parameters.

Chronic therapy typically includes furosemide, ACE inhibitors, and digoxin. Furosemide is given orally at a dosage of 1 to 4 mg/kg q8-12h; ACE inhibitors are given at 0.5 mg/kg q24-48h as tolerated. Digoxin therapy is used as a positive inotrope and to depress AV nodal conduction with supraventricular arrhythmias.[32] Digoxin elixir (0.05 mg/mL) is recommended because of the small doses required in ferrets. The recommended starting dosage is 0.01 mg/kg PO q12-24h.[49] Calculated dosages for digoxin are based on lean body weight, usually 70% of body weight. I often begin therapy once daily and then titrate up to twice daily depending on the clinical response and serum digoxin levels. Side effects of digoxin include inappetence, lethargy, vomiting, diarrhea, and arrhythmias.[54] To date, no pharmacokinetic studies of digoxin in ferrets have been published. To measure digoxin levels, serum samples are taken approximately 6 to 8 hours after drug administration.[54] Reference values for dogs and cats are extrapolated to interpret values in ferrets (0.8-2.0 ng/mL). Contraindications for the use of digoxin include significant azotemia, hypokalemia, bradyarrhythmias including AV block, and severe ventricular arrhythmias.[32]

Long-term management includes periodic monitoring for recurrence of CHF and changes in body weight, renal values, and heart rate and rhythm. If CHF recurs with standard therapy protocols, additional diuretics may be used, including thiazide diuretics or potassium-sparing diuretics. Published feline dosages are used, and the dosage is titrated based on clinical response. Close monitoring of electrolytes after beginning more aggressive and mixed diuretic therapy is recommended. In ferrets with CHF receiving steroid therapy for lymphoma, spironolactone should be considered early in the disease process because of its effects on the aldosterone receptor in the distal renal tubule.[40]

The use of antiarrhythmic drugs is not well documented in ferrets. Atenolol titrated to effect can be given for many supraventricular and ventricular arrhythmias. Diltiazem can be used for many supraventricular arrhythmias to either reduce spontaneous occurrence or slow AV nodal conduction.[31] I successfully used intravenous lidocaine in one ferret with ventricular tachycardia; the dose was markedly reduced and then titrated to effect. With this class of antiarrhythmic drugs, close observation for the development of neurologic and gastrointestinal signs is essential.[31]

TABLE 6-2
M-Mode and Doppler Echocardiographic Values for Normal Ferrets*

Parameter	Mean Value ± SD
Interventricular septum end-diastole (IVSd) (cm)	0.36 ± 0.07
Interventricular septum end-systole (IVSs) (cm)	0.48 ± 0.11
Left ventricular free wall end-diastole (LVWd) (cm)	0.42 ± 0.11
Left ventricular free wall end-systole (LVWs) (cm)	0.58 ± 0.99
Left ventricular internal dimension end-diastole (LVIDd) (cm)	0.88 ± 0.15
Left ventricular internal dimension end-systole (LVIDs) (cm)	0.59 ± 0.15
Fractional shortening (%)	33 ± 14
Ejection fraction (%)	69 ± 19
Left atrial diameter (LA) (cm)	0.71 ± 0.18
Aortic diameter (AO) (cm)	0.53 ± 0.10
LA/AO (ratio)	1.33 ± 0.27
Pulmonary artery diameter (cm)	0.48 ± 0.9
Right ventricular free wall end-diastole (cm)	0.12 ± 0.03
Right ventricular internal dimension end-diastole (cm)	0.38 ± 0.10
Aorta maximum velocity (m/sec)	0.89 ± 0.20
Pulmonary artery maximum velocity (m/sec)	1.10 ± 0.14
Mitral valve E velocity (m/sec)	0.70 ± 0.10
Mitral valve A velocity (m/sec)	0.52 ± 0.11
Mitral valve velocity E/A ratio	1.38 ± 0.32

From Stepien RL, Benson KG, Wenholz LJ: M-mode and Doppler echocardiographic findings in normal ferrets sedated with ketamine hydrochloride and midazolam. Vet Radiol Ultrasound 2000; 41:452-456.
*All ferrets were sedated with ketamine and midazolam (0.2 mg/kg).

DILATED CARDIOMYOPATHY

Dilated cardiomyopathy has been described in ferrets and has clinical characteristics similar to those observed in dogs and cats.[13,19,33] The disease results in a dilated left ventricle, right ventricle, or both, with global systolic dysfunction. The cause for the disease in ferrets is not known; in one ferret, it was reported in association with a cryptococcal infection.[19] Lethargy, dyspnea, anorexia, and weight loss are common complaints in the history. Physical examination findings can include hypothermia, heart murmur, tachycardia, pallor, weakness, or ascites. Pleural effusion is seen as an increased inspiratory effort with muffled heart sounds. Pulmonary edema is heard as moist rales and increased respiratory sounds. In many cases, both pulmonary edema and pleural effusion are present simultaneously, resulting in a combination of the clinical signs mentioned.

Echocardiography is used to make a definitive diagnosis of dilated cardiomyopathy. Typical echocardiographic changes are similar to those observed in other species.[6,35,64] The left ventricle appears dilated, with increased end-diastolic and end-systolic dimensions, and the left atrium is typically dilated (Fig. 6-5). Fractional shortening, a commonly used index of systolic function, is reduced. If the right side of the heart is involved, the right ventricle is dilated, right ventricular systolic motion is reduced, and the right atrium is enlarged. In advanced disease, mitral and tricuspid regurgitation secondary to valve annulus dilation are seen. Left ventricular outflow tract velocities can be normal or reduced.

Radiographically, the cardiac silhouette appears enlarged. CHF is seen as pleural effusion or pulmonary edema. If the abdomen is included in the radiograph, hepatomegaly, ascites, or splenomegaly may be present.

A variety of ECG abnormalities may be present, including ventricular premature contractions, atrial premature contractions, atrial tachycardia, ventricular tachycardia, and atrial fibrillation.[35,64]

Therapy for acute clinical CHF was described earlier and includes oxygen, diuretics, nitroglycerin, and pleurocentesis if necessary. The ferret is placed in an oxygen-rich environment and given furosemide at 1 to 4 mg/kg IV or IM. A thoracic radiograph is taken after the animal is assessed as being stable and the degree of pleural effusion is determined. The venodilator nitroglycerin reduces pulmonary edema in the acute management of CHF.[32] The ointment can be placed on a hairless area of skin every 12 to 24 hours. Monitor the response to initial management of heart failure by close observation of the respiratory rate and effort and auscultation of lung sounds. Obtain an initial database, including values for electrolytes, BUN, and creatinine.

After the ferret's condition is initially stabilized, therapy for chronic disease begins with diuretics, ACE inhibitors, and digoxin. Diuretics are reduced to the lowest dose that prevents reaccumulation of pleural effusion and pulmonary congestion. Low-salt diets and exercise restriction are theoretically beneficial in the management of CHF but can be difficult practices to institute. To date, no cases of taurine-responsive dilated cardiomyopathy have been documented in ferrets.

Long-term therapy includes periodic monitoring of thoracic radiographs; ECG findings; plasma BUN, creatinine, and electrolyte concentrations; and serum digoxin levels. Large amounts of data are not available to estimate the prognosis in ferrets with dilated cardiomyopathy. The clinical response to therapy is often good, and in my opinion ferrets tend to respond better to treatment than do dogs or cats with similar echocardiographic findings.

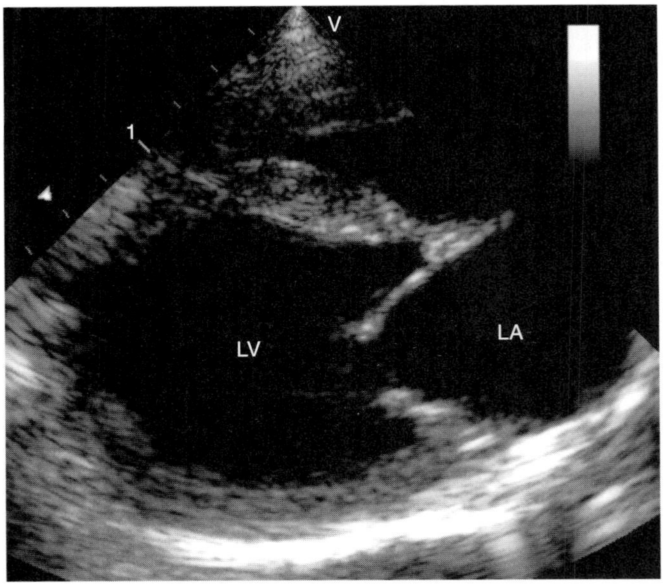

Figure 6-5 Two-dimensional echocardiogram of a ferret with dilated cardiomyopathy. The left ventricle *(LV)* is dilated, with rounding of the left ventricular apex, and the left atrium *(LA)* is enlarged.

HYPERTROPHIC CARDIOMYOPATHY

Hypertrophic cardiomyopathy (HCM) occurs in ferrets, but the clinical characteristics have not been well described, and no reports of HCM have been published. Physiologically, the presence of left ventricular hypertrophy results in impaired filling of the left ventricle (diastolic function). Left ventricular diastolic pressure progressively increases, and the subsequent increase in left atrial pressure results in the development of left-sided CHF.[2] Left ventricular hypertrophy has not been documented secondary to hypertension or hyperthyroidism in ferrets. The course of disease is likely to be similar to that in the feline population, remaining silent until the onset of CHF, thromboembolic events, or sudden death.[2,50]

HCM should be a differential diagnosis in animals with suspected cardiac disease based on auscultation, radiographic findings, or clinical signs of CHF. Echocardiography is used to definitively diagnosis this disease. The entire left ventricle or isolated segments of the left ventricle can be hypertrophied. The left ventricular diastolic and systolic dimensions are reduced, and the fractional shortening is normal or increased. Left atrial enlargement may be present. Systolic anterior mitral valve motion may be seen and is often associated with interventricular septal hypertrophy. Doppler echocardiographic abnormalities can include turbulence in the left ventricular outflow tract secondary to dynamic obstruction and mitral regurgitation.

Treatment is aimed at improving the diastolic efficiency of the left ventricle and relieving signs of CHF.[18] The most commonly used therapeutic agents for the treatment of HCM include β-adrenergic blocking drugs (e.g., atenolol at 3.125-6.25 mg PO q24h) or calcium channel blockers (e.g., diltiazem at 3.75-7.5 mg PO q12h).[55] These drugs reduce heart rate and contractility, resulting in better filling of the left ventricle.[18] Therapy is titrated to achieve an effective reduction in heart rate and clinical improvement. With both medications, side effects include lethargy, inappetence, bradycardia, and hypotension. If clinical signs of CHF are present, treatment with diuretics is recommended (see earlier discussion). Therapeutic monitoring includes periodic echocardiograms to determine the extent of progressive cardiac hypertrophy and atrial enlargement. In those ferrets with CHF, monitor thoracic radiographs, ECGs, and serum biochemical profiles. Thromboembolic disease secondary to cardiac disease in ferrets has not been reported.

VALVULAR HEART DISEASE

Valvular heart disease most commonly occurs in the middle-aged to older ferret and is being recognized with increasing frequency. Clinical signs vary depending on the severity of the underlying disease. Mitral regurgitation is auscultated as a systolic murmur over the left apical region, and tricuspid regurgitation is auscultated in the right parasternal location. A diastolic murmur of aortic insufficiency is rarely heard on physical examination. Femoral pulses can be hyperdynamic with significant aortic regurgitation, but they most often remain normal or reduced with CHF. Labored breathing and moist rales (crackles) are present in ferrets with CHF.

Thoracic radiographs provide a general impression of cardiac size and are required to definitively diagnose CHF. Pulmonary edema is seen as a mixed patchy alveolar and interstitial pattern more prominent in the caudodorsal lung regions. ECG signs vary but may indicate atrial arrhythmias associated with atrial enlargement. Echocardiography shows thickening of the affected valves and atrial enlargement (Fig. 6-6). The left ventricular diastolic dimension is increased, with a normal systolic dimension and preserved fractional shortening. Left ventricular wall thickness is normal. Regurgitation can be identified and quantified with the use of Doppler echocardiography. Aortic regurgitation is a common incidental finding on echocardiograms in ferrets and is rarely clinically significant.

Therapy is recommended if CHF is present or if cardiac enlargement is significant. ACE inhibitors blunt the neurohormonal activation that occurs with advanced cardiac disease and CHF.[32] If there is radiographic evidence of CHF, furosemide is administered. The dose is titrated to effect, and renal values are monitored periodically. Digoxin can be given after the ferret is stabilized on the therapy described. Indications for its use include stabilization of heart rate, positive inotropic effects, and control of supraventricular arrhythmias. The management of CHF was described earlier in this chapter.

Several factors influence the prognosis of ferrets with chronic valvular disease, including renal function, coexisting disease, and cardiac rhythm. Insufficient data are available to predict the prognosis in ferrets with CHF secondary to chronic degenerative valve disease.

MYOCARDITIS

Myocarditis typically manifests as infiltration of the myocardium with inflammatory cells that results in reduced myocardial function, arrhythmias, and fibrous tissue replacement of normal myocardium.[20] Causes of myocardial inflammation include systemic vasculitis and parasitic, autoimmune, bacterial, and viral disorders. A *Toxoplasma*-like organism has been described as causing multifocal myocardial necrosis.[63] Aleutian disease can cause fibrinoid necrosis and mononuclear cell infiltration in arterioles of the heart.[11] Because of the presence of cytokines and other inflammatory factors, systemic

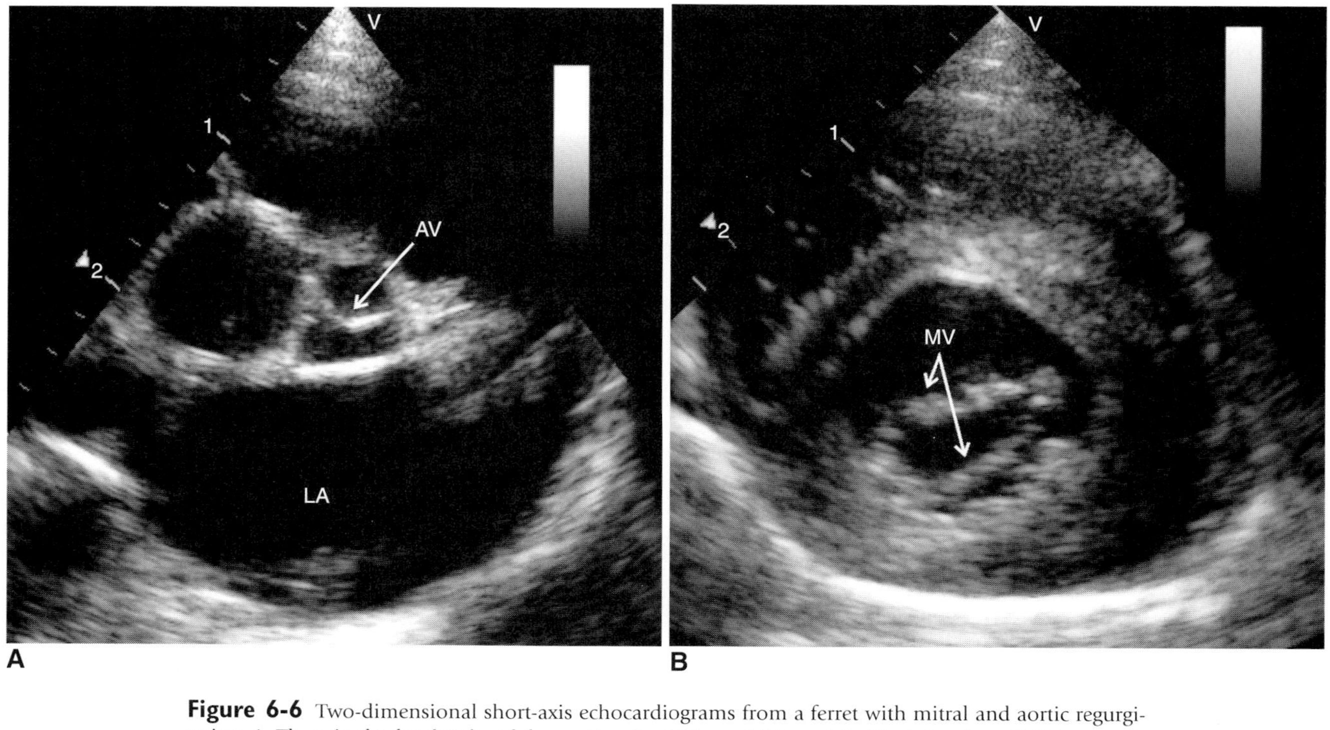

Figure 6-6 Two-dimensional short-axis echocardiograms from a ferret with mitral and aortic regurgitation. **A,** The mitral valve *(MV)* and the aortic valve *(AV)* are thickened. **B,** The left atrium *(LA)* is severely dilated.

inflammatory diseases, including sepsis, can result in a reduction of myocardial function.

The diagnosis of myocarditis requires histologic evaluation of the myocardium, making antemortem verification difficult. This disease should be suspected if arrhythmias and acute myocardial dysfunction are found in the presence of a multisystemic illness. The primary therapeutic goal is directed at the underlying cause of the systemic disorder. Cardiovascular support, including diuretics or antiarrhythmic agents, may be necessary.

NEOPLASIA

Neoplasia involving the myocardium or pericardium has not been reported in ferrets. Lymphoma, a common tumor found in ferrets, can involve the cranial mediastinum. Ferrets with a cranial mediastinal mass are often presented because of dyspnea associated with the presence of pleural effusion.[14] Ultrasonography is useful to rule out the presence of cardiac disease and to visualize any mass that may be present. Fine-needle aspiration of the tumor, or in some cases cytologic examination of the fluid, can be used to make a diagnosis.

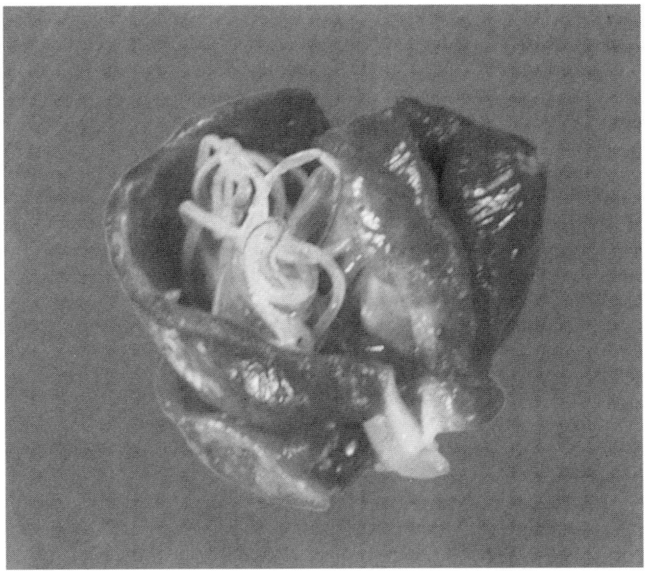

Figure 6-7 Adult *Dirofilaria immitis* in the heart of a ferret.

HEARTWORM DISEASE

Natural and experimental infections with the canine heartworm, *Dirofilaria immitis,* have been reported in ferrets.[3,7,34,37,45] Ferrets living or originating in an endemic area are most susceptible to infection. The susceptibility and life cycle of this parasite have been studied in ferrets and are similar to those of heartworm in dogs; however, because of the small size of ferrets, the clinical presentation more closely resembles that of infected cats.[61] The life cycle begins when a ferret is bitten by a mosquito containing infective (L3) *D. immitis* larvae, which are deposited in the subcutaneous tissues. Larvae migrate to the vascular system and can be found within the small pulmonary arteries (L5). Microfilaria have been reported in ferrets, in both natural and experimental infections. Microfilaria are present in 50% to 60% of infected animals.[62]

Ferrets can be severely affected by the presence of only a single worm. With natural infections, worm burdens ranging from 1 to 21 worms have been reported.[34,37,45] The worms can be found within the pulmonary arteries, right side of the heart, and vena cava. Because of the ferret's small size, infection with a small number of worms can cause mechanical obstruction to blood flow, resulting in clinical signs of right-sided heart failure. In dogs, the host response to living worms within the pulmonary vasculature can include pneumonitis, granuloma formation, pulmonary endarteritis, thromboembolism, and pulmonary hypertension. However, these classic histopathologic changes have not been identified in ferrets, possibly because of the low worm numbers and their primary location within the right side of the heart.

Necropsy reveals heartworms present in the right atrium, right ventricle, cranial vena cava, and pulmonary arteries (Fig. 6-7). Right ventricular and right atrial enlargement develops secondary to pulmonary hypertension and mechanical obstruction. Thickening of the tricuspid valve may result from chronic damage caused by the presence of worms. Pleural effusion, ascites, and congestion of abdominal organs may be present. Microfilaria may be seen in alveolar capillaries and larger vessels. On histopathologic examination, calcified worms, thrombosis, pulmonary endarteritis, and congestion are typically seen. Chronic passive congestion of the liver and renal hemosiderosis are reported. Aberrant larval migration has not been reported in ferrets. The presence of black feces in the colon has been reported but is not a consistent finding.[34,45,49]

Clinical signs in affected ferrets include coughing, lethargy, weakness, and dyspnea. Signs of right-sided heart failure, including pleural effusion and ascites, may be present. Hypothermia is a common finding on physical examination. Sudden cardiac death occurs most likely from pulmonary artery obstruction.[34,45] Thoracic radiographs should be obtained and may show pleural effusion and cardiomegaly (Fig. 6-8). Enlargement of the right atrium, caudal vena cava, and right ventricle are commonly seen. Unlike in dogs, radiographic peripheral pulmonary artery changes are not severe in ferrets, probably because the worms reside primarily in the right side of the heart and in the main pulmonary artery.[34,45,60] Angiographic findings in ferrets experimentally inoculated with *D. immitis* have been published.[60] Common findings include right-sided heart enlargement and filling defects in the right side of the heart, pulmonary artery, and vena cava. Although angiography can be a useful test in the diagnosis of heartworm disease, its clinical use is limited by technical inexperience and the requirement for specialized equipment. Echocardiography is a superior test because it is noninvasive and more widely available. Echocardiographic examination can identify the presence of intracardiac parasites. The worms may be visualized in the pulmonary artery, right ventricle, and right atrium. Right ventricular and right atrial dilation may be seen.[52] The presence of pulmonary hypertension should be also suspected and can be diagnosed with the use of Doppler echocardiography.[26]

Diagnosis of heartworm disease is based on clinical signs, radiographic and echocardiographic findings, and results of heartworm blood testing. Microfilaria are seen in only about 50% of infected ferrets. The antigen tests used most commonly to diagnose heartworm infection are enzyme-linked

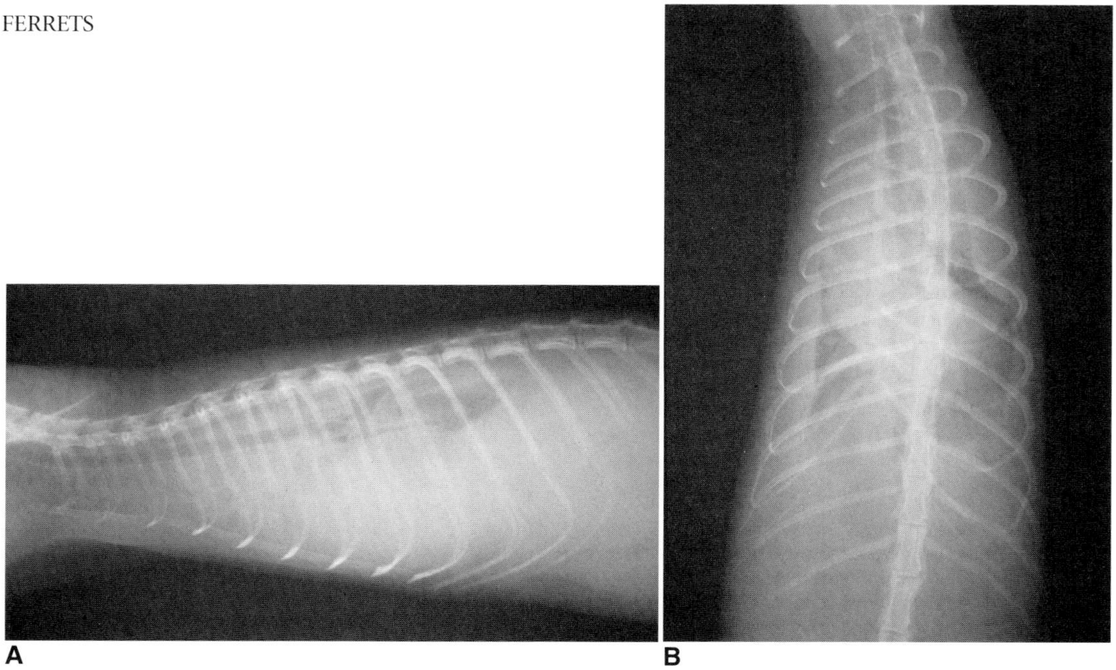

Figure 6-8 Lateral (A) and ventrodorsal (B) radiographs of a ferret with pleural effusion secondary to heartworm disease.

immunosorbent assays (ELISA).[55] Antigen is shed by adult female heartworms into the circulation. Because antigen testing detects only female worms, there is less likelihood of positively identifying ferrets with low worm burdens. Studies are needed to further evaluate the sensitivity and specificity of heartworm testing in ferrets.

Successful therapy for heartworm disease depends on early, accurate detection. The current recommended treatment protocol is as follows (N. Antinoff, DVM, personal communication, 2003). (1) In animals that are symptomatic and microfilaremia positive, administer microfilaricidal therapy with ivermectin (50 µg/kg SQ q30d) until clinical signs resolve and microfilaremia is absent. (2) Give adulticide therapy with melarsomine (Immiticide, Rhone Merieux, Athens, GA) in a two-stage protocol. The first stage consists of a single dose of 2.5 mg/kg IM; the second stage is given 1 month later and consists of two injections (each 2.5 mg/kg IM) given 24 hours apart. Transient swelling and pain at the injection site commonly occur. During the treatment period, management of pleural effusion with diuretics may be necessary. Prednisone (0.5 mg/kg PO q12-24h) is recommended throughout this period and until clinical signs resolve completely. Strict cage rest for 4 to 6 weeks after treatment is essential. Perform a follow-up ELISA for heartworm antigen approximately 3 months after adulticide therapy, and then repeat testing at monthly intervals until the results are negative. If antigen test results remain positive, further diagnostic tests (radiographs, echocardiography) may be necessary to determine whether heartworm infection persists. Most ferrets become seronegative within 4 months after successful adulticide therapy.

Recommend preventive therapy for those ferrets previously infected with heartworm disease and for all ferrets in heartworm-endemic areas. Ivermectin can be given orally once a month; one quarter of the smallest-size canine or feline ivermectin oral tablet (yield, approximately 14-17 µg) (Heartgard-Feline and Heartgard-30, Merck & Co. Inc., Whitehouse Station, NJ) is adequate for ferrets. Because the drug deteriorates once the pill is broken, the remainder of the pill must be discarded.

PART II **OTHER DISEASES**

James K. Morrisey, DVM, Diplomate ABVP

ALEUTIAN DISEASE

Aleutian disease is caused by a parvovirus and was first reported as a disease of mink in the 1940s.[17] Mink that are homozygous for the Aleutian (blue) gene are most severely affected, thus giving the disease its name. The disease in mink is an immune complex–mediated disorder that causes hypergammaglobulinemia. Deposits of immune complexes in various organs are responsible for the clinical signs, which include glomerulonephritis, bile duct proliferation, arteritis, and progressive wasting. In persistently infected mink, other clinical signs are infertility, abortion, and neonatal interstitial pneumonitis.[23] Affected animals are immunosuppressed and are more susceptible to other infections, such as influenza, viral enteritis, and distemper. The disease was first seen in ferrets in the late 1960s.[27,29]

There are several strains of the Aleutian disease virus (ADV) in mink, and they vary in the immune response elicited and therefore in virulence. Although the mink virus can infect ferrets, at least three separate viral strains that are distinct from the mink ADV have been documented in ferrets.[38,46] Because the hypervariable capsid region of the ferret ADV strains is similar to that of the mink virus, these ferret strains are thought to be mutant strains of the mink ADV.[51] Mink can be infected with ferret ADV, but the virulence is lower.[11,39,46]

Clinical Signs

In ferrets that were experimentally infected with mink or ferret strains of ADV, infection persisted for up to 180 days, but the clinical signs that are seen in naturally infected ferrets did not develop.[28] The clinical signs in naturally infected ferrets can vary. Some ADV-infected ferrets die in good body condition without any clinical signs.[11] Most ferrets show signs of a chronic wasting disease, with varying degrees of progressive weight loss, weakness, ataxia, and posterior paresis. Central nervous system (CNS) signs can include tremors, convulsions, and paralysis.[43,58,67,68] Hepatomegaly, splenomegaly, pallor, and melena are also consistent findings. In a recent report, respiratory signs including acute dyspnea were described.[65] Ferrets infected at older ages usually show fewer clinical signs; however, ferrets can be infected for years before clinical signs become apparent. Most reported cases were in ferrets between 2 and 4 years of age.

Clinical pathologic findings in infected ferrets can also vary. The most consistent findings are hypoalbuminemia and hypergammaglobulinemia. Protein electrophoresis of plasma samples from these animals usually demonstrates gamma globulins amounting to 20% to 60% of the total protein concentration (Fig. 6-9). Rare cases with normal protein fractions have been recorded.[65] Because the immune complexes damage internal organs, other biochemical abnormalities, such as azotemia and high liver enzyme concentrations, may be present. Anemia of chronic inflammation has also been reported.[44]

Diagnosis

A presumptive diagnosis can be made based on the history, clinical signs, and a high gamma globulin concentration. Antemortem diagnosis can be made on the basis of a positive serum titer coupled with hypergammaglobulinemia or histologic evidence of associated lymphoplasmacytic inflammation in tissue biopsy samples. At present, available serologic tests for ADV testing include the counterimmunoelectrophoresis (referred to as CIEP or CEP) test (United Vaccines, Inc, Madison, WI) and an ELISA (Avecon Diagnostics Inc., Bath, PA). Immunofluorescent antibody tests have also been performed but currently are not available commercially.

The CIEP test was developed for use in mink and is the standard screening test in mink for all ADV strains. It is used routinely in ferrets and has been shown to be an effective method of serologically identifying ferrets with ADV antibodies.[43,58,67,68] Results are reported as positive, negative, or "no test," which means that an interference with test results has occurred in the sample. Usually results from retesting of "no test" samples are clearly positive or negative. Recently an ELISA test has been developed and is available commercially for testing of blood (serum/plasma) or saliva samples. A Quick-Check point-of-care test (Avecon) is also available for in-house testing of saliva or blood samples or client testing of saliva samples. To date, no studies have been published about the specificity and sensitivity of either ELISA test in ferrets, nor has a comparative study of the CIEP and ELISA methods in ferrets been reported. Therefore, results must be interpreted in light of clinical signs and results of other diagnostic tests.

The presence of ADV antibody in a ferret is not necessarily diagnostic of disease. In serologic surveys of large pet ferret populations, 8.5% and 10% of ferrets surveyed were antibody positive without clinical signs of disease.[23,67] Also, immunocompetent adult ferrets experimentally infected with ferret ADV can develop persistent infection without clinical disease. As in mink, ferrets probably develop persistent, nonprogressive infection as well as nonpersistent, nonprogressive infection with ADV.[4,44] Ferrets infected with these forms of ADV could be seropositive without clinical disease.

At necropsy, gross changes in ferrets with Aleutian disease include hepatomegaly, splenomegaly, lymphadenopathy, and thymic enlargement. A positive diagnosis is made by demonstrating lesions consistent with ADV infection on histopathologic examination, such as periportal hepatitis with aggregates of lymphocytes, plasmacytes, and neutrophils. Bile duct hyperplasia and periportal fibrosis are common findings, and mild membranous glomerulonephrosis may also be seen. In the CNS form of the disease, perivascular cuffing in the brain and spinal cord and lymphoplasmacytic meningitis may be present.

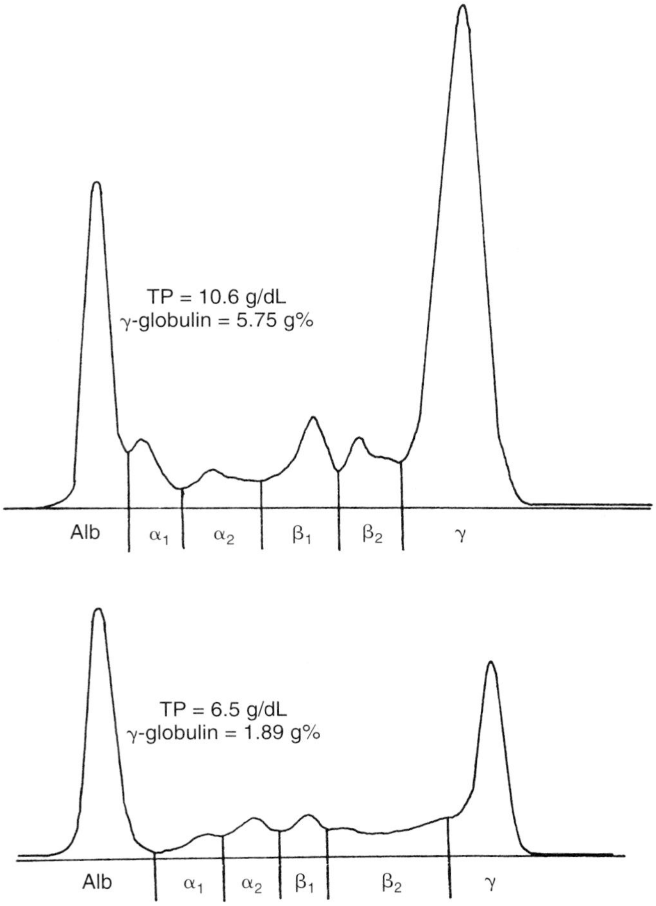

Figure 6-9 Serum protein electrophoretograms from two ferrets with syndromes associated with Aleutian disease. *Top,* Ferret 1: Notice the pronounced hypergammaglobulinemia. The gamma globulin fraction *(γ)* equals 54% of the total protein concentration. *Bottom,* Ferret 2: The gamma globulin fraction equals 29% of the total protein concentration. Hypergammaglobulinemia is the hallmark of Aleutian disease virus infection. *Alb,* Albumin; *TP,* total protein. *(From Palley LS, Corning BF, Fox JG, et al: Parvovirus-associated syndrome [Aleutian disease] in two ferrets. J Am Vet Med Assoc 1992; 201:100-106.)*

Although DNA of ADV can be detected by in situ hybridization, currently this is not a practical screening method.[21]

Treatment and Prevention

No definitive treatment exists for ADV infection in ferrets. In mink, immunosuppressive therapy with cyclophosphamide has been used to control infection for up to 16 weeks, but viral titers did not change in treated animals.[9] Treatment of infected mink kits with gamma globulin–containing ADV antibody decreased mortality rates.[1] In ferrets with clinical disease, supportive care, use of antiinflammatory agents, and immunosuppressive therapy with prednisone or cyclophosphamide should be considered. No vaccine exists for Aleutian disease, and vaccination is probably contraindicated given the immune-mediated nature of the disease. In mink farms, testing by CIEP and removal of animals that test positive has been effective in eradicating the disease[10]; testing and removal could be considered as a control method in ferret colonies and shelters as well.

SPLENOMEGALY

Splenomegaly is a very common clinical finding in ferrets older than 1 year of age. A variety of conditions can cause splenomegaly, including extramedullary hematopoiesis (EMH), neoplasia, hypersplenism, and heart disease. Splenic torsion, abscess, and rupture are rare in ferrets. Splenomegaly may be a normal finding, unrelated to any disease state. Often, splenomegaly is present concurrently with diseases such as adrenal disease and insulinoma, but it is usually an incidental finding and unrelated to these diseases. In some ferrets, the spleen is so enlarged and pendulous that the animal has difficulty lifting its abdomen off the ground. In most cases I have seen, the enlarged spleen was of little or no clinical significance.

The normal ferret spleen is quite large for the size of the animal, measuring approximately 5 cm in length, 2 cm in width, and 1 cm in thickness. The spleen may enlarge slightly with age in ferrets, for reasons that are poorly understood.[11] Chronic immune stimulation or compensation for erythroid bone marrow insufficiency may play a role. More research is needed to determine if splenomegaly is indicative of other disease problems.

The most common cause of splenomegaly in ferrets is EMH. This appears grossly as a smooth, dark red spleen. The cause of this syndrome is unknown, although compensation for myeloid insufficiency has been suggested.[15] Most ferrets with EMH do not show evidence of anemia or other hematologic deficiencies. Splenic lymphoproliferation and resultant splenomegaly in response to chronic immune stimulation has also been suggested as a cause. In mice, evidence exists that chronic infection with *Helicobacter felis* induces this change; a similar situation may exist in ferrets.[12]

Although hemangioma, hemangiosarcoma, and other tumors can occur, lymphoma is the most common neoplasia of the ferret spleen. On gross examination, a spleen with lymphoma often has irregular borders and texture as well as white to tan nodules on the surface and within the parenchyma. Splenic neoplasia often involves other organs, such as the liver and intestinal lymph nodes.

Hypersplenism is rare in ferrets. This disease involves destruction of one or more blood cell lines by the reticuloendothelial system within the spleen. Affected ferrets have blood dyscrasias such as anemia, leucopenia, thrombocytopenia, or pancytopenia. The bone marrow may be normal or hypercellular. Clinical signs are associated with the predominantly decreased blood cell count and include weakness, pallor, petechiae, and secondary infections. Diagnosis is made on the basis of abnormal CBC findings coupled with cytologic results indicating a normal to hypercelluar bone marrow and no other sign of blood loss, infection, or neoplasia. Results of radiographs and plasma biochemical analyses are usually normal but help to rule out other possible causes of disease. The relationship of EMH to hypersplenism is unclear. In one report, ferrets with anemia of undetermined cause responded to splenectomy, but the histologic appearance of the spleen was found to be that of EMH.[15] Two of these ferrets developed systemic disease (lymphoma and multifocal granulomatous disease) within 4 months after splenectomy.

In the diagnostic approach to an enlarged spleen in a ferret, perform a thorough examination with particular attention to palpation of the spleen. With EMH, the spleen is usually of normal shape and consistency with regular borders; neoplasia of the spleen may cause irregular borders and palpable lumps within the spleen. Take care in palpation, because some diseases cause the spleen to be more friable, and splenic rupture is possible. Radiographs may be helpful to define the borders of the spleen and to evaluate for other abnormalities that may be associated with the splenomegaly, such as hepatomegaly, cardiomegaly, and other systemic problems.

Aspiration or biopsy can best determine the cause of splenomegaly. Splenic aspiration with a 22-or 25-gauge needle and a 3-mL syringe can usually be performed in the awake ferret. Distracting the ferret with sweet substances (e.g., offering Nutri-Cal [Tomlyn, Buena, NJ] by syringe) is helpful. On cytologic examination of an aspirate, EMH typically shows a mixed population of mature and immature red cells (see Chapter 38), whereas lymphoma or other lymphoproliferative disease shows a predominant or homogenous population of lymphocytes. Many clinicians prefer surgical biopsy of the spleen, because the cellular architecture of the spleen is maintained and the entire spleen and other abdominal organs can be examined during surgery.

Ultrasonography of the spleen should be used to evaluate for areas of altered echogenicity. Typically the spleen is of uniform echogenicity with EMH, whereas with neoplasia the splenic parenchyma appears mottled. If the splenic parenchyma is irregular, a diagnostic sample should be obtained by ultrasound-guided aspiration. Biopsy of the spleen is best performed surgically or endoscopically. Do not use percutaneous biopsy equipment because it is too large and too long for use in ferrets.

Treatment of splenomegaly depends on the cause. No treatment is known or required for EMH; however, if the spleen has become so large that movement is hampered, removal may be warranted. Do this cautiously, because anemia can result. Splenectomy is recommended for hypersplenism, rupture, torsion, infection, or neoplasia of the spleen. Ferrets with peripheral lymphomas do not necessarily benefit from splenectomy.

ANEMIA

As in other species, anemia in ferrets is caused by decreased production of erythrocytes, destruction of existing erythrocytes, or blood loss. The normal hematocrit of ferrets (46%-61%) is higher than that of other species, and mild anemia may go unrecognized unless clinicians keep this fact in mind. Erythrocyte numbers are also higher; values can be as high as 17.4×10^6 cells/μL.[47] As in other species, hemoglobin concentration and mean cell volume can be used to characterize the anemia, respectively, as normochromic or hypochromic and as normocytic, macrocytic, or microcytic. Normal reticulocyte counts in ferrets can be as high as 10% (see Chapter 38). Reticulocyte counts higher than 12% indicate a regenerative response. Examination of the bone marrow is indicated in any ferret with a nonregenerative anemia that does not respond to treatment within 3 to 6 days.

Decreased production of erythrocytes can be caused by chronic disease or inflammation, bone marrow suppression, or neoplasia. Anemia of chronic disease, also called *anemia of chronic inflammation,* can develop with any long-term illness. It results from decreased iron availability, decreased erythrocyte survival, or decreased response to the anemia.[66] Cytokines secreted during inflammation mediate the response and cause a nonregenerative, normocytic, normochromic anemia. In animals with this type of anemia, results of bone marrow examination are usually normal. In pet ferrets, hyperestrogenemia resulting from an ovarian remnant or from adrenal disease is the most common cause of bone marrow suppression. Chronic estrus as a cause of hyperestrogenemia is much less common in the United States than previously was the case, because pet ferrets are typically spayed before purchase. Neoplasia that affects the bone marrow (e.g., leukemia, myeloma) can suppress erythroid series production because the marrow is replaced by tumor or fibrosis.[30] This typically results in a normocytic, normochromic anemia with a low reticulocyte count. Systemic neoplasia can also cause an anemia of chronic disease.

Erythrocytes can be destroyed by immune-mediated disease, toxins, parasites, or septicemia. Idiopathic, immune-mediated hemolytic anemia has not been documented in ferrets, and diagnosis would be difficult because ferret antibody–specific reagents for the Coombs test are not available. No viral diseases or blood parasites that elicit immune-mediated hemolysis of red blood cells are known to exist in ferrets. Heavy-metal toxicosis and certain drugs are possible causes of hemolytic anemia. Zinc toxicosis as a cause of hemolytic anemia in a ferret has been documented.[59] This type of anemia is uncommon in ferrets, but it may be underdiagnosed because of the inherent difficulties in identifying the toxic agents.

Anemia secondary to blood loss can be caused by trauma, bleeding lesions, parasites, or hemostatic disorders. Trauma is common in ferrets because of their inquisitive nature, and hemorrhage can be internal or external. Bleeding ulcers develop commonly with gastritis caused by *Helicobacter mustelae* infection, gastrointestinal foreign bodies or trichobezoars, or other causes (e.g., chronic use of nonsteroidal antiinflammatory drugs). Parasitism is a less common cause of anemia in ferrets, although coccidiosis in young ferrets or flea infestation could be severe enough to cause anemia. Hemostatic disorders such as thrombocytopenia can develop from estrogen toxicity. Other coagulopathies, such as rodenticide poisoning and disseminated intravascular coagulation, can also occur.

To diagnose anemia in ferrets, obtain a complete history, perform a thorough physical examination, and submit samples for a CBC, reticulocyte count, and, if indicated, bone marrow examination. A plasma biochemical panel, radiographs, and an abdominal ultrasound examination may be helpful, depending on the differential diagnosis established from the history, physical examination, and CBC results. Pay particular attention to the red blood cell values and the reticulocyte count.

Tailor the treatment of the anemia to the specific cause. Specific supportive care can include one or more fresh whole blood transfusions, iron dextran therapy, hemoglobin solutions, and erythropoietin. Ferrets lack blood types and transfusion reactions are difficult to induce, even with repeated transfusions between the same animals. Indications for transfusion in a ferret are a low packed cell volume (PCV), worsening clinical signs, the specific cause of the anemia, and the possibility of continued blood loss. Base the decision to transfuse a ferret on its clinical status and the PCV. Consider a transfusion in a ferret with acute blood loss if the PCV falls to less than 25%. If the anemia has developed gradually, the ferret may tolerate a lower PCV, although its clinical status may benefit from a transfusion if the PCV is less than 25%. Remember to take the volume of blood extracted for diagnostic tests into account when determining the need for a transfusion.

The blood volume required for transfusion can be estimated by the following formula:

$$BV_{donor} = BV_{recipient} \times [(PCV_{post} - PCV_{pre})/PCV_{donor}]$$

where BV is blood volume in milliliters (calculated as 8% of the body weight in kilograms) and PCV_{post} is the desired PCV after transfusion. The value of PCV_{post} is ideally within the reference range, but more often it is 5% to 10% higher than the pretransfusion PCV (PCV_{pre}). A simpler method is to administer 10% to 20% of the recipient's blood volume in a single transfusion given over at least 4 hours. A filter is advised to prevent clots from being administered. Donor blood is collected in sodium citrate or acid-citrate-dextran (ACD). If citrate is used, 0.1 mL of citrate is used for each 0.9 mL of blood collected; for ACD, 1 mL of ACD per 6 mL of blood is recommended.[24] Long-term storage of ferret blood is possible with the use of typical mammalian storage media but is not currently practiced. Whole ferret blood is also commercially available through Marshall Farms (Marshall Pet Products, Inc., Wolcott, NY).

Because they are economic and generally safe, oral iron supplements are preferred for treatment in small animals. Ferrous salts are absorbed better than ferric salts. A total daily dosage of 15 mg/kg, divided two or three times, is recommended in small animals.[22] Continue treatment for several weeks after the anemia resolves to replenish whole-body iron stores. Hemoglobin substitutes, such as Oxyglobin solution (hemoglobin glutamer-200 [bovine]) (Biopure Corporation, Cambridge, MA) are safe and efficacious in ferrets if whole blood is unavailable. The dosage is 11 to 15 mL/kg administered intravenously or intraosseously over 4 hours.[41] This drug has colloidal properties and should be administered slowly in normovolemic animals and in animals with kidney disease, heart disease, or risk of pulmonary edema. Side effects include discoloration of serum or plasma, skin, mucous membranes, sclera, and urine, which is nonpathogenic and transient. Plasma or serum biochemical values may be affected by this discoloration, so a blood sample for these tests should be submitted before Oxyglobin is administered. Although erythropoietin is rarely indicated, it can be used in ferrets with chronic renal failure at 100 U/kg three times weekly until the PCV is stabilized, and then twice weekly.

IBUPROFEN TOXICOSIS

Ibuprofen toxicosis has been documented in many ferrets[8,48] and has been seen in several ferrets at the Animal Medical Center (New York, NY). Prostaglandin inhibition by ibuprofen and other nonsteroidal antiinflammatory drugs can cause altered renal blood flow, ulceration of the gastrointestinal tract, and platelet dysfunction. Clinical signs include vomiting, CNS depression, anorexia, diarrhea, and melena. Severe overdose can cause renal failure, resulting in azotemia and oliguria or anuria. Gastrointestinal signs develop as early as 2 to 6 hours after ingestion; renal signs may develop within 12 hours after ingestion or as long as 5 days later.[42] Seizures can occur with massive overdosage.

Treatment depends on the clinical signs, time elapsed since ingestion, electrolyte imbalances, and azotemia. Treatment is directed at preventing absorption (if possible), managing bleeding ulcers, and maintaining renal perfusion and electrolyte balance. Induction of emesis is effective only within the first 30 to 60 minutes after ingestion, although activated charcoal may be beneficial if given within the first few hours. Intravenous fluids (0.45% NaCl and 2.5% dextrose) should be administered even if no signs of renal compromise are apparent. To control hemorrhage and hypotension, electrolyte solutions, colloids, and transfusions may be needed. Gastrointestinal protectants, such as ranitidine (24 mg/kg q8h), cimetidine (5-10 mg/kg q8-12h), omeprazole (0.7 mg/kg q24h), or sucralfate (25 mg/kg q8h), are helpful in controlling ulceration.

REFERENCES

1. Aasted B, Alexandersen S, Hansen M: Treatment of neonatally Aleutian disease virus (ADV) infected mink kits with gammaglobulin containing antibodies to ADV reduces the death rate of mink kits. Acta Vet Scand 1988; 29:323-330.
2. Atkins CE, Gallo AM, Kurzman ID, et al: Risk factors, clinical signs, and survival in cats with a clinical diagnosis of idiopathic hypertrophic cardiomyopathy: 74 cases (1985-1989). J Am Vet Med Assoc 1992; 201:613-618.
3. Blair LS, Campbell WC: Suppression of maturation of *Dirofilaria immitis* in *Mustela putorius furo* by single dose of ivermectin. J Parasitol 1980; 66:691-692.
4. Bloom ME, Race RE, Wolfinbarger JB: Identification of a nonvirion protein of Aleutian disease virus: mink with Aleutian disease have antibody to both virion and nonvirion proteins. J Virol 1982; 43:608-616.
5. Bone L, Battles AH, Goldfarb RD, et al: Electrocardiographic values from clinically normal, anesthetized ferrets (*Mustela putorius furo*). Am J Vet Res 1988; 49:1884-1887.
6. Calvert C, Brown J: Use of M-mode echocardiography in the diagnosis of congestive cardiomyopathy in Doberman pinschers. J Am Vet Med Assoc 1986; 189:293-297.
7. Campbell WC, Blair LS: *Dirofilaria immitis*: experimental infections in the ferret (*Mustela putorius furo*). J Parasitol 1978; 64:119-122.
8. Cathers TE, Isaza R, Oehme F: Acute ibuprofen toxicosis in a ferret. J Am Vet Med Assoc 2000; 216:1426-1428.
9. Cheema A, Henson JB, Gorham JR: Aleutian disease of mink: prevention of lesions by immunosuppression. Am J Pathol 1972; 55:543-546.
10. Cho JG, Greenfield J: Eradication of Aleutian disease of mink by eliminating positive counter immunoelectrophoresis reactors. J Clin Microbiol 1978; 7:18-21.
11. Daoust PY, Hunter DB: Spontaneous Aleutian disease in ferrets. Can Vet J 1978; 19:133-135.
12. Enno A, O'Rourke JL, Howlett CR, et al: MALT-oma-like lesions in the murine gastric mucosa after long-term infection with *Helicobacter pylori*-induced gastric lymphoma. Am J Pathol 1995; 147:217.
13. Ensley PK, Van Winkle T: Treatment of congestive heart failure in a ferret (*Mustela putorius furo*). J Zoo Anim Med 1982; 13:23-25.
14. Erdman SE, Brown SA, Kawasaki TA: Clinical and pathologic findings in ferrets with lymphoma: 60 cases (1982-1994). J Am Vet Med Assoc 1996; 208:1285-1290.
15. Erdman SE, Xiantang L, Fox JG: Hematopoietic diseases. *In* Fox JG, ed. Biology and Diseases of the Ferret, 2nd ed. Philadelphia, Lippincott Williams & Wilkins, 1998, pp 231-246.
16. Fox JG: Normal clinical and biologic parameters. *In* Fox JG, ed. Biology and Diseases of the Ferret. Philadelphia, Lea & Febiger, 1988, pp 159-173.
17. Fox JG, Pearson RC, Gorham JR: Viral diseases. *In* Fox JG, ed. Biology and Diseases of the Ferret, 2nd ed. Philadelphia, Lippincott Williams & Wilkins, 1998, pp 355-374.
18. Fox PR: Feline cardiomyopathies. *In* Fox PR, Sisson D, Moise NS, eds. Textbook of Canine and Feline Cardiology: Principles and Clinical Practice, 2nd ed. Philadelphia, WB Saunders, 1999, pp 896-923.
19. Greenlee PG, Stephens E: Meningeal cryptococcosis and congestive cardiomyopathy in a ferret. J Am Vet Med Assoc 1984; 184:840-841.
20. Haas GJ: Etiology, evaluation, and management of acute myocarditis. Cardiol Rev 2001; 9:88-95.
21. Haas L, Lochelt M, Kaaden OR: Detection of Aleutian disease virus DNA in tissues of naturally infected mink. J Gen Virol 1988; 69:705-710.
22. Harvey JW, French TW, Meyer DJ: Chronic iron deficiency anemia in dogs. J Am Anim Hosp Assoc 1982; 18:946-960.
23. Hillyer EV: Cardiovascular diseases: Part II. *In* Hillyer EV, Quesenberry KE, eds. Ferrets, Rabbits, and Rodents: Clinical Medicine and Surgery. Philadelphia, WB Saunders, 1997, pp 71-76.
24. Hoefer HL: Transfusions in exotic species. Prob Vet Med 1992; 4:625-635.
25. Hollenberg NK: Control of renal perfusion and function in congestive heart failure. Am J Cardiol 1988; 62:72E-76E.
26. Johnson L, Boon J, Orton EC: Clinical characteristics of 53 dogs with Doppler-derived evidence of pulmonary hypertension: 1992-1996. J Vet Intern Med 1999; 13:440-447.
27. Kenyon AJ, Howard E, Buko L: Hypergammaglobulinemia in ferrets with lymphoproliferative lesions (Aleutian disease). Am J Vet Res 1967; 28:1167-1172.
28. Kenyon AJ, Kenyon BJ, Hanhn ED: Protides of the Mustelidae: immunoresponse of mustelids to Aleutian mink disease virus. Am J Vet Res 1978; 39:1011-1015.
29. Kenyon AJ, Magnano T, Helmboldt CF, et al: Aleutian disease in the ferret. J Am Vet Med Assoc 1966; 149:920-924.
30. Kisseberth WC, MacEwen EG: Complications of cancer and its treatment. *In* Withrow SJ, MacEwen EG, eds. Small Animal Clinical Oncology, 2nd ed. Philadelphia, WB Saunders, 2001, pp 198-218.
31. Kittleson MD: Diagnosis and treatment of arrhythmias (dysrhythmias). *In* Kittleson MD, Kienle RD, eds. Small Animal Cardiovascular Medicine. St Louis, Mosby, 1998, pp 449-494.
32. Kittleson MD: Management of heart failure. *In* Kittleson MD, Kienle RD, eds. Small Animal Cardiovascular Medicine. St Louis, Mosby, 1998, pp 149-194.
33. Lipman NS, Murphy JC, Fox JG: Clinical, functional and pathologic changes associated with a case of dilatative cardiomyopathy in a ferret. Lab Anim Sci 1987; 37:210-212.
34. Miller WR, Merton DA: Dirofilariasis in a ferret. J Am Vet Med Assoc 1982; 180:1103-1104.

35. Moise NS, Dietze AE, Mezza LE, et al: Echocardiography, electrocardiography, and radiography of cats with dilated cardiomyopathy, hypertrophic cardiomyopathy, and hyperthyroidism. Am J Vet Res 1986; 7:1477-1485.
36. Moise NS, Fox PR: Echocardiography and Doppler imaging. *In* Fox PR, Sisson D, Moise NS, eds. Textbook of Canine and Feline Cardiology: Principles and Clinical Practice, 2nd ed. Philadelphia, WB Saunders, 1999, pp 130-172.
37. Moreland AF, Battles AH, Nease JH: Dirofilariasis in a ferret. J Am Vet Med Assoc 1986; 188:864.
38. Murakami M, Matsuba C, Une Y, et al: Nucleotide sequence and polymerase chain reaction/restriction fragment length polymorphism analyses of Aleutian disease virus in ferrets in Japan. J Vet Diagn Invest 2001; 13:337-340.
39. Ohshima K, Shen DT, Henson JB, et al: Comparison of the lesions of Aleutian disease in mink and hypergammaglobulinemia in ferrets. Am J Vet Res 1978; 39:653-657.
40. Opie LH: Diuretics. *In* Opie LH, Hersh BJ, eds. Drugs for the Heart, 5th ed. Philadelphia, WB Saunders, 2000, pp 83-104.
41. Orcutt C: Oxyglobin administration for the treatment of anemia in ferrets. Exotic DVM 2001; 2.3:44-46.
42. Owens-Clark J, Dorman CD: Toxicities from newer over-the-counter drugs. *In* Bonagura JD, ed. Kirk's Current Veterinary Therapy XIII: Small Animal Practice. Philadelphia, WB Saunders, 2000, pp 227-230.
43. Oxenham M: Aleutian disease in the ferret. Vet Rec 1990; 126:585.
44. Palley LS, Corning BF, Fox JG, et al: Parvovirus-associated syndrome (Aleutian disease) in two ferrets. J Am Vet Med Assoc 1992; 201:100-106.
45. Parrott TY, Greiner EC, Parrott JD: *Dirofilaria immitis* infection in three ferrets. J Am Vet Med Assoc 1984; 184:582-583.
46. Porte HG, Porter DD, Larsen AE: Aleutian disease in ferrets. Infect Immun 1982; 36:379-386.
47. Quesenberry KE: Basic approach to veterinary care. *In* Hillyer EV, Quesenberry KE, eds. Ferrets, Rabbits, and Rodents: Clinical Medicine and Surgery. Philadelphia, WB Saunders, 1997, pp 14-25.
48. Richardson JA, Balabuszko RA: Ibuprofen ingestion in ferrets: 43 cases. J Vet Emerg Crit Care 2001; 11:53-59.
49. Rosenthal K: Ferrets. Vet Clin North Am Small Anim Pract 1994; 24:1-21.
50. Rush JE, Freeman LM, Fenollosa NK, et al: Population and survival characteristics of cats with hypertrophic cardiomyopathy: 260 cases (1990-1999). J Am Vet Med Assoc 2002; 220:202-207.
51. Saifuddin M, Fox JG: Identification of a DNA segment in ferret Aleutian disease virus similar to a hypervariable capsid region in mink Aleutian disease parvovirus. Arch Virol 1996; 141:1329-1339.
52. Sasai H, Kato T, Sasaki S, et al: Echocardiographic diagnosis of dirofilariasis in a ferret. J Small Anim Pract 2000; 41:172-174.
53. Smith SH, Bishop SP: The electrocardiogram of normal ferrets and ferrets with right ventricular hypertrophy. Lab Anim Sci 1985; 35:268-271.
54. Snyder PS, Atkins CE: Current uses and hazards of the digitalis glycosides. *In* Kirk RW, Bonagura JD, eds. Kirk's Current Veterinary Therapy XI: Small Animal Practice. Philadelphia, WB Saunders, 1992, pp 689-693.
55. Stamoulis ME, Miller MS, Hillyer EV: Cardiovascular diseases. *In* Hillyer EV, Quesenberry KE, eds. Ferrets, Rabbits, and Rodents: Clinical Medicine and Surgery. Philadelphia, WB Saunders, 1997, pp 63-76.
56. Stepien RL, Benson KG, Forrest LJ: Radiographic measurement of cardiac size in normal ferrets. Vet Radiol Ultrasound 1999; 40:606-610.
57. Stepien RL, Benson KG, Wenholz LJ: M-mode and Doppler echocardiographic findings in normal ferrets sedated with ketamine hydrochloride and midazolam. Vet Radiol Ultrasound 2000; 41:452-456.
58. Stewart JD, Rozengurt N: Aleutian disease in the ferret. Vet Rec 1993; 133:172.
59. Straube EF, Schuster NH, Sinclair AJ: Zinc toxicity in the ferret. J Comp Pathol 1980; 90:355-361.
60. Supakorndej P, Lewis RE, McCall JW: Radiographic and angiographic evaluations of ferrets experimentally infected with *Dirofilaria immitis*. Vet Radiol Ultrasound 1995; 36:23-29.
61. Supakorndej P, McCall JW, Jun JJ: Early migration and development of *Dirofilaria immitis* in the ferret, *Mustela putorius furo*. J Parasitol 1994; 80:237-244.
62. Thomas WP, Gaber CE, Jacobs GJ, et al: Recommendations for standards in transthoracic two-dimensional echocardiography in the dog and cat. Echocardiography Committee of the Specialty of Cardiology, American College of Veterinary Internal Medicine. J Vet Intern Med 1993; 7:247-252.
63. Thornton RN, Cook TG: A congenital toxoplasma-like disease in ferrets (*Mustela putorius furo*). N Z Vet J 1986; 34:31-33.
64. Tidholm A, Jonsson L: A retrospective study of canine dilated cardiomyopathy (189 cases). J Am Anim Hosp Assoc 1997; 33:544-550.
65. Une Y, Wakimoto Y, Nakano Y, et al: Spontaneous Aleutian disease in a ferret. J Vet Med Sci 2000; 62:553-555.
66. Waner T, Harrus S: Anemia of inflammatory disease. *In* Feldman BF, Zinkl JG, Jain NC, eds. Schalm's Veterinary Hematology, 5th ed. Philadelphia, Lippincott Williams & Wilkins, 2000, pp 205-209.
67. Welchman D de B, Oxenham M, Done SH: Aleutian disease in domestic ferrets: diagnostic findings and survey results. Vet Rec 1993; 132:479-484.
68. Wolfensohn HHL: Aleutian disease in laboratory ferrets. Vet Rec 1994; 134:100.

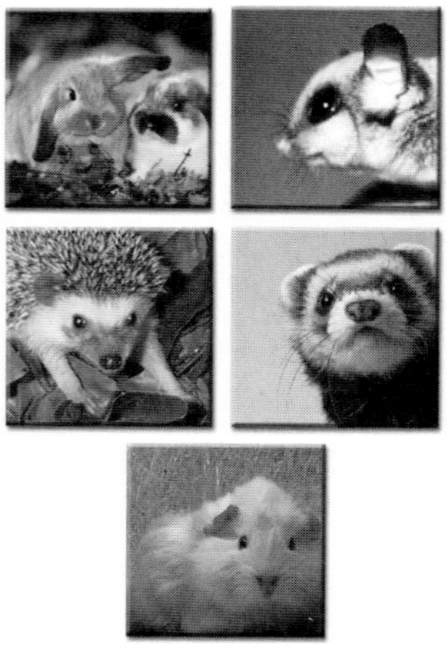

CHAPTER 7

Respiratory Diseases

Karen L. Rosenthal, DVM, MS, Diplomate ABVP

There are few causes of respiratory disease in pet ferrets. Canine distemper virus (CDV) and human influenza virus are the most common causes. Both are transmitted by aerosol exposure. Infection with CDV should be suspected in any unvaccinated, exposed ferret showing compatible clinical signs. Infection with CDV is distinguished from influenza by the clinical history, the presence of compatible clinical signs, and the physical examination findings. No specific treatment is available for CDV infection in ferrets, and the mortality rate is almost 100%. Influenza has a 7- to 14-day course and in adult ferrets is associated with a low mortality rate. Bacterial pneumonia is not a common diagnosis in ferrets. Ferrets with pneumonia exhibit typical clinical signs, such as labored breathing, dyspnea, cyanotic mucous membranes, increased lung sounds, nasal discharge, fever, lethargy, and anorexia. Pulmonary mycoses are also uncommon in pet ferrets. Ferrets that have severe traumatic injuries, such as from a fall from a high-rise building, can develop pneumothorax or diaphragmatic hernia.

CANINE DISTEMPER VIRUS

Canine distemper virus is a ribonucleic acid virus in the family Paramyxoviridae.[18] Although different strains of the virus vary in virulence, canine distemper is typically a fatal disease in ferrets. It is one of the most prevalent viral diseases of dogs,[18] and because it is ubiquitous, ferrets risk being exposed to this virus. Reservoirs of CDV include members of the families Canidae, Mustelidae, and Procyonidae.

The virus is most commonly transmitted by aerosol exposure.[2] Direct contact with conjunctival and nasal exudates, urine, feces, and skin can also cause infection.[15] Ferrets shed virus in all body excretions, and shedding begins about 7 days after exposure.[2] Fomites are also implicated in transmission; on gloves, the virus is viable for up to 20 minutes.[15] Once in a ferret's body, the virus appears to spread by viremia.[26] The incubation period in ferrets is 7 to 10 days.[15]

History and Physical Examination

Infection with CDV should be suspected in any unvaccinated, exposed ferret showing compatible clinical signs. Unvaccinated ferrets of any age are equally susceptible to this disease. In dogs, pyrexia develops 3 to 6 days after infection with CDV and is soon followed by anorexia and a serous nasal discharge.[2] A serous ocular discharge then appears; this discharge quickly becomes mucopurulent.

In ferrets, the first sign of disease is usually a rash on the chin. The skin around the lips and chin becomes swollen and then crusty. These changes can be accompanied by a dermatitis on the anus and inguinal area (Fig 7-1),[15] which is orange-tinged in some ferrets. Other clinical signs are anorexia, depression, pyrexia, photophobia, blepharospasm, and abundant mucopurulent ocular and nasal discharge. Brown crusts may form on the face, and the eyelids may adhere to each other. Hyperkeratosis of the footpads is common. Vomiting and diarrhea, which are seen in dogs with CDV,[18] are uncommon in ferrets.

Coughing may then ensue.[18] The respiratory system is the preferred site for the virus to replicate.[26] Secondary bacterial infections, which are responsible for many of the severe respiratory symptoms and death, are caused by the immunosuppressive effects of the virus.[32]

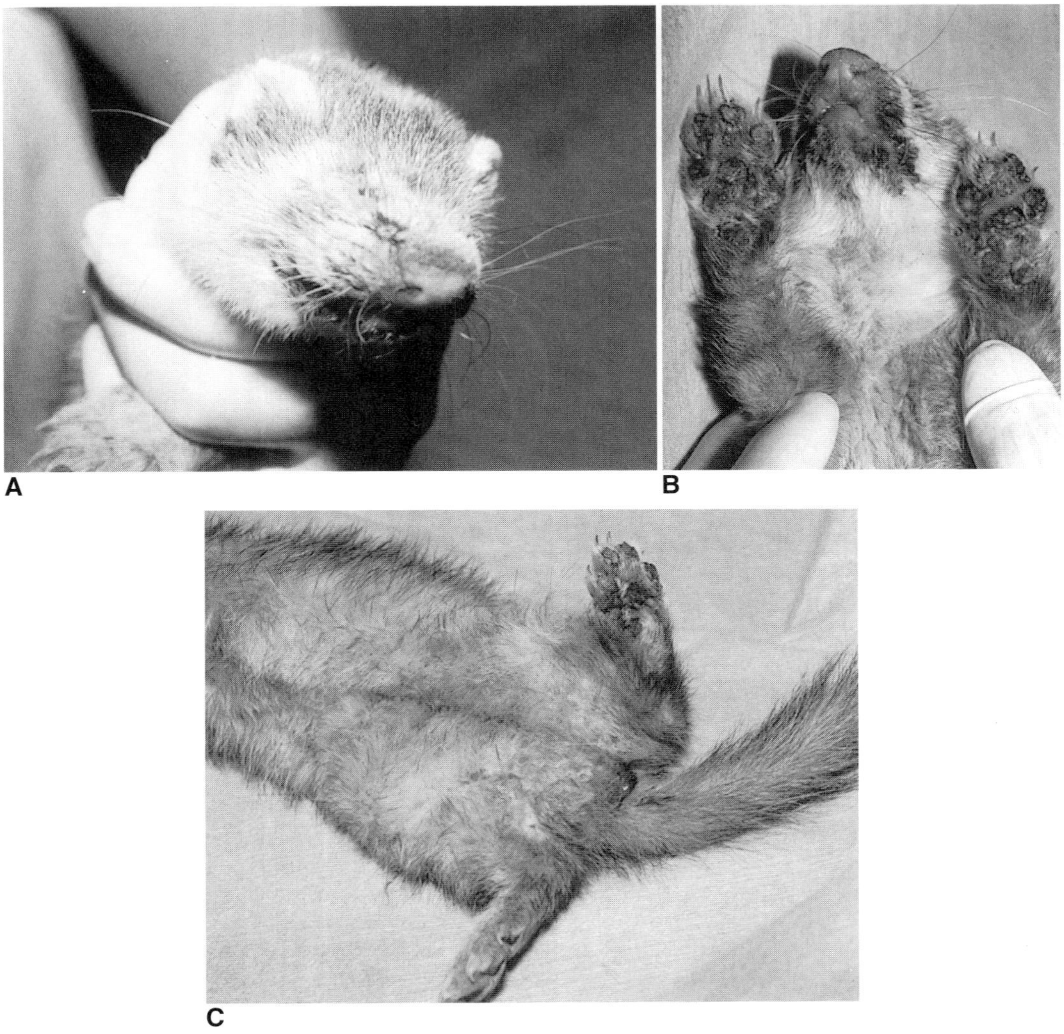

Figure 7-1 Young ferret infected with CDV. A, The eyes are encrusted shut with mucopurulent exudate. B, Dermatitis, excoriations, and crusting around the lips and chin; hyperkeratosis of the footpads. C, Dermatitis in the inguinal area.

Seizures and blindness are common in dogs with CDV infection,[32] and neurologic signs may manifest without previous systemic signs.[2] In ferrets with advanced CDV infection, incoordination, torticollis, and nystagmus can be present.[2]

Diagnosis

Diagnosis of CDV infection is based on history of exposure to the virus, observation of clinical signs, a positive result on fluorescent antibody testing, and positive histopathologic results. Nonspecific test results can include leukopenia and radiographic evidence of lung congestion or consolidation.[2,32] A plasma sample can be submitted to measure an antibody titer against CDV. However, because both infected and vaccinated ferrets can have a positive titer, a positive result is not diagnostic of disease. In practical terms, if a ferret that has not been vaccinated has a positive titer, this test can confirm CDV infection.

Perform a fluorescent antibody test on conjunctival smears, mucous membrane scrapings, or blood smears to identify CDV antigen in cells.[15,18] This test is useful only in the first few days of disease, and false-negative results are possible. Modified live viral strains used for vaccination do not interfere with this test.[32]

Clinical signs of infection with CDV initially can resemble those of influenza. However, within 1 to 2 days, the nasal and ocular discharge turns from serous to mucopurulent, and dermatitis develops around the chin and lips. This dermatitis, when present with other clinical signs typical of CDV, is pathognomonic for CDV infection. Also, ferrets infected with CDV tend to be much sicker than those with influenza. Further distinctions are made in Table 7-1.

A positive postmortem diagnosis can be made by fluorescent antibody staining of imprints from lymph nodes, bladder epithelium, and cerebellum.[2] Histopathologic examination of affected cells can also confirm the disease. Inclusion bodies of CDV are usually intracytoplasmic but can be intranuclear. Inclusions are generally found in the epithelial cells of the trachea, urinary bladder, skin, gastrointestinal tract, lymph nodes, spleen, and salivary glands.[15] Diffuse, interstitial pneumonia may be

TABLE 7-1
Clinical Distinctions Between Canine Distemper Virus and Influenza Virus Infections

Clinical Findings	Canine Distemper Virus	Influenza
Nasal and ocular discharge	+++ (Mucopurulent)	++ (Mucoserous)
Sneezing	+	+++
Coughing	+	+++
Pyrexia	+++ (>40°C)	++†
Dermatitis (chin, lips, inguinal)	+++	—
Footpad hyperkeratosis	++	—
Central signs	+*	—
Outcome	Almost 100% fatal	Self-limiting‡

Frequency of clinical signs: +, may be present; ++, common; +++, usual presentation; —, absent.
*Central nervous system signs seen in advanced stages of disease (rarely the only signs).
†Pyrexia occurs early in the course of disease and may be resolved by the time of presentation.
‡Influenza virus infection can be fatal in neonates.

present. In the central nervous system, inflammatory cell invasion with demyelination is observed.[2]

Treatment

No specific treatment exists for CDV infection in ferrets, and the mortality rate is almost 100%. Euthanasia of affected ferrets is usually the most humane option. Palliative treatment consists of supportive care and antibiotics for secondary bacterial infections.

Prevention

Vaccination is the best way to prevent CDV infection in ferrets (see Chapter 2). Start vaccinations at 6 or 8 weeks of age for kits from nonimmune or immune dams, respectively, and then continue vaccinating every 3 to 4 weeks until the kits are 14 weeks old. Revaccinate yearly. Avoid multivalent canine vaccines, which can be associated with adverse effects.

Over the past few years, anecdotal reports have noted anaphylactic reactions in ferrets after vaccination. Most of these reactions occur after vaccination with canine distemper vaccines. The reactions usually happen within 30 minutes after vaccination, with clinical signs of vomiting, diarrhea, pale mucous membranes, weak pulses, tachycardia, and lethargy. The true incidence and cause of vaccine reactions, and the susceptibility of ferrets to these reactions, are not known. If a reaction occurs, treat the ferret for anaphylactic shock with parenteral fluids, steroids, antihistamines, and even oxygen therapy. It is prudent to suggest that a ferret owner not leave the hospital for up to 30 minutes after CDV vaccination in the event that a reaction occurs. Recently the United States Department of Agriculture has approved a new vaccine for CDV in ferrets, PureVax (Merial, Athens, GA). This product differs from previous vaccines because it is based on recombinant technology. The incidence of anaphylactic reactions with PureVax in ferrets may therefore decrease (see Chapter 2).

If an outbreak of CDV occurs in a group of susceptible ferrets, remove all affected animals and immediately vaccinate healthy ferrets. However, vaccinating nonimmunized ferrets may not stop infection and death in the face of an outbreak.[15]

CDV is relatively labile and its infectivity is destroyed by heat, drying, detergents, and disinfectants.[32] Routine cleaning and disinfection procedures effectively destroy CDV on hard surfaces.

INFLUENZA

Several strains of human influenza virus, from the family Orthomyxoviridae, can infect ferrets.[10,23] In ferrets, as in people, influenza primarily causes upper respiratory disease. The different strains of influenza virus vary in virulence, which accounts for the difference in severity of clinical signs.[4,30]

Influenza virus is transmitted by aerosol droplets from ferret to ferret or from human to ferret. The virus can also be transmitted from ferrets to human beings.[23] The virus can be transmitted beginning at the height of pyrexia and continuing for the next 3 to 4 days.[31]

History and Physical Examination

Ferrets contract this disease after being exposed to infected people or other infected ferrets. All ferrets are susceptible to influenza, although the disease is typically more severe in neonates than in older ferrets. After a short incubation period, the body temperature increases and then decreases approximately 48 hours later.[10,15,23,29] Bouts of sneezing, eye watering, and a mucoid or mucopurulent nasal discharge are common. Clinical signs can appear within 48 hours of exposure.[10,23] Affected ferrets may become lethargic and anorexic,[31] and photophobia and conjunctivitis may be present.[4] Neonates develop a much more severe upper respiratory tract infection than adults, and death may ensue from lower airway obstruction.[6,30]

Clinical signs involving the lower respiratory tract are less common than those of the upper respiratory tract. Infection of the lower respiratory tract is usually confined to the bronchial epithelium[30] and results from secondary bacterial infection. Death can ensue from secondary pulmonary infection with Lancefield group C hemolytic streptococci.[23] Neonates are more likely than older ferrets to develop bronchiolitis and pneumonia[10] and to die from lower respiratory tract infection.[30]

Influenza virus can infect the cells of the intestinal mucosa and cause a limited enteritis.[16] The potential for hepatic dysfunction has been described in ferrets infected experimentally with influenza.[22] Hearing loss has also been associated with influenza infection in ferrets.[28]

Diagnosis

A diagnosis of influenza is based on the presence of clinical signs typical of infection, a history of exposure to infected individuals, isolation of the virus from nasal secretions, and a high antibody titer.[23] See Table 7-1 for the differences in presentation of ferrets infected with influenza and those with CDV. Experimentally, an enzyme-liked immunosorbent assay can detect antibodies against influenza A and can be used to rapidly establish a serologic diagnosis.[7] Antibodies against influenza virus have been detected within 3 days after infection.[24]

A transient leukopenia can be seen with this disease. Increases in concentrations of blood urea nitrogen, creatinine, alanine aminotransferase, potassium, and albumin have been reported in infected ferrets, but plasma biochemical values are usually within reference ranges.[22]

Treatment

Influenza has a 7- to 14-day course in adult ferrets and is associated with a low mortality rate. Most ferrets can be treated at home. Instruct owners to offer favorite foods, chicken or beef broth, or specialized diets (e.g., Eukanuba Maximum-Calorie, The Iams Company, Dayton, OH). Force-feed and offer water by syringe as needed. If necessary, use a pediatric cough suppressant without alcohol (at the pediatric dosage on a per weight basis), an antihistamine such as diphenhydramine (2-4 mg/kg PO q8-12h), or both for symptomatic therapy. To relieve nasal congestion, intranasal delivery of phenylephrine can be effective.[5]

The antiviral medication amantadine (6 mg/kg PO q12h) (Symmetrel; ENDO Pharmaceuticals, Chadds Ford, PA) has been experimentally effective in treating ferrets with influenza.[15] Another antiviral medication, zanamivir (12.5 mg/kg as a one-time intranasal dose) (Relenza; GlaxoSmith Kline, Research Triangle Park, NC), has been shown to prevent influenza infection.[12] Because they are a good model to study influenza infection in people, ferrets are frequently used as experimental subjects to develop new anti-influenza drugs.[34] Anti-influenza drugs used in humans may therefore be used to treat pet ferrets. Antibiotics can be used to control secondary bacterial infections of the respiratory tract. In neonates, death typically results from secondary bacterial infections; antibiotic therapy may thus reduce neonate mortality.[19]

The use of aspirin to control fever is of questionable merit because fever is an important host defense mechanism. Ferrets given aspirin have a lowered body temperature, but they shed more virus and their viral levels decrease less rapidly than those of ferrets not treated with an antipyretic. This suggests that fever is instrumental in restricting the severity of infection.[20,30]

Prevention

Controlling influenza rests mainly on preventing exposure of susceptible ferrets to infected individuals. Newborn ferrets are completely protected from disease by milk-derived antibodies in immunized dams.[21] Experimentally, ferrets remain resistant to infection from the same influenza strain 5 weeks after primary infection.[15]

Vaccinating ferrets against influenza virus is not generally recommended for several reasons. Influenza is a relatively benign disease in ferrets, and the wide antigenic variation of the virus makes vaccination difficult. Also, vaccination seems to confer only short-term immunity.[15] However, if giving a vaccine, use a live rather than an inactivated vaccine. Live vaccines induce a greater protective effect and are more likely to stimulate local antibody production.[13]

PNEUMONIA

Pneumonia is not a common diagnosis in ferrets. Viral causes of pneumonia include CDV and influenza virus. Aleutian disease virus, a parvovirus, is associated with interstitial pneumonia in mink kits[1] and should be considered as a possible cause of pneumonia in young ferrets. Respiratory syncytial virus has been shown to cause rhinitis and infection in the lungs in ferrets, but clinical signs of pneumonia have not been seen.[27]

Bacterial pneumonia is characterized by a suppurative inflammatory process that affects the bronchial tree, the lung lobes, or both. Reported primary bacterial pathogens that cause pneumonia in ferrets are *Streptococcus zooepidemicus, S. pneumoniae,* and groups C and G streptococci. Gram-negative bacteria such as *Escherichia coli, Klebsiella pneumoniae,* and *Pseudomonas aeruginosa* have been isolated from ferrets.[14] Other bacteria that have been isolated from the lungs of ferrets include *Bordetella bronchiseptica* and *Listeria monocytogenes.*

Pneumocystis carinii is known to infect the lungs of ferrets. Latent infections can become active with immune suppression.[3,8] Diagnosis is based on identifying the organism in a tracheal or lung wash.[17] Treatment recommendations for *P. carinii* pneumonia, based on those for dogs, include pentamidine isethionate or trimethoprim-sulfamethoxazole.[17]

Neither exogenous nor endogenous lipid pneumonia has been reported in ferrets. Two cases of mild lipid pneumonia have been documented on histologic examination of ferrets at necropsy at the Animal Medical Center (New York, NY) (K. Quesenberry, personal communication, 2003). In these ferrets, the pneumonia was most likely endogenous, and other disease processes were present. Although exogenous lipid pneumonia has not been documented in ferrets, exercise caution when treating animals with a mineral oil–based preparation for gastrointestinal disease (e.g., trichobezoar). Chronic aspiration of mineral oil products has been associated with lipid pneumonia in cats and people.[9,25]

History and Physical Examination

Ferrets with pneumonia exhibit typical clinical signs such as labored breathing, dyspnea, cyanotic mucous membranes, increased lung sounds, nasal discharge, fever, lethargy, and anorexia. Fulminant pneumonia leading to sepsis and death has been reported.[14,17]

Diagnosis

A diagnosis of pneumonia is based on the clinical signs, radiographic findings, and results of supportive diagnostic tests.

Results of the complete blood count (CBC) may reveal leukocytosis caused by a neutrophilia with a left shift.[17] In young ferrets with evidence of interstitial pneumonia, positive results of serologic tests and high concentrations of gamma globulins may support a diagnosis of Aleutian mink disease.

Early in the disease, radiographs may show an interstitial pattern that changes to an alveolar pattern as the pneumonia progresses (Fig. 7-2). If aspiration pneumonia is present, dependent lung lobes are primarily involved. Marked bronchial patterns suggest primary airway disease.[17]

Microbial cultures of tracheal or lung wash samples are invaluable in establishing a diagnosis and in treating ferrets with pneumonia. Submit samples for both bacterial and fungal culture. Along with culture, cytologic analysis of the collected fluid and debris is instrumental in establishing a diagnosis. Cytologic assessment of tracheal wash samples from a ferret with pneumonia typically reveals septic inflammation and degenerating neutrophils.[17] Results may also suggest the severity, cause, and chronicity of disease.

Treatment

Treat ferrets with pneumonia with good supportive care, including fluid therapy, force-feeding, and oxygen therapy as needed as well as with antimicrobials tailored according to test results. First-line antibiotics to consider before the results of culture and sensitivity testing are known are the quinolones, trimethoprim-sulfa, chloramphenicol, or the cephalosporins.[17] Combination antibiotic therapy may be indicated.

The prognosis depends on the cause of pneumonia and response to treatment. Most ferrets with bacterial pneumonia respond to antibiotic therapy and supportive care.

PULMONARY MYCOSES

Pulmonary mycoses are uncommon in pet ferrets. Because ferrets in the United States are usually indoor pets, exposure to mycotic spores, which are mainly found in the soil, is unlikely.

History and Physical Examination

Not all animals with mycoses exhibit signs consistent with pulmonary disease. If lesions develop in the lungs, animals usually cough. Other signs consistent with a mycotic infection are wasting, lethargy, anorexia, lymph node enlargement, lameness, ocular and nasal discharge, and draining tracts unresponsive to antibiotic therapy.[11,33] The prognosis for ferrets with pulmonary mycoses is poor.

Blastomycosis

Blastomycosis, caused by *Blastomyces dermatitidis,* is endemic in the southeastern United States, the Mississippi River Valley, and the Ohio River Valley.[33] Experimentally, the incubation period is 5 to 12 weeks. The mycelial phase is found in the soil, and the yeast form is found in the tissues. Diagnosis is made on the basis of a history of travel to an endemic region, clinical signs consistent with disease, results of cytologic assessment, positive periodic acid–Schiff reaction, or culture of *B. dermatitidis.* Amphotericin B and ketoconazole or itraconazole are recommended for treatment.[33] Base dosages on those used for cats.

Coccidioidomycosis

Coccidioides immitis, the causative agent of coccidioidomycosis, is endemic in the southwestern United States and parts of

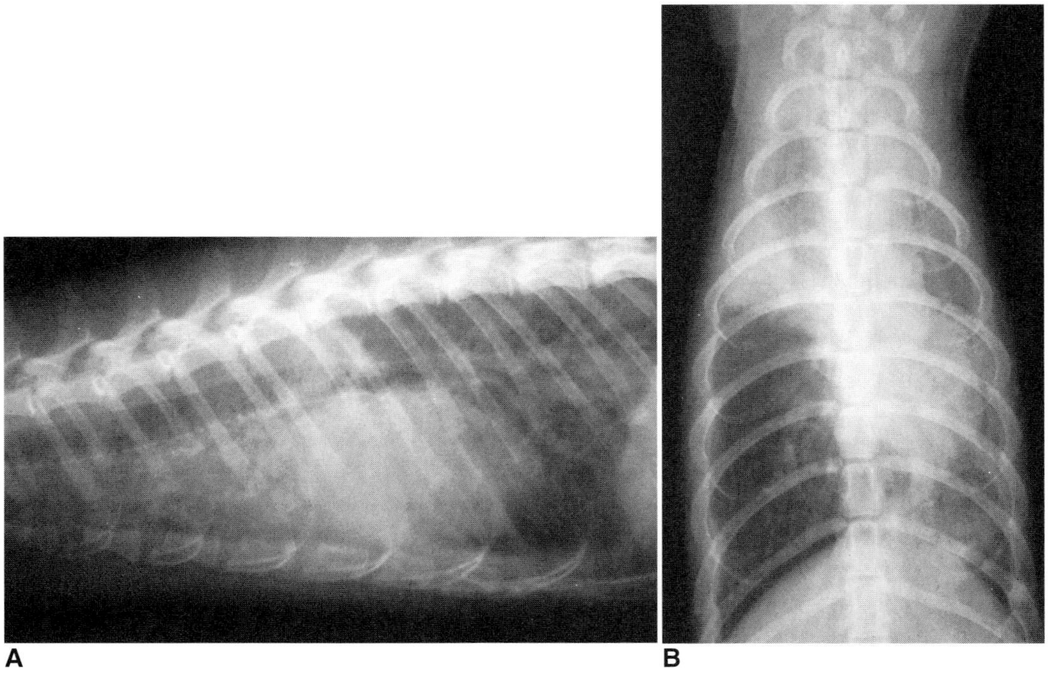

Figure 7-2 Lateral (A) and ventrodorsal (B) radiographs of a ferret with bacterial pneumonia.

Latin America. Primary infection develops after a susceptible host inhales the mycelia. Once in the host, spherules form and then produce endospores.[11,33] Pulmonary signs develop 1 to 3 weeks after infection. Diagnosis of this disease is based on identifying the spherules on cytologic examination; they appear as refractile, double-walled bodies.[33] Recommended treatment, which is based on that for cats with coccidioidomycosis, includes the use of amphotericin B and ketoconazole or itraconazole.[11,33]

OTHER CAUSES OF RESPIRATORY SIGNS

Differential diagnoses for tachypnea, dyspnea, and respiratory distress are similar to those for other small animals. After the history and physical examination, chest and abdominal radiography is the most important tool to differentiate the causes of lower respiratory tract symptoms. The recommended diagnostic approach to dyspnea is presented diagrammatically in Fig. 7-3.

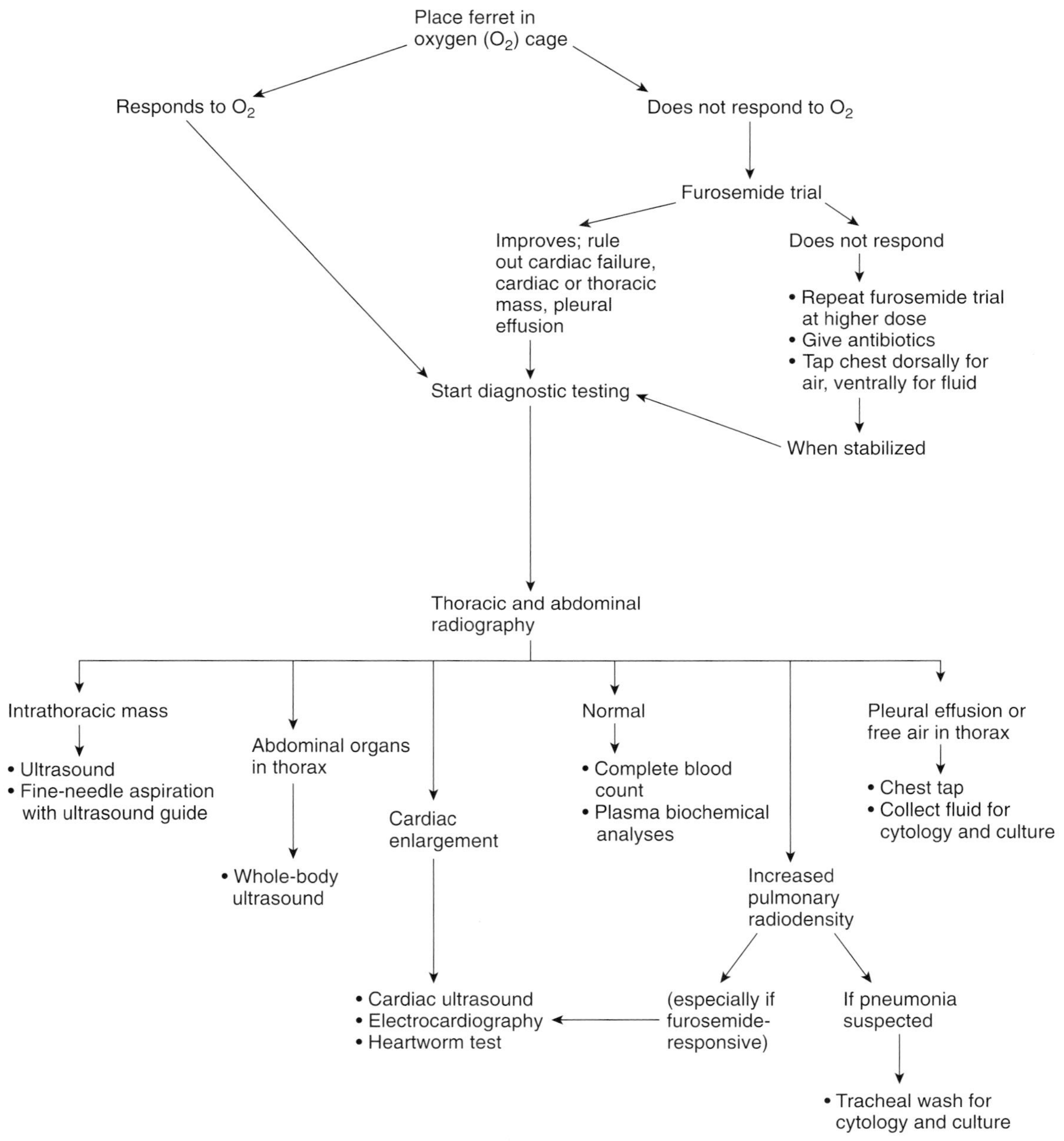

Figure 7-3 Diagnostic approach to dyspnea. The approach recommended here is the most conservative one. Thoracic radiographs (even one view can be very helpful) may be possible to obtain before the ferret is fully stabilized with the use of supplemental oxygen administered by face mask, with or without isoflurane, to reduce stress.

As mentioned previously, ferrets that have severe traumatic injuries, such as from a fall from a great height, can develop pneumothorax or diaphragmatic hernia. Approach these animals as you would a dog or cat with the same injuries.

REFERENCES

1. Alexandersen S, Larsen S, Aasted B, et al: Acute interstitial pneumonia in mink kits inoculated with defined isolates of Aleutian mink disease parvovirus. Vet Pathol 1994; 21:216-228.
2. Appel M: Canine distemper virus. *In* Appel M, ed. Virus Infections of Carnivores. New York, Elsevier Science, 1987, pp 133-139.
3. Bauer NL, Paulsrud JR, Bartlett MS, et al: *Pneumocystis carinii* organisms obtained from rats, ferrets, and mice are antigenically different. Infect Immun 1993; 61:1315-1319.
4. Buchman CA, Swarts JD, Seroky JT, et al: Otologic and systemic manifestations of experimental influenza A virus infection in the ferret. Otolaryngol Head Neck Surg 1995; 112:572-578.
5. Chen KS, Bharaj SS, King EC: Induction and relief of nasal congestion in ferrets infected with influenza virus. Int J Exp Pathol 1995; 76:55-64.
6. Collie MH, Rushton DI, Sweet C, et al: Studies of influenza virus infection in newborn ferrets. J Med Microbiol 1980; 13:561-571.
7. de Boer GF, Back W, Osterhaus AD: An ELISA for detection of antibodies against influenza A nucleoprotein in humans and various animal species. Arch Virol 1990; 115:47-61.
8. Dei-Cas E, Brun-Pascaud M, Bille-Hansen H, et al: Animal models of pneumocystosis. FEMS Immunol Med Microbiol 1998; 22:163-168.
9. de Souza HJM, dos Santos AE, Ferreira AMR, et al: Chronic lipidic pneumonia in a cat. Feline Pract 1998; 26:16-19.
10. Doggart L: Viral disease of pet ferrets. Part II. Aleutian disease, influenza, and rabies. Vet Tech 1988; 9:384-389.
11. DuVal-Hudelson KA: Coccidioidomycosis in three European ferrets. J Zoo Wildl Med 1990; 21:353-357.
12. Fenton RJ, Clark A, Potter CW: Immunity to influenza in ferrets. XIV: Comparative immunity following infection or immunization with live or inactivated vaccine. Br J Exp Pathol 1981; 62:297-307.
13. Fenton RJ, Morley PJ, Owens IJ, et al: Chemoprophylaxis of influenza A virus infections, with single doses of zanamivir, demonstrates that zanamivir is cleared slowly from the respiratory tract. Antimicrob Agents Chemother 1999; 43:2642-2647.
14. Fox JG: Bacterial and mycoplasmal diseases. *In* Fox JG, ed. Biology and Diseases of the Ferret, 2nd ed. Philadelphia, Lippincott Williams & Wilkins, 1998, pp 321-354.
15. Fox JG, Pearson RC, Gorham JR: Viral diseases. *In* Fox JG, ed. Biology and Diseases of Ferrets, 2nd ed. Philadelphia, Lippincott Williams & Wilkins, 1998, pp 355-374.
16. Glathe H, Lebhardt A, Hilgenfeld M, et al: Intestinal influenza infection in ferrets [in German]. Arch Exper Veterinarmed 1984; 38:771-777.
17. Hawkins EC: Pulmonary parenchymal diseases. *In* Ettinger SJ, Feldman EC, eds. Textbook of Veterinary Internal Medicine, 5th ed. Philadelphia, WB Saunders, 2000, pp 1061-1091.
18. Hoskins JD: Canine viral diseases. *In* Ettinger SJ, Feldman EC, eds. Textbook of Veterinary Internal Medicine, 5th ed. Philadelphia, WB Saunders, 2000, pp 403-430.
19. Husseini RH, Collie MH, Rushton DI, et al: The role of naturally-acquired bacterial infection in influenza-related death in neonatal ferrets. Br J Exp Pathol 1983; 64:559-569.
20. Husseini RH, Sweet C, Collie MH, et al: Elevation of nasal viral levels by suppression of fever in ferrets infected with influenza viruses of differing virulence. J Infect Dis 1982; 145:520-524.
21. Husseini RH, Sweet C, Overton H, et al: Role of maternal immunity in the protection of newborn ferrets against infection with a virulent influenza virus. Immunology 1984; 52:389-394.
22. Kang ES, Lee HJ, Boulet J, et al: Potential for hepatic and renal dysfunction during influenza B infection, convalescence, and after induction of secondary viremia. J Exp Pathol 1992; 6:133-144.
23. Marini RP, Adkins JA, Fox JG: Proven or potential zoonotic diseases of ferrets. J Am Vet Med Assoc 1989; 195:990-994.
24. McLaren C, Butchko GM: Regional T- and B-cell responses in influenza-infected ferrets. Infect Immunol 1978; 22:189-194.
25. Midulla F, Strappini PM, Ascoli V, et al: Bronchoalveolar lavage cell analysis in a child with chronic lipid pneumonia. Eur Respir J 1998; 11:239-242.
26. Pearson RC, Gorham JR: Viral disease models. *In* Fox JG, ed. Biology and Diseases of the Ferret, 2nd ed. Philadelphia, Lippincott Williams & Wilkins, 1998, pp 487-498.
27. Prince GA, Porter DD: The pathogenesis of respiratory syncytial virus infection in infant ferrets. Am J Pathol 1976; 82:339-352.
28. Rarey KE, DeLacure MA, Sandridge SA, et al: Effect of upper respiratory infection on hearing in the ferret model. Am J Otolaryngol 1987; 8:161-170.
29. Ryland LM, Gorham JR: The ferret and its diseases. J Am Vet Med Assoc 1978; 173:1154-1158.
30. Smith H, Sweet C: Lessons for human influenza from pathogenicity studies with ferrets. Rev Infect Dis 1988; 10:56-75.
31. Squires S, Belyavin G: Free contact infection in ferret groups. J Antimicrob Chemother 1975; 1:35-42.
32. Swango LJ: Canine viral diseases. *In* Ettinger SJ, ed. Textbook of Veterinary Internal Medicine, Philadelphia, WB Saunders, 1989, pp 298-311.
33. Taboada J: Systemic mycoses. *In* Ettinger SJ, Feldman EC, eds. Textbook of Veterinary Internal Medicine, 5th ed., Philadelphia, WB Saunders, 2000, pp 453-476.
34. Yoshimoto J, Yagi S, Ono J, et al: Development of anti-influenza drugs: II. Improvement of oral and intranasal absorption and the anti-influenza activity of Stachyflin derivatives. J Pharm Pharmacol 2000; 52:1247-1255.

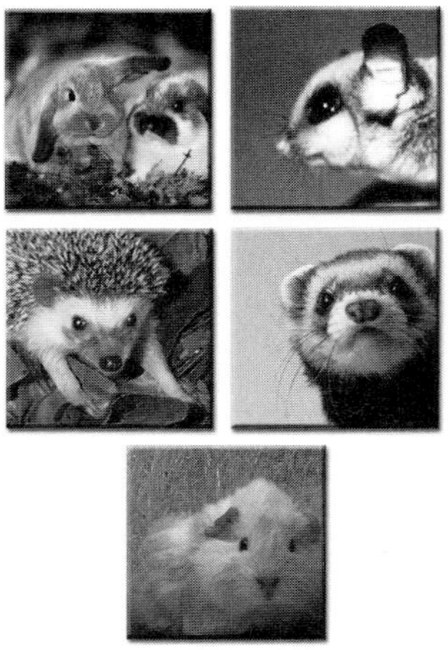

CHAPTER 8

Endocrine Diseases

Katherine E. Quesenberry, DVM, Diplomate ABVP, and
Karen L. Rosenthal, DVM, MS, Diplomate ABVP

PANCREATIC ISLET CELL TUMORS

Pancreatic islet cell tumors are very common in middle-aged and older ferrets. Islet cells are made up of at least four cell types: the beta or B cells, which secrete insulin; the alpha or A cells, which secrete glucagon; the delta or D cells, which secrete somatostatin; and the F (or P) cells, which secrete pancreatic polypeptide. These islet cells, arranged into groups as the islets of Langerhans, make up the endocrine pancreas and comprise only 2% of the total pancreatic tissue.[27] Although tumors of other islet cells also occur, most islet cell tumors in ferrets are beta cell tumors. Beta cell tumors, or insulinomas, produce excessive amounts of insulin, resulting in hypoglycemia. The clinical signs associated with hypoglycemia in ferrets usually prompt their owners to seek veterinary care.

Pathophysiology

Pancreatic beta cell tumors increase basal insulin secretion. Additionally, the tumor cells fail to respond to normal inhibitory stimuli and release excessive amounts of insulin in response to normal provocative stimuli.[33] Continuous hyperinsulinemia sustains the metabolic effects of insulin; thus hepatic gluconeogenesis and glycogenolysis are inhibited, and peripheral uptake of glucose by tissue cells is increased. In normal animals, a low blood glucose concentration triggers the glucoreceptors in the hindbrain and hypothalamus, inducing the release of glucagon, cortisol, epinephrine, and growth hormone.[24] These hormones increase the blood glucose concentration by stimulating gluconeogenesis and glycogenolysis in the liver and by inhibiting peripheral use of glucose. This feedback mechanism is ineffective in animals with insulinomas; the hyperglycemic effects of glucagon, epinephrine, cortisol, and growth hormone are inhibited, and the blood glucose concentration continues to decrease.[24,36]

Clinical signs of hypoglycemia correlate with the rate of decline of the blood glucose concentration and the duration and degree of hypoglycemia.[24] Clinical signs can be categorized as either neuroglucopenic or adrenergic manifestations or a combination of both. Cells in the nervous tissue uptake glucose by diffusion; uptake is not insulin dependent.[35] Because cells in the central nervous system have a high metabolic rate and glucose is the primary energy source, hypoglycemia results in neuroglucopenic signs. When these cells are deprived of glucose, clinical signs of mental dullness, lethargy, ataxia, seizures, and coma result. Prolonged, severe hypoglycemia can result in cerebral hypoxia and, possibly, irreversible cerebral lesions.[35] Adrenergic manifestations occur when the blood glucose concentration rapidly decreases. Catecholamines are released and sympathetic tone increases, resulting in tachycardia, hypothermia, tremors, muscle fasciculations, nervousness, and irritability.[24]

History and Physical Examination

Although pancreatic beta cell tumors are seen in ferrets between the ages of 3 and 8 years, clinical signs are most common in ferrets between 4 and 5 years of age. Both male and female ferrets are affected with no apparent sex predilection.

The history varies from an acute onset of clinical signs to a chronic course of weeks to many months. Most ferrets with insulinoma will have a vague history of weakness and lethargy. The appetite may be normal or decreased, and weight loss may be observed. The owner often notices ataxia or pronounced weakness, particularly in the hind legs. Clinical signs are often intermittent, with normal activity and demeanor between periods of weakness.

In acute hypoglycemic episodes, an owner may describe an episode of collapse during which the ferret is depressed, minimally responsive, and recumbent. The episode may last from several minutes to several hours and ends with spontaneous recovery or after the owner administers an oral sugar solution or syrup. Ferrets are occasionally presented for examination while in this collapsed state. Owners may describe the ferret's eyes as appearing "glazed" during these episodes. The ferret may also paw at its mouth or exhibit pronounced ptyalism. The number of collapse episodes may vary from one to several over a period of days to months; episodes may be isolated occurrences or increase in frequency over time.

Physical examination findings vary. Weight loss and musculoskeletal weakness are commonly present, and animals are lethargic. Clinical findings consistent with other disease problems (e.g., hair loss or thinning, skin masses, and cardiac arrhythmias) are often present in ferrets with insulinoma. Adrenal neoplasia, lymphoma, various skin tumors, and cardiomyopathy are common concurrent problems. Occasionally ferrets with islet cell tumors may appear physically normal and have no discernible clinical signs. In these animals, pancreatic nodules may be found during abdominal exploratory surgery, most commonly for adrenal tumors. On histologic examination of biopsy samples, these nodules are usually confirmed as islet cell hyperplasia or tumors.

Diagnostic Testing

Determining blood glucose and insulin concentrations A presumptive diagnosis of beta cell tumor is based on the history, clinical signs, and documented hypoglycemia. At the initial physical examination, check the blood glucose concentration with either a strip glucose measurement method (Chemstrip bG, Boehringer Mannheim, Gaithersburg, MD) or a digital glucometer such as the Accu-Chek III (Boehringer Mannheim). These glucometers are manufactured for use by human diabetic patients and are very convenient and easy to use. However, clinical experience in ferrets shows that blood glucose concentrations measured by these systems sometimes are 10 to 20 mg/dL lower than actual glucose concentrations. If the glucose concentration measured by one of these methods is low, collect a blood sample to submit for laboratory measurement of blood glucose and insulin concentrations. Testing serial blood samples or after a carefully monitored fast (4-6 hours is sufficient) may be necessary to confirm hypoglycemia.

In ferrets, blood glucose concentrations lower than 60 mg/dL support a diagnosis of insulinoma. The reference range for resting blood glucose concentration in ferrets is 94 to 207 mg/dL; normal fasting blood glucose level is 90 to 125 mg/dL (see Table 2-2). In a study of 57 ferrets with confirmed insulinoma, all had blood glucose concentrations less than 60 mg/dL.[6] Ferrets that are seen when profoundly weak or comatose commonly have blood glucose concentrations in the range of 20 to 40 mg/dL. Some ferrets with insulinoma adjust to chronic low blood glucose concentrations. These ferrets may appear clinically normal, yet their blood glucose concentrations are in the 40 to 50 mg/dL range.

In addition to documented hypoglycemia, absolute insulin concentrations are used as the basis for a presumptive diagnosis of insulinoma. Insulin secretion should be inhibited when the blood glucose concentration drops below 60 mg/dL.[27] If hypoglycemia is present, submit a sample for both insulin and glucose measurement. Always immediately spin and separate the plasma before submitting the sample. If not separated, glucose concentration will artifactually decrease because of red blood cell metabolism. Insulin concentration is affected by a delay in plasma separation as well.[18] Hypoglycemia concurrent with a high blood insulin concentration supports the diagnosis of insulinoma. A normal insulin concentration concurrent with hypoglycemia is also seen in animals with insulinomas. In studies of dogs with insulinoma, 23% to 32% had insulin values in the normal range.[27] However, if the insulin concentration is low in an animal with hypoglycemia, insulinoma is unlikely. In any ferret with hypoglycemia, always consider other differential diagnoses for low blood glucose concentration, such as starvation or poor nutritional status, liver disease, or sepsis. Ferrets may be inappropriately treated for insulinoma on the basis of one low blood glucose concentration when in actuality another disease process is present.

The reference range for serum insulin concentrations in normal ferrets is 5 to 35 μU/mL (36-251 pmol/L; Table 8-1). (Values expressed as conventional units [μU/mL] can be converted to SI units [pmol/L] by multiplying by the conversion factor 7.175.[26]) Reference intervals for insulin previously reported in ferrets are 4.6 to 43.3 μU/mL (mean, 14.1 μU/mL) or 33 to 311 pmol/L (mean, 101 pmol/L).[30] Ferrets with suspected insulinoma may have insulin values that vary from within the reference range up to 279 μU/mL (2000 pmol/L). Reported insulin values in ferrets with insulinomas have ranged from 108 to 1738 μU/mL (773-12,470 pmol/L).[11,19,20,28] Reported reference intervals for the insulin/glucose ratio in ferrets are 3.6 to 34.1 μU/mg (4.6 to 44.2 pmol/mmol).[29]

If the insulin concentration of a ferret with suspected insulinoma is within the reference range, repeat the insulin assay at a later date or serially measure blood glucose concentrations to demonstrate a consistent pattern of hypoglycemia. Alternatively, measure the blood glucose and insulin concentrations after a 4- to 6-hour fast. In a study of six ferrets with confirmed insulinoma, the mean blood glucose concentration after a 4-hour fast was 44 mg/dL, and the mean fasting insulin level was 58 μU/mL (416 pmol/L).[31]

TABLE 8-1
Reference Values for Endocrine Tests in Ferrets

Hormone	Sex	Values
Insulin (pmol/L)*		36-251 (5-35 µU/mL)
Cortisol (nmol/L)†		25.9-235 (mean ± SEM, 73.8 ± 7)
Thyroxine (µg/dL)‡	♂	1.01-8.29 (mean, 4.5)
	♀	0.71-2.54 (mean, 1.38)
Tri-iodothyronine (ng/mL)‡	♂	0.45-0.78 (mean, 0.61)
	♀	0.29-0.73 (mean, 0.53)
Mean thyroxine (µg/dL)§	♂	2.53 at 0 hours; 3.37 at 2 hours; 3.97 at 4 hours; 3.45 at 6 hours

*Reference range from the Clinical Endocrinology Laboratory, College of Veterinary Medicine, University of Tennessee, Knoxville, TN (courtesy Jack W. Oliver, DVM, PhD).
†Administration of cosyntropin, 1 µg/kg IM generally caused a three- to fourfold increase in plasma cortisol concentration.[45]
‡Data from Garibaldi BA, Pequet-Goad ME, Fox JG: Serum thyroxine (T_4) and tri-iodothyronine (T_3) radioimmunoassay values in the normal ferret. Lab Anim Sci 1987; 37:544–547.
§Mean thyroxine at baseline (0 hours) and 2, 4, and 6 hours after intravenous administration of 1 IU of thyroid-stimulating hormone (n = 8 intact males). Data from Heard DJ, Collins B, Chen DL, et al: Thyroid and adrenal function tests in adult male ferrets. Am J Vet Res 1990; 51:32–35.

In the past, the insulin/glucose, glucose/insulin, and amended insulin/glucose ratios were sometimes used to distinguish normal animals from those with disease. However, these ratios are not specific and have a high incidence of false-positive results, and their use is no longer advocated.[7,24,27,32] False-positive results can occur in dogs with liver disease, sepsis, and non–islet cell tumors, especially in the presence of hypoglycemia.[24] Because of the lack of specificity of insulin and glucose ratios and the possibility of normal serum insulin concentration, serum glucose testing is the most reliable method of establishing a tentative diagnosis of insulinoma in dogs.[7]

In other species, provocative tests are sometimes used to diagnose insulinoma. These tests include administering glucagon, glucose, leucine, tolbutamide, or calcium, which act as secretogogues; epinephrine stimulation tests; oral glucose tolerance tests; and calcium-infusion tests.[24,27] However, these tests have not proved superior to simple measurement of insulin and glucose concentrations,[15] and severe and prolonged hypoglycemia may result.[24,35] To my knowledge, these tests have not been used in ferrets.

Hematologic and biochemical analysis In any ferret with a suspected insulinoma, submit blood samples for a complete blood count and plasma biochemical analysis. Increases in alanine aminotransferase and aspartate aminotransferase concentrations are common and may reflect hepatic lipidosis caused by chronic hypoglycemia or liver metastasis of the pancreatic islet cell tumor. Hematologic abnormalities that are sometimes present include leukocytosis, neutrophilia, and monocytosis.[6]

Radiography and abdominal ultrasonography Radiographic results are usually unremarkable except for splenomegaly. Lung metastases have not been seen in ferrets with insulinoma. Because of their small size, discrete insulinomas are rarely detected by abdominal ultrasound examination. However, ultrasonography is sometimes useful from a prognostic standpoint and in presurgical evaluation. Hepatic lipidosis or hepatic infiltrates, which may indicate liver metastasis, can be detected by ultrasound. If any abnormalities are detected, biopsy the liver at surgery for histologic examination.

Other diagnostic tests If any clinical signs of concurrent disease are present, perform the appropriate diagnostic tests to confirm the diagnosis. This is especially critical in ferrets with cardiomyopathy because these ferrets are often poor anesthetic risks.

Management

Ferrets with insulinomas can be managed medically or surgically. The choice of therapy depends on the severity of clinical signs, the age of the ferret, and the owner's preference. Medical therapy to alleviate clinical signs of hypoglycemia can begin once a presumptive diagnosis of insulinoma is made.

Medical management Medical therapy effectively controls clinical signs of hypoglycemia but does not stop progression of the tumor. Prednisone and diazoxide are used singly or in combination, depending on the severity of clinical signs, in conjunction with dietary management. Prednisone increases peripheral blood glucose concentration by inhibiting glucose uptake by peripheral tissues and increasing hepatic gluconeogenesis. Ferrets with mild to moderate clinical signs of hypoglycemia often can be managed with prednisone therapy alone, in doses ranging from 0.5 to 2 mg/kg q12h PO. Except in very small ferrets, a minimum dose of 1 mg is usually needed to control clinical signs. Gradually increase the prednisone dosage as needed. Depending on the owner's preference, prescribe either the oral suspension of prednisolone or the 1-mg tablets of prednisone. Make sure that the oral suspension is not a generic form that contains alcohol, which can cause unwanted side effects.

Diazoxide (Proglycem, Baker Norton Pharmaceuticals, Inc., Miami, FL) is a benzothiadiazide diuretic that inhibits insulin release from the pancreatic beta cells, promotes glycogenolysis and gluconeogenesis by the liver, and decreases cellular uptake of glucose. Add diazoxide (5-10 mg/kg q12h PO) to the therapeutic protocol when clinical signs of hypoglycemia cannot be controlled with prednisone alone. If possible, decrease the prednisone dose to 1 to 1.25 mg/kg q12h PO when adding diazoxide. If a low dosage does not effectively control clinical signs, the diazoxide dosage can be gradually increased to a maximum of 30 mg/kg q12h. Side effects associated with diazoxide treatment include vomiting and anorexia.[24] The major disadvantage of diazoxide therapy is the expense of the commercial suspension. Although compounding pharmacists can make suspensions of diazoxide from tablets, the concentration of the resultant suspension cannot be guaranteed.

Instruct owners to feed their ferrets frequently and to avoid prolonged periods without food. Recommended diets include meat-based, high-protein cat or ferret food. Avoid foods with a high sugar or carbohydrate (cereal) content. Unless a ferret shows signs of hypoglycemia, instruct owners not to give simple sugars such as honey or corn syrup because these foods can stimulate insulin secretion, precipitating a hypoglycemic episode soon thereafter.

Somatostatin, a natural polypeptide hormone secreted by the pancreas, suppresses insulin secretion. Octreotide, a somatostatin analog (Sandostatin, Sandoz Pharmaceuticals Corp., East Hanover, NJ), is sometimes used in dogs for the treatment of insulinoma.[37] We have used somatostatin in the treatment of one ferret with equivocal results.

Medical management is usually effective in controlling clinical signs for periods of 6 months to 1.5 years. Ferrets treated medically commonly show progressive severity of clinical signs, and gradually increasing dosages of medications are usually needed. Older ferrets (≥6 years) and ferrets with concurrent complicating diseases such as cardiomyopathy or lymphosarcoma are the primary candidates for medical therapy. Owners sometimes elect medical therapy over surgical therapy for other reasons (e.g., because of the expense of or their opposition to surgery).

Treatment of a hypoglycemic episode Mild to moderate hypoglycemic episodes can often be treated successfully by the owner. Owners of ferrets with insulinoma should always have honey, corn syrup, or other liquid sugar products readily available. Instruct owners how to recognize the signs of hypoglycemia and how to administer the sugar product with a syringe. If the ferret has an acute hypoglycemic episode, instruct the owner to rub honey or corn syrup on the gingiva, taking care not to be bitten. If the ferret is having seizures, instruct the owner not to place his or her hands or objects in the ferret's mouth to avoid being bitten. Once the ferret improves, the owner should feed the ferret some of its regular diet, then bring the ferret in for examination.

Ferrets that have hypoglycemic episodes that do not respond to oral sugar solutions or that have continuous seizures require hospital treatment. Administer a slow intravenous bolus of 50% dextrose (0.25-2 mL) until the ferret responds. If the ferret remains comatose or is having seizures, establish an intravenous catheter, give shock therapy with intravenous fluids and dexamethasone, and begin a continuous infusion of 5% dextrose.

Always give intravenous 50% dextrose slowly and at the minimal amount to control clinical signs. A rapid increase in blood glucose concentration can overstimulate the tumor, resulting in the release of massive amounts of insulin and subsequent severe hypoglycemia that requires treatment with more intravenous dextrose. This can become a vicious cycle, with progressive worsening of rebound hypoglycemia.[35] Therefore the goal of therapy is to correct clinical signs, not to correct hypoglycemia. Once the ferret becomes more alert, begin enteral feedings and corticosteroid therapy.

Closely monitor ferrets that have seizures or that are comatose as critical patients on continuous dextrose infusion. Rarely, anticonvulsant therapy (e.g., diazepam 1-2 mg intravenously titrated to effect; repeat as necessary up to 5 mg) is needed to control seizures until supportive therapy becomes effective. Follow anticonvulsant protocols used for dogs and cats in status epilepticus, making sure that addressing the hypoglycemia is the first priority.

Surgical therapy Surgical therapy remains the treatment of choice for ferrets younger than 6 years of age or for those suspected of having concurrent adrenal disease. Surgical therapy is usually not curative but may stop or slow progression of the insulinoma. In dogs with insulinoma, those treated surgically have a longer life span than those treated with medical management alone.[24] Also, higher preoperative insulin concentrations were associated with significantly shorter survival times in dogs[7]; however, this finding has not been confirmed in ferrets. In one study, the median survival time of 53 ferrets treated for insulinoma (50 with and 3 without surgery) was 17 months.

Preoperative considerations include placing an indwelling intravenous catheter at least 1 to 2 hours before surgery and infusing maintenance fluids with added 5% dextrose. Fluid therapy is needed before and during surgery to maintain systemic blood pressure and pancreatic perfusion, thus decreasing the risk of pancreatitis.[37] Fast ferrets minimally (3-6 hours) before surgery to prevent severe hypoglycemia. If possible, schedule surgery early in the day so that fasting time is minimal and animals can be closely monitored in the immediate postoperative period. Check the blood glucose concentration with a rapid measurement test before, during, and immediately after surgery.

One or two pancreatic nodules are usually found at surgery, but as many as seven to nine nodules may be present. Nodulectomy, partial pancreatectomy, or both are performed depending on the number and location of the pancreatic nodules (see Chapter 12). In ferrets, metastasis at the time of surgery is uncommon; however, when it does occur, it is usually to regional lymph nodes, the spleen, or the liver.[6,11,31] Routinely biopsy the liver in ferrets with insulinoma to check for liver metastasis. Also obtain biopsy specimens from the spleen and any lymph nodes that are enlarged or appear abnormal. Examine the adrenal glands carefully for abnormalities because concurrent adrenal disease is common.

Ferrets usually recover quickly from surgery, and, unlike dogs, complications related to pancreatic surgery (e.g., pancreatitis) are rare. Withhold food and water for 12 to 24 hours after surgery in routine cases, and gradually introduce water and then food over the subsequent 6 to 12 hours. Many ferrets that undergo stress from surgery manifest clinical signs of *Helicobacter mustelae* infection. Therefore consider treating prophylactically for *Helicobacter* infection with triple therapy (ampicillin IV initially, then amoxicillin, metronidazole, and bismuth subsalicylate perorally; see Chapter 3). Maintain fluid administration with 5% dextrose until the ferret is eating.

While the ferret is hospitalized after surgery, monitor the blood glucose concentration at least twice daily. Many ferrets become euglycemic immediately after surgery, whereas others remain hypoglycemic or are borderline euglycemic. Occasionally, a ferret may become hyperglycemic after insulinoma surgery. Hyperglycemia is typically transient in these ferrets, resolving within 2 to 3 weeks, and usually does not require treatment. Monitor blood glucose concentrations in these ferrets periodically until hyperglycemia resolves. Rarely, ferrets that have undergone radical pancreatectomy become diabetic after surgery.

Most ferrets that have been treated surgically require medical management for recurrent hypoglycemia within 2 to 6 months after surgery. In one study, only 14% of ferrets remained euglycemic after surgery.[6] Therefore in any ferret that has had surgery for insulinoma, recheck the blood glucose concentration 7 to 14 days after surgery and at 2- to 3-month intervals thereafter. Repeat measurements of serum insulin concentrations are also recommended.

Histology Insulinomas in ferrets are usually malignant,[6] as they are in dogs.[32] However, beta cell adenomas or hyperplasia

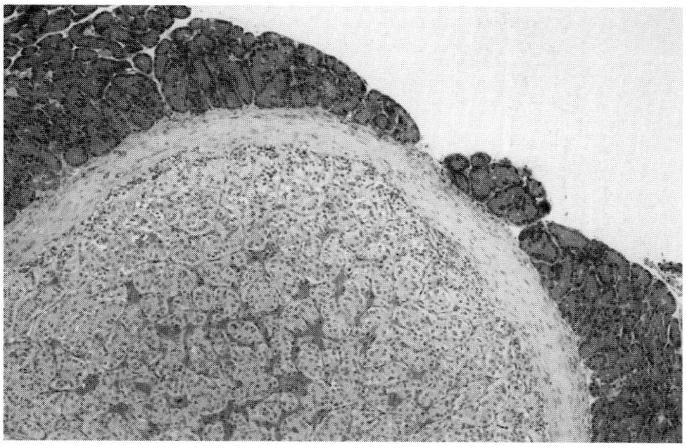

Figure 8-1 Photomicrograph of a ferret pancreas with beta cell adenoma of the pancreatic islets (insulinoma). An encapsulated pale mass is composed of nests of pale-staining, uniform-sized epithelial cells supported by a fibrovascular stroma. The cells have morphologic and tinctorial properties compatible with islet cells. There is a uniformly dense fibrous capsule separating the tumor from the exocrine pancreas. Hematoxylin and eosin stain, ×20. *(Courtesy Dr. James Walberg.)*

are common, sometimes in combination with carcinoma (Fig. 8-1). In dogs, the morphologic characteristics of endocrine neoplasms do not reflect their malignancy,[32] and malignancy is determined by the presence or absence of metastasis.[7]

Immunohistochemical staining has shown that a small percentage of tumors produce other peptide hormones, including somatostatin, glucagon, and pancreatic polypeptide.[1,11] Chromagranin A and neuron-specific enolase are useful neuroendocrine markers for immunohistochemical staining of all islet cell tumors, including those that are insulin negative. The clinical significance of non–insulin-producing tumors in ferrets is not well understood.

ADRENAL GLAND DISEASE

Adrenocortical disease has been recognized for almost 15 years as a common malady affecting pet ferrets in the United States.* It is typically seen in middle-aged to older ferrets and is most commonly characterized by hair loss in both sexes and by vulvar enlargement in female ferrets. Clinical signs of adrenocortical disease in ferrets differ from those of classic Cushing's disease in dogs; moreover, plasma cortisol concentrations are rarely increased in ferrets. Instead, the concentrations of estradiol, 17-hydroxyprogesterone, or one or more of the plasma androgens may be increased as a result of adrenocortical hyperplasia, adenoma, or adenocarcinoma.

The underlying cause of the pathologic changes in the adrenal glands of these ferrets is unknown. It is tempting to speculate that premature neutering has a role.[49] In support of this, studies in some strains of mice have shown that gonadectomy at an early age can lead to adrenocortical nodular hyperplasia or neoplasia of one or both adrenal glands. These glands hypersecrete estrogens or androgens.[10,22,50] During embryologic development, ovaries and adrenal glands develop in close anatomic relation to one another. Both arise in intimate association in the urogenital ridge.[2] Small nests of undifferentiated gonadal cells may be carried with the adrenal glands during migration and come to rest under the adrenal gland capsule. With an appropriate stimulant (i.e., gonadectomy with resultant unopposed pituitary gonadotropin activity), these undifferentiated cells in the adrenal gland may transform into cells that are functionally similar to gonadal tissue cells.

Like mice that undergo gonadectomy during the first few days of life, most commercially raised ferrets in the United States undergo ovariohysterectomy or castration before they are 6 weeks of age. Therefore adrenocortical hyperplasia and tumors in ferrets possibly develop as a result of metaplasia of undifferentiated gonadal cells in the adrenal capsule.

Other possible causes of adrenal gland disease in ferrets may be related to the husbandry of ferrets in the United States compared with that of ferrets in other parts of the world. For example, adrenal disease in ferrets is uncommon in Great Britain. Ferrets in the United States are typically fed prepared food (e.g., commercial ferret or cat food), whereas ferrets in Great Britain eat whole prey. Also, ferrets in the United States are mostly kept indoors, whereas those in Great Britain are often kept outdoors and thus are exposed to natural photoperiods. Finally, the ferret population in the United States is more inbred than that in Great Britain.

History and Physical Examination

Progressive alopecia is the most common historic finding. Hair loss typically begins in the late winter or early spring and may continue until the ferret is partially or completely bald. Occasionally, the hair coat may fully regrow during the fall. During the next winter or spring, alopecia commonly begins again. This sequence can recur over a period of 2 to 3 years until the hair does not regrow. Spayed female ferrets with adrenocortical disease frequently have a history of vulvar enlargement, with or without a mucoid discharge. Male ferrets may have a history of dysuria, urinary blockage, or both.

Most ferrets reported with adrenocortical disease are female.[46] Many owners are aware that an enlarged vulva in a female ferret is a cause for concern. The vulva enlarges normally during estrus, and many owners know that prolonged estrus can result in estrogen-induced bone marrow toxicosis. Thus, although the disease is reported more frequently in females than in males, this may be caused by a presentation bias rather than an actual sex predilection and may not reflect the true incidence of disease.

In one study, the average age at which signs of adrenal disease are first observed by ferret owners was approximately 3.5 years.[46] A smaller study has reported an older age distribution for this disease.[39]

Alopecia is the most common clinical manifestation of adrenocortical disease and develops in both male and female ferrets (Fig. 8-2). More than 90% of ferrets with adrenal gland disease have some extent of hair loss. The hair epilates easily. Alopecia is usually symmetrical, beginning on the rump, the tail, or the flanks and progressing to the lateral trunk, dorsum, and ventrum. Document these patterns of alopecia in the medical record for comparison as the disease progresses.

In more than one third of ferrets with adrenal gland disease, owners report the ferret as pruritic. Pruritus usually accompanies hair loss, but in some ferrets pruritus is the only clinical sign.

*References 13, 17, 25, 34, 39, 42, 46, 52.

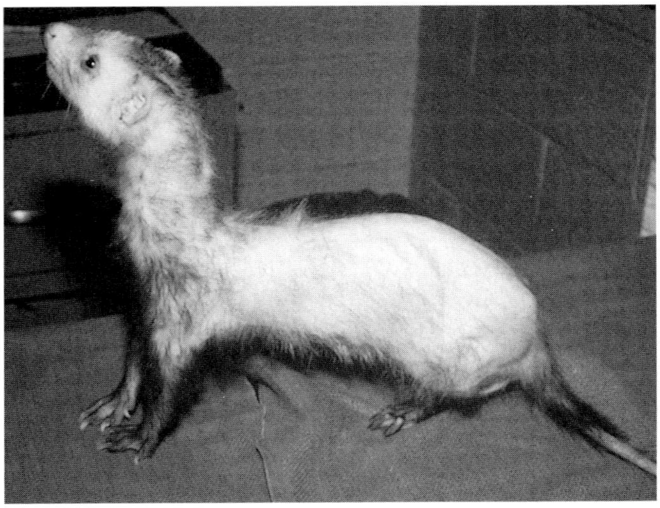

Figure 8-2 The typical pattern of hair loss in a ferret with an adrenocortical tumor.

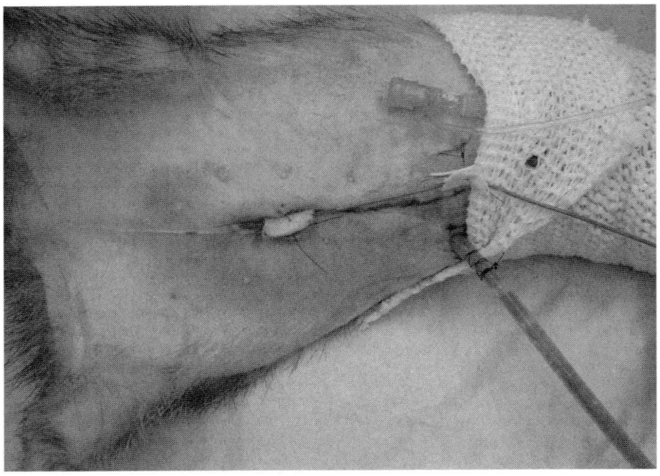

Figure 8-4 A male ferret with a urethral catheter and peritoneal drain in place after surgery for a ruptured prostatic abscess associated with a right adrenal tumor. The ferret had severe stranguria and was catheterized with a 3.5-Fr red rubber catheter. At surgery, a right adrenal tumor was removed and a peritoneal drain was placed because of a septic abdomen from the ruptured abscess. The ferret recovered well after surgery with intensive care and antibiotic therapy.

Pruritus is most frequently observed on the dorsum between the shoulder blades. The skin is often erythematous in these areas.

More than 70% of female ferrets with adrenal gland disease have an enlarged vulva (Fig. 8-3).[46] The vulva can be slightly to grossly enlarged and become turgid and edematous, resembling the vulva of a jill in estrus. A seromucoid discharge may be present, and results of cytologic examination may show localized vaginitis. The perivulvar skin may appear dark and bruised.

Partial or complete urinary blockage in male ferrets is occasionally associated with adrenocortical diseases.[8,43] Affected ferrets have dysuria or stranguria. Periurethral cysts develop in the region of the prostate (possibly originating from hormone-responsive cells) and cause urethral narrowing. Because of the urethral narrowing, passing a urinary catheter into the bladder of these ferrets can be difficult (see Chapter 2). A ferret with a urethral blockage may have a life-threatening metabolic derangement; therefore these cases usually constitute an emergency. In some ferrets, removing the diseased adrenal tissue and draining the cysts resolves the urinary blockage within 1 or 2 days. In others, the prostatic tissue is infected and aggressive surgical treatment along with antibiotic and hormonal therapy are necessary (Fig. 8-4; see Chapter 12).

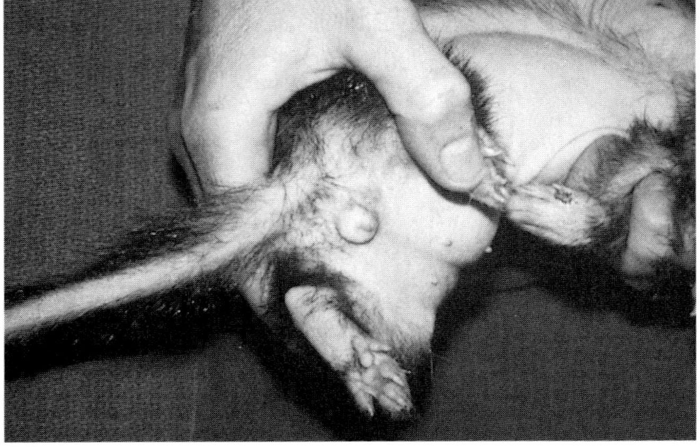

Figure 8-3 An enlarged vulva and hair loss in a female ferret with adrenocortical disease.

On physical examination, enlarged adrenal glands are sometimes palpable. The left adrenal gland is more easily identified than the right. The left gland is usually engulfed in a large fat pad cranial to the left kidney. It may feel like a small, firm, round mass. Because the right gland has a more cranial location and is under a lobe of the liver, it is more difficult to palpate. Enlarged mesenteric lymph nodes may be palpable.

The spleen may be palpably enlarged, but it usually has smooth borders and is not painful. In some instances, the texture of the spleen is irregular and knobby. In most older ferrets, an enlarged spleen is an incidental finding on physical examination (see Chapter 6).

Clinical Pathology and Diagnostic Testing

The presumptive diagnosis of adrenal gland disease is based on history, clinical signs, and results of imaging techniques and steroid hormonal assays. Diagnosis is confirmed by histologic examination of adrenal tissue obtained during surgical biopsy or adrenalectomy.

Results of the complete blood count are usually unremarkable. Rarely, adrenocortical disease is associated with nonregenerative anemia. If disease is severe or prolonged, pancytopenia may be present. These changes mimic those in ferrets with estrogen-induced bone marrow toxicosis (see Chapter 4). In ferrets with anemia and pancytopenia, a packed cell volume less than 15% carries a grave prognosis.

Results of the biochemical profile are also usually within reference ranges. The concentration of alanine aminotransferase is occasionally high, but the association of this finding with

adrenal gland disease is unknown. Because insulinomas are also common in older ferrets, hypoglycemia from a pancreatic beta cell tumor (insulinoma) may be present. A urinalysis is not helpful in diagnosing adrenal gland disease.

Radiographs are generally not helpful in diagnosing this disease. An enlarged adrenal gland rarely displaces other organs or calcifies; therefore organ displacement and mineralized glands are not visible radiographically. Lung metastasis of adrenal gland tumors is very rare. However, radiographs are useful as a screening tool for other conditions such as heart disease or splenomegaly.

Abdominal ultrasound is useful for detecting enlarged adrenal glands. The size, side of enlargement, and architecture can often be determined.[5,23,38,40] Abdominal ultrasound is also useful for detecting concurrent diseases, such as renal or hepatic disease, metastasis from a pancreatic insulinoma, or enlarged lymph nodes. Theoretically, computed tomographic or magnetic resonance imaging scans of the abdomen of ferrets can demonstrate adrenal gland abnormalities. Currently, however, these imaging techniques are rarely used because of cost and availability.

Ancillary diagnostic tests Several diagnostic tests used in dogs with adrenocortical disease are not useful in ferrets. The adrenocorticotropic hormone (ACTH) stimulation test and the dexamethasone suppression test cannot be used to diagnose adrenal disease in ferrets. Both normal ferrets and those with adrenal disease respond equally well to an ACTH stimulation test. This is probably because most ferrets with this disease do not produce abnormally high concentrations of cortisol.[45] Plasma concentrations of ACTH and alpha-melanocyte stimulating hormone in ferrets with adrenal disease are similar to those of normal ferrets, suggesting that adrenal disease in ferrets is independent of ACTH and alpha-melanocyte stimulating hormone.[48] Urinary cortisol/creatinine ratios were higher in 12 ferrets with adrenocortical tumors than in 51 clinically normal ferrets.[15] In dogs, the urinary cortisol/creatinine ratio is a sensitive but not a specific indicator of hyperadrenocorticism. Further studies are needed to evaluate urinary cortisol/creatinine ratios in ferrets with diseases other than hyperadrenocorticism.

Measuring serum concentrations of steroid hormones is a reliable means of diagnosing adrenal disease in ferrets. Hormone panels that measure estradiol, androstenedione, and 17-hydroxyprogesterone in serum samples are commercially available (Clinical Endocrinology Laboratory of the Department of Comparative Medicine at the University of Tennessee [www.vet.utk.edu/diagnostic/endocrinology.html]). In a normal neutered ferret, these steroids are found in minute quantities, whereas in ferrets with adrenal disease, the serum concentrations of one or more of these compounds may be high.[44] In Table 8-2, reference ranges are given for androstenedione, dehydroepiandrosterone sulfate, estradiol, and 17-hydroxyprogesterone in intact female and neutered ferrets.

Differential diagnosis An intact female ferret or one with an ovarian remnant may display an enlarged vulva and alopecia, resembling a ferret with adrenal disease. Several methods are used to differentiate the two conditions. In one method, human chorionic gonadotropin (100 IU IM) is administered and then repeated in 7 to 10 days. If the ferret is intact or if an ovarian remnant is present, the vulva usually decreases in size. Alternatively, measuring steroid hormone concentrations may help differentiate the two conditions. If the concentrations of androgens such as androstenedione, dehydroepiandrosterone sulfate, or 17-hydroxyprogesterone are high, then an adrenal tumor is likely. If only the estradiol concentration is high, then either condition may be present. An ultrasound examination of the abdomen of a female ferret may differentiate between an adrenal tumor and an intact genital tract. Surgery is the definitive method to confirm the presence of ovarian tissue or an abnormal adrenal gland.

Some ferrets, particularly males, exhibit seasonal alopecia of the tail. After several weeks, the hair typically regrows. This condition does not appear related to an adrenal tumor.

TABLE 8-2
Serum Concentrations of Steroid Hormones in Intact and Neutered Normal Ferrets and Ferrets with Adrenal Disease

	Neutered Ferrets*			Intact Female Fitch Ferrets (n = 11)‡	
		Normal Ferrets (n = 26) (13 male, 13 female)			
Steroid Hormone	Adrenal Disease Mean	Mean	Reference Range†	Mean	Reference Range
Androstenedione (nmol/L)	67 (n = 25)	6.6	<0.1–15	58.3	20–96
Dehydroepiandrosterone sulfate (μmol/L)	0.03 (n = 27)	0.01			
Estradiol (pmol/L)	167 (n = 28)	106	30–108	165.5	122–210
17-Hydroxyprogesterone (nmol/L)	3.2 (n = 20)	0.4	<0.1–0.8	7.7	2.3–13.1

*Data from Rosenthal KL and Petersen ME.[44]
†Reference ranges currently in use by the Clinical Endocrinology Laboratory, College of Veterinary Medicine, University of Tennessee, Knoxville, TN. Courtesy Jack W. Oliver, DVM, PhD.
‡Ramer J and Oliver JW, unpublished data.

Possible Concurrent Abnormalities

Pancreatic beta cell tumors and adrenal gland disease are both seen in older ferrets and often occur concurrently. However, it is not known if a correlation exists between the two diseases. An insulinoma is diagnosed on the basis of clinical signs in conjunction with low blood glucose and high insulin concentrations and the finding of pancreatic disease at surgery. Medications (prednisone and diazoxide) used to control the clinical signs of insulinoma do not appear to interfere with therapy of adrenal disease. If adrenalectomy is elected, pancreatic beta cell tumors can be debulked simultaneously.

Many ferrets with adrenal disease have splenic enlargement. Histopathologic examination of the spleen usually shows extramedullary hematopoiesis. Infrequently, neoplasia, including lymphoma and hemangiosarcoma, causes splenic enlargement. Nodular hyperplasia is also seen. In any ferret with an enlarged spleen that undergoes adrenalectomy, biopsy the spleen at the time of surgery (see Chapter 6).

Middle-aged and geriatric ferrets frequently have heart disease, which can be clinical or subclinical (see Chapter 6). Before surgery, evaluate all older ferrets for subclinical heart disease to prevent decompensation that can accompany the effects of anesthesia or fluid administration.

Lymphoma is also common in ferrets. Abnormal nodes can be found incidentally during a diagnostic workup or during abdominal exploratory surgery. At surgery, obtain biopsy samples of any abnormal subcutaneous or mesenteric lymph nodes.

Management

The two treatment modalities for adrenocortical tumors are surgically removing or debulking an affected adrenal gland(s) or medical management. Surgical removal is the preferred treatment for ferrets, as it is for dogs with adrenocortical tumors.[21] With medical management, the growth of the adrenal tumor may not stop but clinical signs may regress either temporarily or permanently.

Surgical therapy Preoperative testing of a ferret with an adrenal tumor can include a complete blood count, biochemical profile, abdominal and thoracic radiographs, and abdominal and cardiac ultrasound examination. Withhold food for 4 to 6 hours before surgery. If a ferret is suspected of having an insulinoma, place an intravenous catheter during most or all of this fasting period to provide intravenous fluid support with added dextrose. Otherwise, place an intravenous catheter at induction.

Adrenalectomy techniques are described in Chapter 12. Fully explore the abdomen before addressing the diseased adrenal gland(s). Other structures to be examined include the liver, the lymph nodes, the pancreas, the kidneys, and the spleen. Because bilateral adrenal gland disease can be present, examine, palpate, and compare both adrenal glands.

Perform a unilateral adrenalectomy if only one adrenal gland is diseased.[53,54] If both glands are diseased, a subtotal adrenalectomy, with total removal of one gland and partial removal of the other, is indicated (see Chapter 12). Total bilateral adrenalectomy is rarely done.

After surgery, give the ferret maintenance and replacement fluids as needed. Unless concurrent gastrointestinal surgery was performed or complications develop, feed the ferret soon after surgery. Ferrets rarely need postoperative corticosteroid replacement therapy after simple unilateral adrenalectomy. If the ferret had a concurrent insulinoma or has had a subtotal adrenalectomy and appears very lethargic after surgery, consider giving prednisone at a physiologic dosage for 2 to 3 days after surgery. If a total or subtotal bilateral adrenalectomy has been performed, monitor electrolyte concentrations closely after surgery. Give sodium dexamethasone phosphate (4 mg/kg IV) followed by maintenance corticosteroid and mineralocorticoid supplementation as needed.

Medical management At present, medical management of adrenal gland disease is aimed at moderating clinical signs rather than curing the condition. Consider medical management if an owner cannot afford surgery or if a ferret is a poor surgical candidate, has bilateral adrenal tumors that cannot be totally resected, or has recurrent disease in the remaining gland after previous unilateral adrenalectomy. Several medical strategies are used to decrease the clinical signs of adrenal disease. Drug therapy includes mitotane, androgen receptor blockers, aromatase inhibitors, and gonadotropin-releasing hormone (GnRH) analogs. However, medical therapy is not always successful, and predicting which ferret will respond to a particular medication is not possible. Numerous attempts with different classes of medications may be needed to find a drug that is effective.

Mitotane Mitotane, or o,p′-DDD (Lysodren, Bristol-Myers Squibb Oncology, Princeton, NJ), is effective in dogs for treating pituitary-dependent hyperadrenocorticism. However, this form of hyperadrenocorticism has not been recognized in ferrets, which may explain why treatment with mitotane is rarely successful in ferrets with adrenocortical tumors. Mitotane treatment does not reliably produce resolution of clinical signs in ferrets with adrenocortical tumors. Moreover, if clinical signs do resolve, they typically recur when mitotane is discontinued.

Use caution when administering mitotane, and warn the owners of potential deleterious side effects associated with this drug. In ferrets, the primary danger associated with mitotane administration is severe hypoglycemia that can develop after several days of therapy in animals with concurrent insulinoma. This can occur even in ferrets that show no clinical signs or laboratory results suggestive of insulinoma before mitotane treatment. Mitotane possibly lowers endogenous cortisol concentrations sufficiently to decompensate ferrets with subclinical insulinoma. Instruct owners how to recognize an episode of hypoglycemia and how to treat their ferret appropriately (see the section on insulinoma earlier in this chapter). Dispense prednisone to be used as a "rescue" therapy if needed.

Mitotane treatment, although not curative, may be palliative and therefore is useful in certain cases. The mitotane dose that has been used for ferrets is 50 mg once daily for 1 week, after which a maintenance dose of 50 mg every 2 to 3 days is given. A compounding pharmacist can prepare 50-mg capsules of mitotane; however, the capsules must be given whole, without being opened, and thus can be difficult to administer. Offer the ferret a small amount of Nutri-Cal (Tomlyn, Buena, NJ) or Linatone (Lambert Kay, Cranbury, NJ) immediately after administering a capsule to encourage swallowing.

Although it is not useful for tracking effectiveness of mitotane therapy, the ACTH stimulation test can be used to monitor decreases in adrenal cortisol levels. With most types of medical therapy, regression of clinical signs is the easiest way to monitor treatment response. Submitting serial serum samples for an adrenal androgen panel can be used to objectively measure response to treatment.

Ketoconazole Because of its ability to inhibit the steroid biosynthetic pathway at several steps, ketoconazole is used in the treatment of adrenocortical disease in other species.[47] However, it is not effective in ferrets.

Androgen receptor blockers Androgen receptor blockers reverse the signs of adrenal disease but do not inhibit the growth of an abnormal adrenal gland. Theoretically, these compounds act at the receptor site to block the actions of androgens. In human medicine, these drugs are used to treat men with benign prostatic hyperplasia or prostatic carcinoma.[3,4,9,30] Like all medical therapies used in ferrets with adrenal disease, androgen receptor blockers are effective in some, but not all, ferrets. Some practitioners suggest that, because these drugs are used mainly to treat men, androgen receptor blockers should be used primarily in male ferrets. Flutamide (Eulexin, Schering Corporation, Kenilworth, NJ) and bicalutamide (Casodex, AstraZeneca Pharmaceuticals LP, Wilmington, DE) have been used in ferrets with adrenal disease. Flutamide has been used in ferrets for behavioral research.[51]

Aromatase inhibitors Another class of drugs that can depress the signs of adrenal disease in ferrets is the aromatase inhibitors. One drug that has been used is anastrozole (Arimidex, AstraZeneca Pharmaceuticals LP). This drug specifically inhibits aromatase, the enzyme that catalyzes the final step in estrogen production. In people treated with continued dosing of anastrozole, plasma concentrations of estradiol decrease approximately 80% from baseline.[14,41] Anastrozole has little or no effect on central nervous system, autonomic, or neuromuscular function.

Gonadotropin-releasing hormone analogs GnRH analogs are a class of compounds that are widely used in human medicine to treat prostatic cancer, endometriosis, and breast cancer. In ferrets, these compounds have been used to control the signs of adrenal disease. There are two general types of analogs: GnRH agonists and GnRH antagonists.

During short-term or intermittent therapy, GnRH agonists have the same stimulatory action as GnRH, but long-term therapy suppresses gonadotropin release and downregulates the receptors. This downregulation of receptors is the mode of action of the agonists. An injectable GnRH agonist used in ferrets is leuprolide acetate (Lupron Depot, TAP Pharmaceuticals Inc., Lake Forest, IL).

GnRH antagonists are being studied in people for treatment of the same diseases as are agonists. Theoretically, antagonists should be more effective than agonists at a much lower dosage. In human medicine, an antagonist called abarelix is being evaluated to determine its ability to inhibit the action of GnRH. This or similar drugs may eventually replace GnRH agonists in the treatment of ferret adrenal disease.

Adrenal Histopathology

On histopathologic examination, adrenal gland disease is described as adrenocortical hyperplasia, adenoma, or carcinoma.[46]

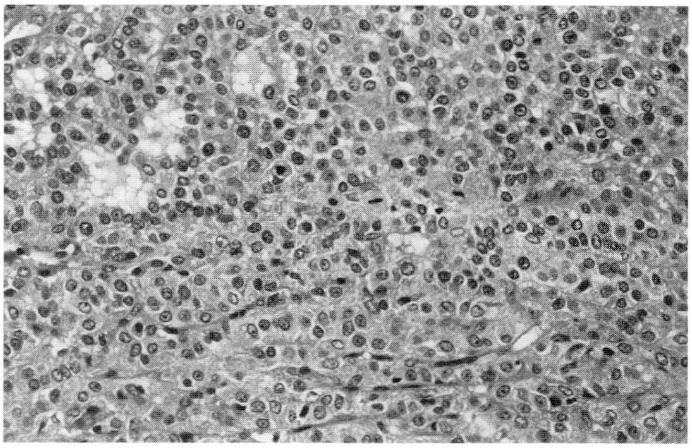

Figure 8-5 Photomicrograph of a liver section from a ferret with hepatic metastasis of an adrenocortical tumor. This tumor is composed of packets or cords of large, pale-staining epithelial cells occasionally with vacuolated cytoplasm. The cells are supported by a delicate fibrous stroma. There is a high mitotic index. Hematoxylin and eosin stain, ×40. *(Courtesy Dr. James Walberg.)*

Although adenomas appear to be most common, the clinical behavior of these tumors and hyperplasia is usually identical. Metastasis is uncommon; however, some tumors locally invade the vena cava or liver (Fig. 8-5). Very rarely, carcinomas can metastasize to the lungs.

Pheochromocytomas occur uncommonly in ferrets (see below).

Prognosis

The prognosis with surgical treatment is good in the hands of an experienced and skilled surgeon. In most ferrets, the associated clinical signs resolve after the diseased adrenal gland has been removed (Fig. 8-6). Later complications of surgical treatment include recurrence of adrenal tumor because of metastasis (rare) or the development of an adrenocortical tumor in the remaining adrenal gland.

Because the results of medical treatment are equivocal, the prognosis with medical treatment is unpredictable. If the effects of the adrenal disease are only cosmetic (alopecia), then the prognosis for life is good. The prognosis worsens if prostatic disease, bone marrow suppression, or tumor-related mechanical interference with the vena cava develops, or if the tumor metastasizes.

PHEOCHROMOCYTOMAS

Pheochromocytomas occur rarely in ferrets.[12] Pheochromocytomas arise from the adrenal medulla and produce excessive amounts of catecholamines. Clinical signs are primarily associated with the effects of catecholamines on the cardiovascular system. In clinical cases seen at the Animal Medical Center in New York City, several ferrets exhibited clinical signs consistent with those seen in dogs with pheochromocytomas: tachycardia, dyspnea, and cardiovascular collapse (K. Quesenberry, personal observation, 2002). High blood pressure is a common finding in other species; however, blood pressure was not measured in

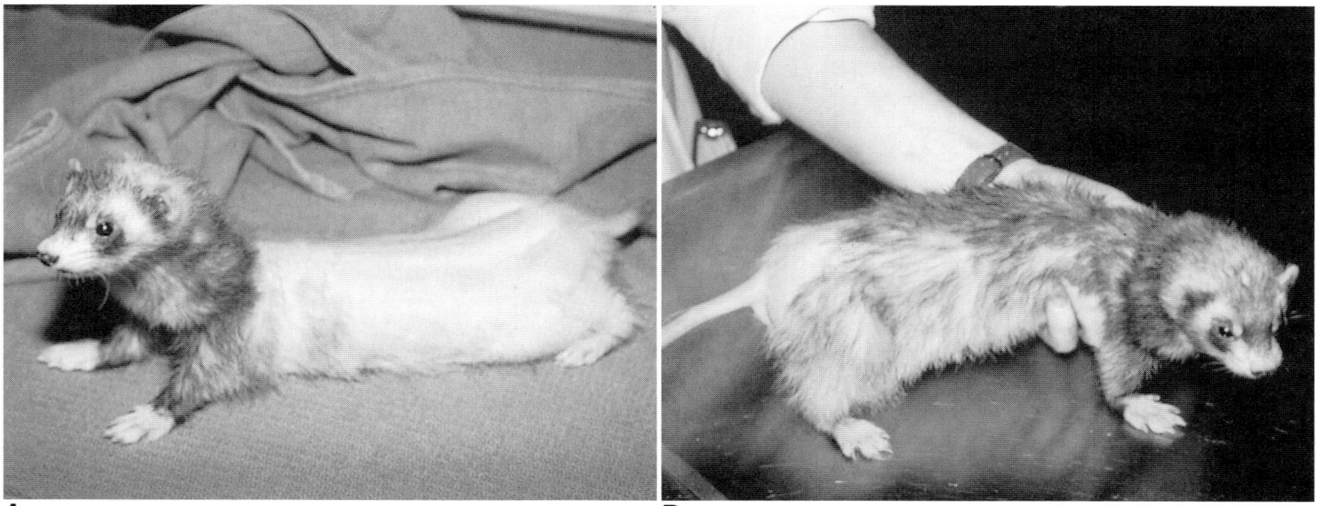

Figure 8-6 A, Four-year-old spayed female ferret with a left adrenocortical tumor. B, The same ferret 2 months after left adrenalectomy. Hair regrowth is almost complete except on the feet, rump, and tail. The hair never fully regrew on the tail. *(Courtesy Dr. Holly Mullen.)*

these ferrets. Histologic diagnosis of a pheochromocytoma is confirmed by immunohistochemical staining. Animals with pheochromocytomas respond poorly to chemotherapy, and surgical excision is the treatment of choice. Prognosis in ferrets with pheochromocytomas is poor.

DIABETES MELLITUS

History and Physical Examination

Spontaneous diabetes mellitus is very uncommon in ferrets. Most ferrets develop iatrogenic diabetes from aggressive pancreatectomy to debulk beta cell tumor nodules. The clinical signs of diabetic ferrets are similar to those of other species. The severity of signs depends on the severity and chronicity of the disease. Affected ferrets are polyuric and polydipsic and may lose weight despite a good appetite. They often appear lethargic, especially if a metabolic derangement such as ketoacidosis is present.

The findings on physical examination are often unremarkable. Ferrets may be thin and have a distended urinary bladder.

Clinical Pathology and Diagnostic Testing

The diagnosis of diabetes mellitus in ferrets is based on some or all of the following: compatible clinical signs (polyuria/polydipsia), a history of recent insulinoma surgery, repeated high blood glucose concentrations, low blood insulin concentration, and normal to high blood glucagon concentration.

In diabetic ferrets, a profound hyperglycemia is usually present. Although a blood glucose concentration of 400 mg/dL or higher is suspicious for diabetes, repeated high blood glucose measurements are needed to confirm consistent hyperglycemia. In uncomplicated diabetes, results of the biochemical analysis are usually unremarkable. However, the same metabolic derangements that are present in other mammals with complicated diabetes can occur in ferrets. Results of the complete blood count are usually normal. However, if a concurrent bladder infection is present, the white blood cell count may be high. A consistent glucosuria is present and, in severe cases, ketones are detected. As with other animals with diabetes, ferrets with diabetes can have an active urine sediment.

Although radiography and ultrasound are not useful for diagnosing diabetes mellitus, they can be used to screen for other conditions such as splenomegaly, hepatic enlargement, and cardiac disease.

Ancillary diagnostic tests Diabetes mellitus in ferrets can be caused by a lack of insulin, insulin resistance, or a glucagonoma. Insulin concentration is routinely measured in ferrets with insulinomas. This test is preferably performed by a diagnostic laboratory that has validated the test for ferrets. Theoretically, a low insulin concentration concurrent with hyperglycemia can confirm the diagnosis of diabetes mellitus. A normal or high insulin concentration could represent either insulin resistance or the presence of a glucagonoma. Therefore measuring glucagon concentration can be an important indicator in ferrets with hyperglycemia. Unfortunately, routine measurement of glucagon concentration is difficult because it must be performed in a laboratory that has validated the assay for ferrets.

Treatment

Treatment of diabetes mellitus depends on the severity of hyperglycemia and other metabolic disturbances. Institute insulin therapy in ferrets if the blood glucose concentration is higher than 300 mg/dL on repeated measurements. Follow the treatment principles used for dogs and cats. Unfortunately, success is limited in tightly regulating the blood glucose concentrations of these ferrets. In hospitalized animals, measure serial blood glucose concentrations while administering insulin twice daily. Use neutral protamine Hagedorn insulin, starting it at an empirical dose of 0.5 to 1 U insulin per ferret twice daily. Increase or decrease the insulin dose as dictated by the blood glucose concentration. Monitor the urine for the presence of glucose and ketones.

After the blood glucose concentration is stabilized between 125 and 200 mg/dL, discharge the ferret to its owner with a prescribed insulin regimen. Some ferrets receive Ultralente insulin, which may have a longer period of action than neutral protamine Hagedorn insulin, in an effort to give injections only once per day. Instruct owners to check for the presence of ketones and glucose in the urine with urine dipsticks. If no glucose is detected in the urine, instruct the owner not to give the next dose of insulin. If trace amounts of glucose are found, the insulin dose is not changed. If the amount of glucose in the urine is large, then the insulin dose is increased slightly. Most diabetic ferrets are difficult to regulate. Realistically, the goal is to have negative ketones and a small amount of glucose in the urine.

Prognosis

Many ferrets that develop iatrogenic hyperglycemia immediately after insulinoma surgery may be transient diabetics. Their prognosis as it relates to diabetes is good because the hyperglycemia usually normalizes without treatment during the first 1 to 2 weeks after surgery. Occasionally, the diabetes spontaneously resolves after 4 to 6 weeks of treatment. The prognosis is worse or, at best, unpredictable for ferrets with diabetes mellitus that occurs spontaneously or is detected weeks to months after insulinoma surgery. Blood glucose concentration is usually difficult to regulate in these animals.

THYROID DISEASE

Clinical hyperthyroidism and hypothyroidism have not been reported in ferrets. One report of medullary thyroid carcinoma diagnosed at necropsy was not a confirmed functional hyperthyroid ferret antemortem.[12] Normal resting values for thyroxine and tri-iodothyronine and results of thyroid-stimulating hormone testing reported in one study of normal intact male ferrets are presented in Table 8-1.[16]

Suspected pseudohypoparathyroidism was reported in a 1.5-year-old neutered male ferret.[55] Pseudohypoparathyroidism, a hereditary condition in people, results from a lack of response to circulating parathyroid hormone rather than hormone deficiency. The ferret was seen because of intermittent seizures, and results of diagnostic tests revealed low serum calcium, high serum phosphorus, and high serum parathyroid hormone concentrations. The ferret responded to long-term treatment with dihydrotachysterol, a vitamin D analog, and calcium carbonate.

REFERENCES

1. Andrews GA, Myers NC III, Chard-Bergstrom C: Immunohistochemistry of pancreatic islet cell tumors in the ferret (*Mustela putorius furo*). Vet Pathol 1997; 34:387-393.
2. Arey LB: Developmental Anatomy, 7th ed. Philadelphia, WB Saunders, 1965, pp 321-324.
3. Ayub M, Levell MJ: Suppression of plasma androgens by the antiandrogen flutamide in prostatic cancer patients treated with zoladex, a GnRH analogue. Clin Endocrinol 1990; 32:329-339.
4. Belanger A, Labrie F, Dupont A, et al: Endocrine effects of combined treatment with an LHRH agonist in association with flutamide in metastatic prostatic carcinoma. Clin Invest Med 1988; 11:321-326.
5. Besso J, Tidwell AS, Gliatto JM: Retrospective review of the ultrasonographic features of adrenal lesions in 21 ferrets. Vet Rad Ultrasound 2000; 41:345-352.
6. Caplan ER, Peterson ME, Mullen HS, et al: Diagnosis and treatment of insulin-secreting pancreatic islet cell tumors in ferrets: 57 cases (1986-1994). J Am Vet Med Assoc 1996; 209:1741-1745.
7. Caywood DD, Klausner JS, O'Leary TP, et al: Pancreatic insulin-secreting neoplasms: clinical, diagnostic, and prognostic features in 73 dogs. J Am Anim Hosp Assoc 1988; 24:577-584.
8. Coleman GD, Chavez MA, Williams BH: Cystic prostatic disease associated with adrenocortical lesions in the ferret (*Mustela putorius furo*). Vet Pathol 1998; 35:547-549.
9. Couzinet B, Pholsena M, Young J, et al: The impact of a pure anti-androgen (flutamide) on LH, FSH, androgens and clinical status in idiopathic hirsutism. Clin Endocrinol 1993; 39:157-162.
10. Fekete E, Woolley G, Little CC: Histological changes following ovariectomy in mice: dba high tumor strain. J Exp Med 1941; 74:1-8.
11. Fix AS, Harms CA: Immunocytochemistry of pancreatic endocrine tumors in three domestic ferrets (*Mustela putorius furo*). Vet Pathol 1990; 27:199-201.
12. Fox JG, Dangler CA, Snyder SB, et al: C-cell carcinoma (medullary thyroid carcinoma) associated with multiple endocrine neoplasms in a ferret (*Mustela putorius*). Vet Pathol 2000; 37:278-282.
13. Fox JG, Pequet-Goad ME, Garibaldi BA, et al: Hyperadrenocorticism in a ferret. J Am Vet Med Assoc 1987; 191:343-344.
14. Goss P, Gwyn K: Current perspectives on aromatase inhibitors in breast cancer. J Clin Oncol 1994; 12:2460-2470.
15. Gould WJ, Reimers TJ, Bell JA, et al: Evaluation of urinary cortisol:creatinine ratios for the diagnosis of hyperadrenocorticism associated with adrenal gland tumors in ferrets. J Am Vet Med Assoc 1995; 206:42-46.
16. Heard DJ, Collins B, Chen DL, et al: Thyroid and adrenal function tests in adult male ferrets. Am J Vet Res 1990; 51:32-35.
17. Hillyer EV: Ferret endocrinology. *In* Kirk RW, Bonagura JD, eds. Current Veterinary Therapy 11: Small Animal Practice. Philadelphia, WB Saunders, 1992, pp 1185-1188.
18. Jane Ellis M, Livesey JH, Evans MJ: Hormone stability in human blood. Clin Biochem 2003; 36:109-112.
19. Jergens AE, Shaw DP: Hyperinsulinism and hypoglycemia associated with pancreatic islet cell tumor in a ferret. J Am Vet Med Assoc 1989; 194:269-271.
20. Kaufman J, Schwarz P, Mero K: Pancreatic beta cell tumor in a ferret. J Am Vet Med Assoc 1984; 185:998-1000.
21. Kintzer PP, Peterson ME: Mitotane treatment of 32 dogs with cortisol-secreting adrenocortical neoplasms. J Am Vet Med Assoc 1994; 205:54-61.
22. Krishna Murthy AS, Brezak MA, Baez AG: Postcastrational adrenal tumors in two strains of mice: morphologic, histochemical, and chromatographic studies. J Natl Cancer Inst 1970; 45:1211-1222.
23. Kupersmith DS, Bauck L: Hyperadrenocorticism in a ferret: diagnosis (using ultrasound) and treatment. J Small Exotic Anim Med 1991; 1:66-68.
24. Leifer CE, Petterson ME, Matus RE: Insulin-secreting tumor: diagnosis and medical and surgical management in 55 dogs. J Am Vet Med Assoc 1986; 188:60-64.
25. Lipman NS, Marini RP, Murphy JC, et al: Estradiol-17beta-secreting adrenocortical tumor in a ferret. J Am Vet Med Assoc 1993; 203:1552-1555.
26. Lundberg G, Iverson C, Radulescu G: Now read this: the SI units are here. JAMA 1986; 255:2329-2339.

27. Lurye JC, Behrend EN. Endocrine tumors. Vet Clin North Am Sm Anim Pract 2001; 31:1083-1110.
28. Luttgen PJ, Storts RW, Rogers KS, et al: Insulinoma in a ferret. J Am Vet Med Assoc 1986; 189:920-921.
29. Mann FA, Stockham SL, Freeman MB, et al: Reference intervals for insulin concentrations and insulin:glucose ratios in the serum of ferrets. J Small Exotic Anim Med 1993; 2:79-83.
30. Marcondes JA, Minnani SL, Luthold WW, et al: Treatment of hirsutism in women with flutamide. Fertil Steril 1992; 57:543-547.
31. Marini RP, Ryden EB, Rosenblad WD, et al: Functional islet cell tumor in six ferrets. J Am Vet Med Assoc 1993; 202:430-433.
32. Mehlhaff CJ, Peterson ME, Patnaik AK, et al: Insulin-producing islet cell neoplasms: surgical considerations and general management in 35 dogs. J Am Anim Hosp Assoc 1985; 21:607-612.
33. Meleo K: Management of insulinoma patients with refractory hypoglycemia. Probl Vet Med 1990; 2:602-609.
34. Mor N, Qualls CW, Hoover JP: Concurrent mammary gland hyperplasia and adrenocortical carcinoma in a domestic ferret. J Am Vet Med Assoc 1992; 201:1911-1912.
35. Nelson RW: Insulin-secreting islet cell neoplasia. *In* Ettinger SJ, Feldman EC, eds. Textbook of Veterinary Internal Medicine. 4th ed. Philadelphia, WB Saunders, 1995, pp 1501-1509.
36. Nelson RW, Foodman MS: Medical management of canine hyperinsulinism. J Am Vet Med Assoc 1985; 187:78-82.
37. Nelson RW, Salisbury SK: Pancreatic beta cell neoplasia. *In* Birchard SJ, Sherding RG, eds. Saunders Manual of Small Animal Practice. Philadelphia, WB Saunders, 1994, pp 257-262.
38. Neuwirth L, Collins B, Calderwood-Mays M, et al: Adrenal ultrasonography correlated with histopathology in ferrets. Vet Radiol Ultrasound 1997; 38:69-74.
39. Neuwirth L, Isaza R, Bellah J, et al: Adrenal neoplasia in seven ferrets. Vet Radiol Ultrasound 1993; 34:340-346.
40. O'Brien R, Paul-Murphy J, Dubielzig RR: Ultrasonography of adrenal glands in normal ferrets. Vet Radiol 1996; 37:445-448.
41. Plourde PV, Dryoff M, Dukes M: Arimidex: a potent and selective fourth-generation aromatase inhibitor. Breast Cancer Res Treat 1994; 30:103-111.
42. Rosenthal KL: Adrenal gland disease in ferrets. Vet Clin North Am Small Anim Pract 1997; 27:401-418.
43. Rosenthal K, Peterson M: Clinical case conference: stranguria in a castrated male ferret. J Am Vet Med Assoc 1996; 209:462-464.
44. Rosenthal K, Peterson M: Plasma androgen concentrations in ferrets with adrenal gland disease. J Am Vet Med Assoc 1996; 209:1097-1102.
45. Rosenthal KL, Peterson ME, Quesenberry KE, et al: Evaluation of plasma cortisol and corticosterone responses to synthetic adrenocorticotropic hormone administration in ferrets. Am J Vet Res 1993; 54:29-31.
46. Rosenthal KL, Peterson ME, Quesenberry KE, et al: Hyperadrenocorticism associated with adrenocortical tumor or nodular hyperplasia in ferrets: 50 cases (1987-1991). J Am Vet Med Assoc 1993; 203:271-275.
47. Saadi HF, Bravo EL, Aron DC: Feminizing adrenocortical tumor: steroid hormone response to ketoconazole. J Clin Endocrinol Metab 1990; 70:540-543.
48. Schoemaker NJ, Moi JA, Lumeij JT, et al: Plasma concentrations of adrenocorticotrophic hormone and alpha-melanocyte-stimulating hormone in ferrets (*Mustela putorius furo*) with hyperadrenocorticism. Am J Vet Res 2002; 63:1395-1399.
49. Schoemaker NJ, Schuurmans M, Moorman H, et al: Correlation between age at neutering and age at onset of hyperadrenocorticism in ferrets. J Am Vet Med Assoc 2000; 216:195-197.
50. Sharawy MM, Liebelt AG, Dirksen TR, et al: Fine structural study of postcastrational adrenocortical carcinomas in female CE-mice. Anat Rec 1980; 198:125-133.
51. Weaver C, Baum M: Differential regulation of brain aromatase by androgen in adult and fetal ferrets. Endocrinology 1991; 128:1247-1254
52. Weiss CA, Scott MV: Clinical aspects and surgical treatment of hyperadrenocorticism in the domestic ferret: 94 cases (1994-1996). J Am Anim Hosp Assoc 1997; 33:487-493.
53. Weiss CA, Williams BH, Scott JB, et al: Surgical treatment and long-term outcome of ferrets with bilateral adrenal tumors or adrenal hyperplasia: 56 cases. J Am Vet Med Assoc 1999; 215:820-823.
54. Wheeler J, Bennett RA: Ferret abdominal surgical procedures. Part I. Adrenal gland and pancreatic beta-cell tumors. Comp Contin Ed Pract Vet 1999; 21:815-822.
55. Wilson GH, Greene CE, Greenacre CB: Suspected pseudohypoparathyroidism in a domestic ferret. J Am Vet Med Assoc 2003; 222:1093-1096.

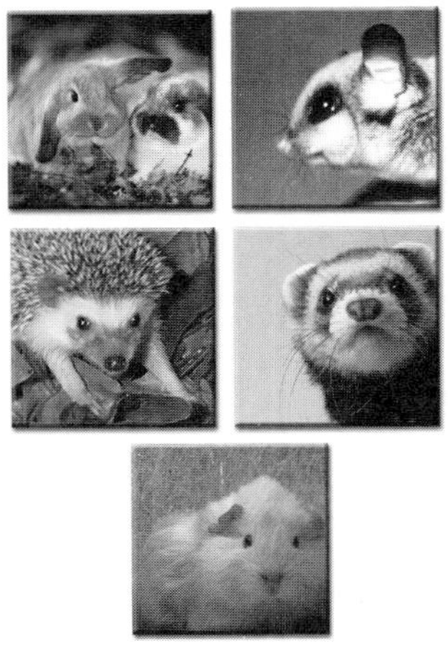

CHAPTER 9

Neoplasia

Bruce H. Williams, DVM, Diplomate ACVP, and Charles A. Weiss, DVM

With the exception of routine vaccinations, neoplasms and accompanying paraneoplastic syndromes are the most common reason ferrets are seen for veterinary care. The probability is good that most ferrets will develop a neoplasm of the endocrine system during the "golden age" for tumors (4 to 6 years) and excellent that some type of neoplasm will become evident over the course of a lifetime. In ferrets from American bloodlines, the incidence of three neoplasms—adrenocortical neoplasia, insulinoma, and malignant lymphoma—exceeds the incidence of all other neoplasms combined.

The increasing popularity of ferrets as both pets and laboratory animals over the past decade has facilitated the compilation of impressive data on neoplasms that provide a fairly accurate look at the distribution of neoplasia in this species* and establish that neoplasia is much more common in ferrets than previously indicated. Our review focuses primarily on the occurrence, diagnosis, treatment, and prognosis of clinically significant neoplasms in the ferret, with emphasis on nonendocrine neoplasms. Incidence data for this review were taken from an archive of 1525 neoplasms (Table 9-1) compiled over a 10-year period at the Armed Forces Institute of Pathology (Washington, DC) and a commercial pathology laboratory with a high prevalence of ferret submissions (Accupath, Potomac, MD).

One tenet should be considered by all veterinarians dealing with ferrets and their neoplasms—a ferret is not a cat or a dog. The clinical behavior, prognosis, and paraneoplastic syndromes in ferrets are often far different than those seen with similar neoplasms in dogs or cats. Insulinoma in the ferret is a neoplasm that rarely metastasizes to distant organs and may be associated with prolonged survival, as opposed to the same neoplasm in dogs and cats, which metastasizes widely and results in short survival times. Adrenocortical carcinoma, a neoplasm that is prone to metastasize widely in the dog, metastasizes only late in the course of disease in ferrets and, with early removal, warrants a good prognosis. Mast cell tumors, often malignant (and fatal) in the dog, are invariably benign and associated with a good prognosis in ferrets. Practitioners who extrapolate diagnostic and therapeutic options from comparable syndromes in more traditional pet species may find themselves in difficult and unexpected situations.

ETIOLOGY

Although the last decade has brought us tremendous information on the frequency and distribution of neoplasia, there is still little definitive information on the cause of neoplasm formation in ferrets. Many theories abound, but few have supportive evidence. The most common theories are as follows:

1. Genetic (familial) predisposition. Genetic or chromosomal aberrations have yet to be studied in domestic ferrets, but the tremendous incidence of neoplasia in American bloodlines of ferrets compared with their European counterparts certainly lends credence to this widely held belief. Fox et al.[16] document a syndrome of multiple neoplasms in an adult ferret that closely resembles multiple endocrine neoplasia type 2 in humans, a condition caused by a genetic mutation.
2. Infectious agents. Suspicious cluster outbreaks of malignant lymphoma in laboratory colonies and rescue operations[1,12] have sparked the investigation of a possible viral cause for

*References 2, 5, 10, 24, 26, 35, 36.

TABLE 9-1

Distribution of Neoplasia in Ferrets Based on 1525 Cases Submitted to the Armed Forces Institute of Pathology (1990-2000)

System	Tumor Type	Site	No.
Endocrine	Islet cell tumor	Pancreas	382
	Adrenocortical adenoma	Adrenal cortex	129
	Adrenocortical carcinoma	Adrenal cortex	251
	Adrenocortical carcinoma (metastatic)	Liver	11
		Spleen	3
		Mesenteric node	1
		Mesentery	1
	Leiomyosarcoma, low-grade	Adrenal gland	20
	Teratoma	Adrenal gland	4
	Malignant lymphoma	Adrenal gland	1
	Pituitary adenoma	Pituitary gland	1
Hematolymphatic	Malignant lymphoma	Multicentric	50
		Peripheral node	37
		Mesenteric node	17
		Spleen	16
		Peripheral blood	14
		Skin	9
		Intestine	9
		Abdominal	4
		Thymus	4
		Stomach	3
		Liver	3
		Colon	2
		Lung	2
		Bladder	2
		Eye	1
		Palate	1
		Uterus	1
		Kidney	1
	Round cell tumor, NOS	Spleen	2
	Metastatic adenocarcinoma		
	Rectal	Lymph node	1
	Salivary	Lymph node	1
	Gastric	Lymph node	1
	Ceruminous	Lymph node	1
	Myelolipoma	Spleen	1
	Thymoma	Thymus	1
Integumentary	Sebaceous epithelioma/adenoma	Skin, site unspecified	68
		Tail	10
		Leg	8
		Ear	5
		Back	5
		Neck	3
		Head	3
		Face	3
		Abdomen	2
		Chin	1
		Digit	1
	Mast cell tumor	Site unspecified	63
		Leg	7
		Digit	3

TABLE 9-1
Distribution of Neoplasia in Ferrets Based on 1525 Cases Submitted to the Armed Forces Institute of Pathology (1990-2000)—cont'd

System	Tumor Type	Site	No.
		Back	2
		Neck	2
		Chin	2
		Face	1
		Head	1
		Abdomen	1
		Trunk	1
	Apocrine		
	Adenocarcinoma	Prepuce	19
		Vulva	3
		Perianal	3
		Site unspecified	3
		Lymph node	2
		Hip	1
		Thigh	1
		Face	1
		Tail	1
	Adenoma	Prepuce	5
	Cystadenoma	Site unspecified	4
	Squamous cell carcinoma	Site unspecified	4
		Head	2
		Mandible	2
		Abdomen	1
		Mandibular node	1
		Lip	1
	Leiomyosarcoma	Neck	6
		Back	3
		Leg	1
	Lipoma	Site unspecified	5
	Simple mammary adenoma	Mammary	4
	Anal sac carcinoma	Anal sac	2
	Ceruminous gland adenocarcinoma	Pinna	2
	Fibrosarcoma	Site unspecified	2
	Complex mammary adenoma	Mammary	2
	Squamous papilloma	Skin	1
	Eccrine adenoma	Footpad	1
Gastrointestinal	Pancreatic adenocarcinoma	Pancreas	11
	Biliary cystadenoma	Liver	10
	Metastatic adenocarcinoma	Liver	10
	Cholangioma	Liver	7
	Hepatocellular carcinoma	Liver	4
	Cholangiocarcinoma	Liver	2
	Hepatoma	Liver	2
	Malignant neoplasm, NOS	Liver	2
	Round cell tumor, NOS	Liver	2
	Signet ring adenocarcinoma	Stomach, intestine	2
	Tubular adenocarcinoma	Stomach, intestine	2
	Mucinous adenocarcinoma	Stomach, intestine	2
	Pancreatic exocrine adenocarcinoma (metastatic)	Liver	1

Continued

TABLE 9-1
Distribution of Neoplasia in Ferrets Based on 1525 Cases Submitted to the Armed Forces Institute of Pathology (1990-2000)—cont'd

System	Tumor Type	Site	No.
	Carcinoma, NOS	Liver	1
	Pyloric adenocarcinoma	Stomach, intestine	1
	Squamous papilloma	Esophagus	1
Vascular	Hemangiosarcoma	Skin	8
		Subcutis	2
		Spleen	2
		Liver	2
		Peritoneum	1
		Mesenteric node	1
	Hemangioma	Skin	7
		Ear	1
		Pancreas	1
		Spleen	1
		Site unspecified	1
Reproductive	Leiomyosarcoma, low-grade	Ovary	10
		Uterus	3
	Leiomyoma	Uterus	4
		Ovary	1
	Leydig cell tumor	Testis	7
		Ovary	3
	Seminoma	Testis	5
	Granulosa cell tumor	Ovary	4
	Teratoma	Ovary	4
	Sertoli cell tumor	Testis	4
	Sex cord stromal tumor	Ovary	2
	Uterine adenocarcinoma	Uterus	2
	Deciduoma	Uterus	1
	Carcinoma of rete testis	Testis	1
Musculoskeletal	Chordoma	Tail	51
		Cervical	3
		Sacral	1
		Skin	1
	Osteoma	Flat bone	10
	Osteosarcoma	Bone	4
	Rhabdomyosarcoma	Skeletal muscle	1
Nervous	Astrocytoma	Brain	3
	Malignant peripheral nerve sheath tumor	Skin	3
		Eyelid	1
	Schwannoma	Eyelid	2
		Muzzle	1
	Primitive neuroepithelial tumor	Brain	1
	Granular cell tumor	Brain	1
	Meningioma	Brain	1
	Ganglioneuroma	Adrenal gland	1
Urinary	Transitional cell carcinoma	Kidney	4
Special senses	Melanoma	Eye	2
Miscellaneous	Carcinoma, NOS	Site unspecified	2
		Mesentery	1
	Sarcoma, NOS	Skin	6
		Oral cavity	2
		Muscle	4

TABLE 9-1
Distribution of Neoplasia in Ferrets Based on 1525 Cases Submitted to the Armed Forces Institute of Pathology (1990-2000)—cont'd

System	Tumor Type	Site	No.
		Kidney	1
		Mesentery	1
		Lung	2
		Multicentric	1
		Humerus	1
		Mammary gland	1
	Round cell tumor, NOS	Site unspecified	2
		Multicentric	1
		Mesentery	1
		Thorax	1
	Mesothelioma	Abdomen	4
	Malignant mast cell tumor	Multicentric	1

NOS, Not otherwise specified.

this neoplasm in ferrets. Transforming retroviruses are known to be responsible for the development of lymphoma in other species, including humans, cats, and rabbits. Erdman et al.[14] in 1995 demonstrated the transmissibility of this neoplasm between ferrets by using cell-free inocula, furthering this theory, although a prolonged incubation time was required. *Helicobacter mustelae*, a ubiquitous inhabitant of the stomach of ferrets, has been circumstantially incriminated in the development of gastric adenocarcinoma,[15,17,21] which is enhanced when coupled with ingestion of chemical carcinogens as promoters, as well as in the development of gastric B-cell lymphomas.[11]

3. Early neutering. There is widespread speculation that early neutering at 4 to 6 weeks of age, a common practice in the United States, may be responsible for the high incidence of adrenal neoplasia in this country. In Europe and Australia, where this is not practiced, adrenal neoplasia is rarely seen. A recent publication in The Netherlands[31] indicated a link between age at neutering and age at the onset of hyperadrenocorticism; however, it did not show an increased incidence of hyperadrenocorticism in ferrets neutered at an early age.
4. Light cycles. It has been suggested that the ferret's innate sensitivity to light may be upset by Americans' predilection for housing ferrets indoors with artificial lighting. In Europe, where most ferrets are housed outdoors and exposed to natural lighting cycles, the incidence of neoplasia, especially adrenocortical, is greatly decreased.[4]
5. Diet. Theories abound concerning the impact of commercially prepared diets on the development of neoplasms in ferrets. The higher concentration of carbohydrates in commercially available food in the United States has been suggested as a primary cause for the increased incidence of insulinoma compared with rates seen in other countries, where raw whole prey (e.g., rats, mice) are fed as the dietary staple.[4]

INCIDENCE AND BEHAVIOR

Our knowledge of ferret neoplasia grows year by year; however, a few general comments about neoplasia in ferrets are warranted. The data presented here (1525 cases), as well as that reported by others,[2,4,6,8,24] are only an approximation of the distribution of neoplasia in North American ferrets. A number of factors affect the reporting of neoplasms for this species, including the economic status of the owner, proximity to veterinarians experienced in ferret diseases, opportunity for qualified histologic examination, and methods of reporting and retrieval. In spite of these factors, we believe that certain generalizations about the incidence of neoplasia in this species can be made.

Overall, the endocrine system appears to be the most common site of neoplasia in ferrets (see Table 9-1 and reports by Li et al.[24] and Brown[4]). Pancreatic islet cell tumors (insulinomas) are the most common neoplasms overall, with adrenocortical neoplasms the second most common. In these studies, lymphoma was both the most common hematopoietic neoplasm and the most common malignancy. Between 12% and 20% of cases in each study had multiple tumor types, with insulinoma and adrenocortical carcinoma most often seen concurrently.[4,24] However, the presence of multiple tumor types in an individual animal should not be interpreted as a neoplastic syndrome arising from a common tumorigenic mechanism. In a study of 66 cases in which ferrets had multiple concurrent neoplasms,[24] there was no evidence of an association between tumor type and multiplicity. Because endocrine neoplasia is extremely common today in ferret bloodlines in North America, it seems reasonable that multiple tumors would develop over time in middle-aged or geriatric ferrets.

TUMORS OF THE ENDOCRINE SYSTEM

Most neoplasms in domestic ferrets in North America arise in the endocrine system, chiefly as islet cell tumors and adrenocortical tumors. In the neoplasms we reviewed (Table 9-1), endocrine neoplasms accounted for 53% (805 of 1525) of the total. Although these are extremely common neoplasms in ferrets, these neoplasms may be slightly overrepresented because of their relatively obvious symptomatology and their response to surgical excision. Although we briefly discuss these neoplasms, detailed information is presented in Chapter 8.

Insulinoma

Islet cell tumors, known as insulinomas because of their secretion of this glucose-regulating hormone, are the most common neoplasm in our review (25% [382 of 1525]; see Table 9-1) as well as in reports by Li et al.[24] (21%) and Brown[4] (38%). In these studies, the average age of ferrets with islet cell tumors was 5 years; there is no sex predilection.

Insulinoma in the ferret progresses differently than in the dog and cat, in which it is highly malignant with marked metastatic potential and a short survival time. In ferrets, surgical removal may result in a prolonged disease-free state.

Therapeutic approaches for the treatment of insulinoma in ferrets are reviewed in Chapter 8. Surgical excision is the preferred course of treatment for symptomatic animals with hypoglycemia. In a recent clinical study,[36] partial pancreatectomy resulted in the longest disease-free intervals and survival times (365 and 668 days, respectively), followed by simple nodulectomy (234 and 456 days, respectively). Medical treatment alone resulted in a mean disease-free interval of 22 days and a mean survival time of 186 days. Owners should be informed of the potential for recurrence of clinical signs of the disease, even with surgery.

Adrenocortical Neoplasms

The second most common neoplasm in ferrets occurs in the adrenal cortex (see Table 9-1). Our review included 380 "true" neoplasms of the adrenal cortex (129 adenomas, 251 carcinomas; 25% of overall neoplasms). Furthermore, 439 cases of adrenocortical hyperplasia, which present with identical symptoms, were also identified. The average age of ferrets with adrenal disease was 4.8 years, which is consistent with reports by Brown[4] and Weiss et al.[35] The cause of the high incidence of adrenal disease in ferrets is currently unknown and a subject of great speculation; however, recent reports[4,30,31,34] suggest that anterior pituitary hyperfunction may have a key role in the development of these lesions.

The combination of cutaneous, behavioral, and reproductive signs exhibited by most ferrets with adrenal disease contributes significantly to the frequency of their presentation for treatment (see Chapter 8). The differentiation of hyperplasia, adenoma, and carcinoma is difficult to make on the basis of clinical signs or laboratory findings and is usually based on histologic examination. Although early literature reports suggested an increased incidence of neoplasia in the left adrenal cortex (perhaps because its comparative ease of removal), results of our survey indicate that the distribution of adrenocortical neoplasms approaches 50% (1:1.06, left vs right). A total of 16% (60 of 380) of adrenal neoplasms in this review were bilateral, either at presentation or over time, including those cases in which a hyperplastic lesion was seen in one gland and a neoplasm in the other.

Although a wide range of medical and surgical approaches exists for removal of adrenal neoplasms (see Chapter 8), some personal observations are warranted at this point. Surgical excision of proliferative adrenocortical lesions (to include neoplasia and the more common finding of cortical hyperplasia) is the treatment of choice. Medical treatment at this time should be restricted to the amelioration of clinical signs in nonsurgical candidates. There is currently no evidence that medical treatment inhibits the progression of these lesions or diminishes the risk of metastatic disease or hemoperitoneum associated with large neoplasms.

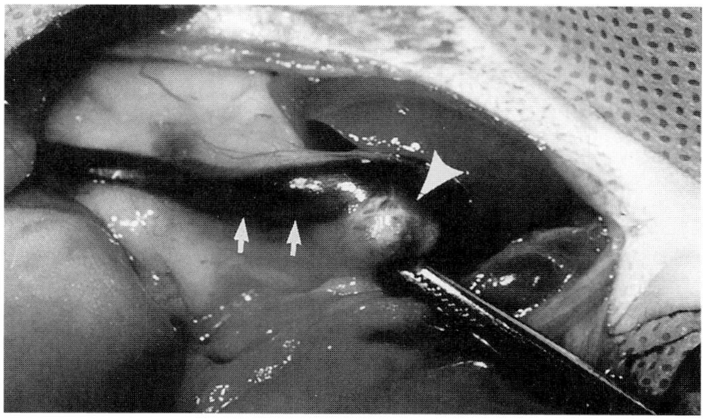

Figure 9-1 Carcinoma of the right adrenal gland (*arrowhead*) in a ferret, demonstrating the proximity between these neoplasms and the caudal vena cava (*arrows*).

Because of its proximity to the vena cava (Fig. 9-1), surgical excision of the right adrenal gland is often a significant challenge for most practitioners. In my practice (C.A.W.), we have achieved excellent results with a wide array of techniques, including liquid nitrogen cryosurgery (584 cases) and carbon dioxide laser (48 cases). In ferrets in which the neoplasm occludes the vena cava by 50% or more, en bloc excision of the neoplasm and the affected section of vena cava may also be performed. This procedure should be approached with care because postsurgical death may occur in ferrets with rapidly growing invasive malignancies that have not yet developed adequate collateral venous return. In such cases, obstruction of venous return leads to hypoxic damage and infarction in multiple organs.

Although common, adrenal carcinoma in the ferret, as opposed to the dog and cat, has low metastatic potential. In this review, only 6% (15 of 267) of ferrets with adrenal carcinoma had evidence of metastasis, primarily to the liver (69% [11 of 16]).

TUMORS OF THE HEMATOLYMPHATIC SYSTEM

Lymphoma (malignant lymphoma, lymphosarcoma) is the most common malignancy in the domestic ferret and the third most common neoplasm overall, following islet cell tumors and adrenocortical neoplasia. Lymphomas most commonly arise spontaneously; however, horizontal transmission of malignant lymphoma in ferrets with cell or cell-free inoculum has been documented.[14] This finding, coupled with the occasional clustering of lymphomas in a single facility, has prompted speculation that lymphosarcoma in the ferret may be the result of a retroviral infection.[12] A viral agent has not yet been isolated from cases of lymphosarcoma in the ferret.

Several variants of lymphoma exist in the ferret. Although various classification schemes for lymphoma exist, including those based on human lymphoma,[1,10,13] the following classification scheme based on broad cell type and distribution is both reproducible and relevant to practitioners.

The most commonly seen form of lymphoma, occurring primarily in older ferrets, is the lymphocytic form. In this variant, the neoplastic cell is a mature, well-differentiated lymphocyte; the lymph nodes are the most affected sites, resulting in peripheral lymphadenopathy, with visceral spread and organ failure occurring late in the course of disease. A second form, the lymphoblastic form, is seen primarily in young ferrets less than 2 years of age. Visceral neoplasms early in the course of disease characterize this form, in which the neoplastic cell is a large, immature lymphocyte. In most cases, the thymus, spleen, and liver are involved, resulting in profound organomegaly. An enlarging thymic neoplasm often results in compression of the lung lobes, dyspnea, and pleural effusion and may often be misdiagnosed as pneumonia or heart disease. A third relatively uncommon form, which is characterized by combinations of peripheral lymphadenopathy, visceral tumors, and the predominant cell type, is a lymphoblast with occasional bizarre karyomegalic or multinucleate forms known as the immunoblastic polymorphous variant.

Terminology involving lymphoma classification can be confusing. *Lymphosarcoma* (malignant lymphoma or lymphoma) denotes solid tissue tumors in organs or lymph nodes throughout the body. However, if neoplastic cells are seen in both the bone marrow and the peripheral blood, a diagnosis of *lymphocytic leukemia* can be made. *Chronic lymphocytic leukemia* indicates a more mature form and the distribution of lymphocytes in the peripheral blood, with total leukocyte counts rarely exceeding normal. *Acute lymphocytic leukemia* suggests lymphoblasts in the bone marrow as well as in the peripheral blood, with leukocyte counts well in excess of normal. True lymphomas are far more commonly seen than leukemias (a ratio of 11:1 in this review).

Clinical Signs and Gross Lesions

Adult (lymphocytic) form Overall, the adult form is the most common variant in ferrets because of its predilection to affect animals over the widest age range (2 to 9 years). Because the neoplastic process is associated with mature lymphocytes, the course of disease is prolonged and longer survival times are seen. Owners often notice clinical signs well before the disease state reaches a critical point. Many cases are associated with cycles of illness and apparent recovery, which may be precipitated by treatment with antibiotics or steroids. In most ferrets with lymphocytic lymphoma, generalized lymph node enlargement is the most common sign (Fig. 9-2), but at times animals are seen simply for chronic lethargy, inappetence, and weight loss. Occasionally only a single node may be enlarged at presentation. In the absence of visibly or palpably enlarged nodes, clinical signs are generally vague and nonspecific. In addition to general malaise, gastric ulcers may be seen as a reaction to the stress of chronic disease.

When evaluating node size, practitioners are cautioned not to be misled by the large accumulations of fat that often surround peripheral nodes (especially the popliteal and axillary nodes) of older ferrets, which may be grossly mistaken for generalized lymphadenopathy. The gross appearance of a neoplastic node is a hard lump often described as a marble, whereas fat-encased normal nodes of geriatric animals are usually soft and pliable. A quick needle aspiration of suspect nodes generally yields an answer. If the aspirate is acellular with abundant greasy fat on the slide, the possibility of lymphoma is greatly lessened.

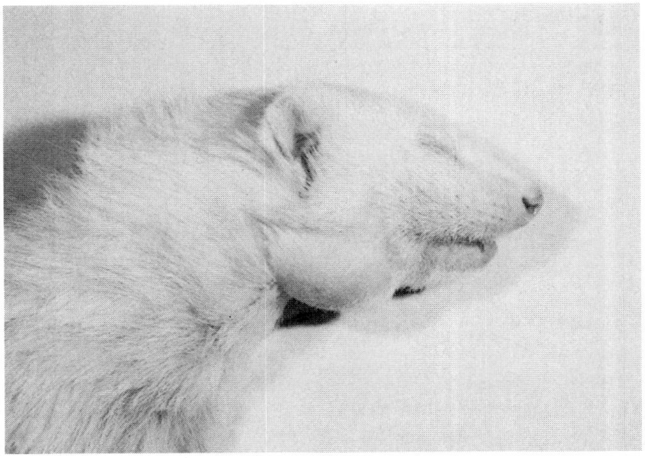

Figure 9-2 Presentation of cervical lymph node enlargement characteristic of adult-onset (lymphocytic) lymphoma.

Juvenile (lymphoblastic) form The infiltration of visceral organs by blastic lymphocytes in the juvenile form results in clinical signs referable to the affected organs. The most common presentation is diffuse enlargement of the liver, spleen, and thymus (Fig. 9-3). Organomegaly of the spleen and liver can be tolerated to a much greater extent in the relatively distensible abdomen than can expansion of the thymus in the bony cage of the thorax. Neoplastic enlargement of the thymus quickly impinges on the ability of the lungs to expand, resulting in exer-

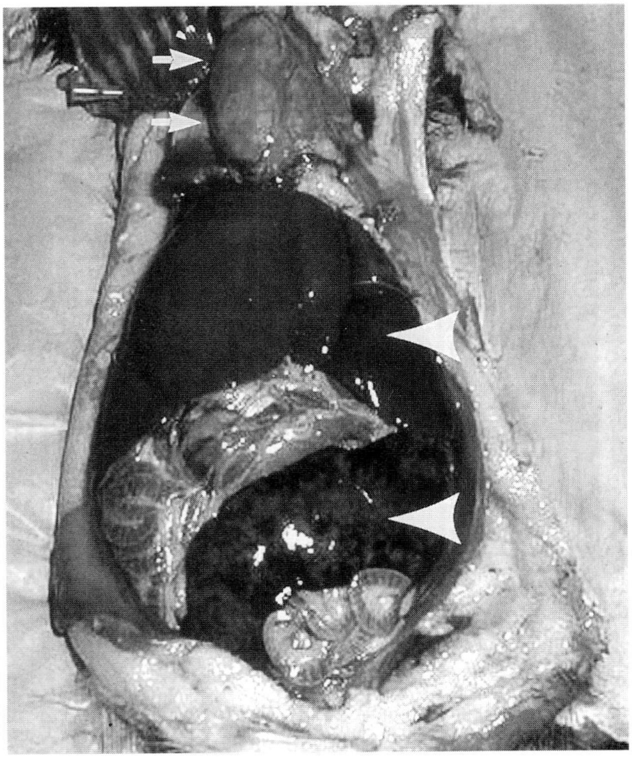

Figure 9-3 Juvenile lymphoma in a 1-year-old ferret. Note thymic mass (*arrows*) and marked hepatosplenomegaly (*arrowheads*) as a result of massive infiltration by this neoplasm.

cise intolerance, increased respiratory rate, dyspnea, and possibly pleural effusion. In such cases, the onset of clinical signs is abrupt because owners may not notice significant impairment until the disease has reached life-threatening proportions. Neoplastic cells may be seen in any organ, including the bone marrow. The incidence of bone marrow infiltration and leukemia is highest in this form of disease. Infiltration of the gastrointestinal tract by neoplastic cells may present vague gastrointestinal signs suggestive of a number of diseases, including a gastric foreign body.

Immunoblastic polymorphous form The progression of the immunoblastic polymorphous form of this disease parallels that of the juvenile form; however, ferrets of all ages can be affected. The combination of immunoblasts, large atypical lymphocytes, Reed-Sternberg–like cells, lymphoblasts, and small lymphocytes has been associated with certain retroviral-associated lymphomas in humans and has given an early clue that ferret lymphomas may be associated with viral infection.[13] This form of lymphoma primarily affects visceral organs, has a short survival time after diagnosis, and is most commonly found in the midwestern United States.

Other forms Cutaneous (epitheliotropic) lymphoma (Fig. 9-4) is of T-cell origin and possesses a mature lymphocytic phenotype and a profound affinity for infiltrate epithelial structures, such as the epidermis and hair follicles. It alone among the ferret lymphomas does not warrant a poor prognosis at onset because prolonged survival times (possibly up to 3 to 4 years) are associated with it, especially in cases in which cutaneous lesions are rapidly surgically excised. Cutaneous lymphoma in ferrets does not necessarily progress to systemic involvement. Epitheliotropic lymphoma is commonly seen in the feet and extremities of ferrets, resulting in grossly swollen, hyperemic, alopecic feet. If untreated, lesions grow in size and multiply. Complete surgical excision of cutaneous lesions may result in prolonged disease-free intervals; chemotherapeutic attempts, both topical and systemic, have generally proved to be unsatisfactory.[22,29]

Mucosa-associated lymphoid tissue lymphomas also have been reported in four ferrets.[11] Considered akin to lymphomas associated with *H. pylori* infection in humans, these neoplasms arise in the stomach of ferrets infected with *H. mustelae*.

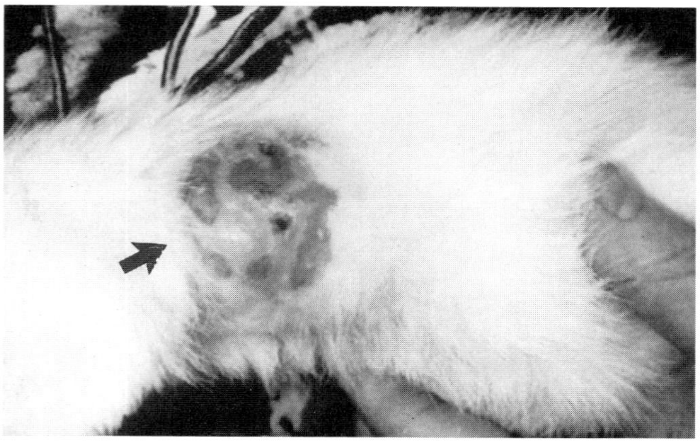

Figure 9-4 Cutaneous lymphoma in a ferret. Surgical excision of this ulcerated neoplasm (*arrow*) was accomplished; despite several recurrences, the ferret was still alive 3 years later.

Diagnosis

Diagnosis of all forms of lymphoma involves direct visualization of neoplastic cells. Excisional biopsy of affected nodes or visceral tumors is best because it allows evaluation of cellular morphology as well as architectural effacement, which may be required in cases composed of well-differentiated lymphocytes. Needle biopsy samples of visceral organs (thymus, liver, spleen) in young animals with suspected juvenile-onset lymphoma may be acceptable for diagnosis. Needle biopsy samples of lymph nodes generally do not yield significant architectural information to confirm a diagnosis of lymphoma.

Avoid biopsy of intraabdominal nodes whenever possible; severe reactive hyperplasia to chronic bowel inflammation may be marked in older ferrets and indistinguishable from lymphoma. Peripheral nodes, such as popliteal and prescapular nodes, are less likely to be affected by local inflammation, and excisional biopsy of these nodes is easily accomplished; complications of this procedure are extremely rare. Definitive diagnosis of lymphoma is best accomplished by a pathologist experienced in the evaluation of ferret lymph nodes because there is often great overlap between the histologic picture of lymphoma and other nonneoplastic causes of lymphadenomegaly.

Aspiration is frequently performed as part of an initial examination, especially when clinical signs point strongly to lymphoma. False readings because of sample preparation, reactive changes, and well-differentiated neoplasms may occur. The possibility of false-negative results is increased when aspirates of visceral organs are obtained.

The cytologic hallmarks of lymphoma are a monotonous population of lymphocytes and the absence of peripheral blood elements. A range of cell size and type, or the presence of other types of white blood cells in aspirated nodes, is not consistent with a diagnosis of lymphoma. In forms of leukemia, bone marrow aspiration may be performed by the proximal femur with an 18- to 20-gauge spinal needle. In most cases of leukemia, the bone marrow is hypercellular and often monomorphic, with a significant decrease or total absence of normal marrow elements.

Pathologists are commonly asked to evaluate splenic aspirates from animals with enlarged spleens. In our experience, at least 95% of these cases are the result of extramedullary hematopoiesis (see Chapter 38). Evidence of erythrocytic precursors and megakaryocytes and abundant peripheral blood should lead to a diagnosis of extramedullary hematopoiesis. Splenic lymphosarcoma is characterized by the presence of a monomorphic population of cells with large nuclei, prominent nucleoli, an absence of erythrocytic precursors, and minimal blood elements. Additionally, mitotic figures should be present.

Results of a CBC and cytologic examination of peripheral blood smears may yield valuable information but are rarely diagnostic for lymphoma. Affected animals may show mild to marked anemia and variable leukocyte counts. Lymphocyte counts may vary widely; levels as high as 90,000/mm^3 may be seen in leukemic cases.[4] Alternatively, older ferrets with chronic disease may become lymphopenic after months or years.[10] Persistently elevated lymphocyte counts should not be used as evidence of lymphoma. As in other species, chronic smoldering infection is the most common cause of lymphocytosis in the ferret. The ubiquitous nature of *Helicobacter* and coronavirus infection in the U.S. ferret population has tremendous potential for inciting this nonspecific change in ferrets. Atypical circulating lymphocytes may occasionally be seen in ferrets with lymphoblastic lymphoma and are more likely to be seen in animals exhibiting lymphopenia.[1,4,10]

Clinical chemistry findings are not considered diagnostic in cases of lymphoma. Abnormalities often reflect only significant replacement of organs by neoplastic infiltrates. Hepatic enzyme concentrations may be elevated in cases of lymphoma. Hypercalcemia has been documented in cases of T-cell lymphomas in ferrets.[1,4,10]

Other clinical tests may yield diagnostic information. Radiographs can be especially valuable, especially in cases of juvenile lymphoma. A large density cranial to the heart, with or without pleural effusion, should immediately raise suspicion of lymphoma in a ferret of any age. Pleural effusion may also be identified by thoracic radiographs; however, effusions may be seen in younger ferrets with other diseases (most commonly cardiomyopathy). Microscopic examination of fluids obtained by thoracocentesis may yield clues to the cause of the effusion. Mature lymphocytes are usually the most prominent cell type in cardiac effusions, and centrifugation of these may yield a cytologic picture identical to that seen with lymphoma. Removal of effusion in some cases may reveal thymic neoplasms (or enlarged hearts) that were previously obscured. Ultrasonography, frequently accompanied by fine-needle aspiration, may also be a useful tool.

Treatment

Ferrets generally tolerate the use of common chemotherapeutic agents in lymphoma protocols well; however, only about 10% experience remission. Several factors may contribute to this apparent lack of success:

1. Concurrent disease. Animals with concurrent adrenal disease or insulinoma, two very common diseases that strike the same age group as most cases of lymphoma, may significantly complicate chemotherapeutic protocols.[4]
2. Inappropriate use of chemotherapeutic agents. Successful chemotherapy often relies on the complex interaction of agents given at specific intervals. The choice of agents based on expense, availability, or ease of administration will affect success rates.
3. Resistance to chemotherapeutic agents. It is well documented that ferrets previously treated with prednisone for other conditions (insulinoma, inflammatory bowel disease, pemphigus) have a diminished response to prednisone when it is subsequently used as part of a chemotherapeutic protocol.[4,38]

It is best to give lymphoma patients a poor prognosis at the outset of chemotherapy. Longer periods of remission have generally been reported in animals with lymphocytic (adult-onset) forms of lymphoma.[4] Because of the variable and generally slow progression of adult-onset lymphomas, it is often difficult to assess the true benefits of chemotherapy. In fact, one group of ferrets survived 2 years (considered the upper limit of remission) with no treatment.[10]

Treatment of lymphoma in ferrets should follow a careful evaluation of the patient's age, concurrent disease and therapy, type of lymphoma, and distribution and staging of tumors. Ferrets with tumors of the stomach, intestine, bone marrow, or liver generally have the poorest response to therapy.[4] Removal of focal lesions (single nodes, spleen, and so on) may be of benefit before initiating chemotherapy.[1,4,10]

Multiple chemotherapeutic protocols have been used in ferrets and are presented in Tables 9-2 and 9-3. The following generalizations and cautionary statements should be noted before chemotherapeutic agents are used in ferrets:

TABLE 9-2
Chemotherapy Protocol I for Lymphoma*

Week	Day	Drug	Dose
1	1	Prednisone	1-2 mg/kg PO q12h and continued throughout therapy
	1	Vincristine	0.025 mg/kg IV
	3	Cyclophosphamide	10 mg/kg PO or SC
2	8	Vincristine	0.025 mg/kg IV
3	15	Vincristine	0.025 mg/kg IV
4	22	Vincristine	0.025 mg/kg IV
	24	Cyclophosphamide	10 mg/kg PO or SC
7	46	Cyclophosphamide	10 mg/kg PO or SC
9	63	Prednisone	Start decreasing the dose gradually to 0 over the next 4 wk

Modified from Brown SA: Ferrets. *In* Jenkins JR, Brown SA, eds. A practitioner's Guide to Rabbits and Ferrets. Lakewood, CO: American Animal Hospital Association, 1993, pp 87-89.

*A CBC should be obtained weekly during therapy (spare the cephalic veins). Stop vincristine if WBCs are <2000 or PCV is <25% and begin antibiotics. Check CBC the following week and resume therapy if rebounding. After therapy is discontinued, continue to monitor CBC results and perform physical examinations at 3-month intervals.

TABLE 9-3
Chemotherapy Protocol II for Lymphoma*

Week	Drug	Dosage
1	Vincristine	0.025 mg/kg IV
	L-Asparaginase	400 IU/kg IP
	Prednisone	1 mg/kg PO q24h and continued throughout therapy
2	Cyclophosphamide	10 mg/kg SC
3	Doxorubicin	1 mg/kg IV
4–6	As weeks 1–3 but discontinue asparaginase	
8	Vincristine	0.025 mg/kg IV
10	Cyclophosphamide	10 mg/kg SC
12	Vincristine	0.025 mg/kg IV
14	Methotrexate	0.5 mg/kg IV

From Rosenthal KE: Ferrets. Vet Clin North Am 1994; 24:19-20.

*Protocol is continued in sequence biweekly after week 14.

1. Chemotherapeutic agents should be used carefully to minimize risks to the patient, technician, and veterinarian. Intravenous chemotherapeutic agents should be administered through a vascular access port[27] or a well-maintained catheter to an anesthetized or sedated ferret. Extravasation of most chemotherapeutic drugs often results in extensive tissue damage and loss of the vein for the remainder of the treatment period.
2. Consultation with a veterinary oncologist and referral should be considered for veterinarians whose experience with these agents is limited.
3. Careful and frequent monitoring of the clinical status and blood values, to include a weekly platelet count and a CBC, should be part of every chemotherapy protocol.

Other chemotherapy agents have been used in the treatment of ferrets with lymphoma in addition to those listed in Tables 9-2 and 9-3. For example, doxorubicin (alone and in conjunction with radiation) has been attempted for treatment of lymphoma in ferrets (2 mg/kg IV q21d for 3-5 treatments).[20]

If traditional multiagent chemotherapy is not an option, palliative therapy often results in a significant decrease in tumor burden for several months. All forms of lymphoma tend to be initially responsive to steroids. Adult-onset forms may show a less significant response to the mature lymphocyte's innate steroid resistance; however, all neoplasms tend to recur over a period of months. When tumors recur, they are steroid resistant. Ferrets that have been receiving prednisone therapy for other diseases (insulinoma, chronic bowel disease) tend to be resistant to definitive and palliative forms of chemotherapy and have shorter mean survival rates.[4,38] A minimum oral dose of prednisone (2.2 mg/kg q24h) should be used and increased as needed to decrease tumor burden and alleviate clinical signs. Fortunately, steroid-induced gastric ulceration is not common in ferrets, even with high-dose regimens.

Adjunct therapy is an important component of lymphoma treatment. Dietary supplementation with a number of high-calorie, high-protein supplements is often necessary for supporting cancer patients. Gerber Second Foods Chicken (Gerber, Inc., Fremont, MI) is well tolerated by most ferrets, may be fed by hand rather than by syringe, and makes an excellent vehicle for the administration of unpalatable medications.[38] Hill's a/d (Hills Pet Products, Topeka, KS) is also widely used, as are a variety of supplements with high-calorie human supplements as a core ingredient, such as Ensure (Abbott Labs, Abbott Park, IL) or Deliver 2.0 (Mead-Johnson Pharmaceuticals, Evansville, IN) combined with any number of additives. Vitamin and mineral supplementation may be required in animals maintained exclusively receiving these types of supplements.[4,38]

If nutritional supplements are administered by syringe, use a rate of 2 to 5 mL q2-3h. Ideally, ill ferrets can be trained to drink gruel from a saucer or bowl, at which time they can be fed every 4 hours.[38] If these products are used for more than 30 days, the ferret's normal ration should be ground up and added to the mixture. This will ensure that all trace mineral and vitamin requirements are met and facilitate the animal's eventual return to normal rations. Ferrets eating a high-quality feline or ferret maintenance diet generally do not need additional mineral or vitamin supplements.[38]

A key to the proper fluid and nutritional support of the ferret patient is the delegation of this activity to the owner to the greatest extent possible. Many ferret owners are capable of giving subcutaneous fluids and hand-feeding ferrets when such activity is required on an around-the-clock basis. Therefore encourage owners to take an active role in nursing as early in the treatment cycle as possible.

Other types of hematopoietic neoplasms, generally arising from cells of leukocytic lineage, are rarely seen. The spleen is the most common site of origin for these neoplasms. Myelolipoma, a benign neoplasm of immature leukocytes admixed with well-differentiated adipocytes, may occasionally present as a space-occupying mass in the spleen but is of no clinical significance.[23] Thymoma, a neoplasm involving the epithelial and mature lymphocytic elements of the thymus, may present as a mass lesion of the anterior thorax and be easily confused with thymic lymphoma. A report of thymoma in two 5-year-old ferrets[33] noted vomiting, lethargy, and dyspnea in both cases. The antemortem diagnosis and treatment of thymomas are challenging, at best.

TUMORS OF THE INTEGUMENTARY SYSTEM

The skin and subcutis are also common sites of neoplasia in ferrets. In this review (see Table 9-1), 275 primary neoplasms of the skin and subcutis were seen, accounting for an overall incidence of 18%. The classification and distribution of cutaneous neoplasia in this collection are consistent with previous reports.[4,24,26] Of the 275 skin neoplasms reviewed, 77 (28%) were malignant, with 67 (87%) of these representing primary malignancy of the skin or subcutis.

Benign tumors of basal cell origin, including sebaceous adenoma and sebaceous epitheliomas (Fig. 9-5), were most prevalent. These warty exophytic neoplasms, which may attain a large size and ominous appearance (largely as a result of self-trauma), are almost invariably benign. In two long-standing cases, squamous cell carcinomas appeared to have arisen in preexisting sebaceous epitheliomas. These neoplasms occasionally caused irritation to the ferret, and self-trauma may result in local inflammation and infection. Surgical excision is curative and should be performed early.

Mast cell tumors are the second most common skin tumor in ferrets. In contrast to the dog and cat, mast cell tumors in ferrets are universally benign and warrant a good prognosis. In the 83

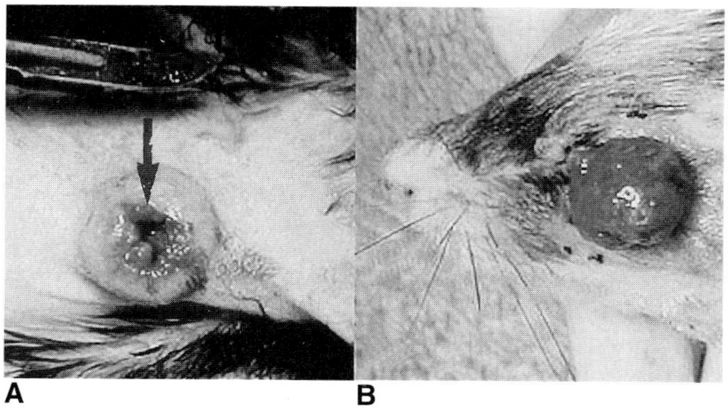

Figure 9-5 Multiple sebaceous adenomas in a ferret on the thorax (**A**) and face (**B**). The neoplasm on the face did not involve the orbit. The center of these neoplasms may occasionally be cavitated because of necrosis (*arrow*). Although impressive in appearance, surgical removal was curative.

cases reviewed, none were considered malignant or showed metastatic potential. These neoplasms are flat, discrete, and have a crusty yellow appearance. Most mast cell tumors in ferrets show minimal infiltration into the dermis and are easily excised; surgical excision is curative. A number of ferrets, however, may show multicentric development of mast cell tumors over time and require additional surgery, but this finding has no prognostic significance.

Neoplasms of apocrine scent glands are the third most common neoplasm seen in the skin and subcutis. These neoplasms are largely restricted to the deeper layers of the skin and subcutis and are often malignant. Apocrine neoplasms are most often seen in areas where scent glands are concentrated (head, neck, prepuce, and vulva). Neoplasms of the prepuce in males are almost exclusively of apocrine scent gland origin. In this review, 19 (79%) of 24 preputial neoplasms (as well as 100% of the less common perianal and perivulvar tumors) were malignant, exhibiting aggressive infiltration of local tissues, metastasis to local nodes, and, occasionally, visceral metastasis. Complete surgical excision of apocrine malignancies is difficult because of their rapid and aggressive growth and the possibility of presurgical metastasis. For this reason, wide excision of all suspected apocrine neoplasms is warranted. In cases of apocrine carcinoma of the prepuce, appropriate surgical treatment may entail amputating the prepuce and a perineal urethrostomy.

Vascular neoplasms of the skin and subcutis occasionally occur in the ferret. In this review, malignant vascular neoplasms (10 cases) of the skin and subcutis were slightly more common than their benign counterparts (eight cases), but all neoplasms were cured after complete surgical excision. Coat color and pigmentation had no prognostic significance for the development of vascular neoplasms because sable animals predominated in both subsets.

Low-grade subcutaneous sarcomas are also occasionally seen in the subcutaneous tissues of the ferret. Although predominantly of smooth muscle origin (10 of 12 in this review), two cutaneous fibrosarcomas were also identified. Most subcutaneous sarcomas are generally low-grade malignancies, with slow rates of growth, low metastatic potential, and a good response to surgical excision. Wide surgical margins should be achieved to ensure complete removal of these infiltrative neoplasms.

Mammary gland neoplasms are rare in domestic ferrets. Six mammary neoplasms were seen in this review, and all were benign (four simple, two complex). Three cases of simple mammary hyperplasia were also observed; similar to that reported previously,[25] two cases were seen in conjunction with adrenal carcinoma.

In this review, other benign neoplasms seen in the skin of ferrets include lipoma (five cases), squamous papilloma (one case), and an adenoma of the eccrine sweat glands of the footpad (one case). Malignant neoplasms include epitheliotropic lymphoma (nine cases), squamous cell carcinoma (six cases), ceruminous gland adenocarcinoma of the ear (two cases), and anal sac carcinoma (two cases).

General guidelines for treatment of cutaneous neoplasms are similar to those prescribed for more traditional pet species. Early surgical intervention is the rule with cutaneous neoplasms; most neoplasms are benign, and most malignancies are low grade and can be successfully treated with early surgical excision with wide margins. Submit sample of all neoplasms for histopathologic evaluation to provide an accurate prognosis. Surgically excise all preputial or perivulvar/perianal neoplasms as early as possible, after careful palpation and radiography, to minimize the opportunity for metastasis.

TUMORS OF THE GASTROINTESTINAL TRACT

Neoplasms of the gastrointestinal tract are common in ferrets and represented 60 primary neoplasms and 83 metastatic neoplasms in this review. The liver, a particularly common site for metastasis, was involved in a total of 71 metastatic neoplasms (including 48 cases of malignant lymphoma, 11 cases of metastatic adrenocortical carcinoma, 10 cases of metastatic adenocarcinoma of unspecified origin, 1 malignant mast cell tumor, and 1 metastatic pancreatic exocrine adenocarcinoma). In contrast to a previous study,[4] metastatic islet cell tumors were not identified.

The liver is also a relatively common site for the development of primary neoplasms. A total of 25 primary neoplasms of the liver were identified, including 17 biliary cystadenoma/cholangiomas, 2 cholangiocarcinomas, 4 hepatocellular carcinomas, and 2 hepatomas. The differentiation of biliary cystadenoma from biliary cyst (a common incidental finding in this species) is made on the basis of one or more of the following factors: presence of clinical symptoms, abnormalities in liver-specific clinical pathology, or expansive growth over time documented by abdominal ultrasound. In several cases, histologically benign biliary cystadenomas (Fig. 9-6) pursued an aggressive course similar to their malignant counterparts, replacing one or more lobes of the liver and ultimately resulting in hepatic failure. Hepatic carcinoma and cholangiocarcinoma in this study consistently resulted in increased concentrations of hepatic enzymes, eventual hepatic failure, and other signs such as profound anemia, hemoperitoneum, and ascites.

In most cases, animals with hepatic neoplasia are seen for nonspecific weight loss, anorexia, and lethargy. A cranial abdominal mass is generally identified by palpation or radiography; clinicopathologic abnormalities are usually mild and nonspecific. Biopsy all hepatic neoplasms, especially those involving

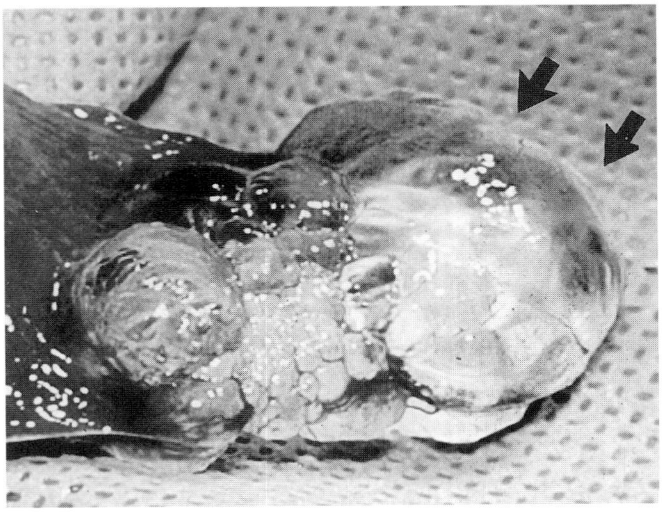

Figure 9-6 Biliary cystadenoma in a ferret. Because of their aggressive nature, these histologically benign tumors *(arrows)* are best treated with lobectomy or, at a minimum, excision with wide surgical margins.

multiple lobes. If the neoplasm is confined to one lobe of the liver, lobectomy is recommended. Because of the aggressive nature of biliary cystadenoma in ferrets, remove any cystic lesion of the liver with wide surgical margins or lobectomy. Neoplasms involving multiple lobes have a poor long-term prognosis; however, survival times of several months or more may be seen with hepatocellular carcinoma. Animals possessing malignancies of the biliary system generally succumb within a short time frame.

The most common neoplasm affecting the gastrointestinal tract is malignant lymphoma (18 primary, 48 secondary in this review). Of the cases in which the gastrointestinal tract was considered the primary site, the intestine was the most common site of origin (9 of 18; 50%), followed by the stomach (3 cases), liver (3 cases), colon (2 cases), and 1 case involving the oral cavity. Lymphoma of the intestine is considered to carry an extremely poor prognosis, is often refractory to treatment, and is associated with the shortest survival times.[4]

Neoplasms of the exocrine pancreas (11 cases in this review) are occasionally seen in the ferret. Most neoplasms exhibit aggressive growth into the surrounding pancreas, but metastasis to distant organs is rare (and only seen in one case in this review). Complete surgical excision may be useful if the neoplasms are discovered early.

Primary neoplasms of the gastrointestinal tract tend to be malignant, with adenocarcinomas arising in the stomach (three cases), intestine (three cases), and rectum (one case). These neoplasms are locally aggressive, often involving multiple layers of the wall with metastasis to local lymph nodes. The predilection of these neoplasms to incite a prominent scirrhous response often results in obstruction and clinical symptoms. This same scirrhous response, however, tends to achieve a type of containment to the neoplasm, allows visualization of the tumor's margins, and facilitates complete excision. The prognosis at this point is affected heavily by the presence or absence of presurgical metastasis.

Tumors of the oral cavity are occasionally seen in ferrets and are usually associated with a poor prognosis. Squamous cell carcinoma appears as an aggressive neoplasm of the gums that invades underlying bone, resulting in tooth loss, disfigurement, and inappetence (Fig. 9-7). One report described treatment of a mandibular squamous cell carcinoma with bleomycin at a dose of 20 U/m^2, which reduced tumor mass.[19] Surgical excision, if attempted, should be attempted early and with wide surgical margins. Various sarcomas, including fibrosarcoma,[4] have been reported in the oral cavity and respond poorly to all forms of treatment.

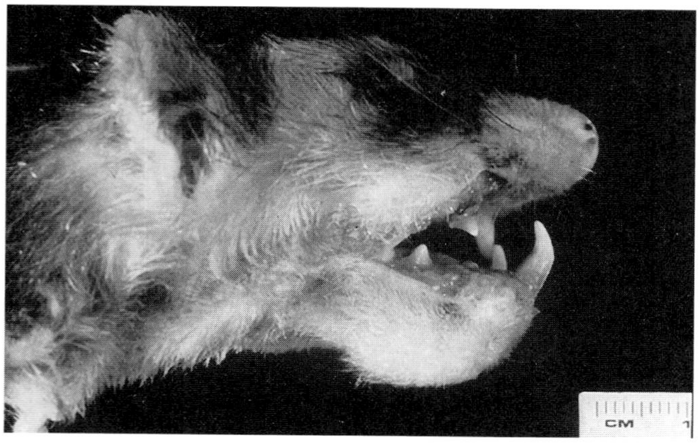

Figure 9-7 Mandibular squamous cell carcinoma in a ferret. There is marked invasion of alveolar bone with tooth loss.

TUMORS OF THE REPRODUCTIVE TRACT

Because of the prevalence of neutering in North American pet ferrets, tumors of the reproductive system are rarely seen in clinical practice. Earlier reports indicated a high prevalence of these neoplasms,[2,8] but the rarity of intact animals in today's pet and laboratory populations has significantly reduced the numbers of the tumors seen. Clinical signs of reproductive neoplasia in ferrets are variable and often nonspecific. Ovarian tumors often result in no overt signs; in a few cases, a failure to breed is noticed. Testicular neoplasms, which commonly arise in retained testes, may result in signs of hyperestrogenism (intact sexual behavior, aggression, prominent musky odor, and poor, greasy hair coat) in affected males. However, with rare exceptions, surgical excision of affected gonads is curative.

In this review, most neoplasms of the ovary and uterine tube were of smooth muscle origin. Although 13 (72%) of 18 were considered malignant based on histologic appearance, evidence of metastasis was not seen and surgical excision was curative.

A total of 13 primary gonadal tumors of the ovary were identified (3 Leydig cell tumors, 4 granulosa cell tumors, 4 teratomas, and 2 sex cord stromal tumors). Ovarian neoplasms are most commonly identified as incidental findings during routine spays. Teratomas may attain a size that is obvious on routine palpation or may be identified by survey radiographs as a result of the presence of bone within the tumor mass. One Leydig cell tumor metastasized to a regional lymph node.

Testicular neoplasms occurred most commonly in cryptorchid testes in this review. Multiple neoplasms may be seen in retained testes, and in one case four distinct neoplasms (interstitial cell, seminoma, Sertoli cell, and a carcinoma of the rete testis) were seen. A total of 17 testicular neoplasms were identified (7 Leydig [interstitial] cell tumors, 5 seminomas, 4 Sertoli cell tumors, and 1 carcinoma of the rete testis). One Sertoli cell tumor metastasized to the liver.

Nonmuscular tumors of the uterine tube are extremely rare in ferrets. One uterine adenocarcinoma and one deciduoma were seen. Implantation sites in female ferrets or even uterine biopsy samples from pseudopregnant animals may be mistaken for uterine carcinoma on histologic examination as a result of the profound atypia of symplasmal cells.

TUMORS OF THE MUSCULOSKELETAL SYSTEM

Neoplasms of the skeletal system are not uncommon in ferrets and generally result in a clinical appearance that is obvious to both owner and practitioner. Tumors of the skeletal muscles, however, are extremely rare; only one example, a rhabdomyosarcoma, was identified (1 of 1524 [<0.07%]).

Chordomas (56 cases in this review) are the most common neoplasm of the musculoskeletal system in the ferret (comprising 79% of the musculoskeletal neoplasms reviewed). They most commonly appear as irregularly round, white-gray, firm, clublike swellings of the tail tip. This low-grade malignancy arising from primitive notochord is most commonly seen at the tip of the tail but may arise in vertebrae in any region of the spinal column.[9] These neoplasms are locally aggressive, destroying the vertebral body in which they arise,[9] but have minimal metastatic potential (with only one report of metastasis after surgical intervention).[39] Radiographs of affected vertebrae reveal a focally extensive vertebral lesion that is both lytic and proliferative.

Chordomas of the tail tip are easily treated by amputation but carry a poor prognosis when affecting other parts of the spinal column. Because of their aggressive nature, extirpation from affected vertebrae is currently not feasible, and eventual loss of function and pathologic fracture will inevitably result. Previous reports of chondrosarcoma of the tail tip, as well as reports that may be obtained from histologic examination of current cases, should be viewed with skepticism.

True tumors of bone (osteomas and osteosarcomas) are occasionally seen in ferrets. Osteomas most commonly arise on flat bones, including the skull and ribs, and progress slowly. Surgical removal may occasionally be accomplished; however, many osteomas regrow when excision is incomplete. Osteosarcomas are rarely reported in ferrets[37] but may arise either on flat or long bones. These malignancies are locally destructive and are best treated by amputation, if possible. Surgeons are cautioned that noncore biopsy samples of malignant bone tumors may result in an errant diagnosis because of the presence of pronounced periosteal reactions overlying the osteosarcomas.

Chondromas and chondrosarcomas, neoplasms of chondrocytic cells, are rare tumors of flat bones that have been occasionally reported but not described in detail.[4,24] Pathologists unfamiliar with the histologic interpretation of ferret tissue sections may confuse this neoplasm with chordoma.

Tumors of skeletal muscle are extremely rare in ferrets. Rhabdomyosarcomas, malignant tumors of skeletal muscle, have been reported[6,24] and one was present in this review. These neoplasms are treatable by radical excision, if possible.

TUMORS OF THE NERVOUS SYSTEM

Neoplasms of the nervous system are rare in ferrets. These tumors can be divided into those of the central nervous system, affecting the brain, and those of the peripheral nervous system, affecting the peripheral nerves and ganglia. Tumors of the central nervous system generally result in neurologic signs, whereas those of the peripheral nervous system result in space-occupying lesions, usually in the subcutis. In this review, neural tumors were seen in only 12 (0.8%) of 1525 neoplasms, with 5 neoplasms in the brain and 7 in the peripheral nerves of the skin and subcutis (see Table 9-1).

Central nervous system tumors are the third most common cause of neurologic signs in ferrets, after insulinoma and bacterial meningitis/encephalitis. Central nervous system neoplasia should only be considered when these two syndromes are conclusively ruled out. Clinical signs associated with these tumors are quite variable and often nonspecific. Lateralizing signs (such as turning toward the side of the lesion), ataxia, cranial nerve deficits, normocellular cerebrospinal fluid, and uncontrolled seizure activity in the presence of a normal blood glucose level are suggestive of, though not specific for, a central nervous system neoplasm.

In this survey, astrocytomas (three cases) were the most common primary brain tumor. These glial neoplasms are generally diagnosed after euthanasia for severe neurologic deficits. They are locally aggressive within the neuropil and resection is not considered feasible.

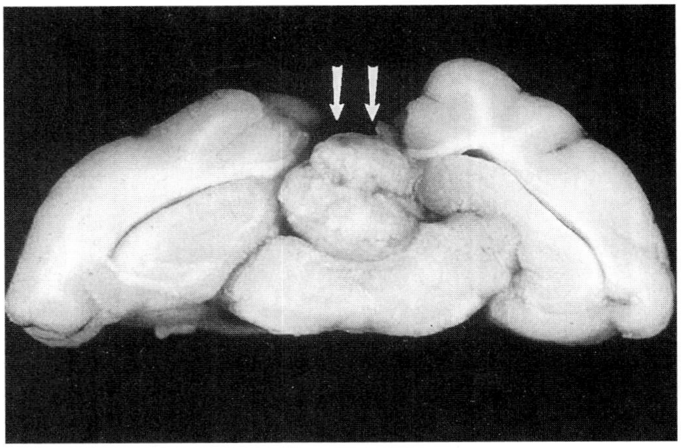

Figure 9-8 Meningioma *(arrows)* in the diencephalon of a ferret. This discrete neoplasm compresses the adjacent cerebrum and brainstem. *(Courtesy Dr. Michael Garner, Northwest ZooPath, Monroe, WA.)*

One granular cell tumor was present in this review. Similar to the only reported case in the literature,[32] this neoplasm presented as a space-occupying mass within the cerebrum and brainstem, which was diagnosed at necropsy in an animal with severe neural deficits, including blindness and seizures. The origin of granular cell tumors in ferrets is currently unknown. Another nonresectable tumor seen in this review that has not been previously reported is a primitive neuroepithelial tumor.

A single meningioma was also observed (Fig. 9-8). This neoplasm was a discrete tumor extending downward from the meninges of the cranium and caused compression and atrophy of the cerebrum and brainstem as well as profound neurologic deficits. This neoplasm has previously been reported only once.[24] Of all of the primary brain tumors, meningiomas show the most promise for surgical excision because they are discrete neoplasms arising from the meninges and, in this limited number of cases, do not infiltrate the neuropil. Antemortem diagnosis is challenging, however.

Neoplasms of the peripheral nervous system carry a significantly improved prognosis over those in the central nervous system because they tend to be restricted to the skin and subcutis. Prognosis is based on the degree of malignancy and infiltration of local tissue. In this review, both benign and malignant peripheral nerve sheath neoplasms were identified. Malignant peripheral nerve sheath tumors as a general rule exhibit rapid growth and tend to infiltrate adjacent tissue to a higher degree than their benign counterparts, rendering complete excision more difficult. In many cases, repeat surgeries are required for a cure. Although these neoplasms may be seen at any site in the body, the tissues of the head (and, interestingly, the eyelid) appear to be a common site of origin (Fig. 9-9). Tumors of nerve sheath origin may be misdiagnosed as fibrosarcoma or leiomyosarcoma when immunohistochemical procedures are not used; however, the prognosis of these three low-grade malignancies is not appreciably different. Schwannoma is a similar neoplasm of perineural cells that generally has a benign course. These tumors should be surgically excised as quickly as possible

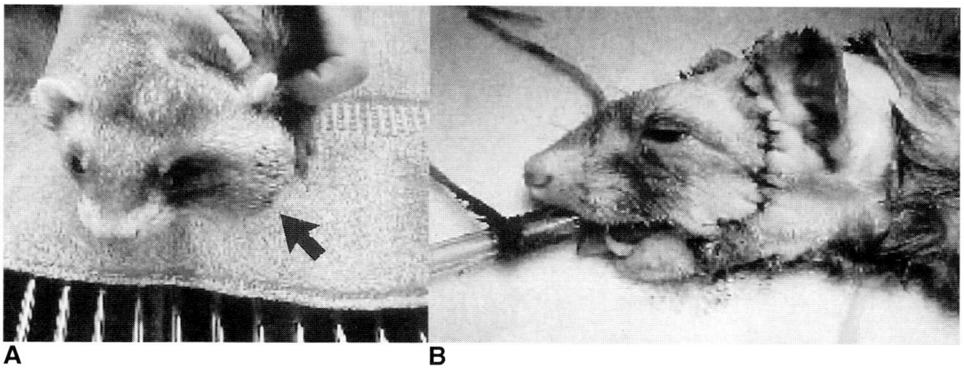

Figure 9-9 Preoperative (A) and postoperative images (B) of a malignant peripheral nerve sheath tumor (*arrow*) in a ferret. The tumor was removed by cryosurgery; however, facial nerve paralysis was encountered after surgery. Recurrence resulted in eventual euthanasia of this patient. *(Courtesy Dr. Darrell Kraft, Woodinville, WA.)*

after diagnosis because growth in areas with high skin tension may result in large defects that are difficult to close.

Ganglioneuromas are rare neoplasms of the peripheral nerve ganglia. The single case reported in this review bears a marked similarity to previously reported cases[24] in which a well-differentiated neoplasm with neurons and glia in a matrix of neural tissue was present in close proximity to the right adrenal gland. Close examination is required to differentiate these nodules from normal ganglia on a histologic basis; however, these tumors tend to be much larger than ganglia—ranging up to 1.5 cm in diameter. Ganglioneuromas have no apparent clinical signs and are often misjudged to be adrenal tumors on gross inspection.

TUMORS OF THE URINARY SYSTEM

Neoplasms involving the urinary system are rare in ferrets. Transitional cell carcinoma of the kidney is the most common; these neoplasms have also been reported in the urinary bladder.[4] In the kidney, transitional cell carcinomas arise in the renal pelvis,[3] eventually causing outflow obstruction and hydronephrosis. Metastasis has not been reported from this site, and unilateral nephrectomy may be curative if early diagnosis is achieved.

In the bladder, transitional cell carcinoma generally results in a poor prognosis. Because the presenting signs are vague, diagnosis is generally achieved only after extensive local invasion has occurred.[4] Dysuria and incontinence may be presenting signs and initially ascribed to cystic prostatic disease or crystalluria. Urinalysis, including the examination of urinary sediment, and contrast radiographic techniques may be helpful to identify this neoplasm; definitive diagnosis is made by surgical biopsy.[4] It is likely that these tumors, once identified, would prove a surgical challenge, especially in the area of the trigone. For unresectable tumors, chemotherapeutic agents that inhibit cyclooxygenase-2 (COX-2) enzymes have shown promise in dogs and may ameliorate clinical signs and prolong life in ferrets; other more traditional agents such as doxorubicin, cisplatin, and cyclophosphamide may also be useful. However, appropriate dosages of all of these agents for the treatment of this and other types of invasive carcinomas have not been defined.

Renal carcinomas and renal adenomas have also been reported in ferrets.[4,24] These unilateral neoplasms of the kidney are most often encountered at necropsy because the majority tend to be slow growing with low metastatic potential. Renal neoplasms generally present as cystic areas on ultrasound examination; however, the high incidence of renal cysts in domestic ferrets would likely preclude further diagnostic workup on the basis of this finding. Renal carcinoma may occasionally result in hemoperitoneum and require emergency nephrectomy.

TUMORS OF THE RESPIRATORY SYSTEM

Neoplasms involving the lung are generally of metastatic origin, although one undescribed primary neoplasm of the lung has been reported.[24] In this review, two cases of malignant lymphoma, one case of metastatic adenocarcinoma, and one poorly differentiated sarcoma of uncertain cause were identified at necropsy. In most cases, pulmonary metastasis of these neoplasms would likely go unnoticed; chemotherapy, however, might be of benefit in metastatic lymphoma.

OTHER MISCELLANEOUS NEOPLASMS

Two neoplasms of structural elements that may be seen in any organ are neoplasms of endothelium and smooth muscle.

Hemangiomas and hemangiosarcomas are occasionally seen in ferrets. In this study, 27 (2%) of 1525 vascular neoplasms were identified, with most arising in the skin or subcutis (18 of 27; 67%). Endothelial neoplasms, however, also were seen in the liver, spleen, pancreas, lymph node, and free-floating in the abdomen. Although 16 of 25 neoplasms showed histologic evidence of malignancy, only one showed evidence of metastasis. Most cutaneous vascular neoplasms are malignant, but they are low-grade malignancies with slow growth and no metastatic potential (Fig. 9-10). Complete excision of these tumors is curative. Rarely, multiple hemangiosarcomas may be seen; however, the prognosis for these cases is no different than that for animals with single neoplasms.

The prognosis, however, for animals with hemangiosarcoma within the abdomen is guarded. These tumors tend to grow more aggressively within abdominal organs and may rupture at any time, seeding the abdomen with metastatic tumors or resulting in fatal hemorrhage. Early surgical intervention should be the rule when the neoplasm is restricted to a single site. An incidence of 22% of hepatic hemangiosarcoma was reported in one colony[7]; the cause of this high incidence is uncertain, and this phenomenon has not been repeated since.

Neoplasms of smooth muscle are extremely common in ferrets. Smooth muscle is a structural component of blood

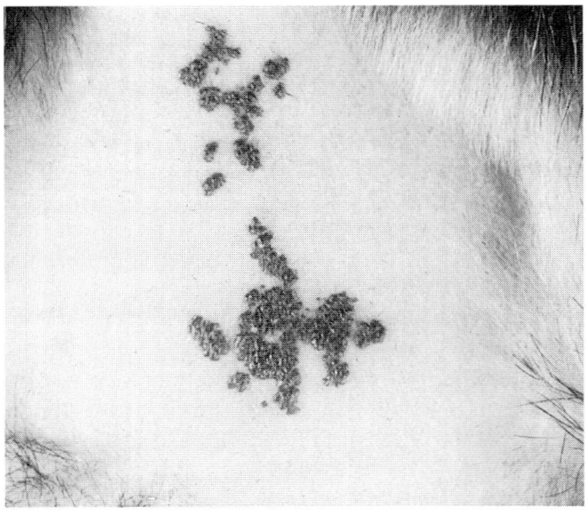

Figure 9-10 Benign cutaneous hemangioma in a ferret.

vessels; erector pili muscles of hair follicles along the dorsal midline and tail; and the predominant muscle in the gastrointestinal, reproductive, and lower urinary tracts. Additionally, smooth muscle is seen in the capsule of the ferret adrenal gland.[18] In this review, 48 (3%) of 1525 of the tumors were of smooth muscle origin: 5 leiomyomas and 43 leiomyosarcomas. The prognosis of a malignant smooth muscle tumor and a benign one, regardless of the site, is similar. Although they may attain a large size, they have little metastatic potential and excision is considered curative at any location.

Leiomyosarcomas of the adrenal capsule are occasionally encountered in ferrets[18] and may result in confusion on the part of the practitioner and the pathologist. These neoplasms may lead practitioners to perform adrenalectomy on normally functioning adrenal glands. The presence of the tumor may also mask the presence of proliferative adrenocortical lesions from the pathologist unless multiple sections at 1 mm or more are examined.

Smooth muscle tumors of the skin are also common findings and likely arise from smooth muscle associated with hair follicles.[28] Surgical excision of these tumors is considered curative and, in general, a good prognosis is warranted.

Leiomyosarcoma is also often seen in association with organs of the reproductive system. The ovary is a common site for development of this neoplasm, and the number of tumors seen would likely be much greater if not for the high frequency of neutering of North American ferrets. As opposed to other domestic species, smooth muscle tumors of the gastrointestinal tract are not common.

Mesotheliomas are uncommon malignancies of ferrets that carry an extremely poor prognosis.[40] These tumors arise in the abdominal cavity and spread extensively before the appearance of clinical signs. The most common clinical sign in affected animals is profound ascites ("malignant" ascites).[40] Abdominocentesis and identification of clusters of atypical mesothelial cells may aid in diagnosis. Because mesothelial cells may be seen in any abdominal tap, take care to prevent misdiagnosis.

Anaplastic neoplasms are those in which the level of cellular differentiation is below that needed to identify a cell of origin. Neoplasms tend to recapitulate their tissue of origin morphologically (e.g., insulinomas look like islets of Langerhans, pancreatic exocrine tumors look like exocrine acini). Sophisticated techniques may yield clues to a tumor cell's origin even if it does not resemble the parent tissue. Immunohistochemical procedures to identify tissue-specific intermediate filaments or ultrastructural analysis of cellular organelles by electron microscopy may identify characteristic organelles for a particular cell type. Today the use of sophisticated techniques at large referral laboratories may help in identifying the origin of a particular neoplasm, thereby enabling the practitioner to develop a strategy for the treatment and prognosis of these tumors. However, many smaller laboratories are not equipped to routinely perform these tests, and a broad diagnosis of poorly differentiated carcinoma, sarcoma, or round cell tumor is often the result.

In this review, the diagnosis of "poorly differentiated" tumors was made only after special staining, immunohistochemical procedures, and electron microscopy were attempted. Even with specialized techniques, a number of malignancies are poorly differentiated enough that they will not disclose information regarding a tissue of origin and are put in broad classifications of epithelial origin (carcinoma) or mesenchymal origin (sarcoma). In some cases, a broad morphologic classification is given (malignant round cell tumor), and in rare instances of extreme anaplasia, even this information cannot be identified and a diagnosis of malignant neoplasm is assigned.

A tissue of origin could not be identified in 32 (2%) of 1525 cases reviewed; however, in 27 of these cases, a broad category of epithelial versus mesenchymal origin was obtained. Even this limited classification has therapeutic importance, because epithelial and round cell tumors tend to be significantly more responsive to chemotherapy than the sarcomas. Sarcomas of the skin were the largest single classification of poorly differentiated tumors but the most responsive to treatment (i.e., surgery.) Because sarcomas of the skin tend to have low metastatic potential, a definitive identification of cell of origin (smooth muscle, skeletal muscle, fibrocyte, etc.) is of little clinical importance. However, the remainder of the poorly differentiated neoplasms generally carry a poor prognosis, especially those present in abdominal organs.

REFERENCES

1. Batchelder MA, Erdman SE, Li X, et al: A cluster of cases of juvenile mediastinal lymphoma in a ferret colony. Lab Anim Sci 1996; 46:271-274.
2. Beach JE, Greenwood B: Spontaneous neoplasia in the ferret *(Mustela putorius furo)*. J Comp Pathol 1993; 108:133-147.
3. Bell RC, Moeller RB: Transitional cell carcinoma of the renal pelvis in a ferret. Lab Anim Sci 1990; 40:537.
4. Brown S: Neoplasia. *In* Hillyer EV, Quesenberry KE, eds. Ferrets, Rabbits, and Rodents: Clinical Medicine and Surgery. Philadelphia, WB Saunders, 1997, pp 99-114.
5. Caplan ER, Peterson ME, Mullen HS, et al: Diagnosis and treatment of insulin-secreting pancreatic islet cell tumors in ferrets: 57 cases (1986-1994). J Am Vet Med Assoc 1996; 209:1741-1745.
6. Chesterman FC, Pomerance A: Spontaneous neoplasms in ferrets and polecats. J Pathol Bacteriol 1965; 89:529-534.
7. Cross BM: Hepatic vascular neoplasms in a colony of ferrets. Vet Pathol 1987; 24:94-95.
8. Dillberger JE, Altman NH: Neoplasia in ferrets: eleven cases with a review. J Comp Pathol 1989; 100:161-176.
9. Dunn DG, Harris RK, Meis JM, et al: A histomorphologic and immunohistochemical study of chordoma in twenty ferrets *(Mustela putorius furo)*. Vet Pathol 1991; 28:467-473.

10. Erdman SE, Brown SA, Kawasaki TA, et al: Clinical and pathologic findings in ferrets with lymphoma: 60 cases (1982-1994). J Am Vet Med Assoc 1996; 208:1285-1289.
11. Erdman SE, Correa P, Coleman LA, et al: *Helicobacter mustelae*–associated gastric MALT lymphoma in ferrets. Am J Pathol 1997; 151:273-280.
12. Erdman SE, Kanki PJ, Moore FM, et al: Clusters of lymphoma in ferrets. Cancer Invest 1996; 14:225-230.
13. Erdman SE, Moore FM, Rose R, et al: Malignant lymphoma in ferrets: clinical and pathological findings in 19 cases. J Comp Pathol 1992; 106:37-47.
14. Erdman SE, Reimann KA, Moore FM, et al: Transmission of a chronic lymphoproliferative syndrome in ferrets. Lab Invest 1995; 72:539-546.
15. Fox JG, Dangler CA, Sager W, et al: *Helicobacter mustelae*–associated gastric adenocarcinoma in ferrets *(Mustela putorius furo)*. Vet Pathol 1997; 34:225-229.
16. Fox JG, Dangler CA, Snyder SB, et al: C-cell carcinoma (medullary thyroid carcinoma) associated with multiple endocrine neoplasms in a ferret *(Mustela putorius)*. Vet Pathol 2000; 37:278-282.
17. Fox JG, Wishnok JS, Murphy JC, et al: MNNG-induced gastric carcinoma in ferrets infected with *Helicobacter mustelae*. Carcinogenesis 1993; 14:1957-1961.
18. Gliatto JM, Alray J, Schelling SH: A light microscopical, ultrastructural and immunohistochemical study of spindle-cell adrenocortical tumors of ferret. J Comp Pathol 1995; 113:175-183.
19. Hamilton TA, Morrison WB: Bleomycin chemotherapy for metastatic squamous cell carcinoma in a ferret. J Am Vet Med Assoc 1991; 198:107-108.
20. Hutson CA, Kopit MJ, Walder EJ: Combination doxorubicin and orthovoltage radiation therapy, single-agent doxorubicin, and high-dose vincristine for salvage therapy of ferret lymphosarcoma. J Am Anim Hosp Assoc 1992; 28:365-368.
21. Lee A: *Helicobacter* infections in laboratory animals: a model for gastric neoplasias? Ann Med 1995; 27:575-582.
22. Li X, Fox JG, Erdman SE: Multiple splenic myelolipomas in a ferret *(Mustela putorius furo)*. Lab Anim Sci 1996; 46:101.
23. Li X, Fox J, Erdman SE, et al: Cutaneous lymphoma in a ferret *(Mustela putorius furo)*. Vet Pathol 1995; 32:55-56.
24. Li X, Fox JG, Padrid PA: Neoplastic diseases in ferrets: 574 cases (1968-1997). J Am Vet Med Assoc 1998; 212:1402-1406.
25. Mor N, Qualls CW Jr, Hoover JP: Concurrent mammary gland hyperplasia and adrenocortical carcinoma in a domestic ferret. J Am Vet Med Assoc 1992; 201:1911-1912.
26. Parker GA, Picut CA: Histopathologic features and post-surgical sequelae of 57 cutaneous neoplasms in ferrets *(Mustela putorius furo L.)*. Vet Pathol 1993; 30:499-504.
27. Rassnick KM, Gould WJ III, Flanders JA: Use of a vascular access system for administration of chemotherapeutic agents to a ferret with lymphoma. J Am Vet Med Assoc 1995; 206:500-504.
28. Rickman BH, Craig LE, Goldschmidt MH: Piloleiomyosarcoma in seven ferrets. Vet Pathol 2001; 38:710-711.
29. Rosenbaum MR, Affolter VK, Usborne AL, et al: Cutaneous epitheliotropic lymphoma in a ferret. J Am Vet Med Assoc 1996; 209:1441-1444.
30. Rosenthal KL, Peterson ME: Evaluation of plasma androgen and estradiol concentrations in ferrets with hyperadrenocorticism. J Am Vet Med Assoc 1996; 209:1097-1102.
31. Shoemaker NJ, Schuurmans M, Moorman H, et al: Correlation between age at neutering and age at onset of hyperadrenocorticism in ferrets. J Am Vet Med Assoc 2000; 216:195-197.
32. Sleeman JM, Clade VL, Brenneman KA: Granular cell tumor in the central nervous system of a ferret *(Mustela putorius furo)*. Vet Rec 1996; 138:65.
33. Taylor TG, Carpenter JL: Thymoma in two ferrets. Lab Anim Sci 1995; 45:363.
34. Wagner RA, Bailey EM, Schnieder JF, et al: Leuprolide acetate treatment of adrenocortical disease in ferrets. J Am Vet Med Assoc 2001; 218:1272-1274.
35. Weiss CA, Williams BH, Scott JB, et al: Surgical treatment and long-term outcome of ferrets with bilateral adrenal tumors or adrenal hyperplasia: 56 cases (1994-1997). J Am Vet Med Assoc 1999; 215:820-823.
36. Weiss CA, Williams BH, Scott MV: Insulinoma in the ferret: clinical findings and treatment comparison of 66 cases. J Am Anim Hosp Assoc 1998; 34:471-475.
37. Wilber J, Williams BH: Osteosarcoma in two domestic ferrets *(Mustela putorius furo)*. Vet Pathol 1997; 34:486.
38. Williams BH: Therapeutics in ferrets. Vet Clin North Am Exotic Anim Pract 2000; 3:131-153.
39. Williams BH, Eighmy JJ, Berbert MH, et al: Cervical chordoma in two ferrets *(Mustela putorius furo)*. Vet Pathol 1993; 30:204-206.
40. Williams BH, Garner MM, Kawasaki TA: Peritoneal mesotheliomas in two ferrets *(Mustela putorius furo)*. J Zoo Wildl Med 1994; 25:240-242.

CHAPTER 10

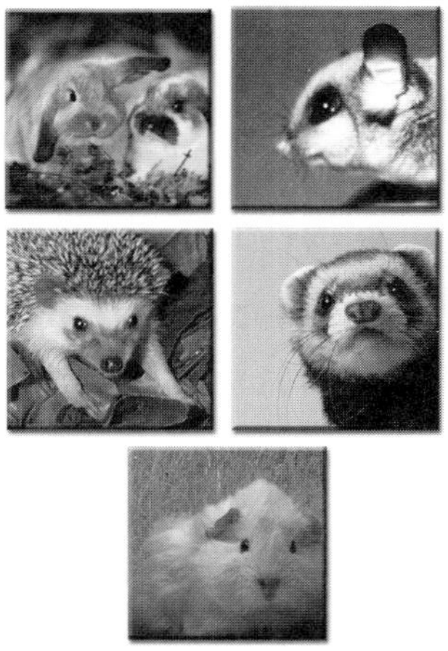

Dermatologic Diseases

Connie Orcutt, DVM, Diplomate ABVP

The initial approach to examining ferrets with dermatologic disease is very similar to that used for other small animals. The signalment (age, sex, and reproductive status) is important in forming the initial list of differential diagnoses. A thorough history should include information on the origin of the ferret, housing, diet, vaccinations, condition of cagemate(s), exposure to other animals, prior or current medical problems, and any skin problems affecting people in the household.

A complete physical examination is extremely important because certain skin conditions are present in conjunction with other clinical signs (e.g., pruritus and alopecia often accompany vulvar swelling in females with adrenal disease). The diagnostic tests performed depend on the refined list of differential diagnoses. Direct microscopic examination of skin scrapings and aural debris aids in diagnosing parasitic diseases. If dermatophytosis is suspected, fungal cultures of the hair and skin samples are indicated. When dealing with wounds and abscesses, a Gram stain of exudate is helpful pending results of bacterial culture and sensitivity testing. With cutaneous or subcutaneous masses, fine-needle aspiration and cytologic evaluation of an impression smear can be done initially, but biopsy is the diagnostic test of choice. With older (>4 to 5 years of age) ferrets, as well as with any ferret suspected of having systemic disease, a complete blood count (CBC), plasma biochemical analysis, and radiographs are important. Other diagnostic tests may include abdominal ultrasonography (e.g., in suspected cases of systemic disease such as adrenal disease or neoplasia) or evaluating plasma androgen levels.

ANATOMY, PHYSIOLOGY, AND HUSBANDRY CONSIDERATIONS

The skin of ferrets contains numerous sebaceous glands. The secretions of these glands sometimes cause the hair coat to have a greasy feel and a characteristic musky odor. Males have more sebaceous glands than do females, and glandular production appears to be under androgenic control.[4,8] Secretions may be so profuse that intact male albino ferrets can appear yellow and dirty. Ferrets do not have well-developed sweat glands and are predisposed to hyperthermia when ambient temperatures are high.[29]

Paired musk-producing glands lateral to the anus store secretions that are expelled when ferrets are agitated, excited, or in estrus. These glands rarely become impacted, but the treatment is the same as for cats. Because most of a ferret's body odor emanates from the dermal sebaceous glands, removing the anal glands does not remove all scent.[4,7] However, neutering does decrease much of the skin odor by reducing androgenic stimulation. Some clinicians do not recommend removing the anal glands unless a specific problem exists.[3]

Ferrets normally have a thick cream-colored undercoat with coarse guard hairs that define the hair coat color. Molting, which usually occurs twice a year, appears to be controlled by hormones responsive to changes in the photoperiod. Estrogens also cause hair loss and weight loss in ferrets.[19] In both intact and neutered ferrets, the hair coat normally thins in response to an increase in the number of daylight hours and in the ambient temperature (simultaneously with the breeding season)—that is, in the late spring in the northern hemisphere.[19] This molt may result in bilaterally symmetric alopecia of the tail, perineum, and inguinal area, or the ferret may lose most of the guard hairs and appear "fluffy." The spring molt is often more marked in females than in males and is usually more pronounced in intact ferrets. In the late fall, a less pronounced molt occurs at the same time as the density of the light-colored undercoat increases. As a result, the hair coat appears lighter during the fall and winter seasons. As the hair thins, red-brown, waxy deposits, often sebaceous secretions, may be visible on the skin. Hair that is shaved during seasonal hair loss may not regrow for several weeks or months. Hair regrowth, such as after shaving for surgery or after treatment of adrenal gland disease, sometimes imparts a bluish appearance to the skin, which may be mistaken for bruising or cyanosis. This apparent discoloration resolves as soon as hairs erupt from the skin. Both sexes accumulate subcutaneous fat beginning with the fall molt and resolving in the spring. As a result, body weight can fluctuate by 30% to 40%.[29]

If dietary requirements are not met, the hair coat can become dry and dull. Providing ferrets with a suitable diet, with or without short-term administration of a fat supplement, usually corrects this problem. Ferrets should be fed high-quality kitten, cat, or ferret food (see Chapter 1). Wild ferrets spend considerable time in underground dens with high humidity. Pet ferrets housed in dry environments (e.g., heated homes in the winter) may scratch or have flaky skin. The use of a cool air humidifier or application of an emollient skin spray have been recommended as treatments.[5]

With the exception of biotin deficiency, nutritional deficiencies are usually not a cause of alopecia.[4] Avidin, an enzyme found in raw egg white, binds biotin and has been reported to cause bilaterally symmetric alopecia in ferrets fed diets containing greater than 10% raw eggs.[8,36] Feeding raw eggs to ferrets is not recommended.

Certain skin or hair problems in ferrets result from self-mutilation or trauma. Ferrets need privacy and should be provided with boxes to hide in or artificial burrows. A ferret with inadequate bedding, nesting, or hiding spots may rub its face on the floor in an attempt to hide and abrade its face. Broken hair shafts can resemble those seen with dermatomycoses.[7] Intact females may pull hair from themselves to use as bedding material.[19] Ferrets can be quite rough during mating and playing and can inflict scratches and bite wounds.

Many pet ferrets are from large breeding farms where animals are tattooed at an early age after neutering. The tattoo is usually inside the pinna and appears as one or two gray or blue dots. On occasion, these dots have been mistaken for skin lesions.

DISEASES

The most common dermatologic lesions in ferrets are those associated with adrenal disease, benign neoplasia, or ear mite infestation. Malignant skin neoplasms, fungal disease, viral disease, and sarcoptic mange are uncommon. Treatment protocols for dermatologic disease, including medication selection and dosages, are often extrapolated from those used for cats.

Ectoparasites

Ferrets are susceptible to most of the ectoparasites that affect dogs and cats. However, other than fleas and ear mites, ectoparasites are rarely seen.

Fleas Flea infestation is occasionally seen in ferrets. As with dogs and cats, *Ctenocephalides* species are usually involved,[15] but *Pulex irritans* can also affect ferrets and other small animals.[6] Fleas are transmitted by direct contact with another animal or a flea-infested environment. Although some ferrets are asymptomatic, clinical signs generally include mild to intense pruritus, especially on the dorsum near the nape of the neck.[7,15,33] With heavy infestations, alopecia may be present on the dorsal thoracic and cervical areas. In addition to self-induced alopecia, ferrets sometimes develop signs of flea bite hypersensitivity, such as papulocrustous dermatitis over the tail base, ventral abdomen, or caudomedial thighs.[18]

Identifying fleas or flea excrement on the animal confirms the diagnosis. Treat the ferret as well as other animals in the household; the environment must also be treated concurrently. None of the treatments discussed below have been approved by the U.S. Department of Agriculture for use in ferrets. Traditional treatment includes flea shampoos, dips, or powders containing pyrethrins, lindane, or carbamates.[18] Toxic reactions occasionally occur with some of these chemicals; pyrethrins are one of the least toxic.[6] Because safe levels have not been established for ferrets,[30] organophosphates are not recommended for topical use in this species.[6] Dichlorvos-impregnated flea collars are also not recommended because they can have toxic effects and can get caught on objects in the environment.[15] Because of the ferret's small body size, use caution when applying any topical medication. Ferrets can ingest sprays and powders while grooming. Be extremely careful when using pesticide dips; some dips can be toxic with prolonged exposure, and ferrets need to be dried and kept moderately warm after dips.[42] When using sprays, first spray a cloth, then rub the cloth on the ferret.

Although newer products that have been developed for flea control in dogs and cats have not been approved for use in ferrets, anecdotal reports of toxicity are uncommon.[6] Topical imidacloprid (Advantage, Bayer Corp., Shawnee Mission, KS) is a flea adulticide that kills on contact. In one study in ferrets, imidacloprid removed the adult flea population and prevented flea reinfestation for 1 week when administered once at a dose of 10 mg/kg and for 3 weeks when administered once at a dose of 0.4 mL 10% imidacloprid.[14] No adverse effects were seen at either dose. Imidacloprid also may have larvacidal activity in the environment.[18] Lufenuron (Program, Novartis Animal Health, Greensboro, NC), an insect growth regulator, kills immature fleas by interfering with chitin production. With this product, there is a lag time of approximately 6 to 8 weeks from the beginning of treatment and the resulting reduced number of adult fleas on the ferret.[6] A dose of 45 mg (half of a cat dose) given orally once a month has been used in ferrets.[6] Fipronil (Frontline, Merial Ltd., Iselin, NJ) is a flea adulticide that also kills ticks. Topical application at half to a full cat dose has been reported anecdotally in ferrets,[6] but the incidence of adverse reactions is unknown. Either imidacloprid or fipronil can be used in conjunction with lufenuron. Selamectin (Revolution, Pfizer, New York, NY) also may be effective (see "Ear Mites" below).

Treatment of the environment is the same as that in households with dogs and cats. Residual chemicals (e.g., microencapsulated formulas of pyrethrins with synergists and diazinon) or methoprene (insect growth retardant preventing fourth instar larva metamorphosis) have been recommended.[18] Potentially less toxic forms of treatment that will also destroy parasites are steam cleaning of carpeting and the application of boric acid salts to the floor or carpet, which desiccate and destroy flea adults and larvae.[6] Prevent pets and humans from coming in contact with any chemicals applied to the environment.

Mites

Ear mites The same ear mite that affects dogs and cats *(Otodectes cynotis)* affects ferrets. The mite is transmitted by direct contact with other infested animals. Ferrets may shake their heads or scratch their ears, but they are more commonly asymptomatic. Other clinical signs vary from inflammation of the external ear canal with accompanying mild pruritus to severe pruritus with excoriations and crusting. Dark brown waxy aural debris is often present; however, this can also be seen in some normal ferrets. The mite is identified by microscopic examination of the aural debris. Although ear mites can reportedly colonize other parts of the body, specifically the perineum,[7] this rarely occurs.

Secondary otitis media or interna with neurologic deficits, most commonly head tilt, has been reported in ferrets with heavy mite infestations.[33] Some authors suggest this syndrome is common in ferrets,[7] but I seldom see this in my practice. Acute onset of head tilt may also result from exuberant ear cleaning with solutions that irritate the vestibular nerve if the tympanic membrane is compromised. Clinical signs in these ferrets generally resolve after treating for mite infestation and any secondary bacterial infection.

To eliminate ear mites, treat all susceptible animals in the household. Gently clean the ears before any treatment, but avoid solutions that can damage the middle ear if the tympanic membrane is ruptured. A common treatment protocol is ivermectin injected subcutaneously at a dose of 0.2 to 0.4 mg/kg repeated every 2 weeks for 3 to 4 treatments. Although this protocol is often successful, some mite infestations are refractory to treatment. Topical treatments include massaging ivermectin into each ear at a dose of 0.5 mg/kg with one half the dose instilled in each ear.[4,35] A topical preparation of thiabendazole, dexamethasone, and neomycin (Tresaderm, Merck Agvet, Rahway, NJ) is also effective.[18] In a study that compared three protocols for treating ear mites in ferrets, results showed that treatment with either the thiabendazole product (2 drops in each ear canal q24h for 7 days, untreated for the next 7 days, then treatment reinstituted for 7 days) or topical ivermectin (1% ivermectin diluted 1:10 in propylene glycol; 0.4 mg/kg divided between each ear canal, then repeated 2 weeks later) was more effective in eliminating mites than parenteral treatment with ivermectin (1% ivermectin diluted 1:4 in propylene glycol; 0.4 mg/kg SC).[33] Topical treatments used alone can fail for several reasons: the ear canal may be too narrow for the medications to penetrate, the ferret may resist treatment, or mites may be present on other areas of the body left untreated.[18] Because of potential toxicity, do not treat with topical and parenteral ivermectin concurrently. Some recommend treating the entire body with flea powder.[18] Take extra care when treating pregnant animals. When high doses of ivermectin were administered to pregnant jills, the rate of congenital defects in kits increased.[18] Thiabendazole is expected to have a wider margin of safety in pregnant animals.[33] Thoroughly clean the environment, including bedding, as part of any treatment protocol.

Selamectin is a semisynthetic avermectin that is approved for use in dogs and cats to control fleas, heartworms, ear mites, and sarcoptic mange mites. Anecdotal reports of use in ferrets at dosages used in cats to treat ear mites have been promising, and reports of adverse effects have been rare.[22] This product is not approved for use in ferrets.

Sarcoptic mange Infestation with *Sarcoptes scabiei,* which also affects dogs and cats, is uncommon in ferrets. This zoonotic parasite is transmitted by direct contact or by fomites. The mite is usually identified by examining a skin scraping; however, false-negative results are possible.

Two different clinical syndromes are seen in ferrets with sarcoptic mange. In the generalized form, clinical signs are focal to generalized alopecia with intense pruritus.[2,18,35] The localized form of the disease, in which only the feet are affected, is seen occasionally. The paws become inflamed, swollen, and crusted and can be very pruritic. In severe cases, the nails may become deformed or even slough; if left untreated, the claws can be lost.[8,18] The layman's term for this form of the disease is *foot rot.*[18]

Treat affected ferrets with ivermectin at an initial dose of 0.2 to 0.4 mg/kg subcutaneously; repeat dosing every 2 weeks until the mites are eradicated. Alternatively, dip the animal once weekly in 2% lime sulfur until 2 weeks after the signs resolve.[39] Disadvantages of lime sulfur dips are discoloration of the fur and the accompanying strong odor. Weekly carbaryl (0.5%) shampoos[18,27,42] or organophosphate dips[37] were previously recommended; however, ivermectin is more effective, simpler to administer, and safer than organophosphates. Use topical or systemic antibiotics for secondary bacterial infections. Treat affected feet with warm water soaks, gentle debridement of crusts, and trimming of diseased claws. Treat all affected animals as well as those in contact with the ferrets, and thoroughly clean cages, bedding, and other materials the ferrets have touched.

Demodectic mange Demodicosis was reported in two ferrets with localized alopecia, yellow discoloration of the skin, and pruritus subsequent to repeated treatment for recurrent ear mite infestations with an ointment containing triamcinolone acetonide.[30] The ferrets had areas of alopecia and seborrhea behind the ears, on the abdomen, in the inguinal area, and on the ventral aspect of the tail. Both ferrets also had a brown ceruminous exudate in the ears. Adult mites and larvae were identified in skin scrapings, biopsy samples, and aural debris.

Both ferrets were dipped in a suspension of 0.0125% amitraz at 7-day intervals for 3 treatments. Two drops of the same solution were instilled in each ear every other day. After this treatment, a few dead mites, but no eggs and no larval stages, were isolated on each ferret. Further treatment consisted of the same protocol every 5 days except that a higher concentration of amitraz (0.025%) was applied to the tail. At the second recheck, all skin scrapings were negative. No adverse signs were reported with this treatment.

Other mite infestations Infestation by the fur mite, *Lynsacarus mustelae,* was reported in 5 ferret kits with ulcerative dermal lesions on the face.[38] Lesions resolved after applying a powder containing permethrin on each kit and cleaning the animals' cage with a permethrin-containing shampoo.

Ticks Ticks can be found on ferrets that are housed outdoors and are reportedly common in ferrets used for hunting (e.g., those in Great Britain).[7,18] Remove ticks from ferrets as from other domestic animals by extracting the entire head from the skin. Because ticks can carry zoonotic diseases, wear gloves and use forceps. Sprays and dips used in cats can be safely used in ferrets.[1] No cases of Lyme disease have been reported in ferrets.

Cutaneous myiasis *Cuterebra* species can cause subdermal cysts in mustelids and have been uncommonly seen in ferrets.[18] Granulomatous masses in the cervical area caused by larval stages of *Hypoderma bovis* are also uncommon.[18] The moving larvae often can be seen through the open pore of the swollen area.

Fly strike, or infestation by the flesh fly *(Wohlfahrtia vigil),* has been reported as a problem by commercial mink and ferret ranchers and by owners who keep ferrets outdoors. Mink kits are attacked during the summer months when 4 to 5 weeks old.[18] Fly eggs laid on the face, neck, or flanks of the kits bore into the skin and cause irritation. Larvae localized in subcutaneous tissues can produce abscesslike lesions.

In any ferret with cutaneous myiasis, remove the larvae intact, if possible, to avoid leaving a nidus of infection or precipitating a systemic response. Debride the wound and use topical antibiotic preparations, with or without systemic antibiotics, to prevent or treat secondary bacterial infections. Allow the wound to heal by second intention.

Viral Disease

Viral disease is a rare cause of dermatopathy in ferrets. Canine distemper virus (CDV) is the important exception. The causative agent, a paramyxovirus, is transmitted by direct contact, aerosol exposure to infected body fluids, or contact with fomites (see Chapter 7). Viremia has been detected 2 days after infection, after which the virus begins replicating in several tissues.[20] By 7 to 10 days after exposure, the ferret becomes anorexic and febrile, blinks as if it is photosensitive, and develops a serous nasal and ocular discharge. Within 10 to 15 days of exposure, a characteristic erythematous and pruritic skin rash develops under the chin, then spreads to the inguinal or perianal region. This generalized dermatitis may be orange tinged and can predispose to secondary pyoderma. The nasal and ocular discharges become mucopurulent, resulting in brown crusts around the face, and the chin, lips, and eyelids can become swollen. A characteristic clinical sign is swelling and hyperkeratosis of the footpads *(hard pad).* Secondary bacterial infections may be observed.

Definitive diagnosis of CDV is difficult. A presumptive diagnosis is based on the presence of distinctive clinical signs as well as a questionable vaccination history. The test of choice to rapidly confirm CDV is a fluorescent antibody test performed on a peripheral blood smear, buffy coat, or conjunctival scraping.[20] In some cases, results of the test can be positive even before the ferret develops pyrexia.[20] Serum antibody titers can also be determined. Because natural immunity to this disease is not seen in ferrets, the titer in an unvaccinated animal should not be high.[9] On histopathologic examination, eosinophilic cytoplasmic and intranuclear viral inclusions are generally widespread in tissues except in skin epithelium and hair follicles, where numbers are fewer.

CDV is a fatal infection in ferrets, although there are anecdotal reports of rare survivors. Death can occur from 12 to 22 days after exposure, with most ferrets dying by 1 week after the onset of clinical signs.[2,9,20] Because of the untreatable and highly infectious nature of this disease, any ferret with a poor vaccination history or suspicious clinical signs should be isolated from other animals. The prognosis is grave, and the only treatment is supportive care.

Fungal Disease

Dermatophytosis Fungal disease involving the skin is uncommon in pet ferrets. Although superficial mycotic skin infections (ringworm) in ferrets are frequently seen by some clinicians,[7] others report them as rare.[2,8] Perhaps this is because of the geographic variation in incidence, which depends on climate. Ferrets are susceptible to infection with both *Microsporum canis* and *Trichophyton mentagrophytes,*[27] although the former is more often described.[2,8] *M. canis* can be transmitted by direct contact or by fomites and is reportedly associated with overcrowding and exposure to cats.[27] Clinical disease is more common in kits and young ferrets and occurs as a seasonal, self-limiting infection.[2,8,17] Dermatophytosis may affect ferrets of any age secondary to immunosuppressive disease (Fig. 10-1). As with dogs and cats, dermatophytosis in ferrets is a zoonotic disease.[17,27]

Skin and hair lesions in ferrets with dermatophytosis are similar to those reported in other species. Dermatologic lesions can begin with small papules that spread peripherally. These can lead to large circumscribed areas of alopecia and inflammation involving all parts of the body. The skin becomes thickened, erythematous, and hyperkeratotic with superficial crusts, and hair shafts may appear broken. Accompanying pruritus leads to excoriation and sometimes secondary pyoderma.

Although clinical signs may be suspicious (especially if other animals or people in the household have skin lesions), dermatophytosis is definitively diagnosed by results of a mycotic culture of a skin scraping or hair sample. Also, fungal organisms can sometimes be appreciated on histologic examination of skin

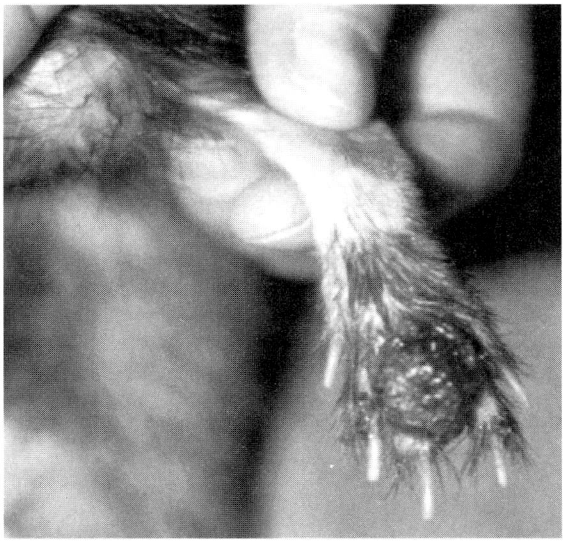

Figure 10-1 Fungal pododermatitis in a 7-year-old male ferret with systemic lymphosarcoma. Cytologic examination of a fine-needle aspirate showed pyogranulomatous inflammation with intralesional fungal hyphae, and a fungal culture grew *Microsporum nanum.*

biopsy samples. *M. canis* may fluoresce, but *Trichophyton* species do not.[7,17] Although some clinicians describe microscopic visualization of fungal arthrospores in skin and hair scrapings that have been mixed with 10% potassium hydroxide,[17] others have not found this method useful.[7]

Many authors report spontaneous remission of clinical signs of dermatophytosis in ferrets.[8,17,27] However, in ferrets that are treated, start by shaving the hair around the lesions. Topical treatments include keratolytic shampoos, povidone-iodine scrubs, and antifungal medications. Griseofulvin has been used at a dosage of 25 mg/kg PO q24h for 21 to 30 days.[8] As with cats, monitor the CBC results every 2 weeks while the ferret is receiving treatment.

Disinfect the entire environment to eliminate infectious spores, which can remain contagious for up to 2 years. Methods of decontaminating the environment include applying dilute (1:10) bleach or chlorhexidine, steam cleaning carpets, changing air conditioning filters, cleaning heating ducts, and vacuuming with prompt disposal of vacuum bags. Treat all animals in the household.

Other fungal infections Systemic mycoses with skin manifestations have been reported infrequently in ferrets. However, systemic mycoses should be included on a list of differential diagnoses for persistent draining tracts and skin eruptions that are unresponsive to antibiotic therapy, especially if other systemic signs are evident (e.g., pneumonia, weight loss, or gastrointestinal signs).[35] *Blastomycosis dermatitidis* was reported in a ferret with pneumonia and an ulcerated lesion with a persistent draining tract in the metacarpal pad.[23] Treatment included oral ketoconazole and intravenous amphotericin B. Infection with *Coccidioides* species was described in a ferret with pyrexia, pneumonia, and a persistent draining tract in the stifle that was nonresponsive to antibiotic therapy.[11] Ketoconazole was used for treatment. Mucormycosis, caused by infection with *Absidia corymbifera*, was reported in ferrets raised for fur in New Zealand.[17]

Bacterial Disease

Ferrets can incur bite wounds while playing, mating, or fighting and can sustain puncture wounds from chewing on objects. These wounds can become infected, resulting in superficial or deep pyoderma, abscesses, or cellulitis. Abscesses can involve the anal glands or remnants of these glands (Fig. 10-2). Causative organisms that are reported most often are *Staphylococcus* and *Streptococcus* species[2,8]; others reported include *Corynebacterium*, *Pasteurella*, and *Actinomyces* species and hemolytic *Escherichia coli*.[16] Abscesses usually become walled off, causing few systemic signs, but in some instances the affected ferret may be febrile and have leukocytosis.

A tentative diagnosis may be reached by examining a Gram stain of discharge aspirated from an abscess. Definitive diagnosis is determined by aerobic or anaerobic bacterial culture and sensitivity testing of the exudate or infected tissue. By sterile technique, lance, excise or debride, and flush abscesses. Place drains in the wound or stent bandages over the wound for wet-to-dry changes. Begin treatment with a broad-spectrum systemic antibiotic while awaiting culture results.

Actinomycosis, or *lumpy jaw*, has been rarely reported in ferrets.[16] *Actinomyces* species are gram positive, anaerobic to microaerophilic bacteria. Infection occurs when bacteria enter

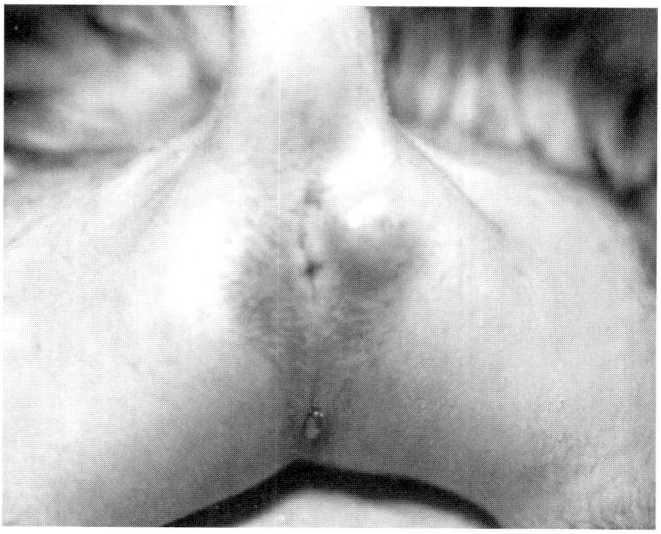

Figure 10-2 Anal gland abscess in a ferret. Anal sacculectomy was performed, and the abscess contents were submitted for aerobic culture. No bacteria were isolated.

wounds to the oral mucosa or are swallowed or inhaled. Actinomycosis is a common opportunistic infection associated with human and feline immunodeficiency virus and feline leukemia virus infections. Clinical signs include cervical masses with sinus tracts containing thick, yellowish-green, purulent material. Reportedly, masses occasionally become large enough to cause dyspnea. Similar clinical signs have been seen with mixed gram-negative bacterial populations isolated from submandibular abscesses.[2] A subcutaneous *Actinomyces*-related granuloma was reported in a ferret with lymphoma.[12] As with any abscessed area, surgically debride and drain lesions. Rely on results of bacterial culture and sensitivity testing for antimicrobial therapy. Empirical treatments that have been suggested for actinomycosis include administering high doses of penicillin or tetracycline.[16]

Neoplasia

A retrospective study of neoplastic diseases in 574 ferrets (1968-1997) reported a 14% incidence of neoplasia involving the integumentary system, making this the third most common system affected.[26] In a literature search of 214 cases of primary neoplasms of the integumentary system in ferrets, benign lesions were predominant, with mast cell tumors, basal cell tumors, and sebaceous cell tumors being the most common.[24] Several of the tumor types described below appear very similar clinically; excisional biopsy should be performed whenever a skin mass is detected. For additional information, see Chapter 9.

Mast cell tumors In ferrets, mast cell tumors generally involve the skin and are benign, being composed predominantly of well-differentiated mast cells and resembling cutaneous mastocytomas of domestic cats.[40] Visceral involvement and malignant behavior of mast cell tumors are rare.

In two retrospective reviews of neoplasia in ferrets, cutaneous mast cell tumors represented 21% to 24% of all neoplasms involving the integumentary system.[24,26] Although mast cell tumors can occur anywhere on the body, they are most common

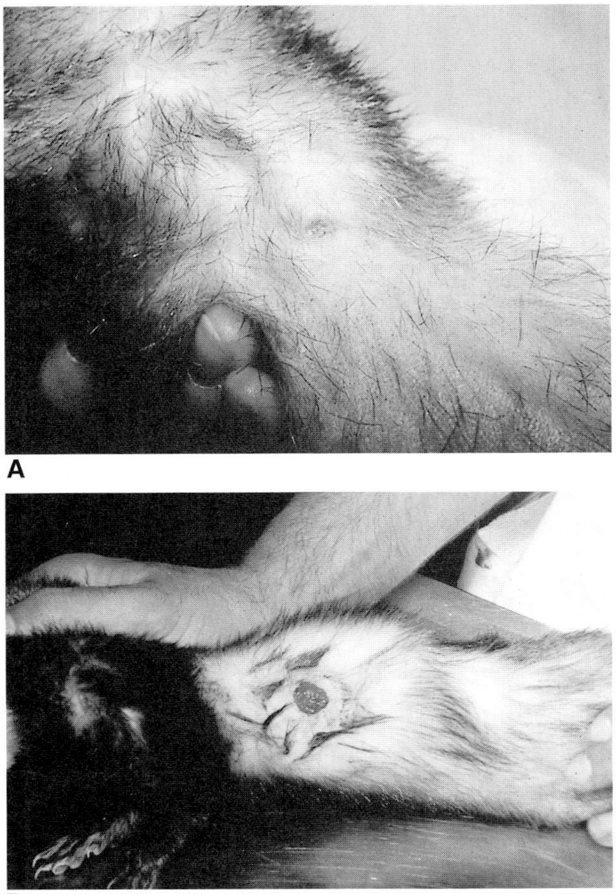

Figure 10-3 A and B, Mast cell tumors on two ferrets. The smaller, erythematous, plaquelike lesion (A) is more typical of the gross appearance of these tumors. Occasionally, mast cell tumors present as larger, ulcerated dermal masses (B).

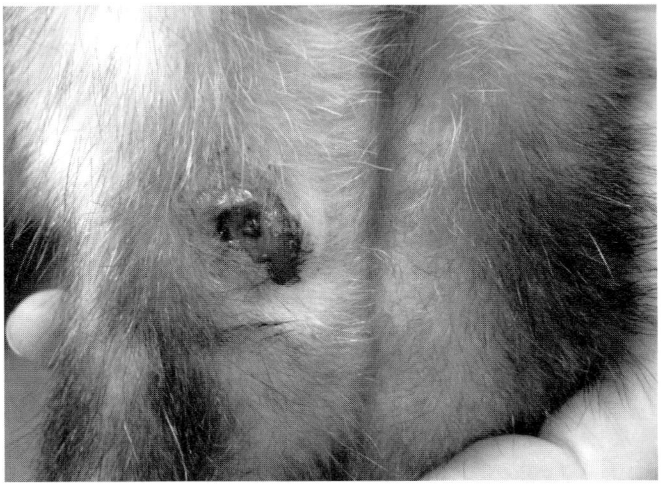

Figure 10-4 This ulcerated lesion on a 4-year-old female neutered ferret involved tissue near the right inguinal mammary gland. The lesion was excised, and the histopathologic diagnosis was sebaceous gland epithelioma.

on the head, neck, shoulders, or trunk. Mast cell tumors usually appear as single or multiple raised, well-circumscribed, hairless nodules that can vary in size from 0.2 to 1 cm. They are often hyperemic (Fig. 10-3). Tumors may be ulcerated or covered with a black, crusty exudate. Some affected ferrets are brought for care because their owners notice this crusty material even though the tumor underneath is still very small and barely raised from the skin surface. Because mast cell tumors are often associated with pruritus, the ulcers may be caused by self-excoriation.

Surgical biopsy provides the definitive diagnosis, but analysis of an aspirate of the mass may reveal mature mast cells. I have not seen any systemic effects from degranulation of mast cells in ferrets after manipulating the dermal mass. Surgical resection is generally curative.[32,35] Some authors describe spontaneous resolution and recurrence of lesions.[2,13,35] New mast cell tumors occasionally develop in the same ferret over time.

Basal cell tumors, sebaceous adenomas, epitheliomas, and cystadenomas In a retrospective study of 57 cutaneous neoplasms diagnosed by biopsy in ferrets, the incidence of basal cell tumors was 58%.[32] Another review reported a 20% incidence.[24] These tumors, which arise from the pluripotential basal cells of the epidermis, have been variably named basal cell tumors, sebaceous cell tumors, or basosquamous-sebaceous tumors.[24] Tumors of basal cell origin can develop anywhere on the body and are usually benign (see Chapter 9).[24,32] Most basal cell tumors are sharply defined, firm, white to pink lesions that are pedunculated or plaquelike and sometimes ulcerate. Recurrence of a basal cell tumor excised from the tail was reported in one ferret, but no other recurrences or metastases have been reported.[32]

Other benign neoplasms include sebaceous adenomas, epitheliomas, and cystadenomas. All these contain neoplastic cells that appear primarily as sebaceous cells.[24] Sebaceous cell tumors, which can develop anywhere on the ferret's body, can be verrucous, inflamed, or ulcerated and up to 3 cm in diameter (Fig. 10-4).[24] In my clinical practice, the prevalence of sebaceous cell tumors in ferrets is nearly that of mast cell tumors and, clinically, the two tumor types often look very similar. In some cases, both tumor types can be present in the same ferret (Fig. 10-5).

Squamous cell carcinoma Squamous cell carcinoma is relatively uncommon in ferrets but has been reported at several anatomic sites, including the cranium, lip, digit, tarsus, thigh, foot pads, and trunk. Both discrete and metastatic forms have been reported.[2,8,21,24,31] These tumors tend to be firm, gray to white, single or multiple nodules or plaques in the skin that occasionally ulcerate. Local invasion is typical, and tumors may metastasize to local lymph nodes and distant organs.[24] I have seen a 5-year-old neutered female ferret with a large, thickened, erythematous, ulcerated perianal squamous cell carcinoma that was nonresectable. The ferret had a second mass in the right inguinal area with an enlarged right inguinal lymph node.

Whenever possible, surgically excise any masses. In most cases, no recurrence of neoplasia after surgical resection has been reported,[31,40,41,43] but length of follow-up for some of the ferrets is unclear.[24] In other cases, tumors have recurred very quickly after excision.[21] Melphalan and bleomycin were tried unsuccess-

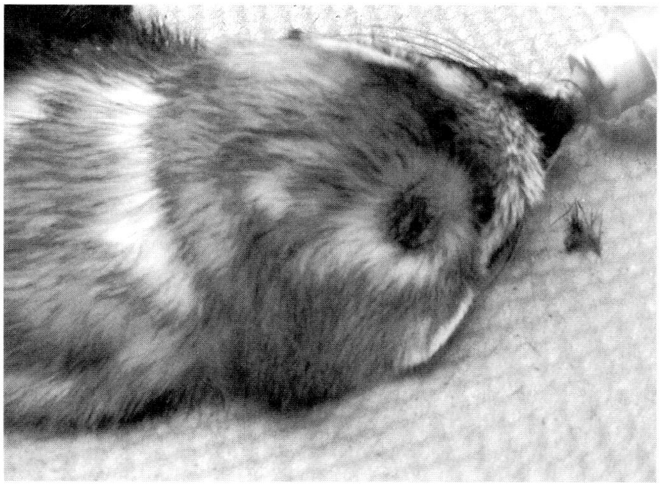

Figure 10-5 This raised, ulcerated dermal mass on a ferret was actually composed of two distinct lesions. Histopathologic diagnosis was sebaceous epithelioma and mast cell tumor.

fully in the treatment of two ferrets with squamous cell carcinoma.[21,31] The prognosis for this tumor type is generally poor.

Adenocarcinoma Adenocarcinomas involving adnexal structures of the skin are reported in ferrets; however, they are relatively uncommon.[2,32] Sebaceous and sweat gland adenocarcinomas were diagnosed in geriatric, captive black-footed ferrets (*Mustela nigripes*).[2] I have seen a slow-growing, broad-based, elevated skin mass on the lateral tail of a young intact male ferret. On excisional biopsy, the mass was identified as a sweat gland adenocarcinoma with local infiltration. Within 2 months, the tumor had metastasized to the deep tissues of the right thigh and perianal area (Fig. 10-6) and a sublumbar mass (possible lymphadenopathy) was seen on radiographs. Two months later, the ferret died suddenly of unknown cause.

Most adenocarcinomas of apocrine scent glands develop in the perineal area. In one report, an infiltrative cutaneous and subcutaneous mass over the anal gland was described in a 7-year-old neutered male ferret.[32] This tumor was excised, and no recurrence or metastasis was reported. A perineal adenocarcinoma with metastasis to an internal iliac lymph node was reported in a black-footed ferret.[32]

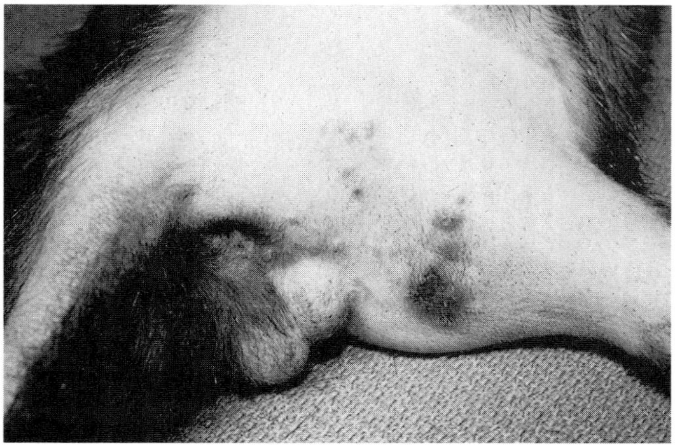

Figure 10-6 Sebaceous gland adenocarcinoma in a ferret. This tumor recurred after resection and spread rapidly.

In a 6-year-old intact male ferret, a 2-cm mass surrounding the preputial orifice was described. Because the tumor was inoperable, the ferret was euthanatized.[32] A well-differentiated adenocarcinoma of sweat gland or preputial gland origin was reported in a male ferret with an acute, fluctuant swelling of its prepuce.[28] This tumor recurred rapidly after each of multiple excisions as well as after radiation therapy and metastasized to the inguinal area. Surgical excision of tumors involving the prepuce may necessitate penile amputation and urethrostomy (see Chapter 12).[15]

Cutaneous lymphoma Cutaneous (epitheliotrophic) lymphoma occasionally occurs in ferrets,[22,25,34] and it should be included in the differential diagnosis of ferrets with chronic pruritus, dermatitis, or alopecia. Cutaneous lymphoma of T-cell origin was diagnosed in an 8-year-old neutered female ferret with generalized progressive, pruritic dermatitis.[34] In a spayed female ferret with severe swelling of all four paws, erythematous skin, and malformed nails, epitheliotropic lymphoma was diagnosed by histopathologic examination of a biopsy sample.[22] After initially responding to medical treatment, this ferret developed systemic lymphoma and was euthanatized. Lymphoma involving the prepuce was reported in a 6-year-old intact male ferret.[32] The tumor presented as a 2-cm ulcerated mass on the prepuce; the inguinal lymph node was also involved.

Other neoplasms involving the skin or subcutis Hemangiomas have been reported in two middle-aged female ferrets.[32] Both hemangiomas were well-circumscribed dermal masses, with one tumor on the pinna and the other in the dorsal lumbar area. No recurrence or metastasis of the masses was reported after resection.

In a review of 57 cutaneous neoplasms in ferrets, six fibromas and two fibrosarcomas were described.[32] There was no site predilection, and the affected ferrets ranged in age from 10 months to 4.5 years. Both tumor types were described as well-circumscribed dermal or subcutaneous masses. In ferrets that were followed up after excision, neither recurrence nor metastasis of either type was reported.

Other cutaneous or subcutaneous tumors in ferrets include hemangiosarcoma,[32] rhabdomyosarcoma,[32] neurofibroma,[24,32] neurofibrosarcoma,[24] histiocytoma,[10,24] myxosarcoma of the subcutis,[24] myelosarcoma,[24] leiomyosarcoma,[35] and papillary cystadenoma.[10]

Endocrine Disease

Endocrine disease, primarily adrenal gland disease, is a very common cause of dermatopathy in ferrets. In fact, adrenal gland disease is the most common cause of progressive and sustained alopecia, often with pruritus, in neutered ferrets (see Chapter 8). Affected ferrets may also develop a strong odor from androgenic stimulation of sebaceous glands in the skin. Other causes of alopecia in both intact and neutered ferrets are estrus, retained ovarian remnants, granulosa cell tumors, luteomas, and fibrosarcomas of ovarian remnants.[4] Hyperestrogenism can be associated with alopecia in female ferrets during estrus (see Chapter

4).[3,7] No clinical cases of hypothyroidism in ferrets have been documented.

REFERENCES

1. Bell JA: Parasites of domesticated pet ferrets. Compend Contin Educ Pract Vet 1994; 16:617-622.
2. Besch-Williford CL: Biology and medicine of the ferret. Vet Clin North Am Small Anim Pract 1987; 17:1155-1183.
3. Brown SA: Preventative health program for the domestic ferret. J Small Exotic Anim Med 1991; 1:6-11.
4. Brown SA: Commonly encountered non-neoplastic disorders of the domestic ferret. Proceedings of the Atlantic Coast Veterinary Conference, Atlantic City, NJ, 1993.
5. Brown SA: Ferret grooming.Veterinary Information Network. Available at: http://www.vin.com/Members/SearchDB/misc/m05000/m01076.htm. Accessed February 24, 2002.
6. Brown SA: Flea control for ferrets. Veterinary Information Network. Available at: http://www.vin.com/Members/SearchDB/misc/m05000/m01077.htm. Accessed February 24, 2002.
7. Burke TJ: Skin disorders of rodents, rabbits, and ferrets. *In* Kirk RW, Bonagura JD, eds. Kirk's Current Veterinary Therapy XI: Small Animal Practice. Philadelphia, WB Saunders, 1992, pp 1170-1175.
8. Collins BR: Dermatologic disorders of common small nondomestic animals. *In* Nesbitt GH, ed. Topics in Small Animal Medicine: Dermatology. New York, Churchill Livingstone, 1987, pp 272-276.
9. Davidson M: Canine distemper virus infection in the domestic ferret. Compend Contin Educ Pract Vet 1986; 8:448-453.
10. Dillberger JE, Altman NH: Neoplasia in ferrets: eleven cases with a review. J Comp Pathol 1989; 100:161-176.
11. Duval-Hudelson KA: Coccidioidomycosis in three European ferrets. J Zoo Wildl Med 1990; 21:353-357.
12. Erdman SE, Moore FM, Rose R, et al: Malignant lymphoma in ferrets: clinical and pathological findings in 19 cases. J Comp Pathol 1992; 106:37-47.
13. Erik S, Robinette J, Basaraba R, et al: Mast cell tumors in three ferrets. J Am Vet Med Assoc 1990; 196:766-767.
14. Fisher MA, Jacobs DE, Hutchinson MJ, et al: Efficacy of imidacloprid on ferrets experimentally infested with the cat flea, *Ctenocephalides felis*. Second International Flea Control Symposium. Compend Contin Educ Pract Vet Suppl 2001; 23(4A): 8-10.
15. Fisher PG: Urethrostomy and penile amputation to treat urethral obstruction and preputial masses in male ferrets. Exotic DVM 2002; 3.6:21-25.
16. Fox JG: Bacterial and mycoplasmal diseases. *In* Fox JG, ed. Biology and Diseases of the Ferret, 2nd ed. Baltimore, Lippincott, Williams & Wilkins, 1998, pp 321-349.
17. Fox JG: Mycotic diseases. *In* Fox JG, ed. Biology and Diseases of the Ferret, 2nd ed. Baltimore, Lippincott Williams & Wilkins, 1998, pp 393-403.
18. Fox JG: Parasitic diseases. *In* Fox JG, ed. Biology and Diseases of the Ferret, 2nd ed. Baltimore, Lippincott Williams & Wilkins, 1998, pp 375-391.
19. Fox JG, Bell JA: Growth, reproduction, and breeding. *In* Fox JG, ed. Biology and Diseases of the Ferret, 2nd ed. Baltimore, Lippincott Williams & Wilkins, 1998, pp 211-227.
20. Fox JG, Pearson RC, Gorham JR: Viral diseases. *In* Fox JG, ed. Biology and Diseases of the Ferret, 2nd ed. Baltimore, Lippincott Williams & Wilkins, 1998 pp. 355-374.
21. Hamilton TA, Morrison WB: Bleomycin chemotherapy for metastatic squamous cell carcinoma in a ferret. J Am Vet Med Assoc 1991; 198:107-108.
22. Kelleher SA: Skin diseases of ferrets. Vet Clin North Am Exotic Anim Pract 2001; 2:565-572.
23. Lenhard A: Blastomycosis in a ferret. J Am Vet Med Assoc 1985; 186:70-72.
24. Li X, Fox JG: Neoplastic diseases. *In* Fox JG, ed. Biology and Diseases of the Ferret, 2nd ed. Baltimore, Lippincott Williams & Wilkins, 1998, pp 405-447.
25. Li X, Fox JG, Erdman SE, et al: Cutaneous lymphoma in a ferret *(Mustela putorius furo)*. Vet Pathol 1995; 32:55-56.
26. Li X, Fox JG, Padrid PA: Neoplastic diseases in ferrets: 574 cases (1968-1997). J Am Vet Med Assoc 1998; 212:1402-1406.
27. Marini RP, Adkins JA, Fox JG: Proven or potential zoonotic diseases of ferrets. J Am Vet Med Assoc 1989; 195:990-994.
28. Miller TA, Denman DL, Lewis GC: Recurrent adenocarcinoma in a ferret. J Am Vet Med Assoc 1985; 187:839-841.
29. Moody KD, Bowman TA, Lang CM: Laboratory management of the ferret for biomedical research. Lab Anim Sci 1995; 35:272-279.
30. Noli C, can der Horst HH, Willemse T: Demodicosis in ferrets *(Mustela putorius furo)*. Vet Q 1996; 18:28-31.
31. Olsen GH, Turk MAM, Foil CS: Disseminated cutaneous squamous cell carcinoma in a ferret. J Am Vet Med Assoc 1985; 186:702-703.
32. Parker GA, Picut CA: Histopathologic features and post-surgical sequelae of 57 cutaneous neoplasms in ferrets (*Mustela putorius furo* L.). Vet Pathol 1993; 30:499-504.
33. Patterson MM, Kirchain SM: Comparison of three treatments for control of ear mites in ferrets. Lab Anim Sci 1999; 49:655-657.
34. Rosenbaum MR, Affolter VK, Usborne AL, et al: Cutaneous epitheliotropic lymphoma in a ferret. J Am Vet Med Assoc 1996; 209:1441-1444.
35. Rosenthal K: Ferrets. Vet Clin North Am Small Anim Pract 1994; 24:1-23.
36. Ryland LM, Bernard SL: A clinical guide to the pet ferret. Compend Contin Educ Pract Vet 1983; 5:25-32.
37. Ryland LM, Gorham JR: The ferret and its diseases. J Am Vet Med Assoc 1978; 173:1154-1158.
38. Schoemaker NJ: Selected dermatologic conditions in exotic pets. Exotic DVM 1999; 1.5:5.
39. Scott DW, Miller WH, Griffin CE: Dermatoses of pet rodents, rabbits and ferrets. *In* Scott DW, Miller WH, Griffin CE, eds. Small Animal Dermatology, 6th ed. Philadelphia, WB Saunders, 1995, pp 1417-1456.
40. Symmers WStC, Thomson APD: A spontaneous carcinoma of the skin of a ferret (*Mustela furo* L.). J Pathol Bacteriol 1950; 62:229-233.
41. Symmers WStC, Thomson APD: Multiple carcinomata and focal mast-cell accumulations in the skin of a ferret (*Mustela furo* L.), with a note on other tumours in ferrets. J Pathol Bacteriol 1953; 65:481-493.
42. Timm KI: Pruritus in rabbits, rodents and ferrets. Vet Clin North Am Small Anim Pract 1988; 18:1077-1091.
43. Zwicker GM, Carlton WW: Spontaneous squamous cell carcinoma in a ferret. J Wildl Dis 1974; 10:213-216.

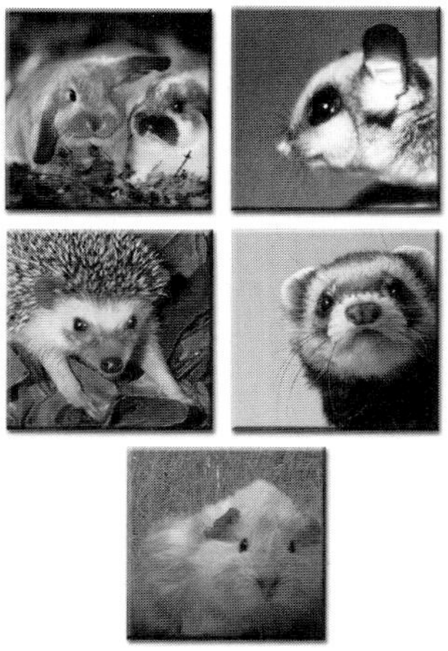

CHAPTER 11

Musculoskeletal and Neurologic Diseases

Natalie Antinoff, DVM, Diplomate ABVP

Primary neurologic and musculoskeletal disorders are not common in pet ferrets. Clinical signs that appear to be caused by primary neurologic disease, particularly posterior paresis, are frequently manifestations of systemic illness. Therefore, a thorough and accurate history-taking and physical examination supported by radiography and laboratory testing are essential to establishing a diagnosis, treatment plan, and prognosis. Fracture management is covered in Chapter 35.

POSTERIOR PARESIS, ATAXIA, AND SEIZURES

Ferrets with neurologic or systemic disease may present with posterior paresis, ataxia, or both. *Posterior paresis*, used here, is synonymous with rear leg weakness. Generalized weakness in ferrets is often more pronounced in the rear legs and may be mistakenly attributed to primary neurologic disease. A ferret that is weak loses the normal upward arch in its back, so that the long axis of its body becomes parallel to the ground when it is standing or walking.

A common cause of posterior paresis or ataxia is hypoglycemia secondary to a pancreatic beta cell tumor, or insulinoma (see Chapter 8). Hypoglycemia can also result from food deprivation or anorexia, vomiting, sepsis, neoplasia, severe hepatic disease, or any metabolic disorder.

Cardiac disease, hypoxia, anemia, and toxin ingestion can result in weakness, ataxia, or central nervous system (CNS) depression.[4,32] Ibuprofen toxicosis has been reported to cause neurologic signs including ataxia, depression, coma, and tremors.[31] Proliferative bowel disease can be associated with ataxia.[11] Discomfort caused by splenomegaly, a caudal abdominal mass, inguinal or sublumbar lymphadenopathy, cystic calculi, peritonitis, prostatic enlargement, or urinary obstruction may mimic ataxia or posterior paresis when severe.

Primary neurologic problems reported as causing posterior paresis or ataxia in ferrets include intervertebral disc disease,[15] plasma cell myeloma,[24] and chordoma[41] involving the spinal column. Infection with Aleutian disease virus has been associated with posterior paresis, urinary incontinence, and tremors (see later discussion and Chapter 6). Potential differential diagnoses for posterior paresis and ataxia in other species, such as thromboembolism, CNS trauma, infection, and other neoplasms, must always be considered. Spinal cord lymphoma is rare but can be associated with pathologic vertebral fracture (Fig. 11-1).

Urinary and fecal incontinence may accompany posterior paresis. Seizures are a common neurologic presentation in middle-aged and older ferrets. Probably, the most common cause is hypoglycemia secondary to insulinoma. Prolonged seizure activity can also result in hypoglycemia. Other potential causes of seizures include toxin ingestion; CNS infection, inflammation, trauma, and neoplasia; and metabolic disturbances such as hepatic or renal failure. Idiopathic epilepsy has not been reported in ferrets.

Diagnosis

Record the medical history and perform a complete physical examination, auscultating carefully for cardiac murmurs or arrhythmias. Ferrets may normally have a respiratory sinus arrhythmia. Palpate for peripheral pulses to evaluate the strength of contraction and to determine the presence of dropped or extra beats. Check mucous membranes for evidence of cyanosis. Palpate the abdomen carefully to detect discomfort, an abdominal mass, urinary calculi, or a distended urinary bladder.

If you suspect primary neurologic disease, perform a complete neurologic and orthopedic examination.[27] Characterize the signs as diffuse or focal, acute or chronic, progressive or static; localize the lesion to areas of brain or spinal cord.[22] Evaluate reflexes and palpate for spinal cord pain or hyperesthesia. The ocular menace response in ferrets is normally diminished or absent.

Evaluate results of a complete blood count (CBC) and plasma biochemical analysis in any ferret with neurologic signs to rule

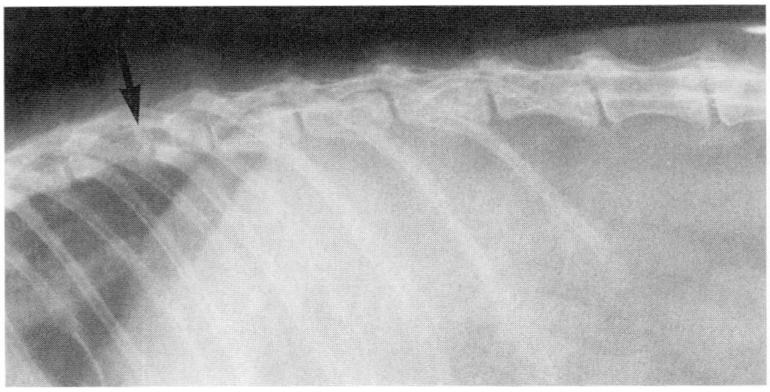

Figure 11-1 Lateral myelogram of a ferret, showing thinning of the dye column at L1 to L2 and a vertebral fracture with compression at T11 *(arrow)*. This was a pathologic fracture associated with spinal cord lymphoma. The ferret had 14 thoracic vertebrae.

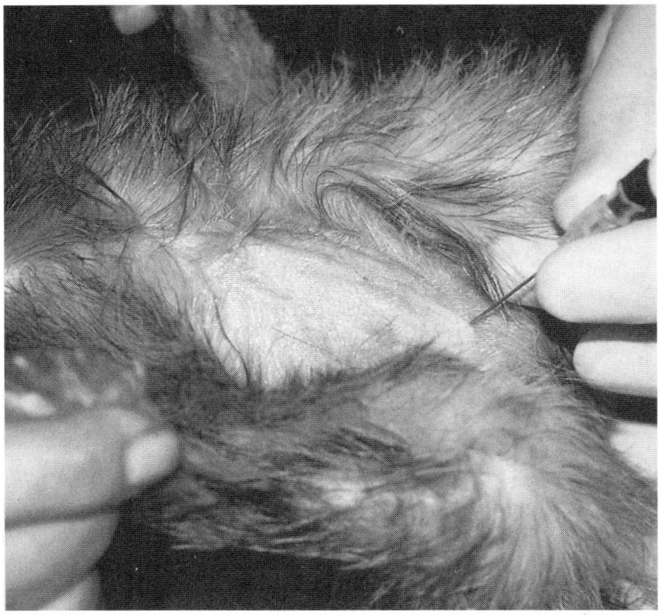

Figure 11-2 Lumbar cerebrospinal fluid tap in a ferret. The rear legs are extended forward to widen the intervertebral space.

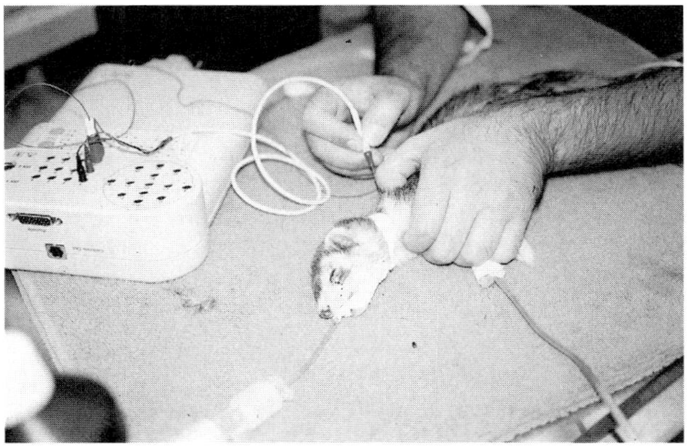

Figure 11-3 Electromyelography and nerve conduction velocity study in a ferret. Results can be compared with those from the contralateral limb, if unaffected, or from another ferret.

out a metabolic or infectious component. Check the blood glucose concentration immediately to minimize artifactual decreases caused by sample shipment or failure to separate plasma or serum from red blood cells. Correct any underlying abnormalities, and reassess the animal for changes in neurologic status. Perform whole-body radiography and, if you suspect cardiac disease, perform echocardiography.

For signs that can be localized to the CNS, perform computed tomography (CT) or magnetic resonance imaging (MRI), if available. Administer intravenous contrast medium to enhance brain lesions. For CT scanning, use 2.2 mL/kg of 400 mg/mL iodinated contrast medium (iothalamate sodium, Conray 400; Mallinckrodt Inc., St. Louis, MO); for MRI, use 0.2 mL/kg of gadolinium-diethylenetriamine pentaacetic acid (Gd-DTPA).[39]

If signs are localized to the spinal column, take spinal radiographs to look for possible fractures or bone abnormalities, such as proliferative or lytic lesions. Myelography is useful for localizing lesions of the spinal cord and determining a site for surgical approach, if needed (see Fig. 11-1). If possible, perform a spinal tap to obtain a sample of cerebrospinal fluid (CSF) for analysis. Sites for CSF tap and myelography are the atlanto-occipital and the lumbar (L5-L6) regions. Use a 22- or 20-gauge spinal needle, as in canine and feline myelography (Fig. 11-2); a suggested contrast medium is iohexol at 0.25 to 0.5 mL/kg.[40] Treatment with one intravenous dose of prednisolone sodium succinate or methylprednisolone sodium succinate (10-30 mg/kg), may help in preventing seizures and minimizing the progression of existing CNS edema.[5,35] Some spinal lesions may be amenable to surgical resection or stabilization; many, however, carry a poor prognosis.

For clinical signs localized to peripheral nerves or muscular defects, consult with a veterinary neurologist to perform electromyelography (EMG) and nerve conduction velocity (NCV) studies (Fig. 11-3). Although normal values for ferrets have not been published, comparison of values from the contralateral limb (in unilateral disease) or from another, unaffected ferret will aid in interpreting the results.

Treatment

Treatment of posterior paresis, ataxia, and seizures in ferrets is tailored to the diagnosis. Follow the standard treatment regimens used for dogs and cats when managing a similar condition in a ferret.

In any seizing ferret, the initial treatment must be directed toward arresting seizure activity (Fig. 11-4). Check the blood glucose concentration immediately in any animal presenting with seizures or ataxia. If the glucose level is lower than 60 mg/dL, give an intravenous bolus of 50% dextrose solution at a dose of 2 to 4 mL/kg or titrate to effect,[21] and begin a dextrose drip infusion adequate to maintain normoglycemia while further diagnostic testing is done. Some ferrets require as much as 10% to 12.5% dextrose added to intravenous fluids to achieve normoglycemia. Administer prednisone or prednisolone to hypoglycemic patients to enhance hepatic gluconeogenesis and inhibit glycogenolysis. If an insulinoma is suspected, initiate additional therapy as indicated (see Chapter 8).

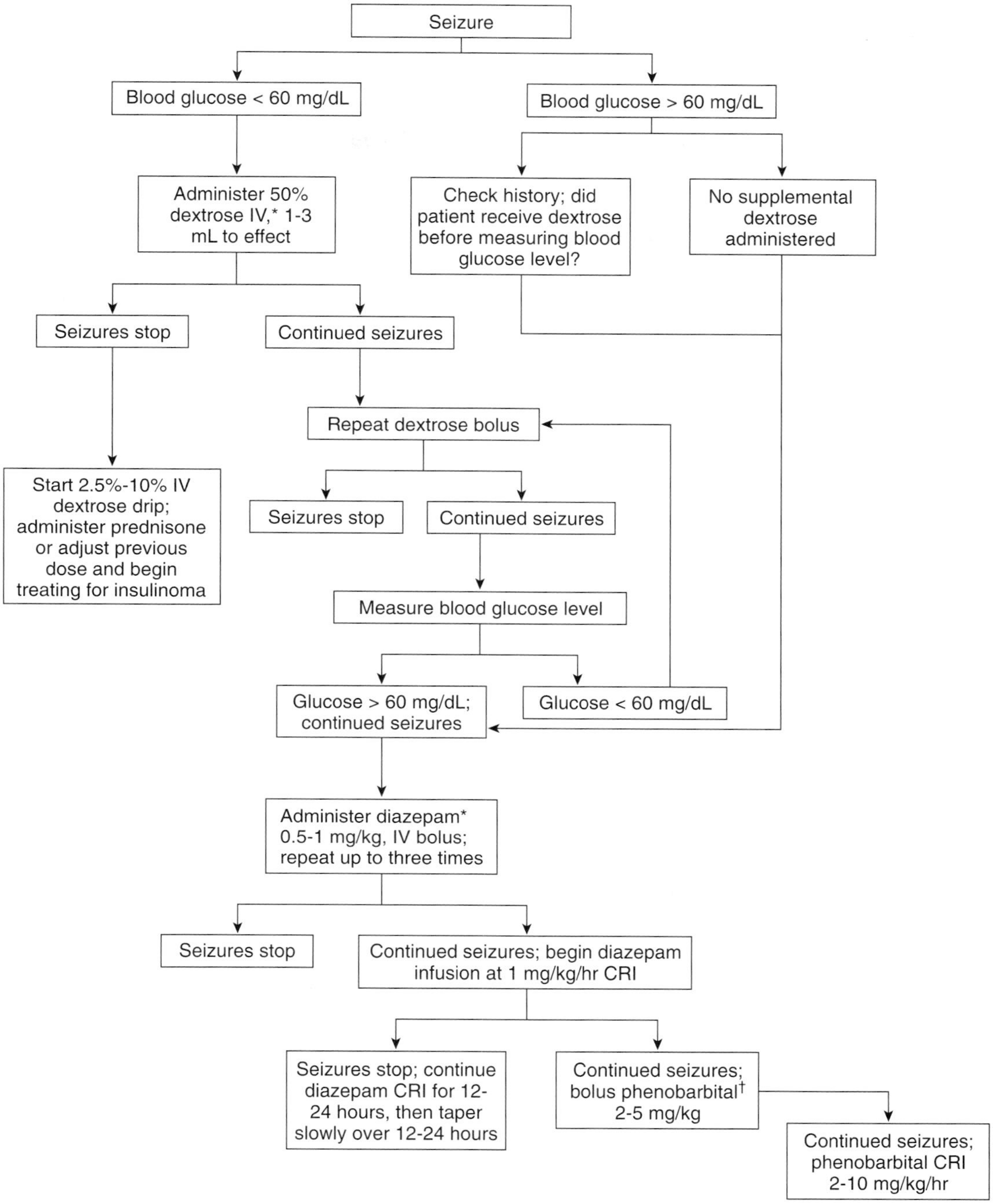

Figure 11-4 Flow chart for treatment of seizures in ferrets. *IV,* Intravenous; *CRI,* continuous rate infusion. *If intravenous access is not available, consider intraosseous catheter placement. Glucose and diazepam may be given orally or rectally. †If seizures are prolonged, consider corticosteroids and mannitol for central nervous system swelling of cerebral edema.

If seizures persist and the blood glucose concentration is normal (or has been restored to normal), begin aggressive seizure management. Administer diazepam (0.5-1.0 mg/kg) intravenously[28]; if venous access is not readily available, administer diazepam intramuscularly, intranasally (for more rapid absorption), or rectally. Repeat up to three times to arrest seizure activity. If grand mal or focal seizures persist, begin a constant-rate infusion of diazepam (0.5-1.0 mg/kg per hour added to IV fluids).[28] If cerebral edema is suspected, administer prednisolone sodium succinate or methylprednisolone sodium succinate (10 mg/kg IV) or dexamethasone sodium phosphate (1-2 mg/kg IV) and mannitol (0.5-1.0 g/kg IV over 20 minutes).[28] Once there have been no seizures for 12 to 24 hours, taper the diazepam infusion slowly over the next 12 to 24 hours. If diazepam does not control the seizures, initiate phenobarbital (2-10 mg/kg per hour) as a constant rate infusion.[28] Phenobarbital and diazepam can be administered concurrently. Once seizures are controlled, depending on their cause, use oral phenobarbital (1-2 mg/kg PO q8-12 h) if necessary for long-term seizure management.[28] Potassium bromide can also be used for seizure control; administer at 70 to 80 mg/kg per day if used alone or at 22 to 30 mg/kg per day in combination with phenobarbital.[28] Check blood levels of phenobarbital within 2 to 3 weeks after starting therapy; potassium bromide levels may not reach a steady state for 60 to 90 days. Adjust dosages based on blood levels.

Physical therapy is an important but often overlooked adjunct treatment. For ferrets with paresis or paralysis, and for those debilitated or recumbent from seizures or metabolic disorders, begin passive range-of-motion exercises three to four times daily for affected limbs (Fig. 11-5). This is essential to prevent contracture. Gently massage muscles to enhance blood flow. Implement active exercise as early as possible to preserve muscle tone and stimulate neural return.

CANINE DISTEMPER

Canine distemper virus in the late stage affects the CNS of ferrets, although initial signs are usually localized to the respiratory and gastrointestinal tracts and to the skin (see Chapter 7).[13] Ferrets are highly susceptible to canine distemper virus and may seem to recover from the acute phase only to die later from the neurotropic form of the disease. Affected ferrets can exhibit salivation, muscle tremors, seizures, and coma.[13] The disease is almost 100% fatal, and infected animals may be a source of infection to other ferrets.[13] Protect ferrets from distemper by vaccination (see Chapter 2).[43]

RABIES

Although reports of rabies in ferrets are rare, ferrets are susceptible to this disease. Clinical signs include anxiety, hyperactivity, lethargy, paresthesia (exaggerated grooming of a focal area), ataxia, and posterior paresis, sometimes followed by ascending paralysis.[13,25] In experimentally induced rabies in ferrets, the mean incubation period was 28 to 33 days, and the mean morbidity was 4 to 5 days.[25,26] In one study, virus was detected in the salivary glands of 63% and in saliva of 47% of the rabid ferrets.[26] You should suspect rabies in any unvaccinated ferret with clinical signs of neurologic disease and a history of exposure to rabid animals. A killed vaccine is approved for yearly use in ferrets (Imrab 3, Rhone Merieux, Athens, GA) but may not be considered protective if the vaccinated animal bites a human (see Chapter 2). In many states, any ferret with suspected rabies that is involved in a biting incident must be euthanatized and tested appropriately. Be aware of local or state laws that may affect you or your clients, and educate ferret owners at the time of vaccination.

ALEUTIAN DISEASE

Ferrets can be infected with Aleutian disease virus (ADV), a parvovirus that infects mink and ferrets. The virus is shed in saliva, urine, and feces, and infection occurs by inhalation or ingestion. Clinical signs vary from mild incoordination to posterior ataxia, ascending paresis, persistent tremors, and quadriplegia.[33,37] In one outbreak, clinical signs developed as soon as 24 hours or as long as 90 days after exposure.[37] The most significant biochemical abnormality is a hypergammaglobulinemia, with serum gamma globulin concentrations increased to greater than 20% of the total serum protein concentration. However, not all affected ferrets have high gamma globulin concentrations.[33,38] Histopathologic changes involving the brain and spinal cord include perivascular cuffing with lymphocytes and sometimes plasma cells, nonsuppurative meningitis, astrocytosis, mononuclear cell infiltration, and focal malacia.[33,38]

If you suspect Aleutian disease in a ferret, submit a blood sample for antibody testing by counterimmunoelectrophoresis (United Vaccines, Madison, WI) or an enzyme-linked immunosorbent assay (ELISA) (Avecon Diagnostics, Bath, PA; www.avecon.com). An in-house test kit is also available to test saliva samples (Avecon). Tentative diagnosis is based on a positive result of ADV testing, a high gamma globulin concentration, and the presence of compatible clinical signs. Disease is confirmed at necropsy in suspected ferrets by demonstration of the presence of lymphocytic and plasmacytic infiltrates on

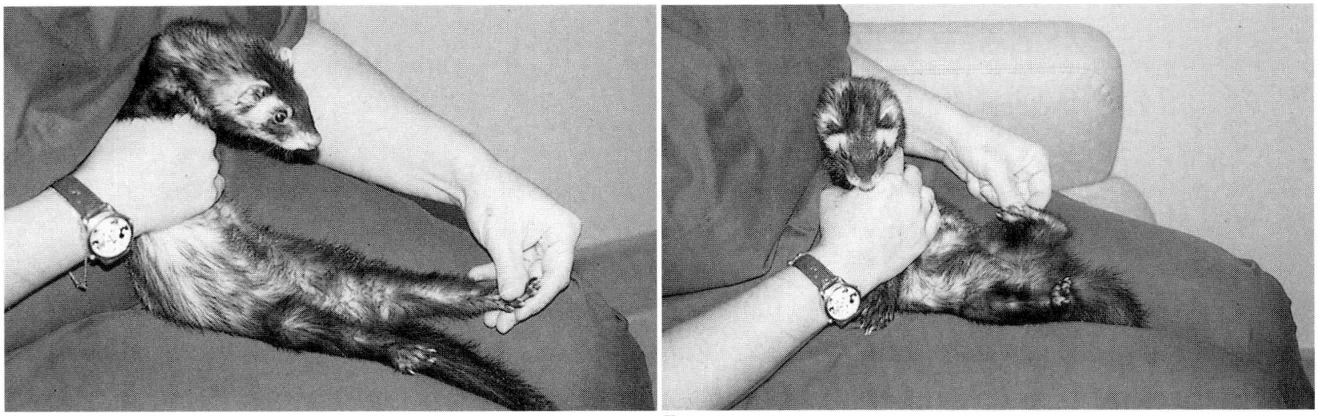

A B

Figure 11-5 A and B, Passive range-of-motion exercises to prevent contracture of the limbs performed on a ferret with hindlimb paresis.

histologic examination of tissue samples. Some infected ferrets may be asymptomatic but remain persistently infected, or the disease may be self-limited and nonpersistent.[38] The overall incidence of Aleutian disease in ferrets appears to be low; in one serologic study of 446 ferrets, the incidence of seropositive animals was 8.5%.[38] Treatment consists of supportive care and isolation of suspected animals from unaffected ferrets (see also Chapter 6).

EXTENSOR RIGIDITY/HYPERREFLEXIA

In a small number of ferrets, a progressive ascending dysfunction of the spinal nerves has been observed. Neurologic signs may begin as paresis or paralysis but more often are seen as an extensor rigidity and hyperreflexia of the rear limbs (Fig. 11-6). Some of these ferrets are presented with clinical signs and exposure history consistent with epizootic catarrhal enteritis (see Chapter 3). This condition may be progressive, but it may also completely regress. I have seen one ferret progress to a complete recovery after severe extensor rigidity that persisted for more than 14 days. The ferret lived for 2 years after recovery, and no spinal or brain lesions were present at necropsy. The pathophysiology of the neurologic signs is not known.

CHORDOMA AND CHONDROSARCOMA

Chordomas are tumors that arise from remnants of notochord.[16] In ferrets, these tumors develop most commonly at the tip of the tail,[1,6,7,16,18] but they have also been described in the cervical region.[41] Ferrets with cervical chordoma can present with posterior paresis and ataxia localized to the area of the lesion.[41] In such cases, perform spinal radiography and myelography to identify a site for surgical approach. Depending on location, these tumors may be amenable to surgical resection; however, the one reported case of recurrence and metastasis of a chordoma in a ferret was that of a cervical chordoma that had been surgically excised.[41] In the tail, chordomas appear as lobulated, firm, nonencapsulated, ulcerated masses at or near the last caudal vertebra. Microscopically, these tumors consist of lobules of physaliphorous cells with areas of well-differentiated bone or cartilage throughout.[7,18,41]

Chondrosarcoma of the tail has also been described in ferrets.[16,17] Clinical and morphologic descriptions are almost identical to those of chordoma. Differentiation must be made on the basis of immunohistochemical staining, with positive uptake of low-molecular-weight cytokeratin occurring in chordoma but not in chondrosarcoma.[7,18]

In ferrets with any distal tail mass, amputate several vertebrae proximal to the lesion. In cases of chordoma and chondrosarcoma, this is considered curative. Recurrence has not been reported.

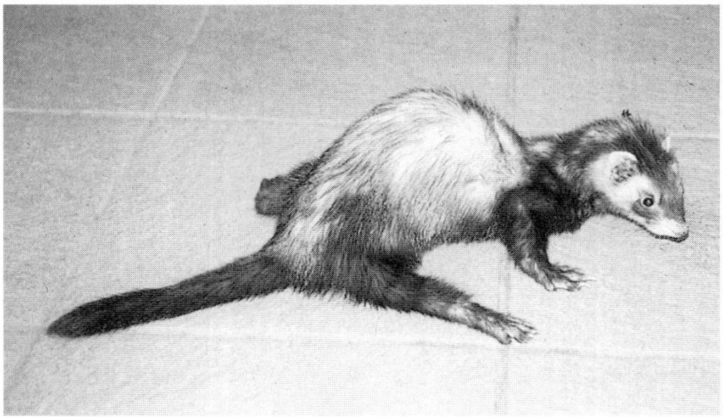

Figure 11-6 Ferret with extensor rigidity and hyperreflexia. The cause of this syndrome is unknown.

OSTEOMA

In ferrets, osteomas of the skull can arise from the zygomatic arch, parietal bone, or occipital bone.[16,19,20,34] An osteoma presents as a firm, dense, bony mass arising from one of the bones of the skull. Although they are benign neoplasms, clinical signs are related to physical displacement or compression of normal structures.[19,20,29,34] Obtain radiographs of any bony swelling to evaluate the extent of the lesion and the bone of origin. Biopsy may be difficult without surgical removal of the mass because of the extreme density of the tumor. The Jamshidi needle biopsy technique has been described.[30] Histopathologic evaluation usually reveals compact lamellar bone, bony trabeculae, and mild to moderate osteoblastic and hematologic activity.[19,20,34] Surgical removal is the treatment of choice and is usually curative if excision is complete.[20]

MISCELLANEOUS DISEASES

Systemic mycoses, which may contribute to CNS depression and lethargy, have been reported in ferrets.[8,9] *Cryptococcus* species have been identified as a cause of meningitis in ferrets, including one that died from congestive heart failure after being treated with steroids for intervertebral disc disease.[9] Blastomycosis has also been identified in ferrets, with multifocal granulomatous meningoencephalitis described in one ferret with systemic blastomycosis.[9,23] I have diagnosed a case of disseminated histoplasmosis in a ferret with fungal organisms present in the brain at necropsy. Diagnose these diseases on the basis of clinical signs, radiographic changes, and isolation of the causative organism. Impression smears of draining tracts or CSF may be useful in identifying the organism.

The only primary CNS neoplasm reported in a ferret was a granular cell tumor (sometimes called myoblastoma) in the cerebrum. Presenting signs included progressive head tilt, ataxia, and circling, followed by refractory seizures.[36] Consider intracranial neoplasia in a ferret with lateralizing, progressive CNS signs or seizures.

Pregnancy toxemia is most common in young, primiparous jills late in gestation. Although hypocalcemia, hypophosphatemia, and ketosis may develop, neurologic signs are rare unless hepatic lipidosis is so severe that encephalopathy is present.[2]

An eosinophilic granulomatous infiltrate in the choroid plexus was reported in a ferret with diffuse eosinophilic gastroenteritis and multisystem involvement.[12] Toxoplasmosis has been identified in ferrets; most likely, it developed after exposure to cat feces or raw meat.[3,4,10] Copper toxicosis has been reported and was believed to be congenital in two ferrets,[14] and iniencephaly in a litter of ferrets has also been described.[42] Other congenital anomalies probably occur but have not been reported.

REFERENCES

1. Allison N, Rakich P: Chordoma in two ferrets. J Comp Pathol 1989; 100:161-176.
2. Batchelder MA, Bell JA, Erdman SE, et al: Pregnancy toxemia in the European ferret (*Mustela putorius furo*). Lab Anim Sci 1999; 49:372-379.
3. Bell JA: Parasites of domesticated pet ferrets. Compend Contin Educ Pract Vet 1994; 16:617-620.
4. Besch-Williford C: Biology and medicine of the ferret. Vet Clin North Am Small Anim Pract 1987; 17:1155-1183.
5. Dewey CW, Budsberg SC, Oliver JE: Principles of head trauma management in dogs and cats: part II. Compend Contin Educ Pract Vet 1993; 15:177-193.
6. Dillberger JE, Altman NH: Neoplasia in ferrets: eleven cases with a review. J Comp Pathol 1989; 100:161-176.
7. Dunn DG, Harris RK, Meis JM, et al: A histomorphologic and immunohistochemical study of chordoma in 20 ferrets. Vet Pathol 1991; 28:467-493.
8. DuVal-Hudelson KA: Coccidioidomycosis in three European ferrets. J Zoo Wildl Med 1990; 21:353-357.
9. Fox JG: Mycotic diseases. *In* Fox JG, ed. Biology and Diseases of the Ferret, 2nd ed. Baltimore, Lippincott Williams and Wilkins, 1998, pp 393-403.
10. Fox JG: Parasitic diseases. *In* Fox JG, ed. Biology and Diseases of the Ferret, 2nd ed. Baltimore, Lippincott Williams and Wilkins, 1998, pp 375-391.
11. Fox JG, Murphy JC, Ackerman JI, et al: Proliferative colitis in ferrets. Am J Vet Res 1982; 43:858-864.
12. Fox JG, Palley LS, Rose R: Eosinophilic gastroenteritis with Splendore-Hoeppli material in the ferret. Vet Pathol 1992; 29:21-26.
13. Fox JG, Pearson RC, Gorham JR: Viral chlamydial diseases. *In* Fox JG, ed. Biology and Diseases of the Ferret, 2nd ed. Baltimore, Lippincott Williams and Wilkins, 1998, pp 335-374.
14. Fox JG, Zeman DH, Mortimer JD: Copper toxicosis in sibling ferrets. J Am Vet Med Assoc 1994; 205:1154-1156.
15. Frederick MA: Intervertebral disc syndrome in a domestic ferret. Vet Med Small Anim Clin 1981; 76:835.
16. Goad MEP, Fox JG: Neoplasia in ferrets. *In* Fox JG, ed.: Biology and Diseases of the Ferret. Philadelphia, Lea & Febiger, 1988, pp 274-288.
17. Hendrick MJ, Goldschmidt MH: Chondrosarcoma of the tail of ferrets. Vet Pathol 1987; 24:272-273.
18. Herron AJ, Brunnert SR, Ching SV, et al: Immunohistochemical and morphologic features of chordomas in ferrets. Vet Pathol 1990; 27:284-286.
19. Jensen WA, Myers RK, Liu CH: Osteoma in a ferret. J Am Vet Med Assoc 1985; 187:1375-1376.
20. Jensen WA, Myers RK, Merkley DF: Diagnostic exercise: a bony growth of the skull in a ferret. Lab Anim Sci 1987; 37:780-781.
21. Kirk RW, Bistner SI, Ford RB, eds: Handbook of Veterinary Procedures and Emergency Treatment, 5th ed. Philadelphia, WB Saunders, 1990, pp 133-145.
22. Lawes INC, Andrews PLR: The neuroanatomy of the ferret brain. *In* Fox JG, ed. Biology and Diseases of the Ferret, 2nd ed. Baltimore, Lippincott Williams and Wilkins, 1998, pp 71-102.
23. Lenhard A: Blastomycosis in a ferret. J Am Vet Med Assoc 1985; 186:70-72.
24. Methiyapun S, Myers RK, Pohlenz JFL: Spontaneous plasma cell myeloma in a ferret. Vet Pathol 1985; 22:517-519.
25. Niezgoda M, Briggs DJ, Shadduck J, et al: Pathogenesis of experimentally induced rabies in domestic ferrets. Am J Vet Res 1997; 58:1327-1331.
26. Niezgoda M, Briggs DJ, Shadduck J, et al: Viral excretion in domestic ferrets (*Mustela putorius furo*) inoculated with a raccoon rabies isolate. Am J Vet Res 1998; 59:1629-1632.
27. Oliver JE, Lorenz MD: Handbook of Veterinary Neurology, 2nd ed. Philadelphia, WB Saunders, 1993.
28. Plumb DC: Veterinary Drug Handbook, 4th ed. Ames, Iowa State University Press, 2002.
29. Pool RR: Tumors of bone and cartilage. *In* Moulton J, ed. Tumors in Domestic Animals, 2nd ed. Los Angeles, University of California Press, 1978, pp 91-99.
30. Powers BE, LaRue SM, Withrow SJ, et al: Jamshidi needle biopsy for diagnosis of bone lesions in small animals. J Am Vet Med Assoc 1988; 193:205-210.
31. Richardson JA, Balabuszko RA: Ibuprofen ingestion in ferrets: 43 cases. J Vet Emerg Crit Care 2001; 11:53-59.
32. Rosenthal K: Ferrets. Vet Clin North Am Small Anim Pract 1994; 24:1-23.
33. Rozengurt N, Stewart S, Sanchez S: Diagnostic exercise: ataxia and incoordination in ferrets. Lab Anim Sci 1995; 45:432-434.
34. Ryland LM, Gogolewski R: What's your diagnosis? J Am Vet Med Assoc 1990; 197:1065-1066.
35. Shores A: Spinal trauma: pathophysiology and management of traumatic spinal injuries. Vet Clin North Am Small Anim Pract 1992; 22:859-888.
36. Sleeman JM, Clyde VL, Brennerman KA: Granular cell tumour in the central nervous system of a ferret (*Mustela putorius furo*). Vet Rec 1996; 138:65-66.
37. Une Y, Wakimoto Y, Nakano Y, et al: Spontaneous Aleutian disease in a ferret. J Vet Med Sci 2000; 62:553-555.
38. Welchman D deB, Oxenham M, Done SH: Aleutian disease in domestic ferrets: diagnostic findings and survey results. Vet Rec 1993; 132:479-484.
39. Westbrook C, Kaut C: MRI in Practice, 2nd ed. Oxford, Blackwell Science, 1998.
40. Widmer WR, Blevins WE: Veterinary myelography: a review of contrast media, adverse effects, and technique. J Am Anim Hosp Assoc 1991; 27:163-176.
41. Williams BH, Eighmy JJ, Berbert MH, et al: Cervical chordoma in two ferrets. Vet Pathol 1993; 30:204-206.
42. Williams BH, Popek EJ, Hart RA, et al: Iniencephaly and other neural tube defects in a litter of ferrets. Vet Pathol 1994; 31:260-262.
43. Wimsatt J, Jay MT, Innes KE, et al: Serologic evaluation, efficacy, and safety of a commercial modified-live canine distemper vaccine in domestic ferrets. Am J Vet Res 2001; 62:736-740.

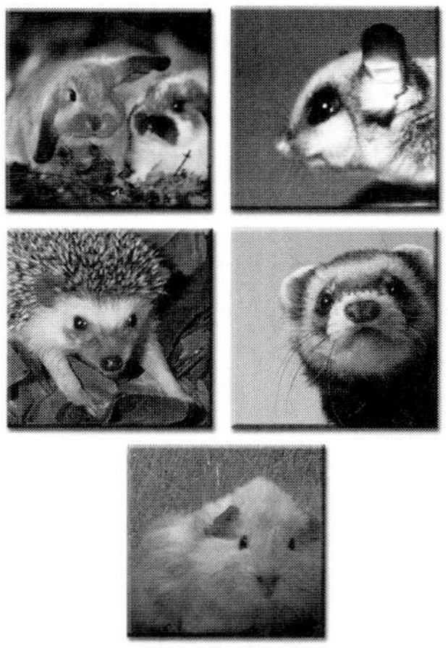

CHAPTER 12

Soft Tissue Surgery

Lori Ludwig, VMD, MS, Diplomate ACVS, and
Sean Aiken, DVM, MS, Diplomate ACVS

Soft tissue surgical procedures in domestic ferrets are similar to those performed in other small animal species treated in a veterinary practice. This chapter describes those soft tissue surgical procedures that are particular to ferrets. Because ferrets may be afflicted with surgical diseases similar to those of other small mammal species, a basic small animal surgery text should be used in conjunction with this chapter to provide a complete understanding of surgical conditions of ferrets.

When performing surgical procedures in ferrets, the availability of some specialized equipment will make surgery on these animals fun and rewarding. Microsurgical instrumentation and magnifying loupes greatly simplify surgical procedures (Fig. 12-1). The surgical suite should be stocked with a variety of synthetic absorbable suture material ranging in size from 4-0 to 6-0. Equip the surgical preparation area, surgical suite, and recovery area with devices needed to maintain the ferret's body temperature throughout the anesthetic procedure. Circulating hot-water blankets, warm-air circulators, and warm-water bottles may be used. Heat lamps can burn the patient and should be used with caution in ferrets. When performing an exploratory laparotomy, place an adherent plastic surgical sheeting (Ioban, 3M Healthcare, St. Paul, MN) over the abdomen after standard surgical draping to act as a water barrier. This aids in keeping the patient warm and dry and can eliminate the need for towel clamps.

Many of the surgical procedures described here are performed during an exploratory laparotomy. For this procedure, make a ventral midline incision beginning at the xiphoid and extending to the pubis (in the female) or to just cranial to the prepuce and extending parapreputial if needed (in the male). Ferrets have relatively thin skin and little subcutaneous tissue, so a light touch with the scalpel blade is warranted. The linea alba of ferrets is a wide, thin structure that is easily identified (Fig. 12-2, *A*). Gently grasp the linea with forceps and lift it away from the abdominal contents before penetrating the abdomen with a No. 15 scalpel blade. Extend the initial incision in the linea with scissors or a scalpel blade (Fig. 12-2, *B*). Be extremely cautious when penetrating the abdominal cavity or extending the incision to avoid damaging dilated or enlarged organs. Also, use caution when extending the incision in the linea cranially so as not to penetrate the diaphragm. Most ferrets have significant abdominal fat deposits that may obscure intraabdominal organs. Remove the falciform fat, as is done in other species, before exploring the abdomen. To help gain exposure to the abdominal cavity, use small Balfour retractors with moistened gauze sponges. As with any exploratory laparotomy, use a thorough and systematic approach to examine the entire abdominal cavity. After completing the procedure, close the linea with 3-0 or 4-0 monofilament suture material (polydioxanone [PDS], polypropylene, or nylon) in a simple continuous or interrupted pattern. Close subcutaneous tissues with fine absorbable suture material. Cyanoacrylic tissue glue can be used instead of skin sutures to support the skin closure by applying the material after opposing the skin edges. Do not place tissue glue within the subcutaneous tissues because it elicits a foreign body reaction.

GASTROINTESTINAL SYSTEM

Salivary Mucocele Resection

Ferrets have five pairs of salivary glands: parotid, mandibular, sublingual, molar (buccal), and zygomatic.[10] Although mucoceles are uncommon, they have been reported in ferrets.[1,17,18] The zygomatic and molar (buccal) glands are most commonly

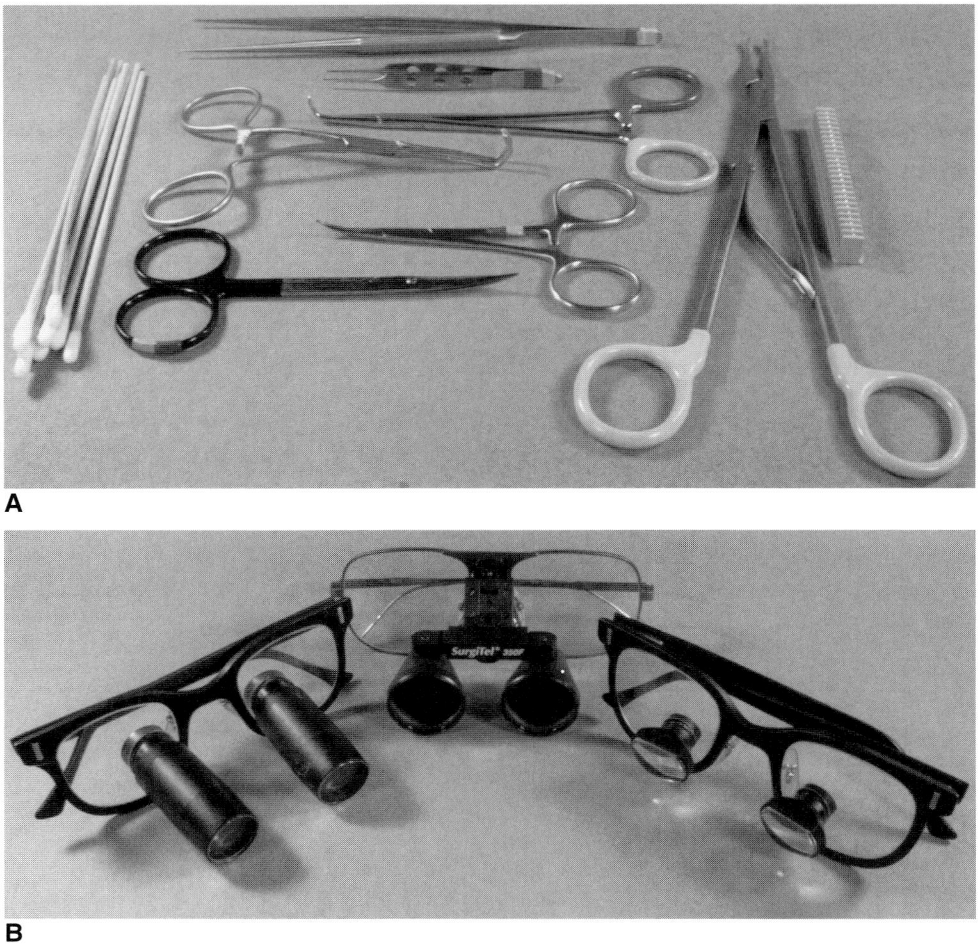

Figure 12-1 **A,** Specialized surgical instruments. *Middle column, from the top:* Vascular forceps, Bishop-Harmon forceps, right angle forceps, neonatal Satinsky forceps, mosquito forceps, iris scissors. *Left:* Cotton-tipped applicators. *Right:* Vascular clips and applicator. **B,** Surgical magnifying loupes. *Left to right:* Custom 4.5× magnification, adjustable 3.5× magnification, custom 2.5× magnification at working focal lengths of 18 to 21 inches.

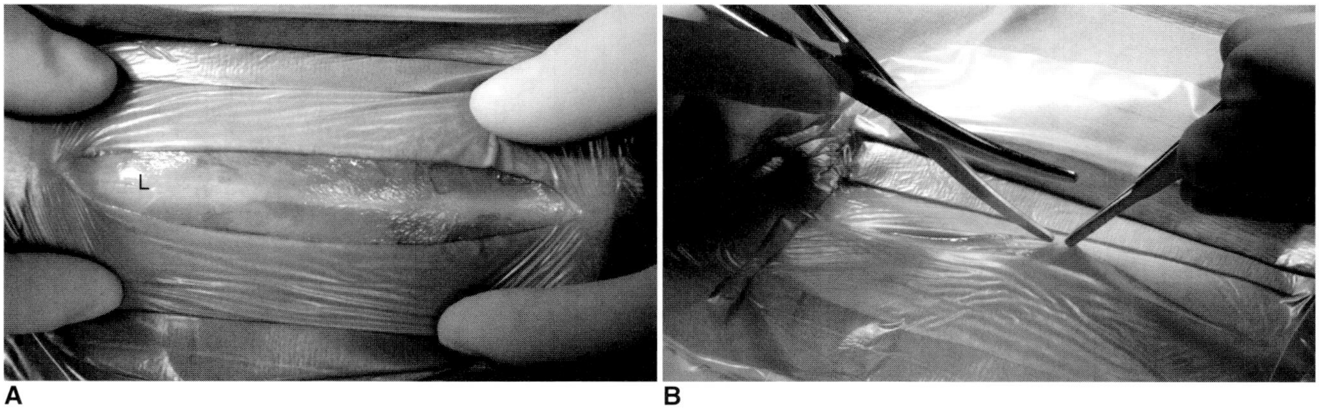

Figure 12-2 **A,** Approach to ferret exploratory laparotomy. Note the wide linea alba *(L)* and minimal subcutaneous fat. The adherent plastic sheeting is applied to the ventral abdominal skin to keep the ferret dry and warm during the surgical procedure. **B,** Approach to ferret exploratory laparotomy by extending the incision in the linea alba with fine scissors. Note that the abdominal wall is elevated to prevent damage to the underlying abdominal organs.

affected. Affected ferrets are presented with unilateral facial or periorbital swelling, and a fine-needle aspirate of the mass reveals a thick, mucoid fluid. Marsupialization or aspiration may provide temporary relief from the swelling, but curative treatment should be aimed at surgical removal of the involved gland or glands. A thorough knowledge of the regional anatomy is required so that all of the involved glandular material is removed. As described in dogs, the zygomatic arch can be partially resected to facilitate exposure of the zygomatic gland. Although there are few reports of mucoceles in ferrets, the prognosis appears to be good after surgical removal of the affected gland.[1,17,18]

Intestinal Surgery

One of the most common surgeries performed in ferrets is removal of ingested foreign material from the stomach and small intestine. Foam rubber sponges, rubber objects, and cork are the most common foreign bodies removed.[19] Most ingested foreign material becomes lodged in the small intestine or stomach, but esophageal foreign bodies have been reported.[5,19] Trichobezoars (hairball foreign bodies) may result from normal or excessive grooming behavior and tend to lodge in the stomach.[19] Although vomiting may not be as frequent as in other domestic species,[19] clinical signs in ferrets with foreign body obstruction are similar to those of other small animal patients with gastrointestinal obstruction. These signs include vomiting, diarrhea, anorexia, and pawing at the mouth (bruxism). Foreign bodies in the intestinal tract may also be discovered during exploratory laparotomy in ferrets that have no clinical signs attributable to intestinal obstruction. Ferrets that are presented with intestinal foreign bodies are usually young (mean age, 22 months), whereas ferrets presenting with trichobezoars tend to be older (mean age, 43 months).[19]

Physical findings depend on the duration of illness. The ferret may be lethargic and dehydrated, or it may simply show signs of weight loss. On physical examination, the foreign body may be detected as a painful or nonpainful, palpable intestinal mass. Holding the ferret upright during abdominal palpation may aid in localizing intestinal foreign bodies located in the stomach and proximal small intestine. Survey radiographs may show loops of small intestine dilated with gas or fluid, dilation of the stomach, or a radiodense foreign body. On abdominal ultrasound examination, fluid-filled loops of intestine may be seen proximal to the obstruction. As with other species, surgery to relieve an intestinal foreign body obstruction is considered an emergency procedure and should be done as soon as the ferret is rehydrated and stabilized.

Esophageal foreign bodies are rare and should be treated as recommended in other small animal species. If possible, remove the foreign body by endoscopy or by advancing it into the stomach for retrieval by gastrotomy. An esophagotomy may be performed through a right lateral thoracotomy, but this procedure can be complicated by postoperative leakage or stricture formation.[5]

Most intestinal foreign bodies can be retrieved during an exploratory laparotomy. The ferret intestine lacks a distinct ileum; instead, the jejunoileum extends from the duodenojejunal flexure to the ascending colon.[10] Evaluate the entire intestinal tract, as multiple foreign bodies may be present, and perform a gastrotomy or enterotomy as in other small animals. Because ferret intestinal tissue is very thin and fragile, gentle tissue handling is needed to prevent iatrogenic damage to the intestines (Fig. 12-3). Isolate the intestinal surgery site from the abdominal cavity with moistened sponges. To minimize contamination of the abdominal cavity, use pediatric Doyan intestinal clamps or sterile bobby pins to occlude the intestinal lumen proximal and distal to the intended enterotomy site.

For a gastrotomy, stabilize the stomach with full-thickness stay sutures of 4-0 nylon before making an incision. Close the gastrotomy incision in one or two layers by using a simple interrupted or continuous suture pattern with 4-0 or 5-0 monofilament absorbable or nonabsorbable suture material. For an enterotomy, use a sharp No. 15 or No. 11 scalpel blade to make the incision, and then extend the incision with fine scissors. Close the enterotomy incision with 4-0 or 5-0 monofilament suture in a simple interrupted pattern. The lumen diameter of the jejunum is very small, so careful tissue handling is required to minimize the chance of intestinal strictures. As with any intestinal surgery, copiously lavage the abdominal cavity with sterile saline solution and change the instruments and gloves before abdominal closure.

Unless treatment is indicated by signs of peritonitis or sepsis, discontinue antibiotic administration 12 hours after surgery. Water can be offered as soon as 12 hours after surgery, and food should be offered after 12 to 24 hours. Continue intravenous fluid therapy until the ferret is eating well. Overall, the prognosis is very good, but possible complications include intestinal leakage and peritonitis as well as stricture formation with possible reobstruction.

Liver Biopsy

A liver biopsy should be done routinely during an exploratory laparotomy to help diagnose suspected or unsuspected liver disease such as hepatic lipidosis, lymphosarcoma, or metastatic neoplasia. At surgery, palpate all liver lobes thoroughly. If all lobes have a similar appearance and palpate similarly, then a random liver biopsy is indicated. If a section of liver is protruding, a guillotine suture can be used. For this technique, place a preformed encircling ligature of 4-0 monofilament absorbable suture material around the protruding section of liver. Tighten the ligature until it has crushed through the hepatic parenchyma (Fig. 12-4). After completing several throws in the knot, excise the sample 1 to 2 mm distal to the ligature with Metzenbaum scissors or a scalpel blade.

If a specific area of the liver is of interest, then the tissue sample can be obtained by the transfixation method or with a 6-mm skin biopsy punch. For the transfixation method, place a ligature through the liver lobe approximately 8 to 10 mm from its edge. Tighten the ligature to crush through the parenchyma of half of the desired biopsy specimen. Make an additional throw at a right angle to the first ligature, tightening the ligature to crush the parenchyma for the second half of the specimen. Remove the sample 1 to 2 mm distal to the crushed area with a scalpel blade or Metzenbaum scissors. If the area of interest does not lie near the edge of the liver lobe, a 6-mm biopsy punch can be used. Push the biopsy punch through the liver parenchyma in the desired area, making sure not to penetrate the opposite surface of the liver (Fig. 12-5). Use extra caution if the biopsy site is close to the hilus so that no more than one half of the thickness of the liver lobe is penetrated. Remove the biopsy punch and separate the biopsy sample from the liver with scissors, being careful not to crush the sample. Control bleeding

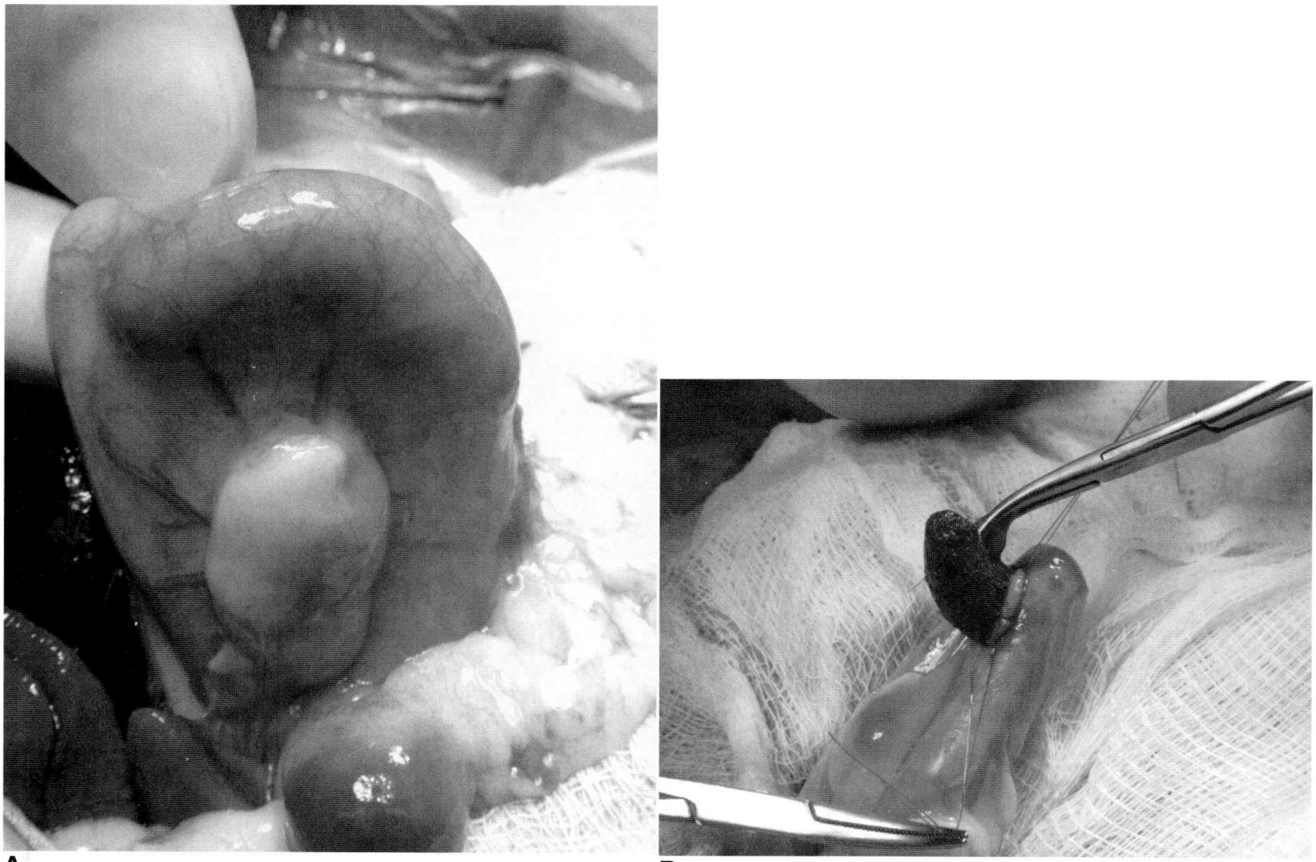

A B

Figure 12-3 A, Gastric foreign body in a ferret. The object was palpated during a routine exploratory laparotomy for an unrelated problem. B, Removal of a gastric trichobezoar through a gastrotomy incision in a ferret. Note the stay sutures supporting the stomach and the sponges isolating the area to protect against contamination by intestinal contents.

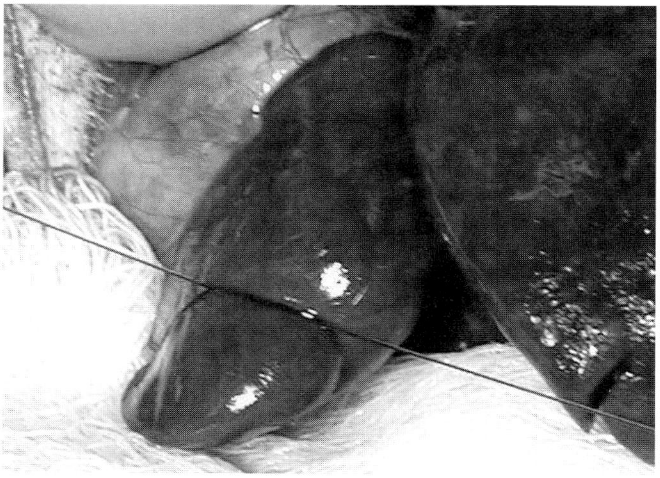

Figure 12-4 The guillotine liver biopsy technique is performed by placing a ligature around the area of interest at the edge of a liver lobe and slowly tightening the knot. The biopsy specimen is then divided approximately 2 mm distal to the encircling ligature.

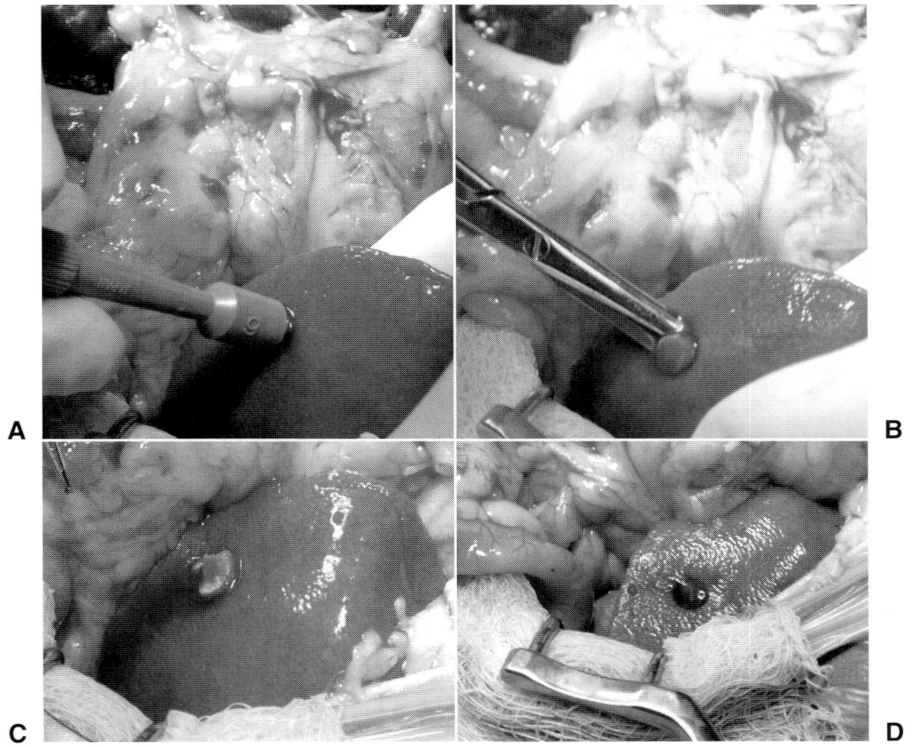

Figure 12-5 The punch liver biopsy technique allows a more selective biopsy. **A,** A 6-mm skin biopsy punch is pushed through the liver parenchyma without penetrating the capsule on the opposite side of the liver lobe. **B,** After removing the biopsy punch, the biopsy sample is separated from the liver with fine scissors, being careful not to crush the sample. **C,** The defect is filled with absorbable hemostatic sponge and digital pressure is applied for 5 minutes. **D,** The hemostatic sponge may be removed or left in place to be absorbed. If bleeding continues, the liver capsule can be sutured with fine absorbable suture material in a cruciate pattern.

either by filling the defect with gelatin sponge hemostatic material and applying digital pressure for 3 to 5 minutes or by suturing the liver capsule with a fine absorbable monofilament suture in a cruciate pattern.

Gallbladder Surgery

Choleliths are rare in domestic species and may be found occasionally in ferrets. Choleliths have been found incidentally in ferrets during exploratory abdominal surgery for other conditions and have been observed at surgery as an explanation for anorexia, fever, and depression. In four cases seen at The Animal Medical Center, choleliths were observed in older ferrets (mean age, 6.5 years; range, 5 to 8 years). Liver enzyme concentrations were elevated in only one of the four ferrets.

The biliary system of ferrets is similar to that of other domesticated animals and is composed of three hepatic ducts feeding into a common bile duct (Fig. 12-6). The gallbladder empties into the cystic duct, which joins the central hepatic duct to beome the common bile duct. The main pancreatic duct joins the common bile duct before it empties into the duodenum at the major duodenal papilla.[21]

Choleliths can be located in the gallbladder, or they can obstruct the common bile duct. Therefore thoroughly examine the biliary tree during exploratory abdominal surgery. If the choleliths are located in the common bile duct, attempt to retropulse the stones by gently milking them backward into the gallbladder with your fingertips. Alternatively, make an incision in the antimesenteric border of the duodenum at the level of the major duodenal papilla. Cannulate the common bile duct with a 25-gauge catheter, and flush the stones into the gallbladder. Once the stones are in the gallbladder, check the common bile duct for patency by flushing the duct with a 3.5-Fr catheter. If it is patent, perform a standard cholecystectomy (as in other domestic species) to prevent recurrent cholecystitis.[16] Gently elevate the gallbladder from the hepatic surfaces of the right medial and quadrate liver lobes with sterile cotton-tipped applicators (Fig. 12-7). Use hemostatic sponges on the liver surface to control hemorrhage. After dissecting the gallbladder and cystic duct to the level of the central hepatic duct, double-ligate the cystic duct with fine nonabsorbable suture material or vascular clips and transect it. Submit sections of the gallbladder for bacterial culture and histopathologic examination, and submit the gallstones for crystallographic analysis. To date, all ferrets with gallstones have had a histologic diagnosis of cholecystitis, with one of four ferrets having a positive bacterial culture. All choleliths have been composed primarily of bile pigment and bile salts.

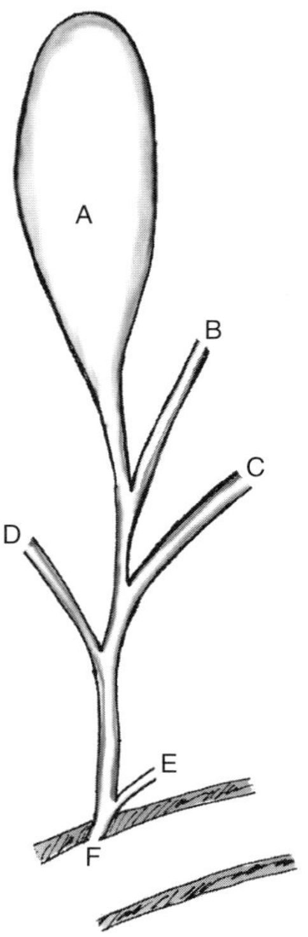

Figure 12-6 The biliary tree and gallbladder. **A**, Gallbladder; **B**, central hepatic duct; **C**, left hepatic duct; **D**, right hepatic duct; **E**, main pancreatic duct; **F**, major duodenal papilla entering the duodenum approximately 2.75 cm distal to the pylorus. *(From Poddar S: Gross and microscopic anatomy of the biliary tract of the ferret. Acta Anat 1977; 97:121-131.)*

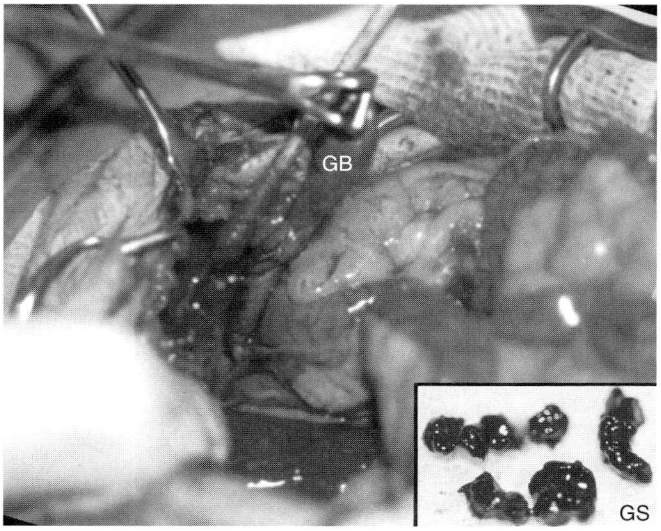

Figure 12-7 Intraoperative view of the gallbladder *(GB)* and biliary tree of a ferret with gallstones. Note that the gallbladder is being elevated from the underlying liver lobes with a cotton-tipped applicator and is grasped with a Babcock forceps. The gallbladder is then ligated at its base, where the cystic duct joins the central hepatic duct. *Inset:* Gallstones *(GS)* that were removed with the gallbladder.

ENDOCRINE SYSTEM

Surgery of the Adrenal Gland

Adrenal neoplasia is common in ferrets, especially neoplasia of the cortex (see Chapter 8). Cortical hyperplasia, adenomas, and carcinomas secreting estrogen and other steroid hormones are the most common tumor types.[2,18] Other types of adrenal gland neoplasia have been reported, including spindle cell tumors, pheochromocytomas, teratomas, and myelolipomas.[13]

Adrenocortical disease in ferrets is not Cushing's disease. Instead of secreting excess cortisol, affected adrenal glands produce estrogens and androgens.[14,23,27] The most common clinical sign associated with adrenocortical disease is alopecia that begins on the tail and progresses cranially along the dorsum, flanks, and body.[12,28,29] Affected females often present with enlarged vulvas, and affected males may show sexual behavior or present with stranguria or urinary obstruction secondary to an enlarged prostate or paraurethral cysts.

Ferrets typically are presented with clinical signs at 3 to 4 years of age (range, 1 to 7.5 years.) One retrospective study found that adrenocortical disease occurred more commonly in females; however, others have found an equal distribution between the sexes.[25,28,29] Most ferrets with adrenocortical disease have been neutered before 6 weeks of age, and the disease rarely occurs in sexually intact ferrets.[25] Some have speculated that there is an association between adrenocortical disease in ferrets and neutering at an early age. This association is postulated to be caused by loss of negative gonadal feedback to the release of gonadotropin-releasing hormone (GnRH) from the hypothalamus, resulting in persistent stimulation of the adrenal cortex by luteinizing hormone (LH) and follicle-stimulating hormone (FSH). Results of one study in ferrets found a correlation between age at neutering and age at onset of adrenocortical disease.[26] However, more studies are needed to prove a cause-and-effect relationship.

Diagnosis of adrenocortical disease in ferrets begins with recognition of clinical signs. Differential diagnoses include seasonal hair loss, external parasites, extended estrus, ovarian remnants, nutritional deficiencies, and pheochromocytoma.[2] Physical examination may reveal a mass palpable cranial to the kidney. Abdominal ultrasound is used to identify an enlarged adrenal gland(s), determine if the disease is unilitaeral or bilateral, and screen for the presence of other disease processes in abdominal organs. The diagnosis can be confirmed with an adrenal hormone panel that measures plasma concentrations of several steroids such as 17-hydroxyprogesterone, androstenedione, and estradiol.[23] Before surgery, a complete blood count and plasma biochemical analysis should be performed on each patient to evaluate for any abnormalities that may need to be addressed. Commonly, hypoglycemia is detected as a result of concurrent insulin-secreting tumors. In all ferrets with adrenocortical disease, measure the blood glucose concentration immediately before surgery and provide dextrose supplementation in intravenous fluids as needed.

Although medical management is effective in some cases, surgery is the treatment of choice for most ferrets with adrenal neoplasia. For the surgical approach, make a ventral midline incision, extending the incision caudally from the xiphoid as needed to allow thorough examination of the abdomen. Evaluate all organs systematically, because splenomegaly, lymphoma, and gastric foreign bodies may also be found concurrently. Islet cell tumors are found in approximately 25% of patients with adrenal neoplasia.[25,28,29] In male ferrets, carefully palpate the prostate gland for cystic enlargement. In females, inspect the ovarian and uterine stumps.

The adrenal glands are often embedded in fat and lie at the cranial pole of the kidneys (Fig. 12-8). Normal adrenal glands are whitish-pink, 2 to 3 mm wide, and 6 to 8 mm long.[18,20] Remember that not all diseased adrenal glands are enlarged, and palpation of the glands alone is not enough to evaluate for disease. If the entire gland is not visible, use mosquito hemostats and cotton-tipped applicators to carefully dissect the thin layer of peritoneum and fat surrounding the gland to free it. On the right side, incise the hepatorenal ligament and use it to retract the caudate lobe of the liver cranially. Yellow-brown discoloration, the presence of cysts, or enlargement is an indication for removal of the gland.

Left adrenalectomy is most commonly indicated and is usually easy. Begin sharp and blunt dissection caudal to the gland and continue in a craniolateral direction. Take care not to disrupt the capsule of the gland. Control hemorrhage of large vessels with cautery or hemostatic clips (Fig. 12-9). The phrenicoabdominal (adrenolumbar) vein is first encountered at the craniolateral aspect of the gland as it courses over the gland's ventral surface. Ligate this vessel with suture or small hemostatic clips. After dissecting the caudal, lateral, and cranial aspects of the gland, lift the gland by grasping tissue along its lateral aspect. Examine the area where the phrenicoabdominal vein enters the vena cava for soft tissue invasion. If no invasion is detected, ligate the vein with clips or suture and remove the gland.

The need for complete right adrenalectomy has been reported in 15% to 20% of cases.[2,25] Right adrenalectomy is often more difficult because of adherence of the gland to the wall of the vena cava and the greater potential for vascular invasion. At surgery, have magnifying loupes, microsurgical instruments, and vascular clamps available for use. Begin dissecting around the gland, as described for left adrenalectomy. If the tumor is small and extends lateral to the cava, often it can be almost completely freed from the wall of the cava with gentle dissection. If so, place hemostatic clips between the gland and the cava and resect the gland. However, if the gland cannot be freed from the vena cava because of tumor invasion, or if it is located mostly on the dorsal aspect of the vessel, this technique is often unsuccessful for complete removal. In these cases, place a small vascular clamp (neonatal Satinsky) on the vena cava for either partial or total occlusion of the vessel (Fig. 12-10). Then remove the gland with a portion of the caval wall and suture the defect with 9-0 or 10-0 nylon suture in a simple continuous pattern. If only a small defect is created, a simple interrupted pattern can be used. The time that the cava is occluded should be limited, although one author has reported occlusion of up to 1 hour without complications.[31] Before releasing the clamp, place a piece of gelatin sponge over the suture line. Mild oozing is usually observed from the incision line, and gentle pressure can be applied to the area with a cotton-tipped applicator. If hemorrhage is severe, replace the clamp and identify and suture the area of bleeding.

With extensive vascular invasion of the cava, resection and anastomosis of the cava may be needed. Some have reported successful outcomes with complete ligation of the vena cava[29]; presumably, the ferrets had enough collateral circulation to allow survival. However, predicting whether a ferret will survive complete ligation at surgery is impossible, and mortality rates may be high. Because delicate surgical procedures can be performed that allow preservation of the cava, these should be attempted before ligation. Cryosurgery, laser surgery, and radiosurgical ablation of the right adrenal gland have been reported anecdotally. A disadvantage of these techniques is that the tissue is not available for histopathologic evaluation. In addition, it may be difficult to evaluate how completely the adrenal gland has been destroyed. Concerns about thermal damage to the vena cava also exist.

Bilateral gland involvement has been reported in 16% to 68% of ferrets with adrenocortical disease.[22,25,29] In one study, 32% of ferrets with unilateral adrenal disease presented an average of

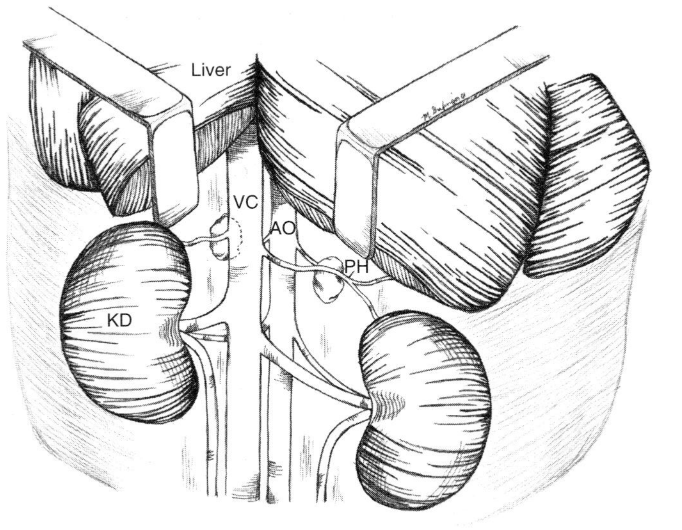

Figure 12-8 Normal adrenal anatomy. The hepatorenal ligament has been incised to allow retraction of the caudate liver lobe and visualization of the right adrenal gland. The right adrenal gland is adhered to the wall of the caudal vena cava *(VC)*. If neoplastic, it often extends dorsally along the vessel wall (indicated by *dashes*.) *AO*, Aorta; *KD*, kidney; *PH*, phrenicoabdominal vein.

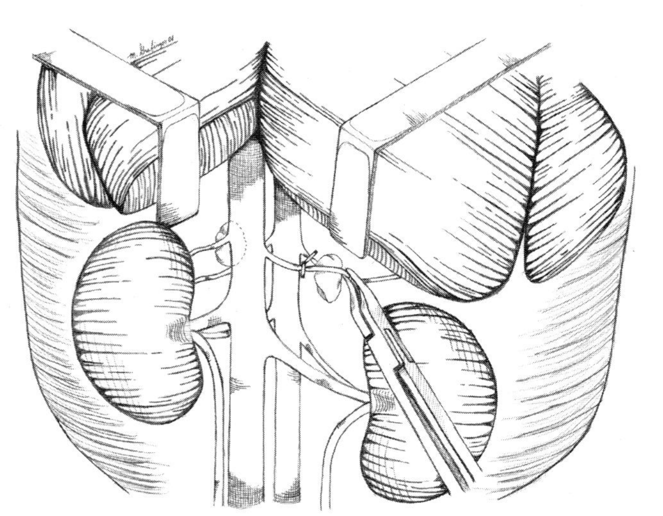

Figure 12-9 Left adrenalectomy is usually simple because of the distance of the gland from the caudal vena cava. Hemostatic clips are useful for ligating the phrenicoabdominal vein as it courses from lateral to medial over the ventral surface of the gland.

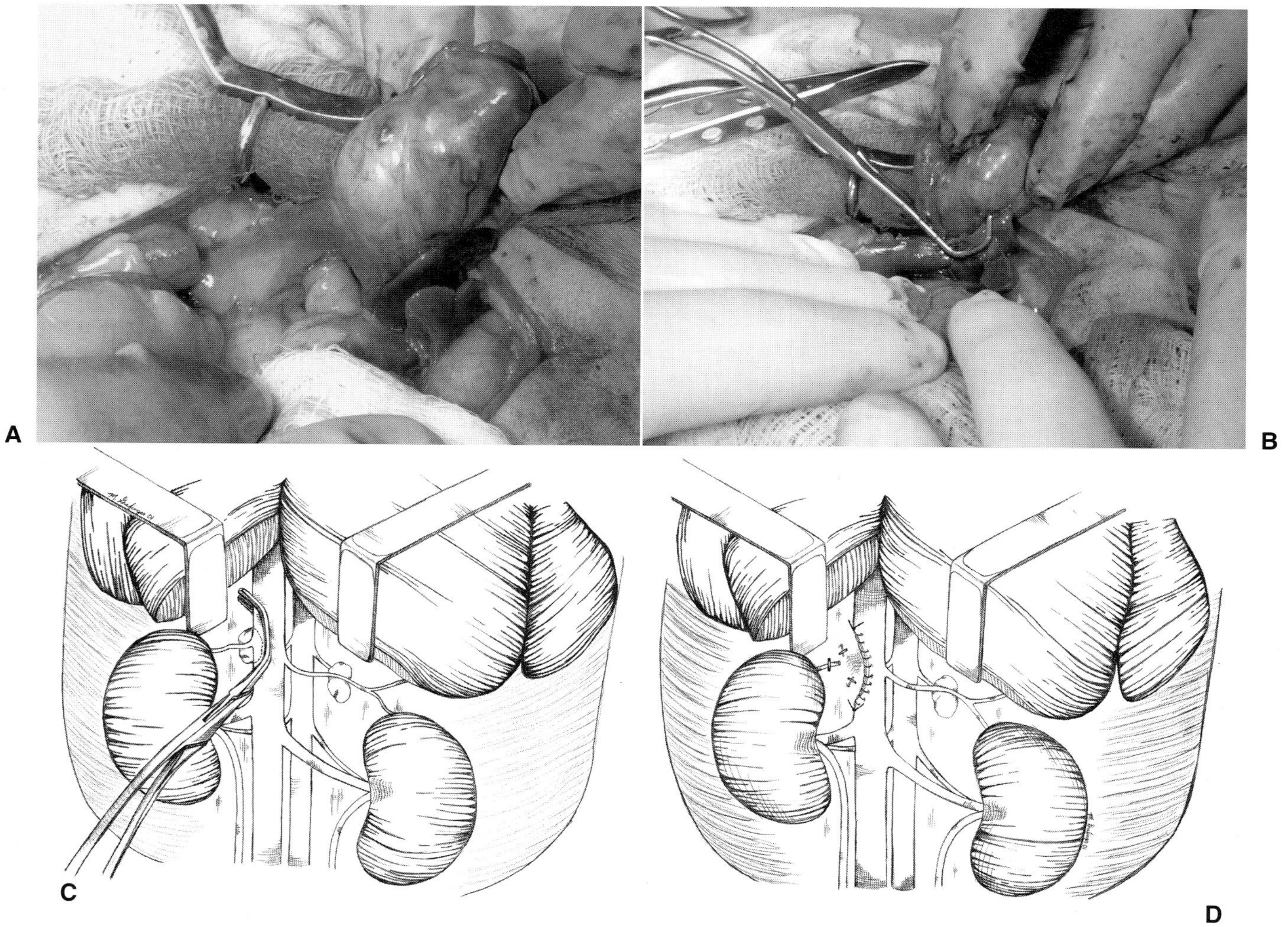

Figure 12-10 A, Large right adrenal mass attached to the caudal vena cava. B, Neonatal Satinsky clamp is applied to the vena cava around the base of the mass to result in partial occlusion of the caudal vena cava. C, Application of the Satinsky clamp. The wall of the caudal vena cava can be incised at this point to remove tumor that is invading the vessel, or it can be resected with the adherent right adrenal mass. D, Closure of the vena cava with simple continuous suture pattern. The lumen of the vena cava has been preserved. Hemoclips have been used to ligate small vessels and the phrenicoabdominal vein.

11 months after the first surgery with disease of the contralateral gland.[29] Subtotal adrenalectomy, with complete removal of one gland and partial removal of the other, is indicated for bilateral disease.[18,29] Often, the left adrenal is completely removed and the right is debulked by freeing it from surrounding tissue and placing a hemostatic clip or crushing suture across a portion of the gland to allow for removal of 50% to 75%.[2] Another method involves incising the capsule and shelling out the contents of the gland.[18] Subtotal adrenalectomy usually does not result in the need for long-term postoperative steroid therapy.[29]

Complications after surgery include hypoglycemia, hypothermia, hypotension, anemia, hypoadrenocorticism, heart failure, and renal failure. If recovery from surgery is slow or the ferret appears depressed, collect a blood sample to measure the packed cell volume and blood glucose and electrolyte concentrations. Also, assess pulse quality and measure systolic blood pressure. Continue intravenous crystalloids, supplementing the fluids with dextrose as required. If hypotension is refractory to crystalloid therapy, a colloid bolus (hetastarch, 5 mL/kg) may be helpful. Vasopressors such as dopamine are a last resort.

If anemia is present, abdominocentesis is indicated. If a small amount of blood is aspirated from the abdomen, place an abdominal wrap and administer a blood transfusion or blood substitute (Oxyglobin [Biopure, Cambridge, MA] at 15 mL/kg) as needed. If a large amount of blood is found on abdominocentesis, a second exploratory surgery may be indicated. However, this is rarely the case. If hemorrhage was minimal at surgery but a hemoperitoneum or severe bruising is observed after surgery, a coagulopathy or disseminated intravascular coagulation may be responsible. A prothrombin time and partial thromboplastin time should be measured and whole blood given if values are abnormal (see Chapter 6). If hypoadrenocorticism is suspected, administer dexamethasone at 0.5 mg/kg initially, or begin therapy with a physiologic dosage of prednisone (0.2 mg/kg per day). If hyperkalemia is detected after surgery, blood urea nitrogen and creatinine concentrations should be measured to evaluate renal function. Renal failure can result from prolonged hypotension during or after surgery, renal vein thrombosis associated with surgery involving the vena cava, or disseminated intravascular coagulation. If no evidence of renal failure is present but the patient is hyperkalemic and hyponatremic, mineralocorticoid supplementation may be necessary.

In most cases, postoperative recovery is uneventful and the ferret is fed as soon as it is fully awake. In females, the vulvar swelling usually regresses within 2 weeks.[31] Complete hair regrowth may take 1 to 6 months. Histopathologic analysis usually reveals hyperplastic or adenomatous changes. Carcinomas have been reported in up to 30% of cases, and ferrets with bilateral disease may have a combination of benign and malignant changes.[28,29] Metastasis of carcinomas is rare; however, local and vascular invasion may necessitate removal of adjacent organs. Mortality rates in the immediate postoperative period are reported to range from less than 2% to 13%; most commonly, perioperative death results from heart disease.[12,25,28,29]

Pancreatic Surgery

Insulin-secreting pancreatic islet cell tumors (also known as pancreatic beta-cell tumors or insulinomas) are one of the most common neoplastic diseases of ferrets (see Chapter 8). Ferrets typically are presented at 5 years of age, but the disease can be seen as early as 2 years of age.[6,9] Clinical signs are associated with hypoglycemia and include lethargy, weakness, ataxia, and, less commonly, seizures. Ptyalism is a frequent complaint and may be a result of nausea.[31] Because adrenal disease commonly occurs in ferrets of this age, clinical signs such as hair loss and vulvar swelling may also be observed. Diagnosis is based on clinical signs associated with hypoglycemia (see Chapter 8). A resting or a 4- to 6-hour fasting blood glucose concentration lower than 60 mg/dL is indicative of an insulinoma.[22] A high plasma insulin level obtained during an episode of hypoglycemia is definitive. If the insulin level is in the reference range, a high insulin/glucose ratio may be diagnostic.[6] Abdominal ultrasonography is usually unsuccessful at detecting pancreatic nodules but may be effective in ruling out other diseases that can result in hypoglycemia, such as neoplasia or severe liver disease. Not all ferrets with hypoglycemia have an insulinoma: other differentials for hypoglycemia include sampling error, starvation, malabsorption, sepsis, and hypoadrenocorticism. At present, surgery is the recommended treatment for ferrets with insulinomas.[6,30] Although surgery is not curative, it provides a definitive diagnosis, allows for evaluation of concurrent disease, and may result in a prolonged disease-free interval and survival.[9,30]

Anatomy of the pancreas in ferrets is similar to that of dogs and cats. The common pancreatic duct empties into the duodenum at the major duodenal papilla with the bile duct. An accessory pancreatic duct is also occasionally present. The blood supply to the pancreas comes from three sources (Fig. 12-11). The right limb is supplied by the cranial and caudal pancreaticoduodenal vessels, and the left limb is supplied primarily by a branch from the splenic artery.

At surgery, fully explore the abdomen to assess any adrenal gland abnormalities, enlarged lymph nodes, or evidence of metastasis to the liver or spleen. Evaluate each limb of the pancreas by visually inspecting and gently palpating both the ventral and dorsal surfaces. The body of the pancreas can be inspected only on its ventral surface. Insulin-secreting tumors can appear as readily visible masses that are discolored or as small nodules (less than 1 mm diameter) that are firm on palpation. Magnification loupes are ideal for locating small nodules. Multiple nodules involving more than one lobe of the pancreas are common. For large masses or multiple nodules on one lobe, perform a partial pancreatectomy, which allows for more complete removal of the tumor and may increase survival.[30] Create a window on either side of the pancreatic limb to be removed, and free the limb from the surrounding omentum or mesoduodenum. Tighten a 4-0 PDS or Monocryl (Ethicon, Johnson and Johnson Healthcare, Piscataway, NJ) suture around the base of the limb, allowing a margin of at least 5 mm from the last visible nodule (see Fig. 12-11). Transect the limb distal to the ligature, and close the rent in the omentum or mesoduodenum with small suture in a simple continuous pattern. Take care during dissection to avoid the pancreaticoduodenal vessels, because damage to these vessels may result in necrosis of the duodenum. A cotton-tipped applicator often can be used to bluntly free the pancreas from these vessels. Preserve the body of the pancreas to avoid damaging the pancreatic duct. Remove nodules in the body of the pancreas by gently teasing the tumor away from the surrounding pancreas (nodulectomy). If more than one limb is affected, perform a partial pancreatectomy on the limb that contains most of the masses. Remove the nodules on the remaining limb by nodulectomy. Use a mosquito hemostat and cotton-tipped applicators to bluntly free the nodules from the surrounding tissue. Hemorrhage usually is minimal and does not require suturing. If enlarged lymph nodes are found, remove them and submit samples for histopathologic evaluation. Biopsy the spleen or any affected liver lobes, or remove them if indicated.

Maintain an intravenous catheter after surgery, and check the blood glucose concentration during recovery. If the glucose concentration is less than 70 mg/dL, administer intravenous fluids with 2.5% or 5% dextrose as needed. Monitor the blood glucose concentration every 12 to 24 hours during hospitalization. Occasionally, the blood glucose concentration remains low for 1 to 3 days or longer after surgery. Postoperative pancreatitis is uncommon, and food may be offered within 12 hours after surgery. Rarely, diabetes mellitus requiring insulin supplementation develops after a large pancreatic resection. Check the blood glucose concentration 10 to 14 days after surgery and every 3 to 4 months thereafter.

Histopathologic analysis may reveal hyperplasia, adenoma, or adenocarcinoma, but these findings do not dictate prognosis, because recurrence of disease and clinical signs is almost always inevitable. Prognosis is affected by the duration of clinical signs and the presence of metastasis at surgery.[9] The longer the duration of clinical signs before surgery, the worse the prognosis. Prognosis is not affected by the number of nodules present or by persistence of hypoglycemia after surgery.[6,9] Mean disease-free intervals after surgery are reported to range from 284 to 365 days.[9] If hypoglycemia recurs, ferrets can be successfully managed medically with frequent feedings and prednisone, diazoxide, or both for extended periods. Average survival times of ferrets treated surgically have been reported to range from 563 to 668 days.[6,9,30]

Splenectomy

Splenomegaly is a common finding on abdominal exploration and is usually benign (Fig. 12-12). The most common cause of splenomegaly in ferrets is extramedullary

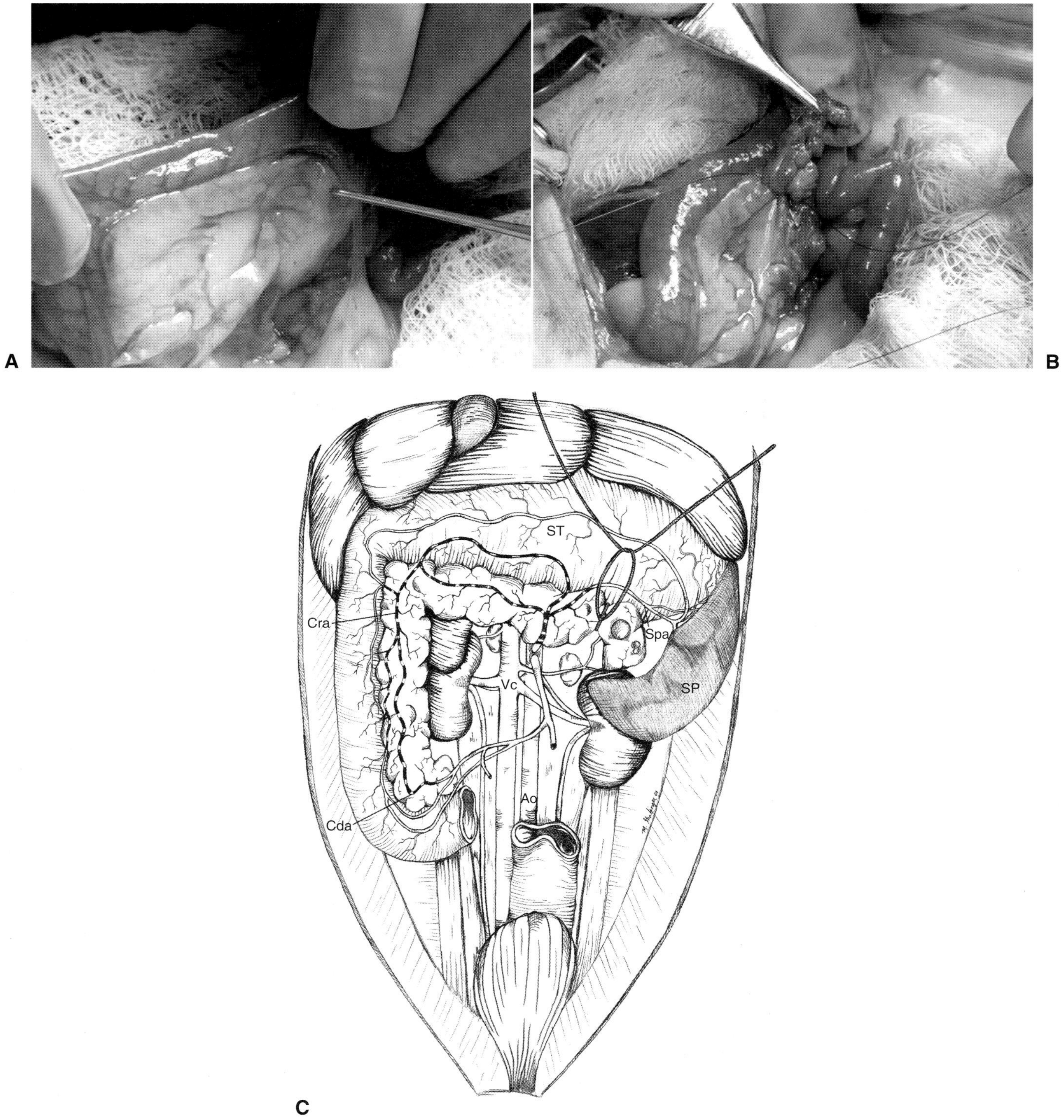

Figure 12-11 A, Pancreatic insulinoma at the tip of the left limb of the pancreas. B, Partial pancreatectomy. The surrounding mesentery has been dissected free from the left limb of the pancreas and a 4-0 PDS ligature is used to ligate the pancreas proximal to the mass. C, Diagram of guillotine suture for partial pancreatectomy with normal pancreatic anatomy. Note the shared blood supply of the pancreas with the spleen and duodenum. *Vc,* Vena cava; *Ao,* aorta; *SP,* spleen; *ST,* stomach; *Spa,* splenic artery; *Cra,* cranial pancreaticoduodenal artery; *Cda,* caudal pancreaticoduodenal artery.

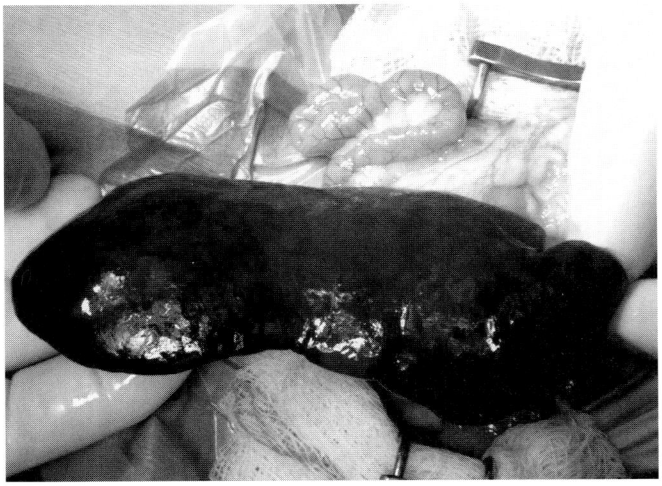

Figure 12-12 Enlarged spleen at abdominal exploratory.

hematopoiesis.[4] Neoplastic conditions associated with splenomegaly include lymphosarcoma, mast cell tumor, hemangiosarcoma, adrenal neoplasia, and insulinoma.[4,11,32] Cardiomyopathy, Aleutian disease, eosinophilic gastritis, and idiopathic hypersplenism have also been reported as causes of splenic enlargement. Splenic sequestration of red blood cells, seen with isoflurane anesthesia, can result in both splenomegaly and a significant reduction in the hematocrit and plasma protein concentration.[15] Within 45 minutes after termination of anesthesia, these variables return close to baseline values.

Ferrets with splenomegaly should be evaluated for underlying disease conditions before splenectomy is considered. Ultrasound-guided fine-needle aspiration or TruCut needle soft tissue biopsy (Allegiance Healthcare Corporation, McGraw Park, IL) can help determine whether primary splenic disease is present. Splenectomy is indicated for primary splenic or metastatic neoplasia, idiopathic hypersplenism, or severe splenic enlargement that interferes with abdominal visceral function. Because the spleen is a major site of erythropoiesis in ferrets, splenectomy should not be taken lightly, and the potential consequences of surgery need to be carefully considered.

Splenic biopsy techniques are the same as for liver biopsy. Small, absorbable suture material (e.g., 4-0 PDS) can be placed in a cruciate or mattress pattern to control hemorrhage. Sutures tend to hold better in the spleen than in the liver because of the relatively thick splenic capsule. Although partial splenectomy is rarely indicated, it can be done for benign processes that result in excessive splenic enlargement. For this procedure, ligate and divide the vessels supplying the portion of spleen to be removed. Place a clamp across the area to be removed, and close it to crush the tissue. Place a thoracoabdominal stapling device (U.S. Surgical Corporation, Norwalk, CT) in the crushed area after the clamp is removed. After the staples are fired, transect the spleen distal to the stapler and release the stapler. Control any subsequent hemorrhage with hemoclips or mattress sutures. As an alternative to a stapling device, place mattress sutures through the spleen proximal to the crushing clamp to control hemorrhage. Close the splenic capsule in a simple continuous pattern before removing the clamp.

Total splenectomy involves ligation of all vessels supplying the spleen. Double-ligate the splenic artery and vein, being careful to avoid damaging the pancreas in this area. Stay close to the spleen when ligating the short gastric vessels, to avoid damaging the stomach. Hemoclips can be used instead of suture material to control hemorrhage, but stapling devices used in other small animals (Autosuture LDS, U.S. Surgical) are too large for use in ferrets.

UROGENITAL SYSTEM

Nephrectomy

Nephrectomy is indicated in cases of unresolved hydronephrosis, chronic bacterial nephritis, and neoplasia. As in other domestic species, the kidneys of ferrets are located in the retroperitoneal space. However, the large amount of retroperitoneal fat in ferrets often obscures their visibility. For nephrectomy, the surgical approach is through a ventral midline incision. Isolate the involved kidney with moistened sponges, and open the peritoneum over the kidney to access the retroperitoneal space. Grasp the kidney and apply gentle traction while using cotton-tipped applicators to isolate the renal vessels and ureter. Although it is simpler to perform, do not mass-ligate the renal artery and vein; instead, individually dissect and double-ligate the renal artery and vein close to the aorta and vena cava, respectively. The vessels may be double-ligated with hemostatic clips or fine 4-0 or 5-0 suture material. Dissect the ureter along its retroperitoneal course all the way to the urinary bladder. Then ligate and transect the ureter as close to the urinary bladder as possible without damaging the nerves that run in the lateral ligament of the bladder. Lavage the abdominal cavity and close it routinely.

Cystotomy

Like other domestic species, ferrets can suffer from cystic and urethral calculi. Magnesium ammonium phosphate is the most common type of urolith found in ferrets and can be associated with pregnancy in jills. The history and clinical signs of urolithiasis in ferrets are similar to those of other small animal species and may be characterized by stranguria, hematuria, recurrent urinary tract infections, or urinary tract obstruction. Surgery to remove calculi is indicated to relieve clinical signs and for quantitative crystallographic stone analysis.

Cystotomy in ferrets is similar to the procedure performed in other small animal species. Make a caudal midline abdominal incision (in females) or a parapreputial skin incision with a midline abdominal incision (in males). After locating the bladder, pack the abdominal cavity with moistened sponges to limit contamination. Choose a ventral location on the bladder that is relatively devoid of blood vessels as the incision site. Using fine suture material, place stay sutures on either side of the planned incision line. The urinary bladder in normal ferrets is very thin, so take care when applying traction to the stay sutures. After making the incision, remove the calculi and thoroughly inspect and lavage the bladder. Flush the urethra with a small, soft catheter to ensure that no calculi remain. Submit the calculi for stone analysis, and submit a crushed specimen of the calculi and a small section of the bladder wall for bacterial culture and sensitivity testing. Close the cystotomy incision with fine (4-0 or 5-0) synthetic absorbable suture material in either a simple interrupted or a simple continuous pattern. Check the bladder for leakage by using a syringe and a 25-gauge needle to infuse sterile saline solution. If leakage is observed, add a continuous inverting suture layer over the initial sutures. Lavage the abdomen thoroughly and close routinely.

Perineal Urethrostomy

Because of recurrent urethral calculi, distal strictures, or neoplasia, a perineal urethrostomy is occasionally indicated in a ferret. The anatomy of the ferret penis and urethra most closely resembles that of dogs. The site of the urethrostomy should be located caudal (proximal) to the os penis and the site of obstruction and ventral to the anus. Magnification with surgical loupes greatly simplifies the procedure. Place the ferret either in dorsal recumbency with the pelvic area elevated or in ventral recumbency within a perineal stand. Aseptically prepare the perineal region and caudal abdomen. If possible, place a urethral catheter in the anesthetized ferret before surgery. This can be difficult because of the small urethral diameter, the hook-shaped os penis, and the relative difficulty of extruding the penis from the prepuce (see Chapter 4). Make a skin incision approximately 1 cm cranial (ventral) to the anus. This exposes the urethra and the cavernous tissue. If a urethral catheter is present, palpate the catheter and make a 1-cm longitudinal incision along the ventral aspect of the urethra. If a urethral catheter cannot be placed, make the incision ventrally, taking care not to stray laterally and incise the cavernous tissue. Open the urethra, and a place a larger urethral catheter proximally to assist in locating the lumen and mucosa. Use simple interrupted sutures of 5-0 or 6-0 synthetic absorbable monofilament suture material to close the urethral mucosa to skin. After surgery, confine the ferret for at least 2 weeks, and prevent self-trauma with an Elizabethan collar if necessary. Remove the sutures after 2 weeks if possible; otherwise, the absorbable sutures may be left in place to dissolve.

Paraurethral/Prostatic Cysts

Prostatic disease in ferrets is usually associated with adrenal gland neoplasia. Ferrets are presented with a history of stranguria and, potentially, urinary obstruction. Alopecia, pruritus, and other clinical signs associated with hyperadrenocorticism may also be observed. Differential diagnoses for stranguria include urinary calculi, infection, neoplasia of the urinary tract or prostate, and prostatic cysts or hyperplasia.[24] Initial diagnostic tests should include a urinalysis and culture and an abdominal ultrasound examination to evaluate the urinary tract, prostate, and adrenal glands. Additional diagnostic tests, such as measurements of plasma concentrations of adrenal hormones, may also be helpful. If the bladder is distended and cannot be expressed, a urinary catheter should be passed with the ferret anesthetized. If urethral catheterization is unsuccessful, perform cystocentesis with a 25-gauge needle. Alternatively, a tube cystostomy can be placed and maintained after adrenalectomy until prostatic inflammation resolves.

Treatment involves an abdominal exploratory and adrenalectomy. At surgery, aspirate the prostatic or paraprostatic cyst with a small-gauge needle (Fig. 12-13). The fluid contained within the cyst is often green and viscous, and a sample should be submitted for bacterial culture and sensitivity testing. Because multiple cysts may be present, aspirate multiple sites. If the cysts are small, aspiration may be the only treatment required. For larger cysts (more than 2 cm in diameter), remove a portion of the cyst wall for biopsy and to allow complete drainage of all cavitations. The cyst can then be omentalized. Theoretically, omentalization provides continued drainage of the cyst, aids in adhesion formation, and enhances immune function to fight against infection. "Pack" a portion of the omentum into the cyst cavity and suture it to the cyst wall with 4-0 absorbable suture.[3] Place three to four sutures, being careful to avoid disrupting the blood supply to the omentum. Express the bladder to check for leakage of urine from the cyst. If leakage is observed, place more omentum into the cyst, and partially close the opening into the cyst with suture. If leakage is still seen, a transurethral catheter or tube cystostomy will need to be maintained for 1 to 2 days after surgery until the communications with the urethra are sealed. Usually, the prostate decreases in size and the cysts regress within 1 to 2 days after adrenalectomy. Histologic findings in ferrets with prostatic cysts have revealed squamous metaplasia and prostatitis caused by keratin, squamous cells, and cellular debris. These changes are believed to be caused by adrenocortical disease and associated high levels of circulating estrogens or androgens.[7,24] Often secondary bacterial infection is present, resulting in large prostatic abscesses.

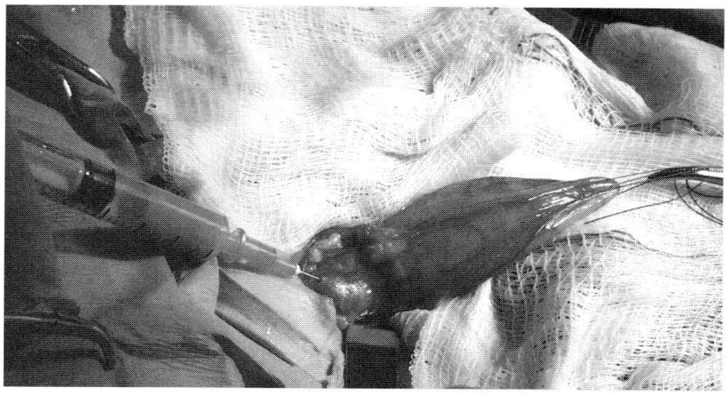

Figure 12-13 Fluid is aspirated from a prostatic cyst. This ferret presented for urinary obstruction. A large left adrenal mass was found and resected.

Ovariohysterectomy

Because most pet ferrets in the United States are spayed at breeding farms before they are 8 weeks of age, ovariohysterectomy is not a common procedure in veterinary practice. Intact female ferrets remain in estrus with high circulating estrogen levels until they are stimulated to ovulate through breeding or artificial stimulation. Spaying of intact pet ferrets is recommended to prevent life-threatening bone marrow suppression caused by chronically high estrogen levels.

For ovariohysterectomy, make a ventral midline incision about 1 cm caudal to the umbilicus. The uterus of ferrets is bicornuate and can be found just dorsal to the bladder. Because of the large amount of body fat, the ovarian vessels may be difficult to locate. Completely ligate the ovarian pedicles and uterine body with 3-0 or 4-0 absorbable suture material. Close the linea routinely with 3-0 or 4-0 absorbable suture.

Ovarian Remnant

In a spayed female ferret, clinical signs of estrus (swollen vulva) are usually caused by adrenal neoplasia. Occasionally, these signs result from a remnant of ovarian tissue inadvertently left behind during prior ovariohysterectomy. Signs typically occur in ferrets younger than 2 years of age, which is younger than in ferrets with adrenal disease. If it is uncertain whether a ferret has an ovarian remnant, administer 100 IU of human chorionic gonadotropin (hCG) intramuscularly. If an ovarian remnant is present, vulvar swelling should subside within a few days. If the vulvar swelling is associated with adrenal disease, vulvar size will not change.[22] Before abdominal exploratory surgery, evaluate the ferret for anemia and thrombocytopenia, which result from estrogen toxicity. At surgery, the remnant typically is found just caudal to the kidneys.[18] A thorough exploration is necessary, because more than one remnant may be present. Ovarian remnants, which may have been dropped during the previous ovariohysterectomy and revascularized, can be found in any part of the abdominal cavity. Vulvar swelling should resolve 1 to 5 days after removal of the remnant.

Pyometra

Because most ferrets are spayed at an early age, pyometra is uncommon. Clinical signs suggestive of pyometra include vulvar discharge, lethargy, and anorexia. Polyuria and polydipsia are not commonly reported. The treatment for pyometra is ovariohysterectomy combined with fluid and antibiotic therapy. Before surgery, submit a blood sample for a complete blood count to evaluate for bone marrow suppression associated with hyperestrogenism. Ovariohysterectomy is routine. At surgery, exteriorize the uterus and place a moistened laparotomy sponge in the abdomen to prevent contamination. Remove the sponge and lavage the stump before closing the abdomen. Treat with a broad-spectrum antibiotic to cover the organisms associated with pyometra in ferrets, including *Staphylococcus, Streptococcus,* and *Corynebacterium* species and *Escherichia coli*.[18] Stump pyometra may be seen with ovarian remnants or adrenal gland disease. In these cases, remove the remnant or adrenal gland in addition to resecting the stump.

Castration

Ferrets should be castrated by 6 to 8 months of age to reduce aggressive behavior, decrease musky odor, and protect against testicular neoplasia. Castration can be performed as it is in cats, with an incision in the scrotum over each testicle. An open or a closed technique can be used, and the spermatic cord can be ligated with a "self-tie" technique (vas deferens to vessels) or with 4-0 chromic gut suture. Leave the incisions open to heal by secondary intention. Alternatively, make a prescrotal incision and exteriorize both testicles through the same incision. With this technique, close the subcutaneous tissue with 4-0 or 5-0 absorbable suture, and close the incision with either intradermal or skin sutures.

Preputial Masses

Masses involving the prepuce are uncommon in male ferrets and usually are found incidentally on physical examination (Fig. 12-14). However, occasionally they result in urethral obstruction. These masses are typically benign adenomas, although adenocarcinomas have been reported.[13] Adenomas can be removed simply by marginal excision and reconstruction of the preputial orifice with 5-0 suture material. Adenocarcinomas must be

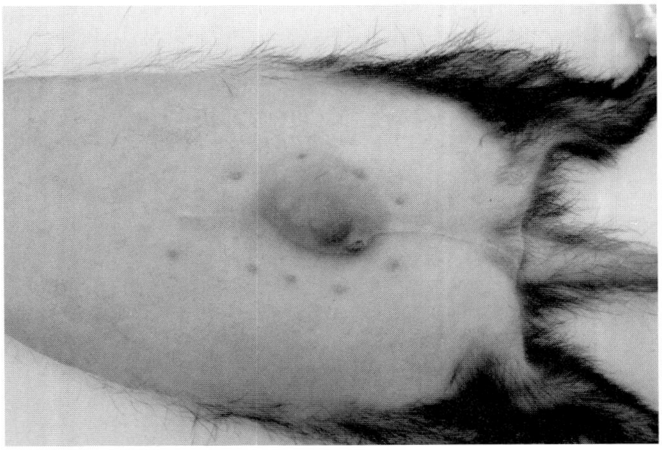

Figure 12-14 Male ferret with a subcutaneous mass cranial to the prepuce. Although these masses are usually benign adenomas, adenocarcinomas have been reported.

resected more aggressively, possibly requiring surgical removal of the prepuce. In these cases, a partial penile amputation is required to prevent exposure damage to the penis, with diversion of urine flow by a perineal urethrostomy.

Anal Sacculectomy

Anal sacculectomy (descenting) is mainly performed in conjunction with early neutering at ferret breeding farms, but it may be done at any age. Removal of the anal sacs may decrease the musky odor in neutered ferrets, but some odor associated with the glands in the perianal region will remain.[8] Also, body odor is primarily caused by sebaceous secretions of the skin, which increase during breeding season (see Chapter 1). The anal sac openings are located at the anocutaneous junction at the 4- and 8-o'clock positions. Magnification is of great assistance in locating the anal sac openings and during the surgical procedure. Identify the opening of the anal sac and grasp it with fine mosquito forceps. Incise the skin 1 to 2 mm around the anal sac opening with a No. 15 scalpel blade. Use a scraping motion with the blade to remove glandular tissue, skin, and subcutaneous tissue surrounding the duct and sac. Dissection of the gland is initially difficult because of the close association of the surrounding glands, but, after a few millimeters, a tissue plane exposing the yellow-white surface of the anal sac will become evident. Continue to dissect the anal sphincter muscle from the anal sac until the entire sac is freed, and then remove the intact sac without spilling the contents. If any of the anal sac tissue remains after surgery, fistulous tracts will develop. If bleeding is observed that does not quickly stop with digital pressure, small blood vessels may need to be ligated or coagulated. Lavage the defect, and either close the opening with a single subcuticular suture using 5-0 synthetic absorbable suture material or leave it open to heal by secondary intention.

REFERENCES

1. Bauck LB: Salivary mucocele in two ferrets. Mod Vet Pract 1985; 66:337-339.

2. Beeber NL: Surgery in pet ferrets. *In* Bojrab MJ, ed. Current Techniques in Small Animal Surgery. Baltimore, Williams & Wilkins, 1998, pp 763-769.
3. Bray JP, White RAS, Williams JM: Partial resection and omentalization: a new technique for management of prostatic retention cysts in dogs. Vet Surg 1997; 26:202-209.
4. Brown SA, Rosenthal KL: Causes of splenomegaly in ferrets. Vet Med 2000; 95:599.
5. Caligiuri R, Bellah JR, Collins BR, et al: Medical and surgical management of esophageal foreign body in a ferret. J Am Vet Med Assoc 1989; 195:969-971.
6. Caplan ER, Peterson ME, Mullen HS, et al: Diagnosis and treatment of insulin-secreting pancreatic islet cell tumors in ferrets: 57 cases (1986-1994). J Am Vet Med Assoc 1996; 209:1741-1745.
7. Coleman GD, Chavez MA, Williams BH: Cystic prostatic disease associated with adrenocortical lesions in the ferret *(Mustela putorius furo.)* Vet Pathol 1998; 35:547-549.
8. Creed JE, Kainer RA: Surgical extirpation and related anatomy of the anal sacs of the ferret. J Am Vet Med Assoc 1981; 179:575-577.
9. Ehrhart N, Withrow SJ, Ehrhart EJ, et al: Pancreatic beta cell tumor in ferrets: 20 cases (1986-1994). J Am Vet Med Assoc 1996; 209:1737-1740.
10. Evans HE, An NQ: Anatomy of the ferret. *In* Fox JG, ed. Biology and Diseases of the Ferret, 2nd ed. Baltimore, Williams & Wilkins, 1998, pp 19-69.
11. Ferguson DC: Idiopathic hypersplenism in a ferret. J Am Vet Med Assoc 1985; 186:693-695.
12. Lawrence HJ, Gould WJ, Flanders JA, et al: Unilateral adrenalectomy as a treatment for adrenocortical tumors in ferrets: five cases (1990-1992). J Am Vet Med Assoc 1993; 203:267-270.
13. Li X, Fox JG: Neoplastic diseases. *In* Fox JG, ed. Biology and Diseases of the Ferret, 2nd ed. Baltimore, Williams & Wilkins, 1998, pp 405-447.
14. Lipman NS, Marini RP, Murphy JC, et al: Estradiol-17β-secreting adrenocortical tumor in a ferret. J Am Vet Med Assoc 1993; 203:1552-1555.
15. Marini RP, Callahan RJ, Jackson LR, et al: Distribution of technetium 99m-labeled red blood cells during isoflurane anesthesia in ferrets. Am J Vet Res 1997; 58:781-785.
16. Martin RA: Liver and biliary system. *In* Slatter DH, ed. Textbook of Small Animal Surgery, 2nd ed. Philadelphia, WB Saunders, 1993, pp 645-659.
17. Miller PE, Picket JP: Zygomatic salivary gland mucocele in a ferret. J Am Vet Med Assoc 1989; 194:1437-1438.
18. Mullen HS: Soft tissue surgery. *In* Hillyer EV, Quesenberry KE, eds. Ferrets, Rabbits, and Rodents: Clinical Medicine and Surgery. Philadelphia, WB Saunders, 1997, pp 131-144.
19. Mullen HS, Scavelli TD, Quesenberry KE, et al: Gastrointestinal foreign body in ferrets: 25 cases (1986-1990). J Am Anim Hosp Assoc 1992; 28:13-19.
20. Neuwirth L, Collins B, Calderwood-Mays M, et al: Adrenal ultrasonography correlated with histopathology in ferrets. Vet Radiol Ultrasound 1997; 38:69-74.
21. Poddar S: Gross and microscopic anatomy of the biliary tract of the ferret. Acta Anat 1977; 97:121-131.
22. Rosenthal KL: Ferrets. Vet Clin North Am Small Anim Pract 1994; 24:1-23.
23. Rosenthal KL, Peterson ME: Evaluation of plasma androgen and estrogen concentrations in ferrets with hyperadrenocorticism. J Am Vet Med Assoc 1996; 209:1097-1102.
24. Rosenthal KL, Peterson ME: Stranguria in a castrated male ferret. J Am Vet Med Assoc 1996; 209:62-64.
25. Rosenthal KL, Peterson ME, Quesenberry KE, et al: Hyperadrenocorticism associated with adrenocortical tumor or nodular hyperplasia of the adrenal gland in ferrets: 50 cases (1987-1991). J Am Vet Med Assoc 1993; 203:271-275.
26. Shoemaker NJ, Schuurmans M, Moorman H, et al: Correlation between age at neutering and age at onset of hyperadrenocorticism in ferrets. J Am Vet Med Assoc 2000; 216:195-197.
27. Wagner RA, Dorn DP: Evaluation of serum estradiol concentrations in alopecic ferrets with adrenal gland tumors. J Am Vet Med Assoc 1994; 205:703-707.
28. Weiss CA, Scott MV: Clinical aspects and surgical treatment of hyperadrenocortism in the domestic ferret: 94 cases (1994-1996). J Am Anim Hosp Assoc 1997; 33:487-493.
29. Weiss CA, Williams BH, Scott JB, et al: Surgical treatment and long-term outcome of ferrets with bilateral adrenal tumors or adrenal hyperplasia: 56 cases (1994-1997). J Am Vet Med Assoc 1999; 215:820-823.
30. Weiss CA, Williams BH, Scott MV: Insulinoma in the ferret: clinical findings and treatment comparison of 66 cases. J Am Anim Hosp Assoc 1998; 34:471-475.
31. Wheeler J, Bennett RA: Ferret abdominal surgical procedures: part I. Adrenal gland and pancreatic beta-cell tumors. Compend Contin Educ Pract Vet 1999; 21:815-822.
32. Wheeler J, Bennett RA: Ferret abdominal surgical procedures: part II. Gastrointestinal foreign bodies, splenomegaly, liver biopsy, cystotomy, and ovariohysterectomy. Compend Contin Educ Pract Vet 1999; 21:1049-1057.

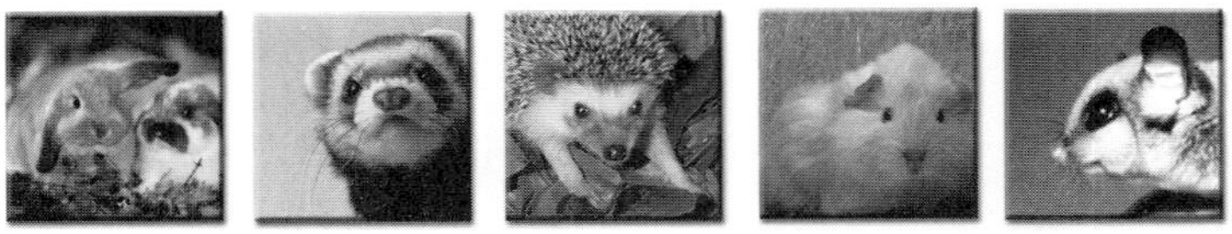

SECTION

TWO

RABBITS

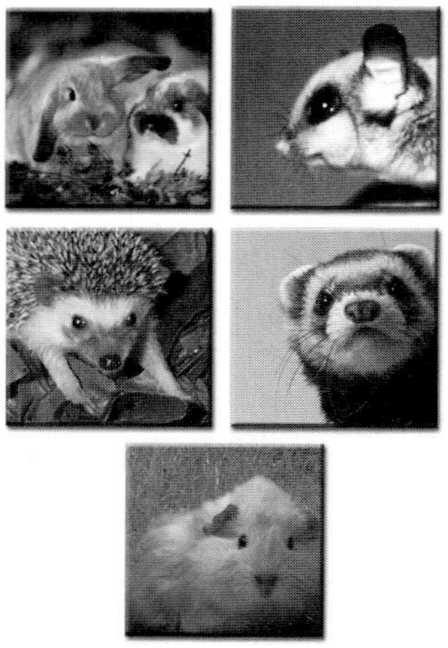

CHAPTER 13

Basic Anatomy, Physiology, and Husbandry

Thomas M. Donnelly, BVSc, Diplomate ACLAM

TAXONOMY AND SIMILARITIES TO RODENTS

The Swedish naturalist Karl von Linne, who established the systematic classification of plants and animals, recognized the similarity of rabbits and rodents. He assigned them to a taxonomic group called Glires. Later naturalists designated Glires as the mammalian order Rodentia. Within this order they grouped rabbits, hares, and pikas in the suborder Duplicidentata because they possessed a second pair of incisor teeth in the upper jaw. Rodents, having only a single pair of upper incisors, were grouped in the suborder Simplicidentata. Subsequent classification in the 20th century resulted in the designation of Duplicidentata as the mammalian order Lagomorpha. We now restrict the order Rodentia to the larger group of mammals with only one pair of upper incisors, such as squirrels, rats, mice, and guinea pigs. The discovery of a new fossil *(Tribosphenomys minutus)* and recent morphologic and molecular evidence suggest that the relationship of rodents and lagomorphs is closer than suspected[27] and their similarities are not an example of convergent evolution.[31] The term *Glires* is again being used to describe the infraclass that encompasses these two orders.

In both rabbits and rodents, the anterior incisors in the upper and lower jaws are modified to form chisel-like cutting organs.[36] The incisors remain permanently sharp from gnawing. Enamel is deposited on the front surface of these teeth only. The back surface is composed of dentin, and because enamel is harder than dentin, the front surface wears down more slowly. Also, teeth are absent between the last incisor and the first cheek tooth. This toothless space is known as the *diastema*.

BREEDS AND VARIETIES

Domestic rabbits are divided into fancy breeds and fur breeds. The fur group is divided into normal fur, Rex, and Satin breeds. The normal fur breeds have a coat made up of an undercoat and projecting guard hairs; the Rex breeds have short guard hairs that do not appear above the level of the undercoat; and the Satin breeds have an abnormal hair fiber that produces a sheen.[39] The term "variety" describes a color (e.g., black, blue, steel grey, tortoiseshell) within a breed.

Body conformation and ear size vary widely among breeds of rabbits, and rabbit fanciers have coined some unusual terms to describe body shape and fall of ear. They refer to the small and chunky body of a dwarf rabbit, like a cobblestone, as "cobby." The long and lean body of a Belgian hare is "racy," and the giant rabbits are "mandolin-shaped" because of the high, curved top line over their hindquarters.[41] Most breeds of rabbits have upright ears, which can be long or short. However, some breeds have ears that hang downward; we know these as "lops."

SKIN AND SCENT-MARKING GLANDS

Rabbit skin is very delicate compared with that of other exotic pet species, dogs, and cats. Unless care is taken when clipping fur before surgery, the skin can be easily torn or ripped. Because rabbit fur is so fine, clipping requires fine clipper heads that are not normally used with cats or dogs. The hair of rabbits grows in periodic orderly waves originating on the ventrum and spreading dorsally and caudally. This is most noticeable when hair grows back after clipping for surgery.

Female rabbits have a large fold of skin over the throat known as the *dewlap*. Breeding does pull fur from this area to line their nests before kindling. In older breeding does, the dewlap can be large and easily mistaken for an abscess. Moist dermatitis often develops in this area.

Rabbits do not have footpads; instead, coarse fur covers their toes and metatarsal areas. When a rabbit is sitting, undisturbed, the plantar surface of the lower hindlimb, from the toes to the hock, is in contact with the ground. Heavy rabbits housed on wire floors often develop an ulcerative pododermatitis of this area called *sore hocks*. The claws of rabbits are very sharp, and a rabbit picked up without appropriate support of its hindquarters can inflict painful scratches on the handler.

Rabbits are strongly territorial, and both sexes have three glands used in scent-marking behavior: the *chin glands*, which are specialized submandibular glands opening onto the underside of the chin; the *anal glands*; and a pair of pocket-like perineal glands called the *inguinal glands*. The size of the glands and the degree of marking are androgen dependent and are related to the level of sexual activity. Males mark more frequently than do females; dominants of both sexes mark more frequently than subordinates; and dominants mark most in the presence of subordinate rivals. Under natural conditions, both bucks and does on their own territory, surrounded by their own odor and that of their clan, win two thirds of all aggressive encounters.[30]

SENSE ORGANS AND NERVOUS SYSTEM

As is expected from an animal subject to predation, the sense organs of rabbits are well developed. Rabbits are sensitive to catecholamines and have evolved for flight rather than fight. Temperature, heart rate, and respiratory rate significantly increase in a frightened animal.

Eyes

Prince[37] described the anatomy and physiology of the rabbit eye in great detail in the old but not outdated text, *The Rabbit Eye in Research*.

The rabbit cornea is large, occupying 30% of the globe, and the eyes are directed more laterally than those of most mammals. These two features give rabbits a panoramic field of vision to detect predators readily. However, their eyes cannot visualize the small area beneath the mouth, and rabbits depend on the sensitivity of the lips and vibrissae to discriminate food.

As in most rodents and other lagomorphs, the lens is spherical and large. The ciliary body is small and poorly developed. These two features suggest that rabbits have a limited need for alternation of near and far focus (i.e., accommodation).

The optic nerve is above the horizontal midline of the eye, and retinal examination of this nerve involves looking upward into the eye. Retinal vessels spread out horizontally from the optic disc; also, rabbits have a depression or physiologic cup in their optic disc, as do dogs. Rabbits do not have a tapetum lucidum.

During anesthesia, the third eyelid moves well across the cornea. Behind it and separated from the deep part of the cartilage is the harderian gland, which has a small, white upper lobe and a large, pink lower lobe. The lower lobe is also known as the deep gland of the nictitating membrane. This gland occasionally prolapses,[19] similar to cherry eye in dogs.

A few millimeters posterior to the limbus and under the bulbar conjunctiva, the rectus dorsalis muscle is visible. Putting an anchoring suture under or around this muscle is possible and serves to stabilize the globe during surgery; in other species, dissection is necessary to find an extraocular muscle.

In rabbits, the primary channel for return of venous blood from the head, including that from the eye, is the external jugular vein.[37] In contrast, the primary drainage of the eye and head in humans is via the internal jugular vein. In other species, such as dogs, significant anastomoses exist between the branches of the internal and external jugular veins. In rabbits, such anastomoses are minor, and ligation or chronic catheterization of the external jugular vein results in swelling and protrusion of the eyeball for about 24 hours, after which its normal appearance returns.[18] The same pattern of vascularity also applies to the arterial blood supply of the rabbit's eyes, but ligation of the external carotid artery results in ipsilateral ocular necrosis.

Rabbits, like rodents, have an extensive orbital venous plexus. Because of possible severe hemorrhage, enucleation of the eye is difficult in rabbits compared with species such as dogs.

The nasolacrimal drainage system provides a conduit for tears from the lacrimal lake to the nasal cavity. In rabbits, a single ventral lacrimal punctum (about 3-4 mm ventral to the lid margin), canaliculus, sac, duct, and nasal meatus form this drainage system for each eye. The diameter of the nasolacrimal duct is small and narrows in two places where it changes course. These two sites, the proximal maxillae and the base of the upper incisor, are important in the development of obstruction.[25] Dacryocystitis and nasal duct obstruction often cause epiphora, one of the most common ocular problems seen in rabbits.

See also Chapter 39 for a discussion of ophthalmologic conditions in rabbits.

Ears

The pinnae represent a large portion of the total body surface in rabbits, approximately 12% in New Zealand white rabbits. The pinnae are highly vascular; when heated, they have the largest arteriovenous shunts in the body. In large-eared rabbits, the vessels are easily accessible for venipuncture. However, in small-eared rabbits such as dwarf breeds, venipuncture of the ear veins can lead to vasculitis, vascular necrosis, and sloughing of portions of the ear pinna. During surgery, the ears are a good site to obtain noninvasive measurements such as blood oxygenation and systemic arterial pressure.[16] However, blood pressure in the central ear artery is about 10 mm Hg less than in the common carotid artery.

MUSCLES AND SKELETON

Bones of rabbits are relatively delicate compared with their muscle mass. The skeleton represents only 7% to 8% of body weight in rabbits, whereas the skeletal muscle comprises more than 50% of the body weight.[3,10] Fractures, especially of the tibia, are always a potential problem. In comparison, the skeleton of a cat constitutes 12% to 13% of body weight. However, the dry matter and percentage of calcium are higher in the bones of rabbits than in those of cats.[1] Rabbits have powerful hind legs that can kick violently. If rabbits are not securely held when picked up, their kicking can result in a vertebral fracture (almost always at the seventh lumbar vertebra) and damage to the spinal cord. Proper handling of a rabbit is essential if injury to the rabbit and the handler is to be prevented.

The number of thoracic (T) and lumbar (L) vertebrae varies from 12T/7L in 44% of rabbits, 13T/6L in 33%, and 13T/7L in 23%.[15] The spinal cord ends within the second sacral vertebra (S2) in 79%, within the first sacral vertebra (S1) in 19%, and within the third sacral vertebra (S3) in 2% of rabbits.[15]

In countries where rabbit meat is commonly eaten, clients may present a headless carcass that they suspect to be that of a cat. The color of the muscles distinguishes the two: rabbit muscles are pale pink, whereas those of cats are deep red. There are also skeletal differences, most noticeably between the scapula and pelvis. The infraspinous fossa of rabbits is sharply triangular, whereas that of cats is more rounded; also, the suprahamate process of the acromion is truly hook-shaped in rabbits (Fig. 13-1), whereas it is blunted in cats. The acetabulum of rabbits is formed by the ilium, the ischium, and a small accessory bone, the os acetabuli, which excludes the pubis. In other animals, the acetabulum comprises the ilium, the ischium, and the pubis. Good drawings of these differences are found in Okerman's *Diseases of Domestic Rabbits.*[32]

The trochanteric fossa of the femur is a good site for intraosseous catheter placement and is easily located by palpating the prominent greater trochanter.

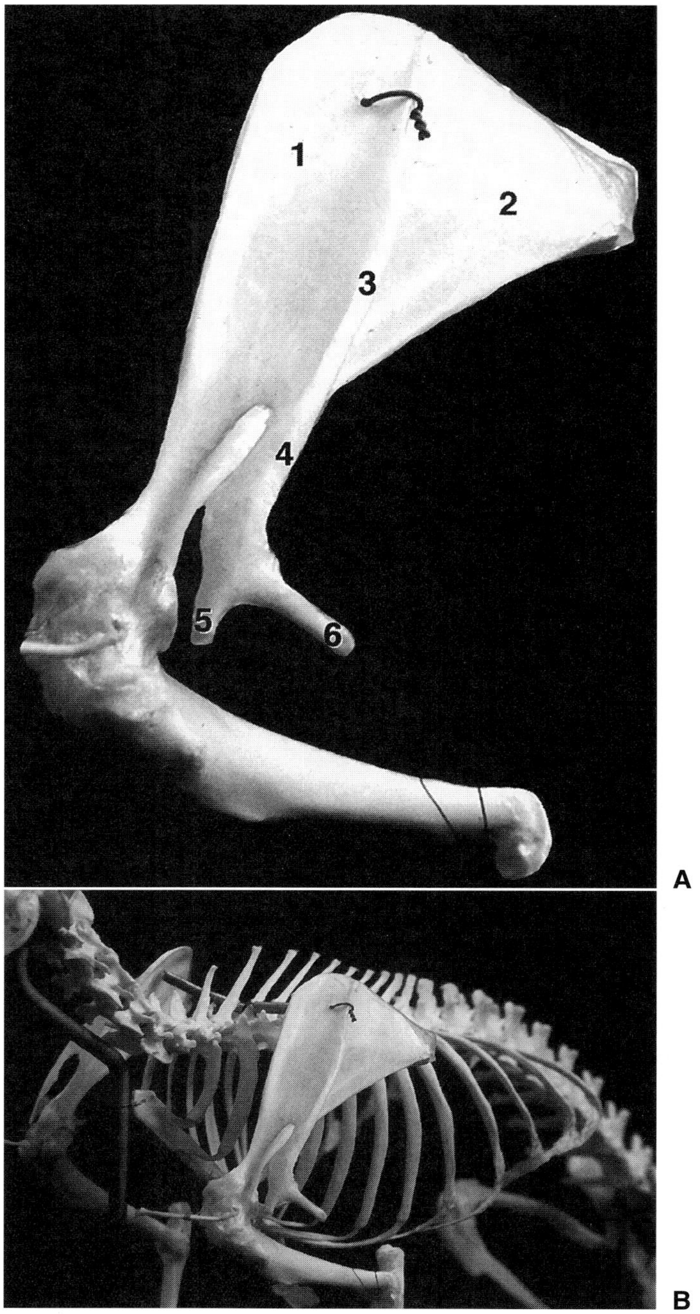

Figure 13-1 A, Lateral aspect of the left scapula of a rabbit. *1,* Supraspinous fossa; *2,* infraspinous fossa; *3,* spine of the scapula; *4,* acromion; *5,* hamate process; *6,* suprahamate process. **B,** Skeleton of a rabbit showing the relationship of the left scapula to other bones.

DIGESTIVE SYSTEM

The definitive reference on the anatomy and physiology of the digestive tract of rabbits is Cheeke's *Rabbit Feeding and Nutrition.*[5] Most of the information described in this section is from Cheeke's book unless otherwise noted.

Teeth

Rabbit teeth grow continuously and are known as hypsodont or open-rooted teeth (see Chapter 34). Instead of a true dental root, there is a very long crown. The dentin layer is relatively thin, and teeth are easily fractured during dental procedures. The periodontal ligament provides a weaker attachment apically than is seen in carnivores. Rabbits shed a set of nonfunctional deciduous teeth perinatally, and their permanent teeth are completely erupted by 3 to 5 weeks of age. The dental formula is: $2\ (I^2_1,\ C^0_0,\ P^3_2,\ M^3_3) = 28$.

Rabbits have four upper and two lower incisors. The smaller upper incisors, or peg teeth, are caudal to the larger incisors. Incisors are worn to proper length because the lower incisors rest between the large upper incisors and the peg teeth. Maxillary or upper incisors grow at approximately 2 mm per week, and mandibular or lower incisors grow at 2.4 mm per week.[22] Incisor malocclusion, in which the lower incisors project in front of the upper incisors, is seen commonly in pet rabbits. One cause is mandibular prognathism, which is analogous to brachiocephalic syndrome in dogs, and consequently dwarf rabbits present most often with this problem.

The premolar and molar teeth as a group are known as the cheek teeth. The last upper molar tooth is very small, so functionally there are five pairs of grinding teeth on each side of the jaw. The upper and lower cheek teeth meet in a relatively level occlusal surface. Deep enamel folds in the cheek teeth create sharp ridges for grinding of coarse material.

Oral Cavity

The mouth opening in rabbits is small, and the upper lip has a divided groove that continues by curving right and left to the nostrils—hence, the expression, "harelip."

The muscles of the jaws extend both forward and backward. This confers a deceptively large appearance to the oral cavity, which is actually smaller than the size of the jaws suggests. Because the articular process forming the temporomandibular joint is elongated longitudinally, the mandible can move forward, backward, and vertically but less so from side to side.

Endotracheal intubation for anesthesia is difficult in rabbits because of their small mouth, large cheek teeth and tongue, and deep oral cavity. Relaxation of the jaw musculature signifies that the animal is sufficiently anesthetized for intubation. During intubation, it is easy to traumatize the oral and respiratory structures unless care is taken.[8]

Abdominal Cavity

The abdominal cavity of rabbits is large. The gastrointestinal tract is relatively long, and its contents can make up 10% to 20% of the body weight. This is an important consideration when the appropriate dose of intravenous anesthetics is being determined. Because of their size, the two most striking organs are the stomach and cecum.

Stomach

The stomach serves as a reservoir for much of the ingested feed. It typically contains 15% of the alimentary tract ingesta, and food and fecal pellets are almost always present. The stomach is thin-walled and often appears ruptured at necropsy because of gas distention during autolysis. However, the cardia and pylorus are well developed. Rabbits are unable to vomit because of the anatomic arrangement of their cardia and stomach, and their pylorus is easily compressed by the duodenum, which exits at an acute angle. Gastric distention or compression due to a furball, gas, or hepatomegaly contributes to pyloric compression and prevents emptying.

Small Intestine

The duodenum and jejunum have a relatively small lumen. The terminal portion of the ileum ends in the cecum and is expanded as the rounded sacculus rotundus. This structure has a minute honeycombed external appearance owing to the presence of a large number of lymph follicles, and it is sometimes referred to as the *ileocecal tonsil*. It is also a common site of foreign body impaction.[20] The small intestine is shorter in rabbits than in other species and makes up about 12% of the total gastrointestinal tract volume. Peyer's patches are absent from the duodenum and the first half of the ileum. No correlation exists between the number of Peyer's patches and intestinal length, and surgeons or pathologists may see only three to nine Peyer's patches in the first quarter of the jejunum and last quarter of the ileum.[28]

Large Intestine

Rabbits have a large, thin-walled, coiled cecum that holds about 40% of the ingesta (Fig. 13-2). It ends in a thick-walled, pale vermiform appendix that is characterized, like the sacculus rotundus, by abundant lymphatic tissue. The cecum is the largest and most prominent organ in the abdominal cavity of rabbits. It folds onto itself three times as it constricts around most of the inner surface of the abdominal cavity wall. The cecal contents are generally semifluid.

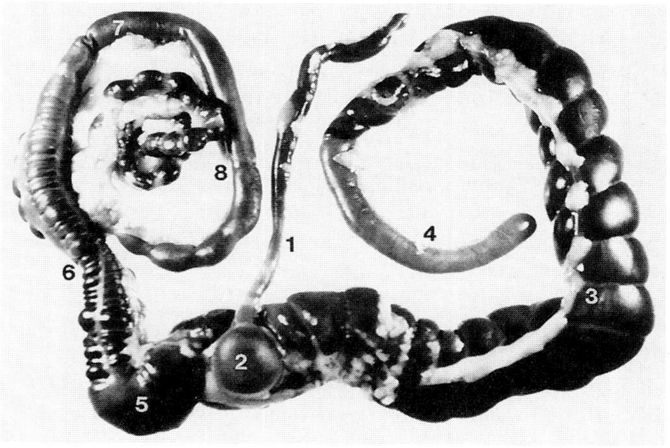

Figure 13-2 Dissected large intestine of a rabbit. *1*, Ileum; *2*, sacculus rotundus; *3*, body of cecum (note the long spiral fold along its length); *4*, vermiform appendix; *5*, ampulla coli; *6*, proximal colon; *7*, fusus coli; *8*, distal colon. *(Courtesy Douglas F. McBride, DVM.)*

Sacculations and bands characterize the colon, which starts from an area of the cecum known as the *ampulla coli*. The proximal colon is separated from the distal colon by the *fusus coli*, a thickened section of colon heavily supplied with ganglionic cell aggregates. The fusus coli acts as a pacemaker that controls the contractions for excreting the two types of feces.

Muscular contractions in the colon cause fiber particles to separate from the nonfiber components of the gut contents. Peristaltic contractions rapidly move fiber through the colon for excretion in the hard feces. Antiperistaltic contractions move fluids and particles retrograde through the colon into the cecum, where they are retained for fermentation. At intervals, the cecum contracts and its fermentation contents are expelled through the colon and consumed directly from the anus by the rabbit. Thus, the products of bacterial growth are made available to the rabbit either by direct absorption or by consumption of the cecal contents. This latter process is known as *coprophagy* or *cecotrophy*. The consumed cecal contents are called *soft feces, night feces*, or *cecotropes*. These appear as a cluster of soft pellets rather than as the single pellets typical of hard feces. A mucilaginous membrane that acts as a barrier to the low pH of the stomach surrounds cecotropes and permits reabsorption in the small intestine (see Chapter 15).

Pancreas, Liver, Gallbladder, and Spleen

Although the pancreas of rabbits is closely associated with the duodenum, it is diffuse and often difficult to differentiate from surrounding mesentery.

Rabbits have a small, circular hepatic lobe known as the *caudate lobe*, which has a narrow attachment or stalk to the dorsal hilar region of the liver. This stalk is prone to displacement, and torsion of the caudate lobe has been infrequently reported.[13]

From a midline approach, the gallbladder is deceptively deep within the abdominal cavity. Like dogs, rabbits have separate openings for the bile duct and the pancreatic duct in the duodenum. Similar to most nonmammalian species, rabbits secrete mainly biliverdin rather than bilirubin in their bile.

Gut-associated lymphoid tissue constitutes about 50% of the total lymphoid tissue mass. Therefore, the spleen is relatively small compared with that of other species. The frequency of accessory spleens in rabbits is 9%.[14]

RESPIRATORY SYSTEM AND THYMUS

Rabbits are obligate nasal breathers. This characteristic has important clinical and anesthetic consequences. Mouth breathing is a poor prognostic sign, and inflammation of the upper respiratory tract increases the risk of anesthetic mortality in nonintubated animals.

The thymus persists into adult life in rabbits. It retains considerable size, lies ventral to the heart, and extends forward to the thoracic inlet.

The thoracic cavity of the rabbit is relatively small; in contrast, the abdominal cavity is large, and the rabbit breathes primarily by contraction of the diaphragm. These characteristics allow for an efficient method of artificial respiration: suspend the rabbit horizontally in midair, holding the forelimbs in one hand and back legs in the other hand, and gently rock the rabbit from a head-up to a head-down position every 1 to 2 seconds.

CARDIOVASCULAR SYSTEM

As with many other organs, the size of the rabbit's heart is directly related to its body size. Because the size of the heart limits blood volume, the tissues cannot be supplied with oxygen by means of increased ventricular volume pumped out in one beat. Instead, heart frequency remains the major modifying variable, and consequently, heart rates are higher in smaller animals than in larger ones. In rabbits, the heart rate can vary from 180 to 250 beats/min. Despite the small size and rapid contraction rate of the rabbit heart, quantitative Doppler-echocardiographic methods have been validated to evaluate structural and functional abnormalities (see Chapter 21).[24,33,42]

Rabbits have a relatively small heart, which accounts for about 0.3% of body weight. The right atrioventricular valve is unique because it is composed of two, rather than three, cusps. The rabbit aorta has a rhythmic contraction that is neurogenic in origin.

The veins have thin walls and are susceptible to hematoma formation, which can be avoided through the judicious use of Teflon catheters and gentle pressure. Muscle swellings in the pulmonary artery make this vessel thicker and more muscular in rabbits than in any other species. Pulmonary hypertension causes death from anaphylaxis; at necropsy, severe constriction of the pulmonary arteries and dilatation of the right side of the heart are observed.

The erythrocyte count varies between 5 and 8 million/mm^3, and erythrocytes show marked anisocytosis. Polychromasia is found in 1% to 2% of erythrocytes. A feature of rabbit blood is the occurrence of numerous thornapple-shaped erythrocytes in the blood smear. The erythrocytes include a large number of reticulocytes (1%-7%) in adult animals and even higher numbers in young rabbits.

Leukocyte counts in rabbits vary considerably because of diurnal fluctuations, nutrition, and differences in sex, age, and breed. The differential count in one healthy rabbit can fluctuate considerably if repeated over a period of 1 month. The neutrophils of rabbits are comparable to those of large domestic animals and humans and are called heterophils or pseudoeosinophils because of their many small eosinophilic-staining granules (see Chapter 38). There is a large variation in lymphocytes according to age and nutritional condition.

Overall, variations in hematologic values due to breed are not as pronounced as those due to the individual physiology, nutrition, age, and sex of the animal.

URINARY SYSTEM

Most mammalian kidneys are multipapillate, but those of rabbits and rodents are unipapillate. Only one papilla and one calyx enter the ureter directly.

The plasticity of the rabbit urinary system has not been fully recognized. Rabbits from Australian desert zones have large kidneys with powerful urine-concentrating ability, small adrenal glands, and low levels of circulating aldosterone. Rabbits from Australian alpine zones have small kidneys (at least 25% less in weight than those of desert rabbits), large adrenal glands, and high levels of circulating aldosterone.[29] At necropsy, the most striking difference is in the size of the renal medulla. In the desert-dwelling rabbits, which live on a high-fiber, high-salt, low-protein plant diet and have limited access to water, the medulla is long. In contrast, in alpine rabbits, which enjoy a high-protein diet of lush grasses that are low in sodium, the renal medulla is short. Probably, the main reason rabbits have been so preeminent in successfully colonizing diverse geographic regions is that their urinary system has the capacity to vary its developmental pattern under different environmental conditions and with different digestive strategies.

The serum calcium level of rabbits is unusual and is not regulated in a narrow range but reflects the level of dietary calcium. Urine is a major route of calcium excretion, which varies directly with the serum calcium level. Whereas the fractional urinary excretion of calcium in most mammals is less than 2%, the range for rabbits is 45% to 60%. Increases in dietary calcium directly increase urinary calcium excretion. The consistency of the urine is often thick and creamy because of a white calcium carbonate precipitate. Prolonged intake of a diet high in calcium results in calcification of the aorta and kidney. High vitamin D intake intensifies this effect.[4,21]

The color of normal rabbit urine varies from yellow to red because it contains pigments that have not yet been identified. Certain types of feed, such as alfalfa or the tropical legume *Leucaena,* seem to increase the intensity of the pigmentation.[6] Because of this discoloration, rabbit owners often erroneously report the presence of blood in their pet's urine.

PUBERTY AND BREEDING LIFE

The age at which rabbits attain sexual maturity varies considerably according to the breed. However, if the biologic pattern of growth is plotted graphically, puberty occurs just after the maximal rate of growth. On the growth velocity curve, sexual maturity occurs at the point at which growth is still taking place but its rate is decelerating rapidly. Therefore body weight is more important than age in determining sexual maturity. Small breeds develop more rapidly and are mature at 4 to 5 months of age. Medium-sized breeds mature at 4 to 6 months and large breeds at 5 to 8 months of age.[35] Does mature earlier than do bucks, which do not achieve optimal sperm production and reserves until 40 to 70 days after puberty. Among New Zealand white rabbits, females reach maturity at approximately 5 months of age and males at 6 to 7 months. The reproductive life of a rabbit again depends on its breed but is about 5 to 6 years for the buck and up to 3 years for the doe.

FEMALE REPRODUCTIVE SYSTEM

Anatomy and Physiology

The reproductive tract of a doe lacks a uterine body; instead, each of two separate uterine horns has its own opening into the vagina (Fig. 13-3). If a cesarean section is performed, the surgeon must remove the fetuses through separate incisions in each horn. The mesometrium is a major fat storage site, and identification and ligation of the uterine vessels can be difficult.

Like cats and ferrets, rabbits are induced ovulators and do not have an estrous cycle. However, does vary in their sexual receptivity, so that a certain rhythm can be detected. In domestic rabbits, this rhythm has been reported as having intervals of 4 to 6 days. Ovulation occurs after coitus or after the injection of luteinizing hormone. The time of ovulation in induced ovulators varies among species. In rabbits, it is 10 hours after copulation, compared with 30 hours in cats and ferrets.

Female Sexual Behavior

Sexual receptivity in a doe is characterized by lordosis, a reverse bending or flattening of the back, raising of the pelvis, or presenting of the perineum in response to attempts by a buck to mount. Similar behavior is seen in cats. Generally, female rabbits are hyperactive and brace themselves when touched. When not receptive, does do not allow males to mount. Depending on cage space, nonreceptive behavior often takes the form of running away, cornering, biting, and vocalizing.

In natural conditions, rabbits exhibit distinct breeding seasons that are influenced by both day length and temperature. In the northern hemisphere, rabbits in natural conditions exhibit their highest conception rate in spring and their lowest rate in autumn. When environmental conditions are controlled, male rabbits mate at any time. Maximal sexual receptivity in does is often accompanied by enlargement of the vulva, which also becomes reddish-purple and moist. Although females will almost invariably mate in this condition, they also occasionally mate even when these changes have not occurred. Vaginal smears do not provide useful information. The most reliable indicator is lordosis that occurs when the female is firmly clasped in the lumbar region. Ovulation occurs between 10 and 13 hours after copulation. To ensure successful ovulation, many breeders give a single intravenous injection of 100 IU of human chorionic gonadotropin to does after mating to induce ovulation. Transportation of female rabbits may also result in spontaneous ovulation, with a resultant pseudopregnancy that lasts approximately 18 days.

Pregnancy and Nursing Behavior

The gestation period in rabbits varies with the breed but is approximately 30 to 32 days. Litter size depends on the breed as well as on parity. Primiparous animals tend to produce smaller litters. Small breeds such as the Dutch-belted produce small litters of 4 or 5 kits, whereas larger breeds such as the New Zealand white produce large litters of 8 to 12 kits. Mammary glands are found in the axillary, thoracic, abdominal, and inguinal areas. Although textbooks describe a total of eight glands, on average five glands are in the axillary area, six to seven in the thoracic area, seven to eight in the abdominal area, and six to eight in the inguinal area.[17]

Does usually give birth in the early morning. A few hours to days before kindling, rabbits pull fur from their abdomen, sides, and dewlap to make a nest. Although the underlying skin can look inflamed, this is normal behavior. The kits are born blind, helpless, and hairless and remain in the nest for about 3 weeks. Does nurse only once a day for 3 to 5 minutes. However, during this brief period, a young rabbit may drink 20% of its body weight. A healthy, well-fed litter bursts out of the fur nest like popcorn when the nest is examined. Olfactory cues are critical during the nursing period: a gland in the region of the nipple

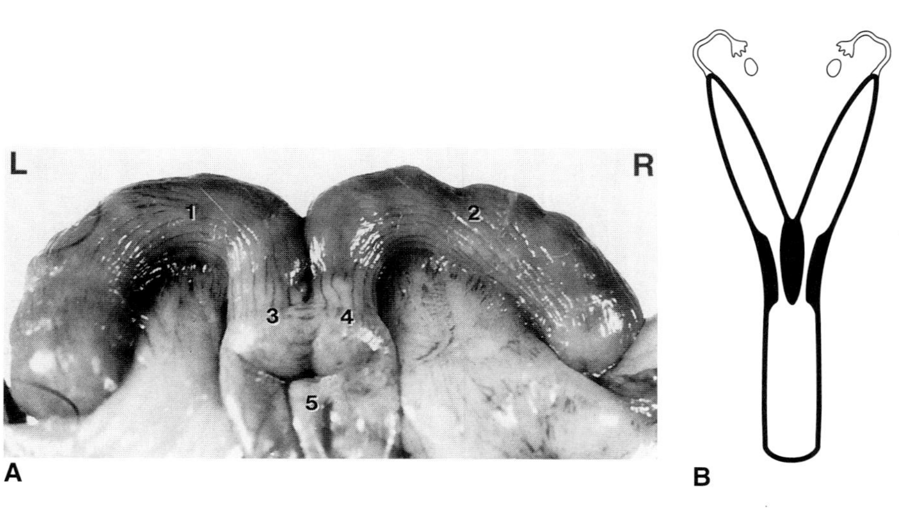

Figure 13-3 **A,** Dorsal surface of a dissected postparturient rabbit uterus. Note the abundant mesometrial fat, which makes identification and ligation of uterine vessels difficult. *L,* Left; *R,* right; *1,* left uterine horn; *2,* right uterine horn; *3,* left cervix; *4,* right cervix; *5,* vagina. **B,** Diagram of a doe's reproductive system, showing two uterine horns and two cervices.

produces a pheromone that attracts kits. Does mark kits with chin and inguinal gland secretions, and they are openly hostile to young that are not their own. They harass young from their own colony but hotly pursue and kill young from other colonies. Does will attack and kill kits smeared with an odor from other rabbits.[29] Successful cross-fostering requires that kits are healthy and have the energy to suckle and that their scent is camouflaged by placing them on the bottom of the litter pile and rubbing them in the nest bedding.[11]

Hand-rearing of Baby Rabbits

Pet baby rabbits may require hand-rearing because of the death of the mother or because of poor nursing, which often occurs with a doe's first litter. Most wild rabbits (including Eastern cottontail rabbits *[Sylvilaglus floridanus]* in the United States) that a person brings into the clinic are probably not abandoned or orphaned. Unlike nursing cats and dogs, nursing does leave their nest, returning only once or twice a day to care for the young. Unless the wild neonate is injured, it should be left undisturbed in the nest.

Immediate support and evaluation of the neonatal pet rabbit is a priority. Baby rabbits are very susceptible to hypothermia. Warming of the neonatal rabbit is critical if its body temperature drops to less than 97°F (36°C). A rabbit can be warmed by immersing it in a warm (100°F [37.8°C]) bath and gently massaging it while keeping its head above the water. Because warming can worsen any dehydration, the neonate may require administration of isothermic (100°F [37.8°C]) lactated Ringers solution (10-15 mL/100 g body weight SC).

Despite warming and fluid administration, weak neonates are often unable to nurse from a teat or syringe and require tube-feeding. I prefer nasal gastric tubing and attempt to provide about 4 mL of rabbit milk replacement formula for newborns. The volume is then increased appropriately for weight gain and body size. Tube feeding permits control of how much milk the neonate receives and avoids the problem of aspiration of milk into the lungs.

Numerous studies have looked at the quantity and composition of milk produced by lactating does. Neither breed nor pregnancy status affects milk composition. However, the stage of lactation significantly affects the major components of milk, except lactose (Fig. 13-4).[12] Rabbit's milk is higher in protein, fat, and ash than that of other species except rats (Fig. 13-5). The milk of both rabbits and rats is high in fat and protein but low in carbohydrates.[26]

Several recipes for rabbit milk replacer have been published (Table 13-1).[40] Milk replacer for neonatal and young rabbits is commonly a combination of Esbilac or KMR (Kitten Milk Replacer) and Multi-Milk (all available from PetAg Inc., Hampshire, IL; www.petag.com). Try to prepare enough fresh milk replacer daily to allow for 1 day of feeding, and keep it refrigerated between feedings. Rabbit breeders and wildlife rehabilitators often like to add a probiotic and infant multivitamin drops to the rabbit milk replacer; however, their effectiveness has not been established.

Although does feed their young only once a day, try to feed neonates three times a day to reduce bloat yet still provide

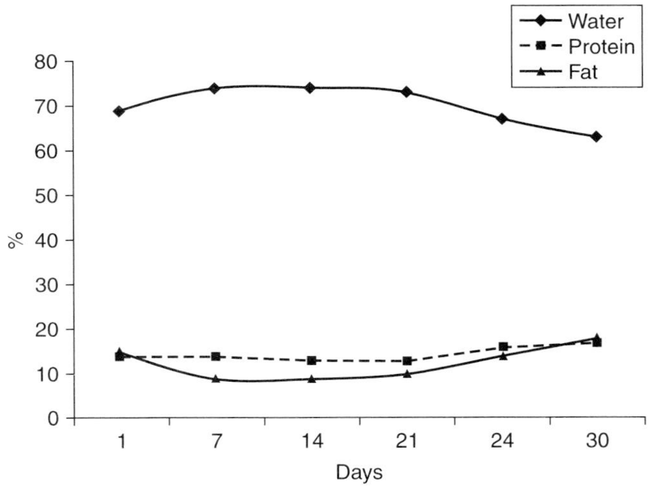

Figure 13-4 The composition of rabbit milk according to day of lactation. *(Data from El-Sayiad GHA, Habeeb AAM, El-Maghawry AM: A note on the effects of breed, stage of lactation and pregnancy status on milk composition of rabbits. Anim Prod 1994; 58:153-157.)*

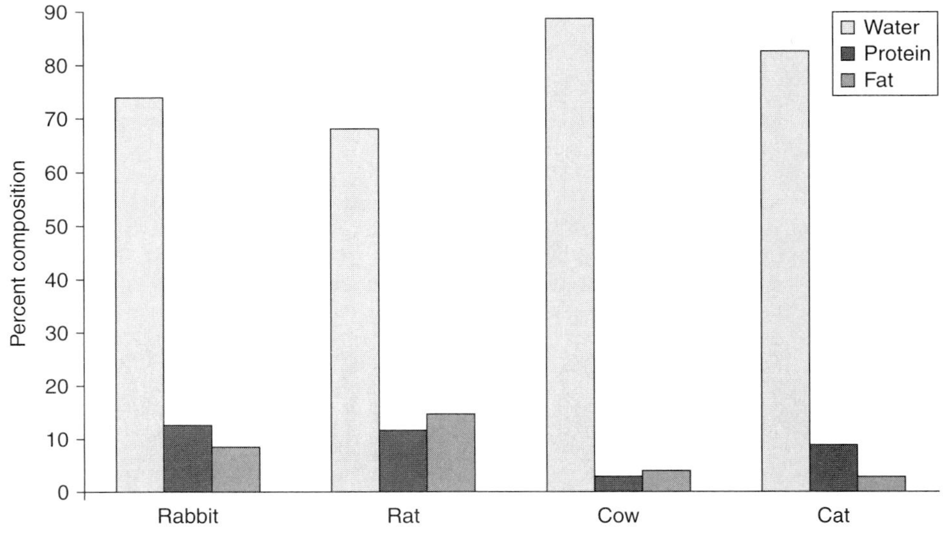

Figure 13-5 The composition of rabbit milk compared with milk of other species. *(Data from McNitt JI, Cheeke PR: Rabbit Production, 7th ed. Danville, IL, Interstate Printers & Publishers, 1996.)*

TABLE 13-1
Recipes for Rabbit Milk Replacer

Cheeke's Milk Replacer[26]	Taylor's Milk Replacer 1[40]	Taylor's Milk Replacer 2[40]	Taylor's Milk Replacer 3[40]	Taylor's Milk Replacer 4[40]
1 part evaporated milk 1 part water Add to 1 cup of mixture: 1 egg yolk 1 Tbsp corn syrup	1 part Esbilac powder $^1/_4$ part heavy cream 1 part water	2 parts KMR liquid 1 part Multi-Milk powder	6 parts Esbilac 4 parts Multi-Milk powder	1 part Esbilac 1 part Multi-Milk powder $1^1/_2$ parts water

adequate calories. Baby rabbits can take 2 to 3 days before they settle into a feeding pattern. I find it helpful to record body weights daily (or at every feeding time), as well as the amount of milk replacer consumed at each feeding. A neonate that drinks a small amount of milk replacer at one feeding may be greedy at the next.

Neonatal rabbits require stimulation of the anogenital region to urinate and defecate. This can be done by gently stroking the anogenital area with a warm, wet, cotton-tipped applicator or gauze sponge. If the rabbits develop normally, this procedure is no longer necessary after 1 week of growth.

Neonatal rabbits depend totally on milk up to day 10. They can digest a small amount (5%) of solid feed by day 15, and by day 20 coprophagy is taking place and solid feed represents most of the feed intake.[2] Hand-raised rabbits may take slightly longer to achieve these time points. By day 21, rabbits should be nibbling on hay and eating small amounts of solid feed. By day 28, rabbits should not be drinking milk replacement but can be offered water from a bottle.

MALE REPRODUCTIVE SYSTEM

Unlike most other placental mammals but similar to marsupials, rabbits have two hairless scrotal sacs cranial to the penis. They do not have an os penis. The testes descend at about 12 weeks of age, and the inguinal canals do not close. The technique of choice for castration must take into account measures to prevent inguinal herniation. Male rabbits have very small nipples that are not apparent under their fur.

Male Sexual Behavior and Reproduction

Bucks show a constant libido after puberty. Initiation of copulation in rabbits is confined to basic patterns such as sniffing, licking, nuzzling, reciprocal grooming, and following the doe. Bucks may also exhibit tail-flagging and enurination, the emission of a jet of urine at a partner during a display of courtship. Experienced males usually initiate copulation within minutes or even seconds after a receptive female is introduced. Inexperienced males generally require longer.

The species-specific copulatory patterns of the male are related to ovulation and corpus luteal function of the female. Copulatory behavior of bucks may be understood by considering that the doe ovulates spontaneously after coitus. The stimulus of coitus is necessary only for ovulation and not for the maintenance of the corpus luteum, which always follows ovulation. Bucks rapidly mount receptive females and accomplish intromission after a series of rapid copulatory movements. Reflex ejaculation follows immediately on intromission. The copulatory thrust is generally so vigorous that the buck falls backward or sideways and may emit a characteristic cry. Vigorous bucks may attempt to copulate again within 2 to 3 minutes. A problem often encountered in male rabbits trained to use artificial vaginas is a reduced ability to induce lordosis during natural mating attempts. These conditioned bucks may become lazy. They fail to grasp and apply pressure to the flanks of the female when attempting to copulate and thus fail to induce lordosis.

Bucks deposit semen into the anterior vagina, and the sperm pass individually through the cervical mucus. This pattern also occurs in sheep, cattle, and humans. If a rabbit is inseminated during an active corpus luteal phase (e.g., early pregnancy, pseudopregnancy), sperm transport does not take place. During this period, when blood progesterone levels are increasing in rabbits (as in humans), the cervical secretions are thick and mucoid and inhibit sperm transport.

BEHAVIOR

The behavior of wild and domestic rabbits is very similar. The major difference is their response to confinement: wild rabbits do not adapt well to cages, often fail to breed, and exhibit abnormal behavior not seen under natural conditions. Other wild lagomorphs (e.g., hares) resist domestication and cannot be raised successfully in cages. In contrast, domestication of rabbits has resulted in an animal that is not stressed by confinement and has a more placid disposition toward humans while retaining most of the behavioral repertoires of its wild ancestors.[39]

Eating and Drinking Behavior

Field studies of wild rabbits indicate that they are selective feeders with a wide food range. They prefer to eat tender, succulent plant parts as the major portion of their diet and consume small quantities of coarse roughage to stimulate gastrointestinal motility. Rabbits chew their food thoroughly, with highly organized tongue movements and up to 120 jaw movements per minute.[9] Nutritional studies have shown that laboratory rabbits also adapt to a high-roughage diet. Wild rabbits can consume a large volume of fiber without the need for a large gut because of the rapid digestive time. Furthermore, the small, herbivorous gut does not interfere with the ability for swift evasion of carnivorous predators.

The primary feeding times for rabbits are in the early morning and at night, with coprophagy commencing 3 to 8 hours after eating.[5] Rabbits like sweet materials and select diets containing molasses or sucrose over similar diets without added sugar.[5] This preference can be used to advantage when an anorectic rabbit is encouraged to eat. Most pet owners feed their rabbits commercial pelleted diets because they are convenient and balanced in their formulation. Most of these diets are alfalfa-based and low in fiber. When pet rabbits are fed a diet of unlimited low-fiber pellets, they can become obese and develop chronically soft stools. Food restriction is practiced in some research laboratories to avoid these problems: New Zealand white rabbits weighing 2 to 3 kg are fed 100 to 120 g of pelleted diet per day. Food restriction in pet rabbits can lead to fur-pulling and gnawing of carpets, furniture, shoes, and, sometimes fatally, electrical wires. Boredom and destructive behavior can be avoided by supplementing the diet with fresh grass, timothy or other hay, and a variety of vegetables and by providing gnawing toys such as a small log from an untreated fruit tree. High-fiber, timothy-based pellets are available (Oxbow Pet Products, Murdock, NE; www.oxbowhay.com). This type of pelleted diet helps to prevent obesity and ensures a high dietary fiber intake.

Compared with other animals, rabbits have a high water intake. A rabbit's average daily water intake is 50 to 150 mL/kg of body weight; a 2-kg rabbit drinks about as much water daily as does a 10-kg dog.[7] When food is withheld from rabbits, they develop polydipsia, and after 3 days of food deprivation they can increase their water intake by 6.5 times.[3] With water deprivation, food consumption declines; after 3 days of deprivation, anorexia results.[7]

Group Behavior

A unique aspect of rabbit behavior is the ability to form large groups or warrens. Rabbits are the only leporid that live in large, stable groups, sometimes numbering several hundred animals.[34] Although rabbits dig burrows that serve as a primary haven and restrict their home range, they are active above ground, moving around, hopping, running, chasing, and playing. Rabbits also engage in "amicable" activities such as lying together, grooming, and nuzzling. These activities may occupy a considerable portion of the activity each day.[23]

HUSBANDRY

Rabbits can be kept indoors or outdoors. An indoor pet rabbit can be either caged most of the time and let out for supervised exercise or given free range of a house. Space to move around is important, and rabbits should always have the minimal space required to indulge in hopping. Owners of house rabbits will attest to the fact that rabbits climb onto objects if they have the opportunity.

Because rabbits are a quarry for carnivores, they seek hiding places when frightened. In the wild, the burrow is the primary haven, but other above-ground hiding places are used in emergencies. If a pet rabbit is given free range in a house, it should still have a cage or box in which to escape.

Rabbits generally have clean habits, depositing their feces and urine in the same place each time. They can be trained to use a litter tray if they are constantly placed in the litter tray every few minutes when first acquired. However, adult bucks deposit strong-smelling feces in scattered places to mark their territory. Male house rabbits that are not castrated will mark their territory with a strong-smelling secretion by rubbing their chins on furniture, carpets, and household goods.

Rabbits like to chew and scratch objects found in a home; two of the greatest hazards are electrical cords and poisonous plants. Electrical wires should be placed out of reach of rabbits. The decorative house plant dumbcane *(Dieffenbachia seguinae)* and the ornamental shrub oleander *(Nerium oleander)* are poisonous to rabbits.[5,6]

Divide the cage area that a rabbit occupies into two functional spaces: a space for lying and sleeping and a space for activities. An indoor rabbit that has free range only requires a cage large enough for it to stretch out when lying on its side. A cage with a plastic bottom and a wire top is suitable because it can be easily cleaned and is well ventilated. Cover the base of the cage with a layer of straw or shavings that are changed daily. Glass terrariums used for reptiles are not suitable for rabbits because they are poorly ventilated. If two or more pet rabbits are kept indoors, each animal should have its own cage. Fighting can result if two rabbits are kept in the same cage.

Pet rabbits can be housed in the same space with different pets if the other animals adapt to the rabbits. Pet birds such as parakeets cohabitate well with rabbits; well-behaved dogs also tolerate pet rabbits; cats are often unpredictable and generally should not be left alone with rabbits. Pet guinea pigs are often kept in the same household as rabbits, but this is not a good practice. Rabbits can carry *Bordetella bronchiseptica* without any ill effects, but this organism is pathogenic for guinea pigs.

Outdoor rabbits should be housed in properly constructed hutches that provide shade and shelter from wind and cold below 39.2°F (4°C). Plans for the construction of hutches are available from libraries, feed manufacturers, and agricultural extension agents; assembled cages are available from farm supply stores or mail order houses that advertise in rabbit breeding journals. Professional and trade journals in laboratory animal science also advertise caging, but such caging is generally the most expensive. Space to move around in the hutch is important, and the space required for a rabbit to complete three hops is the minimum recommended length.[23] A fully grown New Zealand white rabbit moves forward 1.5 to 2.0 m in three hops. The hutch should also be tall enough for a rabbit to stand up on its hind legs. Laboratory rabbits have been observed to climb onto raised platforms and shelves placed 2 m above the cage floor; these have been used successfully for rabbit housing.[23]

With the use of a grazing ark, indoor and hutch rabbits can feed on lawn. The ark can be a mesh top from an indoor rabbit cage or a solid frame with wire mesh (Fig. 13-6). Move the grazing ark every day to a fresh area of grass. Provide a shaded area within the ark, and peg the ark down so that the rabbit cannot tip it upward. Weed killers used on lawns can be poisonous to rabbits.

Does primarily dig burrows, and only pregnant or pseudopregnant females attempt to dig very deep tunnels.[23,32] If rabbits are kept in gardens or lawn areas, provide appropriate borders with 30-cm concrete plates or wire mesh to prevent unwanted escapes. Penned rabbits often dig shallow holes in which they lie or sleep; this behavior can be redirected if fresh, green food is hidden in a heap of hay or a pile of soil for rabbits to root out.

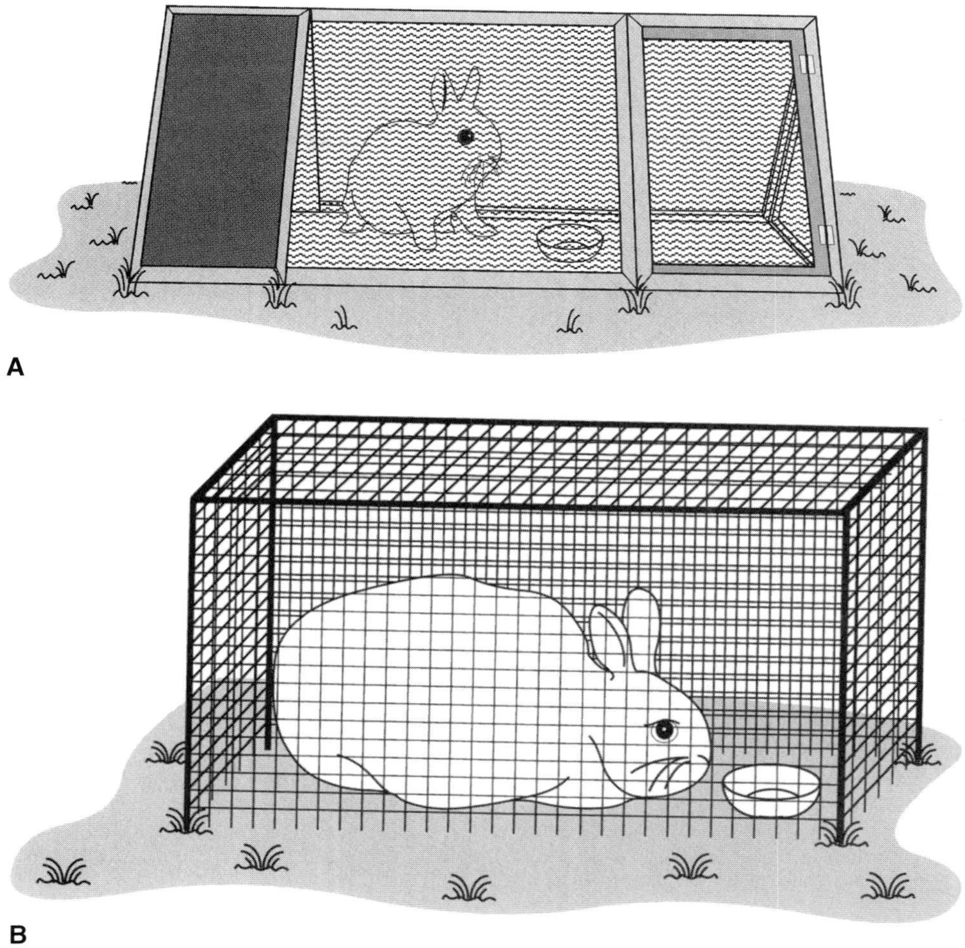

Figure 13-6 **A,** A grazing ark can be constructed from a solid frame and wire mesh. **B,** Alternatively, the metal lid from an indoor rabbit's cage can be used as a small grazing ark.

Rabbits tolerate cold better than heat. Because they do not possess brown fat, they shiver when exposed to cold. Shivering works well in the short term, and rabbits can tolerate cold weather if properly acclimatized and sheltered. Rabbits are unusually sensitive to temperatures higher than 82.4°F (28°C) and have little protection against high ambient temperatures. They cannot sweat except through sweat glands confined to the lips; also, they pant ineffectively, and when sufficiently dehydrated, they stop panting. Rabbits do not increase water intake when the ambient temperature becomes high; heat actually seems to inhibit drinking. Rabbits can tolerate a water loss equivalent to 48% of their body weight. In contrast, when water loss reaches 11% to 14% of body weight in dogs, circulatory failure occurs. Although rabbits use their ears to dissipate heat, they actively seek shade and burrow to conserve water and to shelter themselves from heat. The pulse rate of rabbits increases only mildly in response to an increase in body temperature. Shelter from direct sunlight is essential in the design of any rabbit housing.

The response of rabbits to high and low ambient temperatures is also important during transportation. The risk of mortality is greater in hot weather or in the presence of excessive indoor heating than in cold weather.

REFERENCES

1. Abdalla KEH, Abd El-Nasser M, Ibrahim IA, et al: Comparative anatomical and biochemical studies on the main bones of the limbs in rabbit and cat as a medicolegal parameter. Assist Vet Med J 1992; 26:142-153.
2. Alus G, Edwards NA: Development of the digestive tract of the rabbit from birth to weaning. Proc Nutr Soc 1977; 36:3A.
3. Brewer NR, Cruise LJ: Physiology. *In* Manning PJ, Ringler DH, Newcomer CE, eds. The Biology of the Laboratory Rabbit, 2nd ed. San Diego, Academic Press, 1994, pp 63-70.
4. Buss SL, Bourdeau JE: Calcium balance in laboratory rabbits. Miner Electrolyte Metab 1984; 10:127-132.
5. Cheeke PR: Rabbit Feeding and Nutrition. Orlando, FL, Academic Press, 1987.
6. Cheeke PR, Patton NM, Lukefahr SD, et al: Rabbit Production, 6th ed. Danville, IL, Interstate Printers & Publishers, 1987.
7. Cizek LJ: Relationship between food and water ingestion in the rabbit. Am J Physiol 1961; 201:557-566.

8. Conlon KC, Corbally MT, Bading JR, et al: Atraumatic endotracheal intubation in small rabbits. Lab Anim Sci 1990; 40:221-222.
9. Cortopassi D, Muhl ZF: Videofluorographic analysis of tongue movement in the rabbit (*Oryctolagus cuniculus*). J Morphol 1990; 204:139-146.
10. Cruise LJ, Brewer NR: Anatomy. *In* Manning PJ, Ringler DH, Newcomer CE, eds. The Biology of the Laboratory Rabbit, 2nd ed. San Diego, Academic Press, 1994, pp 47-61.
11. Donnelly TM, Kelsey SF, Levine DM, et al: Control of variance in experimental studies of hyperlipidemia using the WHHL rabbit. J Lipid Res 1991; 32:1089-1098.
12. El-Sayiad GHA, Habeeb AAM, El-Maghawry AM: A note on the effects of breed, stage of lactation and pregnancy status on milk composition of rabbits. Anim Prod 1994; 58:153-157.
13. Evering W, Edwards JF: Hepatic lobe deformity in a rabbit. Lab Anim 1992; 21:14-16.
14. Fox RR, Weisbroth SH, Crary DD, et al: Accessory spleens in domestic rabbits (*Oryctolagus cuniculus*): 1. Frequency, description, and genetic factors. Teratology 1976; 13:243-251.
15. Greenaway JB, Partlow GD, Gonsholt NL, et al: Anatomy of the lumbosacral spinal cord in rabbits. J Am Anim Hosp Assoc 2001; 37:27-34.
16. Herrold EM, Goldweit RS, Carter JN, et al: Noninvasive laser-based blood pressure measurement in rabbits. Am J Hypertens 1992; 5:197-202.
17. Hluchy S: The anatomical structure of the mammary gland of the rabbit [in Slovakian]. Acta Zootechnica 1995; 50:121-126.
18. Hoyt RF Jr, Powell DA, Feldman SH: Exophthalmia in the rabbit after chronic external jugular catheter placement. Contemp Top Lab Anim Sci 1994; 33:A19.
19. Janssens G, Simoens P, Muylle S, et al: Bilateral prolapse of the deep gland of the third eyelid in a rabbit: diagnosis and treatment. Lab Anim Sci 1999; 49:105-109.
20. Jenkins JR: Rabbits. *In* Jenkins JR, Brown SA, eds. A Practitioner's Guide to Rabbits and Ferrets. Lakewood, CO, American Animal Hospital Association, 1993, pp 1-42.
21. Kamphues J, Carstensen P, Schroeder D, et al: Effects of an increasing supply of calcium and vitamin D on calcium metabolism in rabbits [in German]. J Anim Physiol Anim Nutr 1986; 56:191-208.
22. Lobprise HB: Dental and oral disease in lagomorphs. J Vet Dent 1991; 8:11-17.
23. Love JA: Group housing: meeting the physical and social needs of the laboratory rabbit. Lab Anim Sci 1994; 44:5-11.
24. Magid NM, Opio G, Wallerson DC, et al: Heart failure due to chronic experimental aortic regurgitation. Am J Physiol 1994; 267:H556-H562.
25. Marini RP, Foltz CJ, Kersten D, et al: Microbiologic, radiographic, and anatomic study of the nasolacrimal duct apparatus in the rabbit (*Oryctolagus cuniculus*). Lab Anim Sci 1996; 46:656-662.
26. McNitt JI, Cheeke PR: Rabbit Production, 7th ed. Danville, IL, Interstate Printers & Publishers, 1996.
27. Meng J, Wyss AR, Dawson MR, et al: Primitive fossil rodent from Inner Mongolia and its implications for mammalian phylogeny. Nature 1994; 370:134-136.
28. Militaru M, Turcu D, Militaru D, et al: Lymphoid structures in the rabbit intestine: distribution, histology and ultrastructure. [Romanian.] Lucrari Stiintifice, Universitatea de Stiinte Agronomice Bucuresti. Seria C, Medicina Veterinara 1994; 37:59-69.
29. Myers K, Parer I, Richardson BJ: Leporidae. *In* Walton DW, Richardson BJ, eds. Fauna of Australia. Vol. 1B: Mammalia. Canberra, Australian Government Publishing Service, 1989, pp 917-931.
30. Mykytowycz R: Territorial marking by rabbits. Sci Am 1968; 218:116-126.
31. Novacek MJ: Mammalian phylogeny: shaking the tree. Nature 1992; 356:121-125.
32. Okerman L: Diseases of Domestic Rabbits, 2nd ed. Oxford, Blackwell Scientific, 1994.
33. Okin PM, Donnelly TM, Parker TS, et al: High-frequency analysis of the signal-averaged ECG: correlation with left ventricular mass in rabbits. J Electrocardiol 1992; 25:111-118.
34. Parer I: The population ecology of the wild rabbit (*Oryctolagus cuniculus* [L]), in a Mediterranean-type climate in New South Wales. Aust Wildl Res 1977; 4:171-205.
35. Patton NM: Colony husbandry. *In* Manning PJ, Ringler DH, Newcomer CE, eds. The Biology of the Laboratory Rabbit, 2nd ed. San Diego, Academic Press, 1994, pp 47-61.
36. Popesko P, Rajtova V, Horak J: A Colour Atlas of the Anatomy of Small Laboratory Animals. Vol. 1: Rabbit, Guinea Pig. London, Wolfe Publishing, 1992.
37. Prince JH: Anatomy and Histology of the Eye and Orbit in Domestic Animals. Springfield, IL, Charles C Thomas, 1960.
38. Prince JH: The Rabbit Eye in Research. Springfield, IL, Charles C Thomas, 1964.
39. Sandford JC: The Domestic Rabbit, 5th ed. Oxford, Blackwell Science, 1996.
40. Taylor KH: Orphan rabbits. *In* Gage LJ, ed. Hand-rearing Wild and Domestic Mammals. Ames, Iowa State Press, 2002, pp 5-12.
41. Williams CSF: Practical Guide to Laboratory Animals. St Louis, Mosby, 1976.
42. Young MS, Magid NM, Wallerson DC: Echocardiographic left ventricular mass measurement in small animals: anatomic validation in normal and aortic regurgitant rabbits. Am J Noninvasive Cardiol 1990; 4:145-153.

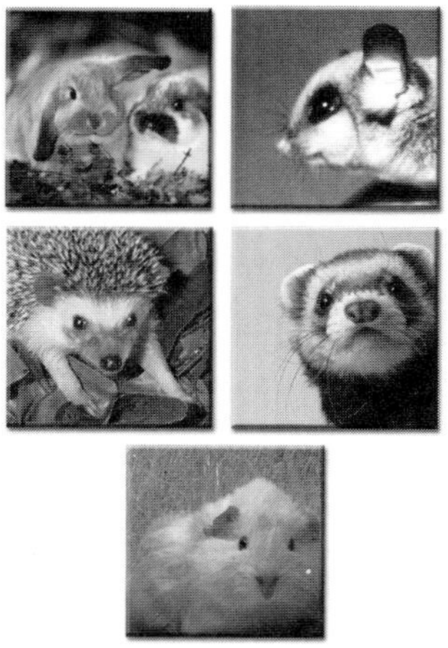

CHAPTER 14

Basic Approach to Veterinary Care

Douglas R. Mader, MS, DVM, Diplomate ABVP

Veterinary practices capable of handling dogs and cats can easily adapt to treating rabbits. A few procedures require special attention, and most of these focus on handling. A properly trained staff will provide the best possible care.

HOUSING

Housing requirements can be readily met. Hospitalized rabbits can be kept in stainless steel cages designed for dogs and cats or specially designed hutch cages. It is wise to place a thick towel on the bottom of the cage to prevent the rabbit from slipping on the smooth surface and injuring its back. A rubberized mat can provide the same traction and has the added benefit of allowing urine and feces to fall through, preventing soiling of the patient.

A rabbit hutch can be easily and inexpensively constructed or purchased from pet or feed stores. Hutch cage units can also be adapted for use as tabletop cages with built-in catch pans or can be suspended with wire, as is commonly done in multianimal rabbitries. Cage floors should be constructed of 14-gauge wire mesh. The mesh openings should be rectangles no greater than 1×2.5 cm. This opening size facilitates cleaning, allows feces to drop through the floor, and is not so large that a rabbit might accidentally get its foot stuck. A portion of the floor should be solid so there is a place to rest and help prevent the rabbit's hocks from becoming sore. A block of wood or soft plastic works well. Rabbits like to chew on these substances, which is good for their teeth. However, keep in mind that wood is difficult to sanitize and is not permitted in facilities regulated by the U.S. Department of Agriculture.

Keep a supply of good-quality feed available for hospitalized rabbits. Rabbits can be finicky eaters, so check with the owner before hospitalizing a rabbit to find out what foods the rabbit prefers. If the diet is poor, it may be necessary to offer the rabbit some of the food to which it is accustomed while gradually introducing a more appropriate diet. A rapid change of diet, even a change from a poor diet to a proper one, may cause gastrointestinal upset and anorexia (see Chapter 15).

Fresh water should always be available. Consult the owner to learn what type of watering system the rabbit uses. Rabbits easily learn to drink from sipper bottles. These should be cleaned daily. If water crocks are used, they should be made of a heavy ceramic so they are not easily tipped over. Bowls with high sides are recommended because rabbits tend to hang their dewlaps in the water when they drink. If the sides of the bowl are too low, this chronic wetting can lead to "wet dewlap" disease, which is an easily preventable moist dermatitis that is most often associated with colonization by *Pseudomonas* species.

HANDLING, RESTRAINT, AND PHYSICAL EXAMINATION

Rabbits have a relatively delicate skeleton that accounts for only 8% of their total body weight; the skeleton of cats of comparable size is 13%. In contrast, the muscles of rabbits are extremely strong and well developed for running. As a result, an improperly handled rabbit that kicks out or struggles is at risk of fracturing its long bones and spine.

Rabbits should never be picked up by their ears. Rather, grasp them by the scruff with one hand and support their hindquarters with the other. Never let a rabbit's rear legs dangle while carrying it. A gentle patient can be lifted with one hand between the front legs (covering the chest) and the second hand supporting the rear quarters.

When transporting a rabbit for any distance, tuck its head under your arms as if you were carrying a football (Fig. 14-1). With its head and eyes covered, the rabbit remains quiet and relaxed. This hold gives the handler extra security if the rabbit struggles or kicks.

During the examination, cover the table with a nonslip surface. If a rabbit is placed on a slippery surface, such as stainless steel, it may slip and kick while trying to gain its footing and possibly break its back. To avoid this, cover the table with a large, heavy towel before placing the rabbit down. Smaller hand towels are easily kicked off the table, making the examination even more difficult than if a bare table were used. This technique also shows clients that you are taking special precautions with their pets.

During the examination, always maintain control of the rabbit (Fig. 14-2). A rabbit may jump off the table for no apparent reason. One method of restraint involves holding the rabbit with your forearm around it and tucking it into your abdomen as you stand against the table's edge. With this method, one hand is free to examine the patient, palpate the abdomen, and use any clinical instruments. When you are finished with one side, gently turn the patient end to end with two hands and examine the opposite side. If a two-handed palpation is required, tuck the rabbit's hindquarters into your abdomen and, with its nose facing away from you, hold on with both hands while palpating.

To examine the abdomen, gently roll the rabbit onto its back and cradle it like a baby in one arm, using your hand to support the rear legs (Fig. 14-3). The other hand is then free to do the examination. This position is also recommended to take a rectal temperature. With your free hand, gently insert the lubricated probe into the rectum. Avoid using a glass thermometer because it can easily break if the rabbit struggles. Electronic pediatric rectal thermometers are inexpensive, sturdy, and safe and record the patient's temperature more rapidly and accurately than glass thermometers.

Perhaps the most difficult part of the physical examination is the evaluation of the rabbit's oral cavity. Rabbits do not like to have their mouths touched or manipulated, and chemical restraint may be necessary for a thorough examination. An assistant is usually needed to help with restraint using the method described for a two-handed palpation. Have the assistant stand at the other side of the examination table so that the rabbit is facing you.

If an assistant is not available, roll the rabbit up in a soft towel to facilitate examination and provide the necessary restraint without causing undue force. Commercial rabbit restraint devices are available. Although effective, the hard restraining devices made of plastic or stainless steel appear excessive to owners. A less visually offensive alternative is the nylon cat bag used in most small animal practices. A cat bag is especially useful when a rabbit must be restrained to collect laboratory samples or perform minor procedures (Fig. 14-4).

A cursory oral examination is possible using your hands. Digitally palpate the jaws and lips. Gentle retraction of the lips allows access to the buccal area, the incisors, and the interdental region.

The oral cavity can be accessed by several methods. Readily available instruments in a dog and cat practice, such as an otoscope cone, can be inserted through the interdental area to examine the tongue, hard palate, and molars. Use a dedicated ear cone because the rabbit's sharp incisors will damage the outside, excoriating the surface and rendering it unusable for aural examinations.

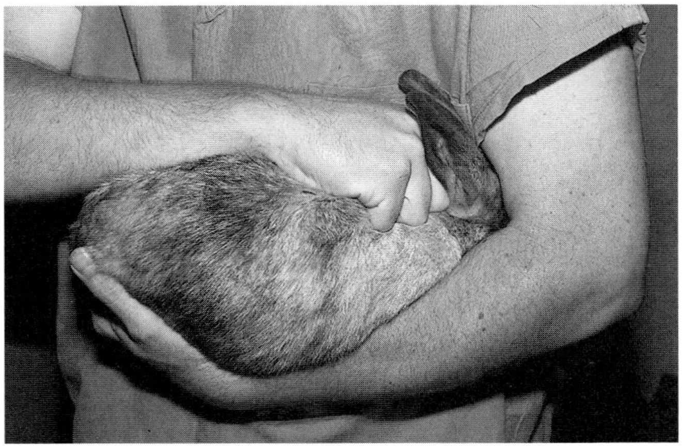

Figure 14-1 Proper technique for carrying a rabbit. Its head is tucked under one arm, and the back and feet are supported with the other.

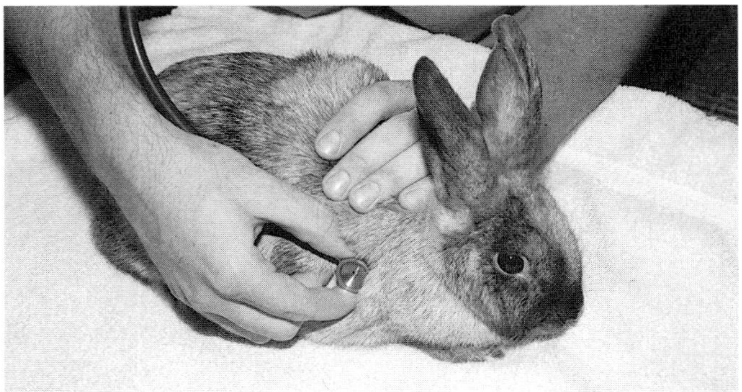

Figure 14-2 Place a thick towel on the examination table to provide traction for the patient. A slippery surface is a source of alarm for the rabbit. In addition, maintain control of the rabbit by keeping your free hand on the patient at all times.

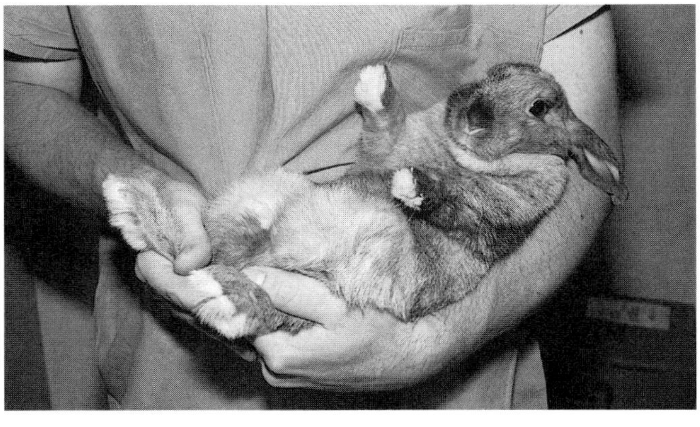

Figure 14-3 Cradling a rabbit for examination of the abdomen.

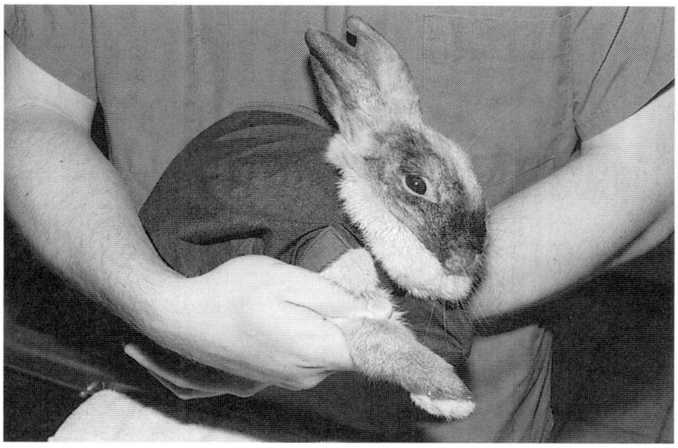

Figure 14-4 Nylon cat restraint bags have zippers that allow handlers to gain access to necessary veins for blood sampling or intravenous catheter placement.

Another tool for oral examination is a stainless steel oral speculum made for use in birds. Insert the narrow end of this instrument between the interdental region of the rabbit's mouth and gently turn it until the mouth gapes open. If a larger field of view is needed, the speculum can be slowly inserted to its next larger size. Examination can be enhanced with the use of a small light source, such as a transilluminator or penlight (Fig. 14-5).

Several instruments are currently marketed for rabbit oral examinations and rabbit dentistry. These are existing instruments that have been either slightly modified or simply described differently for new uses. Vaginal and nasal specula, either with or without an attached light source, are excellent tools for examining the oral cavity of a rabbit. These products are available through exotic specialty catalogues or general veterinary instrument distributors.

If available, a comprehensive oral examination can be performed with a small rigid endoscope. If imaging is available, photos can be taken that document oral pathology for the records and be used in client education (see Chapters 34 and 36).

Be systematic and thorough when performing a physical examination and always follow the same procedure. Collect appropriate physical data such as body temperature, pulse rate, and respiratory rate. Start at the nose and work backward or follow any pattern to which you are accustomed. Special areas of concern in rabbits are the ears (mites are a common problem), the teeth (malocclusion and overgrown molars), and the hocks (chronic abrasions from cage floors).

When placing a rabbit back in its cage, always return it caudal end first (i.e., its head is facing you when you release it) (Fig. 14-6). This technique decreases the chance that the rabbit will kick when it is released. When a rabbit is released head first, its first reaction when its front feet are on the cage floor is to kick away. If the rabbit does not have its footing, it can easily slip and injure its back. Placing a rabbit into its cage is one of the most common causes of vertebral injury.

Chemical Restraint

Chemical restraint is sometimes needed to perform a thorough oral examination, position the patient for radiography, or collect laboratory samples. Isoflurane or sevoflurane anesthesia may be useful in facilitating these procedures and in minimizing patient stress. Depending on the procedure, gas anesthesia may be preceded by a parenterally administered preanesthetic such as midazolam (1 mg/kg IM).

A combination of ketamine hydrochloride (25 mg/kg)/midazolam (1 mg/kg), administered intramuscularly, also produces excellent relaxation and anesthesia for minor procedures. A lower dose of ketamine (5-15 mg/kg) administered intramuscularly in combination with midazolam (1 mg/kg) is also useful as a preanesthetic. There are many published injectable dosages with drugs used alone or in combination. See Chapter 33 for more details.

For longer procedures the rabbit should be maintained on a volatile anesthetic such as isoflurane or sevoflurane. Anesthesia can be administered by face mask; alternatively, and preferably, the patient can be intubated.

Intubation is a difficult procedure in rabbits because of the deep, caudal placement of their glottis. However, with practice, the veterinarian can intubate most rabbits by using a blind

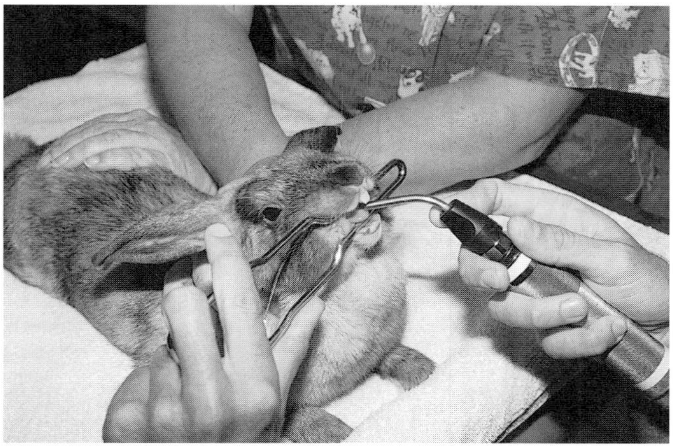

Figure 14-5 A large metal avian speculum and light source are used to examine the oral cavity of a rabbit.

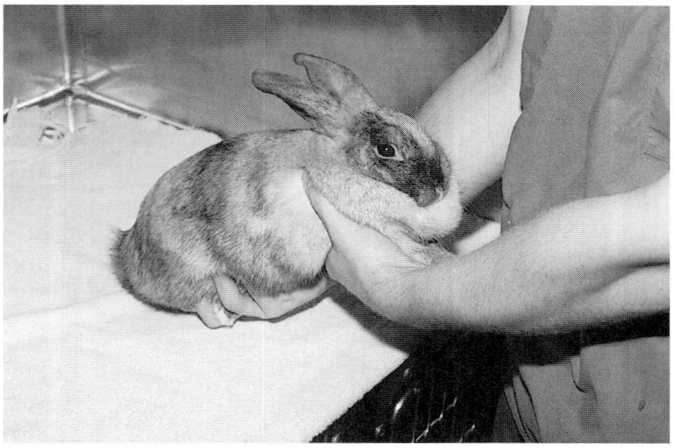

Figure 14-6 Proper placement of a rabbit back into its cage, rear end first.

technique or with the aid of either a curved neonatal laryngoscope, an otoscope cone and a stylet, or a small rigid endoscope. See Chapter 33 for a detailed description of the techniques. Intubation is recommended for any involved or prolonged procedures. Premedication with injectable drugs decreases the concentration of anesthetic gas needed and allows smoother induction.

CLINICAL TECHNIQUES

Venipuncture

Several different venipuncture sites can be used for blood collection in rabbits. These include the marginal ear vein, the central ear artery, the jugular vein, the cephalic vein, and the lateral saphenous vein. The marginal ear vein and the central ear artery are readily accessible even in the small Dutch breeds (Fig. 14-7). However, a possible sequela of ear venipuncture is thrombosis of the vein, with subsequent sloughing of the skin. This is most common in breeds with small ears and very small veins. In addition, even with the best technique, hematoma and bruising may occur. This is objectionable to most owners.

For venipuncture from one of the ear vessels, shave or gently pluck the fur over the vessel. Rub or tap the area with your finger to dilate the vessel. Clean the skin with a mild soap or an alcohol wipe. If the vessel is not yet dilated, hold the ear in your hand for a few minutes, or wrap a warm cloth around the ear. Penetrate the vessel with a small 25- or 27-gauge needle. Allow the blood to drip from the needle hub and catch it in an appropriate collection tube (Fig. 14-8). The use of a syringe or vacuum tube generally collapses the vessel; however, these instruments can be used on rabbits with larger pinna.

Rabbits have accessible cephalic veins; however, small breeds have a short antebrachium, and the vessels can be difficult to locate and hold off. When easily visible, these veins are a good site for venipuncture. If intravenous catheter placement is a part of the therapeutic plan, these vessels should be saved for that purpose and an alternate site for venipuncture should be chosen.

An easy site for venipuncture is the lateral saphenous vein (Fig. 14-9). This vein is readily accessible as it courses from

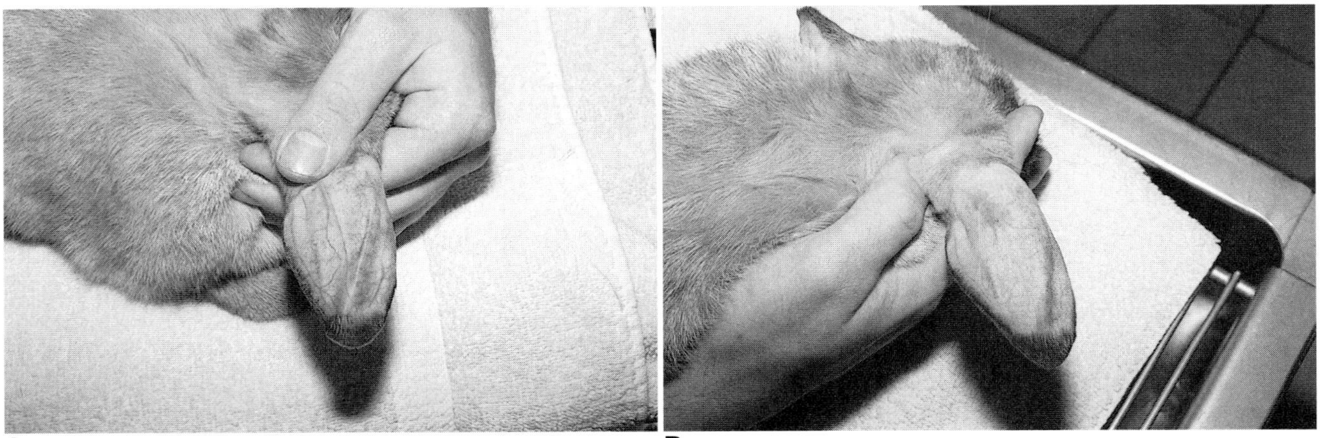

A B

Figure 14-7 Ear vessels in a rabbit. **A,** The central ear artery or marginal ear veins can be used for collecting blood samples. **B,** Even with the best technique, hematomas can develop. Owners may find this unacceptable.

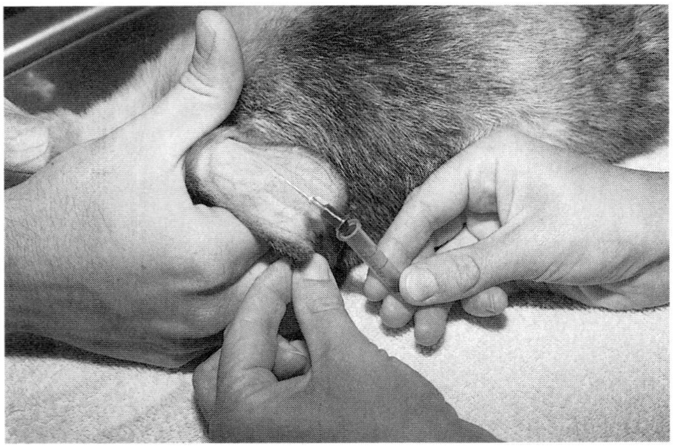

Figure 14-8 Collecting a small blood sample from the central ear artery of a rabbit.

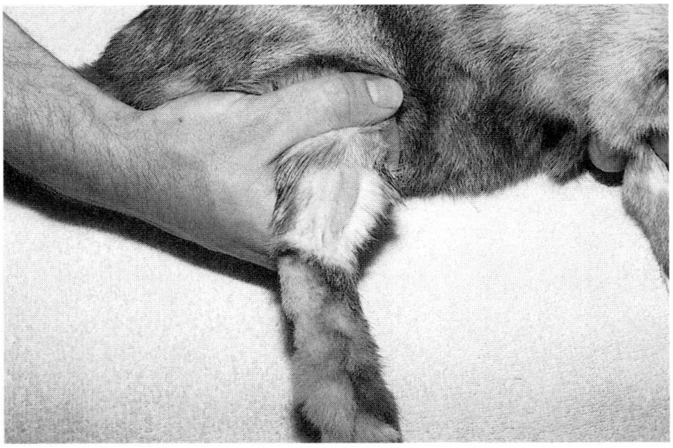

Figure 14-9 Lateral saphenous vein of a rabbit.

medial to lateral diagonally across the lateral aspect of the tibia. Blood can be withdrawn quickly and easily from this vein, especially in large rabbits. For venipuncture, the rabbit is restrained on its side, with the assistant holding off the vein just above the hock joint.

Rabbits have large paired jugular veins. Several methods are suggested for jugular blood collection, but to facilitate the blood draw and minimize stress for the patient, some form of sedation is often necessary. Shave and prepare the neck area over the midtrachea cranial to the thoracic inlet. With the patient in dorsal recumbency, have the assistant hold the rabbit on the table with its head over the edge, grasping the rabbit's body with one hand and pulling the front feet back toward the rear with the other. Take the rabbit's head with your free hand and gently tip it back to expose the ventral neck region. In all but the most grossly obese rabbits, the jugular veins should be readily apparent (Fig. 14-10). Large amounts of blood can be readily collected from this position.

Jugular venipuncture can be done without sedation in calm rabbits. For this technique, restrain the rabbit as you would a cat, with the rabbit held at the edge of a table, the front legs held down, and the head extended up. Pluck or shave the fur from the jugular furrow to enhance visibility of the vein. This technique may be difficult in does with large dewlaps. Use your thumb to push the dewlap ventrally and hold off the jugular vein at the same time. This technique should expose a short section of neck (and raised jugular vein) above the dewlap.

Cardiocentesis is commonly used in research for collection of large blood samples or for exsanguination under anesthesia. However, this method should not be used in clinical patients for blood collection because of the inherent risks of myocardial damage, cardiac tamponade, and death.

Reference ranges for hematologic and plasma biochemical values are presented in Tables 14-1 and 14-2.

Cystocentesis

Urinalysis is a useful diagnostic tool in rabbits. Interpreting samples is often difficult because of the sometimes heavy but normal mineral or pigment content of the urine. Samples can be collected by cystocentesis with a method similar to that used in cats. Cystocentesis can be done without tranquilizers in most rabbits.

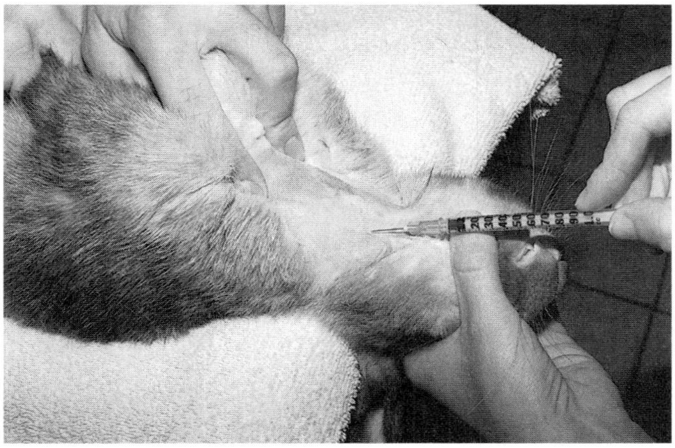

Figure 14-10 Two-person jugular venipuncture in a rabbit.

TABLE 14-1
Reference Ranges for Hematologic Values in the Rabbit

Erythrocytes	5.1-7.9 × $10^6/\mu L$
Hematocrit	33%-50%
Hemoglobin	10.0-17.4 g/dL
Mean corpuscular volume	57.8-66.5 μm^3
Mean corpuscular hemoglobin	17.1-23.5 pg
Mean corpuscular hemoglobin concentration	29%-37%
Platelets	250-650 × $10^3/\mu L$
Leukocytes	5.2-12.5 × $10^3/\mu L$
Neutrophils	20%-75%
Lymphocytes	30%-85%
Monocytes	1%-4%
Eosinophils	1%-4%
Basophils	1%-7%

Adapted from Quesenberry KE: Rabbits. *In* Birchard SJ, Sherding RG, eds. Saunders Manual of Small Animal Practice. Philadelphia, WB Saunders, 1994, p 1346.

TABLE 14-2
Reference Ranges for Serum Biochemistry Values in the Rabbit

Serum protein	5.4-8.3 g/dL
Albumin	2.4-4.6 g/dL
Globulin	1.5-2.8 g/dL
Glucose	75-155 g/dL
Blood urea nitrogen	13-29 mg/dL
Creatinine	0.5-2.5 mg/dL
Total bilirubin	0.0-0.7 mg/dL
Cholesterol	10-80 mg/dL
Total lipids	243-390 mg/dL
Calcium	5.6-12.5 mg/dL
Phosphorus	4.0-6.9 mg/dL
Sodium	131-155 mEq/L
Potassium	3.6-6.9 mEq/L
Chloride	92-112 mEq/L
Bicarbonate	16-38 mEq/L
Amylase	166.5-314.5 U/L
Alkaline phosphatase	4-16 U/L
Alanine aminotransferase	48-80 U/L
Aspartate aminotransferase	14-113 U/L
Lactic dehydrogenase	34-129 U/L

Adapted from Quesenberry KE: Rabbits. *In* Birchard SJ, Sherding RG, eds. Saunders Manual of Small Animal Practice. Philadelphia, WB Saunders, 1994, p 1346.

Have an assistant stretch the patient by holding the scruff in one hand and the rear legs in the other. After appropriate preparation of the antepubic region, collect the urine with a small-diameter needle (23- to 25-gauge) attached to a sterile 6-mL syringe.

TABLE 14-3
Reference Ranges for Urinalysis Values in the Rabbit

Urine volume	
Large	20-350 mL/kg per day
Average	130 mL/kg per day
Specific gravity	1.003-1.036
Average pH	8.2
Crystals present	Ammonium magnesium phosphate, calcium carbonate monohydrate, anhydrous calcium carbonate
Casts, epithelial cells, or bacteria present	Absent to rare
Leukocytes or erythrocytes present	Occasional
Albumin present	Occasional in young rabbits

From Quesenberry KE: Rabbits. *In* Birchard SJ, Sherding RG, eds. Saunders Manual of Small Animal Practice. Philadelphia, WB Saunders, 1994, p 1346.

TABLE 14-4
Values for Constituents of Rabbit Cerebrospinal Fluid

Constituent	Concentration
Glucose	75 mg/dL
Urea nitrogen	20 mg/dL
Creatinine	17 mg/dL
Cholesterol	33 mg/dL
Total protein	59 mg/dL
Alkaline phosphatase	5.0 U/dL (Kings-Armstrong)
Carbon dioxide	41.2-48.5 mL%
Sodium	149 mEq/L
Potassium	3.0 mEq/L
Chloride	127 mEq/L
Calcium	5.4 mg/dL
Magnesium	2.2 mEq/L
Phosphate	2.3 mg/dL
Lactic acid	1.4-4.0 mg/dL
Nonprotein N	5.6-16.8 mg/dL

From Weisbroth SH, Flatt RE, Kraus AL: The Biology of the Laboratory Rabbit. New York, Academic Press, 1974, p 65.

After collection, analyze the sample with standard techniques. Normal urinalysis values are presented in Table 14-3.

Cerebrospinal Fluid Tap

The collection of cerebrospinal fluid may be indicated to help diagnose neurologic disease. Anesthesia, not sedation, is mandatory. The techniques are similar to those used in cats. The best site to collect spinal fluid is the cisterna magna.

Position the rabbit in lateral recumbency with the head flexed toward the chest. Shave the fur on the nape of the neck from the occipital protuberance to the level of the third cervical vertebra and laterally past the margins of the atlas.

The cranial margins of the wings of the atlas and the occipital protuberance are the landmarks for needle placement. A 22-gauge, 1.5- to 3.5-inch spinal needle should enter the skin midway between these points and be directed toward the patient's nose. A stylet is usually not necessary because of the relatively small size of most rabbits. After the needle has penetrated the dura and arachnoid membranes, watch carefully for the appearance of spinal fluid. After placement is confirmed, attach a manometer or syringe and proceed with diagnostic tests. Normal values for constituents of cerebrospinal fluid in rabbits are presented in Table 14-4.

TREATMENT TECHNIQUES

Intravenous Catheters

Many hospitalized rabbits can be treated effectively with maintenance fluids administered subcutaneously. However, rabbits that are azotemic, in shock, or critically ill should be given fluids intravenously. All the vessels mentioned for venipuncture can also be used for venoclysis. Simple injections are easily administered into the cephalic or the saphenous veins. Prolonged infusions, such as those used with fluid therapy, should be given by indwelling catheters.

Although small-bore intravenous catheters can be used for the marginal ear veins, sloughing of the ear tips can occur even with the short-term placement of catheters. This may result from chemical phlebitis caused by solutions or medications infused into the delicate ear veins, mechanical irritation from the catheter itself, or aggressive taping of the catheter to the ear.

Larger veins, such as the cephalic, the saphenous, and the lateral thoracic veins in does are better suited for catheter placement (Fig. 14-11). Large jugular catheters can be inserted, but the insertion procedure often requires sedation or anesthesia.

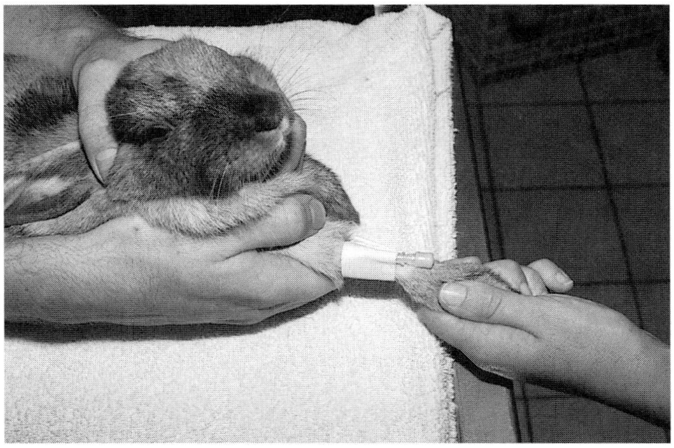

Figure 14-11 An intravenous catheter placed in the cephalic vein of a rabbit.

Intraosseous Catheters

In an emergency or when a rabbit is severely dehydrated and its peripheral veins are collapsed, fluids can be administered intraosseously. Intraosseous catheters are best placed in the greater trochanter of the femur or the tibial crest.

With the rabbit sedated, clip the fur over the selected site and prepare the skin for surgery. Wearing a sterile glove, palpate the top of the greater trochanter or the tibial crest with your finger. Pass the needle (the size of which depends on the size of the patient but can vary from 18 to 23 gauge and from 1 to 1.5 inches in length), anterograde, parallel to the long axis of the femur, and into the medullary cavity. Flush the needle gently with sterile saline solution and attach a male adapter. Apply an antimicrobial ointment to the insertion site and place a light dressing over the entire unit. Occasionally a bone plug will clog the needle. This can be prevented by using a stylet (made of orthopedic wire) or purchasing a dedicated intraosseous catheter needle.

Replacement and maintenance fluids are administered by slow drip into this needle. When the patient has been adequately rehydrated, the intraosseous catheter can either be replaced with an intravenous catheter or removed.

Most rabbits tolerate peripheral catheters. An Elizabethan collar is occasionally needed to prevent a rabbit from chewing or pulling a catheter out. Avoid using collars in very sick or stressed animals if possible.

Fluid selection and the principles of fluid therapy are similar to those used for other small mammals. Calculate the quantities of maintenance fluids on the basis of the normal water consumption of adult rabbits, which is 100 to 150 mL/kg per day. Divide the total calculated fluid volume into three equal treatments administered over a 24-hour period or give fluids by continuous infusion.

Injection Techniques

Injection techniques in rabbits are similar to those used in cats. Administer subcutaneous injections over the scruff or laterally, just cranial to the hips. Give intramuscular injections into the large lumbar muscles on either side of the spine, just cranial to the pelvis (Fig. 14-12). One person can easily do this by tucking the rabbit under an arm as if carrying it. Before penetrating the skin with the needle, squeeze the rabbit gently with your arm to prevent it from jumping during injection.

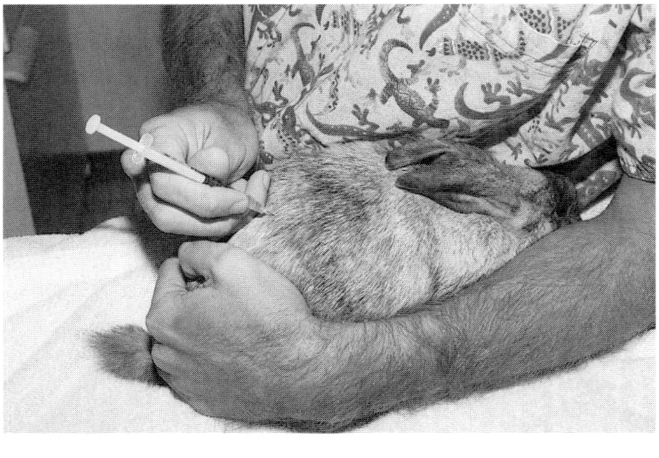

Figure 14-12 An intramuscular injection in the lumbar muscles. Note how the rabbit is cradled in the arms, which helps maintain control during the injection.

Use caution when giving intramuscular injections in the rear leg because of the risk of damaging the sciatic nerve, especially when drugs such as ketamine are used. It is best to give all injections into the cranial aspect of the rear leg in the quadriceps muscle group.

Lacrimal Cannulation

Chronic conjunctivitis is a common sequela to pasteurellosis in rabbits. The lacrimal puncta gets filled with purulent debris or thickened mucus or occludes as a result of chronic inflammation. This needs to be flushed on a regular basis to facilitate clearing the infection.

The rabbit eye has only a single punctum, located midway between the margin of the lower palpebrum and the nictitans near the medial canthus. The opening of the duct is large, between 2 and 4 mm depending on the size of the patient, and may be pigmented.

A topical anesthetic such as proparacaine is administered in the eye. After a few minutes the patient is restrained as previously described. A standard lacrimal cannula or an intravenous catheter (without the stylet) can be used to enter the puncta to flush the duct with saline solution or medication of choice.

Oral Medications

Administering pills to rabbits is difficult. One method involves inserting the pill into the oral cavity by the diastema. If the medication is relatively palatable, such as enrofloxacin, a rabbit may chew and swallow it. Oral medications are best given in suspension form. Many drugs that are available only in tablet form can be made into suspensions for use in rabbits by compounding pharmacists. Alternatively, crush the pill and mix it with jam or a paste nutritional supplement. Place oral medication as far back in the oral cavity as possible to prevent the rabbit from spitting it out.

Clients often find it difficult to administer oral medication to their pet rabbits because most rabbits resist restraint. Teaching the owners to wrap the pet in a towel like a big burrito helps with restraint and will also ensure medication compliance (Fig. 14-13).

Orogastric Tube

An orogastric tube can be inserted by using an oral speculum with an access hole drilled through the center. The speculum is inserted in the back of the mouth behind the incisors. A large-diameter flexible feeding tube is selected that is larger than the diameter of the trachea (to prevent accidental passage into the airway). The tube is lubricated and then passed through the hole in the speculum. Premeasuring the length of the tube from the mouth to the last rib on the left side will give you an idea how far the tube has to pass to reach the stomach (Fig. 14-14). A commercial critical care diet (Critical Care For Herbivores, Oxbow Pet Products, Murdock, NE) can be fed by syringe or orogastric tube.

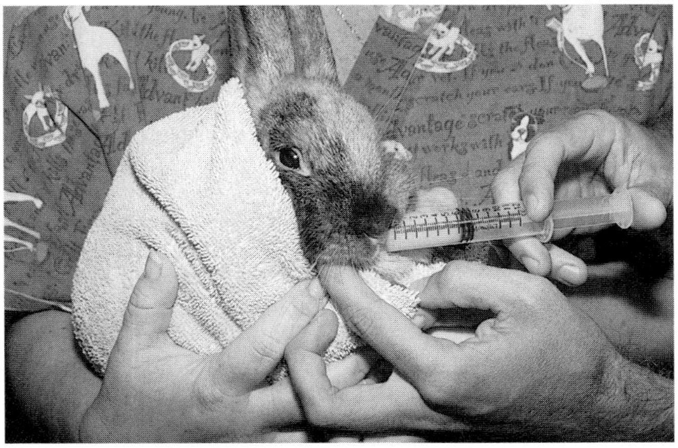

Figure 14-13 The rabbit is wrapped with a towel to keep it under control while receiving oral medication.

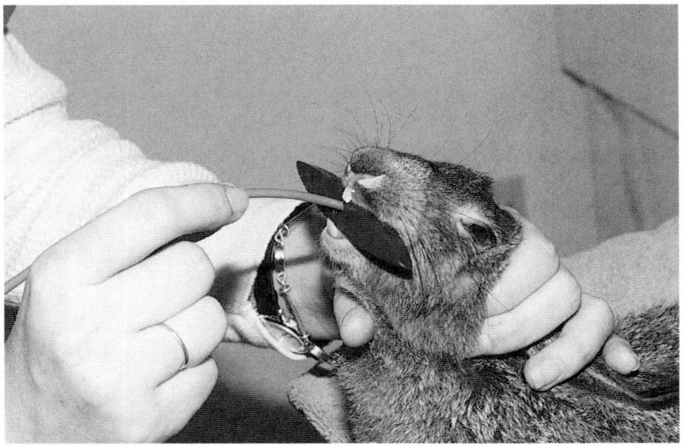

Figure 14-14 An orogastric feeding tube is passed through a hole in the oral speculum. Large-bore feeding tubes should be used to prevent accidental passage through the glottis.

Nasogastric Tube

A nasogastric tube may be used during the management of anorexic rabbits. The technique used for placement is similar to that used in cats. Premeasure an infant nasogastric tube by placing it against the rabbit and estimating the position of the stomach. Mark the end of the tube where it should exit the nasal opening. Place several drops of a topical ophthalmic anesthetic, such as proparacaine (Ophthaine, Solvay Animal Health, Inc., Mendota Heights, MN), into the nasal mucous membranes. After several minutes, introduce the nasogastric tube into the nasal meatus, directing it caudad and dorsally. If the rabbit objects, withdraw the tube and instill more topical drops of anesthetic into the nasal opening.

After passing the tube, secure the tube by applying a piece of butterfly tape and suturing it to the top of the rabbit's head, between the ears. Check the placement of the tube by taking a radiograph of the thorax in a lateral view. Once the tube has been inserted correctly, place an Elizabethan collar on the rabbit to prevent it from pulling the tube out with its feet. Nutritional supplements used must be in liquid form (i.e., banana flavor [i.e., Ensure, Abbott Laboratories, Abbott Park, IL]) so that they can pass easily through the tube.

Vaccinations

There are no routine vaccinations recommended for pet rabbits.

GENERAL REFERENCES

Cheeke PR: Nutrition and nutritional diseases. *In* Manning PJ, Ringler DH, Newcomer CE, eds. The Biology of the Laboratory Rabbit, 2nd ed. San Diego, Academic Press, 1994, pp 321-331.

Harcourt-Brown F: Textbook of Rabbit Medicine. Oxford, Butterworth-Heinemann, 2002.

Harkness JE, Wagner JE: The Biology and Medicine of Rabbits and Rodents, 4th ed. Baltimore, Williams & Wilkins, 1995, pp 13-30.

Krauss AL, Weisbroth AH, Flatt RE, et al: Biology and diseases of rabbits. *In* Fox JG, Cohen BJ, Loew FM, eds. Laboratory Animal Medicine. Orlando, FL, Academic Press, 1984, pp 207-240.

Meredith A, Crossley DA: Rabbits. *In* Meredith A, Redrobe S, eds. BSAVA Manual of Exotic Pets, 4th ed. Gloucester, Great Britain, British Small Animal Veterinary Association, 2002, pp 76-92.

Quesenberry KE: Rabbits. *In* Birchard SJ, Sherding RG, eds. Saunders Manual of Small Animal Practice. Philadelphia, WB Saunders, 2000, pp 1493-1511.

TABLE 15-1
An Evaluation of the Fecal Flora in Adult Rabbits (n = 5)[17]

Microorganism Isolated	Mean ± SD of Log Bacterial Count	No. of Rabbits Harboring Organism
Total count	9.7 ± 0.2	—
Bacteroidaceae	9.6 ± 0.2	5
Eubacteria and anaerobic lactobacilli	5.6 ± 1.0	2
Anaerobic gram-positive cocci	8.3 ± 1.0	5
Bifidobacteria	7.8	1
Streptococci	3.6 ± 0.6	3
Enterobacteriaceae	3.5 ± 1.3	4
Lactobacilli	0	0
Veillonellae	0	0
Clostridia	2.3	2
Spirillaceae	8.6 ± 0.3	5
Staphylococci	3.4	1
Corynebacteria	4.6 ± 0.4	2
Bacilli	0	0
Yeasts	4.3	1

TABLE 15-2
Stomach Contents and pH Values of Rabbits with Diarrhea

	pH		
Stomach Contents	Mucosal Area	Center of Contents	No. of Rabbits
50-100 mL, semifluid to thick food suspension	1-4	1-4	50
80-150 mL, mashed to firm food	1-5	3-7	50

confusing; in many diarrheic samples, no pathogens are detectable, and so-called "enteric" pathogens often are cultured from asymptomatic rabbits. It is suggested that veterinarians instead use anaerobic techniques and test for toxins. Many diarrheas are the result of microbial overgrowth, a dysbiosis (unbalanced flora levels) of the intestine.[1,3,5,8,16]

An important factor in the bacterial pathogenesis of rabbit diarrhea is the establishment of an infective dose of intestinal pathogens. The common rabbit enteropathogens *Escherichia coli* and *Clostridium spiroforme* are not infective as long as their numbers are small. With overgrowth, these organisms become invasive or produce toxins. Factors that further decrease immunity and the host's ability to respond are an inadequate amount of the milk oil, a higher than normal gastric pH, inadequate consumption of fiber, an unbalanced diet (especially one low in fiber, high in protein, and with excessive amounts of carbohydrates), poor sanitation, and stress, especially during the weaning age.[7] The delicate balance of intestinal transport of water is also altered by minor shifts in solute fluxes induced by microfloral changes.

Consumed microorganisms never normally reach an infective dose in the small intestine because they succumb to the antimicrobial factors in the rabbit's stomach. Experimental data show that gastric pH is higher in diarrheic rabbits, with an average pH of 3 to 7, than in normal controls, with a pH of 1 to 2 (Table 15-2).[1]

Normal peristalsis is achieved with the ingestion of a high-fiber diet, which provides a large particle size and results in a latticelike stomach food ball for effective gastric acid penetration. Incomplete penetration of gastric acid may occur with the use of alfalfa meal–based pellets, which have small particle sizes, resulting in the production of a more dense, hard-packed stomach food ball, especially in rabbits with marginal water consumption. A large food ball, often found in the stomachs of the largest and greediest of rabbits, may not allow complete penetration of gastric acid, thus enabling an infective dose of microorganisms to enter the intestine. The normal peristalsis of the small intestine, aided by a high-fiber diet, quickly flushes ingesta into the cecum, reducing transit time for microbial colonization. Low-fiber diets decrease peristalsis, which increases passage time; even with the limited indigenous microflora of the small intestine, large numbers of potentially pathogenic bacteria can quickly proliferate. It is interesting that rabbits digest fiber poorly even though it is a critical dietary component essential to the stimulation of normal peristalsis and the control of gut transit time.

The use of therapeutic antibiotics, especially gram-positive and anaerobic spectrum drugs, may produce a dysbiosis. Experimental oral inocula of *E. coli* and *C. spiroforme* usually do not produce diarrhea unless the stomach pH is neutralized with 10 mL of 10% sodium bicarbonate solution (to raise the gastric pH) or unless antibiotics are administered before the inoculation, reducing the competitive protection of indigenous intestinal flora.[1]

NUTRITION

Pellets

Commercially milled alfalfa meal–based pellets are the predominant feed for rabbits. The fiber content ranges from a low of 10% to 20% to a high of 20% to 22%, with the average content being 15% to 16%. The protein content averages 16% to 18%, with a low of 12% to 14% to a high of 22% to 24%. The feed with higher protein levels, used for maximal growth and weight gains in rabbits raised for meat production, often has a lower fiber content to increase its palatability. However, feeding high-protein and low-fiber feeds also causes increased morbidity and mortality rates from diarrhea. The most successful pellet rations for commercial rabbits have a fiber content of 16% and a reduced protein content of 16%. A fiber content less than 15% may increase the potential for anorexia and diarrhea, and one more than 16% reduces feed palatability. A higher fiber content (18%-22%) helps prevent obesity in pet rabbits and is useful for mature long-term-use laboratory animals. A protein content of up to 18% may be safely fed for achieving extra weight gain in meat production rabbits, for meeting energy requirements during pregnancy and lactation, and for conditioning show rabbits.

Because it is generally lower in protein and calcium and higher in fiber, grass hay (timothy, prairie, oat, brome, etc.) is recommended over legume hay (i.e., alfalfa) for mature pet rabbits. Pelleted diets formulated from timothy hay (Bunny Basic/T, Oxbow Pet Products, Murdock, NE; Forti-Diet Rabbit Timothy Blend Adult Maintenance Formula, Kaytee Products Inc., Chilton, WI) are commercially available for adult pet rabbits. These diets are intended to help prevent obesity, urolithiasis or urinary "sludge," and gastric stasis, and are preferable to alfalfa-based pellets in many adult pet rabbits because they are higher in fiber and lower in calcium. They should not be fed to young growing rabbits.

The free-choice feeding of pellets often increases the incidence of overeating, obesity, and diarrhea. Providing a measured daily pellet intake is the preferred feeding practice for domestic rabbits. An adequate dietary intake for the average adult New Zealand white rabbit (3.6-4.5 kg; 8-10 lbs) should be 120 to 180 g (4-6 oz, approximately $^1/_2$-1 cup) of pellets per day. Sedentary pet rabbits should be fed less ($^1/_8$-$^1/_2$ cup/day, depending on size).

A well-managed rabbitry may feed different protein/fiber ratios varying with age and use of the rabbit. Bucks, dry does, and nonpregnant does may become obese and should be fed lower protein and higher fiber diets. After a positive pregnancy palpation, the quality and quantity of diet are gradually increased over the last trimester. If the doe is stressed and its food intake reduced, pregnancy toxemia, abortion, and dystocia may occur. The energy requirements for lactation are three to four times maintenance needs.

Lactating does and growing young should be fed as much as they will eat each day. A feeding routine is successful when no pellets are left in the food hopper at the next feeding. This can be accomplished by following the "5/5 feeding schedule": 5 days after birth, increase the amount of pellets given by 5 oz (150 g) and by an additional 5 oz each succeeding 5-day period thereafter. Cut back on the number of pellets provided only when excess pellets remain at the next feeding. Waiting 5 days after parturition prevents milk overproduction and reduces the incidence of mastitis ("caked breast"), milk fever, and ketosis. By the time they are 5 days of age, healthy nursing bunnies have developed a full appetite and will depend on a milk diet up to 21 days of age. Increasing the amount of pellets in the doe's diet is continued in 150-g (5-oz) increments each 5 days of the litter's age until the doe is receiving 750 g (25 oz) of pellets (when the bunnies are 3 weeks old). At the age of 3 weeks, the bunnies are starting to crawl and tumble out of their nesting box and begin to nibble at the pellets, decreasing their dependence on their dam's milk. This is a good time to record litter weights as a measure of the dam's milk production (for use in culling and selection breeders).

The rabbit owner must evaluate how much to continue increasing and decreasing the number of pellets by monitoring the amount left in the feeder until the average weaning age of 42 days is reached. At weaning, rabbit owners often move the weanlings to an unfamiliar new cage; this adds further stress to the weaning process. It is less stressful to remove the dam and leave the weanlings in their familiar cage.

Hay

Most show and commercial as well as some pet rabbits do well on a diet of alfalfa meal–based pellets fed daily in measured amounts. However, most pet rabbits, especially older sedentary animals, do better on a limited pellet diet supplemented with hay and a few greens. Some rabbits, especially those of the Angora breeds, fare better on a free-choice hay diet supplemented with a few vegetables.

Fresh greens should be introduced gradually, adding one new food item each week and eliminating any that cause loose stools. A variety of at least three different greens should be fed to help prevent nutritional imbalances. Rabbits with persistent obesity and loose stools may benefit from no pellets, free-choice timothy or grass hay, and 2 cups of fresh mixed greens daily. Vegetables may include collard, mustard, and dandelion greens; carrot, beet, and broccoli tops; alfalfa sprouts, clover, parsley, lettuce, and cabbage. Some pet rabbit owners supplement with 1 to 2 Tbs per 2.3 kg (5 lbs) body weight with high-fiber fresh fruit. Remember most of these vegetables and fruits are high in water content and relatively low in nutritive value. Grains and feeds high in starch and sugar are generally not recommended because of potential complications associated with hindgut carbohydrate overload and diarrhea.

The quality of hay varies tremendously with regions, seasons, and farming techniques, so it is difficult to make general statements regarding the best type of hay and differences in nutritional content. Overall, the most economical and readily available hay is alfalfa.

Alfalfa is a major feed source for many rabbits, especially commercial rabbits, and there is little validity to the contention that alfalfa hay alone is harmful to a healthy rabbit. However, alfalfa hay is high in calcium, and problems with excessive calcium in the urine are seen in some pet rabbits, especially those given excessive vitamin or mineral supplements (see later in this chapter), sedentary obese animals, or geriatric rabbits.

Timothy hay is often suggested to be the best for rabbits and is packaged in small quantities by several feed companies (Oxbow Pet Products; Kaytee Products Inc.). The grain hays, primarily oats and barley, are also available. The clover hays may be musty and dusty. When available, the local grass hays may be the best buy for pet rabbits.

Remember that the dietary requirements vary according to the age and use of a rabbit. A balance of timothy and grass hay and vegetables may be the best diet for some pet rabbits; in contrast, meat production rabbits and most show rabbits do well on a commercially produced alfalfa meal–based pellet (16%-18% protein and 16% fiber) for reproduction, lactation, and growth. Mature laboratory rabbits as well as pet rabbits do better on a higher fiber (18%) and lower protein (14%) diet, which helps reduce obesity, diarrhea, and trichobezoar problems.

The overall best diet for young pet rabbits is a measured daily alfalfa meal–based pellet with a hay supplement provided daily and a treat of "greens," or a free-choice hay diet with vegetable supplement. A similar diet may be offered to mature rabbits, although many rabbitries are now substituting a timothy-based pellet for the alfalfa meal–based pellets.

Other Nutritional Considerations

Other components of rabbit nutrition need to be considered. A dietary fat component of up to 8% increases pellet palatability, especially that of the high-fiber pellets, and helps decrease dustiness and crumbling of pellets.[3] Proper feed storage and quick use prevent rancidity. Synthetic antioxidants and vitamin E are often added to increase shelf life. Excess dietary fat, such as that provided by milk supplements, may increase the incidence of arteriosclerosis, which occurs as whitish-yellow arterial wall plaques especially noticeable in the aorta. Some strains of rabbits have a genetic predisposition to arteriosclerosis and may develop these plaques even on a fat-free diet.[16]

Vitamin A deficiency may result in infertility, resorption, abortion, stillbirth, neonatal death, and central nervous system defects such as hydrocephalus. Conversely, an excess of vitamin A can also cause hydrocephalus when fresh alfalfa pellets, already high in vitamin A, are further supplemented with a vitamin-mineral premix that is high in vitamin A.[3]

The vitamin B complex is adequately synthesized by the hindgut fermentation and the consumption of cecotropes.[14]

Pellets high in calcium or containing excessive vitamin D can occasionally produce gross signs of dystrophic calcification.[11] The normal color and consistency of a rabbit's urine can vary from a clear straw color to cloudy-milky to a reddish-brown, depending on the animal's diet. Rabbits uniquely absorb all the dietary calcium from their intestines and excrete the excess in the urine; this can result in a chalky, cream-colored urine. Excess calcium may cause urinary lithiasis or excessive excretion of calcium "sand," especially when rabbits are overly supplemented with some types of greens, weeds, and vitamin-mineral mixes. Urinary calculi can form in the kidneys, ureters, and urinary bladder (see Chapter 18). Urolithiasis and excessive calciuria are seen most commonly in pet rabbits, probably because of dietary management and their more frequent presentation to veterinarians.

Vitamin E deficiency can cause infertility, resorption, abortion, stillbirth, neonatal death, and muscular dystrophy.[19] Selenium does not seem to be involved as it is in other species with white muscle–type dystrophies.

Some rabbitries suggest providing dietary copper at a supplemented level of 400 ppm to increase weight gain and reduce diarrhea in commercial fryer rabbits.[18]

All commercial feeds should have a mill location and date of manufacture clearly printed on the bag. Optimally, the feed sacks should be stored at 60°F (15.5°C) in a vermin-proof area and fed within 90 days of the milling date. Never purchase more feed than can be used in the shortest convenient period of time. Food older than 6 months has a compromised nutritional quality and reduced shelf life, especially during the hot summer months. Refrigeration should be available for perishable vegetables, greens, and fruits. Grass clippings, weeds, and the outer leaves and tops of vegetables may be contaminated with fertilizers, insecticides, herbicides, feces, and urine that can result in toxicosis, infection, and an unbalanced diet when present in excess. Available greens are often the outer leaves and therefore are more likely to be contaminated. A good rinse in fresh water before feeding is advised. Some greens consist primarily of water and have little nutrient value; thus they should be fed only as a special treat or as an appetite stimulant.

Commercial animal feeds may become contaminated with antibiotics found as a residue in a milling apparatus that was previously used to mix a batch of medicated feed. A few approved commercial rabbit pellet formulations contain low levels of sulfaquinoxaline for coccidia control and low levels of tetracycline for growth stimulation. Remember the legal liabilities of drug administration because rabbits may be used for human consumption and presently there are no governmental approvals for residue withdrawal times. Also, some antibiotics may disrupt the balance of a rabbits intestinal flora, resulting in dysbiosis, anorexia, diarrhea, and death.

Water

Rabbits need access to water at all times. A rabbit can go for several days without feed, relying on coprophagy. However, it cannot endure a lack of water for longer than 24 hours, or less in hot weather. Potable water should be free of harmful contaminants and provided in a manner that minimizes contamination by urine and feces. Check watering devices such as water bottles with drinking tubes and automatic waterers each day to ensure proper operation and availability of water. It may be necessary to train some rabbits that are accustomed to a different watering system how to use automatic devices. The application of a sweet sticky molasses or corn syrup to the surface of the water delivery system helps the animal to find and use automatic waterers. Water bowls are easily contaminated and spilled and need to be cleaned and filled at least daily. The use of heavy clay crocks and bowls containing a heavy round rock reduces tipping. A wet dewlap and resultant "green fur" (*Pseudomonas*-related moist dermatitis) may result in some rabbits that use water bowls.

This overview of the rabbit gastrointestinal system primarily relates to the domestic *Orytolagus* rabbits and does not address the nutritional specifics for wild hares (*Lepus* species), cottontails (*Sylvilagus* species), and pikas (*Ochotona* species), all of which do poorly in captivity. *Rabbit Feeding and Nutrition* by Peter R. Cheeke is an excellent reference for additional information.[3] The dietary requirements for pet, show, meat production, and laboratory rabbits may vary.

REFERENCES

1. Brooks DL: Rabbit gastrointestinal disorders. *In* Kirk RW, ed. Current Veterinary Therapy VIII. Philadelphia, WB Saunders, 1983, pp 654-657.
2. Canas-Rodriguez A, Smith HW: The identification of the antimicrobial factors of the stomach contents of suckling rabbits. Biochem J 1966; 100:79-92.
3. Cheeke PR: Rabbit Feeding and Nutrition. Orlando, FL, Academic Press, 1987.
4. Cheeke PR, Grobner MA, Patton NM: Fiber digestion and utilization in rabbits. J Appl Rabbit Res 1986; 9:25-30.
5. De SN, Bhattacharya K, Sarkar JK: Study of pathogenicity of strains of *Bacterium coli* from acute and chronic enteritis. J Pathol Bacteriol 1956; 71:201-209.
6. Eden A: Coprophagy in the rabbit: origin of "night" faeces. Nature [Lond] 1940; 145:628-629.
7. Gorden RF: The problems of backyard poultry and rabbits. Vet Rec 1943; 55:83-85.
8. Harkness JE, Wagner JE: The Biology and Medicine of Rabbits and Rodents, 3rd ed. Philadelphia, Lea & Febiger, 1989.
9. Hornicke H, Batsch F: Caecotrophy in rabbits: a circadian function. J Mammal 1977; 58:240-242.
10. Huang CM, Mi MP, Vogt DW: Mandibular prognathism in the rabbit: discrimination between single and multifactorial models of inheritance. J Hered 1981; 72:296-298.
11. Kamphues VJ, Carstensen P, Schroeder D, et al: Effect of increasing calcium and vitamin D supply in calcium metabolism of rabbits. J Anim Physiol Anim Nutr 1986; 56:191-208.
12. Kardatsu M, Yoshihara I, Yoshida T: Studies on cecal digestion: II. Study on excretion of hard, soft feces and fecal composition in rabbits. Jpn J Zoo Tech Sci 1959; 29:365-371.
13. Krull WH: Coprophagy in the wild rabbit *Sylvilagus nutalli granger* (Allen). Vet Med 1954; 35:481-483.

14. Kulwich R, Struglia H, Pearson PB: The effect of coprophagy on the excretion of B vitamins by the rabbit. J Nutr 1953; 49:639-645.
15. Lockley RM: The Private Life of the Rabbit. New York, Avon Books, 1975.
16. Manning PJ, Ringler DH, Newcomer CE, eds. The Biology of the Laboratory Rabbit, 2nd ed. New York, Academic Press, 1994.
17. Mitsuoka T, Kaneuchi C: Ecology of the bifidobacteria. Am J Clin Nutr 1977; 30:1799-1810.
18. Patton NM, Harris DJ, Grobner MA, et al: The effect of dietary copper sulfate on enteritis in fryer rabbits. J Appl Rabbit Res 1982; 5:78-82.
19. Ringler DH, Abrams GD: Nutritional muscular dystrophy and neonatal mortality in a rabbit breeding colony. J Am Vet Med Assoc 1970; 157:1928-1934.
20. Smith HW: The antimicrobial activity of the stomach contents of suckling rabbits. J Pathol Bacteriol 1966; 91:1-9.
21. Smith HW: The development of flora of the alimentary tract in young animals. J Pathol Bacteriol 1965; 90:495-513.
22. Smith HW: Observations on the flora of the alimentary tract in young animals. J Pathol Bacteriol 1965; 89:95-122.
23. Taylor EL: Pseudorumination. Vet Med 1940; 35:481-482.
24. Thacker EJ, Brandt CS: Coprophagy in the rabbit. J Nutr 1955; 55:375.
25. Yoshihara T, Kardatsu M: Studies in cecum digestion: IV. Movement of cecal contents in rabbits. Bull Agric Chem Soc Jpn 1960; 24:543-546.
26. Zarrow MX, Denenberg VH, Anderson CO: Rabbit: frequency of suckling in the pup. Science 1965; 150:1835-1836.

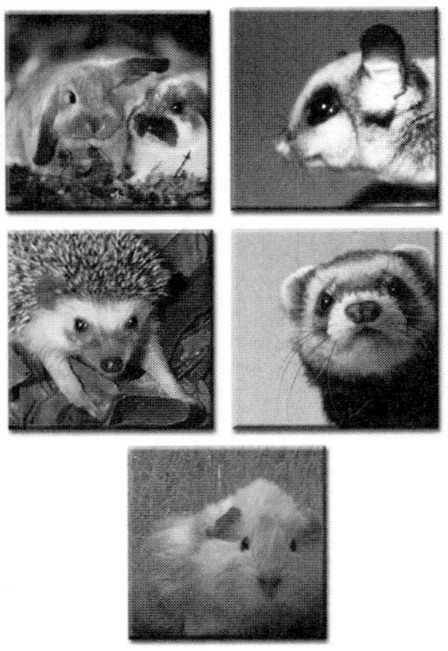

CHAPTER 16

Gastrointestinal Diseases

Jeffrey R. Jenkins, DVM, Diplomate ABVP

The most common clinical problems seen in rabbits involve the gastrointestinal tract. This is true for both pet and laboratory rabbits as well as for rabbits raised for meat and fur. To understand the pathogenesis of diet-related and gastrointestinal diseases of the rabbit, you must first know about the normal anatomic and physiologic aspects of rabbit digestion (see Chapter 15).

CLINICAL ASPECTS OF DIGESTIVE PHYSIOLOGY

Rabbits have a unique digestive physiology. As discussed in Chapter 15, rabbits are herbivores, but their digestive strategy differs from those of other hindgut or cecal fermenters (e.g., horses, guinea pigs) and ruminants. The rabbit's cecum and colon have a well-developed mechanism for selective retention of fine particles and solutes. The result is efficient fermentation of this portion of the diet but remarkably low digestibility of the crude fiber fraction of the diet. The rapid digestive transit allows a high feed intake, increasing the total amount of energy extracted and minimizing the quantity of fiber stored.[11] Digesta is separated in the colon in a process of selective retention of fluid and small particles. Normal peristaltic movements propel the larger, less dense fiber particles through the colon, while contractions of the haustra of the colon move the fluid and small particles (the higher density components) retrograde to the cecum. Small particles and fluid are retained in the cecum, allowing for extensive fermentation. Cecal contents are expelled at intervals and consumed directly from the anus (cecotrophy).[21,40]

Fiber's Role in Rabbit Nutrition

It is thought that plants may have evolved protective mechanisms to guard them from ingestion by predatory herbivorous animals. These protective mechanisms, or "antiquality factors," fall into two groups: metabolic inhibitors and plant structural matter resistant to digestion by animal enzymes. It is the second that is of interest when discussing rabbit digestion. Plant substances may be divided into elements involved with metabolism and elements providing the structural matter of the cell wall. The elements involved with metabolism are digestible by animals;

the structural portions possess unique components that are not. Plant cell walls can be synthesized but not degraded by the plant cell; animal digestive enzymes cannot degrade these structures either. Only bacteria and some fungi have enzymes to degrade these substances, and the use of this material as food by herbivores depends on a symbiotic association with gastrointestinal organisms with the requisite ability to degrade plant structural matter. The storage carbohydrate starch differs from structural cellulose only in the stereochemical linkage of the glucose units (α and β, respectively).[2]

Resistance to digestion arises from several features of the chemical structure. Occurrence of linkages for which no animal enzyme is secreted allows the possibility of fermentation. Microbial enzymes exist that will hydrolyze most glycosidic linkages occurring in plant walls. Polysaccharides will be fermented if the bond is accessible to the enzyme. The galactans that occur in many legumes and their seeds are resistant to animal digestive enzymes but are storage compounds relative to the plant and thus form an exception to the rule that most resistant carbohydrates are in the fibrous elements. Galactans are rapidly fermented and are responsible for flatus. Cellulose and hemicellulose are fermentable to some extent by microorganisms. Cellulose is less digestible than is hemicellulose. The main difference between legumes, such as alfalfa, and grasses is the much higher amount of hemicellulose of different types of grass.[42] Lignin is the main noncarbohydrate component of plant fiber and offers another kind of resistance to biologic degradation. Lignin is an aromatic polymer containing a condensed, continuous carbon-to-carbon linkage system of bonding that offers no possibility of hydrolytic cleavage.

Protective Effects of Fiber

Rabbit diets high in fiber have been shown to have a protective effect against enteritis. The beneficial effect is associated with the indigestible component lignin, commonly known as fiber. The digestible carbohydrate sources do not afford the same protection. Fiber stimulates cecocolic motility, either directly or by a distention effect of the bulk. Conversely, diets low in fiber cause cecocolic hypomotility, which predisposes rabbits to abnormal cecal fermentation and prolonged retention of digesta in the cecum; they also stimulate volatile fatty acid production, alter pH and substrate concentrations, and ultimately produce changes in cecal microflora. Other effects of fiber consumption are indirect. High-fiber diets have a low level of available carbohydrate and thus decrease the risk of enterotoxemia caused by carbohydrate overload of the hindgut. Carbohydrates provide an environment in which pathogens such as *Escherichia coli* and *Clostridium* species proliferate. Glucose, a byproduct of carbohydrate digestion, is necessary for the production of iota toxin by *Clostridium* species.

The pelleted diets fed exclusively to feeder rabbits are high in calories (high in digestible carbohydrate), high in protein, and highly digestible, designed to increase weight gain in growing rabbits raised for their meat. From the previous discussion, the potential for gastrointestinal complications in a rabbit given this diet is obvious.

Rabbit Gastrointestinal Tract Flora

Physiologists and microbiologists generally agree that the most common cecal bacteria are nonsporulated gram-negative bacilli in the genus *Bacteroides*,[12,22] at 10^2 to 10^9/g, and a large anaerobic metachromatic staining bacteria (LAMB) found at 10^8 to 10^{10}/mL of cecal contents.[31] Other bacteria normally present include gram-negative oval and fusiform rods. Coliform bacteria are not isolated from normobiotic animals; if they are present, they represent a very small percentage of the total bacterial population. Large ciliated protozoa, similar to those of the genus *Isotricha* found in ruminants, are present at 10^7/mL.[31] A rabbit-specific ascosporogenous yeast in the *Saccharomyces* family, *Cyniclomyces guttulatulus*, also has been found and identified at 10^6/g.[23] Veterinarians unfamiliar with rabbit fecal and cecal flora commonly mistake this yeast for coccidia on fecal examinations.

Cecotrophy

Cecotrophy is the ingestion of the cecal fermentation product or cecotroph. Both energy and protein levels of a diet affect cecotrophy. With energy deficiency, rabbits consume the total quantity of the produced cecotrophs. During ad libitum feeding, cecotroph intake depends on the protein and fiber levels of the diet. Therefore cecotrophy is greater if a ration is low in protein or high in fiber.[22] The relative composition of feces and cecotrophs is listed in Table 16-1. Cecotrophy is discussed in Chapter 15.

Insulin

Insulin appears to have a minor role in the energy metabolism of rabbits. Rabbits are reported to survive for long periods after pancreatectomy,[5,34,37] and diabetes mellitus is not reported as a clinical disease in rabbits.[24] Diabetes mellitus has been induced in rabbits by treatment with alloxan, a drug that selectively destroys beta cells, in experimental efforts to create a model of human diabetes.[19]

Calcium

Rabbits may have a higher total serum calcium concentration than other mammals. In a study in which rabbits were fed a diet comparable to commercially available diets containing between 0.9 and 1.6 g of calcium per 100 g of feed and between 220 and

TABLE 16-1
Composition of Rabbit Feces and Cecotropes

Component	Feces	Cecotropes
Dry matter (%)	52.7	38.6
Crude protein (%)	15.4	34.0
Ether extract (%)	3.0	5.3
Crude fiber (%)	30.0	17.8
Ash (%)	13.7	15.2
Nitrogen-free extract (%)	37.9	36.7
Gross energy (mJ)	18.2	19.0
Sodium/potassium ratio	0.4	0.6

From Fekete S: Recent findings and future perspectives of digestive physiology in rabbits: a review. Acta Vet Hung 1989; 37:265-279.

560 IU of vitamin D, the mean fractional excretion of calcium was 44%. The fractional excretion of calcium in most mammals is less than 2%.[7] In the rabbit, the absorption of calcium from the gut is not regulated by 1,25-dihydroxyvitamin D (vitamin D_3). Rather, it is believed that parathyroid hormone and calcitonin protect the rabbit from dangerously high serum calcium concentrations, which vary directly with the level of calcium in the diet. Interestingly, the ionized fraction of calcium is comparable to that of other mammals.[7]

DIET-RELATED DISEASES

Nearly all important disease problems in rabbits are directly or indirectly related to diet. Almost every case of enteric disease is related to diet and feeding practices. Even respiratory diseases (e.g., pasteurellosis) are influenced by environmental conditions, particularly the concentration of ammonia in the air from urine, which is associated with the feeding of a high-protein diet. Fur chewing (barbering) and hair-related gastric motility problems (gastric stasis, trichobezoars) are largely a result of dietary inadequacies and may be prevented with proper dietary management. Other diseases, including pregnancy toxemia, abortions, fetal absorption, small litter size, and weak bunnies, usually result from poor nutrition and particularly from inadequate energy intake.

Problems induced by diet and nutrition often involve the disruption of the rabbit's complex hindgut flora and the environment in which it grows. Populations of spore-forming anaerobes, consisting mostly of *Clostridium* species and coliform species such as *E. coli*, increase as the populations of normal organisms decrease. A reduction in the amount of fiber in the diet, an increase in carbohydrate consumption, and disruption of gastroenteric motility frequently lead to alterations in the cecal pH or in the composition of the cecal chyme.

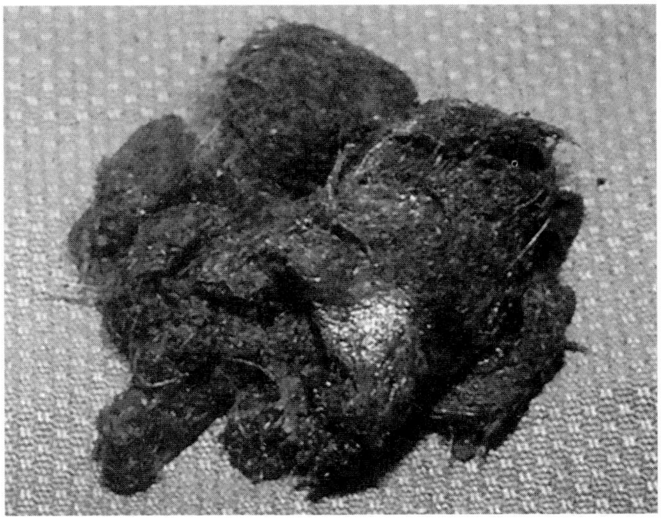

Figure 16-1 Stomach contents of a rabbit with gastric stasis. Note how the hair in the mass is not organized into a true trichobezoar. Most of the mass consists of dehydrated food stuff, primarily hay.

Gastric Stasis Syndrome

Gastric stasis syndrome is common in rabbits and is characterized by anorexia, decreased or no stool production, and a large stomach filled with doughlike contents and, in some cases, hair (Fig. 16-1). Gastric stasis is often associated with a high-carbohydrate/low-fiber diet, stress, lack of exercise, and, in some cases, ingestion of hair. The history most often includes anorexia of 2 to 7 days' duration. Water consumption is often decreased. Rabbits may be alert or depressed, depending on the chronicity of the problem and the hydration status. Weight loss may be noted in some rabbits. Occasionally, a firm, doughlike mass (stomach) can be palpated in the cranial abdomen. Gas may be palpable in the stomach, cecum, or colon. Fecal pellets are significantly reduced or absent, and those that are passed are much smaller than normal.

Radiography may or may not be helpful for diagnosis because the mass of food and hair appears similar to normal ingesta, even with contrast radiography. However, visualization of a large, ingesta-filled stomach on a radiograph of a rabbit that has been anorexic for 4 to 7 days suggests gastric stasis (Fig. 16-2). Furthermore, large amounts of gas in the stomach or intestine may indicate gastric stasis. A definitive diagnosis can be made only with exploratory laparotomy, which is a risky procedure to perform in these patients. Most often a presumptive diagnosis is made on response to treatment.

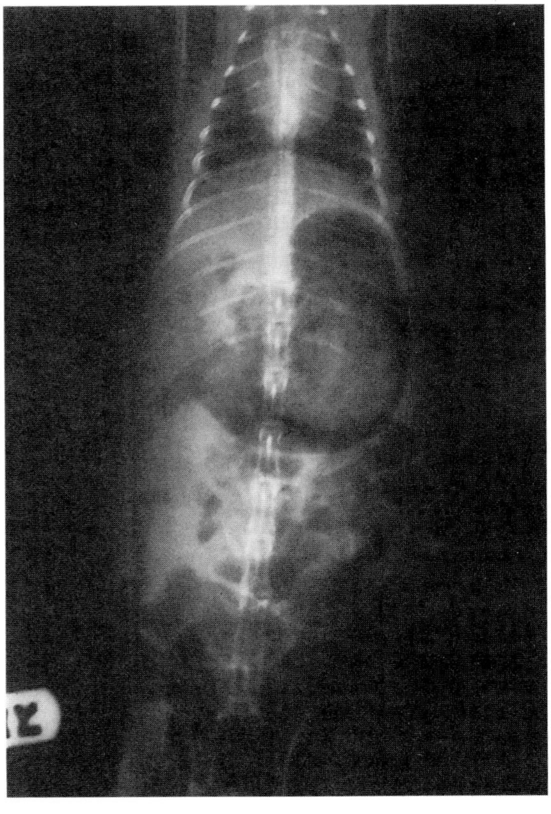

Figure 16-2 Survey radiograph of a rabbit suspected of having gastric stasis. Note the enlarged gas- and ingesta-filled stomach and the large amount of intestinal and cecal gas, which is suggestive of gastrointestinal stasis.

The pathophysiologic characteristics of this syndrome are a change in gastric motility and gastric function that results in the loss of liquid from the material in the stomach. The resultant dehydrated mass of gastric ingesta may not be passed by the rabbit, and its presence leads to clinical changes. The underlying cause of these changes may or may not involve the presence of hair in the rabbit's stomach. This syndrome certainly exists in rabbits that have not ingested large amounts of hair; the material in the stomach may primarily consist of ingested food. Providing rabbits a diet high in fiber has been shown to prevent this syndrome, possibly because the increased fiber component decreases hair accumulation; however, it is more likely that a high-fiber diet stimulates gastrointestinal motility and the creation of a more healthy digestive environment.

The use of a variety of lubricants (e.g., petroleum laxatives, paraffin oil) and protein-digesting enzymes or agents (e.g., pineapple for bromelin, papain) has been advocated for treating this syndrome. However, the response to such treatment is equivocal.

Very good results have been obtained with a medical treatment based on rehydration of the patient, rehydration of the stomach contents, and stimulation of gastric motility. Force-feed fluids (e.g., water, electrolyte solutions, fruit juices) and fruit and vegetable purees (e.g., fruit or vegetable baby food) to rehydrate the rabbit. This is most often done by syringe feeding the rabbit with a curved-tip dental syringe with the tip cut back to allow easy flow of the food. Commercial products are available for this purpose as well (Critical Care for Herbivores, Oxbow Pet Products, Murdock, NE). If indicated in hospitalized animals, administer intravenous or subcutaneous fluids. Administer systemic antibiotics, such as trimethoprim-sulfa (30 mg/kg PO q12h) or enrofloxacin (10 mg/kg PO q12h) to decrease bacterial overgrowth, and metoclopramide hydrochloride (0.5 mg/kg SC q4-8h) to stimulate gastric motility. Do not give motility stimulants if there are clinical signs of an acute abdomen (e.g., gastric dilatation and tympany, painful abdomen, signs of shock). Continue this treatment for 3 to 5 days; the rabbit usually begins eating food by 24 to 48 hours. Rabbits that fail to respond should be reevaluated.

Hepatic lipidosis can develop rapidly in rabbits with a negative energy balance. The hepatic changes occur almost immediately if ketosis develops. Use urine test strips to quickly screen for ketosis in anorexic rabbits. The return of a positive energy balance is the first priority of treatment. Place an intravenous or intraosseous catheter and administer lactated Ringer's solution to correct dehydration. Once the rabbit is hydrated, continue administering glucose-containing crystalloid fluids.

Occasionally, the mass of material in the stomach is so dehydrated that the rabbit fails to respond to medical treatment, and surgical intervention is necessary. However, the prognosis for a successful outcome is greatly reduced in rabbits that are treated surgically. Complications of hepatic lipidosis are a common cause of death in these patients.

Acute Gastric or Intestinal Obstruction

Rarely, a rabbit is seen for an acute onset of abdominal pain and gastric dilatation that is the result of gastric (pyloric) or, more commonly, duodenal obstruction. The most commonly implicated object is a mat of hair. In contrast to the trichobezoars found in the pet cat or ferret, hair found in a rabbit appears to have become matted while still on the coat of the animal rather than in its stomach. Obstruction from carpet fiber or plastic foreign bodies may present similarly. Gastric and intestinal obstructions are life threatening, and affected rabbits must be treated rapidly and aggressively if they are to survive. Treatment consists of the administration of analgesics, such as buprenorphine (0.01-0.05 mg/kg SC, IM q12h) or flunixin meglumine (0.3-2.0 mg/kg SC, IM q12h for no more than 3 days); a shock dose of intravenous or intraosseous crystalloid solution; and short-acting corticosteroids, such as hydrocortisone sodium succinate (10 mg/kg IV; Solu-Cortef, The Upjohn Company, Kalamazoo, MI) or prednisolone sodium succinate (11-25 mg/kg IV; Solu-Delta Cortef, The Upjohn Company). Take radiographs to confirm the location of gas. In some rabbits, a tube can be passed into the stomach for decompression. Most often, this is performed with the patient under isoflurane anesthesia, either while radiographs are being taken or while the rabbit is being prepared for surgery. If obstruction is confirmed, immediate surgery is indicated. A section of the duodenum may be necrotic and thus must be resected. The prognosis in these animals is guarded to poor.

Other Gastrointestinal Foreign Bodies and Cecoliths

A variety of foreign materials can be ingested by rabbits. In addition to those locations already mentioned, foreign bodies may be found at the ileocecal-colonic junction, in the cecum, or in the colon (at the fusi coli, at the end of the sacculated portions of the colon). Rabbits with gastrointestinal foreign bodies most often are seen with intermittent abdominal pain, gas, or diarrhea. Much less common in rabbits are cecoliths and cecal phytobezoars. Some foreign bodies can be identified on radiographic survey films. Contrast studies may be helpful, but their interpretation may be complicated by the presence of intestinal, cecal, and colonic gas and by the recirculation of barium through the ingestion of cecotrophs. Exploratory surgery is required for both diagnosis and correction in most cases (see Chapter 22).

ENTERITIS COMPLEX AND ENTEROTOXEMIA

Enteritis complex, with signs ranging from soft stool and diarrhea to enterotoxemia, sepsis, and death, is one of the most common diseases of rabbits in clinical practice. Pathogenic bacteria and the factors that allow them to proliferate are the usual causes. These factors involve diet, antibiotics, stress, and genetic predisposition to gut dysfunction. Simple cases of enteritis, resulting in soft or pasty stool, may be caused by minor disruption of cecal flora, pH, or motility. Simple correction of the diet, the addition of fiber in the form of hay, and removal of stress often correct the problem.

Enterotoxemia in rabbits, which is characterized by more significant dysbiosis than is enteritis, is caused by the iota-like toxin from *Clostridium spiroforme*. Other *Clostridium* species, especially *C. difficile* and *C. perfringens*, have also been reported but are now not thought to be the cause of the disease.[36] Newly weaned animals (3-6 weeks of age) are most often affected, and they have the greatest mortality rate. This group of rabbits may develop enterotoxemia from simple exposure to *C. spiroforme*. This is likely because these young rabbits have an undeveloped population of normal gastrointestinal flora and a high gastric pH, which allows the proliferation of *C. spiroforme*. Adult rabbits are more resistant and generally require some dietary, environmental, or other stress for the dysbiotic state to be induced and growth of the bacteria allowed. Rapid multiplication of *C. spiroforme* results in significant alteration of the rabbit's normal cecal flora. Nursing does with enterotoxemia can develop a so-called milk enterotoxemia that is thought to be caused by *Clostridium* endotoxin produced in the does' cecum and passed to the bunnies in their milk.

In acute disease, rabbits become anorexic and markedly depressed. Diarrhea is brown and watery and soils the perineum and rear legs. It may contain blood or mucus. As the disease progresses, affected rabbits become hypothermic and moribund, and they die after 24 to 48 hours. Occasionally, a chronic form of the disease characterized by intermittent diarrhea, anorexia, and weight loss is seen. Postmortem findings in these rabbits include petechial and ecchymotic hemorrhages on the serosal surface of the cecum. The appendix and proximal colon may also be involved. Various amounts of gas throughout the intestinal tract, cecum, and colon result from ileus. Hemorrhages, pseudomembranes, or mucus may be present on the mucosa of the cecum and proximal colon.

Mucoid Enteritis

Mucoid enteritis is a disease of and one of the major causes of morbidity and mortality in young rabbits 7 to 14 weeks of age. It is characterized by anorexia, lethargy, weight loss, diarrhea, cecal impaction, and excessive production of mucus by the cecum. Its cause is unknown; however, studies have convincingly established the relation between bacterial dysbiosis and hyperacidity of the cecum and the symptoms of mucoid enteritis.[31] Alterations in cecal pH resulting from changes in the production or absorption of volatile fatty acids or from vigorous fermentation of carbohydrates can destabilize the cecal microbial population and stimulate mucus production within the cecum and colon. Feeding a diet high in fiber and low in simple carbohydrates is preventative.

Dysbiosis Caused by Treatment with Antibiotics

Other factors involved in the development of enteritis include antibiotic administration and stress. Some antibiotics suppress normal flora, allowing pathogens to proliferate. Clindamycin, lincomycin, ampicillin, amoxicillin, amoxicillin-clavulanic acid, cephalosporins, many penicillins, and erythromycin can induce enteritis in rabbits. Epinephrine-mediated inhibition of gut motility is believed to be the cause of stress-induced enteritis.

Treatment of Enteritis

Treatment of rabbits with severe enteritis, enterotoxemia, and mucoid enteritis consists of aggressive supportive care and efforts aimed at increasing cecal and colonic motility, discouraging the growth of pathogenic bacteria and the production of toxins, and supporting the growth of normal flora. Administration of cholestyramine (Questran, Bristol Laboratories, Princeton, NJ), an ion exchange resin capable of binding bacterial toxins, at a dosage of 2 g in 20 mL water q24h by gavage, has been reported to prevent death in rabbits with clindamycin-induced enterotoxemia[32] and has proven effective in my practice. Antimicrobial drugs have limited value in treatment of the disease and are used primarily as supportive therapy. *C. spiroforme* has been shown to be sensitive to vancomycin, bacitracin, metronidazole, and penicillin G.[8] The use of metronidazole (20 mg/kg IV, PO q12h) has been reported to reduce the number of deaths from enterotoxemia. Correction of dehydration and maintenance of normal hydration are of paramount importance, and administration of intravenous or intraosseous fluids often is indicated. In my experience, use of motility-stimulating drugs (e.g., metoclopramide) and giving a diet high in fiber (force-fed, if necessary) yield the most favorable results.

Prevention of Enterotoxemia

To prevent enterotoxemia, maintain optimal husbandry and minimize stress. Feed a good-quality grass hay and limit or remove pellets from the diet. If fed, a pelleted diet should contain no less than 18% to 20% fiber and should be limited to less than one third cup per 5 lb (2.3 kg) of body weight. Avoid sudden changes in the diet. Make hay available to weanling rabbits from 3 weeks of age; avoid early or forced weaning.

Bacterial Enteritis

Colibacillosis Enteritis caused by exposure to or overgrowth of gram-negative enteric bacteria is less common than enterotoxemia. The most common bacterial enteritis is colibacillosis caused by pathologic strains of *E. coli*. Strains of *E. coli* have been divided into four major groups on the basis of virulence and pathogenesis: enterotoxigenic *E. coli* (ETEC), enteroinvasive *E. coli* (EIEC), enteropathogenic *E. coli* (EPEC), and enterohemorrhagic *E. coli* (EHEC). Diarrhea in rabbits is most often caused by a strain similar to EPEC, which causes chronic diarrhea in human infants. This strain, called rabbit enteropathogenic *E. coli* (rabbit EPEC), also referred to in the literature as rabbit diarrhea *E. coli* (RDEC-1), is considered an attaching and effacing *E. coli* (AEEC) because of its capability of attaching and effacing the intestinal microvillous border with adhesin or adhesion factor.[37] AEEC strains include both EPEC and certain strains of EHEC bacteria. EPEC strains do not express the high levels of shiga toxin that are characteristic of EHEC strains, but all AEEC strains have a common genetic code to produce factors necessary to produce attaching and effacing lesions. These genes are present in *Citrobacter rodentium* and certain strains of *Hafnia alvei* as well.

E. coli–related diarrhea in postweaning rabbits may be caused by a variety of different serotypes that belong to the rabbit EPEC group. Morbidity and mortality rates vary; signs range from mild diarrhea and weight loss to death, and the mortality rate can be 50% or greater. Those animals that recover may have retarded growth. *E. coli*–related diarrhea in neonatal rabbits is most common between 1 and 14 days of age. The diarrhea is typically watery and stains the abdomen and perineum yellow. The morbidity and mortality rates within a litter approach 100%. Subsequent litters of the doe may have passive immunity. The disease process is limited to the cecum and colon. The cecal wall may be inflamed with longitudinal "paintbrush" hemorrhages. In severe cases, intussusception and rectal prolapse may be present. Presumptive diagnosis may be based on isolation of *E. coli* from stool or tissue samples from affected animals; however, nonpathogenic *E. coli* routinely proliferates in any rabbit with dysbiosis. Confirmation of the diagnosis requires histologic examination of tissues and observation of *E. coli* attachment to the intestinal cells. Serotyping of *E. coli* isolated from rabbits is not available to clinical veterinarians and remains a tool of research only. Biotyping may be available from some laboratories.

Treat individual rabbits with appropriate antibiotics, guided by the results of culture and sensitivity testing. Use trimethoprim-sulfa combination antibiotics (30 mg/kg PO q12h) or enrofloxacin (10 mg/kg PO q12h) until culture and sensitivity test results are obtained. Positive results may be obtained with early treatment.

Proliferative enteritis, proliferative enteropathy, proliferative enterocolitis The obligate intracellular bacteria *Lawsonia intracellularis*, previously referred to as intracellular *Campylobacter*-like organisms, has been reported as a cause of enterocolitis in rabbits both alone and in association with a EPEC strain of *E. coli* distinct from the prototypic RDEC-1 strain.[41] These intracellular bacteria are gram negative, curved to spiral shaped, and found free in the apical cytoplasm of intestinal epithelial cells. The disease is most often characterized as an acute diarrhea disease of rabbits 2 to 4 months of age (weanlings). Proliferative enteritis (PE) or enteropathy is an enteric disease that develops in many animals. Much of the literature focuses on the disease in swine and hamsters. In addition, PE has been reported in rats and guinea pigs; ungulates other than swine, including white-tailed deer, sheep, and horses; carnivores, including arctic foxes, dogs, ferrets, and nonhuman primates; and birds (ratites). The disease is not an important problem in these other species.[41] Histologic findings in these cases most often show a proliferative ileitis, with or without proliferative colitis, characterized by epithelial hyperplasia and mucosal inflammation. Similar disease in pigs and ferrets has been shown to be caused by a similar but distinctively different bacterium, *Desulfovibrio desulfuricans*.[25,35] Treatment of *L. intracellularis* in rabbits is challenging. Antibiotics used to treat *L. intracellularis* in other species include those of the macrolide family (e.g., tylocin, erythromycin, and lincomycin). These antibiotics are not recommended for use in rabbits. Chloramphenicol is generally efficacious and is administered at 30-50 mg/kg PO, SC q12h for 7 to 14 days. Florfenicol (NuFlor, Schering-Plough Animal Health Corp., Union, NJ) is a new antibiotic that may be useful as an antimicrobial agent in rabbits, but its efficacy and potential side effects in this species need to be evaluated.

Tyzzer's disease Tyzzer's disease is caused by *Clostridium piliforme* (formerly *Bacillus piliformis*[20]), a motile, gram-variable, spore-forming, obligate intracellular bacterium. The disease occurs in many rodents and other mammalian species in addition to rabbits. Stress (produced by overcrowding, unsanitary conditions, high temperatures, or breeding) may be an important component of this disease. Clinical signs of Tyzzer's disease include watery diarrhea, depression, and death. Morbidity and mortality rates may be especially high in weanling rabbits. Older rabbits can have a more chronic form of the disease develop that results in chronic weight loss. Postmortem examination of rabbits with Tyzzer's disease may show the characteristic foci of necrosis in the liver and degenerative lesions of the myocardium. More often, the intestinal wall is edematous, with areas of necrosis in the mucosa of the proximal colon. Treatment is palliative once clinical signs have been observed. The intracellular location of the bacteria may contribute to the difficulty in treating affected animals. If exposed animals are treated early (if they are isolated from affected animals, good hygiene is promoted, and supportive care and a high fiber diet are provided), they may not develop the disease. Once symptoms of the disease develop, treatment may be unsuccessful. Prevention of the disease depends on good husbandry. Bacterial spores are killed with a 0.3% sodium hypochlorite solution or with heating to 173°F (80°C) for 30 minutes. There is no vaccine available for Tyzzer's disease.

Other bacterial enteritides Other causes of enteritis include *Salmonella* and *Pseudomonas* species. Salmonellosis is not common but can cause disease with both high morbidity and mortality rates. The disease is well studied in rabbits, and the rabbit is used as a model of salmonellosis in humans.[26] The species and serovar most often associated with salmonellosis in rabbits is *S. typhimurium*; however, other species and serovars have been reported.[4] Transmission of the disease is most often associated with contaminated food or water. Affected rabbits usually develop sepsis, which quickly leads to death; however, diarrhea may occur as well. Postmortem findings are consistent with septicemia and include vascular congestion of organs and diffusely distributed petechial hemorrhages. Lymph nodes and gut-associated lymphoid tissue may be edematous and contain similar foci of necrosis.

I have seen an epidemic of lethal diarrhea in rabbits associated with *Pseudomonas aeruginosa*, which was isolated from the watering system. The morbidity rate associated with this outbreak was low to moderate, but the mortality rate in affected animals was high.

VIRAL DISEASES OF THE DIGESTIVE TRACT

Papillomatosis

Rabbit oral papillomatosis is a benign disease caused by a papillomavirus. Lesions consist of small white growths on the ventral surface of the tongue but only rarely elsewhere in the mouth. Early lesions are sessile, later becoming rugose or pedunculated and, ultimately, ulcerated. The lesions can exceed 4 to 5 mm at their greatest dimension but are typically smaller (1-3 mm). Lesions may persist as long as 145 days, but they usually disappear within weeks. In one study, oral papillomas were seen in 31% of New Zealand white rabbits (n = 51) examined from two local sources. Structural antigens of papillomavirus were detected by the peroxidase-antiperoxidase technique in cells of the stratum spinosum that contained basophilic intranuclear inclusions. Homogenates of papillomas hemagglutinated mouse red blood cells and also induced papillomas on the ventral surface of tongues, but not the conjunctiva or vulva, of susceptible rabbits. The same oral papilloma homogenate induced fibromas in neonatal hamsters. Homogenates of hamster fibromas did not cause lesions on tongues of susceptible rabbits.[45]

Rabbit Enteric Coronavirus

In 1980, a coronavirus was found to be the cause of diarrhea in rabbits.[30] Further research has shown that this virus affects rabbits 3 to 10 weeks of age, but it has also been found in clinically normal adult rabbits. Clinical signs in naturally occurring outbreaks include lethargy, diarrhea, abdominal swelling, and death. Pleural effusion and cardiomyopathy in rabbits have also been associated with coronavirus-like particles.[38] The disease is associated with high rates of morbidity and mortality; in one described outbreak, 40% to 60% of rabbits were affected. Death occurred in almost 100% of these animals within 24 hours of the onset of clinical signs.[15] Necropsy findings include fluid cecal contents, and histopathologic examination reveals atrophy of intestinal villi. Tentative diagnosis of this disease is based on clinical history, clinical signs, necropsy findings, and results of histopathologic analysis. The virus agglutinates red blood cells; evidence of hemagglutination activity in the feces therefore supports a tentative diagnosis. The diagnosis is confirmed by demonstration of the virus in feces or cecal contents.

Rotavirus

Infections in animals caused by rotavirus alone may be only mildly pathogenic; in rabbits, however, the virus is associated with very high morbidity but variable mortality rates. Although poorly studied in pet rabbits, antibodies to rotavirus as well as the virus itself have been found in the feces of rabbits from commercial rabbitries throughout the world. Severity of diarrhea associated with rotavirus infection varies widely and is likely influenced by synergy with various microorganisms associated with the infection. Severe anorexia, dehydration, and mucoid or greenish-yellow watery diarrhea have been reported. Rabbits between 30 and 80 days of age are most often affected. The mortality rate in young rabbits with naturally occurring infections may be as high as 80%. In experimental studies, rotavirus caused soft or fluid feces in some rabbits, but in most animals, diarrhea did not develop at all.[9] One study showed that a strain of rotavirus induced diarrhea, depression, anorexia, and death; however, results of the experiment was not reproducible.[16,17] The clinical signs of naturally occurring infections involving rotavirus and other agents include marked congestion and distention of the intestines and cecum and petechial hemorrhages in the small intestine and colon. Histologic lesions include moderate to severe villous atrophy, with the most severe lesions found in the ileum. Apical enterocytes on the tips of villi are swollen, rounded, and desquamating, and the tips may be denuded. The lamina propria is usually infiltrated with lymphocytes and, occasionally, with neutrophils. Diagnosis is established on the basis of the results of histopathologic examination of the intestine, isolation of the virus, or demonstration of antibodies. Clinical signs and gross pathologic findings alone are not diagnostic.[15] The prevention and control of rotavirus infection is complicated by its highly infectious nature. Reduction of stress (by cessation of breeding, reducing crowding, removal of socially dominant animals, and addition of fiber to the diet) along with appropriate treatment of concurrent disease and improved hygiene should reduce mortality rates.

Rabbit Calicivirus Disease (Rabbit Viral Hemorrhagic Disease) and European Brown Hare Syndrome

Caliciviral diseases in rabbits include rabbit calicivirus disease (RCD), previously referred to as rabbit hemorrhagic disease, and European brown hare syndrome. Although these two syndromes are very similar, European brown hare syndrome is associated with diarrhea and has now been shown to be caused by a different calicivirus. RCD was first identified in China in angora rabbits imported from Europe in 1984. Since then, RCD has been reported in parts of Asia and Europe, including the Czech Republic, Germany, France, Italy, Korea, and Spain. Investigations suggest the disease spread from country to country through shipments of contaminated rabbit meat and infected live rabbits. The first report of RCD in the western hemisphere was in 1988, when the disease was detected in domestic rabbits in the Mexico City area. The outbreak was traced to a shipment of 18 metric tons of frozen rabbit carcasses from China that had been delivered to a supermarket chain outside Mexico City. In 1989, the Mexican government began a control and eradication program that included quarantine of infected farms; prohibition of movement or sale of rabbits, voluntary destruction of diseased rabbits; and cleaning, disinfecting, and repopulating premises after a 2-month waiting period. The campaign was successful. Mexico is the only country to succeed in eradicating RCD.

The first reported occurrence of RCD in the United States was confirmed in 2000. The disease occurred in a backyard rabbitry of 27 pet rabbits in Iowa. The origin of the outbreak is unknown. In 2001, The U.S. Department of Agriculture's Foreign Animal Disease Diagnostic Laboratory confirmed RCD in a rabbitry in Utah and in a captive exotic animal facility in New York. The origins of these infections have not been determined as of yet; however, there is some thought that the New York outbreak may have originated from products containing rabbit meat from China used to feed carnivorous animals at the facility.

The disease, caused by a calicivirus,[15] targets rabbits older than 2 months of age; younger rabbits are clinically unaffected. Transmission is horizontal, with fecal-oral spread being the major route. However, fomites such as water sipper tubes, feed, and utensils can transmit the virus. The virus enters the rabbit through the conjunctiva, nasal passages, or traumatized tissue. The course of the disease is acute, with the duration of incubation only 1 to 2 days. RCD is highly infectious and has traditionally been associated with both high morbidity rates (70%-80%) and high mortality rates (100%). The number of rabbits affected during outbreaks peaks in 2 to 3 days, and the disease course may last only 7 to 13 days. Initially, affected rabbits are febrile and show signs of depression, lethargy, and anorexia. Some may show signs of tachypnea, cyanosis, abdominal distention, and constipation or diarrhea. At the end stage of the disease, the rabbit becomes hypothermic and recumbent and may have convulsions or epistaxis. Because of the rapid course of the disease, signs may not be noticed, and the affected rabbit is found dead. Surviving rabbits exhibit depression, anorexia, and fever that may last for 2 to 3 days.

Hematologic testing often shows a lymphopenia and a gradual decline in the number of thrombocytes. In most moribund rabbits, prothrombin and thrombin times are prolonged; paracoagulation tests with protamine sulfate give a strong positive reaction, and fibrin degradation products can be detected. Gross pathologic changes are associated with viremia, and acute disseminated coagulopathy is associated with deep venous thrombosis. Congestion and hemorrhage may be seen in most organs but is most pronounced in the lungs. The liver is pale, and periportal necrosis with a fine reticular pattern is observed; a segmental catarrhal enteritis is often identified.[15] A presumptive diagnosis may be made on the basis of data in the history, clinical signs, and pathologic findings. Definitive diagnosis requires demonstration of the virus by electron microscopic examination of tissues or with hemagglutination, immunoenzyme, or immunofluorescence tests. The virus is inactivated by 0.5% sodium hypochlorite or 1% formalin. However, the RCD virus may be changing, adapting to its new rabbit host (A. Smith, personal communication, 2003). This could result in the virus behaving more as calicivirus diseases in other species and infected rabbits surviving longer and more rabbits becoming carriers of the virus.

A tissue-derived vaccine inactivated with formaldehyde has been shown to be safe and efficacious in preventing rabbit RCD.[15] No vaccine is available in the United States. Antisera also have been shown to be protective against the disease. Suspected cases of RCD or European brown hare virus should be reported to local agricultural authorities.

PARASITIC DISORDERS OF THE GASTROINTESTINAL TRACT

Coccidia

Coccidia are the most common parasites of the rabbit's gastrointestinal tract and are a common cause of illness. All rabbit coccidia are members of the genus *Eimeria*. Twelve species are reported to infect rabbits (Table 16-2). Only one species, *E. stiedae*, which attacks the liver, is found outside the intestinal tract. Very often, two or more species of coccidia are present in diseased rabbits; the precise role of the different species as pathogens is therefore not clearly defined. The presence of only a few coccidial oocysts does not rule out coccidiosis or confirm the diagnosis because many rabbits are subclinically infected with coccidia.

Hepatic coccidia *E. stiedae*, the coccidium responsible for hepatic coccidiosis, is ubiquitous in open rabbitries in which rabbits are not treated preventatively with coccidiostats. Infection results from ingestion of sporulated oocysts that undergo

TABLE 16-2
Comparison of *Eimeria* Species Infecting Rabbits

Species	Mean Size of Oocyst (μm)	Shape	Distinguishing Characteristics	Part of Digestive Tract Affected	Prepatent Period (days)	Pathogenicity
E. stiedae	37 × 20	Ellipsoidal	Smooth, light yellow wall; wide, thin micropyle; no residual body in oocyst; sporocyst with terminal knob (stiedae body)	Bile duct, epithelium	15-18	Variable
E. irresidua	38 × 26	Ovoid	Smooth, light yellow wall; prominent micropyle; small residual body; variable	Small intestine	7-8	Significant
E. magna	35 × 24	Ovoid to ellipsoidal	Dark yellow-brown wall; prominent micropyle with lipping; large residual body	Jejunum	6-7	Significant (serious diarrhea)*
E. media	31× 18	Ellipsoidal	Smooth, thick, light-pink wall; micropyle; large residual body	Small, large intestines	6-7	Moderate
E. perforans	21 × 15	Ellipsoidal	Smooth, colorless wall; indistinguishable micropyle; small residual body	Small intestine	5	Slight (nonpathogenic)*
E. exiqua	15 × 13	Ovoid	Smooth wall; indistinguishable micropyle; no residual body	—	—	—
E. intestinalis	27 × 18	Ellipsoidal	Smooth, yellow wall; micropyle; large granular residual body	Ileum	10	Significant (very pathogenic)*
E. matsubayashii	25 × 18	Ovoid	Smooth, light-colored wall; no residual body	Small intestine, cecum	7	Slight
E. nagpurensis	23 × 13	Barrel-shaped	Smooth, colorless wall; no micropyle; no residual body	—	—	—
E. neoleporis	39 × 20	Elongate ellipsoidal	Smooth, yellow wall; distinct micropyle; no residual body; sporocysts	Small intestine, cecum	12	Significant
E. coecicola	29 × 18	Ellipsoidal	Smooth, light yellow-brown wall; prominent micropyle; no residual body	Jejunum, ileum	9-10	Significant (nonpathogenic)*
E. flavesceus	32 × 21	Broadly ellipsoidal	Smooth, light yellow wall; prominent micropyle; no residual body	Lower small intestine, cecum, colon	9	Significant (very pathogenic)*

Modified from Pakes SP, Gerrity LW: Protozoal diseases. *In* Manning PJ, Ringler DH, Newcomer CE, eds. The Biology of the Laboratory Rabbit, 2nd ed. San Diego, Academic Press, 1994, p 206.
*From Økerman L: Diseases of Domestic Rabbits, 2nd ed. Oxford, Blackwell Scientific, 1994.

excystation in the duodenum. Liberated sporozoites penetrate the intestinal mucosa and move to bile epithelial cells, where they undergo schizogony. Merozoites invade contiguous epithelial cells and undergo gametogeny, which develop into microgametes and macrogametes. After being fertilized by a microgamete, the macrogamete develops into an oocyst. Oocysts rupture from the epithelial cells and are passed in the bile and, eventually, in the feces.[28] In mild infections, the symptom is unapparent retardation of growth; however, the disease may be fatal, especially in young rabbits. Heavily infected rabbits show signs related to the interference of hepatic function and the blockage of bile ducts. Infected rabbits become anorexic and debilitated; diarrhea or constipation may be noted in the terminal stages of the disease. The abdomen is occasionally enlarged and icterus is observed. On radiographs, the liver may appear enlarged and ascites may be present. On postmortem examination, the liver is enlarged and has yellowish-white, nodular, abscesslike lesions of varying size, some of which are within a fibrous capsule. The gallbladder often is enlarged by exudate. Diagnosis is based on the identification of oocysts in a sample of bile, by histologic examination, or by fecal examination.

Intestinal coccidia The most important species of intestinal coccidia are *E. perforans, E. magna, E. media,* and *E. irresidua,* with *E. perforans* being the most common. Infection is by ingestion of sporulated oocysts. Although rabbits are cecotrophic, it is generally accepted that cecotrophs eaten from the anus do not contain infectious oocysts. Clinical signs vary widely depending on the age of the rabbit, the organism involved, the degree of infection (i.e., the number of oocysts ingested), and the relative susceptibility of the animal (determined by factors such as age, stress, and diet). Infections are usually not apparent. Clinical signs are most often seen in young rabbits. Weight loss, mild intermittent to severe diarrhea that may contain mucus or blood, and dehydration may be observed. Animals with severe diarrhea may develop intussusception. Death most often is attributed to dehydration and secondary bacterial infections. Postmortem examination reveals lesions in the small or large intestine, depending on the agent involved. The epithelium of the intestine may be ulcerated. The presence of the organism (or organisms) in fecal samples or scrapings of the intestine supports a presumptive diagnosis. Definitive diagnosis is based on histologic findings.

Numerous agents have been used to prevent and treat intestinal and hepatic coccidiosis. Sulfa drugs appear to be the most effective. The addition of sulfadimethoxine to the diet in an amount to ensure intake of 75 mg/kg for 7 days or 0.02% sulfamerazine sodium to the drinking water is safe and efficacious.[39] In my experience, sulfadimethoxine (15 mg/kg PO q12h for 10 days) and trimethoprim-sulfa combinations (30 mg/kg q12h PO for 10 days) have similarly proved effective. Amprolium 9.6% in drinking water (0.5 mL per 500 mL) also is effective. The major role of chemotherapeutic agents may be limiting multiplication until immunity develops. Once a rabbit is infected, it is rare for it to show clinical signs of coccidiosis, and immunity resulting from mild infections may be lifelong.[39] Research studies have shown that suckling rabbits vaccinated orally or with a spray dispersion into the nest box with a precocious line of *E. magna* were protected from challenge.[14,18] Prevention depends on keeping rabbits in hygienic conditions and avoiding infected feces or feces-contaminated food and water.

Cryptosporidia

Cryptosporidium parvum may cause a discrete and transitory diarrhea in young rabbits, peaking at 30 to 40 days, that may lead to growth retardation. Clinical signs include diarrhea lasting 3 to 5 days, decreased appetite, depression, lethargy, exhaustion, and dehydration. *C. parvum* infects the intestinal tract, especially the ileum and the jejunum. The organism apparently does not cause disease in adults. Atrophy of villi of the ileum in young rabbits was observed histologically.[36] Currently, no effective treatment for cryptosporidiosis is recognized.

Other Protozoa

Several nonpathogenic flagellates may be found in the feces of rabbits. They occur more commonly in animals with diarrhea. *Giardia duodenalis* occurs rarely in the anterior region of the small intestine of rabbits and is not considered pathogenic. Other nonpathogenic protozoa found in the cecum and colon include *Monocercomonas cuniculi* and *Retortamonas cuniculi,* which are flagellates from the cecum; large ciliated protozoa found in the cecum that are similar to those of the genus *Isotricha* in ruminants; and *Entamoeba cuniculi,* which is commonly found in the cecum and colon of rabbits.[39]

Helminths

Nematodes *Passalurus ambiguus* is the common pinworm of domestic rabbits, although *P. nonanulatus* also is reported. Occurrence is widespread in both wild and domestic rabbits; however, the presence of even relatively large numbers of pinworms is nonpathogenic. The adult parasite is found in the anterior portion of the cecum and colon. Adult worms are grossly visible in the lumen of the cecum and large intestine and when they are passed with fresh feces. Infection is through the ingestion of infected eggs. Juvenile stages are found in the mucosa of the small intestine and cecum. Pinworms are commonly seen during routine surgical procedures such as ovariohysterectomy. Diagnosis is made by identification of adult worms or by demonstration of the parasite's eggs in the feces.

The rabbit stomach worm, *Obeliscoides cuniculi,* a member of the family *Trichostrongylidea,* is found in the stomach of North American rabbits that have the opportunity to graze on grass or where fresh grass is used as a feed. Eggs of the parasite are passed in feces, and larvae hatch in 30 hours. Infectious, third-stage larvae develop in approximately 6 days. The larvae penetrate the gastric mucosa, where they develop into adults. Eggs may be found in feces as soon as 16 to 20 days after infection, and shedding continues for 61 to 118 days. Rabbits do not typically show signs of the infection. Large numbers of the parasite may cause general malaise, anorexia, and a decrease in weight gain. Pathologic changes are limited to the stomach. On gross examination, the mucosa is thickened and has an irregular "cobblestone" appearance, with excess mucus on the surface. Adult worms are pink and may be seen in the gastric mucus. Eggs of *O. cuniculi* are thin shelled and oval.[27]

Treatment of helminthic infections with a variety of drugs has been successful. The benzimidazoles are effective in greatly reducing, if not eliminating, pinworms. Thiabendazole (110 mg/kg PO for one treatment, followed by 70 mg/kg PO q4h for eight doses) showed 99% efficacy in the treatment of *O. cuniculi* with no ill effects.[27] I have obtained good results with thiabendazole, 50 mg/kg PO repeated in 10 to 14 days, and fenbendazole (Panacur, Hoechst-Roussel Agri-Vet Co., Somerville, NJ), 10 to 20 mg/kg PO repeated in 10 to 14 days. I have used ivermectin (Ivomec 1%, Merck AgVet, Iselin, NJ), 0.4 mg/kg SC repeated in 10 to 14 days, to treat rabbits with *O. cuniculi* infection, with no side effects and apparent good success. However, I have not observed the same in the treatment of *P. ambiguus* infection. My experience mimics that of studies showing the administration of ivermectin at doses of 0.4, 1.0, and 2.0 mg/kg to be ineffective against *P. ambiguus*.[44] Piperazine (200 mg/kg PO repeated in 14 days) can be used to treat individual rabbits, or it can be given in drinking water (100 mg/100 mL of water for 1 day repeated in 10 days) to treat large numbers of animals. My experience is that this treatment is effective in most cases but is not as reliable as fenbendazole.

Cestodes and trematodes The rabbit's gastrointestinal tract is host to five species of cestodes: *Cittotaenia variabilis, Mosgovoyia pectinata americana, M. perplexa, Monoecocestus americana,* and *Ctenotaenia ctenoides. C. variabilis* is found in domestic rabbits, whereas the other species are most often found in wild rabbits in North America and Europe.[1,3] Adult parasites are found in the small intestine. The life cycles for some species are not well known; however, oribatid mites or ants are thought to act as intermediary hosts.

Trematode parasites of the rabbit gastrointestinal tract include *Hasstilesia tricolor* and *Fasciola hepatica. H. tricolor* is not associated with disease but most often is found incidentally at necropsy, or the ova are found on fecal examination. Adult *H. tricolor* are found in the small intestine of wild rabbits; the intermediary hosts are small terrestrial snails. *F. hepatica* occurs in rabbits that graze in wet pasture or along the banks of streams in endemic areas. These rabbits also may act as a reservoir for the parasite. Adult forms are found in the gallbladder and bile ducts. Signs of infection include cachexia, poor coat, lethargy, and death. Eggs of the fluke may be found on examination of feces, or the adult form may be found at necropsy. Treatment of cestode and trematode parasites consists of the administration of a single dose of praziquantel (5-10 mg/kg PO; Droncit, Miles Animal Health, Shawnee Mission, KS). Prevent these parasites by not feeding rabbits grass from wet meadows.

NEOPLASIA

Neoplasms of the gastrointestinal tract include adenocarcinoma and leiomyosarcoma of the stomach, leiomyoma and leiomyosarcoma of the intestine, papilloma of the sacculus rotundus, papilloma of the rectal squamous columnar junction, and bile duct adenoma and carcinoma. Metastatic neoplasia, most commonly uterine adenocarcinoma, often involves the gastrointestinal tract. Surgical resection is the treatment of choice for many of these tumors. If diagnosed early, intestinal masses can be resected with good success.

Rectal papillomas (cauliflower-like, fungating masses arising from the anorectal junction) appear to be benign and are not related to the papillomas of skin or the oral cavity. Removal of these lesions often is curative.

Bile duct adenoma and adenocarcinoma occasionally occur in pet rabbits. These tumors often are multiple and consist of interlocking cysts filled with thick, viscous, myxoid fluid. A variety of noxious stimuli, particularly infection with *E. stiedae*, may be causative factors. Antemortem diagnosis in some rabbits is based on the results of radiography and ultrasound. Surgical removal often is not practical. Metastatic disease is most often miliary and carries a grave prognosis.[45]

AFLATOXICOSIS

Aflatoxins are secondary metabolites of fungi, produced primarily by *Aspergillus flavus* and *A. parasiticus*. When feed that contains aflatoxins is ingested, a complex metabolic pathway is created for removing this toxin from the body. There are four different aflatoxins produced by *Aspergillus*; AFB_1, B_2, G_1, and G_2, but the aflatoxin of main concern is aflatoxin B_1 because of its role in carcinogenesis. In its natural state, aflatoxin B_1 is not toxigenic. It becomes harmful when it enters the body and is recognized as a foreign substance and is metabolized initially to B8,9-epoxide by cytochrome P450 subfamilies and specific isoforms. A major detoxification pathway that the body uses is the conjugation of B8,9-epoxide with glutathione. This process is catalyzed by glutathione-S-transferase. Aflatoxin B_1-8,9-epoxide and AFB_{2a} are intermediates of the most active metabolite, AFB-dihydrodiol. The production of AFB-dihydrodiol is an attempt made by the body at detoxification. This pathway is used to a lesser extent. The epoxide is converted into a dihydrodiol because of the actions of epoxide hydrolase. Aflatoxin B-dihydrodiol is further metabolized to form AFM_1, AFQ_1, and AFP_1, which form glucuronides and sulfate conjugates that are excreted in the urine and feces.[10] The LD_{50} for aflatoxins in rabbits is among the lowest for any species studied.[13] Levels of aflatoxin B_1 greater than 100 ppm in the diet of rabbits have been shown to be associated with morbidity and death.[33] In one outbreak of aflatoxicosis in angora rabbits, affected animals had anorexia, dullness, and weight loss followed by jaundice in terminal stages. Death occurred within 3 to 4 days of the appearance of clinical signs. On postmortem examination, livers were moderately to severely congested, icteric, and were hard to cut. Gallbladders were distended and had inspissated bile. Liver sections showed degenerative changes of hepatic cells along with dilatation and engorgement of sinusoids. Bile ducts had mild to severe periportal fibrosis. Focal areas of pseudolobulation and regenerative foci were also predominant. The level of aflatoxin B_1 in feed samples from various farms submitted at the time of the investigation varied from 90 to 540 μg aflatoxin B_1/kg of feed. Withdrawal of feed and supplementary therapy resulted in gradual disappearance of signs and death.[29]

REFERENCES

1. Andrews CL, Davidson WR: Endoparasites of selected populations of cottontail rabbits (*Sylvilagus floridanus*) in the southeastern United States. J Wildl Dis 1980; 16:395-401.
2. Armstrong DG, Cook H, Thomas B: The lignin and cellulose contents of certain grassland species at different stages of growth. J Agric Sci 1950; 40:39-99.
3. Boag B: The incidence of helminth parasites from the wild rabbit *Oryctolagus cuniculus* (L.) in eastern Scotland. J Helminthol 1985; 59:61-69.
4. Bolton AJ, Osborne MP, Stephen J: Comparative study of the invasiveness of *Salmonella* serotypes *typhimurium, choleraesuis* and *dublin* for Caco-2 cells, Hep-2 cells and rabbit ileal epithelia. J Med Microbiol 2000; 49:503-511.

5. Brewer NR: Biology of the rabbit—X. Synapse 1991; 24:9.
6. Brewer NR: Biology of the rabbit—XVI. Synapse 1991; 24:27-29.
7. Buss SL, Bourdeau JE: Calcium balance in laboratory rabbits. Miner Electrolyte Metab 1984; 10:127-132.
8. Carman RJ, Wilkins TD: In vitro susceptibility of rabbit strains of *Clostridium spiroforme* to antimicrobial agents. Vet Microbiol 1991; 28:391-397.
9. Castrucci G, Frigeri F, Ferrari M, et al: Comparative study of rotavirus strains of bovine and rabbit origin. Comp Immunol Microbiol Infect Dis 1984; 7:171-178.
10. Cheeke PR: Natural Toxicants in Feeds, Forages, and Poisonous Plants, 2nd ed. Danville, IL, Interstate Publishers, 1998, pp 87-103.
11. Cheeke PR, Grobner MA, Patton NM: Fiber digestion and utilization in rabbits. J Appl Rabbit Res 1986; 9:25-30.
12. Cheeke PR, Patton NM, Lukefuhr SD, et al: Rabbit Production, 6th ed. Danville, IL, Interstate Printers and Publishers, 1987.
13. Clard JD, Jain AV, Hatch RC: Experimentally induced chronic aflatoxicosis in rabbits. Am J Vet Res 1980; 41:1841-1845.
14. Coudert P, Licois D, Provot F, et al: *Eimeria* sp. from the rabbit (*Oryctolagus cuniculus*): pathogenicity and immunogenicity of *Eimeria intestinalis*. Parasitol Res 1993; 79:186-190.
15. DiGiacomo RF, Mare CJ: Viral diseases. *In* Manning PJ, Ringler DH, Newcomer CE, eds. The Biology of the Laboratory Rabbit, 2nd ed. San Diego, Academic Press, 1994, pp 171-204.
16. DiGiacomo RF, Thouless ME: Age-related antibodies to rotavirus in New Zealand rabbits. J Clin Microbiol 1984; 19:710-711.
17. DiGiacomo RF, Thouless ME. Epidemiology of naturally occurring rotavirus infections in rabbits. Lab Anim Sci 1986; 36:153-156.
18. Drouet-Viard F, Coudert P, Licois D, et al: Vaccination against *Eimeria magna* coccidiosis using spray dispersion of precocious line oocysts in the nest box. Vet Parasitol 1997; 70:61-66.
19. Duff GL, McMillan GC: The effect of alloxan diabetes on experimental cholesterol atherosclerosis in the rabbit. I. The inhibition of experimental cholesterol atherosclerosis in alloxan diabetes. II. The effect of alloxan diabetes on the retrogression of experimental cholesterol atherosclerosis. J Exp Med 1994; 89:611-630.
20. Duncan AJ, Carman RJ, Olsen GJ, et al: Assignment of the agent of Tyzzer's disease to *Clostridium piliforme* comb. nov. on the basis of 16S rRNA sequence analysis. Int J Syst Bacteriol 1993; 43:314-318.
21. Ehrlein HF, Reich M, Schwinger M: Colonic motility and transit of digesta during hard and soft faeces formation in the rabbit. J Physiol 1983; 338:75-86.
22. Fekete S: Recent findings and future perspectives of digestive physiology in rabbits: a review. Acta Vet Hung 1989; 37:265-279.
23. Forsyth SJ, Parker DS: Nitrogen metabolism by the microbial flora of the rabbit caecum. J Appl Bacteriol 1985; 58:363-369.
24. Fox JG, Cohen BJ, Loew FM: Laboratory Animal Medicine. Orlando, FL, Academic Press, 1984.
25. Fox JG, Dewhirst FE, Fraser GJ, et al: Intracellular *Campylobacter*-like organism from ferrets and hamsters with proliferative bowel disease is a *Desosulfovibrio* sp. J Clin Microbiol 1994; 32:1229-1237.
26. Hanes DE, Robl MG, Schneider CM, et al: New Zealand white rabbit as a nonsurgical experimental model for *Salmonella enterica* gastroenteritis. Infect Immunol 2001; 69:6523-6526.
27. Hofing GL, Kraus AL: Arthropod and helminth parasites. *In* Manning PJ, Ringler DH, Newcomer CE, eds. The Biology of the Laboratory Rabbit, 2nd ed. San Diego, Academic Press, 1994, pp 231-257.
28. Kraus AL, Weisbroth SH, Flatt SH, et al: Biology and disease of rabbits. *In* Fox JG, Cohen BJ, Loew FM, eds. Laboratory Animal Medicine. Orlando, Academic Press, 1984, pp 207-240.
29. Krishna L, Dawra RK, Vaid J, et al: An outbreak of aflatoxicosis in Angora rabbits. Vet Hum Toxicol 1991; 33:159-161.
30. LaPierre J, Marsolais G, Pilon P, et al: Preliminary report on the observation of a coronavirus in the intestine of the laboratory rabbit. Can J Microbiol 1980; 26:1204-1208.
31. Lelkes L, Chang CL: Microbial dysbiosis in rabbit mucoid enteropathy. Lab Anim Sci 1987; 37:757-764.
32. Lipman NS, Weischedel AK, Conners MJ, et al: Utilization of cholestyramine resin as a preventative treatment for antibiotic (clindamycin)-induced enterotoxemia in the rabbit. Lab Anim 1992; 26:1-8.
33. Makkar HPS, Singh B: Aflatoxicosis in rabbits. J Appl Rabbit Res 1991; 14:218-222.
34. Manning PJ, Ringler DH, Newcomer CE, eds. The Biology of the Laboratory Rabbit, 2nd ed. San Diego, Academic Press, 1994.
35. McOrist S, Gebhart CJ, Boid R, et al: Characterization of *Lawsonia intracellularis* gen. nov., sp. nov., the obligate intracellular bacterium of porcine proliferative enteropathy. Int Syst Bacteriol 1995; 45:820-825.
36. Mosier DA, Cimon KY, Kuhls TL, et al: Experimental cryptosporidiosis in adult and neonatal rabbits. Vet Parasitol 1997; 69:163-169.
37. Økerman L: Diseases of Domestic Rabbits. 2nd ed. Oxford, Blackwell Scientific, 1994.
38. Osterhaus AD, Teppema JS, Van Steenis G: Coronavirus-like particles in laboratory rabbits with different syndromes in The Netherlands. Lab Anim Sci 1982; 32:663-665.
39. Pakes SP, Gerrity LW: Protozoal diseases. *In* Manning PJ, Ringler DH, Newcomer CE, eds. The Biology of the Laboratory Rabbit, 2nd ed. San Diego, Academic Press, 1994, pp 205-229.
40. Sakaguchi E, Kaizu K, Nakamichi M: Fibre digestion and digesta retention from different physical forms of the feed in the rabbit. Comp Biochem Physiol 1992; 102A:559-563.
41. Schauer DB, McCathey SN, Daft BM, et al: Proliferative enterocolitis associated with dual infection with enteropathogenic *Escherichia coli* and *Lawsonia intracellularis* in rabbits. J Clin Microbiol 1998; 36:1700-1703.
42. Sullivan JT: Studies of the hemicellulose of forage plants. J Anim Sci 1966; 5:83-86.
43. Sundberg JP, Junge RE, el Shazly MO: Oral papillomatosis in New Zealand white rabbits. Am J Vet Res 1985; 46:664-668.
44. Tsui TLH, Patton NM: Comparative efficacy of subcutaneous injection doses of ivermectin against *P. ambiguus* in rabbits. J Appl Rabbit Res 1991; 14:266-269.
45. Weisbroth SH: Neoplastic diseases. *In* Manning PJ, Ringler DH, Newcomer CE, eds. The Biology of the Laboratory Rabbit, 2nd ed. San Diego, Academic Press, 1994, pp 205-229.

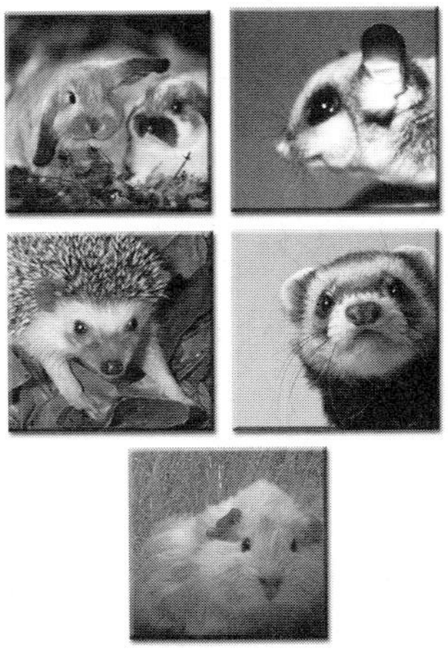

CHAPTER 17

Respiratory Disease and Pasteurellosis

Barbara J. Deeb, DVM, MS

In the first edition of *Ferrets, Rabbits, and Rodents: Clinical Medicine and Surgery,* pasteurellosis was emphasized as the major cause of respiratory disease in rabbits. That is probably still true in many rabbitries. However, in recent years some *Pasteurella*-free rabbitries have been established. In pet rabbits, pasteurellosis is less common than in past years. *Pasteurella multocida* should always be considered but never assumed to be the only cause of respiratory disease in pet rabbits. Differentiation is crucial.

In the first edition, I summarized the work of Webster and Smith in the 1920s. They established *P. multocida* as the cause of a rabbit respiratory infection ("snuffles") in a large colony of rabbits to be used in research. They also studied epidemiology, virulence of *P. multocida* strains, pathogenesis, and control of the infection. Their conclusions and control methods still guide us. They found that some of the rabbits exposed to the agent (1) resisted infection; (2) spontaneously eliminated infection; (3) became subclinical carriers; (4) developed acute disease (bacteremia or pneumonia); or (5) developed chronic disease. These conclusions also may apply to other bacterial causes of respiratory disease.

Respiratory disease in rabbits is often caused by bacterial agents: *P. multocida, Bordetella bronchiseptica, Staphylococcus* species, *Pseudomonas* species, and other bacteria, or occasionally by viral agents. Noninfectious causes include allergens, nasal or thoracic neoplasia, cardiovascular disease, and exposure to respiratory irritants or trauma. Many more studies involving pasteurellosis have been reported than for any other cause of respiratory disease in rabbits. This chapter presents information about these causes, then discusses the diagnosis and differentiation, treatment, and control of respiratory disease in rabbits.

INFECTIOUS CAUSES

Pasteurellosis

Bacterial and cultural characteristics *P. multocida* is a gram-negative, bipolar, nonmotile asporogenous coccobacillus of the family Pasteurellaceae, which includes *Haemophilus, Actinobacillus,* and *Pasteurella* species (i.e., the HAP group). *P. multocida* grows on blood agar and dextrose starch agar but not on MacConkey's agar. Some strains may require fresh blood for growth on nutrient agar, with cultural characteristics influenced by the type of blood used. Colonies grow larger and produce greenish discoloration on media with horse blood. *P. multocida* produces a distinctive odor, which bacteriologists liken to that of indole. Growth occurs under aerobic conditions or in 5% carbon dioxide. Temperature-sensitive and carbon dioxide–sensitive strains may exist. Most isolates require 24 to 48 hours of incubation to become apparent on blood agar, especially if mixed with other bacteria. Blood agar with 2 μg/mL of clindamycin can be used to inhibit other bacteria in mixed cultures. Colonies are convex and smooth but vary in coloration from bluish to greenish iridescence when observed in obliquely transmitted light, and they may vary in mucoid appearance. Colonies of the mucoid strains appear to run together, if their numbers permit. Capsular type A strains have large capsules and produce mucoid colonies, whereas colonies of the type D strains may appear iridescent.

P. multocida strains isolated from rabbits usually have the following biochemical characteristics: oxidase+, catalase±, indole±, hydrogen sulfide–, urease–, ornithine decarboxylase+, hexose+, and carbohydrate fermentation+ for most sugars. These characteristics are useful in distinguishing *P. multocida* from other *Pasteurella* species that may be part of the normal flora.[26]

Serotypes Serologic typing is done with the use of indirect hemagglutination, to identify capsular types A, B, D, E, or F, and the gel diffusion precipitin test, which has been used to describe 16 somatic antigen determinants of lipopolysaccharide. The acriflavine flocculation test is specific for capsular type D strains, whereas a staphylococcal hyaluronidase inhibition test specifically inhibits type A strains. With these tests, most isolates from rabbits were shown to be of type A. Serotypes vary by region, but in the United States, A:12 and A:3 are the most prevalent types.[22]

Okerman and co-workers[24] substantiated the conclusion of Webster and Smith that some strains of *P. multocida* are more pathogenic than others. Capsular type D isolates from rabbits with bacteremia are significantly more pathogenic for mice than are type A isolates from rabbits with rhinitis only. Somatic type 3 isolates are more pathogenic than type 12 isolates.[22]

Sodium dodecyl sulfate-polyacrylamide gel electrophoresis (SDS-PAGE) provides enhancement of differentiation among *P. multocida* isolates from rabbits.[11] Single-primer polymerase chain reaction (PCR) fingerprinting is efficient and reproducible for discriminating *P. multocida* isolates.[10]

Virulence factors Virulence factors of *P. multocida* include adhesions, phagocyte resistance, endotoxin (lipopolysaccharide), exotoxin, and iron regulation. Pili or other adhesion proteins on the outer membrane of some strains of *P. multocida* enhance colonization. Type A strains are more adhesive to respiratory mucosa than are type D strains. Invasion and multiplication of the organism occur because the capsule, largely consisting of hyaluronic acid, which also is present in host tissues, inhibits phagocytosis and complement-activated bactericidal activity of serum (opsonization). Some type D strains, although ingested by phagocytes, resist bactericidal activity. Leukotoxic enzymes also are produced. Growth of some strains of *P. multocida* is regulated by the availability of iron, and most strains produce iron-binding outer membrane proteins, which enhance their survival in iron-poor cavities of the hosts.

Serotype D:1 strain (noncapsulated, fimbriae+, hemagglutination [HA]+, dermonecrotic toxin [now termed *P. multocida* toxin, or PMT]+) was highly adherent to tracheal mucosa, lung, and aorta explants when compared with serotype A:3 (capsulated, fimbriae+, HA–, and PMT–), although A:3 adhered after prolonged incubation. Adhesion to endothelial receptors may explain association of some strains with pneumonia and septicemia.[2]

Endotoxin enhances resistance to bactericidal activity of serum and stimulates the release of inflammatory mediators, such as interleukin-1. In cases of bacteremia, free endotoxin in plasma causes fever and depression and may induce shock. A toxin with characteristics of an exotoxin is produced by some strains of *P. multocida*. PMT of some type D strains enhances attachment and colonization of mucosa. This protein toxin, which is similar to that causing atrophic rhinitis in pigs, also is associated with nasal turbinate atrophy in rabbits. Toxin has been demonstrated for type D[26] and for type A isolates,[15] but it is not clear whether it is the same toxin. Purified PMT induces pneumonia, pleuritis, lymphoid atrophy, and possibly osteoclastic bone resorption in rabbits.[6]

Antibiotic sensitivities Antibiotic sensitivities for 42 isolates of *P. multocida* from rabbits are as follows: 100% were sensitive to chloramphenicol, erythromycin, novobiocin, oxytetracycline, penicillin G, nitrofurazone, and nitrofurantoin; most were resistant to sulfonamides and streptomycin; and all were resistant to lincomycin and clindamycin. In my laboratory, four strains of *P. multocida* from rabbits were resistant to erythromycin and had moderate or intermediate sensitivity to penicillin G but otherwise were sensitive to 16 antibiotics, including several fluoroquinolones and cephalosporins. In my practice, most isolates of *P. multocida* tested on Mueller-Hinton agar with 5% sheep blood have been sensitive to amikacin, chloramphenicol, ciprofloxacin, doxycycline, enrofloxacin, gentamicin, penicillin G, tetracycline, and trimethoprim-sulfa.

Transmission and pathogenesis Transmission of *P. multocida* is by aerosol from acutely affected rabbits, by direct contact, or by fomites.[22] Venereal transmission also occurs with genital infections, and kits may be infected at birth if the doe has genital infection. However, kits usually remain uninfected for several weeks, and the prevalence of infection increases with age and exposure.

P. multocida gains entry to the host primarily through the nares or wounds. If the host does not resist infection, the bacteria colonize the nares and may cause production of nasal exudate. The incubation period is difficult to define because many rabbits are subclinical carriers of infection; however, in experimental studies, rhinitis occurred 1 to 2 weeks after intranasal inoculation of *P. multocida*. Once established in the nasal passages, infection spreads to contiguous tissues (paranasal sinuses, nasolacrimal duct and conjunctiva, eustachian tube and middle ears, trachea, bronchi, and lungs). Hematogenous spread also accounts for infection that reaches the middle ears, lungs, and internal organs.

Most of the Pasteurellaceae are commensal organisms on mucous membranes but exhibit pathogenicity under conditions of immunodeficiency and stress in the host. Nutritional, environmental, managerial, or social changes may predispose to disease, as may concomitant infection and physical or chemical injury to the mucosa. Exposure of mucous membranes to ammonia or dilute acetic acid increases the susceptibility of rabbits to *P. multocida* infection, and stress or hydrocortisone treatment increases pathogenicity. With disseminated pasteurellosis, fever enhances the neutrophil response and increases survival.

The protective role of the humoral immune response to *P. multocida* is unclear. Immunization partially protects against severe disease but does not prevent infection.[22] Antibodies to antigens of *P. multocida* or to cross-reacting antigens of other bacteria may enhance opsonization and phagocytosis. Common epitopes do occur between *P. multocida* and other gram-negative bacteria, notably *Pasteurella, Yersinia,* and *Moraxella* species.

Antibodies to gram-negative core antigens occur in rabbits and increase with age, indicating possible cross-reactive epitopes between *P. multocida* and Enterobacteriaceae and possible protection against pasteurellosis.[28] An *Escherichia coli* J5 bacterin induced antibodies and reduced bacteremia in rabbits challenged with *P. multocida,* but was not protective against colonization.[27] *P. multocida* serotype A:3 was shown to attach to and invade epithelial cells, causing deciliation of ciliated cells and hyperplasia of goblet cells of nasal mucosa; thickening of alveolar septa; swelling of capillary lining cells; and infiltration of inflammatory cells in the lungs.[2,3] Thrombocytosis is a consistent secondary response to *P. multocida* infection; however, it does not appear to be predictive of disease outcome.[29]

Serum with immunoglobulin G (IgG) to *P. multocida* is not bactericidal in vitro or in vivo.[22] Rabbits with chronic and severe infections usually have high IgG titers to *P. multocida*. Also, the secretory immune response (IgA) does not protect against nasal infection,[12] although it may play a role in limiting spread. The protective role of cell-mediated immunity in *P. multocida* infection has not been well studied, but depressed T-lymphocyte function results in severe disease in infected rabbits.

Vaccine strategies No vaccine is currently available for the prevention of pasteurellosis in rabbits. The following vaccine preparations have been evaluated and have *not* prevented nasal infection on challenge: bacteria killed with heat or formalin; potassium thiocyanate extracts; and live but avirulent strains, such as a streptomycin-dependent strain.[22] Characterization of the protein patterns and immunogenic epitopes of *P. multocida* by electrophoresis and immunoblotting indicates that several proteins are consistently recognized by the immune systems of infected rabbits.[13,39] Several antigens associated with virulence have been identified, offering promise for their use in subunit vaccines. Specific antiserum to an outer membrane 87-kDa antigen protected mice against lethal challenge.[30] Cloning and sequencing of subunit proteins associated with virulence (fimbriae, capsule, transferrin binding, hemolysis) may lead to potential vaccine candidates.[1] Immunization with inactivated, purified PMT stimulated a protective response to PMT challenge that was enhanced by coadministration of cholera toxin (CT), a potent adjuvant for the mucosal immune system.[19] When CT was administered with potassium thiocyanate extract (PTE) of *P. multocida,* protective immunity to pasteurellosis was enhanced in rabbits.[32] Intranasal immunization with both inactivated purified PMT and PTE induced a protective response against homologous *P. multocida* challenge.[31] Use of oral or intranasal delivery of microencapsulated antigens (PTE) also enhanced protection, as evidenced by production of anti-PTE IgA and IgG as well as decreasing severity of infection after challenge. Coadministration of CT did not improve protection when used with the microencapsulated PTE.[33]

Clinical and pathologic manifestations The clinical presentation of pasteurellosis in rabbits includes upper respiratory tract disease (rhinitis, sinusitis, conjunctivitis, lacrimal duct infection), otitis, pleuropneumonia, bacteremia, and abscesses of the subcutaneous tissues or internal organs, bones, joints, and genitalia.

Upper respiratory tract disease Upper respiratory tract disease (snuffles) in rabbits is often caused by *P. multocida;* however, predisposing factors influence pathogenicity. Rhinitis and sinusitis are the most common forms of pasteurellosis. A serous nasal discharge precedes the typical white or yellowish mucopurulent discharge associated with *P. multocida.* Exudate adheres to the fur around the nares (Fig. 17-1), and, because rabbits groom the face with their forepaws, to the medial aspects of the forepaws, where it mats and becomes yellowish-gray on drying. Affected rabbits often make audible sonorous noises and have bouts of sneezing, with exudate forcibly expelled from the nares. Conjunctivitis is sometimes a manifestation of upper respiratory tract disease. Infection of the nasal lacrimal duct may extend to the conjunctiva. Exudate occluding the duct causes excessive tearing and scalding of the face, alopecia, and pyoderma.

Auscultation of the trachea and nares reveals rales and rattles caused by exudate in the upper respiratory tract. The origin of these respiratory sounds must be determined so that rales from the lungs are not misinterpreted. Signs of rhinitis may subside or even disappear, with affected rabbits harboring infection in the paranasal sinuses or middle ears. Recovery from acute disease and elimination of infection may occur, but spontaneous recovery from chronic infection is unlikely.

Acute infection of the nares is accompanied by edema and hyperemia of the mucosa. Chronic infection may be accompanied by mucosal erosion and atrophy of the turbinates.

Otitis Extension of the infection from the nares to the middle ears probably occurs through the eustachian tubes. Most rabbits with otitis media also have rhinitis, but some clear the infection from the nares while the middle ears remain infected.[12] Otitis media may be asymptomatic, or, if infection spreads to the inner ear, torticollis, nystagmus, and ataxia can occur. Infection extends to the external ear if the tympanic membrane ruptures. What appears to be accumulation of wax deep in the ear canal may be dried exudate, which, if removed, reveals the typical white, purulent exudate underneath. Exudate may be physically expressed by gentle pressure at the base of the ear, and its origin can be determined by otoscopic examination. Consider otitis media in a rabbit that scratches excessively at the base of the ear but has no external parasites or when an abscess is detected at the base of the ear. A dorsoventral radiograph of the skull aids in diagnosis of otitis media; increased soft tissue opacity caused by the exudate can be visualized within the bulla, and the bone

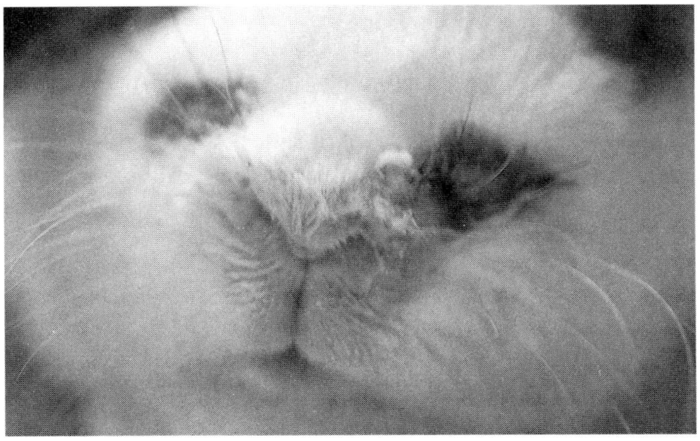

Figure 17-1 Severe rhinitis and nasal exudate in a rabbit infected with *Pasteurella multocida.* Note the exudate around the nares.

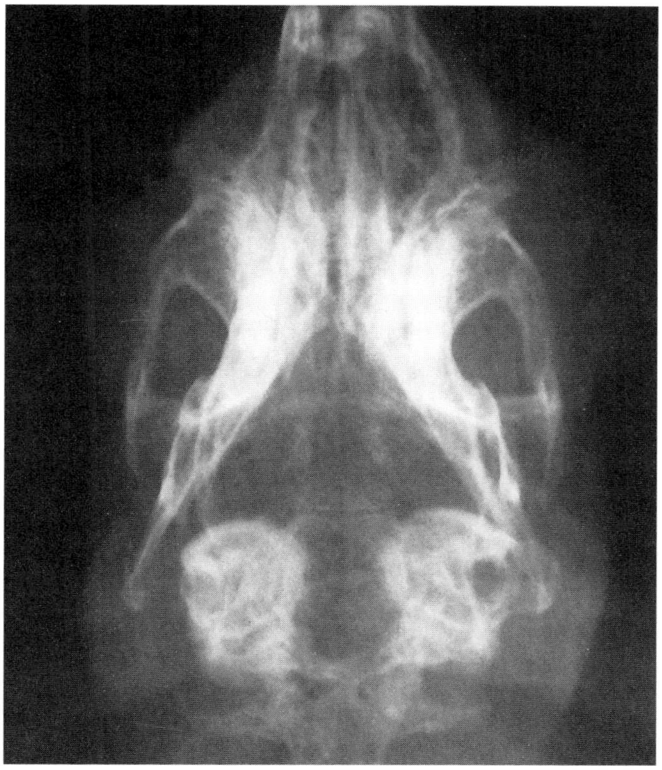

Figure 17-2 Dorsoventral radiograph of the skull of a Holland lop rabbit with exudate in the ear canals. Increased density and thickening of the tympanic bullae indicates bilateral otitis media.

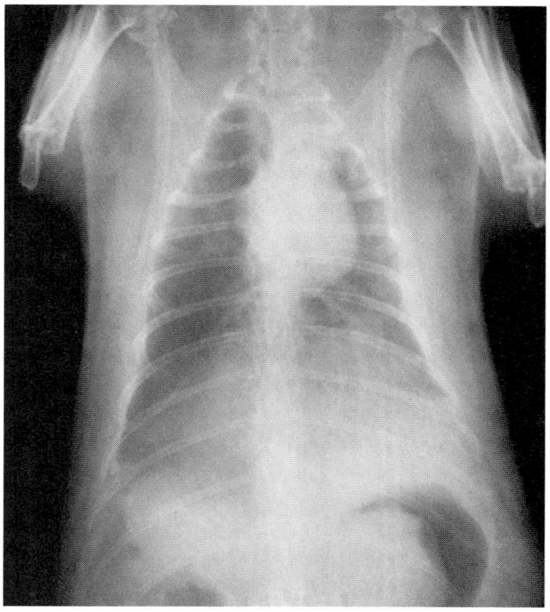

Figure 17-3 Dorsoventral radiograph of the thorax of a rabbit with pulmonary rales resulting from a chronic bronchopneumonia. Note increased peribronchial density.

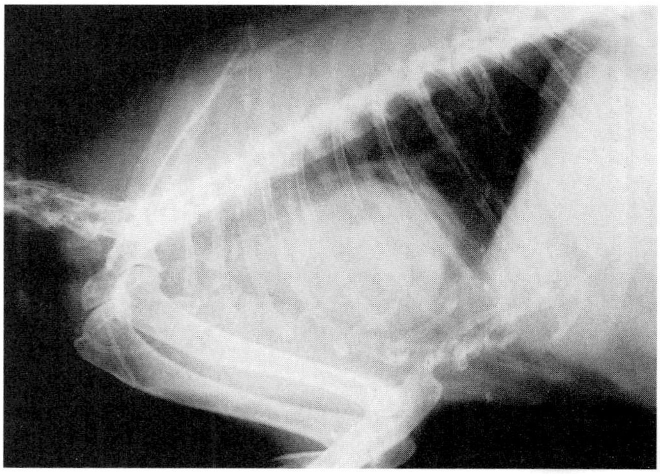

Figure 17-4 Lateral radiograph of the thorax of a rabbit with respiratory distress and bradycardia caused by pericarditis and abscess anterior to the heart. Note dorsal tracheal deviation. *Pasteurella multocida* was isolated from the abscess.

shows thickening (Fig. 17-2). The tympanic bullae are normally thin-walled and hollow.

Bacteremia The more pathogenic strains of *P. multocida* are likely to spread hematogenously, causing acute generalized disease, fever, and sudden death. Pathologic examination may reveal congestion, petechiation, and microscopic abscesses throughout the viscera. Pleuropneumonia is another sequela of hematogenous spread.

Pneumonia, pleuritis, pericarditis Chronic infection within the thoracic cavity may go undetected until long after the acute phase of infection (Fig. 17-3), and it is likely to take the form of pleuropneumonia or pericarditis, with abscesses developing in or around the lungs or heart (Fig. 17-4). Anorexia, weight loss, depression, and rapid fatigue are nonspecific signs, but in rabbits they should arouse suspicion of lower respiratory tract disease. Dyspnea occurs on exertion. Auscultation may reveal areas in the thorax in which lung sounds are absent because of consolidation or abscess. Pulmonary rales must be differentiated from those referred from the upper respiratory tract. Radiographs help to determine the extent of involvement. Rabbits often appear relatively normal, even with minimally functioning lungs.

Pathologically, pasteurellosis in the thorax is characterized by the presence of fibrinopurulent exudate in the airways and on serosal surfaces. Neutrophils (also called heterophils) are the principal inflammatory cells, but macrophages and erythrocytes may be present. Lymphocytic peribronchial and perivascular cuffing also occur.

Abscesses and genital infections Abscesses in subcutaneous tissues, retrobulbar tissues, or the internal organs of rabbits frequently are caused by *P. multocida*. These abscesses are well encapsulated, contain thick white exudate that does not drain, and enlarge slowly. Mandibular abscesses and infections of the hock joints are common. Genital tract infections occur in both males and females; pyometra is common. Occasionally wound infections caused by *P. multocida* result in cellulitis rather than an abscess. Cellulitis is more difficult to treat than an abscess, and antibiotic sensitivity testing becomes even more important.

Abscesses in rabbits tend to appear similar regardless of cause, and not all are caused by *P. multocida.* For example, I have cultured the following organisms in pure culture from abscesses that appeared as described: *Pseudomonas aeruginosa* and *Peptococcus* species from mandibular abscesses, *Staphylococcus aureus* from a pericardial abscess, and *Enterococcus* species from a joint abscess. It is important to document the bacterial pathogen and antibiotic sensitivity and not to assume that the cause is *P. multocida.*

Bordetella bronchiseptica

B. bronchiseptica is a common inhabitant of the respiratory tract of rabbits. The prevalence of infection increases with age, and both nares and bronchi become colonized. There is an inverse relationship between *B. bronchiseptica* and *P. multocida* in rabbitries: weanlings have higher rates of infection with *B. bronchiseptica,* whereas *P. multocida* usually predominates in adults.[12] Experimentally, intranasal inoculation of *B. bronchiseptica* caused serous nasal discharge, bronchopneumonia, and pleuritis in suckling or weanling rabbits.[17] Sinusitis and bronchopneumonia due to *B. bronchiseptica* resulted when local host defense was reduced.[4]

B. bronchiseptica is pathogenic in guinea pigs, dogs, cats, and pigs. It adheres to ciliated mucosa, resists respiratory clearance, induces ciliostasis, and reduces macrophage adherence and phagocytosis.[38] Cytotoxic *B. bronchiseptica* enhances colonization by toxigenic *P. multocida.*[16] Therefore *B. bronchiseptica* is suspected as a copathogen or predisposing factor in *P. multocida* infections. More pathogenic strains of *B. bronchiseptica* may exist. For example, an investigation of upper respiratory tract infections in rabbits from a colony of inbred rabbits showed them free of *P. multocida;* however, the nares were colonized by *B. bronchiseptica,* which was resistant to several commonly used antibiotics (B. J. Deeb and R. DiGiacomo, unpublished data). Clinically, I have seen numerous cases of rhinitis associated with pure cultures of *B. bronchiseptica.* In such cases, selective antibiotic therapy for *B. bronchiseptica* is indicated.

Staphylococcus aureus

S. aureus is often isolated from the nares of both healthy and diseased rabbits. It is probably a secondary agent that increases suppurative inflammation of compromised mucosa. As with *P. multocida* infection, pathogenicity depends on host susceptibility and bacterial virulence. *S. aureus* produces toxins that are lethal for rabbit neutrophils as well as protein A, which binds the crystallizable fragment (Fc) of IgG. By these means, bactericidal mechanisms of the host are blocked.[8]

Disseminated staphylococcosis results in fibrinous pneumonia or abscesses in the lungs or heart. Abscesses caused by *S. aureus* appear similar to those caused by *P. multocida,* but *S. aureus* more often shows in vitro resistance to a variety of antibiotics than does *P. multocida.* Therefore a culture and sensitivity test is advisable if the abscess is in an accessible area. Chloramphenicol, enrofloxacin, and trimethoprim-sulfa combinations are antibiotics of choice for rabbits when a culture specimen cannot be obtained.

Pasteurella Species

Pasteurella species other than *P. multocida* are often cultured from nasal swab samples of rabbits. Unless the organism is present in pure culture and is associated with clinical disease, it is probably a commensal organism rather than a pathogen.

Moraxella catarrhalis

Moraxella catarrhalis, previously known as *Micrococcus, Neisseria,* or *Branhamella catarrhalis,* is a well-represented member of the nasal flora of rabbits. Like *B. bronchiseptica,* it is sometimes isolated from rabbits with rhinitis or conjunctivitis. If isolated in pure culture, the organism may have a role in the disease, probably as an opportunist on unhealthy mucosa. However, unless clinical disease is present, antibiotic therapy is not justified to eliminate *M. catarrhalis* from the nares.

Other Bacteria

Other bacterial agents that have caused pneumonia in rabbits are *Mycobacterium bovis, Mycobacterium tuberculosis, Francisella tularensis, Yersinia pestis, Moraxella bovis, E. coli,* and *P. aeruginosa.* Tularemia is rare in domestic rabbits. *P. aeruginosa* can cause abscesses similar to those of *P. multocida,* as well as septicemia and pneumonia.

Cilia-associated respiratory (CAR) bacillus colonizes ciliated epithelial cells of the respiratory tract and causes chronic respiratory disease in rodents. Although it occurs in rabbits, CAR bacillus induces only mild hyperplasia of ciliated epithelium and inflammatory infiltration.[9,20]

Mycoplasma/Chlamydia

In 1967, I isolated *Mycoplasma pulmonis* from the nasopharynx of rabbits with signs of upper respiratory tract disease. Specimens from the rabbits were not cultured for *P. multocida.* The rabbits were housed in close proximity to rats, which may have been the source of the infection. *M. pulmonis* causes chronic respiratory disease in rats, but the pathogenicity of *M. pulmonis* in rabbits has not been investigated. Isolation of *Mycoplasma* species requires special media and methods and precludes routine examination for these organisms. In 1986, I attempted to isolate *Mycoplasma* species from the nasopharynx and lungs of 52 rabbits from four commercial rabbitries where respiratory disease was endemic. *Mycoplasma* species were not recovered (unpublished data).

Chlamydia species have been isolated from the lungs of domestic rabbits with pneumonia. A mild interstitial pneumonia occurred when the agent was inoculated into the trachea of laboratory rabbits.

Viruses

Viral agents of respiratory disease in rabbits are not well studied; they may be insignificant as pathogens in the respiratory tract, or they may be underreported.[14]

Myxoma virus causes nasal and ocular discharge and dyspnea in protracted cases. However, respiratory disease is not a hallmark of myxomatosis and is not likely to occur in the absence of generalized disease, edema, and tumors. Myxoma virus causes acute hemorrhagic pneumonia.[23]

A herpesvirus has been recovered from the nares of European rabbits with respiratory disease.[14] Rabbits have also developed antibodies to Sendai virus, a paramyxovirus that causes respiratory disease in rodents. However, experimental inoculation did not induce disease in rabbits.

A coronavirus has been implicated in association with pleural effusion and infectious cardiomyopathy.[14] The disease occurred in the 1960s in Scandinavia in rabbits used to propagate *Treponema pallidum*. Because no cases of the disease outside the laboratory environment have been reported, the agent may have been a contaminant of suspensions of testicular cells infected with *T. pallidum*. The target organ of the viral agent was the heart. Clinical signs were those typical of acute viremia and, in survivors, of myocarditis and congestive heart failure.

NONINFECTIOUS CAUSES

Immunologic Causes

Rhinitis, conjunctivitis, and chronic bronchitis resulting from exposure to allergens occur in rabbits. If the allergen cannot be identified and eliminated from the rabbit's environment, corticosteroids or antihistamines are used to reduce and control inflammation. Pasteurellosis or infections with other pathogenic agents must be ruled out. Prolonged use of corticosteroids in rabbits with chronic *P. multocida* infection is contraindicated.

Neoplastic Disease

Carcinoma of the nasal turbinates causes disruption of the normal architecture of the upper air passageways. Sneezing and nasal discharge accompany the disease, which is usually unresponsive to antibiotics.

Thymomas are often seen in both young and adult rabbits (see Chapter 21). These tumors can be of either lymphoid or epithelial origin. Clinical signs include tachypnea and moderate to severe dyspnea. Bilateral exophthalmos is occasionally observed[36] and may be related to interference of vascular return to the heart caused by the mass. Radiographs reveal a rounded, soft tissue opacity cranial to the heart, dorsal tracheal deviation, and caudal displacement of lungs (Fig. 17-5). Removal of a thymoma via median sternotomy has been accomplished.[7]

Metastases may reach the lungs from tumors in other sites in the body (Fig. 17-6). The rabbit becomes increasingly dyspneic with time. Antibiotics and bronchodilators may help relieve respiratory distress caused by neoplasia, but only temporarily.

Cardiovascular Disease

Pulmonary edema, the accumulation of fluid in the interstitial tissue, alveoli, and bronchi, occurs in conjunction with circulatory disorders. Pulmonary edema in rabbits may be fairly common. Cardiomyopathy and arteriosclerosis are often diagnosed in pet rabbits because their life span is extended (more than 10 years is common). Differentiation from infectious processes involves auscultation of the lungs for typical wheezing sounds, radiographic evaluation, ultrasonography, and hematologic testing. If heart murmurs or arrhythmias are detected, an electrocardiogram or echocardiogram is indicated (see Chapter 21). Treat cardiovascular disease with diuretics, bronchodilators, enalapril, and/or digoxin as indicated.

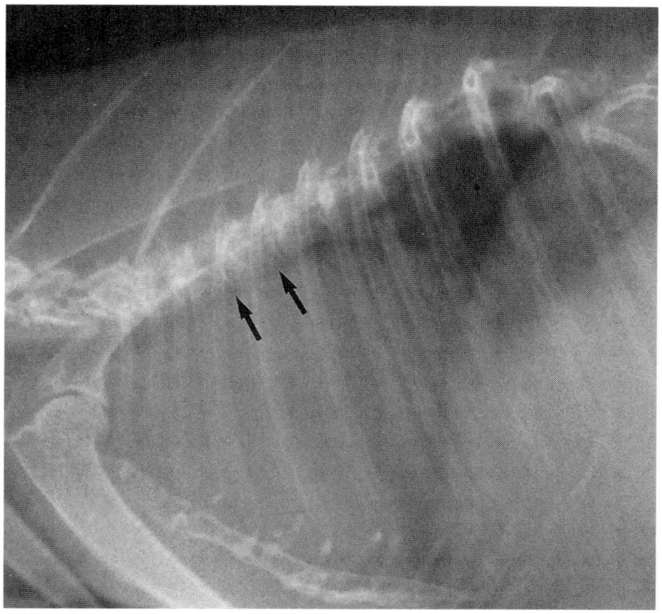

Figure 17-5 Thoracic radiograph from a rabbit with respiratory distress and bilateral exophthalmos, which became pronounced when the rabbit was stressed. A cranial mediastinal mass has caused dorsal tracheal deviation *(arrows)* and border effacement of the cardiac silhouette. The histopathologic diagnosis was thymoma.

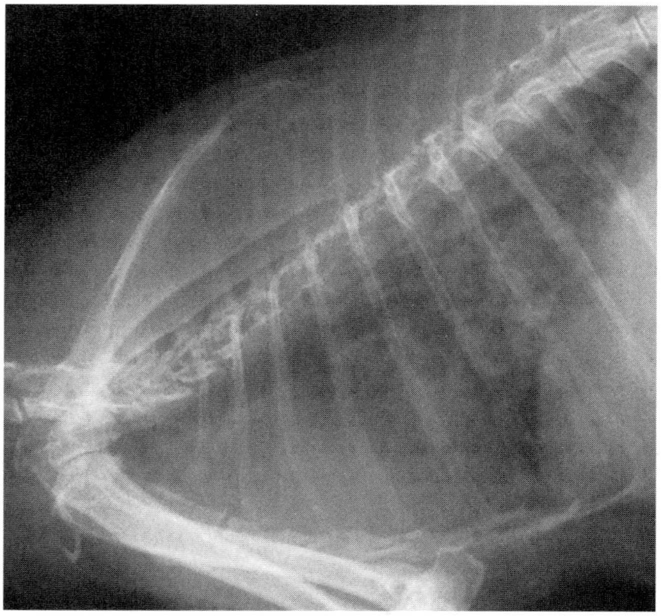

Figure 17-6 Lateral radiograph of the thorax of a rabbit with respiratory distress. Diffuse pulmonary densities resulted from carcinoma metastases.

Traumatic Causes

Traumatic tracheitis may result from endotracheal intubation for inhalant anesthesia. Rabbits maintained for 3 to 4 hours on halothane developed severe necrotizing tracheitis, submucosal edema, and mucosal erosion where the tip of a Sheridan cuffed endotracheal tube touched the trachea. Use a soft, pliable silicone endotracheal tube or face mask when administering gas anesthesia to rabbits.

Irritation to the respiratory tract occurs with aerogenous exposure to chemicals, such as excessive ammonia from urine buildup, cigarette smoke, and possibly vapors from wood shavings used for litter. Such exposure may predispose the mucosa to infection.

Foreign materials can accidentally gain entry to the nares, pharynx, or trachea (Fig. 17-7). Severe upper respiratory tract rales and respiratory distress result. Open-mouth breathing in a rabbit indicates an emergency, sometimes necessitating oxygen therapy and an immediate attempt to find and remove the airway obstruction. Although rabbits do not normally vomit, postmortem examination in my laboratory has confirmed several cases of food aspiration, probably caused by regurgitation.

DIAGNOSIS AND DIFFERENTIATION

Physical Examination

Examine the rabbit's general appearance; look for evidence of nasal discharge, matted forepaws, and dyspnea; note the color of the mucous membranes. Auscultate the heart and lungs, and listen for nasal and pharyngeal sounds. Determine the origin of respiratory rales and whether they are heard primarily on inspiration or expiration. Absence of lung sounds or very loud heart sounds, or both, may indicate replacement of normal lung tissue with abscesses or neoplasia. Heart murmurs or arrhythmias may be detected on auscultation. Bradycardia may be more indicative of cardiomyopathy than tachycardia in a frightened rabbit (normal heart rate is 180 to 220 beats/min).

Although rhinitis, conjunctivitis, or respiratory distress in rabbits is suggestive of pasteurellosis, a causative diagnosis cannot be made on the basis of clinical signs alone.

Hematologic evaluation is recommended, but hematologic values are not always indicative of infection. Neutrophilia or a shift in the normal neutrophil : lymphocyte ratio (about 2 : 3) is suggestive of bacterial infection. Abnormal biochemical values help detect organ failure.

Table 17-1 outlines the differentiation of respiratory disease in rabbits.

Isolation of Bacteria

Isolation of the causative agent from affected tissues requires culture before the use of antibiotics. Once antimicrobial therapy has been initiated, bacteria may be attenuated, if not eliminated, and difficult to grow in vitro. To determine whether a bacterial pathogen is present in the nares, in the case of rhinitis or in screening for *P. multocida*, insert a No. 4 calcium alginate swab 1 to 4 cm into the nares along the nasal septum on both sides (nasal infection may be unilateral). The nasopharynx may be a better site to recover a pathogen, but it is less accessible. A bacterial agent causing rhinitis is likely to be present in almost pure culture from the nares. There is no need to do multiple sensitivity tests on normal nasal flora in a mixed culture.

For various reasons, *P. multocida* is sometimes difficult to recover, and more than one attempt should be made before ruling it out. To maximize success, the swab of the affected tissue should be inoculated directly or within a short period onto a blood agar plate. If the specimen must be transported to a laboratory, Cary-Blair transport medium is recommended. Incubate the culture for at least 48 hours for the best visualization of the slowly growing *P. multocida* colonies. Some strains grow better in 5% carbon dioxide, and some grow better at 93.2°-95.0°F (34° to 35°C), a temperature range that approximates that in rabbit nares. When collecting a swab sample from an abscess for culture, insert the swab against the inner wall of the capsule, because the centers of abscesses are often sterile. Abscesses in rabbits, especially those associated with infected tooth roots, are sometimes caused by anaerobic bacteria, which will not grow on blood agar plates incubated with oxygen.

Serodiagnosis of *Pasteurella multocida*

Because rabbits infected with *P. multocida* develop antibodies but usually remain infected, serologic testing is helpful in detecting internal infections or subclinical carriers. Enzyme-linked immunosorbent assays (ELISAs) have been developed to detect immunoglobulins against *P. multocida*.[26] ELISAs are reliable in

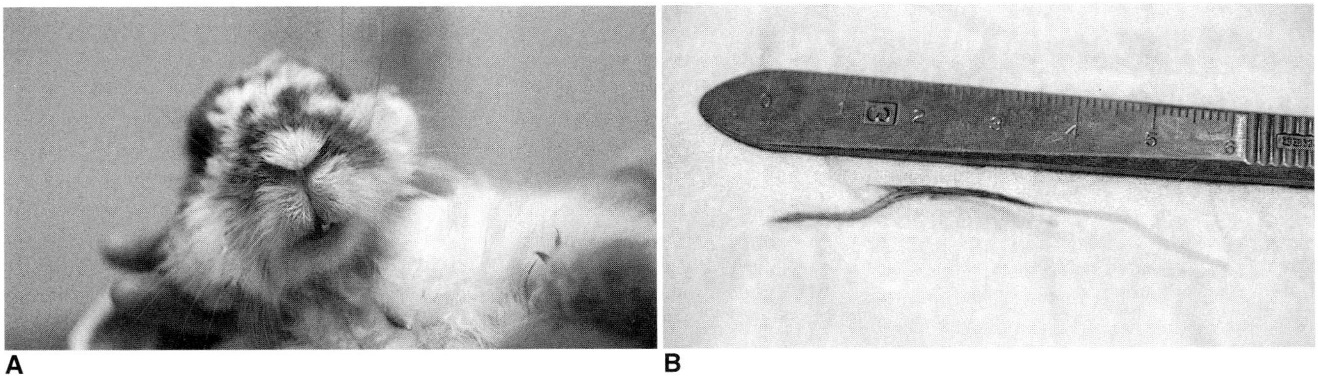

A B

Figure 17-7 A, Upper respiratory tract disease and mouth-breathing in a 6-year-old Holland lop. B, A piece of hay was recovered from the nares 3 weeks after signs appeared.

TABLE 17-1
Differentiation of Respiratory Disease in Rabbits

Procedure/Findings	Diagnosis
Physical examination	
Sneezing, snoring	URT involvement
Nasal discharge	URT involvement
Matted fur on face and forepaws	URT involvement
Fever or normal temperature	URT involvement
Anorexia, weight loss	LRT involvement
Depression, fatigue	LRT involvement
Dyspnea	LRT involvement
Mucous membranes pale or cyanotic	LRT involvement
Fever or hypothermia	LRT involvement
Auscultation	
Nasopharyngeal rales, pulmonary sounds normal	Rhinitis/sinusitis
Pulmonary rales	Bronchopneumonia
Friction sounds	Pleuritis
Absence of sounds	Thoracic mass or masses
Fluid sounds	Pulmonary edema
Loud heart sounds	Thoracic mass/ cardiomegaly
Radiography	
Increased opacity in nasal turbinates/sinuses	Infection
Bronchial pattern	Bronchitis
Effusion line	Pleuritis, neoplasia
Masses (mediastinal or pulmonary), tracheal elevation	Abscess/neoplasia
Generalized increase in pulmonary opacity	Edema
Cardiomegaly	Cardiomyopathy
Lysis of turbinates/bone	Neoplasia/infection
Interstitial pattern	Pneumonia
Other tests	
Culture from nares	—
CBC, serologic testing for *Pasteurella multocida*	—
Guided needle aspiration/cytology	—
Electrocardiogram	—

CBC, Complete blood count; *LRT,* lower respiratory tract; *URT,* upper respiratory tract.

screening for *P. multocida* infection in rabbits[37] (Table 17-2), but the practitioner must understand the limitations of these tests and not misinterpret results. High levels of antibody to *P. multocida* correlate well with chronic infection. The test does not detect antibody very early in infection, because it takes 2 to 3 weeks for the titer to rise substantially. Antibody in a rabbit younger than 8 weeks of age is probably maternally acquired. Sera with antibodies to related bacteria, possibly normal flora, react at low levels in the test, giving false-positive results. Immunosuppression results in decreased antibody and possibly false-negative results. If a serum sample is reactive at a low level, testing of a second sample about 3 weeks later helps in determining whether the antibody level is increasing (early infection), decreasing (maternal antibody or infection eliminated), or remaining about the same (probably because of infection with related bacteria that are not necessarily pathogenic). The ideal test would be one that detects antibody to an antigenic epitope that is unique to *P. multicoda,*[39] present in all strains, and associated with protective antibodies.[21] A 37-kDa antigen was shown to be a major immunogen during *P. multocida* infection in rabbits. Monoclonal antibody against this antigen, used in a capture enzyme immunoassay, was shown to be sensitive and specific in identifying rabbits infected with *P. multocida.*[25]

Imaging

Radiographs of the head are useful in providing information about the nares, sinuses, and middle ears. Careful dorsoventral positioning is necessary for accurate interpretation of radiographs. Comparison with radiographs of the normal respiratory tract is helpful (Fig. 17-8). Increased density in tympanic bullae, nares, or sinuses indicates infection (see Fig. 17-2). Decreased density occurs in advanced infection if atrophic rhinitis and sinusitis exists or if bone lysis has occurred because of nasal carcinoma.

Thoracic radiography helps differentiate pneumonia, cardiovascular disease, and neoplasia. In bronchitis, thickened bronchial walls appear as "doughnuts" when viewed on end. An interstitial or alveolar pattern of increased density occurs with pneumonia (see Fig. 17-3). Cardiomegaly and a generalized increase in pulmonary opacity can be observed in cardiac disease. A mediastinal mass or multiple pulmonary nodules are indicative of neoplasia but could be confused with abscesses (see Figs. 17-4 and 17-6). Ultrasonography offers the advantage of guided needle biopsy of lesions. Thoracocentesis and cytology are indicated if pleural fluids are apparent.

TREATMENT

Identification of the bacterial agent associated with respiratory disease is important but not always possible. Do not assume *P. multocida* is the cause. Other bacterial agents are more likely to have antibiotic resistances.

Studies for determining the effectiveness of various antibiotics in treating *P. multocida* infection usually have involved rabbits with chronic disease. Results of these studies have shown diminution or cessation of clinical signs during treatment for 7 to 14 days but recurrence after treatment was discontinued, as well as a failure to eliminate infection. Infection was eliminated in seven of eight rabbits treated with enrofloxacin (5 mg/kg SC q12h) for 14 days.[5] Enrofloxacin given in the drinking water (50-100 mg/L) before and continuing for 48 hours after inoculation with a virulent strain of *P. multocida* protected rabbits against bacteremia, provided that daily intake of the drug was greater than 5 mg/kg. Kits from enrofloxacin-treated does were free from *P. multocida* infection, although the infection was not eliminated in the does.[34] Ciprofloxacin (20 mg/kg PO q24h) for 5 days

Table 17-2
Antibodies Against *Pasteurella multocida* in Pet Rabbits*

	Interpretation of Optical Density Readings							
	Negative		Suspicious/Equivocal		Positive		Total	
Age (yr)	*n*	URD	*n*	URD	*n*	URD	*n*	URD
<1	44	19	64	16	251	51	359	86
≥1	408	77	309	51	625	98	1342	176
Total (% with URD)	452	96 (21)	373	67 (18)	876	99 (11)	1701	262 (15)

n, Number tested; *URD,* number with nasal and/or ocular discharge (upper respiratory tract disease).
*As determined by an enzyme-linked immunosorbent assay. Data were collected over a 5-year period on sera submitted by veterinarians in the United States; includes only samples for which clinical signs were listed. Tests were performed by Sound Diagnostics, Inc., 1222 NE 145th, Shoreline, WA 98155.

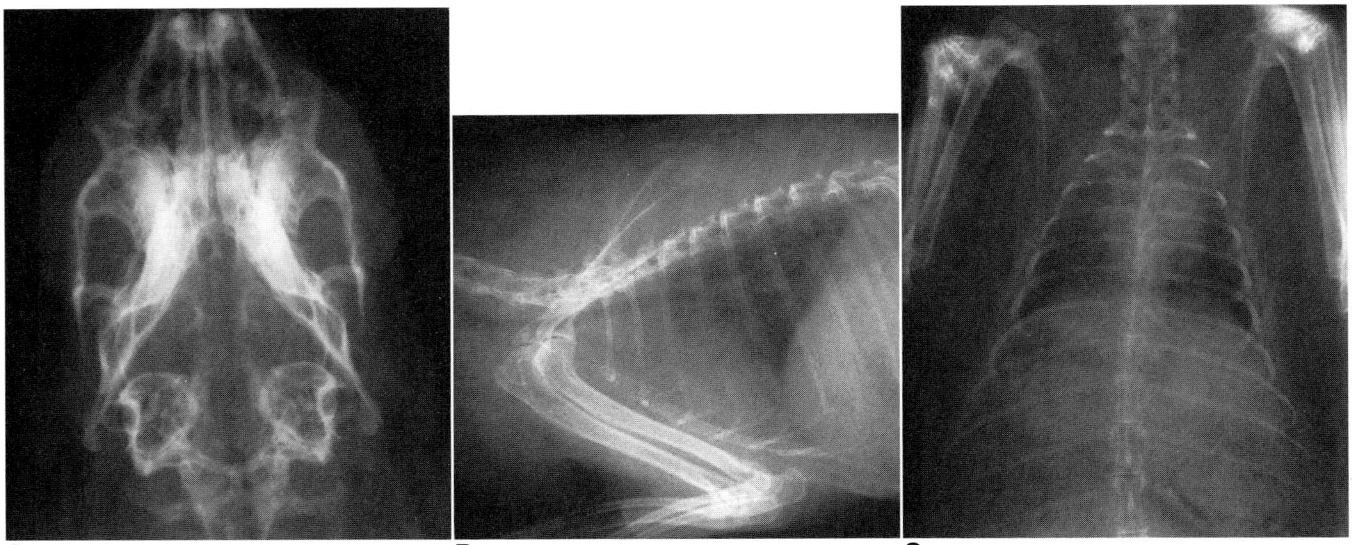

Figure 17-8 Radiographs of a normal 7-year-old rabbit. **A,** Dorsoventral view of the head showing normal turbinates, sinuses, and tympanic bullae. **B,** Lateral view of the thorax showing normal heart and lungs. **C,** Dorsoventral view of the thorax.

eliminated *P. multocida* infection in diseased rabbits.[18] High tissue concentrations of ciprofloxacin were found in kidney, lung, liver, spleen, and muscle. Penicillin (24,000 U/kg) penetrated easily and remained at high levels in the pleural space of rabbits with empyema caused by *P. multocida.*[35] I have had success with some acute pasteurellosis cases and mandibular abscesses using penicillin G benzathine/penicillin G procaine (40,000 IU/kg SC q24h × 2 weeks, then q48h × 2 weeks or longer), and with chronic cases of pasteurellosis using enrofloxacin (5-10 mg/kg PO q12h) or chloramphenicol (50 mg/kg PO q12h) for extended periods (2-3 months). Signs of disease were eliminated and antibody titers diminished. Some owners are willing to use antibiotics in the long term to improve the health and extend the lives of their pets. Adjunct therapy includes instillation of antibiotic drops such as ciprofloxacin ophthalmic drops or gentamicin ophthalmic drops into nares, ear canals, or conjunctival sacs or nebulization with antibiotics. If indicated, lacrimal ducts should be flushed and abscesses surgically removed or lanced and debrided.

Choose an antibiotic based not only on in vitro sensitivity test results but also on the sensitivity of the rabbit's intestinal flora. Enteric dysbiosis can result in fatal enterocolitis or enterotoxemia. Antimicrobial drugs that are less likely to cause this side effect are trimethoprim-sulfa, the fluoroquinolones, chloramphenicol, and tetracyclines. Penicillin given parenterally is less likely to cause dysbiosis than if given orally, and it is the antibiotic of choice for anaerobic infections. The use of any antimicrobial agent in rabbits warrants monitoring. In the event of anorexia, diarrhea, or excretion of abnormal feces, discontinue use of the antibiotic and select a different drug.

CONTROL

Pasteurella-free rabbit colonies were first established by Webster. Webster's methods are still used today and are referred to as "barrier housing."[22] *Pasteurella*-free rabbits are selected by bacteriologic and serologic screening and housed away from

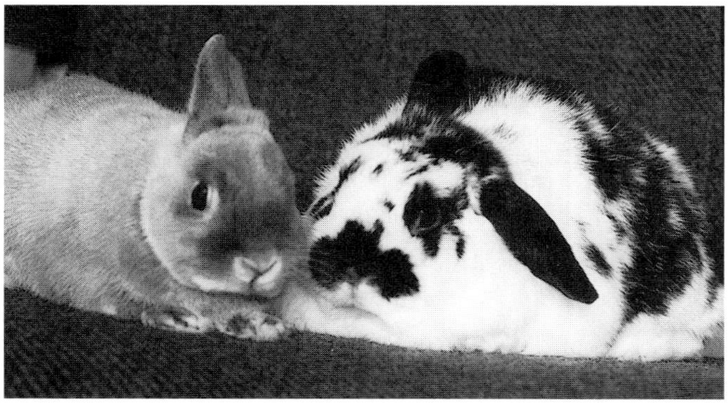

Figure 17-9 This 9-year-old Netherland dwarf lived with chronic but controlled pasteurellosis for years. Its mini-lop companion remained free of pasteurellosis and died when 9 years old from a pulmonary carcinoma.

rabbits of unknown or infected status. Traffic of materials and caretakers from infected to uninfected rabbits is prevented. Cesarean derivation and fostering of kits onto *Pasteurella*-free does is another method of establishing a *Pasteurella*-free colony. Early weaning, with or without the use of antimicrobial drugs for infected does, can yield *Pasteurella*-free weanlings.

Rabbits available at pet stores are not likely to be from *Pasteurella*-free colonies. A rabbit recently acquired from a pet store should be examined, tested for *P. multocida* infection, and, if infected, treated with antibiotics. Elimination of infection may be easier in young rabbits, before disease becomes chronic. If rhinitis is severe and exudate is being expelled by sneezing, isolate the affected animal from other rabbits and ensure that infectious exudate is not spread by fomites. Transmission from rabbits with chronic pasteurellosis is less common than from those acutely affected. Some infected rabbits have lived in relatively close contact with uninfected rabbits and have not transmitted the organism (Fig. 17-9). Germicidal agents that are effective against *P. multocida* include a 10% solution of sodium hypochlorite 5.25%, 1 oz/gal of 2% chlorhexidine diacetate, and 2 mL/gal of 20% benzalkonium chloride; 70% alcohol is not effective. Controlling the spread of infection in the host depends on proper diet, avoidance of stress or changes in ambient temperature, and good husbandry practices, including good ventilation, as well as treatment with antibiotics.

The principles of controlling pasteurellosis also apply to controlling other bacterial infections. In homes where many rabbits reside, new rabbits should be quarantined until their disease status is known. Those with chronic infections can be housed together and cared for after those without disease have received care.

REFERENCES

1. Adler B, Balach D, Chung J, et al: Candidate vaccine antigens and genes in *Pasteurella multocida*. J Biotechnol 1999; 73:83-90.
2. Al-Haddawi MH, Jasni S, Zamri-Saad M, et al: In vitro study of *Pasteurella multocida* adhesion to trachea, lung and aorta of rabbits. Vet J 2000; 159:274-281.
3. Al-Haddawi MH, Jasni S, Zamri-Saad M, et al: Ultrastructural observation of nasal and pulmonary intracellular *Pasteurella multocida* A:3 in rabbits. Vet Res Commun 2000; 24:153-167.
4. Berglof A, Norlander T, Feinstein R, et al: Association of bronchopneumonia with sinusitis due to *Bordetella bronchiseptica* in an experimental rabbit model. Am J Rhinol 2000; 24:225-232.
5. Broome RL, Brooks DL: Efficacy of enrofloxacin in the treatment of respiratory pasteurellosis in rabbits. Lab Anim Sci 1991; 41:572-576.
6. Chrisp CE, Foged NT: Induction of pneumonia in rabbits by use of a purified protein toxin from *Pasteurella multocida*. Am J Vet Res 1991; 52:56-61.
7. Clippinger TL, Bennett RA, Alleman AR, et al: Removal of a thymoma via median sternotomy in a rabbit with recurrent appendicular neurofibrosarcoma. J Am Vet Med Assoc 1998; 213:1140-1143.
8. Cohen JO: *Staphylococcus*. *In* Baron S, ed. Medical Microbiology. New York, Churchill Livingstone, 1991, pp 203-214.
9. Cundiff DD, Besch-Williford CL, Hook RR, et al: Characterization of cilia-associated respiratory bacillus isolates from rats and rabbits. Lab Anim Sci 1994; 44:305-312.
10. Dabo SM, Confer AW, Lu YS: Single primer polymerase chain reaction fingerprinting for *Pasteurella multocida* isolates from laboratory rabbits. Am J Vet Res 2000; 61:305-309.
11. Dabo SM, Confer AW, Montelongo M, et al: Characterization of rabbit *Pasteurella multocida* isolates by use of whole-cell, outer-membrane, and polymerase chain reaction typing. Lab Anim Sci 1999; 49:551-559.
12. Deeb BJ, DiGiacomo RF, Bernard BL, et al: *Pasteurella multocida* and *Bordetella bronchiseptica* infections in rabbits. J Clin Microbiol 1990; 28:70-75.
13. DeLong D, Manning PJ, Gunther R, et al: Colonization of rabbits by *Pasteurella multocida*: serum IgG responses following intranasal challenge with serologically distinct isolates. Lab Anim Sci 1992; 42:13-19.
14. DiGiacomo RF, Maré CJ: Viral diseases. *In* Manning PJ, Ringler DH, Newcomer CE, eds. The Biology of the Laboratory Rabbit, 2nd ed. San Diego, Academic Press, 1994, pp 171-204.
15. DiGiacomo RF, Deeb BJ, Brodie SJ, et al: Toxin production by *Pasteurella multocida* isolated from rabbits with atrophic rhinitis. Am J Vet Res 1993; 54:1280-1286.
16. Dugal F, Bélanger M, Jacques M: Enhanced adherence of *Pasteurella multocida* to porcine tracheal rings preinfected with *Bordetella bronchiseptica*. Can J Vet Res 1992; 56:260-264.
17. Glavits R, Magyar T: The pathology of experimental respiratory infection with *Pasteurella multocida* and *Bordetella bronchiseptica* in rabbits. Acta Vet Hung 1990; 38:211-215.
18. Hanan MS, Riad EM, el-Khouly NA: Antibacterial efficacy and pharmacokinetic studies of ciprofloxacin on *Pasteurella multocida* infected rabbits. Dtsch Tierarztl Wochenschr 2000; 107:151-155
19. Jarvinen LZ, Hogenesch H, Suckow MA, et al: Induction of protective immunity in rabbits by coadministration of inactivated *Pasteurella multocida* toxin and potassium thiocyanate extract. Infect Immunol 1998; 66:3788-3795.
20. Kurisu K, Kyo S, Shiomoto Y, et al: Cilia-associated respiratory bacillus infection in rabbits. Lab Anim Sci 1990; 40:413-415.
21. Lu YS, Lai WC, Pakes SP, et al: A monoclonal antibody against a *Pasteurella multocida* outer membrane protein protects rabbits and mice against pasteurellosis. Infect Immunol 1991; 59:172-180.
22. Manning PJ, DiGiacomo RF, DeLong D: Pasteurellosis in laboratory animals. *In* Adlam C, Rutter JM, eds. *Pasteurella* and Pasteurellosis. London, Academic Press, 1989, pp 263-302.
23. Marlier D, Mainil J, Linde A, et al: Infectious agents associated with rabbit pneumonia: isolation of amyxomatous myxoma virus strains. Vet J 2000; 159:171-178.

24. Okerman L, Spanoghe L, DeBruycker RM: Experimental infections of mice with *Pasteurella multocida* strains isolated from rabbits. J Comp Pathol 1979; 89:51-55.
25. Peterson RR, Deeb BJ, DiGiacomo RF: Detection of antibodies to *Pasteurella multocida* by capture enzyme immunoassay using a monoclonal antibody against P37 antigen. J Clin Microbiol 1997; 35:208-212.
26. Rimler RB, Rhoades KR: *Pasteurella multocida. In* Adlam C, Rutter JM, eds. *Pasteurella* and Pasteurellosis. London, Academic Press, 1989, pp 37-73.
27. Ruble RP, Cullor JS, Brooks DL: Evaluation of commercially available *Escherichia coli* J5 bacterin as protection against experimental challenge with *Pasteurella multocida* in rabbits. Am J Vet Res 1999; 60:853-859.
28. Ruble RP, Cullor JS, Brooks DL: Seroprevalence of antibodies against gram-negative core antigens in rabbits, using an *Escherichia coli* J5 antigen-capture enzyme-linked immunosorbent assay. Am J Vet Res 1999; 60:501-506.
29. Ruble RP, Cullor JS, Brooks DL: The observation of reactive thrombocytosis in New Zealand white rabbits in response to experimental *Pasteurella multocida* infection. Blood Cells Mol Dis 1999; 25:95-102.
30. Ruffolo CG, Adler B: Cloning sequencing, expression and protective capacity of the oma87 gene encoding the *Pasteurella multocida* 87-kilodalton outer membrane antigen. Infect Immunol 1996; 64:3161-3167.
31. Suckow MA, Bowersock RL, Neilsen K, et al: Protective immunity to *Pasteurella multocida* heat-labile toxin by intranasal immunization in rabbits. Lab Anim Sci 1995; 45:526-532.
32. Suckow MA, Bowersock TL, Nielsen K, et al: Enhancement of respiratory immunity to *Pasteurella multocida* by cholera toxin in rabbits. Lab Anim 1996; 30:120-126.
33. Suckow MA, Bowersock TL, Park H, et al: Oral immunization of rabbits against *Pasteurella multocida* with alginate microsphere delivery system. J Biomater Sci Polym Ed 1996; 8:131-139.
34. Suckow MA, Martin BJ, Bowersock TL, et al: Derivation of *Pasteurella multocida*-free rabbit litters by enrofloxacin treatment. Vet Microbiol 1996; 50:161-168.
35. Teixeira LR, Sasse SA, Villarino MA, et al: Antibiotic levels in empyemic pleural fluid. Chest 2000; 117:1734-1739.
36. Vernau KM, Grahn BH, Clarke-Scott HA, et al: Thymoma in a geriatric rabbit with hypercalcemia and periodic exophthalmos. J Am Vet Med Assoc 1995; 206:820-822.
37. Zaoutis TE, Reinhard GR, Cioffe CJ, et al: Screening rabbit colonies for antibodies to *Pasteurella multocida* by an ELISA. Lab Anim Sci 1991; 41:419-422.
38. Zeligs BJ, Zeligs JD, Bellanti JA: Functional and ultrastructural changes in alveolar macrophages from rabbits colonized with *Bordetella bronchiseptica*. Infect Immunol 1986; 53:702-706.
39. Zimmerman TE, Deeb BJ, DiGiacomo RF: Polypeptides associated with *Pasteurella multocida* infection in rabbits. Am J Vet Res 1992; 53:1108-1112.

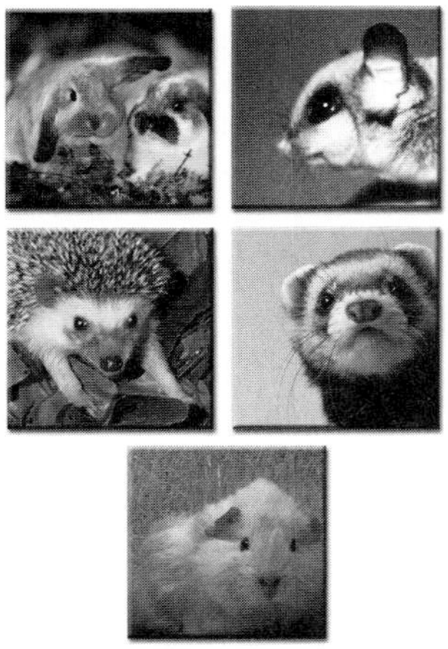

CHAPTER 18

Disorders of the Reproductive and Urinary Systems

Jean A. Paré, DMV, DVSc, Diplomate ACZM, and
Joanne Paul-Murphy, DVM, Diplomate ACZM

DISORDERS OF THE REPRODUCTIVE SYSTEM

Rabbit does are prolific breeders. They reach sexual maturity by 4 to 6 months of age, are induced ovulators, and have serial estrous cycles that last 7 to 14 days until conception. A mildly swollen and congested vulva often accompanies receptivity and should not be mistaken for a vulvitis or vaginitis. Bucks are precocious and may attempt to breed as early as 3.5 to 4 months of age. Spraying is a normal sexual behavior of intact bucks, and sometimes of does, and should not be confused with inappropriate elimination due to urinary tract infection or inflammation. Disorders of the reproductive tract in female pet rabbits are seen less commonly than previously because educated owners typically elect to have their rabbits spayed to prevent uterine disease. Fewer than 6% of all rabbits presented to the University of Wisconsin are diagnosed with reproductive disorders. However, older intact females need to be carefully and regularly monitored for reproductive tract disease, especially neoplasia. Careful abdominal palpation allows for detection of ovarian or uterine enlargement. Any perceived abnormality should be investigated fully and aggressively.

Uterine Adenocarcinoma

Uterine adenocarcinoma is the most common neoplasia of female rabbits.[52] Age is the most important factor in the development of adenocarcinoma, and occurrence is independent of breeding history. Rabbits of certain breeds (tan, French silver, Havana, and Dutch) that are older than 4 years of age have an incidence of 50% to 80%.[2,26,52] With age, the endometrium undergoes progressive changes, a decrease in cellularity, and an increase in collagen content. These changes are associated with the development of uterine cancer.[2] Adenocarcinoma of the uterus is a slowly developing tumor. Local invasion of the myometrium occurs early and may extend through the uterine wall to adjacent structures in the peritoneal cavity; hematogenous metastasis to the lungs, liver, and sometimes brain and bones may occur within 1 to 2 years.[52]

Early clinical signs, such as decreased fertility, small litter size, and an increased incidence of fetal retention or resorption and stillbirths may be recognized in a breeding doe. The first signs observed in many pet rabbits are hematuria or a serosanguineous vaginal discharge. Frank blood in the urine is most pronounced at the end of urination. Cystic mammary glands can develop concurrently with uterine hyperplasia or adenocarcinoma.[22,32] Clinical signs of late-stage adenocarcinoma include depression, anorexia, and dyspnea if pulmonary metastasis has occurred. Ascites may be present. The diagnosis relies on palpation of an enlarged uterus or uterine nodular masses (1 to 5 cm in diameter), or both, in the caudal abdomen. Adenocarcinomas are often multicentric, involving both uterine horns[2,52] (Fig. 18–1). Other causes of uterine enlargement include pregnancy, pyometra, metritis, hydrometra or mucometra, endometrial venous aneurysms, endometrial hyperplasia, and other tumors such as leiomyosarcoma.

Radiography and ultrasound imaging assist in establishing the diagnosis when a caudal abdominal soft tissue mass or uterine enlargement can be identified. Imaging may further allow you to differentiate between potential causes of uterine enlargement, to measure masses, or to scan for multiple nodules. Perform thoracic radiographs to screen for the presence of pulmonary metastasis. Pulmonary involvement carries a grave prognosis. If abdominal masses are identified in the early stages of disease before metastasis occurs, surgical excision with ovariohysterectomy is the treatment of choice. Ovariohysterectomy is curative if the tumor is contained within the uterus. Metastatic disease or local invasion of peritoneal structures may not be macroscopically apparent at laparotomy, and a guarded prognosis is always warranted. Reexamine the rabbit every 3 months for a period of 1 to 2 years after surgery for evidence of abdominal or pulmonary metastases. Successful chemotherapy for this tumor has not been reported.

Prevention is the key to management of this disease. Client education begins at the time of the initial visit for routine health evaluation of the patient. Many veterinarians recommend ovariohysterectomy for pet rabbits before they reach 2 years of age. We prefer to spay rabbits between the ages of 6 and 12 months, because they have less abdominal fat than older rabbits do. Alternatively, thoroughly discuss early clinical signs of the disease with the client and recommend annual or, preferably, semiannual health examinations for intact female rabbits 3 years of age and older.

Endometrial Hyperplasia or Uterine Polyps

Endometrial changes may occur along a continuum—from polyp formation, to cystic hyperplasia, to adenomatous hyperplasia, to adenocarcinoma—as it does in humans.[15,26,32] Uterine hyperplasia is associated with aging, as are cystic and hyperplastic changes in endometrial glands. Other reports, however, have found no association between cystic hyperplasia and uterine adenocarcinoma in rabbits, because adenocarcinomas are associated with senile atrophy of the endometrium.[2]

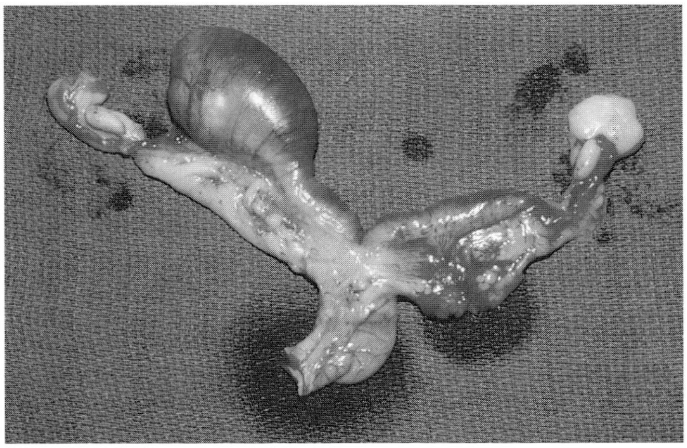

Figure 18-1 Adenocarcinoma of the uterus is often multicentric and involvs both uterine horns.

Clinical signs of endometrial hyperplasia can mimic those associated with uterine adenocarcinoma and include intermittent hematuria, anemia, and a decrease in activity. A firm, irregular uterus sometimes can be detected by palpation. Cystic mammary glands and cystic ovaries can occur concurrently with this condition.[22,32] Radiography and ultrasonography help in the diagnosis of uterine changes. Ovariohysterectomy is the recommended treatment, and a thorough exploration of the abdomen is warranted.

Pyometra and Endometritis

Vaginal discharge, anorexia, lethargy, weakness, and an enlarged abdomen are clinical signs that frequently accompany endometritis or pyometra. Clinical signs of mild endometritis can be subtle, making the condition difficult to diagnose. Rabbits with chronic disease may have no overt clinical signs. The history of a breeding doe often includes a recent parturition, pseudocyesis, or an inability to rebreed. Rabbits with mild endometritis may kindle successfully or have fetal resorptions and stillbirths. Pyometra and endometritis can also develop in nulliparous does. Diagnosis relies on palpation of a doughy and enlarged uterus, best demonstrated radiographically. If the uterus is greatly enlarged, use caution when palpating the abdomen, because the uterine wall becomes very thin and may be friable. Ultrasound imaging can rule out other uterine conditions such as polyps, masses, or cystic changes. Results of a complete blood count may be normal or may show a slight leukocytosis with a heterophilia. Evaluate serum or plasma biochemical values, because chronic inflammation of the uterus has been reported to induce amyloid deposition in the kidneys.[24] Cytologic assessment and a Gram stain of cervical mucus or drainage can assist diagnosis.

Exploratory laparotomy and ovariohysterectomy are the procedures of choice to confirm the diagnosis. Uterine vessels may be engorged and prominent. Multiple adhesions to adjacent viscera often complicate the procedure. Before surgery, obtain a guarded deep vaginal or cervical swab for bacterial culture and sensitivity testing, or take an intraoperative sample for culture. Begin broad-spectrum antibiotic therapy as soon as a sample for culture has been collected. Intravenous fluids are an important component of therapy.

Pasteurella multocida and *Staphylococcus aureus* are frequently isolated from rabbits with pyometra or metritis. Venereal transmission occurs when infected does breed with uninfected bucks, or vice versa. *P. multocida* can localize in the genital tract by hematogenous spread from another location, or a retrograde infection can occur as a result of vaginitis.[12] Ovarian abscesses may occur concurrently with *P. multocida* pyometra.[27] Rare cases of naturally occurring metritis or pyometra have been associated with *Chlamydia* (*Chlamydophila*), *Listeria monocytogenes*, *S. aureus*, *Moraxella bovis*, *Actinomyces pyogenes*, *Brucella melitensis*, and *Salmonella* species.[23,39,47,51] Postpartum metritis can occur in conjunction with hypervitaminosis A, and the delivery of stillborn young and metritis have been associated with uterine torsion.[23]

For a breeding rabbit with mild endometritis, appropriate antibiotic and fluid therapy may be sufficient, but the tenacious and caseous nature of inflammatory exudates in rabbits makes it extremely difficult to achieve adequate drainage of the uterus.

The use of prostaglandins to assist uterine contraction and drainage has not been reported. Ovariohysterectomy is the best choice for treatment of pyometra because of the high incidence of *P. multocida* infections.

Pregnancy Toxemia

Pregnancy toxemia usually occurs during the last week of gestation, when nest-building behavior begins. The exact causes leading to metabolic disturbances and pregnancy toxemia are unknown. It is more common in obese rabbits. Inadequate caloric intake predisposes pregnant rabbits to toxemia, and environmental changes or stress can precipitate the disease. Hair pulling for nesting can contribute to hairball formation and inappetence.[41] Weakness, depression, incoordination, anorexia, abortion, convulsions, and coma are common clinical signs. Signs can progress over 1 to 5 days, or death may occur acutely. Some rabbits are dyspneic, and their breath may have an acetone-like odor. The urine becomes acidic and clear, because the lower pH decreases the concentration of calcium carbonate crystals. Clinical findings that support the diagnosis include acidic urine (pH 5-6), proteinuria, ketonuria, hyperkalemia, ketonemia, hyperphosphatemia, and hypocalcemia. Hepatic lipidosis is a common finding at necropsy.

There is no consistently effective treatment for pregnancy toxemia. Keep the animal warm and administer intravenous or intraosseous fluids. Calcium gluconate and corticosteroids may be helpful if the doe is in shock. In rabbits with trichobezoars, administer metoclopramide or cisapride and oral fluids. Once the rabbit's condition is stabilized, nutritional support must be provided, either by syringe feeding or by a nasogastric or percutaneous endoscopic gastrostomy tube. Pregnancy toxemia carries a very grave prognosis, and treatment is usually unrewarding. The best approach is prevention. Avoid fasting or undernutrition in late pregnancy, and prevent obesity and sudden stress at all times.

Pseudopregnancy

Pseudopregnancy (pseudocyesis, false pregnancy) can occur in rabbits, even in pet does kept singly. Pseudopregnancy typically lasts 16 to 17 days and may be followed by hair pulling and nesting behavior.[40] Mammary development is most pronounced in the first 10 days of false pregnancy, after which involution typically follows.[40] The condition resolves spontaneously but may recur or may lead to hydrometra or pyometra. Ovariohysterectomy is the treatment of choice and ideally would be performed once the mammary tissue has involuted. Hormonal therapy with either progestins or androgens is of unproved effectiveness and should be considered only in rare cases in which does undergo protracted or refractory pseudopregnancy.

Dystocia or Retained Fetuses

Gestation in rabbits averages 31 to 32 days but may be as short as 28 or as long as 36 days. Dystocia is unusual in rabbits, and normal delivery is usually complete within 30 minutes after onset. Rarely, the young are delivered several hours apart. Litter size ranges from 4 to 12 kits. Anterior and breech positions are normal for rabbits. Palpate does 24 hours after delivery to determine whether any fetuses have been retained. A rabbit may be predisposed to dystocia by obesity, large fetuses, a small pelvic canal, or uterine inertia. Signs of dystocia include persistent contractions, straining, and bloody or greenish-brown vaginal discharge. Radiographs may disclose abnormalities in the fetuses or in the width of the pelvic canal. Assistance usually requires gentle manual removal of the fetuses and rapid removal of fetal membranes from them. Oxytocin (1-3 units IM) can assist uterine contraction. If uterine inertia is suspected, give 5 to 10 mL of 10% calcium gluconate orally 30 minutes before administering the oxytocin. Place the doe in a quiet, dark room for 30 to 60 minutes after administration. Cesarean section is indicated if there is no response to the injection of oxytocin, and the prognosis is guarded.

Extrauterine Pregnancy

Extrauterine pregnancy sometimes occurs in does.[1,3,4] Extrauterine implantation of fertilized ova, often on the parietal peritoneum, can lead to the development of near-term fetuses, with subsequent mummification.[4] Mummified fetuses were found free in the abdominal cavity of a healthy doe presented for a routine examination.[3] The uterus and ovaries appeared normal, and the rabbit made an uneventful recovery after surgical removal of the fetuses. Extrauterine pregnancy is usually subclinical in rabbits.[4] False extrauterine pregnancy refers to cases in which fetal implantation occurred in the uterus and fetuses were later expelled into the abdominal cavity as a result of a traumatic event.[4] One rabbit died with three partially mummified, full-sized fetuses free in the abdominal cavity.[1] On postmortem examination, one uterine horn showed evidence of a relatively recent tear. The doe had delivered three kits 3 weeks previously, suggesting that the uterine rupture had occurred at parturition. The possibility of primary extrauterine pregnancy or of false extrauterine pregnancy should be kept in mind when palpable fetuses are present in does that have not undergone timely parturition. Surgery is the treatment of choice.

Abortion and Resorption

Fetal death before 3 weeks of gestation typically resolves as resorption, whereas fetal death after 3 weeks results in abortion. A critical period in gravid does occurs at 3 weeks of gestation because of a temporary reduction in blood flow to the uterus and the changing size and shape of the fetuses. When abortion or fetal resorption is suspected, a thorough history is extremely important. Ask questions such as: Is this the first litter? Is there a prior history of abortion? Have any drugs been administered recently? Has there been a recent change in environment? Are other rabbits aborting? Always check the doe for remaining fetuses. Submit fetuses and placentas for culture and histopathologic examination. Possible causes of fetal resorption or abortion are numerous and include infection, stress, genetic predisposition, trauma, drug use, and dietary imbalances (e.g., deficiencies of vitamin E, vitamin A, and protein). *Listeria* has a predilection for the gravid uterus and should be considered in rabbits with late-term abortion.[51]

Reduced Fertility

One or more factors can contribute to reduction in fertility, including malnutrition (e.g., excess vitamin A, deficiencies of vitamins A, D, or E), heat stress, systemic illness, nitrate contamination of food or water, environmental disturbances, a decrease in daylight, endometrial carcinoma, metritis, or pyometra. Old age, sexual exhaustion, or breeding of rabbits that are too young are additional causes of infertility. Vitamin E deficiency causes myodystrophy, which can lead to abortions, stillbirths, and neonatal deaths. An increased level of creatine phosphokinase supports a diagnosis of hypovitaminosis E and indicates a need for diet supplementation.[39] Hypervitaminosis A can cause fetal resorptions, abortions, and stillbirths. A suppurative metritis may follow the delivery of dead fetuses.[13] Hypovitaminosis A can cause similar reproductive disorders, resulting in poor fertility and weak, hydrocephalic young. The National Research Council recommends vitamin A levels of 1160 IU/kg of diet for gestation, or approximately 20 mg/kg of body weight per day.[49]

Prolapsed Vagina

A prolapsed vagina manifests as a blood-covered mass of swollen and fragile tissue protruding from the vulva. The prolapse may be full of clotted blood. Affected rabbits are depressed or recumbent with an increased respiratory rate or are in shock with cold extremities. Pale mucous membranes or cyanotic ears and mucous membranes indicate severe shock. The hematocrit in such rabbits may be as low as 9%.[50] Treatment is directed at correcting hypovolemic shock and blood loss. Reduce the prolapse under anesthesia, or surgically amputate the tissue if it is necrotic. Prolapses start from the proximal circular part of the vaginal vault just distal to the urethral opening.[50]

Eight cases of vaginal prolapse were described in closely related rabbits during periods of increased sexual activity or receptivity, suggesting a genetic susceptibility.[50]

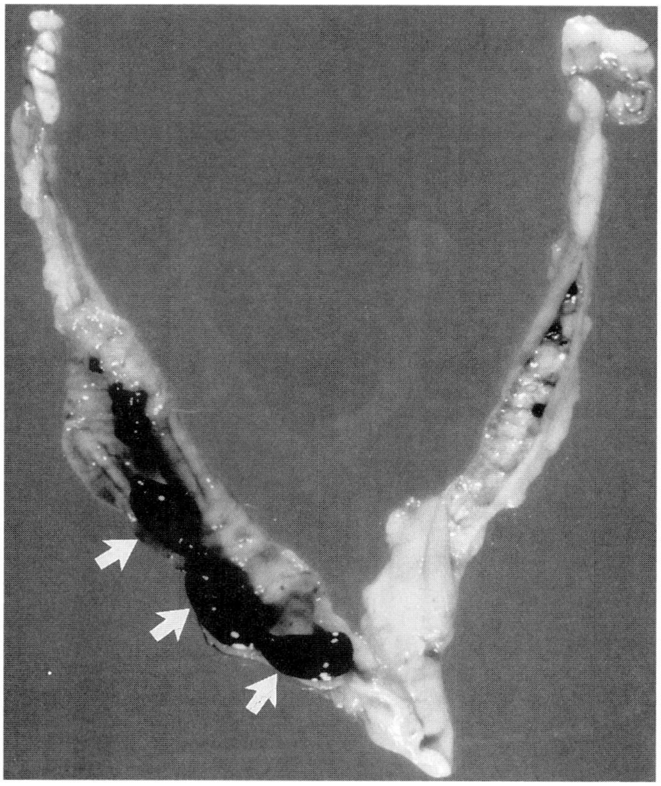

Figure 18-2 Endometrial venous aneurysms in a doe. Cylindrical blood clots *(arrows)* are present within the lumen of the uterine horns. *(Reproduced with the permission of Iowa State University Press.)*

Endometrial Venous Aneurysms

Multiple endometrial venous aneurysms can cause hematuria because of episodic bleeding in the lumen of the uterus. Cylindrical blood clots molded within the uterine horns are typically passed with the urine and are highly suggestive of this condition. Affected does are at high risk for fatal exsanguination from uterine hemorrhage, and ovariohysterectomy should be performed as soon as the animal is stabilized. Endometrial venous aneurysms occur in young does of larger breeds. The condition was reported in three New Zealand white rabbits and confirmed by exploratory laparotomy and histopathologic examination of the uterus.[6] In rabbits with this condition, the uterine horns have multiple, blood-filled endometrial varices (veins) that periodically rupture into the uterine lumen, causing the clinical hematuria (Fig. 18-2). Although the causes have not been elucidated, venous aneurysms in other species are related to congenital defects of the adventitia, increased intraluminal pressure, or trauma.[6]

Hydrometra

Hydrometra is the accumulation of watery fluid in the uterus. It has been described in four unbred sandy half-lop rabbits from the same research colony[37] and in New Zealand white rabbits.[23] Clinical signs include an enlarged, fluid-filled uterus, increased respiratory rate, anorexia, and weight loss. Transabdominal uterocentesis yields clear fluid with a low specific gravity, a low cell count, and a moderate amount of protein.[23] Diagnosis can be supported by radiography and ultrasonography. The rabbits in the published reports were all euthanatized or found dead, and no anatomic abnormalities could be correlated with this condition.[37] Ovariohysterectomy and supportive care are indicated if hydrometra is diagnosed in a pet rabbit.

Uterine Torsion

Torsion of the uterus is rare in rabbits but has been reported in association with pregnancy, hydrometra, or endometritis.[23] Clinical signs include shock, cachexia, and abdominal distention with hydrometra, or a bloody vaginal discharge with endometritis and torsion.[23] The cause of uterine torsion is difficult to identify, and the prognosis is grave. Ovariohysterectomy is the treatment of choice.

Cryptorchidism

In bucks, the testicles have usually descended by 12 weeks of age. Failure of one or both testicles to descend in the scrotal sac by 4 months of age is defined as unilateral or bilateral cryptorchidism. Rabbits, however, do have the ability to retract testicles intraabdominally. Cryptorchid rabbits retain their sexual drive, but fertility is impaired. In true cryptorchid bucks, the scrotal sac of the retained testicle does not develop. If the scrotal sac is present but the testicle cannot be palpated, it has most likely been retracted into the inguinal canal or the abdominal cavity. Neither the causes nor the medical implications of cryptorchidism for rabbits have been adequately investigated. Based on other species, it appears prudent to assume a hereditary pattern for cryptorchidism in at least some rabbits, as well as a potential for the development of testicular neoplasia in untreated affected animals. Cryptorchid rabbits should be castrated, using a standard midline abdominal approach.

Orchitis and Epididymitis

Clinical signs of orchitis include fever, intermittent appetite, and weight loss. The testicles may be enlarged with obvious abscesses, or abscesses may be small and internal, with minimal swelling of the testicles. The epididymis rather than the testis may be infected. An affected breeding buck has low conception rates. Treatment is castration and antibiotic therapy. *P. multocida* is often isolated from exudate or abscessed tissue on bacterial culture. Specific culture for *Treponema* species should also be requested. Male rabbits should be housed separately to prevent bite wounds to the testes or scrotum and other fighting injuries that lead to abscesses.

Testicular Neoplasms

Testicular tumors are rare in rabbits but include seminomas, interstitial cell tumors, Sertoli cell tumors, and teratomas.[38,52] A tentative diagnosis is typically based on palpation of an enlarged, firm or nodular, nonpainful testicle. A definitive diagnosis is achieved with surgical castration and submission of the affected testicle for histopathologic examination. Rarely, tumors are incidentally found on the cut section of an otherwise normal-looking testicle.[54]

Venereal Spirochetosis: *Treponema paraluiscuniculi*

Treponema paraluiscuniculi is the spirochete responsible for rabbit syphilis or vent disease. This is not a zoonotic disease. Transmission between rabbits is by direct and venereal contact. Bucks can spread the disease to several does, and young rabbits can be infected. It is a self-limiting disease, and carriers may be asymptomatic until stress occurs. Lesions first appear on the skin of the perineum and genitalia and begin as areas of redness that progress to edema, vesicle formation, ulcerations, and scabs. The lesions can be painful and can impair breeding activity. Autoinfection can lead to facial lesions around the chin, lips, nostrils, and eyelids. Inguinal lymph nodes may be enlarged. Colony epidemics result in a decreased rate of conception and an increased incidence of metritis, placenta retention, and neonatal deaths.

Clinical signs and distribution of lesions are often diagnostic. Few other skin problems resemble those of rabbit syphilis, but dermatitis, dermatophytosis, acariasis, and myxomatosis are possibilities. Lesions on the nose and lips are often proliferative and scaly and are commonly mistaken for dermatophyte lesions. For a definitive diagnosis, submit a skin biopsy sample and request silver staining. Examine skin scrapings of the lesions by darkfield microscopy to identify the organism. Large rabbitries can benefit from a serologic survey with the microhemagglutination test to screen and verify infected animals. Other serologic tests are available, such as the rapid plasma reagin card test, which is very specific.[14] In rabbitries, the prevalence of *T. paraluiscuniculi* infection increases with parity: often females that have had six or more litters are seropositive, and bucks that have been in a breeding program for 6 to 12 months are also seropositive.[14] Bucks are often asymptomatic carriers and may have small, star-shaped scars on their scrotum.

Rabbits with venereal spirocthetosis are effectively treated with parenteral (never oral) penicillin. Administer penicillin G benzathine–penicillin G procaine at 42,000 to 84,000 IU/kg SC at 7-day intervals for 3 injections,[11] or penicillin G procaine at 40,000 to 60,000 IU/kg IM q24h for 5 to 7 days. Tetracyclines and chloramphenicol can also be effective. Treat all exposed rabbits.

DISORDERS OF THE MAMMARY GLAND

Does usually possess 8 but may have up to 12 mammary glands.[40] Disorders of the mammary glands are mainly inflammatory, infectious, hormonal, or neoplastic and are often accompanied by ovarian or uterine abnormalities, or both.[4]

Septic Mastitis

Mastitis can occur in a lactating doe or in a rabbit in pseudocyesis. Abscesses can develop in the mammary gland independent of lactation. Heavy lactation, poor sanitation, abrasive bedding or caging, or injury to the gland or teat predisposes the doe to mammary infection. Mastitis may occur in conjunction with metritis. Clinical signs may include depression, fever, anorexia, polydipsia, septicemia, and death of the doe or the young. The mammary glands are firm, hot, and swollen, and the skin is discolored red to dark blue. Infection can begin in one gland and spread to other glands. The initial discharge may not be purulent. *Streptococcus* species, *Staphylococcus aureus*, and *Pasteurella* species are most frequently isolated. Suckling kits may die of peracute septicemia, particularly with *S. aureus* mastitis.

Submit samples of exudate or express the gland to obtain samples for bacterial culture. Choose systemic antibiotic therapy based on the results of culture and sensitivity testing. Common antibiotic choices are enrofloxacin or a trimethoprim-sulfa combination. Supportive care includes fluid therapy, application of hot packs, and drainage of abscesses. Surgical excision may be necessary for severe infections. Consider analgesia with buprenorphine if the animal experiences pain. Force-feeding may be necessary if the doe is anorexic. Remove bunnies but do not foster them onto another doe; this is known to transmit infection. Disinfect the environment.

Cystic Mastitis, Mammary Dysplasia, and Mammary Tumors

Noninfectious cystic mastitis occurs in both breeding and nonbreeding does. The affected glands can be are swollen and firm, and a clear to serosanguineous discharge can be expressed from the distended nipples. The glands do not seem painful, and the doe is not depressed. Epithelial hyperplasia, adenosis, papillomatous changes, and cystic mammary glands have been associated with uterine hyperplasia and adenocarcinoma.[22,52] Cystic mammary glands may continue to progress and coalesce, with fibrous connective tissue accumulating around the cysts.[52] Eventually, malignant cellular changes may occur, leading to invasive mammary adenocarcinoma. Metastasis to the regional lymph nodes, lungs, or other organs can occur with adenocarcinoma. Mammary adenocarcinomas are not uncommon in 3- to 4-year-old multiparous does.

Evaluate rabbits with clinical signs of cystic mastitis for infectious mastitis and uterine disease. Fine-needle aspiration and cytology will assist the diagnosis of mammary masses. The treatment for noninfectious cystic mastitis is ovariohysterectomy; clinical signs usually resolve within 3 to 4 weeks after surgery. Partial mastectomy or wide excision of mammary tumors is indicated if malignant changes have occurred. The correlation between mammary and uterine disorders suggests that routine ovariohysterectomy of young, healthy does may reduce the risk of mammary neoplasms at a later age.

Several cases of mammary dysplasia, associated with pituitary adenomas, have been described in older, primiparous New Zealand white rabbits.[43] One or more mammary glands were swollen and firm, with enlarged and discolored teats. Histologically, changes were dysplastic in nature. At necropsy, prolactin-producing acidophil pituitary adenomas were found in affected does.[43]

DISORDERS OF THE URINARY SYSTEM

Disorders of the urinary tract are relatively common in rabbits. Ten percent of pet rabbits presented to the University of Wisconsin over the last 5 years were diagnosed with urinary tract disease. Polyuria and/or polydipsia, incontinence, inappropriate elimination behavior, perineal urine scalding, hematuria, stranguria, and pollakiuria are common presenting complaints. Physical examination and careful abdominal palpation may reveal abnormalities in size, contour, and texture of the kidneys, and uroliths can often be detected within the urinary bladder. Results of a complete blood count and biochemical profile may disclose changes consistent with early or advanced renal insufficiency. Urine voided onto a clean surface may yield useful information, but ideally urine should be collected by cystocentesis, taking care to avoid the voluminous intestinal tract. Gentle manual pressure to the bladder often leads to micturition, and a midstream urine sample can be collected. Urinalysis is useful in assessing renal function and the presence of bacteria, proteinuria, glucosuria, ketonuria, and occult hematuria.

Urolithiasis and Hypercalciuria

Urolithiasis refers to the presence of calculi in the urinary system. Rabbits can have any combination of cystic, urethral, renal, and ureteral calculi (Fig. 18-3). The cause of urolithiasis in rabbits is not fully understood, but several factors are involved, including nutrition, anatomy, and, rarely, infection. Hypercalciuria is a clinical condition seen frequently in pet rabbits. Affected rabbits have a large amount of amorphous, pasty to slightly gritty, calcium "sand" or "sludge" in their bladder (Fig. 18-4). Rabbits have an unusual calcium metabolism in that intestinal absorption of calcium does not directly depend on vitamin D. Although the fractional urinary excretion of calcium is less than 2% in most mammals, the range for rabbits is 45% to 60%. Increases in dietary calcium directly increase the urinary excretion of calcium.[7,10]

Rabbits with either urolithiasis or hypercalciuria often have limited exercise, are fed a free-choice pellet and alfalfa hay diet, and tend to be obese. Frequently, the rabbits have a history of vitamin or mineral dietary supplementation. Clinical signs of urolithiasis include depression, anorexia, weight loss, lethargy, hematuria, anuria, stranguria, a hunched posture, grinding of teeth, and urine scald of the perineum. Urolithiasis in rabbits may also be subclinical. Rabbits with hypercalciuria usually have a thick, creamy urine. Often, voided urine appears only slightly turbid; however, with manual bladder expression, copious amounts of pasty urine are passed. Frequently, a doughlike mass

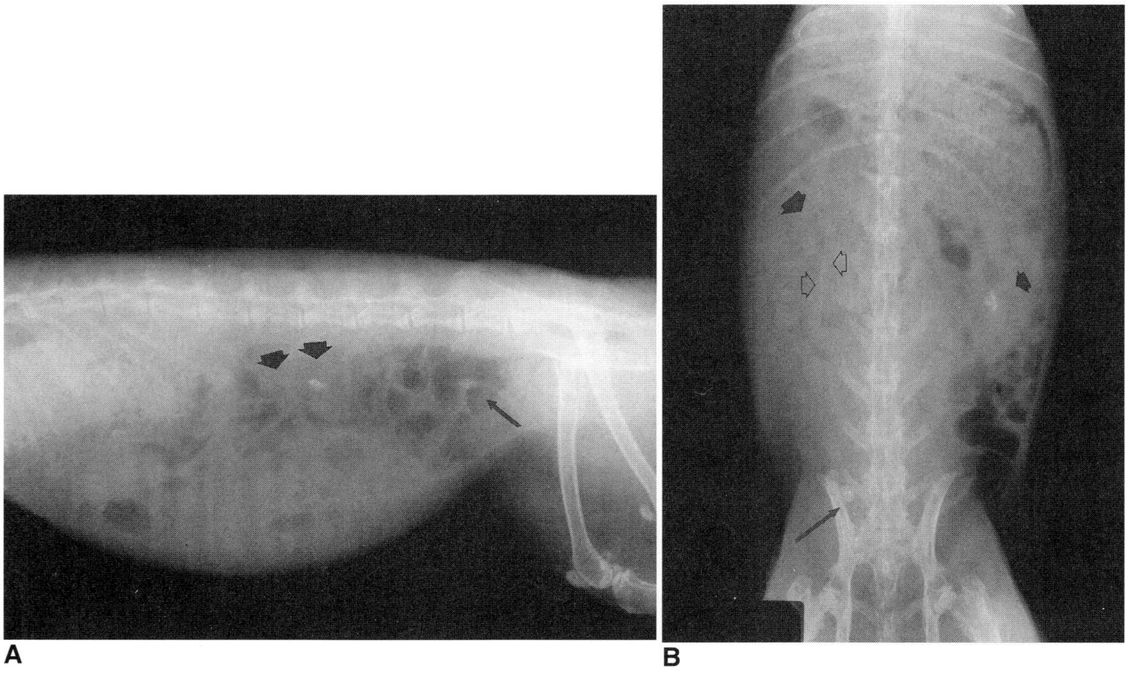

Figure 18-3 Right lateral (A) and ventrodorsal (B) radiographic views of a 6-year-old castrated male rabbit with bilateral nephroliths *(wide arrows)* and right ureteral uroliths *(thin arrows)*. Note the radiopaque sand outlining the right ureter, cranial to the ureteroliths *(open arrows)*.

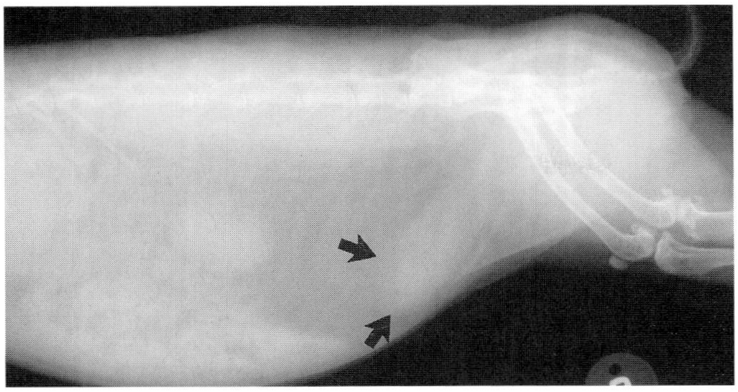

Figure 18-4 Right lateral radiographic view of a 4-year-old neutered male rabbit with a diffusely opaque urinary bladder filled with urinary sand *(arrows)*.

is palpated in the caudal abdomen, or a turgid bladder is evident if urethral obstruction is present. An enlarged kidney or ureter may be palpated if hydroureter or hydronephrosis has occurred (Fig. 18-5).[33] There is a report of a female rabbit with a large cystic calculus that became wedged in the pelvic inlet and indirectly obstructed the bowel.[48]

Confirm the diagnosis of urolithiasis radiographically. A discrete calculus or the presence of homogenous dense material can be seen in the dependent portion of the bladder or completely filling a distended bladder. A small amount of sand in the bladder is a common incidental radiographic finding, especially in older animals, because the presence of amorphous calcium carbonate crystals is normal in rabbits. Close inspection may be needed to identify stones in the kidneys, ureters, or urethra.

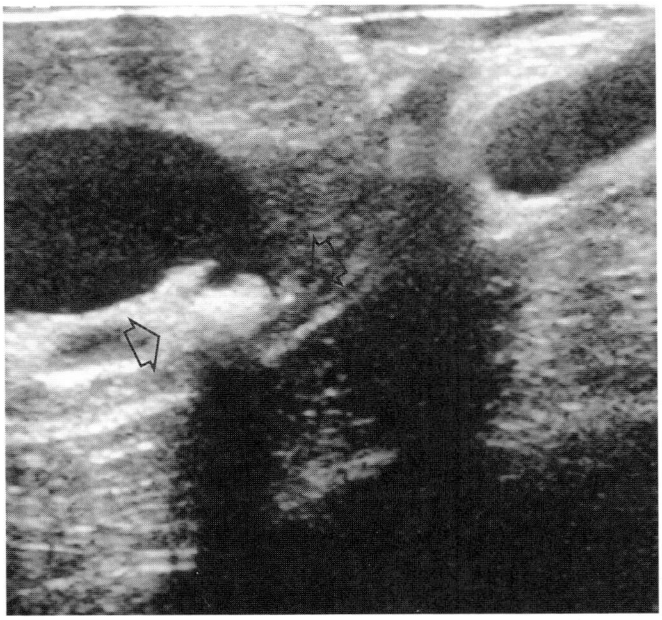

Figure 18-5 Ultrasound image of a rabbit showing marked hydronephrosis and hydroureter caused by uroliths in the distal ureter. Shadow-producing echoic structures, consistent with nephroliths, are present in the kidney *(arrows)*.

Perform ultrasound examination to detect the presence of discrete calculi in a bladder that is distended and diffusely opaque radiographically. Multiple renal cysts may be confused with hydronephrosis; use ultrasound examination to differentiate the two. If renal calculi are present, intravenous pyelography may be performed to evaluate renal function.

Obtain urine for analysis by cystocentesis or free catch. Analysis may reveal crystalluria; numerous calcium oxalate crystals are common, but ammonium phosphate, calcium carbonate, and monohydrate crystals are also frequently observed. Proteinuria and hematuria are common additional findings. If bacteria are identified, submit urine obtained by cystocentesis for culture. *Pseudomonas* species and *Escherichia coli* are bacteria known to cause cystitis. Results of a complete blood count and serum biochemical assay assist in assessing renal function and in developing a prognosis.

Treatment of urolithiasis depends on the location and severity of the lesion. Cystotomy is the treatment of choice for large cystic calculi. The procedure may be difficult because the neck of the bladder is flaccid and extends into the pelvic canal. Preanesthetic drugs such as benzodiazepines induce muscle relaxation and facilitate the passage of surprisingly large vesical calculi into the urethra (Fig. 18-6). The location of the calculus should, therefore, be ascertained immediately preoperatively. Attempts to force small stones out of the urethra during surgery may result in their becoming lodged within the neck of the bladder or in the proximal or distal urethra. Use a surgical spoon to retrieve small stones from the bladder. Flushing and gentle surgical suction can aid removal of fine granular material. Submit the calculi for analysis, and obtain a swabbed sample of the bladder wall for bacterial culture. Perioperative support includes intravenous fluid diuresis, analgesia, and systemic antibiotics. Subsequent radiographic monitoring is helpful because this condition often recurs.

Nephrectomy may be indicated if a calculus in the renal pelvis is causing obstruction and hydronephrosis. A pyelolithotomy or nephrotomy may be considered if function of the affected kidney is still adequate and renal parenchymal damage is minimal. Extracorporeal shock wave lithotripsy has been experimentally applied to rabbit kidneys, but no information is available on a clinical application.[30] Prognosis is guarded for rabbits with either unilateral or bilateral renal calculi.

If hypercalciuria or nonobstructive calculi in the kidney or ureter are identified, consider a nonsurgical approach. Fluids, administered either intravenously or subcutaneously, are necessary to increase the flushing action of the urinary tract. Manually express the bladder daily for 2 to 4 days to encourage the passage of crystals or residual calcium "sand" that may not be voided during normal micturition. A technique similar to voiding that is used in dogs and cats, termed urohydropropulsion,[36] can be used in rabbits for the nonsurgical removal of fine granular or small, smooth cystic calculi. Rabbits must be anesthetized for this procedure. Hold the rabbit in an upright position so that the vertebral column is vertical, and apply steady pressure to the bladder. Administer preanesthetic diazepam to help relax the urethralis muscle; we recommend using intraoperative butorphanol or buprenorphine, because bladder expression is painful. Hematuria is expected to occur for 1 to 2 days after urohydropropulsion.[36]

Dietary changes are an important part of treatment and prevention. The alkaline pH of rabbit urine and the high concen-

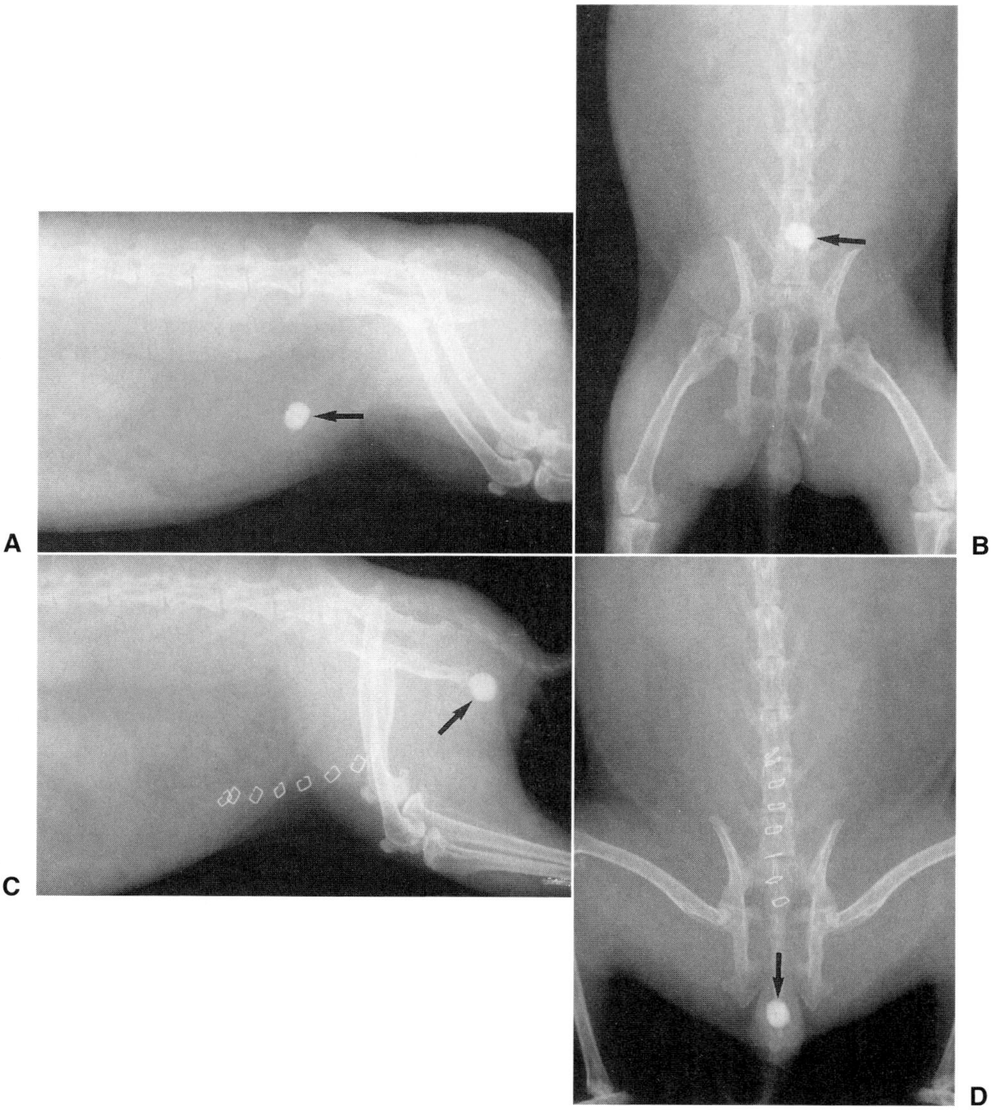

Figure 18-6 Preoperative right lateral (A) and ventrodorsal (B) radiographic views of a 4-year-old male Dutch rabbit, revealing a large radiopaque vesical calculus *(arrows)*. Cystotomy was unsuccessful, because the calculus *(arrows)* moved into the distal urethra (C and D), probably at the time of anesthetic induction. The calculus was removed by a perineal urethrostomy, and recovery was uneventful.

tration of calcium in the urine increase the risk of precipitation of solutes.[28] Decreasing dietary calcium levels directly lowers serum calcium concentration and the amount of calcium excreted in the urine.[10,29] To reduce calcium intake, give grass hay and green vegetables as the primary diet, and use timothy-based pellets. Discontinue any vitamin or mineral supplementation. One investigation determined that a level of 0.22 g of calcium per 100 g of food is necessary for maximal growth[9]; most commercial rabbit pellets contain 0.90 to 1.60 g of calcium per 100 g of food.[7] Consideration should be given to the hardness of drinking water, especially in polydipsic animals. Because many rabbits that develop urolithiasis are overweight, we recommend a decrease in total caloric intake and an increase in exercise. Acidifiers are not effective, because rabbits are herbivores with naturally alkaline urine. Oral potassium citrate may be useful in treating rabbits with calcium oxalate crystals because it reduces urinary calcium ion concentrations.

Renal Failure

Both acute and chronic renal failure can occur in older rabbits. Clinical signs include lethargy, depression, anorexia, polyuria, polydipsia, and perineal urine scalding. Serum creatinine and blood urea nitrogen levels are elevated, as are serum concentrations of calcium, phosphorus, and potassium. Urine specific gravity is isosthenuric. Other findings from urinalysis may include proteinuria, hematuria, pyuria, and cast formation. Submit a urine sample for bacterial culture to screen for infectious causes; blood cultures are indicated if clinical signs of septicemia are concurrent. Indicators of inflammation in the urine (pyuria, proteinuria, hematuria) occur more frequently with acute renal failure and nephritis than with chronic renal failure. Acute renal failure has a better potential for response to treatment, but the prognosis remains guarded. Pyelonephritis in rabbits is often caused by *P. multocida* or *Staphylococcus* species. *Encephalitozoon cuniculi* is a common cause of subclinical, chronic interstitial nephritis. Noninfectious causes of chronic renal disease include hypercalcemia,[20] renal calcinosis resulting from hypervitaminosis D and hypercalcemia,[45] mineralization of the kidneys with interstitial fibrosis caused by excessive presence of vitamin D in the diet,[53] and fatty degeneration in overweight animals. In rabbits with lymphosarcoma, renal involvement is common, often causing marked renomegaly and eventually resulting in renal failure from infiltrative destruction of the cortices.[52]

Treatment should be aimed at promoting diuresis and diminishing the consequences of uremia. Treatment is supportive in cases of chronic renal failure. Achieve diuresis with initial intravenous fluid administration in rabbits with acute or chronic renal failure; follow this with long-term subcutaneous fluid support in chronic renal failure. Antibiotics are indicated if infectious disease is suspected. The dietary changes discussed in the section on urolithiasis are indicated. Consider administering synthetic erythropoietin in rabbits with anemia secondary to chronic renal failure.

Nephrotoxicity

Several compounds are nephrotoxic in rabbits. Therapeutic use of gentamicin can result in acute tubular necrosis.[16,31] Administering fluids and supplemental doses (10 mg/kg SC) of vitamin B_6 during gentamicin therapy may help protect the kidneys.[16] The tiletamine in the tiletamine/zolazepam (Telazo; Fort Dodge Laboratories, Fort Dodge, IA) anesthetic combination is documented to cause nephrotoxicity in rabbits, inducing nephrosis at low doses and severe nonreversible nephrosis at high doses.[5,17]

Renal Cysts

The occurrence of multiple small, subcapsular cysts in the kidneys is an inherited condition of rabbits. The cysts are either of tubular origin or primitive ductules, and the condition is similar to renal cortical dysplasia in humans.[34] Although renal cysts do not create any clinical signs or alter results of renal function tests, they may be detected on ultrasound examination or at necropsy.

Renal Agenesis

Renal agenesis, or congenital absence of one kidney, has been reported as an autosomal recessive mutation in one colony of laboratory rabbits, and a high incidence of this condition has been reported in rabbits of the Havana breed.[34] The condition is seen in both genders. In males, the ipsilateral testicle is often missing as well.[34]

Encephalitozoonosis: *Encephalitozoon cuniculi*

Encephalitozoonosis, or nosematosis, is a common disease of rabbits caused by *E. cuniculi*, a microsporidian, obligate, intracellular protozoan parasite. Transmission is by urine-oral passage, usually from doe to young. The organism is absorbed from the intestines into mononuclear cells and then is distributed to other organs. Spores have a predilection for kidney and brain tissue, where the most common lesions are found (see Chapter 20). Spores appear in the kidney 31 days after inoculation and are excreted in the urine up to 3 months after inoculation.[42]

Infections typically result in nonsuppurative, granulomatous nephritis that may progress to interstitial fibrosis, but the disease is usually subclinical and chronic.[18] At necropsy, numerous small pits and stellate scars may be found on the cortical surface of the kidneys in rabbits with chronic encephalitozoonosis. Clinical signs of incontinence result from central nervous system infection rather than renal lesions. Diagnostic tests and therapeutic options for encephalitozoonosis are discussed in detail with diseases of the central nervous system (see Chapter 20).

Urinary Incontinence

Urinary incontinence can be caused by lumbosacral vertebral fractures or dislocations or by central nervous system lesions from *E. cuniculi* infection. Ovariohysterectomized rabbits can develop urinary incontinence that is responsive to diethylstilbestrol.[8] Rabbits with urinary calculi or hypercalciuria often exhibit urinary incontinence and urine scalding. Clinical signs include a urine-soiled perineum and ulcerations of the vaginal mucosa and intertrigonal pouches, as well as sticky, strong-smelling urine. A positive titer to *E. cuniculi* and additional central nervous system signs support a diagnosis of protozoal infection. Urolithiasis or hypercalciuria can be identified on radiographs. Vertebral fractures can be ruled out on thorough neurologic examination and radiography. A positive response to 0.5 mg of diethylstilbestrol given orally 1 to 2 times per week to spayed females suggests a hormone-responsive urinary incontinence similar to that seen in dogs. Additional differentials include ectopic ureter, urinary tract infection, neoplasia, and pyoderma. Initial supportive care includes daily cleaning of the perineum and topical treatment for dermatitis with a drying agent such as Domeboro astringent solution (Miles Inc., West Haven, CT), in addition to treatment of the primary problem. Older, obese, and/or arthritic rabbits may choose not to urinate in their litter box and appear suddenly "incontinent" to their owner.

Psychogenic Polyuria and Polydipsia

Normal daily water intake for a rabbit is 120 mL/kg or more, and urine output is approximately 130 mL/kg of body weight. Psychogenic polyuria and polydipsia were demonstrated in four laboratory New Zealand white rabbits by excluding other potential causes through a set of diagnostic tests.[44] The causes were not clearly identified, but in some affected rabbits, water consumption decreased after environmental enrichment measures, suggesting that boredom was a contributing factor.[44]

Urinary Bladder Eversion

Transurethral eversion and prolapse of the urinary bladder has been documented in postparturient does, shortly after kindling.[21] Multiple kindlings at a young age, along with other undetermined factors, may predispose to the occurrence of this condition.[21] Surgical reduction by laparotomy was successful in one Hotot doe.

Tumors of the Urinary Tract

Benign embryonal nephromas are common in rabbits of all ages and are usually incidental findings at necropsy. In one report, an extremely large, palpable embryonal nephroma caused obliteration of the kidney and polycythemia.[35] Lymphosarcoma in rabbits often involves the kidneys. Renal carcinoma and leiomyoma have also been reported.

Red Urine

Rabbits can excrete a porphyrin-pigmented urine that often incorrectly suggests hematuria. The urine may be dark brown, dark orange, or red. The unusual urine color is probably caused by a plant pigment and does not affect the rabbit's health. Pigmented urine tends to be intermittent and lasts only 3 to 4 days. It is speculated that dietary compounds, ingestion of pine needles, or antibiotic administration may cause increased pigment levels in rabbit urine. Porphyrin pigments, but not hemoglobin, fluoresce when urine is examined under a Wood's lamp.

True hematuria is determined on examination of a urine sediment and the finding of more than five red blood cells per high-power field; a positive reaction for blood with the use of a urine dipstick also indicates hematuria or hemoglobinuria. Hematuria can originate from the genital tract or from the urinary tract. Blood from the reproductive tract can be associated with adenocarcinoma, polyps, abortion, or endometrial venous aneurysms. Blood originating from the urinary tract can be the result of cystitis, bladder polyps, pyelonephritis, renal infarcts, urolithiasis, or disseminated intravascular coagulation.[19] Lead toxicosis can also cause hematuria, along with renal damage.[25] Blood clots in the urine most likely originate from the genital tract and are particularly suggestive of endometrial venous aneurysms. History, signalment, physical examination, laboratory tests, radiography, and ultrasound examination are helpful in determining the cause.

Hyperpigmented urine has also been associated with urobilinuria, which may appear similar to hematuria except that the test results are negative for blood and positive for urobilinogen.[19] There is one documented report of a New Zealand white rabbit with porphyria.[46] Porphyrias are diseases caused by impaired enzyme function in the heme biosynthesis pathway. No clinical signs were noted in the case reported, but necropsy findings included a pink tinge to the teeth, ultraviolet fluorescence of teeth and femur, and increased uroporphyrin levels in the urine.[46]

REFERENCES

1. Arvidsson A: Extra-uterine pregnancy in a rabbit. Vet Rec 1998; 142:176.
2. Baba N, von Haam E: Animal model for human disease: spontaneous adenocarcinoma in aged rabbits. Am J Pathol 1972; 68:653-656.
3. Beddow BA: Ectopic pregnancy in a rabbit. Vet Rec 1999; 144:624.
4. Bergdall VK, Dysko RC: Metabolic, traumatic, mycotic, and miscellaneous diseases. *In* Manning PJ, Ringler DH, Newcomer CE, eds. The Biology of the Laboratory Rabbit. New York, Academic Press, 1994, pp 335-353.
5. Brammer DW, Doerning BJ, Chrisp CF, et al: Anesthetic and nephrotoxic effects of Telazol in New Zealand white rabbits. Lab Anim Sci 1991; 41:432-435.
6. Bray MV, Weir EC, Brownstein DG, et al: Endometrial venous aneurysms in three New Zealand white rabbits. Lab Anim Sci 1992; 42:360-362.
7. Buss SL, Bourdeau JE: Calcium balance in laboratory rabbits. Miner Electrolyte Metab 1984; 10:127-132.
8. Caslow D: Hormone responsive perineal urine soiling in two female ovariohysterectomized rabbits. Comp Anim Pract 1989; 19:32-33.
9. Chapin RE, Smith SE: Calcium requirement of growing rabbits. J Anim Sci 1967; 26:67-71.
10. Cheeke PR, Amberg JW: Comparative calcium excretion by rats and rabbits. J Anim Sci 1973; 37:450-454.
11. Cunliffe-Beamer TL, Fox RR: Venereal spirochetosis of rabbits: eradication. Lab Anim Sci 1981; 31:379-381.
12. DeLong D, Manning PJ: Bacterial diseases. *In* Manning PJ, Ringler DH, Newcomer CE, eds. The Biology of the Laboratory Rabbit. New York, Academic Press, 1994, pp 131-170.
13. DiGiacomo RF, Deeb BJ, Anderson RJ: Hypervitaminosis A and reproductive disorders in rabbits. Lab Anim Sci 1992; 42:250-254.
14. DiGiacomo RF, Talburt CD, Lukehart SA, et al: *Treponema paraluis-cuniculi* infection in a commercial rabbitry: epidemiology and serodiagnosis. Lab Anim Sci 1983; 33:562-566.
15. Elsinghorst TA, Timmermans HJF, Hendriks HG: Comparative pathology of endometrial carcinoma. Vet Q 1984; 6:200-208.
16. Enriquez JI Sr, Schydlower M, O'Hair KC, et al: Effect of vitamin B_6 supplementation on gentamicin nephrotoxicity in rabbits. Vet Hum Toxicol 1992; 34:32-35.
17. Evans KD, Dillehay DL, Huerkamp MJ, et al: Diagnostic exercise: azotemia in a rabbit (*Oryctolagus cuniculus*). Lab Anim Sci 1996; 46:442-443.
18. Flatt RE, Jackson SJ: Renal nosematosis in young rabbits. Pathol Vet 1970; 7:492-497.
19. Garibaldi BA, Fox JG, Otto G, et al: Hematuria in rabbits. Lab Anim Sci 1987; 37:769-772.
20. Garibaldi BA, Pecquet-Goad ME: Hypercalcemia with secondary nephrolithiasis in a rabbit. Lab Anim Sci 1988; 38:331-333.
21. Greenacre CB, Allen SW, Ritchie BW: Urinary bladder eversion in rabbit does. Compend Contin Educ Pract Vet 1999; 21:524-528.
22. Hillyer EV: Pet rabbits. Vet Clin North Am Small Anim Pract 1994; 24:25-65.
23. Hobbs BA, Parker RF: Uterine torsion associated with either hydrometra or endometritis in two rabbits. Lab Anim Sci 1990; 40:535-536.
24. Hofmann JR, Hixson CJ: Amyloid A protein deposits in a rabbit with pyometra. J Am Vet Med Assoc 1986; 189:1155-1156.
25. Hood S, Kelly J, McBurney S, et al: Lead toxicosis in 2 dwarf rabbits. Can Vet J 1997; 38:721-722.
26. Ingalls TH, Adams WM, Lurie MB, et al: Natural history of adenocarcinoma of the uterus in the Phipps rabbit colony. J Natl Cancer Inst 1964; 33:799-806.
27. Johnson JH, Wolf AM: Ovarian abscesses and pyometra in a domestic rabbit. J Am Vet Med Assoc 1993; 203:667-672.
28. Kamphues J: Calcium metabolism of rabbits as an etiological factor for urolithiasis. J Nutr 1991; 121:S95-S96.
29. Kamphues VJ, Carstensen P, Schroeder D, et al: Effects of increasing calcium and vitamin D supply on calcium metabolism of rabbits. J Anim Physiol Anim Nutr 1986; 17:191-208.
30. Karalezli G, Gögüs O, Bedük Y, et al: Histopathologic effects of extracorporeal shock wave lithotripsy on rabbit kidney. Urol Res 1993; 21:67-70.
31. Kojima T, Kobayashi T, Iwase S, et al: Gentamicin nephrotoxicity in young rabbits. Exp Pathol 1984; 26:71-75.
32. Kraus AL, Weisbroth SH, Flatt RE, et al: Biology and disease of rabbits. *In* Fox JE, Cohen BJ, Loew FM, eds. Laboratory Animal Medicine. New York, Academic Press, 1984, pp 207-237.

33. Lee KJ, Johnson WD, Lang CM, et al: Hydronephrosis caused by urinary lithiasis in a New Zealand white rabbit (*Oryctolagus cuniculus*). Vet Pathol 1978; 15:676-678.
34. Lindsey JR, Fox RF: Inherited diseases and variations. *In* Manning PJ, Ringler DH, Newcomer CE, eds. The Biology of the Laboratory Rabbit. New York, Academic Press, 1994, pp 293-319.
35. Lipman NS, Murphy JC, Newcomer CE: Polycythemia in a New Zealand white rabbit with an embryonal nephroma. J Am Vet Med Assoc 1985; 187:1255-1256.
36. Lulich JP, Osborne CA, Carlson M, et al: Nonsurgical removal of urocystoliths in dogs and cats by voiding urohydropropulsion. J Am Vet Med Assoc 1993; 203:660-663.
37. Morrell M: Hydrometra in the rabbit. Vet Rec 1989; 125:325.
38. Ness RD: Neoplasia in rabbits and guinea pigs. Proceedings of the North American Veterinary Conference, 1998, pp 853-854.
39. Okerman L: Diseases of Domestic Rabbits, 2nd ed. London, Blackwell Scientific Publications, 1994.
40. Patton NM: Colony husbandry. *In* Manning PJ, Ringler DH, Newcomer CE, eds. The Biology of the Laboratory Rabbit. New York, Academic Press, 1994, pp 27-45.
41. Patton NM, Holmes HT, Cheeke PR: Hairballs and pregnancy toxemia. J Appl Rabbit Res 1983; 6:99.
42. Percy DH, Barthold SW: Pathology of Laboratory Rodents and Rabbits. Ames, IA, Iowa State University Press, 1993.
43. Percy DH, Barthold SW: Pathology of Laboratory Rodents and Rabbits, 2nd ed. Ames, IA, Iowa State Press University, 2001.
44. Potter MP, Borkowski GL: Apparent psychogenic polydipsia and secondary polyuria in laboratory housed New Zealand white rabbits. Contemp Topics 1998; 37:87-89.
45. Quimby F, Foote R, Profit-Olstad M, et al: Hypercalcemia, hypercalcitoninism, and arterial calcification in rabbits fed a diet containing excessive vitamin D and calcium. Lab Anim Sci 1982; 32:415.
46. Samman S, Fussell SH, Rose CI: Porphyria in a New Zealand white rabbit. Can Vet J 1991; 32:622-623.
47. Soave OA, Dominguez J, Doak RL: *Moraxella bovis*-induced metritis and septicemia in a rabbit. J Am Vet Med Assoc 1977; 1:972-973.
48. Talbot AC, Ireton VJ: Unusual cause of intestinal blockage in the female rabbit. Vet Rec 1975; 96:477.
49. The National Research Council: Nutrient Requirements of Domestic Animals: Nutrient Requirements of Rabbits, 2nd ed. Washington, DC, National Academy of Sciences, 1992.
50. Van Herck H, Hesp APM, Versluis A, et al: Prolapsus vaginae in the IIIVO/JU rabbit. Lab Anim 1989; 23:333-336.
51. Watson GL, Evans MG: Listeriosis in a rabbit. Vet Pathol 1985; 22:191-193.
52. Weisbroth SH: Neoplastic diseases. *In* Manning PJ, Ringler DH, Newcomer CE, eds. The Biology of the Laboratory Rabbit. New York, Academic Press, 1994, pp 259-292.
53. Zimmerman TE Jr, Giddens WE, DiGiacomo RF, et al: Soft tissue mineralization in rabbits fed a diet containing excess vitamin D. Lab Anim Sci 1990; 40:212-215.
54. Zwicker GM, Killinger JM: Interstitial cell tumors in a young adult New Zealand white rabbit. Toxicol Pathol 1985; 13:232-235.

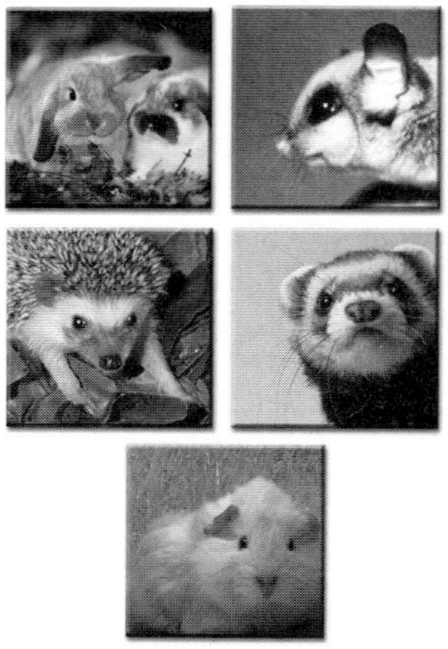

CHAPTER 19

Dermatologic Diseases

Laurie Hess, DVM, Diplomate ABVP

BACTERIAL INFECTIONS

Subcutaneous Abscesses

Subcutaneous abscesses result from traumatic wounds or bacteremia secondary to tooth root abscesses, oral foreign bodies, or upper respiratory tract or urinary tract infections. Often no inciting factor is identifiable.[14,18,19,23] Abscesses usually are soft to firm swellings that gradually enlarge over several days. Although abscesses most commonly develop on the head and limbs, they may be found anywhere in the body. They usually are not painful, are frequently immovable, are minimally inflamed, and often contain thick, caseous exudate. Abscesses may be confined to the subcutaneous space, or they may extend to underlying dermis and bone. Affected rabbits may have no other clinical signs; they may develop inappetence and lose weight (with oral abscesses); or they may become lame (with limb abscesses).

Subcutaneous abscesses are diagnosed by palpation and oral examination. Aspirate subcutaneous swellings with a 22-gauge or larger needle to obtain samples for cytologic evaluation, Gram stain, and both aerobic and anaerobic bacterial culture and sensitivity testing.[18,19] Organisms most commonly isolated from rabbit abscesses are *Staphylococcus aureus, Pasteurella multocida, Pseudomonas aeruginosa, Proteus* spp., and *Bacteroides* spp.[12,22,26,33] Cultures of samples from abscesses are sometimes negative for bacterial growth. However, because bacteria can become resistant to antibiotics, always submit samples for bacterial culture and sensitivity testing, even after antibiotic treatment of recurrent abscesses.[14] In the diagnostic workup of an abscess, include radiographs to determine whether underlying bone is affected. If the animal has an abscess on the head, take a skull radiograph, but also take a thoracic radiograph to check for pneumonia or pulmonary abscesses. Ultrasonography and computed tomography may help delineate abscess margins and are especially helpful with retrobulbar abscesses. Also, submit a blood sample for a complete blood count and plasma biochemical analysis, and submit a urine sample for urinalysis.

Treatment depends on the location and extent of the abscess. Complete surgical excision of the abscess *en bloc,* followed by at least 2 weeks of antibiotic administration based on the results of culture and sensitivity testing, is ideal.[14,18,19,22,23] If joints are affected, amputation of the limb may be necessary. With abscesses that extend into the retrobulbar space, enucleation may be warranted (see Chapter 39). Address all inciting causes, such as foreign bodies or dental disease. If *en bloc* excision is not possible, debride all infected soft tissue and bone. Because the purulent content is usually thick, most rabbit abscesses cannot be treated effectively with drains. Antibiotics do not penetrate the thick abscess capsule and exudate easily, and abscess recurrence is likely, even with antibiotic treatment, if any infected tissue remains after the abscess is debrided. If complete excision is impossible, abscessed tissue should be debrided, flushed with sterile saline solution twice a day, and allowed to heal by second intention. Abscesses also have been successfully treated by packing the completely debrided abscess cavity with antibiotic-impregnated polymethylmethacrylate beads (AIPMMA) (bone cement of a synthetic polymer).[23,26] The beads slowly release antibiotics over days to weeks, providing high local tissue concentrations of drugs with low systemic levels and few systemic side effects (see Chapter 34).

Jaw abscesses are particularly difficult to treat. These abscesses often have fistulas connecting the abscess pocket to teeth roots; abscesses may result from periapical disease causing abnormal tooth growth and destruction of surrounding bone.[33] Bacteria commonly isolated from these abscesses are *Fusobacterium, Prevotella, Peptostreptococcus, Actinomyces,* and *Arcanobacterium* species.[36,37] For treatment, necrotic tissue must be curetted and flushed, infected teeth must be extracted, and the remaining pocket must be packed with AIPMMA beads or a synthetic bone graft particulate (Consil, Nutramax Laboratories, Baltimore, MD) (see Chapter 34). After surgery, systemic antibiotics are given for at least 2 weeks and up to 6 weeks or longer. Successful treatment of jaw abscesses has been achieved with long-term administration of penicillin G benzathine/penicillin G procaine combination at a dosage of 75,000 units SC every other day for rabbits weighing less than 2.5 kg, and 150,000 units SC every other day for rabbits weighing more than 2.5 kg.[35] For rabbits with recurrent abscesses, lifelong antibiotic treatment and repeated surgeries may be necessary.[19] The long-term prognosis for rabbits with abscesses is improved with proper husbandry, including good sanitation and a high-fiber diet.[18]

Mastitis

Rabbit mastitis is most common in heavily lactating does.[19,26] It may be caused by trauma to the teats with secondary bacterial infection from environmental contamination. The most commonly isolated organism in rabbits with suppurative mastitis is *S. aureus*. In young rabbits, this organism also causes exudative dermatitis with pustules, and one virulent biotype can cause high mortality of juvenile rabbits in rabbitries.[18] Other bacteria that cause mastitis include *Pasteurella* and *Streptococcus* species. Teats initially are pink from hyperemia and then turn blue from vascular stasis. Does become depressed, anorectic, septicemic, and febrile, and the condition is often fatal. Treatment includes administration of intravenous fluids and antibiotics, isolation of affected animals to prevent spread of infection, hot packing of infected teats, and surgical debridement of abscessed mammary glands.

Nonseptic cystic mastitis can develop in nonbreeding does (see Chapter 18).[19] Mammary glands are swollen and firm with discolored, distended nipples exuding clear to brown discharge. Glands usually are not painful, and generally does are not systemically ill. This condition often is associated with uterine hyperplasia and uterine adenocarcinoma. The treatment is ovariohysterectomy.

Cellulitis

Cellulitis in rabbits usually occurs acutely and may develop secondary to a respiratory tract infection.[3,18,22,23] Affected rabbits exhibit fevers of 104°-108°F (40° to 42.2°C), and the skin around the head, neck, and chest becomes painful, inflamed, and edematous. Bacteria commonly isolated from these lesions include *S. aureus, P. multocida,* and *Bordetella bronchiseptica*. Treatment involves use of parenteral antibiotics (enrofloxacin, β-lactams, and aminoglycosides) based on the results of culture and sensitivity testing, topical antiseptics (1% chlorhexidine or 10% povidone-iodine), and cool baths. In rabbits that survive, lesions may become necrotic eschars or abscesses requiring surgical debridement.

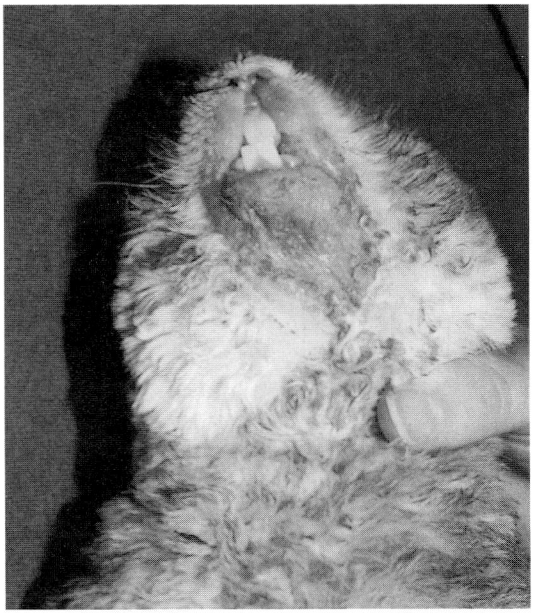

Figure 19-1 Moist dermatitis under the chin of a rabbit secondary to drooling because of dental malocclusion. *(Courtesy Elizabeth Hillyer, DVM.)*

Moist Dermatitis

In rabbits, moist dermatitis usually develops on the chin or ventral neck ("slobbers") or perianally as urine scald ("hutch burn").* Chin or neck lesions can result from excessive drooling secondary to dental disease or from a constantly wet dewlap in rabbits that drink out of a water bowl (Fig. 19-1). Urine scald can be associated with excessive urination or urinary incontinence from renal disease, cystitis, or urinary tract calculi, or with immobility from posterior paresis or obesity (Fig. 19-2). With both types of dermatitis, the skin is inflamed, alopecic, ulcerated, and necrotic. Commonly, *P. aeruginosa* causes a secondary infection and produces pyocyanin pigment that turns the skin green. To determine any underlying cause, the diagnostic workup of rabbits with moist dermatitis includes skull or abdominal radiographs, urinalysis, and a complete blood count and plasma biochemical analysis. Submit samples of exudate or skin for bacterial culture and sensitivity testing. Treat underlying diseases and correct associated environmental factors. Clip the hair over the affected skin and allow the area to dry. Drying agents such as Domeboro Powder (Bayer Inc.,

*References 3, 12, 18, 22, 23, 26.

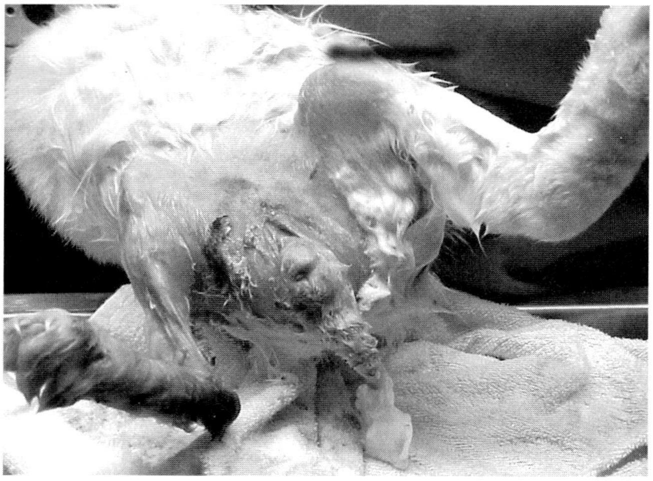

Figure 19-2 Dermatitis secondary to urine scald in a female rabbit. Note the erythematous skin and the ulcerations on the legs. This condition is common in rabbits with cystitis and urinary calculi. *(Courtesy Susan Kelleher, DVM.)*

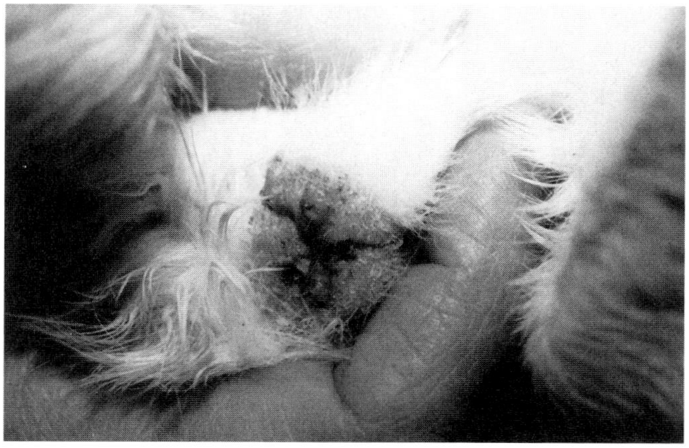

Figure 19-3 Crusty, erythematous, edematous ulcers on the vulva of a rabbit infected with *Treponema paraluis-cuniculi,* the cause of rabbit syphilis. *(Courtesy Karen Rosenthal, DVM.)*

Elkhart, IN) may help. Administer a systemic antibiotic while awaiting the results of culture and sensitivity testing. If obesity is a factor, change the diet of the rabbit to a high-fiber, low-calcium diet, and encourage exercise. Urine scald in grossly obese rabbits may require surgical removal of excess skin folds that interfere with urination; a more conservative approach is to restrict food and encourage exercise to promote weight loss.

Ulcerative Pododermatitis

Ulcerative pododermatitis *(sore hocks)* is a chronic, granulomatous, ulcerative dermatitis of the plantar metatarsal and, occasionally, the volar metacarpal and phalangeal surfaces of the feet. This condition usually results from trauma due to rough, dirty floors or frequent thumping. It also may develop in rabbits with thin plantar fur pads or in large-breed or obese rabbits as a result of pressure necrosis and confinement in small cages with wire floors.[11,19,22,23,26] Lesions start as erythematous decubital ulcers that become infected, usually with *S. aureus,* from contaminated bedding. Infected ulcers develop into abscesses covered with raised, dry, hyperkeratotic, fibrotic scabs. Infection can spread to underlying bone, causing osteomyelitis and sepsis.

For treatment of pododermatitis, submit samples of abscessed tissue for bacterial culture and sensitivity testing and take radiographs of the legs to check for osteomyelitis.[14] Clean wounds with antiseptics, debride necrotic tissue, and bandage the area daily with light dressings, such as Tegaderm (3M Medical-Surgical Division, St Paul, MN), to protect weight-bearing surfaces of the feet. Topical antibiotics, such as silver sulfadiazine (Silvadene Cream 1%, Monarch Pharmaceuticals, Bristol, TN), and systemic antibiotics, selected based on results of culture and sensitivity testing, usually are warranted. Provide solid cage floors and clean, soft, dry bedding. Debride and flush abscessed tissue, and consider packing severe abscesses with AIPMMA beads. Modify the diet of obese rabbits to increase fiber and lower carbohydrates, and encourage exercise. Unilateral pododermatitis unresponsive to treatment may require amputation at midfemur.

Rabbit Syphilis

Rabbit syphilis, also called venereal spirochetosis or "vent disease," is a contagious venereal disease caused by the spirochete *Treponema paraluiscuniculi* (see also Chapter 18).[31] Transmission is through direct contact with infected skin or from dam to kits at birth.[3,14,19] Lesions may appear 3 to 6 weeks after exposure as erythematous, edematous, crusty ulcers around the lips, eyelids, nostrils, philtrum, vulva, prepuce, and perineum (Fig. 19-3).[26] Ulcers usually wax and wane over months. Asymptomatic carrier rabbits may develop lesions if exposed to stress (e.g., overcrowding, poor sanitation).

Rabbit syphilis is diagnosed from clinical signs and identification of the causative organism with silver staining or darkfield microscopy of affected skin.* Rabbit syphilis is usually self-limited; however, autoinfection from perineum to face is possible. Treatment involves administration of parenteral benzathine penicillin G/procaine penicillin G (42,000-84,000 IU/kg SC q7d for 3 treatments) or penicillin G procaine (40,000-60,000 IU/kg IM q24h for 5-7 days).

Necrobacillosis

Necrobacillosis, or Schmorl's disease, is an uncommon skin infection with *Fusobacterium necrophorum,* an anaerobic, filamentous, gram-negative bacterium normally found in the gastrointestinal tract and feces.[14,23] Infection occurs commonly from wound contamination. Abscessed, ulcerated, necrotic lesions may be found around the head, neck, and feet.[3] The causative bacterium may be isolated from anaerobic culture of affected tissue. Lesions should be debrided and flushed, and treatment with antibiotics effective against

*References 3, 14, 19, 23, 26, 31.

anaerobic bacteria, such as penicillin G procaine, should be administered.

FUNGAL INFECTIONS

Dermatophytosis

Dermatophytosis, or ringworm, is a zoonotic, usually self-limiting, often asymptomatic infection of the skin in rabbits, most commonly caused by *Trichophyton mentagrophytes.** Less often, rabbits are infected with *Microsporum* species. Dermatophytosis is more common in young rabbits, possibly because of their incompletely developed immune systems and low levels of fungistatic fatty acids in sebum. Asymptomatic carriers may develop lesions in response to overcrowding, malnutrition, or other infections. Dermatophyte lesions are dry, crusty, hairless areas of skin around the head, legs, feet, and nail beds that may become pruritic, erythematous, and occasionally abscessed. Affected epidermis is hyperkeratotic and acanthotic, with an acute to chronic inflammatory cell infiltrate in the underlying dermis. Dermatophytosis is diagnosed based on growth of the infecting organism on dermatophyte culture medium from hair or skin samples. Fungal mycelia and arthrospores also may be seen on skin scrapings mounted in 10% potassium hydroxide or in skin biopsy samples stained with periodic acid-Schiff stain, Gridley fungal stain, or Gomori's methenamine silver. Fluorescence of mycelia under ultraviolet light from a Wood's lamp is not a reliable method of testing in rabbits, because *T. mentagrophytes* does not fluoresce.

Several methods can be used to treat dermatophytosis in rabbits. For small lesions, clip the hair and apply topical miconazole cream (Conofite, Mallinckrodt Veterinary Inc., Mundelein, IL), clotrimazole cream (Veltrim, Miles Inc., Shawnee Mission, KS), or clotrimazole lotion (Lotrimin Lotion 1%, Schering-Plough Corp., Kenilworth, NJ).[14,18,23] Other topical treatments include twice-daily application of a 10:1 mixture of water and chlorhexidine (Nolvasan, Fort Dodge Laboratories, Fort Dodge, IA), povidone-iodine, or 2% chlorhexidine/2% miconazole shampoo (Malaseb, DVM Pharmaceuticals Inc., Miami, FL).[6,19] Imidazole-containing creams and lotions may be ineffective because they do not penetrate infected hair shafts and follicles.[9] For multiple lesions, clip the entire hair coat, dip the rabbit in lime sulfur solution (LymDyp, DVM Pharmaceuticals), and administer griseofulvin (Grifulvin V Suspension, Ortho Pharmaceutical, Raritan, NJ) (25 mg/kg PO q24h or divided q12h for 30 days).[3,18,26] Use griseofulvin cautiously, because at high doses it can cause bone marrow suppression and panleukopenia.[9] Also, griseofulvin is teratogenic and cannot be given to pregnant does. Owners administering griseofulvin should wear gloves. Ketoconazole (Nizoral, Janssen Pharmaceuticals, Titusville, NJ) (10-15 mg/kg PO q24h) can be administered to rabbits that do not tolerate griseofulvin. Because it inhibits steroid synthesis, do not give ketoconazole to breeding animals. Other drugs used to treat dermatophytosis include itraconazole (Sporanox, Janssen Pharmaceuticals) (5-10 mg/kg PO q24h) and terbinafine (Lamisil, Novartis, Basel, Switzerland) (8-20 mg/kg PO q24h). Continue systemic antifungal treatment for 2 weeks beyond resolution of clinical signs or until monthly fungal cultures are negative twice.[9,19,23] Most treatments last a minimum of 3 to 4 months. Disinfection of the environment also is essential. Vacuum contaminated areas and clean all surfaces with a 1:10 solution of bleach and water. Foggers containing enilconazole or formaldehyde are preferred to steam cleaning for carpets because steam cleaning does not reach a temperature high enough to kill infectious spores.

*References 3, 9, 10, 14, 18, 19, 23, 39.

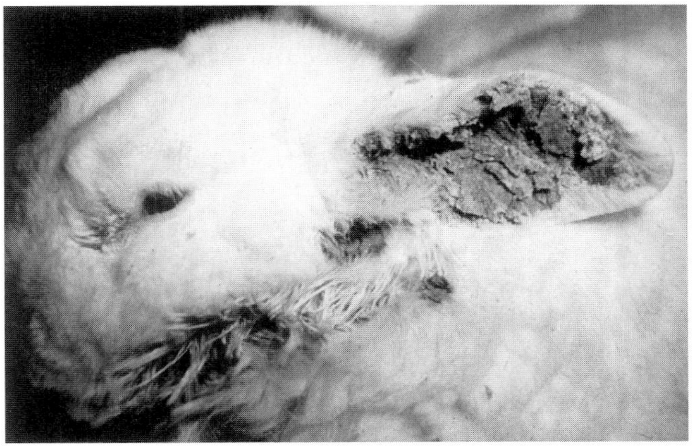

Figure 19-4 Infestation of a rabbit's external ear canal with *Psoroptes cuniculi*. Note the profuse, thick crust that covers areas of inflammation. *(Courtesy Karen Moriello, DVM.)*

Dermatophytes may be hard to eliminate from large rabbit colonies. Success has been achieved by dipping rabbits in 1% copper sulfate solution (cupric sulfate pentahydrate, Sigma Chemical, St Louis, MO).[23] Large numbers of infected rabbits may be sprayed with a solution of metastabilized chlorous acid/chlorine dioxide (MECA, LD Disinfectant, Alcide, Norwalk, CT) diluted 1 : 1 : 10 with activator compound and water, respectively.[10] MECA also may be used to disinfect the environment. Large dermatophyte outbreaks may be treated with griseofulvin-medicated diets (0.825 g griseofulvin per kilogram of diet).[26]

PARASITIC INFECTIONS

Ear Mites

The rabbit ear mite, *Psoroptes cuniculi,* is a large, obligate, nonburrowing parasite with a 3-week life cycle and the ability to survive off the host for up to 21 days. Mite infection can cause inflammation and reddish-brown crusting of the external ear canal, head shaking, ear drooping, and pruritus (Fig. 19-4).* In debilitated rabbits, inflammation and crusting may extend to the face, dewlap, neck, trunk, legs, feet, and perineum. Mites may spread down the ear canal, leading to otitis media and neurologic signs. Rabbits with subclinical infections that are otherwise healthy may only be mildly pruritic for years. *Psoroptes* mites may be identified with the naked eye, otoscope, or microscope. Mites have two to three pairs of legs with jointed pedicles ending in a sucker-shaped bell. Microscopic examination of crust reveals mites, mite feces, mite eggs, inflammatory cells, desquamated epithelial cells, and serum.

*References 3, 14, 19, 19, 22, 23, 26.

Ear mites can be treated with ivermectin (Ivomec, Merck, AgVet Division, Rahway, NJ) (0.4 mg/kg SC q10-14d for 3 treatments).* Less effective treatment methods include topical mineral oil, acaricides, and flea powder.[18,26] Severe pruritus may be treated with a combination of topical thiabendazole, dexamethasone, and neomycin sulfate (Tresaderm, MSD-AGVET, Rahway, NJ). Aural crusts usually resolve after treatment with ivermectin. To prevent reinfection, clean the environment and treat contaminated areas with flea products. Fipronil spray (Frontline, Meriel Limited, Iselin, NJ) has been used in rabbits at 3 mL/kg given every 2 months as a preventative measure in case of poor environmental disinfection.[8] However, fipronil administration has been associated with death in rabbits, and the product's manufacturer does not recommend its use.[28] Although the antiparasitic agent selamectin (Revolution, Pfizer Animal Health, Exton, PA) is not labeled for use in rabbits, studies show that it can be used safely and effectively to treat *P. cuniculi* infestation. It can be administered at 6 or 18 mg/kg twice, 28 days apart, without adverse effects.[29] Also, use any insecticide dips or baths (such as carbaryl, pyrethrin, and lime sulfur-based products) cautiously in rabbits, because shock and death have occurred in association with these products.[14] In rabbits, toxicity of topical drugs used safely in cats and dogs may be related to the thinness of rabbit skin, ingestion of topical products from excessive grooming, hypersensitivity to the drug's vehicle, or absolute overdosage.[3] The act of bathing or dipping rabbits also may induce stress that is exacerbated by overheating, chilling, or the presence of hepatic dysfunction.

Fur Mites

Cheyletiella parasitovorax, the rabbit fur mite, is zoonotic to people, dogs, and cats.[18,21] This mite is often called *walking dandruff*, because it resembles a large, white, mobile dandruff flake.[23] Although *Cheyletiella* can cause subclinical disease, more often it causes a scaly, dry, sometimes pruritic dermatitis with patchy alopecia or broken hairs over the dorsal neck, trunk, hind end, and abdomen.[22,26] In severe infestations, these nonburrowing mites may be visible with the naked eye as clear to white saddle-shapes with inward curving claws and hook-like mouth parts.[14] Their eggs adhere to hair shafts. Histopathologic analysis of affected skin shows hyperkeratosis with an exudate of inflammatory cells (mononuclear phagocytes, plasma cells, lymphocytes, and eosinophils). *Cheyletiella* infection is diagnosed from clinical signs and microscopic identification of mites in skin scrapings, acetate tape preparations, or skin and hair debris that sticks to a flea comb. Treat rabbits infected with *Cheyletiella* with ivermectin (0.4 mg/kg SC q14d for 3 treatments). Other treatments include weekly lime sulfur dips for 3 to 6 weeks or application of carbaryl flea powder appropriate for cats twice weekly for 6 weeks. Dips and flea powder have successfully eliminated mites, but both treatments have been associated with toxicity in rabbits. Disinfect the environment with flea products (i.e., carbaryl 5% dust).

Another mite that causes dermatitis in rabbits is *Leporacarus gibbus* (formerly *Listrophorus gibbus*).[23,25,26,32] Like *Cheyletiella*, this mite attaches to hair shafts; however, its eggs stick more distally on the shaft and are more loosely attached. *Leporacarus* causes moist, sometimes pruritic, alopecic dermatitis affecting the back, groin, and ventral abdomen.[3] Diagnose *Leporacarus* infection by the same methods as those used in rabbits infected with *Cheyletiella*. *Leporacarus* mites are brown and laterally compressed, with short legs and single projections extending from the head. Males have long clasping organs projecting caudally from their body. Treatment is the same as for *Cheyletiella* infection.

Sarcoptes scabiei and *Notoedres cati* occur in both laboratory and pet rabbits.[18,26] These mites cause a crusty, pruritic dermatitis around the head, neck, and trunk. Diagnosis and treatment are the same as for *Cheyletiella* infection.[23]

Demodex cuniculi may occur in rabbits without clinical signs.[23] This mite normally inhabits rabbits' epidermis and hair follicles; it can cause dermatitis in rabbits that are immunosuppressed by other diseases or subject to environmental stress.[15,18]

Fleas

Flea infestation most commonly affects rabbits housed with dogs and cats.[18,19,22,23] Pet rabbits often are infected with the cat flea, *Ctenocephalides felis*, or the dog flea, *Ctenocephalides canis*. Other fleas found on domestic rabbits, especially when they are exposed to wild rabbits, include *Cediopsylla*, *Odontopsyllus*, *Spilopsyllus*, and *Hoplopsyllus* species and *Echnidnophaga gallinacea* (the *sticktight flea*). Flea infection may be manifested as a dull coat, easily epilated hair, and patchy alopecia with pruritus, skin erythema, and crusting, especially on the pinnae and face.[3,14] Fleas not only cause dermatitis but also transmit myxoma virus (discussed later).

Diagnose flea infestation from clinical signs and by identifying fleas and their eggs on the rabbit. Treat flea dermatitis with carbaryl-based flea powder, safe for cats, 1 to 2 times per week. Imidacloprid (Advantage, Bayer Animal Health, Agriculture Division, Shawnee Mission, KS) and the insect growth regulator, lufenuron (Program, Novartis Animal Health Canada, Mississauga, Ontario) have been used topically on rabbits to treat fleas,[21,23] although neither is labeled for use in rabbits. The 10% spot-on topical formulation of imidacloprid (Advantage 40 for cats, 0.4 mL topical solution) has been used safely and effectively to treat flea infestations in rabbits.[34] For rabbits older than 10 weeks of age and weighing less than 4 kg , 0.4 mL is applied to the skin at the base of the neck. Adult rabbits weighing more than 4 kg should receive 0.8 mL in the same site. The environment also must be treated with insect growth regulators and insecticidal sprays, and rabbits must be removed until the environmental products have dried. Borate powder may be used on infected rugs. Permethrin and pyrethrin-based environmental treatments may be ineffective because of flea resistance.

Myiasis

Larvae of *Cuterebra* species, or bot flies, and maggots of dipterid flies may infect rabbits housed outdoors in warm weather.[18,19,23] *Cuterebra* flies are large and have three larval stages that commonly infect wild rabbits and rodents. Adult flies live only a short time to breed. Larvae pupate in the subcutis, causing multiple swellings, especially over the dorsum and in the axillary, inguinal, and ventral cervical regions. Each 1- to 3-cm subcutaneous swelling encapsulates a single larva and has a breathing hole visible at the skin surface.[14,22] Although some rabbits are unaffected by these swellings, others become weak, anorectic, dehydrated, lame, and in shock. *Cuterebra* larvae also

*References 3, 4, 6, 7, 14, 19, 22, 23.

can migrate aberrantly from the nasal passages, eyes, sinuses, and ear canals through the central nervous system, causing neurologic signs.[17,18]

Treatment involves removal of larvae. After preparing the affected skin area for surgery, enlarge each breathing hole with hemostats. Gently remove the larvae through the enlarged openings, ensuring that they are not crushed, because damage to larvae can cause anaphylaxis. After removal of the larvae and debridement of necrotic tissue, the swelling usually resolves. If it does not, or if the skin is abscessed, surgically excise the affected tissue. Antibiotics are essential to prevent secondary bacterial infection. Cuterebrid infection is prevented by fly control and protective screens.

Noncuterebrid maggots, including those of the flesh fly, *Wohlfahrtia vigil*, cause moist dermatitis and matted hair around the perineum, face, and rump.[18,19,23,26] Hundreds of larvae may colonize a single skin area. Maggots cause extensive lesions by feeding on dead tissue.[14,22] Preexisting wounds are not necessary for maggot infection. Perineal dermatitis, urine scald, or skin fold dermatitis secondary to obesity may predispose to maggot infection. Rabbits infested with maggots should be sedated to clean the affected skin, remove the maggots, and debride necrotic tissue. Administer ivermectin (0.4 mg/kg SC q14d for 2 treatments) to kill larvae and an antibiotic with good skin activity, such as trimethoprim-sulfa, to treat secondary bacterial infection. Clean the surgical site daily, apply topical silver sulfadiazene cream (Silvadene Cream 1%, Monarch Pharmaceuticals), and allow the wound to heal by second intention. Rabbits with extensive infestation may initially appear stable after surgery but then die, possibly from secondary infection of necrotic wounds with *Clostridium* species. Penicillin G procaine (30,000-60,000 IU/kg SC q24h for up to 5 days) may be administered to prevent secondary anaerobic bacterial infection.

Blackflies of the Simuliidae family bite rabbits around lips, ears, and nares and transmit viral infections, including myxomatosis (see below).[23] Bites are painful and may become inflamed. Fly control and protective screens prevent blackfly bites.

Ticks

Ticks affect both domestic and wild rabbits. The most common hard (ixodid) tick of rabbits, the continental rabbit tick, *Haemaphysalis leporis-palustris,* has three stages in its life cycle, and rabbits may host each stage.[23,26] Other ixodid ticks that feed on rabbits include *Amblyomma*, *Boophilus* (cattle ticks), *Rhipicephalus*, and *Dermacentor* species. Soft (argasid) ticks, such as *Otobius lagophilus*, *Ornithodoros turicata*, and *Ornithodoros parkeri,* also may parasitize rabbits. Severe tick infestation causes blood loss with a macrocytic, normochromic anemia. Rabbit ticks also may transmit viral infections, such as myxomatosis and papillomatosis (see later discussion), and zoonotic diseases, including tularemia, Lyme disease, and Rocky Mountain spotted fever. Remove visible ticks with forceps, and give ivermectin (0.4 mg/kg SC) to kill any remaining feeding ticks.

Lice

The rabbit louse, *Haemodipsus ventricosus,* rarely occurs on domestic rabbits.[3,12,26] With severe infestation, this blood-sucking parasite causes anemia, weight loss, erythematous papules, hair loss, and pruritus. Lice and their eggs are visible with the naked eye. Infected rabbits may be treated with ivermectin (0.4 mg/kg SC).

Pinworms

Passalurus ambiguus, the common rabbit pinworm, is host-specific.[3] It inhabits the small intestine, cecum, and colon, passing eggs into the feces without causing clinical signs. Severe infections cause perianal pruritus, self-trauma, and, occasionally, rectal prolapse.[13] Diagnose pinworm infection by clinical signs and by identifying ova or adult worms in a fecal smear or fecal float. Treatment is difficult, because eggs passed in contaminated feces often are re-ingested. Usually, infection is only transiently eliminated. Clean the pinworms from the perianal area, and give thiabendazole (50 mg/kg PO) or fenbendazole (10-20 mg/kg PO) in two doses 10 to 14 days apart. Alternatively, administer piperazine directly to individual rabbits (200 mg/kg PO, repeat in 14 days), or give it in food to adult rabbits (0.5 g/kg per day for 2 days) or to juvenile rabbits (0.75 g/kg per day for 2 days).[13,26] Piperazine also may be given in drinking water (100 mg/100 mL of water for 1 day, repeat in 10 days). Environmental cleanup to kill pinworm eggs is difficult.

VIRAL INFECTIONS

Myxomatosis

Myxomatosis is caused by myxoma viruses of the pox family.[18] This disease is transmitted through arthropod bites (mosquito, gnat, fly, flea, fur mite), on spiny thistles and birds' feet, and by direct contact.[14,18,23] Clinical signs depend on the virulence of the viral strain and on the genus and species of the infected rabbit. In *Sylvilagus* species, myxomatosis manifests as benign skin tumors at the site of viral entry (usually at the ear base). Domestic rabbits may exhibit lethargy, fever, anorexia, skin hemorrhages, and seizures with a high mortality rate.[18,19,22,26] Rabbits that survive initial infection may develop purulent blepharoconjunctivitis and erythematous, edematous nodules on the face and perineum.[3,18,23,26] Myxomatosis is diagnosed by clinical signs, histopathologic analysis of affected tissue, and viral isolation. Histopathologic examination of biopsy samples of affected skin shows undifferentiated mesenchymal cells, inflammatory cells, mucin, and edema. Treatment is supportive and often unsuccessful. Insect vectors must be eliminated. Vaccines, including one made from a genetically engineered recombinant virus, have been developed for high-risk rabbitries but are not commercially available.[1]

Rabbit (Shope) Fibroma Virus

Rabbit (Shope) fibroma virus is a Leporipoxvirus that infects many European wild rabbits and cottontails (*Sylvilagus* species); other rabbit species are resistant.[3,23] The natural host of the poxvirus is the eastern cottontail (*Sylvilagus floridanus*). Other *Sylvilagus* species (*S. bachmani, S. nuttalli,* and *S. audoboni*) are refractory to infection. Malignant rabbit fibroma virus, a recently described recombinant virus of Shope fibroma and myxoma virus, is a distinct virus that causes generalized infection, tumors, and immunosuppression that is highly fatal.

Rabbit (Shope) fibroma virus is transmitted by biting arthropods, including fleas and mosquitoes. In cottontails, clinical signs of fibroma virus infection are worse in young rabbits and include large, wartlike tumors of the face, feet, and legs. Diagnosis is based on gross and histopathologic analysis of tumors and on isolation of virus from affected skin. Tumors start as acute inflammation and progress to localized fibroblastic proliferation with infiltration of mononuclear and polymorphonuclear inflammatory cells. The overlying epidermis may become necrotic and slough, or lesions may regress over several months. Treatment involves supportive care and elimination of insect vectors.

Rabbit (Shope) Papillomavirus

The rabbit (Shope) papillomavirus, also called cottontail rabbit papillomavirus, is an oncogenic, DNA virus of the Papovaviridae family that is transmitted by biting arthropods (especially continental rabbit ticks, reduvid bugs, and mosquitoes).[23] This virus causes rough, red, wartlike, keratinized, often pigmented lesions on the ears, eyelids, neck, shoulders, abdomen, and thighs. Lesions in wild cottontail rabbits (*Sylvilagus* species) often are found around the neck and shoulders and in domestic rabbits around the hairless areas of the ears and eyelids.[26] This virus is distinct from the rabbit oral papillomavirus, which causes tongue and oral cavity papillomas in domestic rabbits. In rabbits infected with Shope papillomavirus, lesions may undergo immune-mediated resolution and disappear after months, or they may progress to squamous cell carcinoma that often metastasizes to axillary lymph nodes.[3] The incidence of carcinoma development from viral infection is threefold lower in cottontail rabbits than in domestic rabbits.

Shope papillomavirus is diagnosed by histopathologic analysis of typical gross lesions. In domestic rabbits, affected tissue is hyperkeratotic but rarely contains the inclusion bodies that are characteristic of papillomaviruses. Differential diagnosis must discriminate Shope papillomas from spontaneous, nonviral papillomas. In contrast, in the natural host (*Sylvilagus* species), papillomas usually contain infectious viral particles.

Treatment involves surgical removal of horny papillomas. Control of arthropod vectors helps prevent spread of the disease.

Rabbitpox

Rabbitpox virus, an orthomyxopoxvirus, is a very rare, highly contagious, often fatal infection that is usually seen only among research populations in the United States and The Netherlands.[23] This virus is transmitted by ingestion or inhalation of infected tissue.[26] Affected rabbits die without clinical signs or develop enlarged lymph nodes, fever, and an erythematous rash that progresses to papules and crusty nodules. There may be edema of the face, oral cavity, scrotum, and vulva.[3] Some rabbits develop blepharitis, keratitis, and conjunctivitis. Definitive diagnosis is based on characteristic skin lesions and on virus isolation or fluorescent antibody identification of viral antigen in infected tissue. Histopathologic analysis of lesions shows lymphoid necrosis and mononuclear cell infiltration. Treatment is supportive.

CUTANEOUS NEOPLASIA

Skin tumors unassociated with viral infection are uncommon in rabbits.[14,23] Primary skin tumors include squamous cell carcinoma, basal cell tumor, trichoepithelioma, and sebaceous cell carcinoma. Uterine adenocarcinoma, fibrosarcoma, and connective tissue tumors can metastasize to skin.[27] Lymphosarcoma also occurs in rabbit skin as erythematous, crusty, alopecic plaques confined to the epidermis or extending through the dermis.[20,38] Often, cutaneous lymphosarcoma in rabbits is associated with neoplastic lymphocytes in organs besides the skin (i.e., lymph nodes and lungs). Diagnosis of neoplasia is by microscopic examination of tissue biopsy samples. Tumors are treated by surgical excision or debulking. Chemotherapy generally has been unsuccessful in treating cutaneous lymphoma in rabbits (see Chapter 21).

BEHAVIORAL CAUSES OF SKIN DISEASE

Barbering

Barbering, or hair pulling, occurs when a dominant rabbit pulls a subordinate's hair; it can also be self-induced in rabbits fed low-fiber diets.[18,22,23] Female rabbits self-barber to build nests if they are pregnant, pseudopregnant, or in heat. These rabbits pull hair from their legs and thorax. Occasionally, rabbits groom excessively as a dissociative behavior in response to stress (i.e., overcrowding). Treatment for barbering depends on its cause. Separate dominant and subordinate rabbits, and provide a high-fiber diet or a less crowded enclosure as needed. A change in light cycle or intensity may help.

Self-mutilation after Intramuscular Injection

Two to four days after intramuscular injection of ketamine and xylazine into the caudal thigh, rabbits may mutilate digits on the ipsilateral leg.[2] Self-mutilation is thought to result from perineural drug infiltration around the sciatic nerve, resulting in dysthesia. If this occurs, clean and bandage damaged digits and begin to administer antibiotics. To prevent this syndrome, give ketamine and xylazine separately in different sites, away from the sciatic nerve, such as in the lumbar muscles.

SKIN DISEASE OF UNKNOWN CAUSE

Sebaceous Adenitis

Sebaceous adenitis has been reported in several different breeds and ages of rabbits. All of the affected animals had nonpruritic, scaly, flaky dermatitis that began around the face and neck and progressed to diffuse skin disease.[40] Histopathologic examination of affected tissue showed hyperkeratosis, follicular keratosis, follicular dystrophy, perifollicular fibrosis, and replacement of sebaceous glands with perifollicular lymphocytic infiltrate (Fig. 19-5). No infectious organisms were identified. Various treatments for sebaceous adenitis, including isotretinoin (Accutane, Hoffman-LaRoche Inc., Nutley, NJ), etretinate (Tegison, Hoffman-LaRoche Inc.), prednisone, azathioprine (Imuran, Faro Pharmaceuticals, Bedminster, NJ), griseofulvin, essential fatty acids, and topical propylene glycol, have been tried unsuccessfully. Rabbits with sebaceous adenitis usually die or are euthanized because of the severity of the skin condition.

Ehlers-Danlos–like Syndrome

Ehlers-Danlos syndrome is an inherited skin disorder in humans that is associated with abnormal collagen structure.[36]

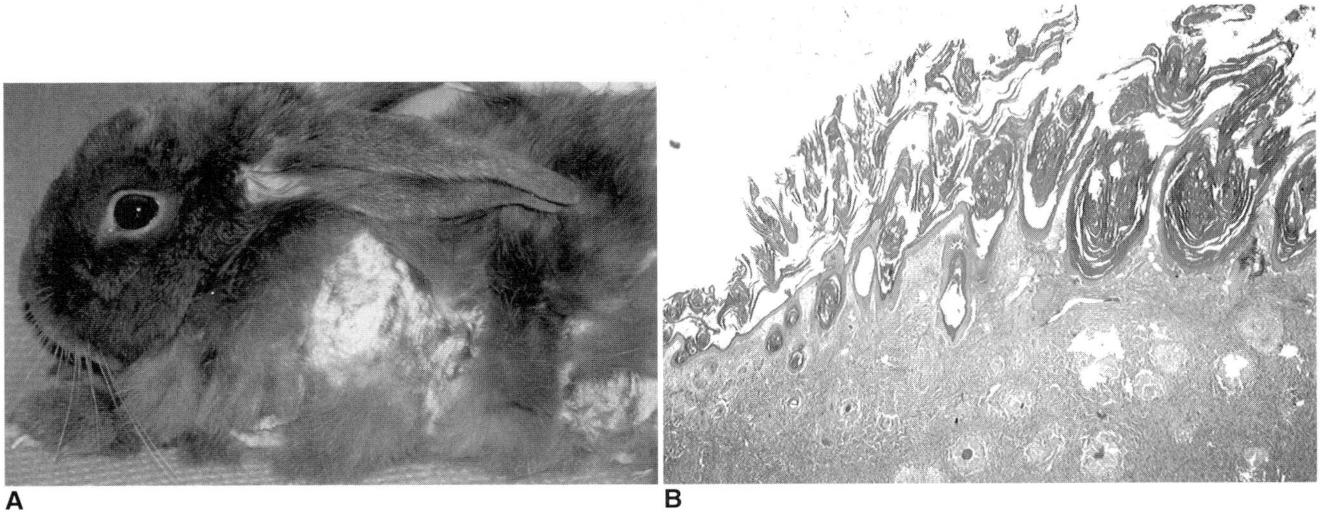

Figure 19-5 **A,** Male rabbit that presented with crusty, thick skin lesions and alopecia involving the thorax, abdomen, inguinal area, and extemities. **B,** Photomicrograph of a skin biopsy sample from this rabbit. Histologically, severe follicular hyperkeratosis and granulomatous perifollicular dermatitis is present, consistent with sebaceous adenitis. No infectious organisms were seen with special stains. (Hematoxylin and eosin stain; ×4.) *(Courtesy Keith Baer, DVM.)*

This syndrome results from mutations in collagen-forming genes or collagen-synthesizing enzymes that cause joint laxity and skin hyperextensibility. An Ehlers-Danlos–like syndrome has been reported in rabbits with markedly fragile skin.[5,16] Electron microscopic examination revealed irregularly shaped dermal fibrils and high variability in dermal cell diameter. Treatment for this syndrome in rabbits is not yet known.

ACKNOWLEDGMENT

I thank Dr. Tom Donnelly for his review and helpful comments.

REFERENCES

1. Barcena J, Morales M, Vasquez B, et al: Horizontal transmissible protection against myxomatosis and rabbit hemorrhagic disease by using a recombinant myxoma virus. J Virol 2000; 74:1114-1123.
2. Beyers TM, Richardson JA, Prince MD: Axonal degeneration and self-mutilation as a complication of the intramuscular use of ketamine and xylazine in rabbits. Lab Anim Sci 1991; 41:519-520.
3. Bourdeau PJ: Dermatology of small mammals: I. Parasitic and infectious skin diseases in rodents and rabbits. Proceedings of the Fourth World Congress of Veterinary Dermatology, 2000, pp 195-200.
4. Bowman DD, Fogelson ML, Carbone LG: Effect of ivermectin on the control of ear mites *(Psoroptes cuniculi)* in naturally infested rabbits. Am J Vet Res 1992; 53:105-109.
5. Brown PJ, Young RD, Cripps PJ: Abnormalities of collagen fibrils in a rabbit with a connective tissue defect similar to Ehlers-Danlos syndrome. Res Vet Sci 1993; 55:346-350.
6. Curtis SK, Brooks DL: Eradication of ear mites from naturally infested conventional research rabbits using ivermectin. Lab Anim Sci 1990; 40:406-408.
7. Curtis SK, Housley R, Brooks DL: Use of ivermectin for treatment of ear mite infestation in rabbits. J Am Vet Med Assoc 1990; 196:1139-1140.
8. Cutler SL: Ectopic *Psoroptes cuniculi* infestation in a pet rabbit. J Small Anim Pract 1998; 39:86-87.
9. Donnelly TM, Rush EM, Lackner PA: Ringworm in small exotic pets. Semin Avian Exotic Pet Med 2000; 9:82-93.
10. Franklin CL, Gibson SV, Caffrey CJ, et al: Treatment of *Trichophyton mentagrophytes* infection in rabbits. J Am Vet Med Assoc 1991; 198:1625-1630.
11. Gentz EJ, Carpenter JW: Neurologic and musculoskeletal disease. *In* Hillyer EV, Quesenberry KE, eds. Ferrets, Rabbits, and Rodents: Clinical Medicine and Surgery. Philadelphia, WB Saunders, 1997, pp 220-226.
12. Harkness JE, Wagner JE: The Biology and Medicine of Rabbits and Rodents, 4th ed. Baltimore, Williams & Wilkins, 1995, pp 143-151.
13. Harkness JE, Wagner JE: The Biology and Medicine of Rabbits and Rodents, 3rd ed. Baltimore, Williams & Wilkins, 1989, pp 168-171.
14. Harvey C: Rabbit and rodent skin diseases. Semin Avian Exotic Pet Med 1995; 4:195-204.
15. Harvey RG: *Demodex cuniculi* in dwarf rabbits *(Oryctolagus cuniculus)*. J Small Anim Pract 1990; 31:204-207.
16. Harvey RG, Brown PJ, Young RD, et al: A connective tissue defect in two rabbits similar to the Ehlers-Danlos syndrome. Vet Rec 1990; 126:130-132.
17. Hendrix CM, DiPinto MN, Cox NR, et al: Aberrant intracranial myiasis caused by larval *Cuterebra* infection. Compend Contin Educ Pract Vet 1989; 11:550-559.
18. Hillyer EV: Dermatologic diseases. *In* Hillyer EV, Quesenberry KE, eds. Ferrets, Rabbits, and Rodents: Clinical Medicine and Surgery. Philadelphia, WB Saunders, 1997, pp 212-219.
19. Hillyer EV: Pet rabbits. Vet Clin North Am Small Anim Pract 1994; 24:25-65.

20. Hinton M, Regan M: Cutaneous lymphosarcoma in a rabbit. Vet Rec 1978; 103:140-141.
21. Hutchinson MJ, Jacobs DE, Bell GD, et al: Evaluation of imidacloprid for the treatment and prevention of cat flea *(Ctenocephalides felis felis)* infestations on rabbits. Vet Rec 2001; 148:695-696.
22. Jenkins JR: Skin disorders of the rabbit. J Small Exotic Anim Med 1991; 1:64-65.
23. Jenkins JR: Skin disorders of the rabbit. Vet Clin North Am Exotic Anim Pract 2001; 4:543-563.
24. Jenkins JR: Soft tissue surgery and dental procedures. *In* Hillyer EV, Quesenberry KE, eds. Ferrets, Rabbits, and Rodents: Clinical Medicine and Surgery. Philadelphia, WB Saunders, 1997, pp 227-239.
25. Kirwan AP, Middleton B, McGarry JW: Diagnosis and prevalence of *Leporacarus gibbus* in the fur of domestic rabbits in the UK. Vet Rec 1998; 142:20-21.
26. Kraus AL, Weisbroth SH, Flatt RE, et al: Biology and diseases of rabbits. *In* Fox JG, Cohen BJ, Loew FM, eds. Laboratory Medicine. San Diego, Academic Press, 1984, pp 207-240.
27. Li X, Schlafer DH: A spontaneous skin basal cell tumor in a black French minilop rabbit. Lab Anim Sci 1992; 42:94-95.
28. Malley D: Use of Frontline spray on rabbits [letter]. Vet Rec 1997; 140:535-536.
29. McTier TL, Hair JA, Walstrom DJ, et al: Efficacy and safety of topical administration of selamectin for treatment of ear mite infestation in rabbits. J Am Vet Med Assoc 2003; 223:322-324.
30. Merchant SR: Zoonotic diseases with cutaneous manifestation: part I. Compend Contin Educ Pract Vet 1990; 12:371-375.
31. Paul-Murphy J: Reproductive and urogenital disorders. *In* Hillyer EV, Quesenberry KE, eds. Ferrets, Rabbits, and Rodents: Clinical Medicine and Surgery. Philadelphia, WB Saunders, 1997, pp 202-211.
32. Pinter L: *Leporacarus gibbus* and *Spilopsyllus cuniculi* infestation in a pet rabbit. J Small Anim Pract 1999; 40:220-221.
33. Remeeus PGK, Verbeek M: The use of calcium hydroxide in the treatment of abscesses in the cheek of the rabbit resulting from a dental periapical disorder. J Vet Dent 1995; 12:19-22.
34. Reuter K, Pospischil R, Endepols S, et al: Flea infestation in exotic pet animals. Suppl Compend Contin Educ Pract Vet 2002; 24:10-13.
35. Rosenfield ME: Successful eradication of severe abscesses in rabbits with long-term administration of penicillin G benzathine/penicillin G procaine. Available at: http:/moorelab.sbs.umass.edu. Accessed on November 11, 2002.
36. Sinke JD, van Dijk JE, Willem SE: A case of Ehlers-Danlos-like syndrome in a rabbit with a review of the disease in other species. Vet Q 1997; 19:182-185.
37. Tyrrell KL, Citron DM, Jenkins JR, et al: Periodontal bacteria in rabbit mandibular and maxillary abscesses. J Clin Microbiol 2002; 40:1044-1047.
38. Vangeel I, Pasmans F, Vanrobaeys M, et al: Prevalence of dermatophytes in asymptomatic guinea pigs and rabbits. Vet Rec 2000; 146:440-441.
39. White SD, Campbell T, Logan A, et al: Lymphoma with cutaneous involvement in three domestic rabbits *(Oryctolagus cuniculus)*. Vet Dermatol 2000; 11:61-67.
40. White SD, Linder KE, Schultheiss P, et al: Sebaceous adenitis in four domestic rabbits *(Oryctolagus cuniculus)*. Vet Dermatol 2000; 11:53-60.

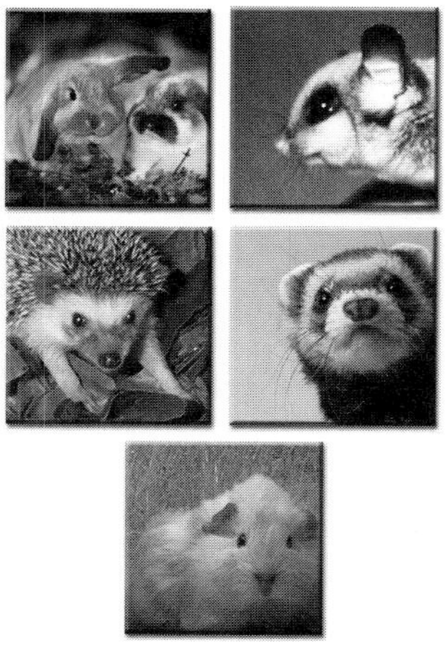

CHAPTER 20

Neurologic and Musculoskeletal Diseases

Barbara J. Deeb, DVM, MS, and
James W. Carpenter, MS, DVM, Diplomate ACZM

ENCEPHALOMYELITIS: HEAD TILT AND ATAXIA

Neurologic diseases are common in rabbits, and recognition of these conditions is becoming more frequent, in part because many pet rabbits are living longer. The causes of neurologic disease have been investigated more thoroughly in recent years, increasing our confidence in diagnosis and possible treatment. The most common causes of neurologic disease in rabbits are pasteurellosis and other bacterial infections, encephalitozoonosis, cerebral larva migrans, cranial or vertebral trauma, heat stress, and toxemia.

Signs of neurologic disease in rabbits include behavioral changes, head tilt (torticollis or wry neck), nystagmus, tremors, paresis, paralysis, and seizures. Head tilt usually is an indication of vestibular dysfunction, which can be central (cerebellum, brain stem) or peripheral (inner ear). Ataxia, paresis, and paralysis can also be caused by central (brain or spinal cord) or peripheral nerve disease. Subtle or overt behavioral changes, such as hyperesthesia, may be caused by central disease; seizures and rolling indicate brain lesions. Differentiation of the causes of encephalomyelitis is challenging. Sometimes more than one cause is present in the same animal.[12]

Otitis Interna

Head tilt resulting from otitis interna has often been described and associated with *Pasteurella multocida* infection. However, other bacterial agents may be the cause of otitis media or otitis interna in rabbits. Infection sometimes spreads from the middle ear to the ear canal (if the tympanic membrane ruptures); or to the inner ear, causing labyrinthitis; and sometimes to the brain, causing severe neurologic signs, including seizures. For a more detailed discussion of pasteurellosis and otitis media, see Chapter 17. Diagnosis of otitis media can be made radiographically (see Fig.17-2). In some cases, rabbits with severe otitis media may have soft tissue swelling at the base of the ear canal, apparently a result of buildup of pus within the ear. The diagnosis of encephalitis related to bacterial extension from the middle ear is made histologically (Fig. 20-1).

Treatment of otitis media and otitis interna should be long term, 4 weeks or longer. Antibiotics do not penetrate well into pus-filled tympanic bullae. We recommend chloramphenicol (50 mg/kg SC, PO q12h) or enrofloxacin (5-10 mg/kg PO q12h) and, if the tympanic membrane is ruptured, topical 0.3% gentamicin or 0.5% enrofloxacin/1.0% silver sulfadiazine otic solution (Baytril Otic, Bayer Corporation, Shawnee Mission, KS). In cases of severe disease, anesthetize the rabbit with isoflurane and gently flush the ear canal with warm saline solution by passing a small, $3^1/_2$-Fr red rubber catheter into the ear canal. Avoid flushing, however, when the tympanic membrane is ruptured.

Encephalitozoonosis

Encephalitozoon cuniculi infection is often associated with neurologic disease in pet rabbits. Rabbits with antibodies to *E. cuniculi* have been exposed to and probably carry the parasite, often as a latent infection, without signs of disease. Signs of neurologic disease caused by *E. cuniculi* include behavioral changes, head

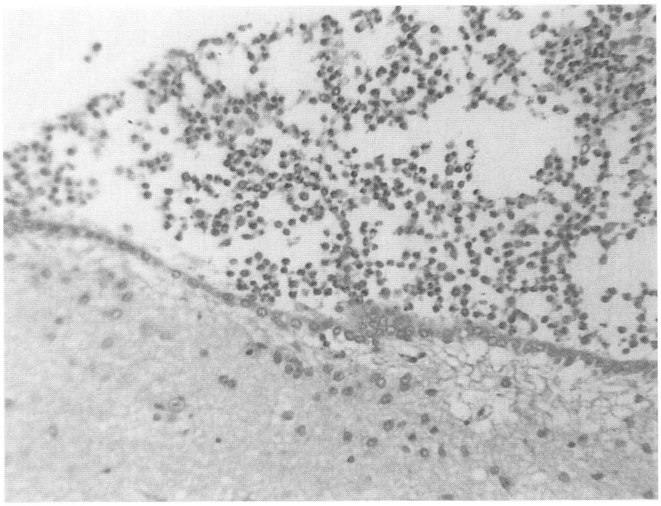

Figure 20-1 Photomicrograph of the midbrain of 1-year-old rabbit that died after a history of otitis media due to *Pasteurella multocida*. The diagnosis was severe suppurative meningoencephalitis with foci of gliosis in the midbrain, consistent with extension of bacterial infection from the ear. *(Courtesy Drs. K. Jackson and M. Garner, Phoenix Central Laboratory, Everett, WA.)*

tilt, nystagmus, ataxia, rolling, or seizures and often follow a stressful event in the rabbit's life (Fig. 20-2).

E. cuniculi is a microsporidian, obligately intracellular protozoan parasite. The infectious stage of any microsporidian organism is a spore (1.0-3.0 × 1.5-4.0 mm for mammalian species), which may be ingested or inhaled. The spore possesses a polar filament (tubule) through which spore contents are injected into a host cell, initiating infection. After entering a host cell, the organism divides within a vacuole. Eventually, infected cells

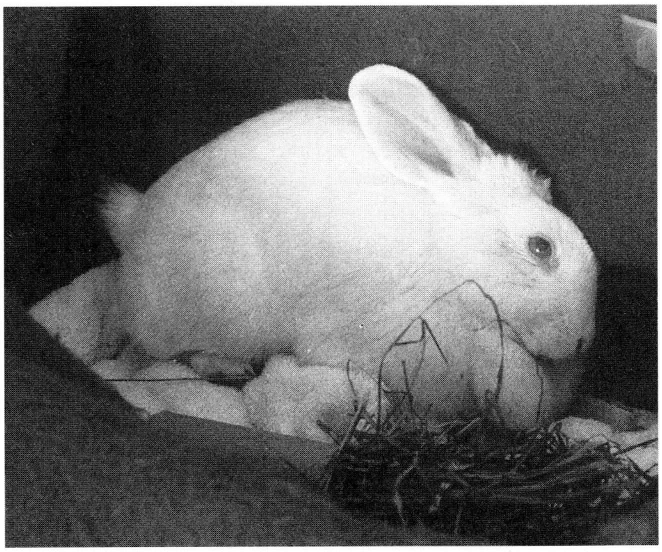

Figure 20-2 New Zealand white rabbit with severe head tilt and rolling caused by encephalitozoonosis. Note the padding in the small recovery container, which allows the animal to lean against a wall for stability and prevents trauma from rolling (see Fig. 20-4).

rupture, releasing spores that then infect other cells, are phagocytosed, or are shed in urine. Organisms are disseminated in the host by macrophages. Vertical transmission is possible.[4,9,24] Spores of *E. cuniculi* are environmentally resistant; dry spores can survive at least 4 weeks at 72°F (22°C).

In 1922, Wright and Craighead[26] first reported *E. cuniculi* as the cause of encephalomyelitis resulting in motor paralysis in rabbits. The organism was later shown to be a cause of head tilt.[16] In the acute stage of infection, lung, kidney, and liver are affected; in chronic cases, brain, kidney, and heart are affected.[7] *E. cuniculi* has been associated with myocarditis, vasculitis, and spinal nerve root inflammation in addition to encephalitis, pneumonitis, hepatitis, nephritis, and splenitis in rabbits.[20] Uveitis with lens rupture due to *E. cuniculi* infection has been documented.[22] Abortion and neonatal deaths have been attributed to encephalitozoonosis. Rabbits with this infection often are asymptomatic, but a wide range of symptomatology is possible, in addition to signs of neurologic disease.

The host responds to *E. cuniculi* infection by making antibodies, which are detectable in serum as early as 2 weeks before spores are detected in urine or tissues.[6] Antibodies peak and spores are excreted by 6 weeks after infection. The duration of excretion may be up to 3 months, and infection probably is terminated by humoral and cell-mediated immunity.[7] Offspring from seropositive dams have antibody up to 4 weeks of age, after which it diminishes. By 8 to 10 weeks of age, antibody titers rise and peak at about 14 weeks.[18] Rabbits naturally infected with *E. cuniculi* had depressed immunoglobulin G (IgG) and elevated IgM responses to experimental infection with other organisms.[5]

Immunocompetent rabbits develop chronic, subclinical infections in a balanced host-parasite relationship (e.g., focal granulomas in brain and kidneys). Antibodies contribute to resistance by inducing opsonization by macrophages and complement-mediated killing. Resistance is T-lymphocyte dependent; animals and humans with $CD4^+$ T-lymphocyte deficiencies are particularly susceptible to microsporidiosis, as are those treated with immunosuppressive drugs.[9] In the 1980s, microsporidial species were found to be associated with disease in human patients with the acquired immunodeficiency syndrome (AIDS).

Currently, the presumptive diagnosis of encephalitozoonosis is made on the basis of signs of neurologic disease together with demonstration of high levels of serum antibodies or demonstration of spores in affected tissues. Various methods are used to measure antibodies to *E. cuniculi* in rabbits. Enzyme-linked immunosorbent assays (ELISAs), indirect immunofluorescence assays, and carbon immunoassays are all suitable for detecting antibodies.[2] Using ELISAs, we (B.J.D. and associates) have demonstrated a significant correlation between high antibody levels and signs of neurologic disease in rabbits (Table 20-1).

Definitive diagnosis of encephalitozoonosis usually requires histopathologic examination. Typical lesions found in the brain are areas of multifocal necrosis, granulomas with perivascular lymphoplasmacytic cuffs, and lymphocytic meningitis (Fig. 20-3). Spores found in tissue are 1.5 × 2.5 mm in size. They are gram positive, stain deep purple with Goodpasture's carbol fuchsin, and are green birefringent when viewed with polarized light. The staining characteristics differentiate *E. cuniculi* from *Toxoplasma gondii*, which is gram negative, nonstaining with Goodpasture's carbol fuchsin, and nonbirefringent.

Benzimidazole anthelmintics (albendazole, cambendazole, oxibendazole, thiabendazole) are active against *E. cuniculi* in

TABLE 20-1

Antibodies against *Encephalitozoon cuniculi* in Pet Rabbits Detected by Enzyme-linked Immunosorbent Assay*

		Interpretation of Optical Density Readings			
		Positive		Negative	
Signs of Disease	Sample Size (*N*)	*N*	%	*N*	%
None	294	144	49	150	51
Head tilt, vestibular dysfunction	459	360	78†	99	22
Ataxia, paresis, paralysis	340	213	63†	127	37
Seizures	52	33	63	19	37
Intraocular lesions	55	41	75†	14	25
Renal signs	79	48	61	31	39

*Data were collected over 5 years on sera submitted by veterinarians in the United States; includes only samples for which clinical signs were listed. Tests were performed by Sound Diagnostics, Inc., 1222 NE 145th St. NE, Shoreline, WA 98155.

†$p < 0.001$.

vitro because of bioenergetic disruptions of membranes and microtubular (tubulin) inhibition of *E. cuniculi.*[10,19] Toxicity appears to be selective for parasites, with no toxicity for the host.[21] Fenbendazole was shown to be effective in preventing experimental infection with *E. cuniculi* and in treating infected rabbits.[23]

Albendazole (400 mg PO q12h) reportedly is the most effective agent against microsporidiosis in humans,[1] and it is thought to be better absorbed from oral administration than are other benzimidazoles. Disseminated *E. cuniculi* infection and renal disease in an AIDS patient were successfully treated with albendazole.[8] Dexamethasone was found to increase plasma levels of albendazole by 50%.[14] Although we do not know the permeability of benzimidazole anthelmintics through the blood-brain barrier, clinical response indicates that they do pass into the brain.

Our current treatment protocol (B.J.D.) for presumptive encephalitozoonosis is as follows: dexamethasone (0.1 mg/kg SC q24h, then at 48h for two more doses), chloramphenicol (50 mg/kg SC q12h × 7 days), oxibendazole (30 mg/kg PO q24h × 7-14 days). If the rabbit has been seizing or rolling, we give diazepam (0.1 mg/kg SC) as necessary. With this regimen we hope to control seizures, reduce inflammation, control potential bacterial infection (always a concern when giving immunosuppressive medications), and limit the spread of *E. cuniculi* organisms in the brain. If serologic testing shows high levels of antibodies to *E. cuniculi*, there is no evidence of otitis media, and the neurologic signs abate, the antibiotic is discontinued and the oxibendazole dose is reduced (to 15 mg/kg q24h × 30-60 days). In some patients, neurologic signs have abated during treatment with oxibendazole and recurred after the drug was stopped. These patients are continued indefinitely on oxibendazole (15-30 mg/kg PO q24h). Treatment of encephalitozoonosis is not always successful, but it has resulted in improvement in many cases (Fig. 20-4); lack of treatment more often leads to euthanasia due to severe neurologic disease.

Some veterinarians have had success with albendazole (30 mg/kg PO q24h × 30 days, then 15 mg/kg PO q24h × 30 days[22] [R. C. Gandolfi, personal communication, 2001]; or 10-15 mg/kg PO q24h × 3 months [C. Harvey, personal communication, 2001]). Fenbendazole (given in medicated feed to achieve a daily dose of 20 mg/kg for 28 days) was also reported to

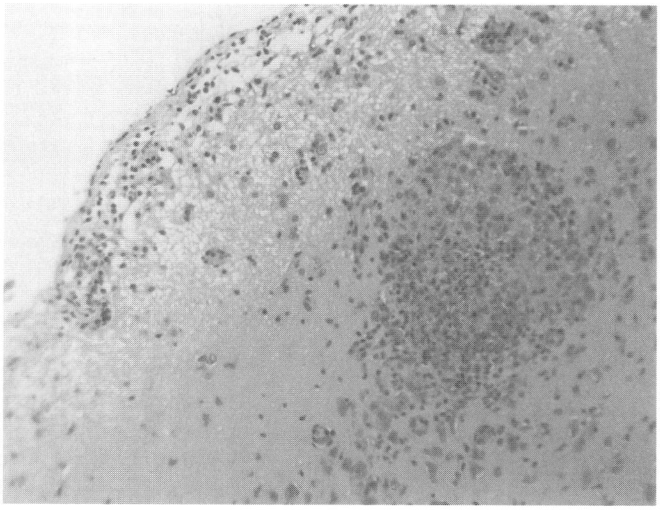

Figure 20-3 Photomicrograph of the brain of a 4-year-old dwarf rabbit that was euthanized because of severe neurologic disease. The diagnosis was severe nonsuppurative meningoencephalitis with microglial nodules and foci of mineralization. Extracellular gram-positive spores were detected within microglial nodules, a finding consistent with encephalitozoonosis. *(Courtesy Drs. K. Jackson and M. Garner, Phoenix Central Laboratory, Everett, WA.)*

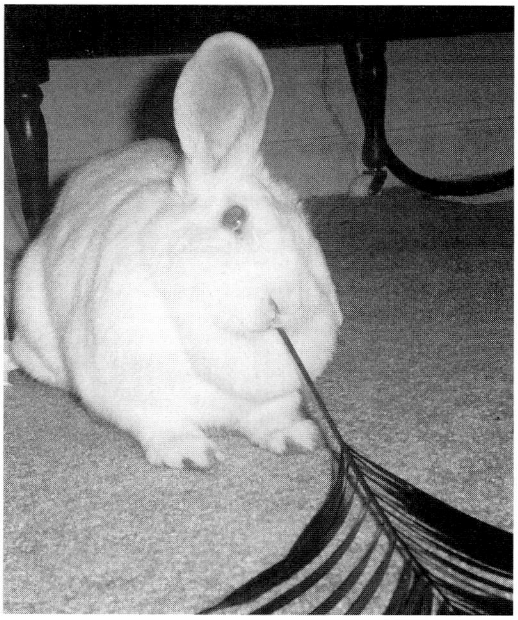

Figure 20-4 After 2 months of treatment with oxibendazole, the rabbit shown in Figure 20-2 still had a slight head tilt but was able to move about freely.

have eliminated parasites from brain tissue of infected rabbits.[23] Fenbendazole can also be given as an oral suspension to pet rabbits at the same dosage used for treatment of *E. cuniculi*.

Control of encephalitozoonosis may be most effectively done in rabbitries, where transmission usually occurs. The acute phase of the disease usually occurs in very young rabbits, and spores are shed in urine until antibodies are produced. Cleaning and sanitation are essential to limit transmission of this infection. Most disinfectants are effective at inactivating spores, including quaternary ammonium compounds, amphoteric surfactants, phenolic derivatives, alcohols, iodophors, and hydrogen peroxide. Feed medicated with fenbendazole may be useful in preventing the spread of infection in rabbitries.

It is possible to select *E. cuniculi* antibody-negative breeders and to develop encephalitozoon-free rabbitries. Even if transmission from rabbit to rabbit is prevented, the possibility exists of transmission of spores from wild rodents.

A simple test to determine whether rabbits are shedding spores in the urine is needed to clarify potential transmission duration time. This information could then guide recommendations of quarantine periods when new rabbits are introduced.

Cerebral Larva Migrans

Cerebral larva migrans due to *Baylisascaris* species is not uncommon in rabbits.[11] Signs of disease associated with cerebral larva migrans are tremors, ataxia, head tilt, and vertical nystagmus, progressing to falling, rolling, paralysis, seizures, and recumbency (Fig. 20-5). Swaying and falling are usually pronounced with cerebral larva migrans, whereas they are seen less often with encephalitozoonosis or otitis interna. Typically, an affected rabbit shows intermittent improvement, followed by more severe signs.

Wild and feral rabbits often present with signs of cerebral larva migrans. The history includes an "out of doors" living environment with possible exposure to eggs of *Baylisascaris procyonis* or *Baylisascaris columnaris*, the roundworms carried, respectively, by raccoons and by skunks. Raccoons deposit feces in or around edible vegetation, feed, hay, and bedding. Eggs in the feces may remain infective for 1 year or longer. Materials contaminated with *Baylisascaris* eggs are ingested by rabbits. Larvae are released in the intestine and migrate through the body; they seem to have a predilection for the central nervous system, causing encephalomalacia (Fig. 20-6). Destruction of brain tissue may be extensive, even from only a few larvae, and it is progressive as the larvae continue to migrate in the brain.

We have had success slowing the progression of presumptive cerebral larva migrans by treatment with oxibendazole (60 mg/kg PO q24h) indefinitely. Signs recurred and progressed when the drug was discontinued. Rabbits with severe posterior paresis can be fitted with an apparatus to permit movement (Fig. 20-7). Those rabbits that are most severely affected are probably best euthanatized.

Advise owners of rabbits to prevent cerebral larva migrans by eliminating access to feed and bedding that is potentially contaminated by raccoon feces.

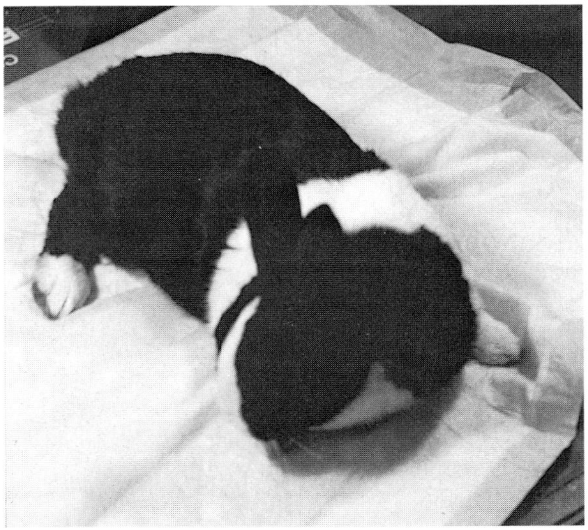

Figure 20-5 Dutch rabbit with clinical signs of cerebral larva migrans (i.e., falling, circling, and finally paralysis).

Toxoplasmosis

Toxoplasmosis is an uncommon cause of neurologic disease in rabbits. Signs include ataxia, tremors, posterior paresis, paralysis, and tetraplegia.[11] In most species, toxoplasmosis is often associated with immunosuppression. This disease can be differentiated from encephalitozoonosis by serologic testing and, histologically, by demonstration of gram-negative spores in brain tissue.

If toxoplasmosis is diagnosed, treat with trimethoprim-sulfa and pyrimethamine or doxycycline. Clindamycin should not be used because it causes dysbiosis and death in rabbits. Prevent toxoplasmosis in rabbits by preventing exposure to feed or bedding contaminated by cat feces.

Viruses

Rabies Rabies has been reported in rabbits, albeit rarely. Between 1971 and 1997, 30 cases of rabies in rabbits were

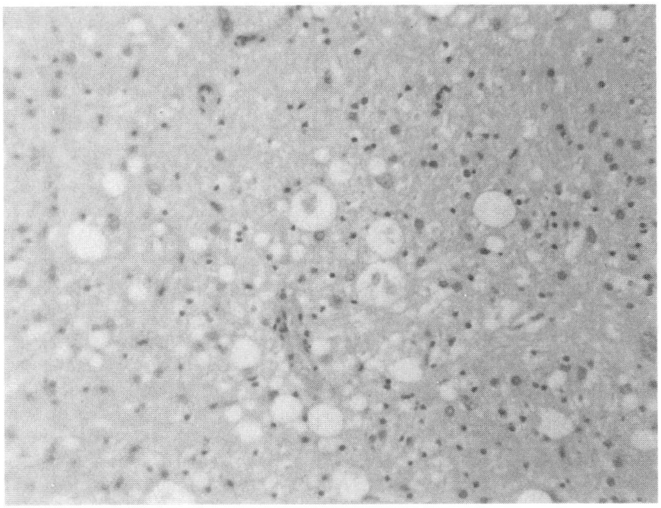

Figure 20-6 Photomicrograph of the brain stem of a once feral rabbit with severe neurologic disease, including seizures. The diagnosis was severe localized nonsuppurative, cavitating encephalitis, consistent with parasite migration (probably *Baylisascaris* species). *(Courtesy Drs. K. Jackson and M. Garner, Phoenix Central Laboratory, Everett, WA.)*

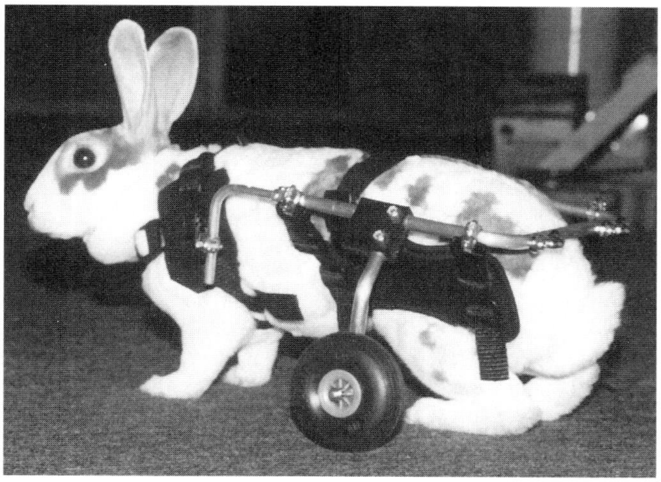

Figure 20-7 Rex rabbit (once feral) with presumptive cerebral larva migrans. It showed tremors and severe ataxia and was fitted with an apparatus permitting daily exercise periods. The rabbit received oxibendazole daily and remained in this condition for longer than 1 year.

reported to the Centers for Disease Control and Prevention.[15] Most of these were privately owned domestic rabbits located in states in which the raccoon variant of rabies was enzootic or epizootic. Rabbits usually develop the paralytic form of rabies. Early signs of rabies in rabbits may be nonspecific and include anorexia, fever, and lethargy.[15]

In one case, neurologic signs included blindness and forelimb paralysis and developed approximately 1 month after exposure. Because no rabies vaccine is approved for use in rabbits in the United States, pet rabbits housed outdoors should be protected from contact with wildlife, especially in areas where rabies is endemic or epizootic.

Herpes Encephalitis caused by herpes simplex 1 resulted in circling and spinning in a 1-year-old rabbit. The diagnosis was confirmed by histologic and electron microscopic demonstration of intranuclear inclusion bodies in neurons and glial cells. The virus was identified by immunocytochemistry and polymerase chain reaction analysis. The source of infection was suspected to be human contact.[25]

Stroke and Trauma

Cerebrovascular accidents have not been documented but often are suspected in older rabbits that develop sudden, unilateral loss of motor function. If other causes of neurologic disease have been ruled out, a diagnosis of stroke can be suggested. Supportive care allows recovery of function in many cases.

Although head trauma is probably not common, a head blow or fall can cause brain damage and neurologic signs that mimic those of encephalitis.

POSTERIOR PARESIS AND ACUTE PARAPLEGIA

Vertebral Fracture or Luxation

The most common cause of acute posterior paralysis is vertebral fracture or luxation (Fig. 20-8). Fractures are more common than dislocations. The most common site of fracture (or luxation) is the lumbosacral region (L7). This injury often results from improper handling, but it can occur in caged rabbits that are startled or frightened. Injury occurs when the heavily muscled hindquarters are allowed to twist about the lumbosacral junction, which acts as a fulcrum in applying leverage to the vertebral column.[11] In addition to paraplegia, neurologic signs may include loss of skin sensation and loss of motor

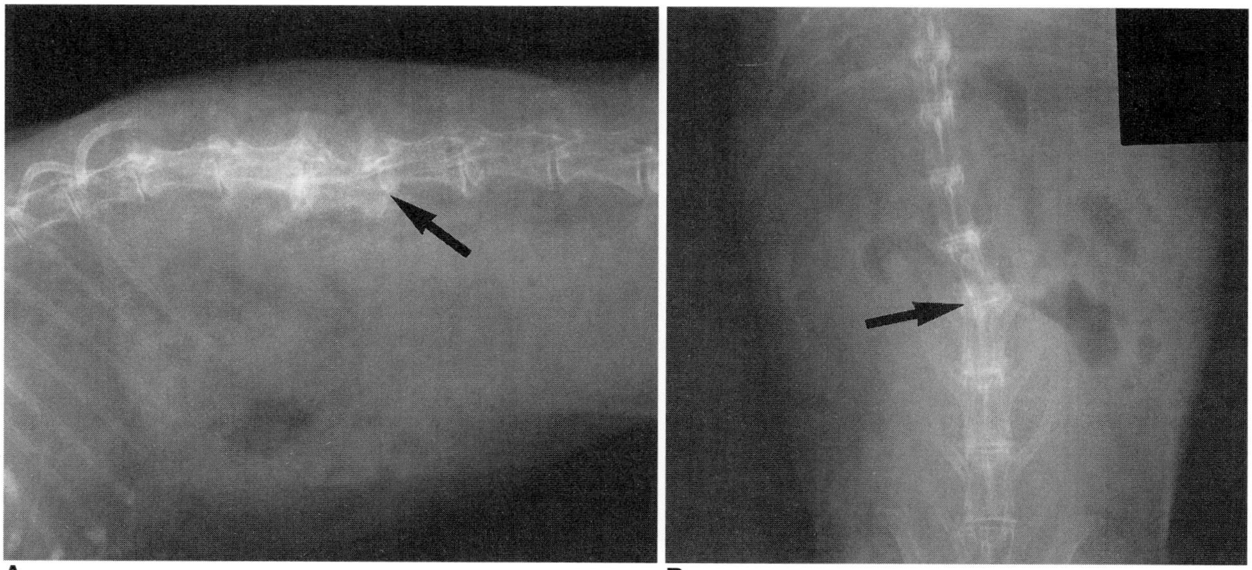

A B

Figure 20-8 A, Lateral and B, ventrodorsal radiographs of an 8-year-old mixed-breed rabbit showing a fracture and luxation of the spine at L3-L4 *(arrow)*. Intervertebral spaces L2, L3, L4, and L5 are compressed. The injury resulted from a fall.

control of the urinary bladder and anal sphincter, depending on the amount of compromise to the spinal cord.

The clinical diagnosis of posterior paresis or paralysis is confirmed radiographically. In acute cases, administer shock doses of methylprednisolone sodium succinate. If treatment is delayed, rabbits with broken backs can become azotemic or uremic because of retention of urine in the urinary bladder. Mildly affected rabbits may respond to conservative medical management, including cage rest for several weeks, if the spinal cord is not transected.

Supportive therapy must include manual expression of the bladder. Some rabbits tolerate the use of a cart to support the hindquarters and continue to lead a life of apparently good quality.[3] Medical therapy depends on the severity of the condition and usually includes administration of nonsteroidal antiinflammatory drugs as long-term antiinflammatory and analgesic treatment.[12]

Meloxicam (Metacam, Boehringer Ingelheim Vetmedica, St. Joseph, MO) is a useful product for long-term therapy and is now available in the United States. Carprofen (2.2 mg/kg PO q12-24h) is available and is helpful. Prednisolone (0.25 mg/kg PO q12h × 5 days) may be used. However, euthanasia is often indicated.

The extrusion of intervertebral disc material into the vertebral canal, particularly in the area of the lumbar spine, also can cause spinal cord compression and paresis. Both of these conditions can be prevented in a physically restrained rabbit by proper support of its hindquarters.

Spondylosis

Spondylosis is common in older pet rabbits. Owners typically report an abnormal gait or inability to hop or groom. Radiographs of the spine reveal spinal exostoses and degenerative changes (Fig. 20-9). Inappropriate urination or incontinence is often associated with spondylosis and results in urine burn in the perineal area. Treatment involves hygiene and antibiotics to control the dermatitis. Rabbits with pain and inflammation due to spondylosis often show remarkable improvement when treated with carprofen (2.2 mg/kg PO q12-24h).

Encephalitozoonosis

E. cuniculi has been associated with paresis (see above).

Splay Leg

Splay leg, a developmental musculoskeletal condition, occurs in pet rabbits ranging in age from a few days to a few months (Fig. 20-10). These rabbits may be unable to adduct one to all four limbs and therefore cannot ambulate effectively.[13] The condition may be relatively mild, allowing some clumsy movement, or so severe that the animal is completely paralyzed. The hind limbs are more commonly affected, with femoral neck anteversions, femoral shaft torsion, and subluxation of the hip. Because this condition is inherited in a simple autosomal recessive pattern, breeding from the affected animal and its parents should be discouraged. Although a few individuals recover some limb function, euthanasia is advisable for most.[3]

SEIZURES/COLLAPSE

Seizures in rabbits have a variety of causes, including encephalitozoonosis, heat stroke, pregnancy toxemia, hypoxia secondary to empyema, pneumonia, metastatic tumor, or azotemia and electrolyte imbalances associated with renal disease. Bacterial encephalitis, primarily caused by *P. multocida*, can also result in seizures in rabbits. Seizures are seen in the terminal stages of diseases such as hepatic lipidosis. Epilepsy is a rare diagnosis in this species, but it has been reported in blue-eyed white rabbits.

E. cuniculi can cause seizures resulting from an inflammatory response to rupture of brain cells.[12] The seizures are sudden in

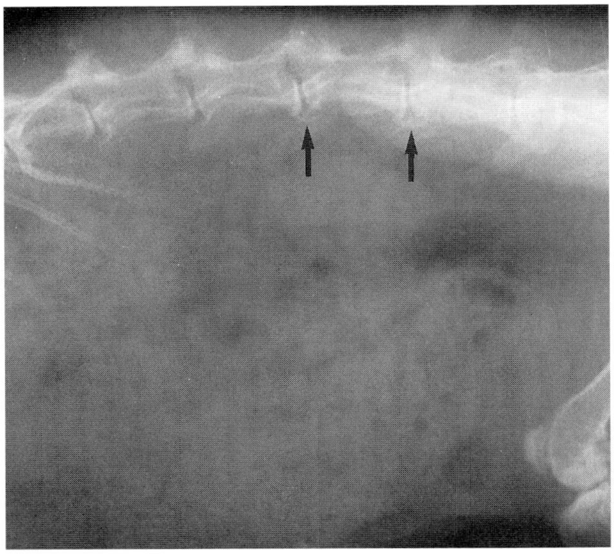

Figure 20-9 Lateral radiograph of a 9-year-old rex rabbit with spondylosis *(arrows)*.

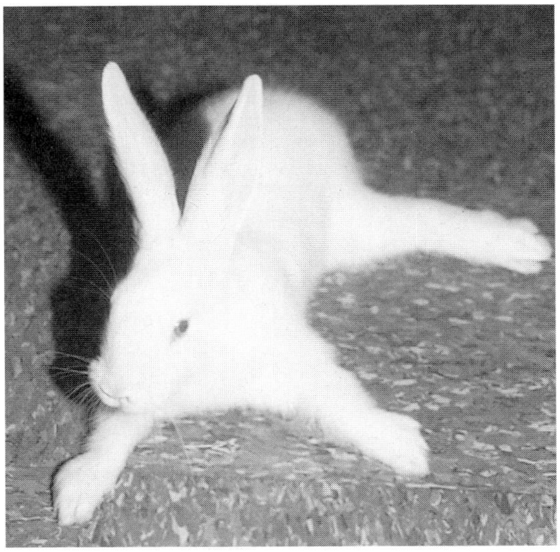

Figure 20-10 Splay leg in a rabbit. *(Courtesy College of Veterinary Medicine, Kansas State University, Manhattan, KS.)*

onset, and affected rabbits are sometimes left blind or comatose. Others recover completely.

Symptomatic treatment is similar to that in other species.[12] Diazepam or midazolam can be given intravenously, intramuscularly, or subcutaneously.

GENERALIZED MUSCULAR WEAKNESS/INCOORDINATION AND OTHER NEUROMUSCULOSKELETAL DISORDERS

Lead Toxicosis

Lead toxicosis can cause neurologic signs in rabbits, including seizures, although anemia, nonspecific anorexia, depression, loss of condition, apparent blindness, and gastrointestinal stasis are more characteristic. Signs result from oxygen deprivation and edema. Lead poisoning should be suspected in rabbits that have the tendency to chew or lick walls or metallic objects. Radiographs showing gastrointestinal metallic densities, the presence of erythrocytes that are nucleated or have basophilic stippling, and blood lead levels greater than 10 µg/dL are diagnostic for lead poisoning.

Treat with calcium disodium ethylenediaminetetra-acetate (CaEDTA, calcium versenate, 25 mg/kg SC q6h × 5 days). Two courses of treatment 1 week apart may be required. Plumbism can be prevented by reducing the exposure of rabbits to lead sources, such as old paints, lead toys, drapery weights, sinkers, battery plates, golf balls, improperly glazed ceramic dishes, plumbing materials, linoleum, tile, and lead smelters.

Heat Stroke

Rabbits are particularly susceptible to heat stroke or heat stress. Neurologic signs may resemble those of pregnancy toxemia, but no evidence of ketosis is present. Signs are accompanied by an elevation in rectal temperature to greater than 105°F (40.5°C). Treatment includes slowly reducing the body temperature by spraying the rabbit or immersing it in tepid water or wrapping it in cool wet towels. Give intravenous fluids and shock doses of corticosteroids if the rabbit is unresponsive; intubation and artificial ventilation may be necessary. Rabbits that recover from heat stroke should be monitored closely for several days for metabolic abnormalities or renal failure. Rabbits with heat stroke usually do not respond well, and the prognosis is poor. Pet rabbits housed outdoors during the summer, when the ambient temperature can exceed 85°F (29°C), require shade, good ventilation, and an adequate supply of cool drinking water.

Pregnancy Toxemia

Pregnancy toxemia can produce neurologic signs in rabbits. Although toxemia is primarily a problem of late gestation, it also occurs in postpartum and pseudopregnant does. Neurologic signs may include weakness, depression, incoordination, convulsions, and coma. Death may occur within a few hours after the signs are first noted. Obesity and fasting are predisposing factors. Treatment for the associated ketosis includes intravenous administration of lactated Ringer's solution and 5% glucose solution. Prevent toxemia by avoiding fasting and preventing obesity in pregnant does and by providing a high-energy diet during late gestation.

Nutritional Deficiencies

Nutritional muscular dystrophy in rabbits is caused by hypovitaminosis E and is characterized by degeneration and necrosis of skeletal muscle myofibers. Rabbits with vitamin E deficiency have increased plasma concentrations of creatine phosphokinase and cholesterol. Prolonged storage of feed adversely affects the vitamin E content. Feeding pet rabbits only fresh feed, or supplementing the diet with an alternative vitamin E source such as wheat germ, should prevent this problem.

Other neurologic and musculoskeletal diseases in rabbits may also have a nutritional base. For example, hypovitaminosis A causes a neurologic disturbance in rabbits that is characterized by circling, convulsions, opisthotonos, and paralysis. Hydrocephalus has been observed in young rabbits born to does with hypovitaminosis A or hypervitaminosis A. Convulsions can occur in rabbits maintained on a diet that is deficient in magnesium, and ataxia or muscular weakness may be a manifestation of hypokalemia. With the current rigid quality-control standards for commercial feed production, confirmed nutritional problems are relatively rare.

Other Causes

A variety of other conditions can cause generalized muscular weakness and incoordination, as well as other neuromusculoskeletal disorders in rabbits. Ulcerative pododermatitis is a relatively common musculoskeletal problem and is discussed in Chapter 19. Neurologic signs in rabbits have also been associated with trauma, cerebral accidents (e.g., strokes suspected in older rabbits), hypocalcemia in lactating does, neoplasia, listeriosis, and other infectious organisms. A variety of heritable disorders causing neuromuscular or skeletal diseases in rabbits have been reported.[17] These include hereditary ataxia (a glycogen storage disorder characterized by neurologic signs such as nystagmus, opisthotonos, and paddling), tremors, syringomyelia, and various skeletal deformities (e.g., achondroplasia).

REFERENCES

1. Beauvais B, Sarfati C, Challier S, et al: In vitro model to assess effect of antimicrobial agents on *Encephalitozoon cuniculi*. Antimicrob Agents Chemother 1994; 38:2440-2448.
2. Boot R, Hansen AK, Hansen CK, et al: Comparison of assays for antibodies to *Encephalitozoon cuniculi* in rabbits. Lab Anim 2000; 34:281-289.
3. Boydell P: Nervous system and disorders. *In* Flecknell PA, ed. Manual of Rabbit Medicine and Surgery. Gloucester, GB, British Small Animal Veterinary Association, 2000, pp 57-61.
4. Couzinet S, Cejas E, Schittny J, et al: Phagocytic uptake of *Encephalitozoon cuniculi* by nonprofessional phagocytes. Infect Immun 2000; 68:6930-6945.
5. Cox JC: Altered immune responsiveness associated with *Encephalitozoon cuniculi* infection in rabbits. Infect Immun 1977; 15:392-395.
6. Cox JC, Gallichio HA: Serological and histological studies on adult rabbits with recent, naturally acquired encephalitozoonosis. Res Vet Sci 1978; 24:260-261.
7. Cox JC, Hamilton RC, Attwood HD: An investigation of the route and progression of *Encephalitozoon cuniculi* infection in adult rabbits. J Protozool 1979; 26:260-265.
8. DeGroote MA, Visvesvara G, Wilson ML, et al: Polymerase chain reaction and culture confirmation of disseminated *Encephalito-*

zoon cuniculi in a patient with AIDS: successful therapy with albendazole. J Infect Dis 1995; 171:1375-1378.
9. Didier ES: Microsporidiosis. Clin Infect Dis 1998; 27:1-8.
10. Franssen FF, Lumeij JT, van Knappen F: Susceptibility of *Encephalitozoon cuniculi* to several drugs in vitro. Antimicrob Agents Chemother 1995; 39:1265-1268.
11. Gentz E, Carpenter JW: Neurologic and musculoskeletal disease. *In* Hillyer EV, Quesenberry KE, eds. Ferrets, Rabbits, and Rodents: Clinical Medicine and Surgery. Philadelphia, WB Saunders, 1997, pp 220-226.
12. Harcourt-Brown F: Neurological and locomotor disorders. *In* Textbook of Rabbit Medicine. Oxford, UK, Butterworth-Heinemann, 2002, pp 307-323.
13. Harkness JE, Wagner JE: The Biology and Medicine of Rabbits and Rodents, 4th ed. Philadelphia, Williams & Wilkins, 1995, pp 293-294.
14. Jung H, Hurtado M, Medina MT, et al: Dexamethasone increases plasma levels of albendazole. J Neurol 1990; 237:279-290.
15. Karp BE: Rabies in two privately owned domestic rabbits. J Am Vet Med Assoc 1999; 215:1824-1827.
16. Kunstyr I, Naumann S: Head tilt in rabbits caused by pasteurellosis and encephalitozoonosis. Lab Anim 1985; 19:208-213.
17. Lindsey JR, Fox RR: Inherited diseases and variations. *In* Weisbroth SH, Flatt RE, Kraus AL, eds. The Biology of the Laboratory Rabbit. New York, Academic Press, 1974, pp 379-382.
18. Lyngset A: A survey of serum antibodies to *Encephalitozoon cuniculi* in breeding rabbits and their young. Lab Anim Sci 1980; 30:558-561.
19. McCracken RO, Stillwell WH: A possible biochemical mode of action for benzimidazole anthelmintics. Int J Parasitol 1991; 21:99-104.
20. Nast R, Middleton DM, Wheler CL: Generalized encephalitozoonosis in a Jersey wooly rabbit. Can Vet J 1996; 37:303-305.
21. Russell GJ, Gill JH, Lacey E: Binding of 3H benzimidazole carbamates to mammalian brain tubulin and the mechanism of selective toxicity of the benzimidazole anthelmintics. Biochem Pharmacol 1992; 43:1095-1100.
22. Stiles J, Didier E, Ritchie B, et al: *Encephalitozoon cuniculi* in the lens of a rabbit with phacoclastic uveitis: confirmation and treatment. Vet Comp Ophthalmol 1997; 7:233-238.
23. Suter C, Muller-Doblies UU, Hatt JM, et al: Prevention and treatment of *Encephalitozoon cuniculi* infection in rabbits with fenbendazole. Vet Rec 2001; 148:478-480.
24. Wasson K, Peper RL: Mammalian microsporidiosis. Vet Pathol 2000; 37:113-128.
25. Weissenbock H, Hainfellner JA, Berger J, et al: Naturally occurring herpes simplex encephalitis in a domestic rabbit (*Oryctolagus cuniculus*). Vet Pathol 1997; 34:44-47.
26. Wright JH, Craighead EM: Infectious motor paralysis in young rabbits. J Exp Med 1922; 36:135-140.

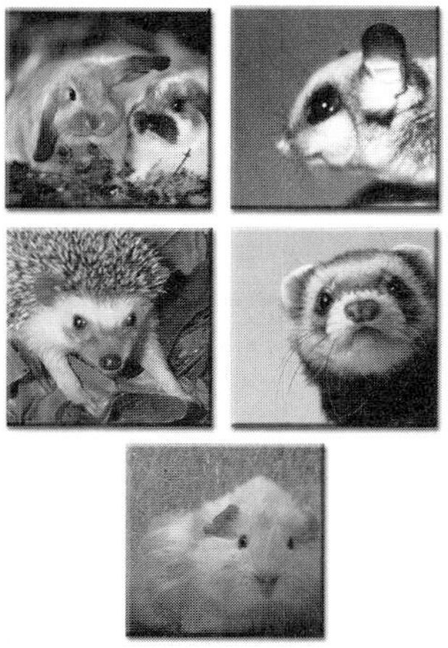

CHAPTER 21

Cardiovascular and Lymphoproliferative Diseases

Part I: Sharon M. Huston, DVM, Diplomate ACVIM (Cardiology)
Part II: Katherine E. Quesenberry, DVM, Diplomate ABVP

PART I **CARDIOVASCULAR DISEASES**

Sharon M. Huston, DVM, Diplomate ACVIM (Cardiology)

CARDIAC DISEASE

Cardiac disease has become increasingly recognized in domestic rabbits. Despite their frequent use as laboratory models for cardiac disease in humans, little is known about the pathogenesis and treatment of naturally occurring heart disease in rabbits. Reports of spontaneous heart disease are sporadic and case numbers are often low. Despite this, a complete cardiac evaluation and systematic approach can lead to a correct diagnosis and successful treatment of rabbits with cardiovascular disease.

Normal Cardiovascular Structure

The rabbit heart differs from that of other small animal species in several ways. The tricuspid valve is composed of two rather than three cusps; the aortic nerve is not associated with chemoreceptors but only with baroreceptors; and the rabbit pulmonary artery and its branches are heavily muscular.[6] Additionally, the myocardium has limited collateral circulation and is therefore predisposed to ischemia mediated by coronary vasoconstriction.[26]

Examination of the Rabbit with Cardiovascular Disease

Information gathered from a thoughtful history and complete physical examination comprise the most important part of the cardiac evaluation.

History A thorough general history, including husbandry, diet, and past or present illnesses, should be obtained for rabbits suspected of having cardiac disease. Tachypnea, dyspnea, syncope, anorexia, weight loss, and malaise may be signs of heart disease in rabbits.

Physical examination Take care to minimize the handling of a rabbit in cardiac distress; a complete physical examination and further diagnostic testing sometimes must be delayed until the rabbit is clinically stable. In rabbits suspected of having cardiac disease or respiratory distress, focus the initial examination on observing the respiratory rate and pattern, obtaining the heart rate and rhythm, auscultating the thorax, examining the mucous membranes, and palpating the pulses. Normal heart rate is 180 to 250 beats/min and normal respiratory rate is 30 to 60 breaths/min.

Rabbits with heart disease may have cyanotic or pale mucous membranes, arrhythmia, or heart murmurs. Rabbits with congestive heart failure often have tachycardia, tachypnea, and labored breathing. Pulses may be irregular or weak. Auscultating the thorax systematically is the most important part of the cardiac examination. It is important to listen over the entire thorax to localize heart murmurs and detect arrhythmias and lung sound abnormalities. A pediatric stethoscope allows better localization of heart sounds in rabbits and is preferred for cardiac auscultation; a larger-diaphragm stethoscope enhances auscultation of the lungs. Auscultatory findings vary among rabbits with congestive heart failure, and these findings are not pathognomonic. The examiner may hear muffled heart and lung sounds with pleural effusion and increased bronchial sounds or crackles with pulmonary edema.

DIAGNOSTIC METHODS

Diagnosis of cardiovascular disease is based on complete history and physical examination findings complemented by appropriate diagnostic tests. Thoracic radiographs, electrocardiography, echocardiography, and routine blood tests are useful in reaching a definitive diagnosis and treatment plan.

Radiography

Thoracic radiography provides critical information in the patient with cardiopulmonary disease, namely cardiac shape and size, pulmonary pattern, vascular pattern, and other thoracic lesions. Congestive heart failure and respiratory disease can be differentiated by evaluating thoracic radiographs. Radiographic findings supporting a diagnosis of cardiac disease are similar to those in other species and include cardiac enlargement, pulmonary vascular enlargement, pulmonary interstitial and alveolar pulmonary pattern of pulmonary edema, and pleural effusion. Figures 21-1 and 21-2 show thoracic radiographs of a normal adult rabbit and a rabbit with heart disease, respectively.

Electrocardiography

Electrocardiography (ECG) is a simple and practical diagnostic test in rabbits with suspected or confirmed cardiac disease. An ECG is critical to diagnose and manage arrhythmias or syncope. The ECG may also be a helpful addition to the cardiac database. To minimize skin trauma, file the alligator-style ECG clips. Normal rabbit rhythm is sinus and does not include respiratory sinus arrhythmia.[33] Recently, normal rabbit ECG values were determined in a novel study of 46 clinically normal domestic rabbits (B. Reusch, personal communication, 2003). ECG reference ranges are summarized in Table 21-1.

Echocardiography

Echocardiography provides a sensitive, accurate, and noninvasive means of assessing the heart. Most rabbits easily tolerate echocardiography, making it a practical diagnostic tool. Because of the rabbit's rapid heart rate and small size, optimal evalua-

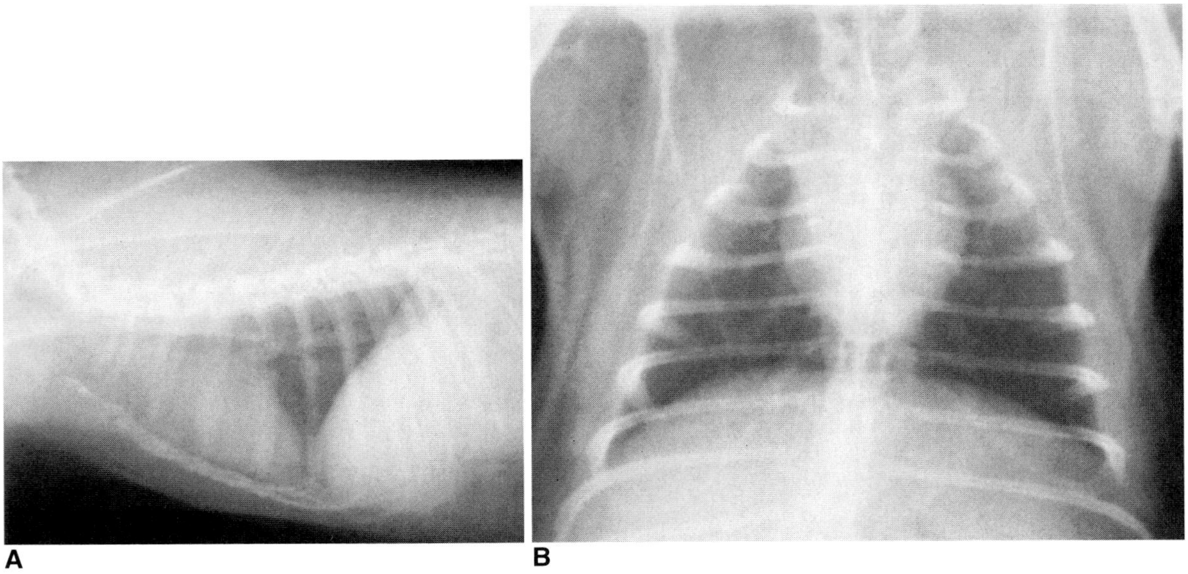

Figure 21-1 Normal thoracic radiographs of a rabbit. **A,** Right lateral projection. **B,** Ventrodorsal projection.

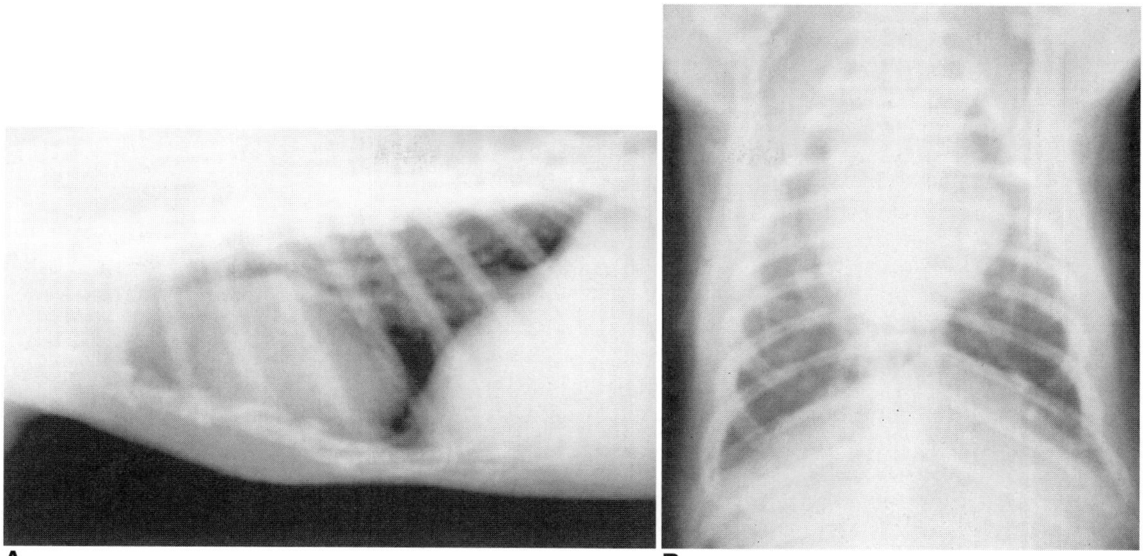

A B

Figure 21-2 Severe, generalized cardiac enlargement in a 9-year-old French lop rabbit. **A,** In the right lateral view, the cardiac silhouette is generally enlarged and can be seen throughout four intercostal spaces. The intrathoracic trachea and carina are dorsally elevated, and the main stem bronchi are compressed and deviated by an enlarged left atrium. The caudal border of the heart is rounded by left atrial and left ventricular enlargement. The cranial border of the heart is rounded, and the trachea is elevated cranial to the carina because of right atrial and ventricular enlargement. **B,** In the ventrodorsal view, an enlarged left auricle is evident as a bulge between the 2- and 3-o'clock positions. The left ventricular apex is rounded by an enlarged left ventricle. An enlarged right atrium is evident as a bulge between the 9- and 11-o'clock positions.

TABLE 21-1
Electrocardiographic Values in Clinically Normal Pet Rabbits

ECG Parameter	Values
Heart rate	198-330 beats/min*
Measurements (lead II)	
P wave	
Duration (width)	0.01-0.05 sec
Amplitude (height)	0.04-0.12 mv
P-R interval	
Duration	0.04-0.08 sec
QRS complex	
Duration	0.02-0.06 sec
R-wave amplitude	0.03-0.039 mv
Q-T interval	
Duration	0.08-0.16 sec
T wave	
Amplitude	0.05-0.17 mv
Electrical axis (frontal plane)	–43 to +80 degrees

From B. Reusch, A. Boswood, A. Petrie, unpublished data.
*This range should be used as a guide; lower values are expected in acclimated rabbits.

tion requires a high-frequency transducer and high frame rate ultrasound machine. Two-dimensional and M-mode echocardiography assess cardiac structure, chamber size, wall thickness, and motion, as well as extracardiac structures, masses, and pleural effusion. Color-flow and spectral Doppler echocardiography assess direction and velocity of blood flow, further defining cardiac conditions. Normal echocardiographic values have been published for several breeds of rabbits reported as study controls (Table 21-2). Sedative drugs used for restraint may affect cardiac measurements.

DISEASES AND MANAGEMENT

Congestive Heart Failure

In rabbits, congestive heart failure is the clinical condition in which pulmonary edema, pleural effusion, or hepatomegaly develops as a result of structural or functional cardiac disease. The goal of therapy is to relieve congestion, control future retention of sodium and fluids, and improve cardiac performance. To this end, numerous management strategies are used during the acute stage. Place the patient in a quiet cage with supplemental oxygen. Administer parenteral furosemide (1-4 mg/kg IV or IM q4-12h) and nitroglycerin 2% ointment ($^1/_8$ inch applied transdermally q6-12h). In a rabbit with pleural effusion, perform therapeutic pleurocentesis if the rabbit is dyspneic.

Long-term therapy of congestive heart failure should include a diuretic (furosemide 1-2 mg/kg PO q8-24h) combined with treatment directed at the underlying precipitating cause. Knowledge of the cardiac disease process is the basis of specific

TABLE 21-2
Echocardiographic Values in Clinically Normal Rabbits

Parameter	Dutch Belted Rabbits* (n = 6)	Japanese White Rabbits† (n = 4)	New Zealand White Rabbits‡ (n = 8)
Body weight (kg)	2.32 ± 0.36	3.0 (mean)	1.5-2.0 (range)
Age (mo)	7 mo (mean)	>13 mo	—
LVEDD (cm)	1.17 ± 0.19	1.69 ± 0.05	1.4 ± 0.2
LVESD (cm)	0.70 ± 0.09	1.15 ± 0.05	—
%FS	39.50 ± 5.39	—	—
IVSD (cm)	0.25 ± 0.05	0.33 ± 0.03	0.3 ± 0.0
LVPWD (cm)	0.31 ± 0.08	0.33 ± 0.03	0.2 ± 0.0
LA (cm)	—	1.05 ± 0.25	—
Ao (cm)	0.67 ± 0.10	1.07 ± 0.12	—
LA/Ao	1.38 ± 0.32	—	—
RADs (cm)	0.61 ± 0.08	—	—
RA/Ao	0.88 ± 0.17	—	—
EPSS (cm)	0.05 ± 0.05	—	—
MVEFS (mm/sec)	70.17 ± 31.82	—	—
RVOT velocity (m/sec)	0.83 ± 0.10	—	—
LVOT velocity (m/sec)	0.65 ± 0.14	—	—
LVET (sec)	0.08 ± 0.01	—	—
VCF (circumference/sec)	4.74 ± 0.45	—	—
MV E (m/sec)	—	0.44 ± 0.12	—
MV A (m/sec)	—	0.46 ± 0.17	—
MV E/A	—	1.0 ± 0.2	—
MV DT (msec)	—	41.3 ± 2.5	—

Values are mean ± SD.

LVEDD, Left ventricular *(LV)* end-diastolic dimension; *LVESD,* LV end-systolic dimension; *%FS,* % LV fractional shortening; *IVSD,* intraventricular septal thickness at end-diastole; *IVSS,* intraventricular septal thickness at end-systole; *LVPWD,* LV posterior wall thickness at end-diastole; *LA,* left atrium; *Ao,* aorta; *LA/Ao,* left atrium to aortic ratio; *RADs,* right atrial dimension in systole; *RA/Ao,* right atria to aorta ratio; *EPSS,* E point to septal separation; *MVEFS,* mitral valve E-F slope; *RVOT,* right ventricular outflow tract; *LVOT,* left ventricular outflow tract; *LVET,* left ventricular ejection time; *VCF,* velocity of circumferential fiber shortening; *MV E,* mitral valve E wave; *MV A,* mitral valve A wave; *MV E/A,* mitral valve E to A ratio; *MV DT,* mitral valve deceleration time.

*Data adapted from Marini RP, Li X, Harpster NK, et al: Cardiovascular pathology possibly associated with ketamine/xylazine anesthesia in Dutch belted rabbits. Lab Anim Sci 1999; 49:153-160. (Rabbits sedated with diazepam.)

†Data adapted from Saku K, Fujino M, Yamamoto K, et al: Cardiac function of WHHL rabbit, an animal model of familial hypercholesterolemia. Artery 1990; 17:271-280. (Rabbits sedated with xylazine and ketamine.)

‡Data adapted from Plehn JF, Foster E, Grice WN, et al: Echocardiographic assessment of LV mass in rabbits: models of pressure and volume overload hypertrophy. Am J Physiol 1993; 265:H2066-H2072. (Rabbits sedated with pentobarbital sodium.)

treatment of the underlying condition. Drug dosages for rabbits are not available for all cardiac medications, but drugs and dosages published for cats or ferrets may be successfully used on a milligram per kilogram basis. Angiotensin-converting enzyme inhibitors such as enalapril maleate (0.25-0.5 mg/kg PO q24-48h, begin q24h) may be beneficial in treating rabbits with congestive heart failure. Digoxin (0.005-0.01 mg/kg PO q24-48h) may benefit rabbits with mitral and bicuspid regurgitation, dilated cardiomyopathy, or supraventricular arrhythmia. If digoxin is used, monitor serum digoxin levels. During acute and chronic management, it is critical that clinical and radiographic signs, hydration status, appetite, and body weight as well as serum blood urea nitrogen, creatinine, and electrolyte concentrations are monitored.

Congenital Heart Disease

Congenital heart disease in rabbits is rarely reported. Ventricular septal defect, diagnosed with echocardiography, has been described.[35] A ventricular septal defect, pulmonary hypertension, and valvular cyst identified at necropsy have been described in a New Zealand white rabbit.[23]

Arrhythmia

Arrhythmias in domestic rabbits have not been reported. However, we have diagnosed arrhythmias in several rabbits that exhibited syncope and an irregular heart beat (Fig. 21-3). In a rabbit with an arrhythmia, base the treatment protocol on ECG

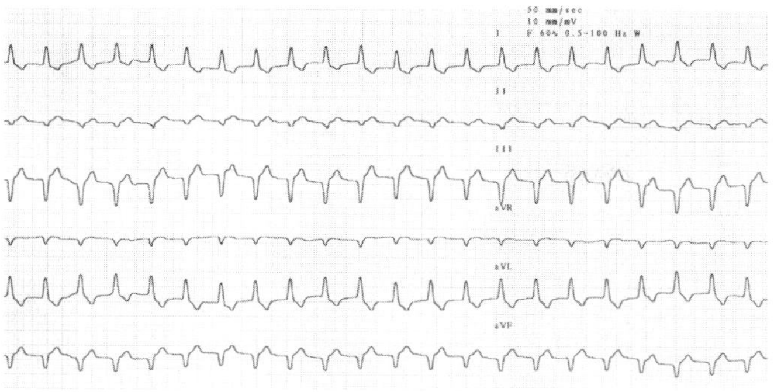

Figure 21-3 Six-lead, simultaneous electrocardiogram in a rabbit with ventricular tachycardia.

findings and clinical signs. Dosages are published for lidocaine, verapamil, atropine, and glycopyrrolate. Other antiarrhythmic drugs may be used at dosages published for cats or ferrets. In a controlled study, glycopyrrolate was more effective than atropine sulfate in increasing heart rate.[32]

Myocardial Disease

Numerous myocardial diseases have been reported in rabbits, and cardiomyopathy is a common postmortem finding in older rabbits.[35] Idiopathic hypertrophic cardiomyopathy and dilated cardiomyopathy have been diagnosed by echocardiography (Fig. 21-4).[33] Vitamin E deficiency produces a muscular dystrophy in which the myocardium may be affected.[3] In experimental studies, myocardial disease has been created through inoculation of *Trypanosoma cruzi*[36] and administration of doxorubicin.[44] Infectious myocardial diseases are rare in pet rabbits. Known infectious organisms include *Pasteurella multocida, Salmonella* species, *Encephalitozoon cuniculi,*[26] and coronavirus.[8] The alpha-agonist drug detomidine has been associated with myocardial necrosis and fibrosis in New Zealand white rabbits.[19] A similar ischemia-mediated process is suggested in association with ketamine/xylazine administration.[26]

Valvular Disease

Mitral and tricuspid insufficiencies are not uncommon and have been identified in pet rabbits.[33] A focal murmur is the most common clinical finding. Valvular disease is diagnosed with

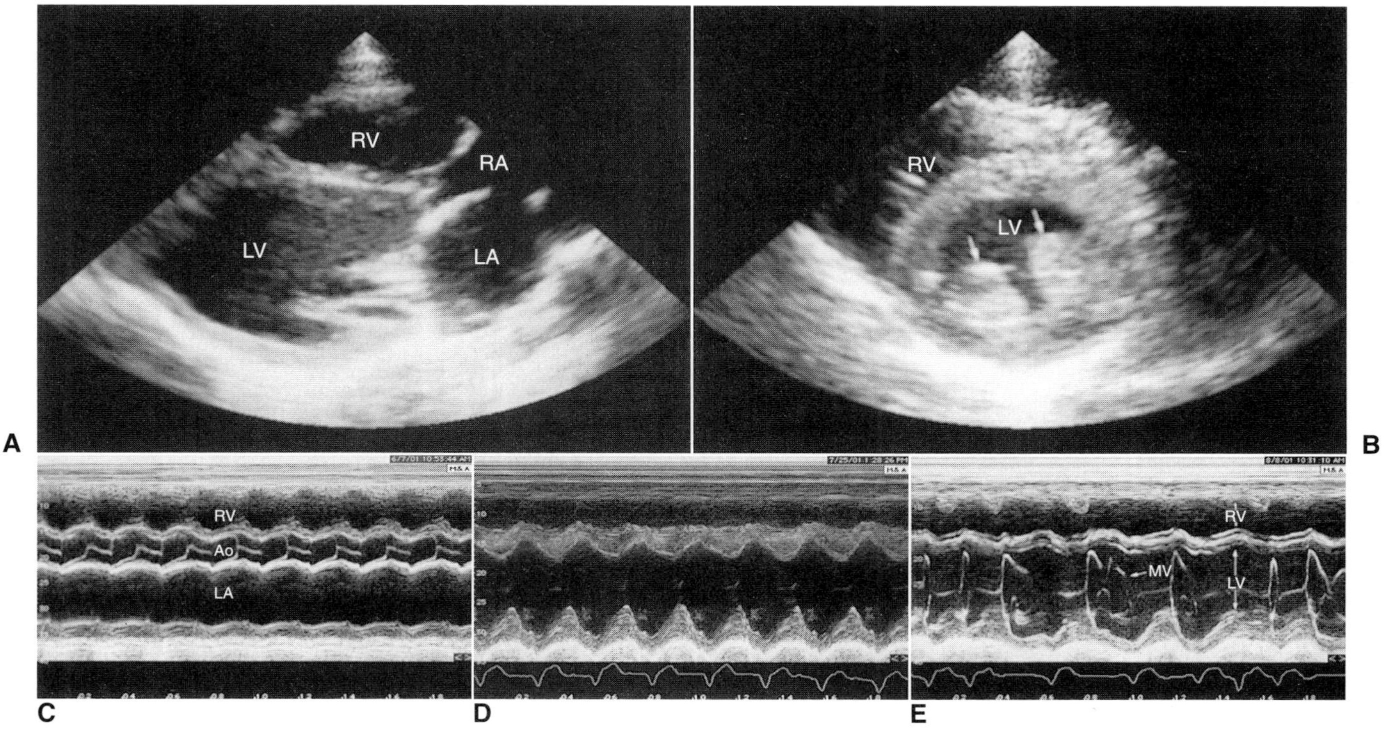

Figure 21-4 Standard echocardiographic views in rabbits with cardiac disease. **A,** Right parasternal, long-axis, four-chamber view. Notice the left and right ventricular dilation in this rabbit with mitral and tricuspid insufficiency. **B,** Right parasternal, short-axis, left ventricle papillary muscles view. Notice the prominence of the left ventricular papillary muscles (*arrows*) in this rabbit with left ventricular hypertrophy. **C,** Parasternal, short-axis M-mode echocardiogram in which the M-mode beam is directed across the right ventricle, aortic valve, and left atrium. Note the dilation of the left atrium. **D,** Parasternal, short-axis, M-mode view of the left ventricle in which the M-mode beam is directed across the right ventricle (*top*) and left ventricle (*bottom*). Notice the dilated left ventricle and the decreased excursion of the septum compared with the posterior wall in this rabbit with cardiomyopathy and ventricular tachycardia. **E,** Parasternal, short-axis M-mode echocardiogram of the left ventricle and mitral valve. Note the irregular rhythm. *LV,* Left ventricle; *LA,* left atrium; *RV,* right ventricle; *RA,* right atrium; *Ao,* aorta; *MV,* mitral valve.

two-dimensional and Doppler echocardiography (see Fig. 21-4). Echocardiographic findings most often include thickening of one or both atrioventricular valves, dilation of cardiac chambers, and turbulent regurgitation of blood detected by Doppler.

Valvular endocarditis, caused by *Staphylococcus aureus,* has been reported in rabbits.[40]

Vascular Disease

Spontaneous arteriosclerosis of the aorta and other arteries has been observed in nearly all rabbit breeds. Clinical signs, if present, may include lethargy, anorexia, and weight loss. The cause is unknown. In rabbits with spontaneous arteriosclerosis, arterial walls and other soft tissues mineralize; the aortic arch and descending thoracic aorta are most commonly affected. Radiopaque vessels, caused by calcification, may be visible on radiographs.[24,38]

Pulmonary hypertension associated with high altitude has been reported in a rabbit.[17] Lesions included right ventricular hypertrophy and pulmonary artery proliferation from hypoxia.

PART II LYMPHOPROLIFERATIVE DISORDERS

Katherine E. Quesenberry, DVM, Diplomate ABVP

Lymphoproliferative disorders are seen occasionally in pet rabbits. Before the 1960s, rare cases of lymphoproliferative disease in domestic rabbits had been reported in the European literature. In 1968, lymphoma was first reported in a domestic rabbit in the United States. In that report, generalized lymphoid neoplasia involving the lymph nodes, liver, spleen, lungs, and gastrointestinal tract was described in a New Zealand white rabbit from a research colony.[43] Since then, lymphoproliferative diseases have been reported in both laboratory and pet rabbits. Most of these cases have involved generalized lymphoma; however, cutaneous lymphoma, leukemia, and thymomas have also been described.

Rabbits are used extensively to study disease pathogenesis in experimental studies of induced lymphoid neoplasia. However, few studies have investigated the cause of naturally occurring lymphoid disorders in rabbits. In one of the first reports, lymphoma was described in a series of rabbits from a breeding farm,[25] leading to speculation that a breed or strain susceptibility exists or an infectious agent is associated with disease.[12,25,43] A strain susceptibility was demonstrated in Wirehair (WH) rabbits[12]; this susceptibility is associated with a single autosomal recessive gene, *ls.* In the WH strain, affected rabbits die at 5 to 13 months of age, usually with generalized lymphoma involving visceral organs and lymph nodes similar to the distribution of organ involvement seen in other domestic animals.[12] This pattern of susceptibility was also thought compatible with vertical transmission of a virus, as occurs with feline leukemia virus. Some have speculated that lymphoma in rabbits is caused by an oncogenic C-type tumor virus, similar to viruses associated with lymphoma in rodents. In an early study, tissues samples from an adult New Zealand white rabbit with generalized lymphoma were examined in an attempt to document the presence of virus.[42] Results of electron microscopic examination, tissue culture, immunodiffusion studies with FeLV antiserum, and immunofluorescent tests were negative for the virus. However, in another study, viruslike particles were demonstrated by electron microscopy in the kidneys of a 7-month-old New Zealand white rabbit with generalized lymphoma.[15]

TYPES OF LYMPHOPROLIFERATIVE DISORDERS

Multicentric Lymphoma

Multicentric lymphoma is the most common type of lymphoproliferative disease in rabbits. It has been reported in several rabbit breeds, including New Zealand white, Japanese white, Dutch, and Netherland dwarf rabbits.[5,16,39,41,42] A hereditary predisposition to lymphoma involving the *ls* recessive gene has been demonstrated in the WH strain of rabbits.[12] Clinically, lymphoma has been observed in a variety of rabbit breeds, including satin, mini lop, and tan breeds. Lymphoma can occur in rabbits of all ages, from animals less than 1 year of age to geriatric animals.* In pet rabbits with lymphoma seen at the Animal Medical Center in New York City, ages have ranged from 2 to 9 years, with most averaging 4 to 5 years.

Both T-cell– and B-cell–origin lymphoma have been documented in rabbits. In a domestic rabbit with lymphoma and lymphocytic leukemia, the neoplasia was of T-cell origin.[41] In a pet Dutch dwarf rabbit, T- and B-cell infiltrates were observed in the skin, lung, kidneys, liver, intestine, and lymph nodes. In this rabbit, the diagnosis was multicentric, T-cell–rich, B-cell lymphoma with cutaneous involvement.[14]

Rabbits with multicentric lymphoma often exhibit nonspecific general signs, such as anorexia, lethargy, emaciation, pallor, diarrhea, and rhinitis. In a 2-year-old rabbit seen at the Animal Medical Center, the presenting clinical sign was severe upper respiratory stridor. At necropsy, lymphoma was present in the nasal turbinates and sinus, stomach, liver, spleen, kidneys, lymph nodes, and bone marrow. Another rabbit with multicentric lymphoma presented with acute onset of hind limb paresis and gastrointestinal stasis. At necropsy, neoplastic cells compatible with large cell lymphoma (immunoblastic) were found in the spleen, kidneys, lungs, cecum, intestines, lymph nodes, and adrenal glands; no lesions were found in the spinal cord.

Laboratory findings depend on the organs involved. Results of plasma biochemical analysis may be unremarkable or reveal increases in concentrations of aspartate aminotransferase, creatine phosphokinase, blood urea nitrogen, and creatinine. Rabbits may be moderately to severely anemic[12,46]; in young rabbits, fluctuating and depressed hematocrit values were considered the best diagnostic tool for early identification of lymphoma.[12] In rabbits with multicentric lymphoma seen at the Animal Medical Center, most had hematocrit levels in the low normal range (30%-33%; reference range, 30%-50%[2]). The white blood cell (WBC) count is often within reference ranges; however, some rabbits with lymphoma have leukemia (see below). In young rabbits with multicentric lymphoma, high WBC counts were less frequent than a relative predominance of lymphoid cells, including immature and atypical cells, representing 80% to 90% of total WBCs. In an 18-month-old rabbit

*References 5, 12-16, 27, 39, 41-43, 46.

seen at the Animal Medical Center, the WBC count was 10,000 cells/μL, with 63% lymphocytes. Lymphoma was present in the bone marrow of this rabbit.

At necropsy, neoplastic lesions are commonly found in the gastrointestinal tract, kidneys, liver, spleen, lymph nodes, adrenal glands, gonads, and bone marrow.* Less common sites of neoplastic infiltrates are the auditory meatus, eye, and heart.[5]

Cutaneous Lymphoma

Cutaneous lymphoma can be either epitheliotrophic lymphoma of T-cell origin (*mycosis fungoides*) with a potential to metastasize to visceral organs, or visceral lymphoma with cutaneous involvement. Several cases of cutaneous lymphoma have been reported in rabbits.[18,46] In a 18-month-old Netherland dwarf rabbit with multiple subcutaneous swellings over the shoulders, cutaneous lymphoma was diagnosed by histologic examination of biopsy samples.[18] At necropsy, no gross or histologic evidence of lymphoma was found in any other organ system, and no viral particles were seen on electron microscopic examination of neoplastic tissue. In another report, three domestic rabbits were diagnosed with cutaneous lymphoma.[46] Two rabbits were young (7 months and 1 year) and the third was 9 years. One young rabbit had erythematous alopecia and hemorrhagic crusts of the chin and ventral neck. At necropsy, neoplastic lymphocytes were found in the skin, lymph nodes, and lungs. In skin sections, the lymphocytes infiltrated the entire dermis and into the epidermis. The second rabbit had bilateral blepharitis that was unresponsive to treatment. At necropsy, superficial and deep lymph nodes were markedly enlarged, and lungs had reddened areas. Lymphocytic infiltrates were found in the skin, lungs, liver, kidneys, and heart. In the skin sections, lymphoid infiltrates were primarily in the subcutis and deep dermis. The third rabbit had nonpruritic alopecia of the left lateral thorax. Cutaneous lymphoma was diagnosed by biopsy of a skin sample; in this rabbit, lymphocytes infiltrated the superficial dermis and epidermis. The rabbit lived for an additional year after diagnosis, with no response to treatment with interferon alpha-2b (see Treatment below). A necropsy was not performed. In all three rabbits, immunologic staining of tissue sections confirmed the lymphoma to be of T-cell origin.

In two cases of cutaneous lymphoma seen at the Animal Medical Center, both rabbits presented because of a subcutaneous mass. In one 7-year-old rabbit, cutaneous lymphoblastic lymphoma was diagnosed by excisional biopsy of a subcutaneous nodule on its dorsal neck. Three more masses developed within 1 month and were excised. The rabbit died 2 months after the first biopsy, and at necropsy, lymphoma was found in the cervical, mesenteric, and thoracic nodes. In a second rabbit, a large, hemorrhagic mass was present on the ventral thorax. This rabbit was euthanatized. On histologic examination, lymphoma involving the skin mass and spleen was diagnosed.

Leukemia

Three cases of lymphoblastic leukemia and one case of myeloid leukemia have been documented in rabbits.[5,10,28,41] In rabbits with lymphoid leukemia, WBCs have ranged from 30,000 to more than 100,000 cells/μL. In all rabbits with lymphoblastic leukemia, neoplastic cells were present in bone marrow, lymph nodes, and other organs typical of stage V lymphoma.

Thymoma/Thymic Lymphoma

Thymomas have been reported in three rabbits,[4,21,45] and we have seen three cases of rabbits with mediastinal masses confirmed as either thymoma or thymic lymphoma. Thymomas are composed of variable mixtures of lymphoid and reticular-epithelial cells. In some cases, the lymphoid cells are small, mature cells; in others, lymphocytes are pleomorphic with prominent nucleoli. Thymic lymphoma denotes lymphoma involving the thymus, with other organ involvement. However, distinguishing thymoma from thymic lymphoma clinically can be difficult.

In all reported and clinical cases, rabbits had a mediastinal mass identified radiographically (Fig. 21-5). In two reported cases and in two of the clinical cases, rabbits had exophthalmos. In these rabbits, eyes could be retropulsed with no evidence of pain, suggesting the exophthalmos was not caused by the presence of a space-occupying mass. Prolapse of the third eyelid was described in one reported case[45] and seen in one clinical case. These signs are consistent with a diagnosis of cranial vena caval syndrome caused by the space-occupying mass compressing the vessels of the anterior thorax and impeding vascular return to the heart.[4] Increased respiratory rate was reported in one rabbit[21] and seen in one clinical case. In one rabbit, hypercalcemia (14.7 mg/dL) was described as a paraneoplastic syndrome, similar to dogs with thymoma.[45] However, because the influence of diet and calcium metabolism on the serum calcium concentration in rabbits was not considered in this case, this conclusion is possibly erroneous.

In two of the clinical cases, rabbits with mediastinal masses also had high WBC counts. In these rabbits, WBCs were 42,000 and 18,000 cells/μL, with more than 70% lymphocytes. On microscopic interpretation of a blood smear of the first rabbit, the cells were characterized as small lymphocytes with cleaved nuclei and scant cytoplasm. A bone marrow aspirate showed no marrow infiltration, confirming the diagnosis of lymphoma. In this rabbit, cytologic examination of an aspirate of the thoracic mass was diagnostic of lymphoma. This rabbit was treated with radiation therapy. In the second rabbit, no further diagnostic tests were performed. Both rabbits were eventually euthanatized. No bone marrow involvement was found at necropsy in either rabbit. On histopathologic examination, the mass in the first rabbit was identified as a thymoma, not thymic lymphoma; therefore the final diagnosis remains in question. The second rabbit was diagnosed as thymic lymphoma.

In all reported and clinical cases except one, rabbits died or were euthanatized within 6 months of diagnosis. In one reported case, the thymoma was successfully excised; this rabbit was euthanatized 9 months after diagnosis because of recurrent appendicular neurofibrosarcoma.[4] In the third clinical case of thymoma, the rabbit was treated with a low dose of prednisone (0.5 mg/kg q24h), with no other therapy. After 1 month, the tumor had not changed in size. The rabbit was euthanatized 5 months later because of labored breathing and poor clinical condition. In the rabbit treated with radiation therapy, the tumor regressed; however, the rabbit was euthanatized 3 months after diagnosis because of lethargy and severe pleural edema. On histologic examination, the mediastinum was markedly fibrotic with

*References 5, 12, 16, 42, 43, 46.

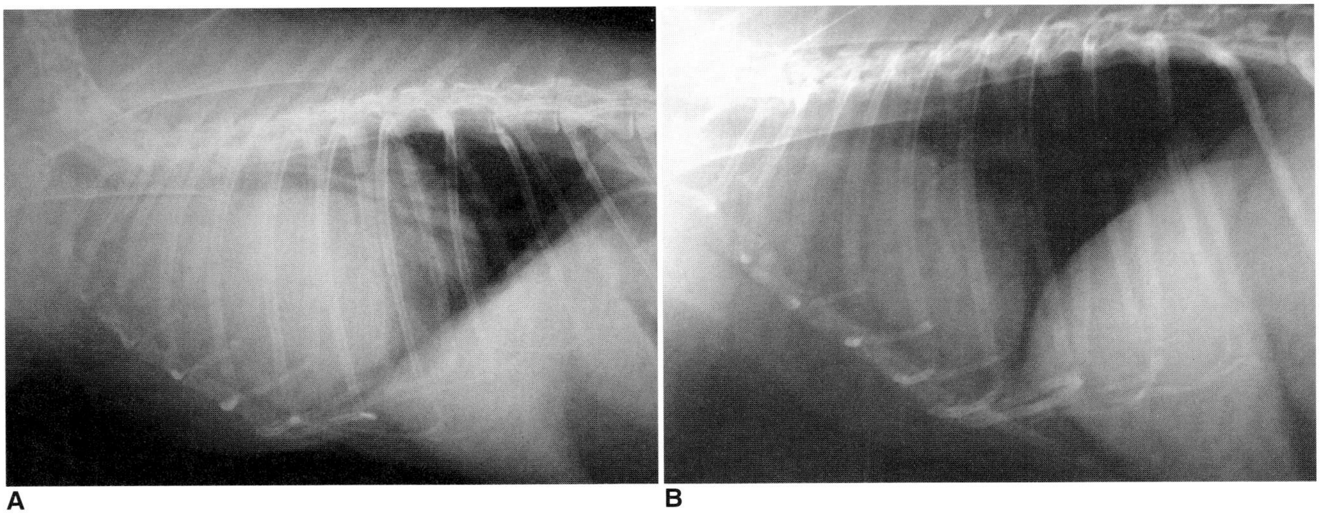

Figure 21-5 Right lateral thoracic radiographs of a mini-lop rabbit with a thymic mass, leukocytosis, and lymphocytosis. At necropsy, the mass was identified histologically as a thymoma. **A,** At presentation, the mass displaced the heart caudally. The normal cardiac silhouette is not visible. **B,** One week after the first dose of radiation therapy. The mass has regressed considerably in size, and the heart is in a more normal position.

sterile granulomatous inflammation and thrombi in mediastinal vessels. Chronic active pyelonephritis was found with numerous *E. cuniculi* organisms in renal tubular cells and lumen.

DIAGNOSIS

The diagnostic workup of a rabbit with a lymphoproliferative disease is similar to that of other small animals. If complete blood count (CBC) results reflect either a high WBC count with lymphocytosis or a normal WBC count with an inverse lymphocyte/neutrophil ratio, repeat the test to confirm the findings. If anemia is found on a routine CBC, consider ruling out possible lymphoma and perform additional tests. Submit a blood sample for a plasma biochemical analysis to look for evidence of multiorgan involvement. Take both thoracic and abdominal radiographs, and perform an abdominal ultrasound examination to visualize architecture of abdominal organs and to identify abdominal masses or enlarged lymph nodes. Submit a bone marrow sample for evaluation, and take a biopsy of any enlarged peripheral lymph nodes or subcutaneous masses. If a thoracic mass is present, perform an ultrasound-guided fine-needle aspiration if possible, and submit the sample for cytologic examination.

TREATMENT

Little information is available on treating rabbits with lymphoproliferative diseases. Much of this information is anecdotal, with protocols based on those used in other small animals. At best, the prognosis with treatment is guarded to poor.

Chemotherapy

Although much information has been published about chemotherapeutic agents in experimental studies in rabbits, only one report describes the use of chemotherapy in a clinical case. As mentioned, a 9-year-old rabbit with cutaneous lymphoma was treated with recombinant human interferon α_{2b} at 1.5 million units per square meter administered subcutaneously three times weekly.[46] After 1 month, no response was seen, and isotretinoin (4 mg/kg q24h on food) was added to the treatment for 2.5 weeks. After 2 months, no change was seen in the lesions, and all treatments were discontinued.

Anecdotal information is available on the use of doxorubicin in pet rabbits. One recommended dose is 1 mg/kg given intravenously over at least a 20-minute period, repeated every 3 weeks. The CVP/COP (cyclophosphamide, vincristine, prednisolone) protocol, with or without doxorubicin and L-asparaginase, has also been recommended.[31] We have used prednisone (0.5 mg/kg q12h for 28 days) in one rabbit that underwent concurrent radiation therapy (see below). This rabbit died with pleural effusion and severe *E. cuniculi* infection.

Because of the lack of information available on the benefits of chemotherapy in rabbits, the potential risks must be considered before treatment. In one study, rabbits that were experimentally infected with spores of *E. cuniculi* were treated with cyclophosphamide (50 mg/kg first dose, then 15 mg/kg weekly for a 12-week period). In these rabbits, clinical signs of encephalitozoonosis developed between weeks 4 and 6, and all rabbits died during week 6. No signs of infection were seen in control rabbits. These results indicate that immunosuppression induced by cyclophosphamide gave rise to lethal encephalitozoonosis. Most likely, the rabbit we treated with prednisone and radiation therapy also developed encephalitozoonosis because of immunosuppression. Other side effects can include severe anemia, enteritis, typhlitis, and nephrotoxicity. In an experimental study of rabbits given daunorubicin or doxorubicin at 3 mg/kg weekly for 10 weeks, cardiotoxicity was documented with daunorubicin but not with doxorubicin.[20] Both drugs produced hemotoxicosis manifested by aplastic anemia. Rabbits treated with doxorubicin exhibited more weight loss and had higher mortality rates than those treated with daunorubicin. A single dose of L-asparaginase at 10,000 IU/kg when given intravenously can induce a hyperinsulinemic, insulin-resistant, diabetic syndrome in rabbits.[22] However, in small animals L-asparaginase is currently given intramuscularly or subcutaneously; therefore route of administration may factor in toxicity. The neurotoxic effects of vincristine have been well studied in rabbits.[11,29,30]

Radiation

No reports describe the use of radiation in treating rabbits with lymphoid disorders. However, rabbits have been used in research studies regarding effects of irradiation on soft tissues.[7,9] We have used radiation therapy to treat one rabbit with a thymoma. The rabbit was given a short course of radiation treatment with 800 rad (8 Gy) per treatment on days 0, 7, and 21. The tumor was considerably smaller after the first treatment (see Fig. 21-5, *B*). However, 1 month after the final treatment the rabbit was euthanatized because of pleural effusion and poor clinical condition. As described previously, fibrotic tissue was found at the tumor site at necropsy, with thrombosis of mediastinal vessels.

Surgical Excision of Cutaneous Tumors and Thymomas

Surgical excision of thymomas has been described in two rabbits. In one rabbit, a right fourth intercostal thoracotomy was performed and the mass was excised. A chest drain was placed, but pneumothorax persisted after surgery and the rabbit was euthanatized.[45] In another rabbit the mass was removed by median sternotomy.[4] A chest drain was kept in place 24 hours, after which it was removed and the rabbit recovered uneventfully. When the rabbit was euthanatized 9 months later, no evidence of tumor recurrence was present.

REFERENCES

1. Bryan J, Olive G, Bergman P: Adriamycin dose, rabbits. Available at http://www.vin.com/Members/SearchDB/Boards/B0195000/B0192906.htm.Accessed May 30, 2003.
2. Carpenter JW, Mashima TY, Rupiper DJ: Exotic Animal Formulary, 2nd ed. Philadelphia, WB Saunders, 2001, p 423.
3. Cheeke PR: Nutrition and nutritional diseases. *In* Manning PJ, Ringler DH, Newcomer CE, eds. The Biology of the Laboratory Rabbit, 2nd ed. San Diego, Academic Press, 1994, p 328.
4. Clippinger TL, Bennett RA, Alleman AR, et al: Removal of a thymoma via median sternotomy in a rabbit with recurrent appendicular neurofibrosarcoma. J Am Vet Med Assoc 1998; 213:1131,1140-1143.
5. Cloyd GG, Johnson GR: Lymphosarcoma with lymphoblastic leukemia in a New Zealand white rabbit. Lab Anim Sci 1978; 28:66-69.
6. Cruise LJ, Brewer NR: Anatomy. *In* Manning PJ, Ringler DH, Newcomer CE, eds. The Biology of the Laboratory Rabbit, 2nd ed. San Diego, Academic Press, 1994, p 56.
7. Danielsson M, Engfeldt B, Larsson B, et al: Effects of therapeutic proton doses on healthy organs in the neck, chest, and upper abdomen of the rabbit. Acta Radiol Ther Phys Biol 1971; 10:215-224.
8. DiGiacoma RF, Mare CJ: Viral diseases. *In* Manning PJ, Ringler DH, Newcomer CE, eds. The Biology of the Laboratory Rabbit, 2nd ed. San Diego, Academic Press, 1994, pp 190-192.
9. Engfeldt B, Larsson B, Naeslund C, et al: Effect of single dose or fractionated proton irradiation on pulmonary tissue and Vx2 carcinoma in lung of rabbit. Acta Radiol Ther Phys Biol 1971; 10:298-310.
10. Finnie JW, Bostock WDE, Walden NB: Lymphoblastic leukaemia in a rabbit: A case report. Lab Anim 1980; 14:49-51.
11. Fiori MG, Schiavinato A, Lini E, et al: Peripheral neuropathy induced by intravenous administration of vincristine sulfate in the rabbit. An ultrastructural study. Toxicol Pathol 1995; 23:248-255.
12. Fox RR, Meier H, Crary DD, et al: Lymphosarcoma in the rabbit: genetics and pathology. J Nat Cancer Inst 1970; 45:719-729.
13. Fox RR, Norberg RF, Meier H: Clinical hematological progression of hereditary lymphosarcoma in rabbits. J Hered 1976; 67:376-380.
14. Gomez L, Gazquez A, Roncero V, et al: Lymphoma in a rabbit: histopathological and immunohistochemical findings. J Small Anim Pract 2002; 43:224-226.
15. Gupta BN: Lymphosarcoma in a rabbit. Am J Vet Res 1976; 37:841-843.
16. Hayden DW: Generalized lymphosarcoma in a juvenile rabbit: a case report. Cornell Vet 1970; 60:73-82.
17. Heath D, Williams D, Rios-Dalenz J, et al: Pulmonary vascular disease in a rabbit at high altitude. Int J Biometeorol 1990; 34:20-23.
18. Hinton H, Regan M: Cutaneous lymphoma in a rabbit. Vet Rec 1978; 103:140-141.
19. Hurley RJ, Marini RP, Avison DL, et al: Evaluation of detomidine anesthetic combinations in the rabbit. Lab Anim Sci 1994; 44:472-478.
20. Klimtova I, Simunek T, Mazurova Y, et al: Comparative study of chronic toxic effects of daunorubicin and doxorubicin in rabbits. Hum Exp Toxicol 2002; 21:649-657.
21. Kostolich M, Panciera RJ: Thymoma in a domestic rabbit. Cornell Vet 1992; 82:125-129.
22. Lavine RL, Dicintio DM: L-Asparaginase-induced diabetes mellitus in rabbits. Diabetes 1980; 29:528-531.
23. Li X, Murphy JC, Lipman NS: Eisenmenger's syndrome in a New Zealand white rabbit. Lab Anim Sci 1995; 45:618-620.
24. Lindsey JR, Fox RR: Inherited diseases and variations. *In* Manning PJ, Ringler DH, Newcomer CE, eds. The Biology of the Laboratory Rabbit, 2nd ed. San Diego, Academic Press, 1994, p 311.
25. Loliger H: Ueber das vorkommen von leukosen beim kaninchen. Berlin u Munchen Tierarztl Wchnschr 1966; 79:192.
26. Marini RP, Li X, Harpster NK, et al: Cardiovascular pathology possibly associated with ketamine/xylazine anesthesia in Dutch belted rabbits. Lab Anim Sci 1999; 49:153-160.
27. Meier H, Fox RR: Hereditary lymphosarcoma in WH rabbits and hereditary hemolytic anemia associated with thymoma in strain X rabbits. Bibl Haematol 1973; 39:72-92.
28. Meier H, Fox RR, Crary DD: Myeloid leukemia in the rabbit (*Oryctolagus cuniculus*). Cancer Res 1972; 32:1785-1787.
29. Muzylak M, Maslinska D: Neurotoxic effect of vincristine on ultrastructure of hypothalamus in rabbits. Folia Histochem Cytobiol 1992; 30:113-117.
30. Ogawa T, Mimura Y, Kato H, et al: The usefulness of rabbits as an animal model for the neuropathological assessment of neurotoxicity following the administration of vincristine. Neurotoxicology 2000; 21:501-511.
31. Ogilvie G, Bennett A, Bergman P. Cutaneous lymphoma in rabbits. Available at http://www.vin.com/Members/SearchDB/Boards/B0047500/B0046942.htm. Accessed May 30, 2003.
32. Olson ME, Vizzutti D, Morck DW, et al: The parasympathetic effects of atropine sulfate and glycopyrrolate in rats and rabbits. Can J Vet Res 1994; 58:254-258.
33. Orcutt CJ: Cardiac and respiratory disease in rabbits. 2000 Proceedings of British Veterinary Zoological Society. Autumn meeting, 2000, pp 68-73.

34. Plehn JF, Foster E, Grice WN, et al: Echocardiographic assessment of LV mass in rabbits: models of pressure and volume overload hypertrophy. Am J Physiol 1993; 265:H2066-H2072.
35. Redrobe S: Imaging techniques in small mammals. Semin Avian Exotic Pet Med 2001; 10:195.
36. Rossi MA: Microvascular changes as a cause of chronic cardiomyopathy in Chagas' disease. Am Heart J 1990; 120:233-236.
37. Saku K, Fujino M, Yamamoto K, et al: Cardiac function of WHHL rabbit, an animal model of familial hypercholesterolemia. Artery 1990; 17:271-280.
38. Shell LG, Saunders G: Arteriosclerosis in a rabbit. J Am Vet Med Assoc 1989; 194:679-680.
39. Shibuya K, Tajima M, Kanai K, et al: Spontaneous lymphoma in a Japanese white rabbit. J Vet Med Sci 1999; 61:1327-1329.
40. Snyder SB, Fox JG, Campbell LH, et al: Disseminated staphylococcal disease in laboratory rabbits (*Oryctolagus cuniculus*). Lab Anim Sci 1976; 26:86-88.
41. Toth LA, Olson GA, Wilson E, et al: Lymphocytic leukemia and lymphosarcoma in a rabbit. J Am Vet Med Assoc 1990; 197:627-629.
42. Ubertini TR: Brief communication: etiological study of a lymphosarcoma in a domestic rabbit. J Natl Cancer Inst 1972; 48:1507-1511.
43. Van Kampen KR: Lymphosarcoma in the rabbit. A case report and general review. Cornell Vet 1968; 58:121-128.
44. Van Vleet JF, Ferrans VJ: Clinical and pathologic features of chronic adriamycin toxicosis in rabbits. Am J Vet Res 1980; 41:1462-1469.
45. Vernau KM, Grahn BH, Clarke-Scott HA, et al: Thymoma in a geriatric rabbit with hypercalcemia and periodic exophthalmos. J Am Vet Med Assoc 1995; 206:820-822.
46. White SD, Campbell T, Logan A, et al: Lymphoma with cutaneous involvement in three domestic rabbits (*Oryctolagus cuniculus*). Vet Dermatol 2000; 11:61-67.

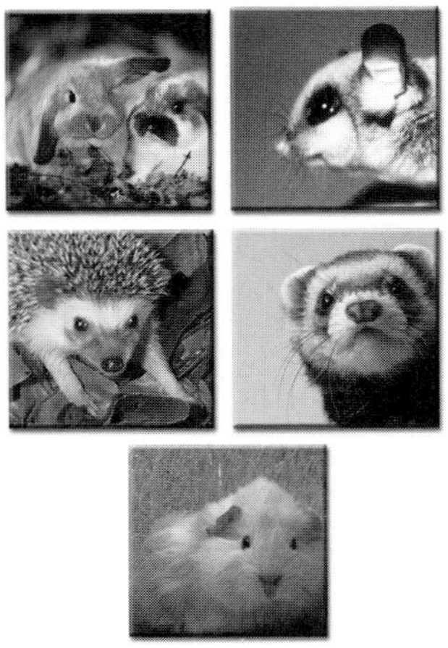

CHAPTER 22

Soft Tissue Surgery

Jeffrey R. Jenkins, DVM, Diplomate ABVP

The intrinsic physiologic and anatomic differences between rabbits and species that are more familiar to veterinarians are substantial. Rabbit behavior, such as reaction to stress and pain and poor acceptance of sutures, dressings, and coaptation devices, is unlike that of other pets.

The behavior of rabbits has a strong influence on their suitability as candidates for surgery. Rabbits are timid and submissive. Rabbits may become anorectic, even to the point of starvation, after a surgical procedure. Rabbits are fractious and may struggle violently if frightened while restrained, resulting in a fractured limb or spine. A frightened rabbit may have very high circulating catecholamine concentrations, which could seriously affect anesthesia. Rabbits are fastidious about their grooming, and this behavior, combined with finely honed incisors, makes it challenging to maintain sutures and dressings after surgery.

The rabbit is a highly specialized herbivore with a posterior fermentation-type of digestive strategy. A highly complex population of gastrointestinal microflora is responsible for normal digestion. The intricate relationship between the microflora and gut motility is affected by several factors, including diet, antibiotics, and stress. The rabbit has both incisors and cheek teeth that grow continuously, which may lead to problems of malocclusion. The oral cavity is long and curved and opens only a few centimeters, which makes intubation difficult. The stomach pH is significantly more acidic than that of a dog or cat. The small intestine of the rabbit has a small luminal diameter and a relatively thick visceral wall. The caudal end of the ileum is modified to form a round, muscular enlargement called the sacculus rotundus, which helps direct ingested material into the cecum or colon. This is a common site of foreign body impaction and a very important structure in normal digestive tract function (Fig. 22-1). The rabbit's cecum is a large, blind-ended sac with a terminal appendix. It is the primary site of fermentation in rabbits and is important in their digestive physiology. The serous membranes of the cecum are extremely thin and delicate compared with those of other sections of the bowel and may tear easily when handled or sutured. The colon has an upper sacculated portion and a lower nonsacculated portion. The sacculated portion of the colon terminates in a highly innervated, conical section located at the root of the mesentery called the fusi coli. This is the most common location for lower-bowel foreign body obstructions

EVALUATION OF THE RABBIT AS A SURGICAL PATIENT

Complete a thorough history, including signalment, diet and appetite, and a complete physical examination, including state of hydration and presence of infection, before surgery. Addressing preexisting problems improves a patient's prognosis for a successful surgery. Make an attempt, through discussion with the owner, observation of the animal, and evaluation of clinical data, to assess the level of stress that the animal is experiencing. Sometimes it is advantageous to postpone surgery until the animal has adapted to its new situation.

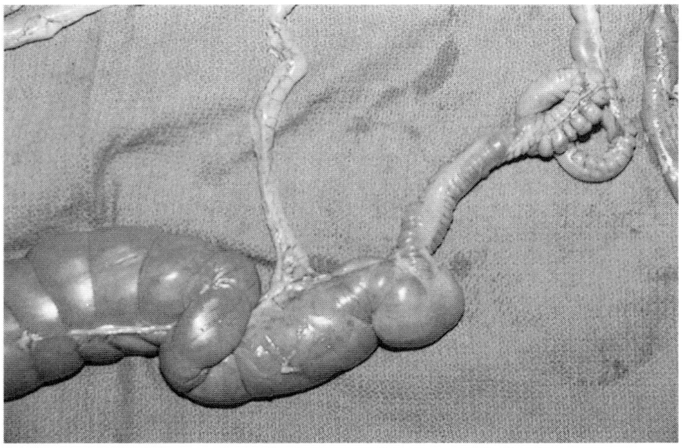

Figure 22-1 The caudal end of the ileum of the rabbit is modified to form a round, muscular enlargement called the sacculus rotundus, which is a common site of foreign body impaction.

EQUIPMENT

Little specialized equipment is required for surgery in rabbits. Appropriately sized Cole-style endotracheal tubes and a short, narrow laryngoscope, or an open-style otoscope and a rigid plastic catheter, are helpful for intubating the rabbit (see Chapter 33 for other intubation techniques). Equipment to monitor heart rate should be capable of measuring rates of 350 to 400 beats/min. A heated surgery table or circulating water blanket, as well as a source of radiant heat at locations where the patient is anesthetized and a device to accurately monitor body temperature, are necessary during long procedures on small patients.

Small (human infant) Balfour retractors enhance abdominal exposure, and malleable retractors serve well to hold viscera out of the way without removing them from the abdomen. An assortment of sterilized stainless steel spoons of various sizes is helpful in removing the stomach contents during gastric exploratory surgery, and mechanical suction is helpful for surgery of the gastrointestinal tract. Skin staples work well for skin closure and cannot be removed by most rabbits.

Vascular clamps (Acland Clinical Microvascular Clamps, S & T Microlab, AG, Neuhausen am Rheinfall, Switzerland; distributed in the USA by Fine Science Tools, Foster City, CA) are used to occlude the flow of blood from vessels during vascular surgery. Microvascular clamps are small, are designed to be used in areas where access is limited, are resistant to slippage, and can withstand pressures of blood flow. Clamp pressure is important when selecting a vascular clamp and is determined by the clamp's closing force (in grams) divided by the area of the wall (vessel or intestine) being compressed between the jaws of the clamp (in square millimeters); the smaller the compressed area, the greater the pressure. These clamps have proved to be safe and effective for occluding blood vessels and have also been used to occlude small-diameter loops of intestine.

PRESURGICAL TREATMENT

I provide food (hay) and water to rabbits up until the time of surgery, although many recommend a fast of more than 6 hours before surgery. Although some authors have suggested that a large volume of food in the rabbit's stomach can cause variations in anesthetic doses,[3] we have not experienced complications from this practice. Begin antibiotic therapy in rabbits with systemic or localized bacterial infections, such as those with upper respiratory tract infections caused by *Pasteurella* species ("snuffles") or with infected wounds. Prophylactic antibiotics may be given if there is a significant chance of bacterial contamination during surgery. Quinolones, trimethoprim-sulfa combinations, sulfa drugs, and aminoglycosides generally do not affect the normal cecal-colic microflora of rabbits. Use caution with β-lactams, macrolides, and other antibiotics that target gram-positive or anaerobic bacteria.

Parenteral fluids are not indicated in routine procedures. When supportive fluid therapy or vascular access is needed, a 20- to 26-gauge indwelling catheter is placed in the cephalic or lateral saphenous vein. Peripheral catheters work well during surgery and in the immediate recovery period. However, some rabbits do not tolerate a catheter when awake and need to have an Elizabethan collar, or the catheter and intravenous line may be covered with split-loom tubing or heavily bandaged to keep the rabbit from chewing on them. Alternatively, an intraosseous catheter may be placed within the greater trochanter. Moving the intravenous line away from the face results in better tolerance in some rabbits (Fig. 22-2).

Steroids are administered only if indicated by the underlying disease process; they usually are not given for routine or elective surgery. Give atropine when indicated (0.1-0.2 mg/kg SC or IM; see also Chapter 33) or glycopyrrolate (0.01-0.02 mg/kg SC) to control bradycardia, salivation, or respiratory secretions. These problems are rare when isoflurane anesthesia is used. Some

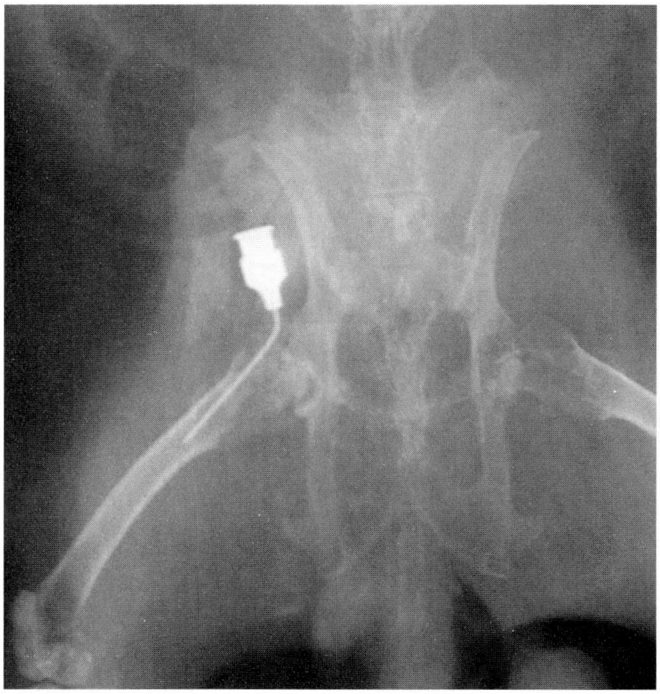

Figure 22-2 Radiographic survey film showing an intraosseous catheter placed in the greater trochanter of a rabbit. This moves the catheter away from the face and is better tolerated by some rabbits.

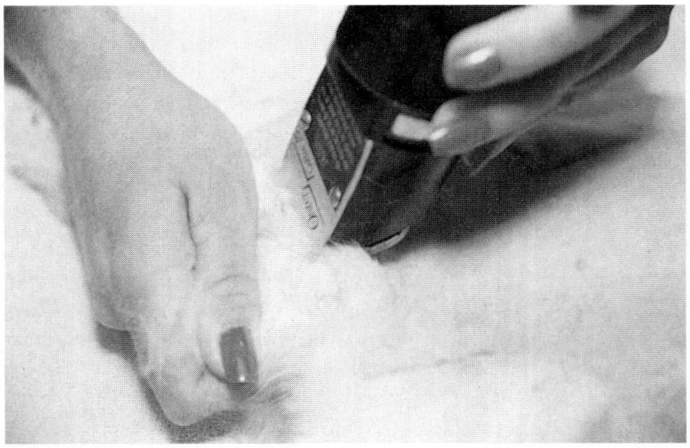

Figure 22-3 When clipping fur from the skin of a rabbit, keep the skin spread flat in front of the blade and hold the clipper close to the skin to prevent nicks and cuts.

rabbits produce atropine esterase, and the dose of atropine may have to be repeated as signs recur.

The combination of thin skin and dense fine fur makes it easy to cut a rabbit when clipping hair or shaving. Keep the skin spread flat in front of the blade, and clip with the blade held flat and close to the skin to minimize nicks and cuts (Fig. 22-3). A fine, No. 40 blade and an unhurried approach help to prevent the fine hair from accumulating between the clipper blades, causing them to jam or cut poorly.

POSTSURGICAL MONITORING

Blood Loss

The blood volume of the rabbit is reported to be approximately 57 mL/kg body weight.[4,6] Most mammalian species experience a drop in arterial pressure and cardiac output with moderate blood loss. Loss of 15% to 20% of the total blood volume causes massive cholinergic release, with tachycardia and intense arterial constriction that redistributes blood away from the gut and skin. In a 4-kg rabbit, this amounts to 34 to 45 mL of blood. An acute blood loss of 20% to 30% of total blood volume, or 45 to 68 mL in a 4-kg rabbit, is critical.

Pain and Analgesics

The very nature of rabbits is the foremost argument for the use of analgesics. A rabbit in pain is inactive, anorectic, and poorly responsive and may grind its teeth. Pain is assumed based on anthropomorphic evaluation of the injury or surgery the animal has experienced. See Chapters 33 and 41 for suggested dosages of analgesics.

SURGICAL TECHNIQUES

Adhesion Formation

Rabbits are used extensively as experimental models for formation of intraabdominal adhesions. Promising research has been published on the use of calcium channel-blocking agents to reduce or prevent adhesion formation in rabbits. In one study, administration of the calcium channel blocker verapamil (Calan, Searle Pharmaceuticals, Skokie, IL), at 200 μg/kg slowly IV or PO immediately after surgery and every 8 hours thereafter for a total of nine doses, was shown to significantly decrease adhesion formation, compared with untreated controls, with no overt evidence of cardiopulmonary compromise, increased infectious morbidity, or failure of wound healing.[10] I have used verapamil in cases in which surgery resulted in damage or irritation of abdominal organs in rabbits, with similar results. Studies of nonsteroidal antiinflammatory drugs[8] and a variety of other drugs or methods to prevent adhesion formation may also have clinical applications in rabbits.

Choice of Suture Material

The biologic and physical characteristics of suture material influence wound healing. Rabbits are more negatively affected by suture than are other mammals because of the caseous, suppurative response of the rabbit's immune system to foreign material and the proclivity to form adhesions. New suture material made from polymers that are removed by hydrolytic degradation are much less reactive and cause fewer and weaker adhesions, in my experience. I prefer monofilament polyglyconate (Maxon, Davis + Geck, Manati, PR) or other similar monofilament synthetic suture for closure of gastrotomy, enterotomy, or colotomy sites, cesarean sections, or other major abdominal surgery. Stainless steel or tantalum clips (Hemoclips, Weck, Research Triangle Park, NC) are excellent for vessel and small pedicle ligation with minimal adhesion formation. A study of laser anastomosis for sutureless closure of the colon of rabbits has been published,[5] and this technique holds potential for the future.

Skin Closures

Rabbits have a great fondness for suture removal and a similarly great dislike of Elizabethan collars. This combination has led to a search for a dependable method of skin closure. All but the smallest rabbits will chew sutures of stainless steel monofilament. Intradermal closures work very well but are time-consuming to place. Cyanoacrylate tissue cement (Vet-Bond, 3M Medical-Surgical Division, St. Paul, MN) is adequate but is occasionally removed by the rabbit. Skin staples are both reliable and well accepted by rabbits and their owners, and they are my preference.

COMMON PROCEDURES

Ovariohysterectomy

The reproductive tract of the female rabbit is unusual, compared with that of the dog or cat. The uterus is bicornate. Each uterine cornua possesses a cervix (there is no uterine body) and is coiled tightly in the caudal abdomen, cranial and just dorsal to the urinary bladder. Long uterine (*tuba uterina*) and infundibular tubes (*infundibulum tubae*) extend between the cornua and the ovary.[7] The uterus is easily exteriorized but is more fragile than that of other species. In a healthy doe, the caudal portion of the broad uterine ligament (*ligamentum latum uteri*), the mesometrium, is a principal fat-storage site, which makes identifying and ligating uterine vessels difficult (Fig. 22-4).

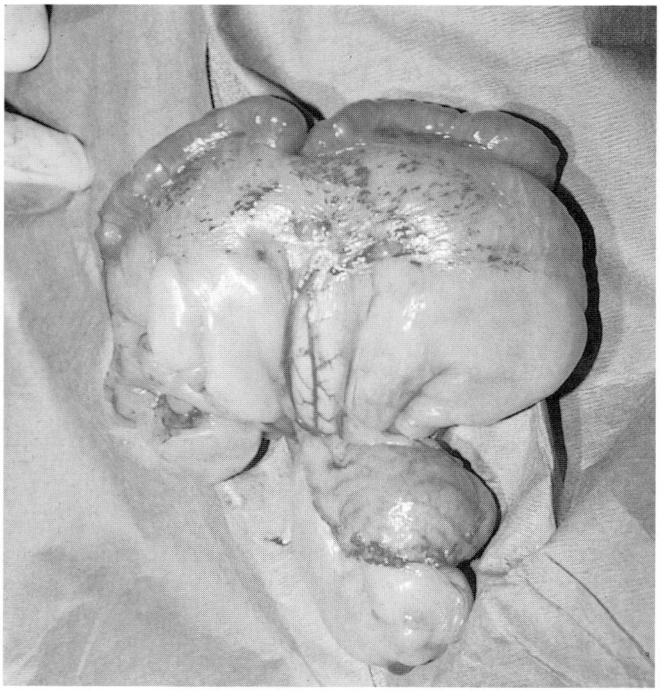

Figure 22-4 The mesometrium of a doe is a primary site of fat storage. This makes identification and ligation of uterine vessels difficult during an ovariohysterectomy.

The urethra of the female rabbit empties into the proximal end of a deep vaginal vestibule. Expression of the bladder with the animal in dorsal recumbency often leads to retrofilling of the vaginal vault. This can be a source of contamination of the peritoneal cavity during uterine surgery. It is also important not to confuse the vaginal vault with the bladder.

With the rabbit anesthetized before surgery, empty the rabbit's bladder by gentle palpation. Shave and prepare the abdominal area, and restrain the rabbit on the surgery table in dorsal recumbency, draped for surgery. Make a 2- to 3-cm midline incision centered over the cranial pole of the bladder, about half the distance between the umbilicus and the cranial rim of the pubis. Lift the narrow linea alba from the abdominal contents as you make a stab incision into the abdomen; be very careful when entering the abdominal wall, because the thin-walled cecum and bladder are often pressed firmly against the ventral abdomen. The uterus typically can be seen as it lies cranial and dorsal to the cranial pole of the bladder and may be lifted through the incision with forceps. A spay (snook) hook is not necessary and may cause damage to the cecum. Follow the uterus to the oviduct and infundibulum. The oviduct is coiled in a large loop that is several times longer than that of a dog or cat; be careful not to leave any portion of it. There are multiple vessels associated with the ovary, but they are smaller than those of many mammals. Carefully identify vessels and double-ligate them with transfixing sutures of chromic gut or synthetic absorbable suture. Hemorrhage is seldom a problem with these vessels. The uterine vessels stand several millimeters off the uterus and may be of significant size in mature does. Double-ligate these vessels with transfixing ligatures to the vaginal serosa. Ligate the uterus just cranial or just caudal to the cervices. Avoid contaminating the abdomen with urine or vaginal contents if a caudal ligature is used. Ligate each uterine horn if removed cranial to the cervix, or carefully ligate at the dorsal vagina if the uterus is removed caudal to the cervices. Closure of the abdomen is routine. Close the skin with surgical staples, an intradermal suture pattern, or tissue cement.

Orchidectomy (Castration)

Sexually active male rabbits (bucks) have obnoxious urine marking behaviors that generally lead to their owners' wanting to have them neutered. Furthermore, bucks may become territorial and possessive about their environment and owners, leading to aggressive behavior.

The rabbit's testes are similar to those of the cat but may move freely from the scrotum to the abdomen through an open inguinal canal. Soft tissue herniation and strangulation of bowel loops is prevented by a large mass of fat associated with the epididymis, which rests in the inguinal canal when the testicle is in the scrotum.

For castration, anesthetize and restrain the buck in dorsal recumbency. Carefully shave the hair from the scrotum and surrounding area, and surgically prepare and drape the area to minimize contamination. Make a 1- to 1.5-cm incision with a No. 15 scalpel blade through the skin and vaginal tunic on the ventral surface of both sides of the scrotum. Remove the testis from the tunic and carefully tear the ligament of the testicle from the tunic with a dry gauze sponge (Fig. 22-5). Pull the testis caudally to expose a section of the vas deferens and the vascular structures of the spermatic cord, then tie them in an overhand knot with a small Mayo needle holder or mosquito forceps. Alternatively, ligate the duct and vasculature with 2-0 to 3-0 synthetic absorbable suture. Cut the duct and vessels distal to the knot or ligature and return the spermatic cord to the inguinal canal in such a way that it may be recovered if bleeding occurs. Return the tunic to the scrotum and repeat the process for the remaining testis. Observe the rabbit for several hours after the surgery for hemorrhage. Complications most often result from overactivity or sexual activity; therefore, I hospitalize castrated rabbits overnight for "cage rest."

GASTROINTESTINAL SURGERY

Gastrotomy

Because of the success of medical management of gastric stasis, I only rarely perform a gastrotomy. Aggressive therapy with parenteral fluids, metoclopramide (Reglan, A. H. Robbins, Co., Richmond, VA) at 0.5 mg/kg q4-8h, syringe feeding, and correction of diet and management practices should be attempted before surgery. Surgery is indicated for rabbits with suspected or known gastric foreign bodies or complete gastric or pyloric obstruction, or for those that fail to show clinical signs of improvement after 3 to 5 days of intensive medical therapy. Rabbits with gastric stasis should receive a thorough workup, and every effort should be made to return the rabbit to a positive energy balance and to correct fluid and electrolyte imbalances before surgery. A common accompanying lesion with gastric stasis or obstruction is hepatic lipidosis, presumably caused by starvation. Correct any negative energy balance, acidosis, and ketosis to reduce complications in these rabbits.[2]

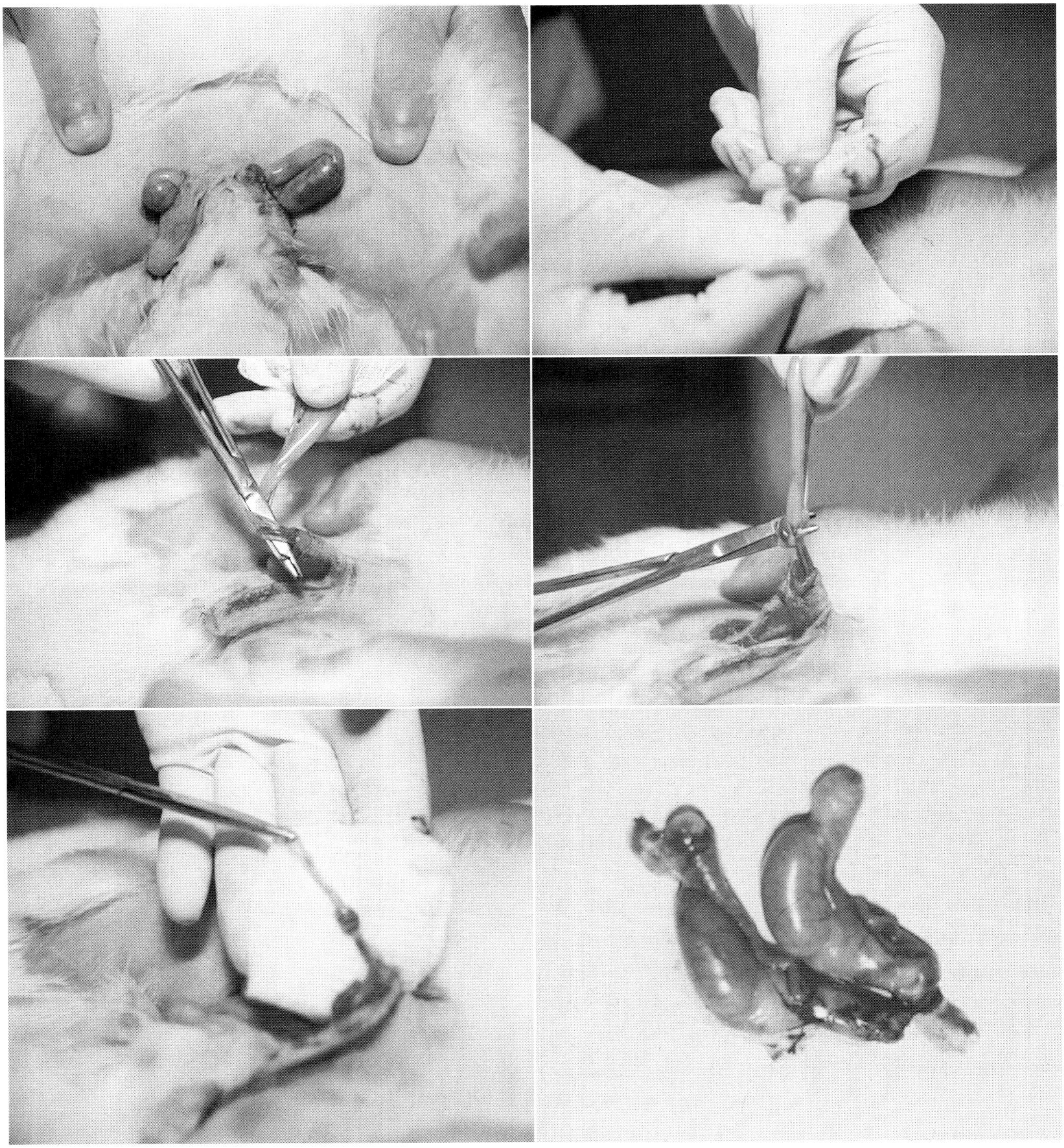

A B C D E F

Figure 22-5 A technique for castration of a rabbit. **A,** The skin and vaginal tunic on both sides of the scrotum are incised, and the testes are removed from the vaginal tunic. **B,** The ligament of the testicle is torn from the tunic with a dry gauze sponge. **C** and **D,** The vas deferens and vessels of the spermatic cord are tied with an overhand knot or ligated. **E,** The testicle is removed by cutting distal to the knot or ligature. **F,** The testes as removed from a castrated rabbit.

In contrast to hairballs in a cat or ferret, the stomach of a rabbit with gastric stasis contains a dehydrated network of food and fur ("felt") that may be so large as to distend the stomach beyond its normal limits. This mass is intertwined and sometimes can be removed in one piece. The stomach of a rabbit without gastric stasis may contain loose hair, which disintegrates when removed. This leads one to suspect that the pathogenesis of the problem is one of abnormal gastric physiologic function rather than simply the presence of hair.

Anesthetize the rabbit, restrain it on a circulating water blanket in dorsal recumbency, shave it from the inguinal to the midthoracic area, and prepare it for aseptic surgery. Place a catheter in the cephalic or lateral saphenous vein for fluid administration and vascular access during surgery. Make a midline incision that is long enough for exploration of the entire gastrointestinal tract, taking care not to damage the stomach or cecum, which may be pressed tightly against the abdominal wall. Drape lap pads moistened with normal saline along the incision line, and use a Balfour retractor to fully expose the abdomen. Explore the abdomen before the gastrotomy to determine if additional lesions are present. Examine the liver carefully; if it is abnormally pale or yellow, do a liver biopsy and submit the sample for histopathologic examination. Place stay sutures in the greater curvature of the stomach and elevate it into the surgical field. Place additional moistened lap pads around the stomach to prevent contamination of the abdomen with gastric contents. Make an incision in the avascular area between the lesser and greater curvatures, and carefully remove the stomach contents or foreign body with a sterile surgical spoon. Rinse the lumen with a small volume of warm saline and examine it for abnormalities, then gently palpate the pylorus for patency. Close the stomach in a two-layer inverting pattern with 3-0 to 4-0 synthetic monofilament suture. Extend the sutures into, but not through, the gastric mucosa. Thoroughly lavage the abdomen with body-temperature isotonic fluids and close it routinely. Pain management is also essential.

Postoperative management is equally critical to the successful outcome of the procedure.[9,11] Supportive therapy to optimize wound healing, prevent further hepatic damage, and promote hepatic regeneration is essential. Furthermore, care must be taken to support the normal gut microflora to prevent complications of stress-induced enteritis complex.

Intestinal Resection, Anastomosis, and Enterotomy

Intestinal resection or enterotomy is most often indicated in rabbits with foreign body ingestion or with trauma to the intestine. Neoplasia and infiltrative intestinal diseases are uncommon and, in my experience, consist mostly of metastatic uterine adenocarcinomas. Successful intestinal surgery in rabbits demands attention to surgical principles. Special attention to preserving the blood supply and luminal diameter must be taken to compensate for the small size of the lumen in relation to visceral wall thickness in the rabbit intestine.[1] The bowel must be handled gently to prevent shock and postoperative ileus.

The preparation of the rabbit for surgery and the abdominal incision are the same as for gastrotomy. Care must be taken not to damage the cecum while making the incision. Examine the entire gastrointestinal tract before the enterotomy. If resection and anastomosis are necessary, ligate the mesenteric and arcade vessels and apply crushing and noncrushing clamps, as is done in other small animals. Vascular clamps, bulldog clamps, or serrefines work well as noncrushing clamps on the small-diameter intestines of rabbits. Incise the intestine at an acute angle to augment the small luminal diameter. I prefer an appositional suture technique with 4-0 to 6-0 synthetic monofilament suture. Occasionally, linear foreign bodies may be accompanied by bowel plication or intussusception. Multiple enterotomy sites may be required to remove these foreign bodies. Longitudinal incisions with transverse closures are sometimes used if the luminal diameter is small (Fig. 22-6). If the abdomen is contaminated during the procedure, lavage with warm saline for several cycles of irrigation and suction before closure.

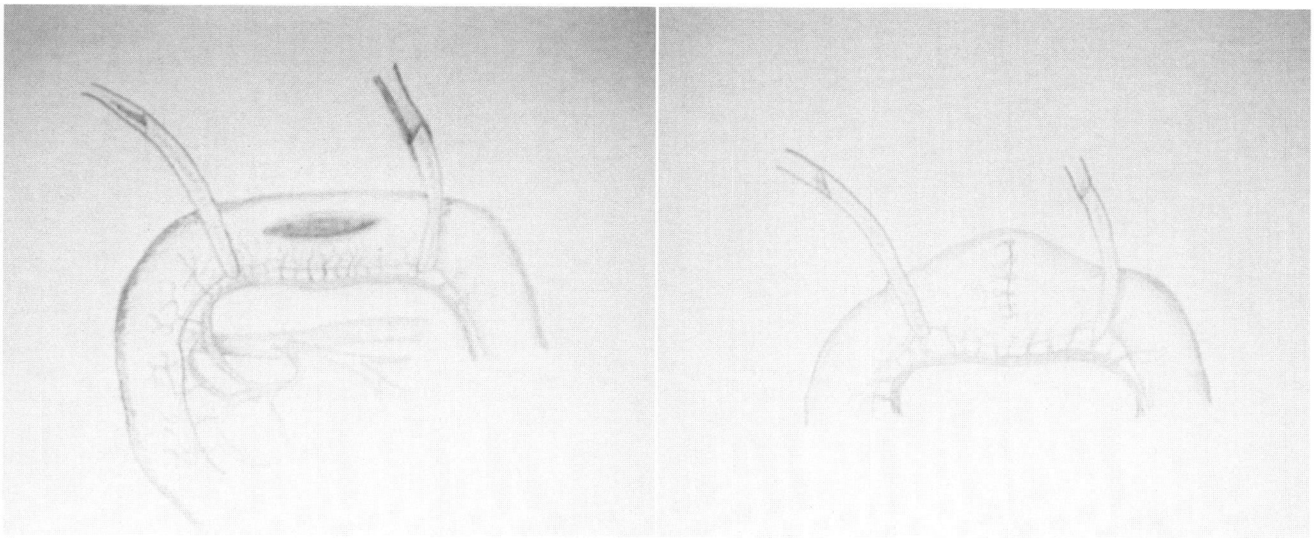

A B

Figure 22-6 A longitudinal incision (A) of the intestine with a transverse closure (B) may help prevent stricture formation in the rabbit if the luminal diameter is small.

Surgery of the Large Bowel

Surgery of the rabbit colon is performed primarily to correct obstructions at the level of the fusi coli. Other indications for surgery of the large bowel include injury resulting from bite wounds, intraluminal trauma resulting from diagnostic or clinical instrumentation, or trauma secondary to accidents during surgery. Many rabbits with these injuries are seen as referral cases, and the condition may have been present for several days before examination. Neoplasia of the lower bowel, with the exception of rectal polyps and metastatic uterine adenocarcinoma, is rare. Several areas of the colon and cecum are thin walled and easily torn, and their suturing characteristics are less than optimal. Surgery at the fusi coli is challenging because of its location at the root of the mesentery. If possible, massage the material causing the obstruction (typically hard feces or cecoliths) past the tight spot and into the descending colon. If bowel must be resected, incise it at an acute angle, as with the small intestine. In the descending colon, make longitudinal incisions and close them transversely to increase luminal diameter. Use an interrupted suture pattern in an appositional or crushing technique for anastomosis of the colon. An inverting suture technique may be used to close lesions of the cecum; I prefer a 4-0 to 6-0 synthetic monofilament suture placed at intervals of 2 to 3 mm. A segment of omentum can be used to reinforce the anastomosis or incision line. Before closure, lavage the abdomen with several cycles of warmed saline containing 10% povidone-iodine/saline solution, followed by suction. Remove any grossly evident ingesta in the abdominal cavity. If the abdominal cavity becomes contaminated, take samples for both aerobic and anaerobic bacterial culture, and treat the rabbit aggressively with antibiotics.

ANORECTAL PAPILLOMA REMOVAL

Anorectal papillomas are cauliflower-like, fungating masses that arise from the anorectal junction. They are benign and are not related to the papillomas of the skin or the oral cavity. Papillomas arise from the rectal squamous columnar junction and protrude from the anus once they have grown to a sufficient size. Removal of these lesions is usually successful.

The tissue of the papilloma is friable and has a tendency to bleed. The mucosal attachment may be stalk-like or broad-based. Removal is facilitated by good exposure of the lesion. Position the rabbit in dorsal recumbency with the pelvis slightly elevated. Have an assistant place and hold a human nasal speculum (veterinary canine vaginal speculum) in the anus. Alternatively, place several stay sutures around the circumference of the anus so that an assistant can provide gentle traction. Remove the papilloma by sharp dissection or electrosurgery, taking care to remove all of the mass to prevent recurrence. Suture the mucosa with a fine, 5-0 to 6-0 absorbable suture material in a simple continuous pattern. Large papillomas may be removed in sections to simplify closure.

URINARY TRACT SURGERY

The kidneys are mobile, accessible, and convenient for biopsy. The urinary bladder of the rabbit is tough but thin walled. When greatly distended, it may rupture easily.

Renal calculi are a common problem in rabbits and a common cause of renal failure. Pyelolithotomy, nephrotomy, or nephrectomy is indicated in these cases. As with a dog or cat, a rabbit with renal calculi must be thoroughly evaluated before surgical correction of the problem is attempted. If renal calculi have resulted in dilation of the proximal ureter and renal pelvis, they may be removed through an incision made at the junction of these structures (pyelolithotomy). This approach to removal of renal calculi does not require occlusion of the renal vasculature and avoids trauma to the renal parenchyma, thereby minimizing deleterious effects on postoperative renal function. In rabbits with substantial renal disease, nephrectomy or nephrotomy is indicated.

Anesthetize the rabbit, shave the ventral abdomen from pubis to midthorax, and prepare the rabbit for aseptic surgery in dorsal recumbency. Make a midline incision that is long enough to explore the abdomen. Take care not to damage the stomach or the cecum, which may be pressed tightly against the abdomen. Drape lap pads moistened with normal saline solution along the incision, and place a Balfour retractor for better visibility of the abdomen. Explore the abdomen to determine if additional lesions are present. Gently remove the cecum, colon, and intestines from the abdomen, and wrap them in moistened gauze to facilitate exposure of the kidney.

Pyelolithotomy

Dissect the kidney free of its peritoneal attachments and rotate it medially, exposing the renal pelvis and proximal ureter. Make an incision over the pelvis and proximal ureter, and remove the calculi. Flush the renal pelvis and calyces with saline to remove small calculi that may remain. Pass a 3.5- to 5-Fr catheter into the bladder through the ureter to ensure patency. Close the incision in the renal pelvis and ureter with 5-0 or 6-0 continuous absorbable suture, lavage the abdomen, and close normally.

Nephrotomy

I have performed sagittal nephrotomy in several rabbits; however, complications, including renal failure, have occurred in some rabbits with this technique. Thoroughly evaluate renal function before performing this surgery. Sagittal nephrotomy is performed as in the dog or cat. Isolate the kidney as described previously. Use serrefines or vascular clamps of appropriate size for temporary vascular occlusion. Divide the kidney along its sagittal plane. Remove renal calculi, and flush the renal pelvis and calyces with saline to remove small calculi that may remain. Pass a 3.5- to 5-Fr catheter into the bladder through the ureter to ensure patency. Press the kidney together and hold it in place for several seconds to allow the two halves to "stick together." Suture the capsule, using 4-0 to 6-0 suture and a simple interrupted pattern and placing sutures every 2 to 4 mm. Remove the vascular clamps and observe the kidney for bleeding. Control minor bleeding by covering the site with absorbable gelatin sponges (Gelfoam, Pharmacia & Upjohn, Kalamazoo, MI). Close the abdomen routinely.

Nephrectomy

Nephrectomy is indicated in rabbits with a diseased or damaged kidney if adequate function remains in the opposite kidney. Expose the kidney as described previously. Use vascular clips to ligate the renal artery, vein, and ureter. Close the abdomen routinely.

ABSCESSES

Rabbits form thick-walled abscesses that contain caseous, purulent discharge in reaction to most bacterial infections. If these abscesses are simply opened and drained, they frequently recur. Therefore, abscesses should be excised with a substantial margin, so that all contaminated tissue is removed. Ligate blood vessels with a small-diameter absorbable suture, and close the skin with surgical staples. Excision of large abscesses may require the use of skin flaps to cover the defect. Complete excision often is not possible with foot or dental abscesses, and aggressive surgical debridement must be used. After debridement, the wound is allowed to granulate in, but the prognosis is poor for a complete cure. The use of antibiotic-impregnated polymethylmethacrylate (AIPMMA) beads in these abscesses has proved to be highly successful when total excision is not an option. Pododermatitis and the resulting osteomyelitis can cripple a rabbit; these lesions are painful, and the rabbit may be reluctant or unable to stand or walk. In these rabbits, consider amputation as an alternative to more conventional treatment of abscesses (see Chapter 35).

DERMOPLASTY AND TAIL AMPUTATION TO CORRECT PROBLEMS OF URINE SCALD

Dermatologic problems that result from urine scald or chronic diarrhea are common in pet rabbits (see Chapter 19). Underlying causes of obesity, dietary indiscretion, urinary tract disease, and spinal cord disease must be addressed; however, correcting the dermatologic problem may depend on preventing urine contamination of the perineal tissues. These problems result from repeated urine or diarrhea contamination of the perineal skin and medial surfaces of the hind legs. In obese rabbits, a large fold of skin and fat may partially cover the genital area, interfering with the passage of urine. Alternatively, the rabbit may be unable to rotate its pelvis during urination or defecation to direct the stream of urine caudally, resulting in urine contamination of the skin of the perineum and legs. These problems are compounded because the urine scald causes increased immobility, which further contributes to the likelihood of urine contamination.

I have used two techniques to correct these problems: dermoplasty of the caudal abdomen to remove the fold of skin that interferes with the passage of urine, and a combination of tail amputation and dermoplasty to lift the genital area dorsally, resulting in passage of urine in a more caudal direction. It must be emphasized that these surgeries are adjunct and salvage procedures; every effort should be made to correct the underlying cause of the problem before surgery is undertaken. However, I have obtained excellent results when I have used these corrective procedures in rabbits.

Use systemic as well as topical antibiotics and protectants before surgery to decrease inflammation and infection in the area. For the skin fold resection, position the rabbit in dorsal recumbency, and shave and prepare the area from the midabdomen to the tail, including the medial thigh region to the stifle. Identify a crescent area of skin cranial to the genital area that, when removed, will eliminate any excessive tissue that protrudes over the genital area (Fig. 22-7). Incise along this crescent of skin, avoiding damage to the lateral abdominal vein, which lies lateral to the nipple and deep to the glandular tissue of the mammary gland. There may be an advantage in removing some or all of the inguinal adipose body, which extends from just cranial to the inguinal mammary gland to the genital area and is a primary location for deposition of adipose tissue. Tissue removal should result in taut skin over the caudal ventral abdomen when the rabbit is in dorsal recumbency but no tension on the incision. I prefer a two-layer closure, with an absorbable suture in the deep layer and staples in the skin.

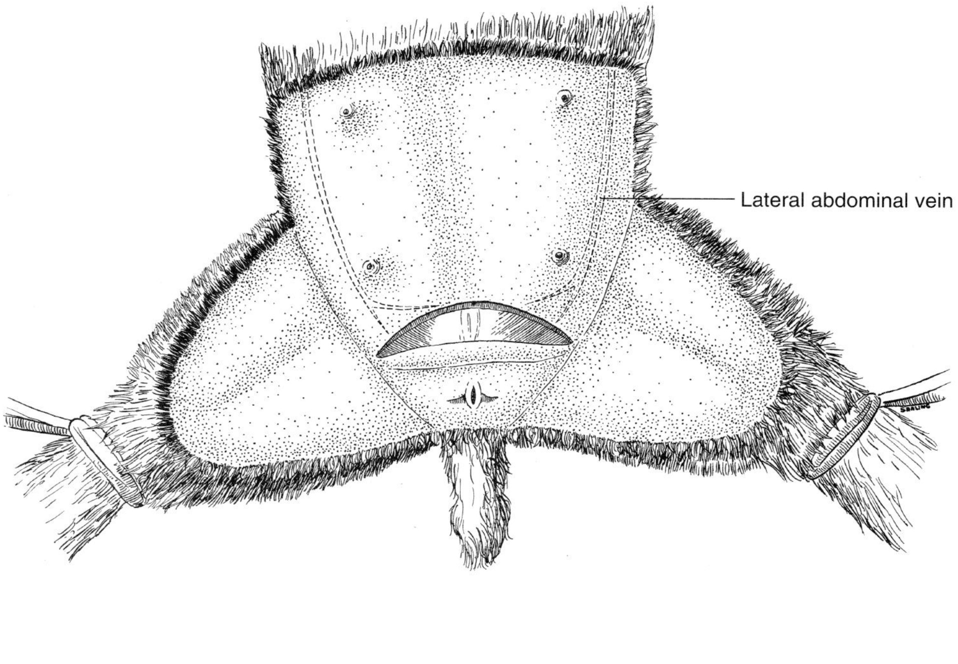

Figure 22-7 Procedure for ventral skin fold resection in a rabbit. A large fold of abdominal skin may interfere with urine passage in an obese rabbit, causing contamination of the surrounding skin and urine scald. A ventral skin fold resection of the caudal abdomen removes a crescent-shaped area of skin, allowing unimpeded passage of urine.

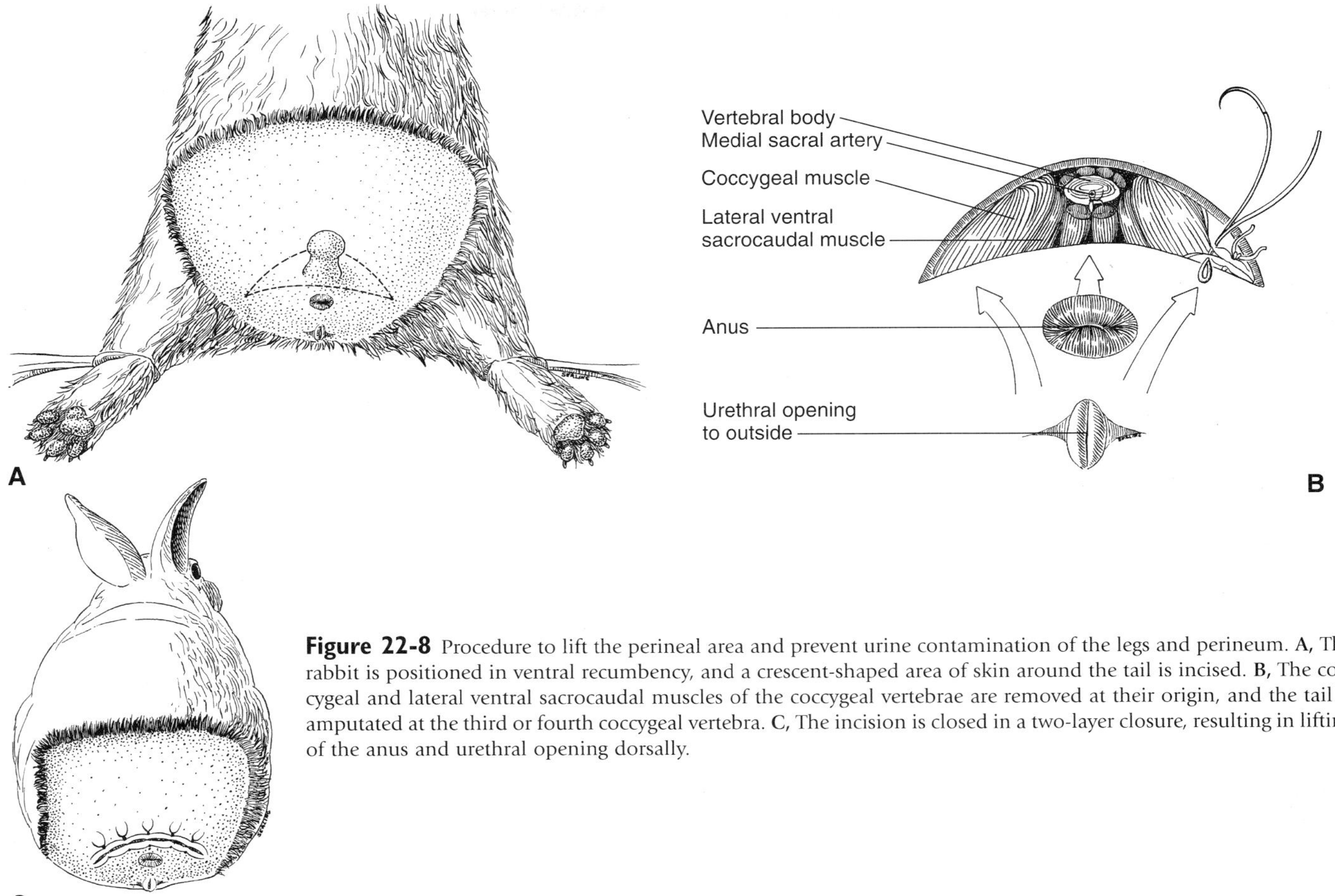

A B C

Figure 22-8 Procedure to lift the perineal area and prevent urine contamination of the legs and perineum. **A,** The rabbit is positioned in ventral recumbency, and a crescent-shaped area of skin around the tail is incised. **B,** The coccygeal and lateral ventral sacrocaudal muscles of the coccygeal vertebrae are removed at their origin, and the tail is amputated at the third or fourth coccygeal vertebra. **C,** The incision is closed in a two-layer closure, resulting in lifting of the anus and urethral opening dorsally.

The second procedure (B. Loudis, personal communication, 2003) is more difficult to perform but is very effective for rabbits that urinate on their legs because of an inability to lift their pelvis and direct the stream of urine away from their legs. Position the rabbit for surgery in ventral recumbency with the rear legs extended behind the rabbit. Shave an area extending 3 to 5 inches from the anus and tail and prepare it for surgery. Delineate a crescent-shaped section of skin that, when removed, will lift the anus and urethral opening to a dorsal position at the caudal-most extreme of the rabbit. The crescent should extend from a point dorsal to the anus, just beyond the dorsal limits of the external anal sphincter muscle on its ventral curvature to immediately dorsal of the tail, and lateral and ventral to the urethral opening (Fig. 22-8). Identify the coccygeal and lateral ventral sacrocaudal muscles of the coccygeal vertebrae and remove them from their insertion. In male rabbits, the retractor penis muscle must also be identified and, in some cases, carefully dissected from its origin. Amputate the tail at the third or fourth coccygeal vertebra, and ligate the medial sacral artery. The coccygeal and retractor penis muscles (if removed) are reattached at or about the dorsocaudal origin of the semitendinosus muscle with polypropylene or strong absorbable suture. Place vertical mattress sutures to position the closure and relieve tension, and close the incision in two layers, as described previously.

REFERENCES

1. Booth HW, Hartsfield SM: Use of the laboratory rabbit in the small animal student surgery laboratory. J Vet Med Educ 1990; 17:16-18.
2. Gillett NA, Brooks DL, Tillman PC: Medical and surgical management of gastric obstruction from a hairball in the rabbit. J Am Vet Med Assoc 1983; 183:1176-1178.
3. Harkness JE, Wagner JE: The Biology and Medicine of Rabbits and Rodents, 4th ed. Media, PA, Williams & Wilkins, 1995.
4. Kozma C, Macklin W, Cummins LM, et al: Anatomy, physiology, and biochemistry of the rabbit. *In* Weisbroth SH, Flatt RE, Kraus AL, eds. The Biology of the Laboratory Rabbit. New York, Academic Press, 1974, pp 50-72.
5. Kuramoto S, Ryan PJ: First sutureless closure of a colotomy: short-term results of experimental laser anastomosis of the colon. Dis Colon Rectum 1991; 34:1079-1084.
6. McGuill MW, Rowan AN: Biological effects of blood loss: implications for sampling volumes and techniques. ILAR News 1989; 31:5-18.
7. Popesko P, Rajtová V, Horák J: A Colour Atlas of Anatomy in Small Laboratory Animals. Vol. 1: Rabbit, Guinea Pig. London, Wolfe Publishing, 1992.
8. Rodgers K, Girgis W, diZerega GS, et al: Intraperitoneal tolmetin prevents postsurgical adhesion formation in rabbits. Int J Fertil 1990; 35:40-45.

9. Sebesten A: Acute obstruction of the duodenum of a rabbit following the apparently successful treatment of a hairball. Lab Anim 1977; 11:135.
10. Steinleitiner A, Lambert H, Kazensky C, et al: Reduction of primary postoperative adhesion formation under calcium channel blockade in the rabbit. J Surg Res 1990; 48:42-45.
11. Wagner JL, Hackel DB, Samsell AG: Spontaneous deaths in rabbits resulting from gastric trichobezoars. Lab Anim Sci 1974; 24:826-830.

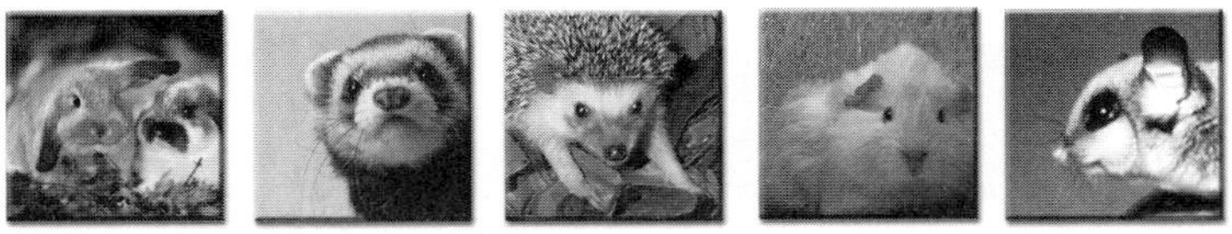

SECTION THREE

GUINEA PIGS, CHINCHILLAS, AND PRAIRIE DOGS

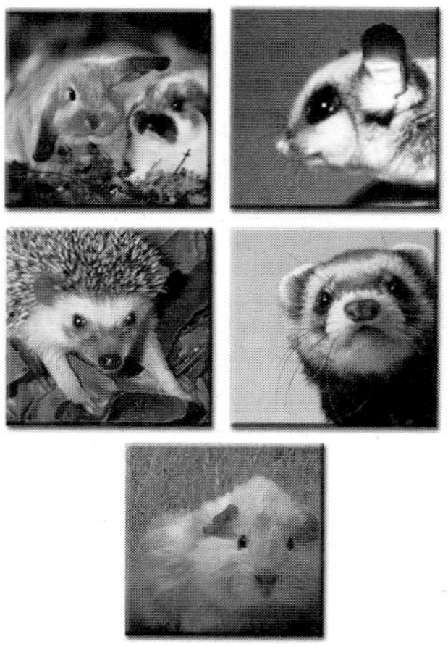

CHAPTER 23

Biology, Husbandry, and Clinical Techniques of Guinea Pigs and Chinchillas

Katherine E. Quesenberry, DVM, Diplomate ABVP, Thomas M. Donnelly, BVSc, Diplomate ACLAM, and Elizabeth V. Hillyer, DVM

Guinea pigs *(Cavia porcellus)* and chinchillas *(Chinchilla laniger)* are hystricomorph rodents from South America (Fig. 23-1). They share many anatomic and physiologic characteristics, and the approach to their veterinary care is similar. Both species are monogastric herbivores with a large cecum, and both produce precocious young after a relatively long gestation period. There are also some important differences between the two species. For example, guinea pigs require a dietary source of vitamin C but chinchillas do not; dystocia is common in guinea pigs but not in chinchillas; and chinchillas require daily dust baths but guinea pigs do not. Both guinea pigs and chinchillas are small, gentle, and lively species that make good pets because they are docile and relatively easy to care for.

This chapter summarizes the information on basic biology, husbandry, and clinical techniques that is relevant to the medical care of these species as pets. Readers who are interested in more detailed descriptions of anatomy and physiology of guinea pigs can find these in the references.[4,27,31] Guinea pigs have been used as laboratory animals for more than 400 years, and abundant information is available about them; less has been published about chinchillas. Much of the information available on chinchillas concerns husbandry and breeding and is found in the lay literature. Information on anatomy and physiology of chinchillas is more difficult to find.

BIOLOGY AND HUSBANDRY OF GUINEA PIGS

Guinea pigs, also known as cavies, were domesticated in South America between 500 and 1000 AD, and possibly as early as 1000 BC.[37] At the time of the Spanish invasion of South America, guinea pigs, known as *cuy*, were raised by the Incas for food and for use in religious ceremonies.[37] Guinea pigs were brought to Europe about 400 years ago. Although they never became popular as a food source outside of South America, they have been raised as pets and laboratory animals ever since.

Several species of wild cavy have been described *(Cavia aperea, Cavia tschudii, Cavia cutleri, Cavia rufescens,* and *Cavia fulgida)*; according to one source, these may all be different varieties of *C. aperea.*[34] Wild cavies are found today in Colombia, Venezuela, Brazil, Argentina, Paraguay, and Peru.[34,37] They inhabit a wide variety of habitats, including grasslands, the forest edge, swamps, and rocky areas. Domestic guinea pigs are still raised by the people of the altiplano; they are often left uncaged to forage for food about the dwellings.[34,37]

Three standard breeds of guinea pigs were originally recognized by the American Rabbit Breeders Association: the American

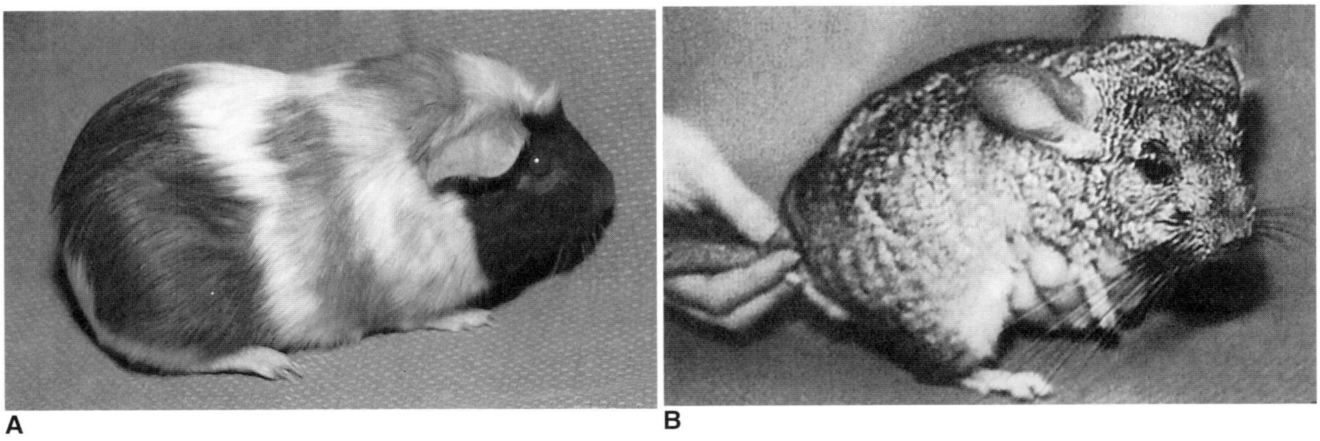

Figure 23-1 A, Normal guinea pig. B, Normal chinchilla, showing method of restraint. *(B, From Hoefer HL: Chinchilla. Vet Clin North Am Small Anim Pract 1994; 24:103-111.)*

(or English), the Abyssinian, and the Peruvian. The American guinea pig has short smooth hair, the Abyssinian has relatively short coarse hair that grows in whorls or rosettes, and the Peruvian has very long (up to 15 cm) silky hair. Currently, the American Cavy Breeders Association (www.acbaonline.com), an organization associated with the American Rabbit Breeders Association, recognizes at least 13 breeds. The more recently recognized breeds include the Texel, which has long hair in ringlets and curls all over its body; the Teddy, which has a short, dense coat with a kinked hair shaft; and the Silkie (or Sheltie), which is similar to the Peruvian except that long hair does not cover its face. Additionally, several new breeds, including hairless breeds, have been developed by cavy breeders. Hairless breeds now available are the Skinny, which is hairless except for the head and lower legs, and the Baldwin, which is born with hair but becomes totally bald at weaning. Coat colors of guinea pigs include white, red, tan, brown, chocolate, and black; coats can be monochromatic, bicolored, or tricolored. A solid color is described as *self*; for example, black self is monochromatic black. The Himalayan color variety has a white body with black or chocolate nose, ears, and feet. Brindle describes a coat of mixed black and white hairs. Agouti guinea pigs have an undercolor that is ticked throughout with another color, similar to wild guinea pigs. Albino guinea pigs are common in a laboratory setting.

Guinea pigs are lively, responsive, and gentle pets, particularly if they are handled frequently while young. They have some peculiarities, however, of which all persons working with them should be aware. First, their response to perceived danger is freeze or flight (rather than fight or flight). If frightened, they tend to become immobile or, alternatively, make an explosive attempt to escape. Second, guinea pigs do not tolerate dietary or environmental changes. Their food preferences are established early in life, and they often refuse to eat if their food is changed in type or presentation. Moreover, they may become depressed or go off feed when hospitalized; therefore, the attitude and food consumption of all hospitalized animals should be monitored carefully. Third, guinea pigs require a dietary source of vitamin C.

Under conditions of good husbandry, guinea pigs are hardy animals with few disease problems. Conversely, inadequacies in diet or husbandry can lead to illnesses that, if not managed early, are difficult to reverse (Fig. 23-2). Sick guinea pigs do not tolerate clinical procedures very well and have been known to go into cardiac and respiratory arrest secondary to the stress of restraint or a diagnostic procedure that would be routine in species such as ferrets. Handle very sick guinea pigs with "kid gloves." Concentrate on providing good supportive care and maintaining caloric intake in a low-stress environment, while working toward a diagnosis and therapy specific to that diagnosis.

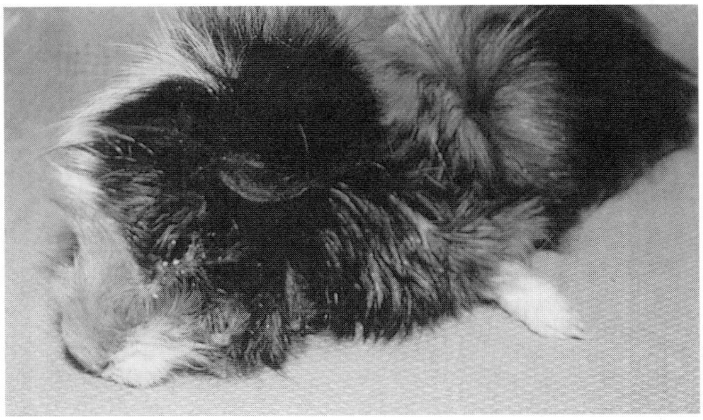

Figure 23-2 Recumbent, very ill guinea pigs have a guarded to poor prognosis. In addition to specific medical therapy, intensive supportive care and force-feeding in a low-stress environment are necessary to help these animals.

Anatomy and Physiology

Guinea pigs have stocky bodies, delicate short limbs, rounded hairless pinnae, and no tails. Males are larger than females, weighing 900 to 1200 g compared with 700 to 900 g for females. Obesity is relatively common in pet animals. The lifespan of pet guinea pigs is typically 5 to 6 years. Wild cavies feed at dawn and dusk; they live in small groups (5 to 10 individuals) in burrows or crevices.[34]

The hair coat of guinea pigs is composed of large guard hairs surrounded by an undercoat of fine hairs. Androgen-dependent sebaceous glands are abundant along the dorsum and around the anus. The sebaceous glands around the anal area are important for marking, and guinea pigs are frequently seen rubbing or pressing the rump against a surface.[4] In older males, excessive accumulation of sebaceous secretions occurs in the skin around the base of the spine, resulting in thick, matted, greasy fur. Breeders may call this a "grease gland." The fur and skin can be cleaned with alcohol. Both male and female guinea pigs have one pair of inguinal nipples (Fig. 23-3).

Guinea pigs have large tympanic bullae. They have 32 to 36 vertebrae; the vertebral formula is C7, T13(14), L6, S2(3), Cd4(6). There are 13 to 14 pairs of ribs, of which the last one or two are cartilaginous. The small cylindrical clavicle attaches laterally to the coracoid process of the scapula and medially to the manubrium. The pelvic symphysis generally remains fibrocartilaginous,[4] and a gap in the symphysis can be palpated at the time of impending parturition. Guinea pigs have four digits on the front feet and three digits on the rear feet; each digit has a short claw that may require periodic clipping in some individuals (Fig. 23-4).

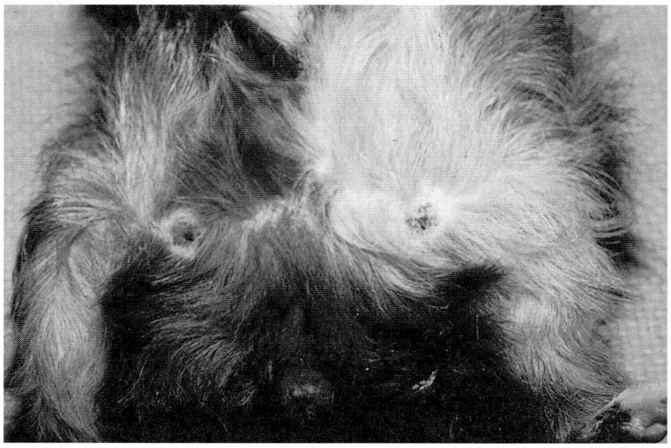

Figure 23-3 Guinea pigs have one pair of nipples in the inguinal area.

The spleen is relatively broad in guinea pigs. The thymus in immature animals is located within the ventral cervical area and the cranial mediastinum; in adults, a thymic remnant may be present in the cranial mediastinum.[4] Guinea pigs, like monkeys, ferrets, and humans, are considered to be corticosteroid-resistant species because steroid administration is not associated with marked changes in thymic physiology or peripheral lymphocyte counts.

Guinea pigs have no laryngeal ventricles, and their vocal folds are small; nonetheless, they command a wide range of vocalizations. The right lung is composed of four lobes (cranial, middle, caudal, and accessory), whereas the left lung is composed of three lobes (cranial, middle, and caudal). In the heart, as in other mammals, the right atrioventricular valve is tricuspid, and the left atrioventricular valve is bicuspid. There is usually one septomarginal trabecula (moderator band) within the lumen of the right ventricle, and there is rarely one within that of the left ventricle.[4]

Gastrointestinal system The dental formula of guinea pigs is $2(I\frac{1}{1}\ C\frac{0}{0}\ PM\frac{1}{1}\ M\frac{3}{3}) = 20$. All teeth are open-rooted and grow throughout life. In animals with dental malocclusion, the maxillary cheek teeth tend to overgrow laterally into the buccal gingiva, and the mandibular cheek teeth tend to overgrow in a medial direction, entrapping the tongue (see Chapter 34). The incisors are normally white, unlike those of many other rodents (Fig. 23-5). Between the incisors and the cheek teeth (premolars and molars) is a gap called the diastema.

Guinea pigs have large tongues and relatively small, narrow oral cavities. The soft palate is continuous with the base of the tongue. The oropharynx communicates with the remainder of the pharynx through a hole in the soft palate called the palatal ostium.[32] Take care when attempting to pass any instrument (such as a feeding tube) that the instrument does not slip to either side of the ostium, where it can damage the vascular soft palate.

Guinea pigs have four pairs of salivary glands—parotid, mandibular, sublingual, and molar—the ducts of which empty into the oral cavity near the molars. The entire alimentary tract measures approximately 2.3 m from pharynx to anus.[20] The stomach is lined with glandular epithelium; unlike the stomachs

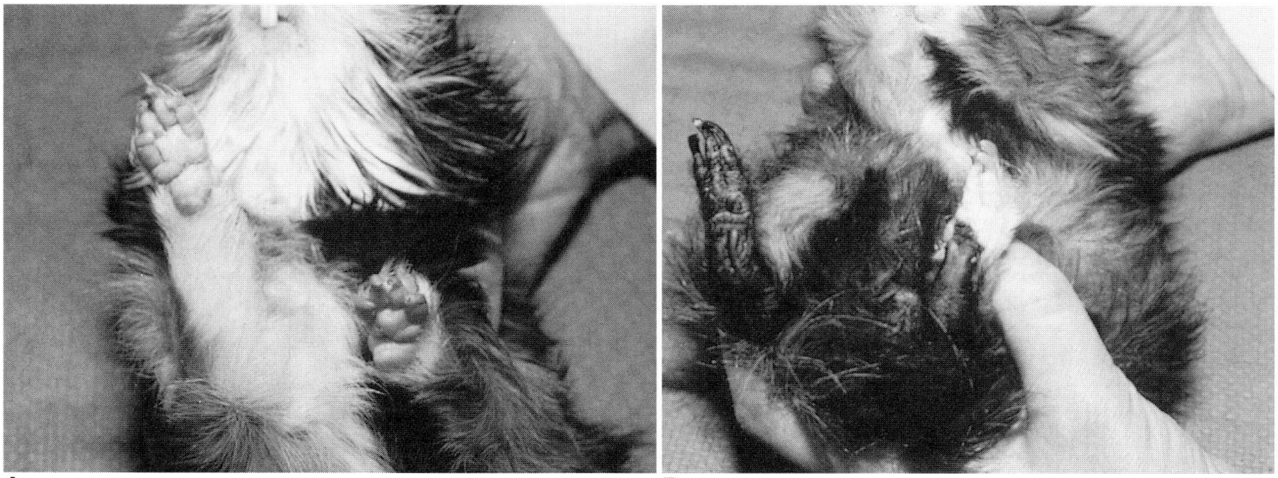

A **B**

Figure 23-4 **A,** Normal forefeet of a guinea pig. **B,** Normal hindfeet of a guinea pig. Each forefoot has four digits, and each hindfoot has three digits.

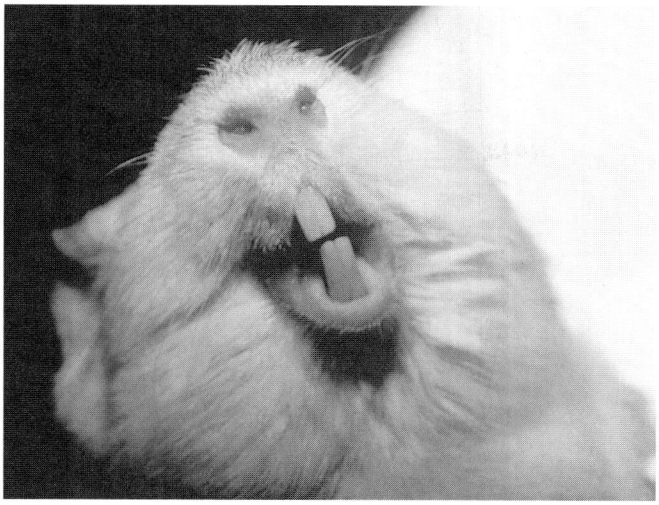

Figure 23-5 Normal incisors in a guinea pig. As in other rodents, the upper incisors are much shorter than the lower ones; in contrast to many other rodents, the incisors are white.

of rats, mice, and hamsters, there is no nonglandular portion.[4] The small intestine is located on the right side of the abdominal cavity, and the cecum occupies the central and left portions. The cecum is a large, thin-walled sac with many lateral pouches that are formed by the action of three taeniae coli (thick, longitudinal muscular bands that run the length of the large intestine). Smooth muscle cells harvested from the taeniae coli of guinea pigs were commonly used in physiologic studies, because they could be obtained easily without damaging the gut. The cecum is 15 to 20 cm long and contains up to 65% of the gastrointestinal (GI) contents.[21] The liver has six lobes—right, medial, left lateral, left medial, caudate, and quadrate. The gallbladder is well developed.

The normal gastric emptying time in guinea pigs is 2 hours. Total GI transit time is approximately 20 hours (range, 8-30 hours); however, when coprophagy is factored in, the total GI transit time is 66 hours.[20]

Guinea pigs perform coprophagy, or cecotrophy, many times per day.[10] They eat the soft cecal feces directly from the anus.[29] Obese or pregnant animals may eat them from the floor, and young, unweaned guinea pigs can be seen eating the dam's droppings. Coprophagy appears to be an important function, although its contribution to the nutritional needs of guinea pigs has not been fully characterized. As in rabbits, coprophagy may be a source of B vitamins and a means of optimizing protein utilization.[7] If coprophagy is prevented, guinea pigs lose weight, digest less fiber, and excrete more minerals in the feces.[7,10]

Geriatric guinea pigs may develop fecal impactions within the anus, perhaps because of a loss of muscle tone or inability to eat feces directly from the anus. According to one author, these impactions are composed of soft, cecal feces, and the harder feces can still pass.[29] These impactions can be relieved by gentle manual expression, which may need to be repeated weekly.

Similar to the GI flora of rabbits, that of guinea pigs is primarily gram-positive.[25] Anaerobic lactobacilli are the predominant bacterial species in the large intestine.[7]

Urogenital system The accessory sex glands of male guinea pigs (boars) include the vesicular glands, prostate gland, coagulating glands, and bulbourethral glands. The vesicular glands are long, coiled blind sacs that lie ventral to the ureters and extend 10 cm into the abdominal cavity.[4] Do not mistake these for uterine horns! The testes are located in the open inguinal canals. Guinea pigs have an os penis. A pouch containing two horny styles (slender projections) is located caudoventral to the urethral opening. During erection, the pouch is everted and the styles project externally.

Female guinea pigs (sows) have paired uterine horns, a short uterine body (12 mm long), and a single os cervicis opening into the vagina. Guinea pigs have a vaginal closure membrane that opens at estrus, at parturition, and, in many animals, at day 26 or 27 of gestation.[38]

The renal pelvis is relatively large and has a single longitudinal renal papilla. The alkaline urine is normally thick and cloudy white or yellow. Like the urine of other herbivores, it contains many crystals.

Sexing Guinea pigs are easily sexed. Boars have obvious scrotal pouches and large testes (Fig. 23-6, *A*). There is a flat area of

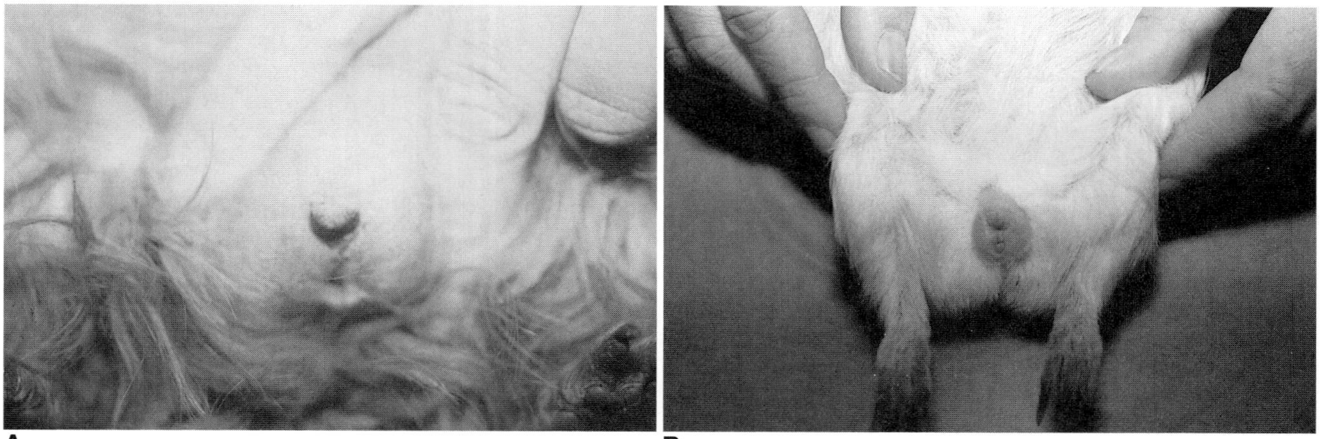

A B

Figure 23-6 **A**, Normal external genitalia of a male guinea pig. **B**, Normal external genitalia of a female guinea pig. Traction on the abdominal skin opens the genitalia slightly to show the transverse slit marking the vaginal opening.

tissue between the urethral opening and the anus, in which a longitudinal shallow slit may be present, marking the junction of the two scrotal pouches on the midline. The penis can be everted from the prepuce by placing gentle pressure at its base.

Sows have a Y-shaped depression in the perineal tissues (Fig. 23-6, *B*). The top branches of the Y point cranially and surround the urethral opening. The vulvar opening lies at the intersection of the branches, and the anus is located at the base of the Y.

In immature males, the penis can be prolapsed out of the prepuce; in immature females, the Y-shaped tissue depression is evident.

Reproduction Reproductive variables for guinea pigs are presented in Table 23-1. Many reported features of the reproductive cycle (e.g., length of estrus and the estrous cycle, timing of postpartum estrus, litter size) vary according to the source, presumably because of variations among strains of guinea pigs. The numbers reported here are compiled from several different sources and are referenced accordingly.

Puberty, defined as age at first conception, occurs at 2 months of age in females and at 3 months in males.[38] Males begin to mount at 1 month of age, and ejaculation is evident by the time they are 2 months old.[13] The peak reproductive period for females is from 3 or 4 months to 20 months of age; pet animals may reproduce until they are 4 or 5 years old.[21]

Guinea pigs are polyestrous and breed year-round in a laboratory setting. The estrous cycle in most females is 15 to 17 days (range, 13-21 days), and ovulation is spontaneous.[21] Fertile postpartum estrus occurs in most females from 2 to 10 hours after parturition.[31] Females show distinct signs of proestrus and estrus. During proestrus, they become more active and may chase their cage mates; they may sway the hindquarters and utter a distinct guttural sound. Estrus lasts 6 to 11 hours, during which time females show lordosis, or the copulatory reflex—an arching and straightening of the back with elevation of the rump and dilation of the vulva. In mature sows, the vaginal membrane is open for approximately 2 days during estrus; it closes after ovulation.

Copulatory plugs Copulation in guinea pigs (and chinchillas) can be confirmed by finding the vaginal (copulatory) plug, a solid mass of coagulated ejaculate that falls out of the vagina several hours after mating. Rodent copulatory plugs are typically hard and rubbery or waxy in consistency and are the exclusive product of male secretions. Copulatory plugs are not restricted to rodents and have been reported in some bats, insectivores, primates, and marsupials.[9]

Voss[33] advanced five possible functions of rodent copulatory plugs. The copulatory plugs may (1) store sperm, (2) prevent sperm leakage, (3) induce pseudopregnancy, (4) effect sperm transport, or (5) prevent later fertilization of the female by other males. Current hypotheses suggest that the primary function of the copulatory plug is chastity enforcement in polygamous breeding rodents. The other functions, especially sperm transport, are regarded as incidental but necessary effects. In guinea pigs, the copulatory plug prevents competing ejaculate from reaching the site of fertilization. This is also the case with chinchillas.

TABLE 23-1
Physiologic Values for Guinea Pigs

Usual life span as pet	5-6 years
Adult weight	Males, 900-1200 g; females 700-900 g
Sexual maturity	Males, 3 mo; females, 2 mo
Type of estrous cycle	Nonseasonally polyestrous
Length of estrous cycle	15-17 days
Ovulation	Spontaneous
Gestation period	59-72 days (average, 68 days)
Litter size	1-13 (2-4 is usual)
Normal birth weight	45-115 g (70-110 g is usual)
Weaning age	21 days (or at 180 g body weight)
Rectal temperature	99.0-103.1°F (37.2-39.5°C)
Average blood volume	70 mL/kg
Heart rate	240-310 beats/min

Pregnancy, parturition, and lactation Similar to the placenta of humans, that of guinea pigs is hemochorial, meaning that the trophoblasts are in contact with maternal blood. The duration of gestation is 59 to 72 days (average, 68 days), depending on the strain of guinea pig, parity of the sow, and litter size. Gestation is typically shorter in primiparous sows and in those with small litters. The fetuses can be palpated as early as 15 days of gestation, although they are more evident at 28 to 35 days of gestation.

Impending parturition is signaled by separation of the pubic symphysis; a gap of 15 mm is palpable about 2 days before parturition and increases in width (up to 25 mm or more) at the time of parturition.[13] This separation may be inadequate in sows that are bred for the first time after 7 or 8 months of age, and dystocia commonly results. Other causes of dystocia include obesity and large fetal size. Suspect dystocia in gravid sows that show depression or a bloody or discolored vaginal discharge; an emergency cesarean section is indicated in most cases (see Chapter 27).

Normal parturition is typically rapid, with only a few minutes between births. Guinea pigs do not build nests. The average litter size varies according to guinea pig strain and management practices, but is typically 2 to 4,[31,38] with a range of 1 to 13 young reported.[38] Birth weights range from 45 to 115 g and are inversely related to litter size[21]; young weighing less than 60 g rarely survive.[13] Although otherwise completely herbivorous, guinea pigs are placentophagic. In addition to the mother, males and other females may also consume the placenta.

Newborn guinea pigs (typically called pups or young, but not piglets) are precocious, meaning that they are fully furred, their eyes are open, and they are able to stand shortly after birth (Fig. 23-7). They are not, however, able to fend for themselves at this time.[38] The pups ideally should receive sow's milk for a minimum of 5 days, and the normal lactation period is 3 weeks.[38] Pups often do not survive if they fail to receive sow's milk for the first 3 to 4 days of life.[13] Guinea pig sows are not very "motherly." They passively allow nursing to occur rather than seek out the young. Lactating sows permit the young of other females to nurse. Licking of the pup's anogenital region by the sow is necessary to stimulate urination and defecation, because voluntary micturition does not occur until the second week of life. The young are weaned at 21 days, or at a weight of 180 g (15-28 days of age).[21]

Orphaned guinea pigs should be fostered to a lactating guinea pig if feasible. If there is no suitable foster mother, the

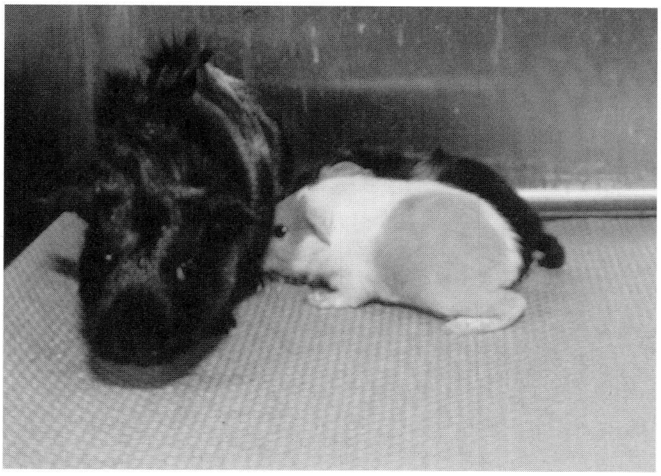

Figure 23-7 One-day-old guinea pig nursing from the dam.

young can be fed from a dropper or pet nurser beginning at 12 to 24 hours after birth. One author recommended feeding the pups every 2 hours until 5 days of age, after which feeding every 4 hours becomes sufficient.[29] The hand-rearing formula should approximate guinea pig milk, which contains 4% fat, 8% protein, and 3% lactose.[13] Evaporated milk mixed with an equal amount of water can be used. Guinea pigs begin nibbling on solid food at 2 days of age, and guinea pig pellets moistened with water or formula can be offered at that time.

Behavior

Guinea pigs are social animals that seek physical contact with other guinea pigs when housed together. They often stand side by side when resting and crowd together at feeders. However, there is little mutual grooming. Hair pulling can be a form of aggression, and hair pulling and ear nibbling of subordinate animals is seen in crowded or stressful environments.[14]

The vocalizations of guinea pigs have been well characterized. Recognized call types include the chutt, chutter, whine, tweet, whistle (single or in long bouts), purr, drr, scream, squeal, chirp, and grunt.[2,14] Many guinea pig owners are familiar with the excited squeals emitted by their pets when a refrigerator door is opened or feeding is imminent.

Husbandry

Housing Housing for guinea pigs should be set up with the knowledge that healthy guinea pigs produce prodigious amounts of feces, often defecate in food and water containers, turn over any unstable container, and are known to inject a premasticated slurry of pellets into the tubes of their sipper bottles. This said, guinea pigs require relatively simple housing.

In a laboratory setting in the United States, the minimum required floor space is 652 cm^2 (101 in^2) per adult animal; however, guinea pigs in a laboratory are often group-housed, and each animal has more than this amount of space. Pets should be provided with at least twice as much floor space. Cages may be constructed of plastic, metal, or wire. Good ventilation is important. If a solid-sided cage, such as an open glass aquarium, is used, change the bedding frequently to minimize ammonia levels in the cage. Guinea pigs do not jump or climb; therefore, the top of the cage does not need to be enclosed. The cage walls should be at least 25 cm (10 in) in height.

The flooring of the cage may be solid or wire mesh, although foot and leg injuries are more common in guinea pigs that are kept on wire. Guinea pig breeders use 12 × 38 mm wire mesh to minimize the potential for leg injuries.[13] Newspaper, shredded paper, wood shavings, and straw may be used for bedding on solid floors. A small, upside-down cardboard box provides shelter within the cage, although some guinea pigs prefer chewing the box to hiding in it.

Place the cage in a quiet area out of direct sunlight. The recommended temperature range for guinea pigs is 65° to 79°F (18° to 26°C).[13] Because of their susceptibility to hyperthermia, guinea pigs are better able to tolerate cool than warm environments and should not be exposed to high temperatures and humidity.

For breeding purposes, guinea pigs are usually housed in a harem-style arrangement with a single boar and 1 to 10 sows in a pen.[13] They can also be housed in pairs. In intensive breeding systems, the sow and young are left in the pen so that the sow can be rebred at the postpartum estrus. However, removal of the sow and young to a nursery area shortly after parturition minimizes trampling and ear chewing of the young by other adults.

Nutrition and feeding Guinea pigs develop dietary preferences early in life and do not adapt readily to changes in type, appearance, or presentation of their food or water. Even a change in the brand of pelleted feed can result in refusal of food. It may be a good idea to expose pets, while they are still young, to small amounts of different guinea pig chows and vegetables so that they become accustomed to variety. Always teach clients about this characteristic of guinea pigs to prevent a potentially dangerous, self-imposed fast by a pet guinea pig that is fed new food.

Wild cavies eat many different types of vegetation. Domestic guinea pigs are also completely herbivorous (with the exception of placentophagy). They digest fiber more efficiently than rabbits do.[7] Interestingly, they do not increase their food intake, as do rabbits and many other species, when cellulose or other fiber is used to dilute the diet. This suggests that satiety in guinea pigs is governed more by distention of the GI tract than by metabolic energy need.[7] A crude protein level of 18% to 20% is adequate for growth and lactation, and the recommended minimum level of crude fiber is 10%.[7]

Guinea pigs require a dietary source of vitamin C (ascorbic acid) because they lack L-gulonolactone oxidase, an enzyme involved in the synthesis of ascorbic acid from glucose. Nonbreeding adult guinea pigs require 10 mg/kg daily of ascorbic acid. Higher levels should be provided for growing and pregnant animals; 30 mg/kg daily is recommended during pregnancy.[13]

The recommended diet for pet guinea pigs consists of guinea pig pellets and grass hay, supplemented with fresh vegetables. Usually, the pellets are offered by free choice, although some clinicians believe that, as with rabbits, a limited quantity of this nutritionally rich food source is best for sedentary adult guinea pigs. Good-quality hay should be available at all times. Guinea pigs enjoy a variety of leafy greens, and these can be offered in handfuls. All fresh foods should be washed and prepared as though for human consumption, and they should be removed from the cage after a few hours if not yet eaten. Fruits, rolled oats, and dry cereals should be offered only in very small quantities, if at all, as treats. Any additions or changes to the diet should be made gradually.

Commercially available guinea pig pellets usually contain 18% to 20% crude protein and 10% to 16% fiber.[13] Pellets are fortified with ascorbic acid; however, approximately half of the initial vitamin C content may be oxidized and lost 90 days after the diet has been mixed and stored at 22°C. Increased storage temperature and humidity accelerate the rate of vitamin C loss. It is best to assume that the pellets contain no vitamin C; instead, supply adequate levels of this important nutrient in the form of vegetables and fruits or in the drinking water. Foods that contain high levels of ascorbic acid are leafy greens (kale, parsley, beet greens, chicory, spinach), red and green peppers, broccoli, tomatoes, kiwi fruit, and oranges. Vitamin C can be added to the water at 1 g/L.[13] In an open container, water with added vitamin C loses more than 50% of its vitamin C content in 24 hours. Aqueous solutions of vitamin C deteriorate more rapidly in the presence of metal, hard water, or heat. Vitamin C is more stable in neutral to alkaline solutions. Water must be changed daily to ensure adequate activity of the vitamin.

TABLE 23-2
Physiologic Values for Chinchillas

Usual life span as pet	10 years (up to 20 years reported)
Adult weight	Males, 400-500 g; females 400-600 g
Sexual maturity	8 months
Type of estrous cycle	Seasonally polyestrous (November to May)
Length of estrous cycle	30-50 days
Ovulation	Spontaneous
Gestation period	105-118 days (average, 111 days)
Litter size	1-6 (2 is usual)
Normal birth weight	30-50 g
Weaning age	6-8 weeks
Rectal temperature	98.6-100.4°F (37-38°C)
Heart rate	100-150 beats/min

BIOLOGY AND HUSBANDRY OF CHINCHILLAS

Chinchillas, like guinea pigs, originated in South America. The name *chinchilla* (little *chincha*) was coined by the Spaniards in the 16th century after the Chincha Indians, who used chinchilla pelts to decorate their ceremonial dress.[18] Chinchilla pelts were also prized by Europeans, and overhunting almost led to extinction of the species in the late 1800s and early 1900s. In the 1920s, 13 chinchillas were transported to California by Matthew Chapman. From these animals are descended most of the chinchillas in the United States today.

Chinchillas are rare in the wild and may be extinct. According to Walker,[34] probably only one species of chinchilla *(C. laniger)* remains in the wild. A short-tailed species, *Chinchilla brevicaudata*, has been described and is recognized by other authors.[36] The native habitat of *C. laniger* is (or was) the Andes mountains of Peru, Bolivia, Chile, and Argentina, where the animals inhabit cool, semiarid, rocky slopes at elevations from 3000 to 5000 m (10,000-16,600 ft) above sea level.[34] Consequently, they have a higher hemoglobin oxygen affinity than other pet rodents and rabbits.

Anatomy, Physiology, and Behavior

Chinchillas have a compact body with delicate limbs, large eyes, large round pinnae, long whiskers, and a bushy tail. They usually weigh between 400 and 600 g, and females tend to be larger than males (Table 23-2). The average life span is 10 years, which is much longer than that of other pet rodents; some chinchillas are reported to have lived 20 years.[34] Chinchillas are gregarious, living in groups of several hundred in the wild.

Chinchillas are quiet, shy, and agile. In the wild, chinchillas live in burrows and rock crevices, and they have long hind limbs and feet adapted for leaping. The long, plumed tail acts as a balance when the animal is sailing through the air. Chinchillas require larger cages than their less active cousins, the guinea pigs, do. In their natural habitat, chinchillas are active at dusk and at night; however, in captivity, they can be active during the day. They readily habituate to humans if handled frequently while young. Flight is their defense mechanism; rarely, they bite. Chinchillas are virtually odorless, although one author reported that frightened animals produced secretions, which gave off an odor similar to that of scorched almonds, from glands inside the anus.[24] Females reportedly may stand up on their hind legs and spray urine at a presumed attacker.

The hair coat is luxurious, soft, and very dense. As many as 60 hairs grow from a single hair follicle.[34] The natural wild-type color is bluish-grey with yellow-white underparts. Breeding has produced color mutations including white, silver, beige, and black (Fig. 23-8). Frequent dust baths are necessary to maintain the health of the fur (see Dust Baths). When frightened, chinchillas can shed patches of fur, a condition known as "fur-slip." The hairless patches take 6 to 8 weeks to fill in, and it may take several months for these patches to become indistinguishable from surrounding fur.

Chinchillas have four toes on front and rear feet, all with small, weak claws. There is no fur on the palmar and plantar

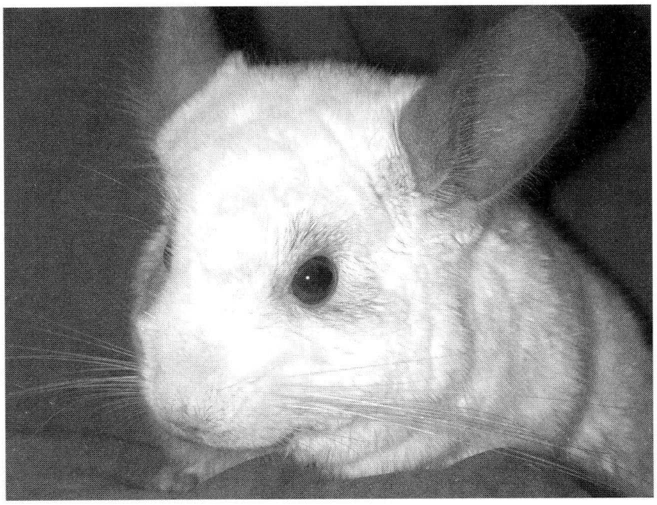

Figure 23-8 A white chinchilla, a color mutation produced by selective breeding. Note the dense, luxurious fur.

regions of the feet. They have very large, thin-walled auditory bullae, which are readily visible on radiographs. The eyes are large and sit in a shallow bony orbit. The iris is densely pigmented with a vertical pupil, both features consistent with the chinchillas' habit of basking in the sun in their high-altitude habitat.[26]

The dental formula of chinchillas is the same as that of guinea pigs: $2(I_1^1\ C_0^0\ PM_1^1\ M_3^3) = 20$. As in guinea pigs, all the teeth are open rooted and grow continuously throughout life. The incisors grow 5 to 7.5 cm (2-3 in) per year and are normally yellow in adult animals. Upper incisors grow faster than lower incisors.[40] The oral cavity is small and narrow. Like guinea pigs, chinchillas have a palatal ostium, an opening in the soft palate through which the oropharynx communicates with the rest of the pharynx.[32]

Chinchillas have a long gastrointestinal tract. The small and large intestines in one adult animal measured 3.5 m (11.5 ft).[40] The cecum is relatively large and coiled; the colon is highly sacculated. The cecum of a chinchilla holds less of the contents of the large intestine than that of a rabbit or guinea pig. According to one study, the cecum of a chinchilla held 23% of the dry matter content from the large intestine; that of a rabbit held 57%, and that of a guinea pig, 44%.[17]

Both guinea pigs and chinchillas produce two types of fecal pellets. One is nitrogen rich, intended for cecotrophy; the other is nitrogen poor, excreted as fecal pellets.

Chinchillas eat mainly at night, ingesting more than 70% of total daily intake during the dark. Fecal excretion is predominantly at night. Mean transit time of food in the gastrointestinal tract is 12 to 15 hours, similar to that of other rodents. However, in contrast to other pet rodents, transit time in chinchillas is not affected by reducing the dietary fiber level.

Urogenital tract, sexing, and reproduction Females have two uterine horns and two cervices.[30,36] The vaginal closure membrane is open only during parturition and for 2 to 4 days during estrus.[38] Chinchillas have three pairs of mammary glands—one inguinal pair and two lateral thoracic pairs.[38] Several reports in the veterinary literature have erroneously stated that chinchillas have two pairs of mammary glands.

Males do not have a true scrotum. Instead, the testes are contained within the inguinal canal or abdomen, and there are two small, moveable sacs next to the anus (postanal sacs), into which the caudal epididymis can drop.[36] The inguinal canal is open. The penis is readily apparent below the anus, from which it is separated by an expanse of bare skin. The penis can be manually everted 1 to 2 cm when flaccid.

The anogenital distance is the best criterion for sexing chinchillas, particularly because the relatively large urinary papilla of a female chinchilla can be confused with a penis (Fig. 23-9). The anogenital distance is greater in male chinchillas than in females; the penis is approximately 1 to 1.5 cm (0.4-0.6 in) cranioventral to the anus. This difference between the sexes is evident even at birth: the urinary papilla is adjacent to the anus in females, whereas the penis is separated from the anus by a narrow band of tissue in males. Eversion of the penis from the urethral orifice confirms the sex of the chinchilla.

Females have a large urinary papilla; at the end of the papilla is the urethral orifice. The structure we call the urinary papilla has been variously called the urethral cone and the clitoris. Immediately caudal to the urinary papilla is the slitlike vulva, which is oriented transversely relative to the craniocaudal axis of the body. The vaginal orifice is difficult to distinguish when closed and is indicated by a slightly raised, semicircular area. When the vaginal orifice is covered by its closure membrane, the urethral orifice can be mistaken as the genital opening. As previously mentioned, the vulva is closed by a membrane except during estrus and parturition. The anus is located immediately caudal to the vulva.

Chinchillas are seasonally polyestrous in the wild and in captivity, usually bearing two litters of young between November and May (breeding season in the northern hemisphere).[34] Age at puberty in males, defined as age at successful conception, is 8 months or older; in females, the average age at puberty is 8.5 months (range, 2-14 months).[36] If conception does not take place during postpartum estrus, the next estrus occurs about 40 days later (see Table 23-2). Estrous cycles range from 30 to 50

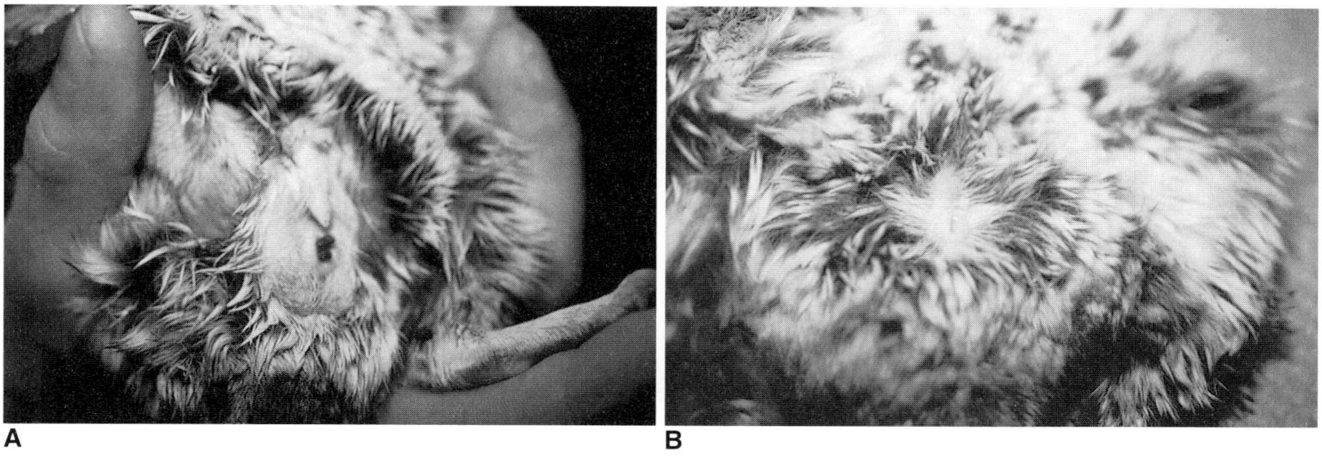

Figure 23-9 **A,** Normal external genitalia of a male chinchilla. **B,** Normal external genitalia of a female chinchilla. Note shorter anogenital distance and presence of the prominent urinary papilla (which can be confused with a penis) in the female. *(Photograph courtesy Dr. Heidi Hoefer.)*

days, with an average of 38 days. An open vulva, often with visible mucus, is an external indication of estrus. There is no vulvar swelling during estrus; rather, there is a change in perineal color, which goes from a dull flesh color to a deep red. The color of the perineum increases dramatically at the time of vaginal perforation and remains intense throughout most of the luteal phase of the estrous cycle.[5]

Chinchillas can be housed in pairs or in polygamous units, with a single male and two to six females. The polygamous units used by breeders are set up with separate cages for the females, each with a rear door onto a common runway used by the male. The male can go through any open door at will, but the females wear collars that prevent exit from their cages. In a polygamous setting, the male is kept out of the female's cage during parturition and raising of young; however, in a pair setting, the male can often remain with the female during this time if she tolerates his presence.[22] Expulsion of a copulatory plug by the female is a sign that mating occurred the day before (see previous discussion of copulatory plugs in guinea pigs).

Gestation averages 111 days (see Table 23-2), and there are usually two young in each litter (range, 1-6).[38] Pet chinchillas have smaller litters and more males per litter than do chinchillas from fur ranches or laboratory colonies.[38] Parturition typically occurs in the early morning, and dystocia is uncommon in well-managed breeding establishments. Although chinchillas do not build nests,[40] the females can learn to use a nest box that, when heated, prevents the first-born young from becoming hypothermic while the rest of the litter are being born.[24] Chinchillas, like guinea pigs, are placentophagic. Blood on the nose and front paws of the female indicates that she has eaten the placenta and the birthing process is over.[24]

Chinchilla young are precocious, weighing 30 to 50 g at birth, and are fully furred with teeth and open eyes. They are able to walk within 1 hour after birth. The dam stands, rather than lying down, while they nurse.[24] If the mother dies after birth, another lactating female will usually accept the newborn young, especially if they are close in age to her own. According to one author, a lactating guinea pig may be an appropriate foster mother in some cases.[35]

Hand-feeding is necessary if a foster mother is not available or if supplemental nutrition is needed for litters of four or more. A formula of equal parts evaporated milk and water can be administered with an eye dropper or pet nurser. One author recommended adding glucose (1 g/15 mL) to this formula.[36] For the first 3 or 4 days, the young should be hand-fed as often as possible during the day, with no more than 4 hours between feedings, and once or twice at night. After this time, the night feedings can be dropped and the intervals between daytime feedings gradually lengthened.[36]

The young of large litters may fight over access to the teats, and it may be necessary to clip the incisor teeth to prevent serious injury to the teats or to siblings. Chinchillas begin to eat solid foods at 1 week of age. To minimize fighting, food bowls should be large enough to accommodate the entire litter simultaneously. Weaning is at 6 to 8 weeks of age.

Husbandry

Housing Chinchillas are very active, acrobatic animals and require a lot of space. According to one author, the enclosure should be at least 2 × 2 × 1 m (6.6 × 6.6 × 3.3 ft), with a wooden nesting box measuring 30 × 25 × 20 cm (12 × 10 × 7 in).[35] Large, multilevel cages that provide sufficient space for climbing and jumping are excellent for housing pet chinchillas. Because chinchillas chew wooden cages, the cage should be constructed of 15 × 15 mm welded wire mesh, with or without an area of solid flooring. Drop pans below the cage facilitate cleaning.

Chinchillas are shy animals, and in captivity they need a place to hide. In the wild, chinchillas conceal themselves in rock crevices. Polyvinyl chloride (PVC) plumbing pipes, especially elbows and Y- and T-sections, make ideal hiding places and can be sanitized in a dishwasher. The pipes should be 10 to13 cm (4-5 in) in diameter. Alternatively, clay pipes of a similar diameter can be used.

Chinchillas can be housed in pairs, colonies, or polygamous units, although colony housing is not advised for breeding chinchillas.[24] Cage setup for polygamous units was described earlier.

Chinchillas do best in a dry environment at relatively cool temperatures. One recommended temperature range for housing chinchillas is 50 to 68°F (10-20°C).[35] Temperatures lower than 65°F (18°C) and relative humidity lower than 50% promote good fur growth.[35] Chinchillas do not tolerate dampness and are prone to heat stroke at environmental temperatures greater than 82° to 86°F (28°-30°C).

Dust baths Access to a dust bath should be provided daily, if possible, or at least several times per week. Sanitized chinchilla dust is available commercially at pet stores. Two commercial dust baths, Blue Cloud and Blue Sparkle, can be obtained from various web-based chinchilla supply stores (e.g., chinworld.com, onestarchinchilla.com). Alternatively, a 9:1 mixture of silver sand and Fuller's earth can be used.[19] Fuller's earth is a variety of kaolin that contains aluminum magnesium silicate. The name is derived from the ancient process of cleaning, or fulling, wool to remove the oil and dirt particles with a mixture of water and earth or clay. Beach or playground sand is not suitable for dust baths.

Some people are allergic to the commercially available powders. It is possible to make a homemade dust bath preparation consisting of perfume-free talc powder (also known as talcum or French chalk) and food-grade cornstarch. Food-grade cornstarch (marketed as Maizena or Mondamin) is best. Avoid using soluble starch, which is potato or corn starch treated with dilute hydrochloric acid. Some breeders eliminate or reduce the amount of cornstarch used for nursing mothers, because the babies get it in their noses and develop rhinitis.[30] More recently, volcanic ash from Mount St. Helens in Washington has become very fashionable. This is a very fine powder; allow access for 3 to 4 minutes.[30]

The dust is placed at a depth of 2 to 3 cm (1 in) in a pan, such as a plastic dishpan, that is big enough for the chinchilla to roll around in. A chinchilla may spend up to an hour dust bathing, rolling, and fluffing its fur.[22] The dust bath can be kept clean and free of feces by removing it from the cage after use. Excessive use of dust baths can lead to conjunctivitis, especially in young chinchillas.

Nutrition and feeding In their natural habitat, the relatively barren areas of the Andes Mountains, chinchillas reportedly feed on any available vegetation, eating in the early morning and the late evening, by holding the food with their forepaws while sitting on their haunches.[34] Chinchillas eat mainly at night. Work by Farmer[11] more than 50 years ago showed the importance of grasses and hays in the diet, and it is recommended that chinchillas be given a high-fiber diet. Despite statements made more than 40 years ago, such as "a great deal of work and clear thinking is required on the nutrition of the chinchilla,"[3] the specific nutrient requirements for chinchillas are still unknown. Commercial chinchilla diets are available (e.g., Chinchilla Deluxe, Oxbow Hay Co., Murdock, NE, www.oxbowhay.com; Mazuri Chinchilla Diet, Mazuri, St. Louis, MO, www.mazuri.com). Some diets marketed for chinchillas are, in reality, mixtures of rabbit, guinea pig, and rodent pellets. As such, they provide a diet supplemented with Vitamin C that is lower in protein and fat than standard rodent chow and has the same fiber content as a rabbit maintenance diet. However, the pellets are longer than rabbit or guinea pig pellets and therefore are easier for the chinchilla to hold. The accepted formula for chinchilla pellets is 16% to 20% protein, 2% to 5% fat, and 15% to 35% bulk fiber.[12,16,35]

Although very little has been published about the nutritional needs of pet chinchillas, it is safe to assume that growing animals and breeding females require more calories and higher levels of calcium, protein, and fat than do nonbreeding chinchillas. Nonbreeding animals do well on a diet of good-quality grass hay supplemented with small amounts of chinchilla or rabbit pellets, fresh vegetables, and grains.[19] One to two tablespoons of pellets daily should be sufficient for a nonbreeding adult animal. A pellets-only diet has insufficient roughage and can predispose the chinchilla to enteritis. Chinchillas consume their food more slowly than rabbits and guinea pigs do.

Limit treats such as grains, dried apples, raisins, figs, hazelnuts, and sunflower seeds to not more than one teaspoon per day. As with guinea pigs, clean and prepare all food as if for human consumption. Any change in diet should be instituted gradually. Abrupt dietary changes will lead to temporary but dramatic (up to 50%) decreases in food intake.

Have clean, fresh drinking water available at all times. Chinchillas can be trained to use automated watering devices in a laboratory setting, or they can do equally well with cage-mounted water bottles. Water in a bowl tends to get dirty quickly and can spill.

Hard foods for gnawing can be offered. These may include porous stones such as pumice; young branches of trees such as elm, ash, maple, and birch; pieces of bark from apple, pear, and peach trees; and young grapevines. Advise the owner to avoid branches from poisonous trees, such as cedar, plum, redwood, cherry, and oleander.

CLINICAL TECHNIQUES FOR GUINEA PIGS AND CHINCHILLAS

Handling and Restraint

Guinea pigs are docile animals that usually need minimal restraint during a physical examination. Most will sit quietly on the examination table while the owner or an assistant places a hand on the rump so that the animal does not back away. To auscultate the heart and lungs and palpate the abdomen, gently pick up the animal in one hand. Turn it over on its back, while supporting it in your hand, to examine the perineal area and genitalia.

Carry a guinea pig by supporting its weight in one hand and cupping its dorsum with the other hand. If the guinea pig is nervous or is not used to handling, keep it in a carrier as much as possible and avoid excessive handling.

Chinchillas tend to be active at dusk and at night; therefore, try to schedule evening appointments. Most pet chinchillas are easy to hold and do not bite; however, even a well-mannered pet will give warning nips if distressed, and if frightened, it will bite. Usually, a hand-tamed chinchilla comes out of its cage willingly; if it does not, it can be lifted out by the examiner or the owner. You must be fast and on target, however, because a scared chinchilla can lose a patch of fur where it is grasped (known as fur-slip). If the chinchilla escapes from the cage and is loose in a room, it can ricochet off walls like a rubber ball—never try to catch a speeding chinchilla by the tail or you might be left holding the skin of the tail and no chinchilla.[30]

When lifting a chinchilla out of its cage, place one hand under the animal's abdomen or around the scruff of the neck, and hold it by the base of the tail with the other hand (Fig. 23-1, *B*). When you carry a chinchilla, hold the base of its tail with one hand to prevent it from jumping. As with transporting rabbits, the head can be tucked under your arm.

If the chinchilla is prone to bite, two people should hold it. One person restrains the chinchilla on a table with one hand under the thorax and one hand holding the base of the tail; the examiner additionally holds the animal by the scruff of the neck.

Physical Examination

The initial examination should involve observing the guinea pig or chinchilla in its cage. Focus on the animal's movement, mentation, and rate and rhythm of breathing. Healthy guinea pigs have an alert demeanor with clear eyes. The animal should react to stimuli by moving or vocalizing; some animals will move very quickly. Healthy guinea pigs usually eat readily when offered treats or greens.

Healthy chinchillas have a spirited curiosity and a curled tail that is carried high. Sick animals are indifferent and have a dull coat; often the perianal area is stained or covered with feces. An animal that flies around the cage in a frenzy when the owner attempts to capture it has not been socialized to people or other chinchillas and will be difficult to examine without sedation.

Begin the physical examination by measuring the animal's weight; this is also a good time to obtain the animal's temperature before it becomes excited or stressed. Next, examine the fur, skin, and mucous membranes. Follow this by auscultating the heart and lungs, and then palpate the abdomen. Check the rectal area for impaction of feces in guinea pigs. Observe the genitalia and note any abnormalities.

Overgrowth of the nails is common in pet guinea pigs. Often a horny growth is present and extends from the footpads, especially in older animals. Trim the nails of guinea pigs and chinchillas with human fingernail clippers or with cat claw clippers. The horny overgrowth can be trimmed back carefully, but avoid causing bleeding.

Examine the oral cavity last; this can be stressful for the guinea pig or chinchilla, and the animal may become excited. Guinea pigs will object to examination of their teeth by squealing, and both guinea pigs and chinchillas may struggle or try to escape. For examination of the guinea pig, have an assistant place one hand on the animal's rump and the other hand around the shoulder and thoracic area. Use a speculum or otoscope to examine the cheek teeth, similar to the method used in rabbits. Chinchillas can be held by an assistant; use both hands to encircle the thoracic area while the animal is restrained on the table, or support the animal's weight in one hand and restrain the forelimbs with the other hand. Healthy chinchillas have yellow incisors because of iron deposition on the enamel.

Blood Collection

Venipuncture in guinea pigs and chinchillas can be difficult. The lateral saphenous and cephalic veins are the most accessible, but they are very small, and only small amounts of blood can be collected from each vein. Shave the fur from the area and wet the skin with alcohol to enhance visibility of the vein. Use an insulin or tuberculin syringe and a small (25- to 27-gauge) needle to prevent collapse of the vein. Venipuncture of multiple veins is often necessary to collect an adequate volume of blood for analysis.

The jugular vein can be used to collect large blood samples; however, the restraint required for blood collection can be very stressful for these animals. Guinea pigs, especially, have short, thick, compact necks, and it is often difficult to locate the jugular vein. For venipuncture, restrain the animal with the forelegs extended down over a table edge and the head and neck extended up (Fig. 23-10). If necessary, shave the fur from the area to enhance visibility of the vein, and use a small (22- to 25-gauge) needle and a 3-mL syringe for blood collection. If the animal shows obvious signs of stress or becomes dyspneic during jugular venipuncture, abort the procedure immediately. Observe the animal closely for several minutes after restraint is removed to see that it recovers. If the animal still appears to be stressed or dyspneic after several minutes, abandon further venipuncture attempts. Jugular venipuncture can also be done after the animal has been anesthetized with isoflurane or chemically restrained with an injectable tranquilizer.

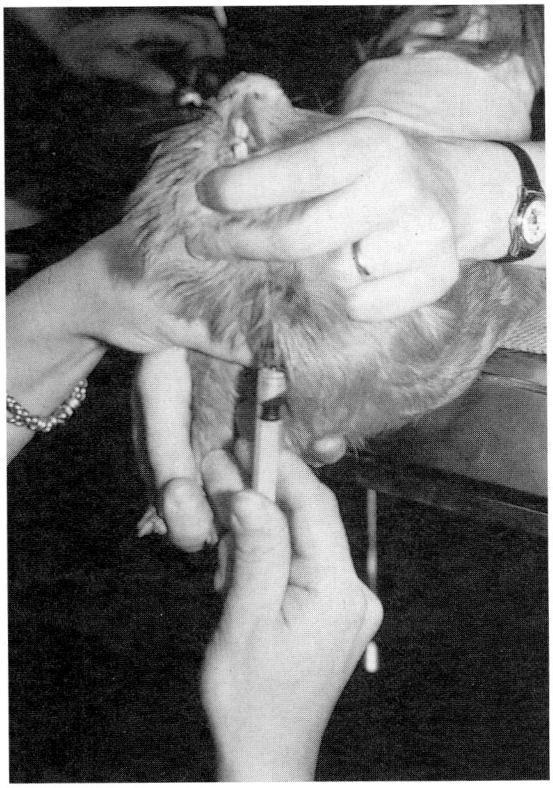

Figure 23-10 Jugular venipuncture in a guinea pig. This positioning and blood collection technique is too stressful for very sick guinea pigs.

Venipuncture of the cranial vena cava can be used, but there is a risk of subsequent traumatic bleeding into the thoracic cavity or pericardial sac.[28] Cardiac puncture is not recommended as a blood collection technique unless it is performed as a terminal procedure during euthanasia, and then only with the animal deeply sedated or under anesthesia.

The blood volume in guinea pigs averages 7 mL/100 g body weight.[31] Approximately 7% to 10% of the blood volume (0.5-0.7 mL/100 g) can be safely collected from a healthy, nonanemic guinea pig. Similar guidelines can be used in chinchillas.

Cystocentesis

Cystocentesis is sometimes necessary in animals with clinical signs of urinary tract disease. The method is similar to that used with other small animals, and a small (25-gauge) needle is used. Anesthesia may be necessary for restraint.

Clinical Laboratory Findings

Reported reference ranges of laboratory values for guinea pigs and chinchillas are given in Tables 23-3 and 23-4, respectively.[6,13,21-23] Published data are readily available for guinea pigs but pertain primarily to laboratory-housed animals, not pets. Published data for chinchillas are sparse. Clinical laboratory values vary according to physiologic state of the animal and laboratory techniques used. Ideally, as for other species, each laboratory should have established reference ranges.

In guinea pigs, alanine aminotransferase activity is low in hepatocytes; therefore, it is not sensitive or specific as a marker of hepatocellular injury.[39] Hypercholesterolemia is common in guinea pigs, often in conjunction with fatty infiltration of many tissues, including the liver. If guinea pig serum is stored in plastic, potassium levels are lower than if glass containers are used.[39]

A unique leukocyte of the guinea pig is the Kurloff cell (see Chapter 38). This mononuclear cell resembles a lymphocyte but contains round or ovoid inclusions termed Kurloff bodies.[31] The origin of Kurloff cells (thymus or spleen) is controversial. The number of circulating cells is variable: Kurloff cells are rare in very young animals, numbers are low in males, and numbers in females are related to the estrous cycle. Kurloff cells are highest in females during pregnancy and may play a role in creating a physiologic barrier between the fetus and the mother.[31]

The cellular distribution of bone marrow in the guinea pig is 26.7% erythroblasts, 63.3% myeloid cells, 4.6% lymphocytes, and 5.4% reticulum cells.[1] The myeloid/erythroid (M/E) ratio is 1.5 : 1[15] to 1.9 : 1.[8]

The normal pH of guinea pig urine is 9.0.[25] The normal pH of chinchilla urine is 8.5; specific gravity often exceeds 1.045.[22]

Treatment Techniques

Intravenous catheters Peripheral intravenous catheters can be used in guinea pigs and chinchillas but are difficult to place because of the small size and fragility of the veins. Use a small (24-gauge or smaller) indwelling catheter, and place the catheter while the animal is under anesthesia. Jugular cutdowns can be done to catheterize the jugular vein if an indwelling catheter is necessary and a peripheral catheter cannot be placed. Venous

TABLE 23-3
Reference Ranges for Hematology and Serum Biochemical Values in Guinea Pigs

Value	Reference Range
Hematocrit (%)	32-50
Hemoglobin (g/dL)	10.0-17.2
Red blood cells ($\times 10^6/\mu L$)	3.2-8.0
Sedimentation rate (mm/h)	1.1-14.0
White blood cells ($\times 10^3/\mu L$)	5.5-17.5
Neutrophils (%)	22-48
Lymphocytes (%)	39-72
Monocytes (%)	1-10
Eosinophils (%)	0-7
Basophils (%)	0.0-2.7
Platelets ($\times 10^3/\mu L$)	260-740
Mean corpuscular volume (μm^3)	71-96
Mean corpuscular hemoglobin (pg)	23-27
Mean corpuscular hemoglobin concentration (%)	26-39
Total protein (g/dL)	4.2-6.8
Albumin (g/dL)	2.1-3.9
Globulin (g/dL)	1.7-2.6
Glucose (mg/dL)	60-125
Blood urea nitrogen (mg/dL)	9.0-31.5
Creatinine (mg/dL)	0.6-2.2
Sodium (mmol/L)	120-152
Potassium (mmol/L)	3.8-7.9
Chloride (mmol/L)	90-115
Calcium (mg/dL)	8.2-12.0
Phosphorus (mg/dL)	3.0-7.6
Alanine aminotransferase (U/L)	25-59
Aspartate aminotransferase (U/L)	26-68
Alkaline phosphatase (U/L)	55-108
Bilirubin (mg/dL)	0.0-0.9
Cholesterol (mg/dL)	16-43

Data from Harkness JE, Wagner JE: The Biology and Medicine of Rabbits and Rodents, 4th ed. Baltimore, Williams & Wilkins, 1995; Manning PJ, Wagner JE, Harkness JE: Biology and diseases of guinea pigs. *In* Fox JG, Cohen BJ, Loew FM, eds. Laboratory Animal Medicine. Orlando, Academic Press, 1984, pp 149-177; Mitruka BM, Rawnsley HM: Clinical Biochemical and Hematological Reference Values in Normal Experimental Animals and Normal Humans, 2nd ed. Chicago, Year Book Medical Publishers, 1981, pp 70-73, 166-177.

access ports are used in many laboratory animals and are an alternative if long-term intravenous therapy is anticipated.

Fluid therapy Supplemental fluids are commonly given subcutaneously into the loose skin of the dorsal neck and upper back areas (Fig. 23-11). Normal daily water intake in the guinea pig is estimated to be 100 mL/kg.[21] Supplemental fluid requirements should be calculated based on this estimation plus additional fluid to compensate for dehydration. The total volume can be divided into two to three daily treatments. Volumes of 25 to 35 mL can be given into each subcutaneous injection site with a 22- to 25-gauge butterfly catheter. Many guinea pigs react to the pain caused by subcutaneous fluid administration and become very stressed. To avoid unnecessary stress, animals that are drinking water can be given oral fluids, unless they are azotemic or moderately to severely dehydrated.

TABLE 23-4
Reported Averages and Reference Ranges for Hematology and Serum Biochemical Values in Chinchillas

Value	Reference Range
Hematocrit (%)	38*
Hemoglobin (g/dL)	11.7-13.5†
Red blood cells ($\times 10^6/\mu L$)	6.6-10.7†
White blood cells ($\times 10^3/\mu L$)	7.6-11.5†
Neutrophils (%)	23-45†
Lymphocytes (%)	51-73†
Monocytes (%)	1-4†
Eosinophils (%)	0.5-2.6†
Basophils (%)	0-1†
Platelets ($\times 10^3/\mu L$)	254-298†
Total protein (g/dL)	5-6
Albumin (g/dL)	2.5-4.2
Glucose (mg/dL)	60-120
Blood urea nitrogen (mg/dL)	10-25
Sodium (mmol/L)	130-155
Potassium (mmol/L)	5.0-6.5
Chloride (mmol/L)	105-115
Calcium (mg/dL)	10-15
Phosphorus (mg/dL)	4-8
Alanine aminotransferase (U/L)	10-35
Aspartate aminotransferase (U/L)	15-45
Alkaline phosphatase (U/L)	3-12
Cholesterol (mg/dL)	40-100

*Data from Williams CSF: Practical Guide to Laboratory Animals. St Louis, CV Mosby, 1976, pp 3-11.
†Hematology ranges represent ranges of average figures compiled from several studies by Douglas W. Stone, DVM, and presented in Merry CJ: An introduction to chinchillas. Vet Tech 1990; 11:315-322. Serum Biochemical data from The Care of Experimental Animals: a Guide for Canada. Ottawa, Canadian Council on Animal Care, 1969, p 438.

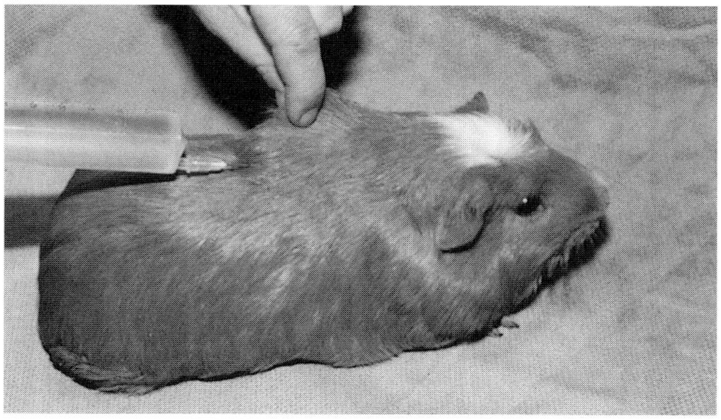

Figure 23-11 Subcutaneous fluid administration in a guinea pig.

Use a Buretrol device (Baxter Healthcare, Deerfield, IL) or an injection pump with either continuous or intermittent infusion for intravenous fluid administration. Monitor fluid volumes closely to avoid overhydration.

Medications Give parenteral medications by subcutaneous or intramuscular injection. The upper back is a common site for subcutaneous injection. The skin in this area is thick in guinea pigs, especially in intact males, and is sometimes difficult to penetrate with a 25-gauge or smaller needle. Give intramuscular injections in the lumbar muscles. Give oral medications and nutritional supplements by squeezing them from a syringe into the side of the mouth. Administration of tablets to chinchillas is possible; because chinchillas are inquisitive, they will usually eat tablets that are hidden in raisins.

Force-feed partially anorectic and anorectic guinea pigs and chinchillas with food supplements such as Critical Care (Oxbow Hay Co.), softened guinea pig pellets, strained baby food vegetables, or a soy-based liquid enteral formula. Give hospitalized guinea pigs parenteral vitamin C daily.

Guinea pigs do not adapt well to changes in their environments or routines and should be hospitalized only if necessary. Hospitalized guinea pigs should be given supportive care in anticipation of decreased appetite and water consumption.

REFERENCES

1. Baranski S: Effect of chronic microwave irradiation on the blood forming system of guinea pigs and rabbits. Aerosp Med 1971; 42:1196-1199.
2. Berryman JC: Guinea-pig vocalizations: their structure, causation and function. Z Tierpsychol 1976; 41:80-106.
3. Bowden RST: Diseases of chinchillas. Vet Rec 1959; 71:1033-1039.
4. Breazile JE, Brown EM: Anatomy. *In* Wagner JE, Manning PJ, eds. The Biology of the Guinea Pig. New York, Academic Press, 1976, pp 53-62.
5. Brookhyser KM, Aulerich RJ: Consumption of food, body weight, perineal color and levels of progesterone in the serum of cyclic female chinchillas. J Endocrinol 1980; 87:213-219.
6. The Care of Experimental Animals: A Guide for Canada. Ottawa, Ontario, Canadian Council on Animal Care: 1969, p 438.
7. Cheeke PR: Nutrition of guinea pigs. *In* Rabbit Feeding and Nutrition. Orlando, Academic Press, 1987, pp 344-353.
8. Dineen JK, Adams DB: The effect of long-term lymphatic drainage on the lympho-myeloid system in the guinea pig. Immunology 1970; 19:11-30.
9. Donnelly TM: Behaviour and reproduction. *In* Rabbits and Rodents: Laboratory Animal Science. Proceedings 142 of the Post-Graduate Committee in Veterinary Science, Sydney, 1990, pp 381-388.
10. Ebino KY: Studies on coprophagy in experimental animals. Exp Anim 1993; 42:1-9.
11. Farmer FA: A study of the dietary requirements of chinchillas. Natl Chinchilla Breeder Can 1951; 5:11-18.
12. Harkness JE: A Practitioners Guide to Domestic Rodents. Denver, American Animal Hospital Association, 1993.
13. Harkness JE, Wagner JE: The Biology and Medicine of Rabbits and Rodents, 4th ed. Baltimore, Williams & Wilkins, 1995.
14. Harper LV: Behavior. *In* Wagner JE, Manning PJ, eds. The Biology of the Guinea Pig. New York, Academic Press, 1976, pp 31-48.
15. Harris RS, Herdan G, Ancill RJ, et al: A quantitative comparison of the nucleated cells in the right and left humeral bone marrow of the guinea pig. Blood 1954; 9:374-378.
16. Hoefer HL: Chinchillas. Vet Clin North Am Small Anim Pract 1994; 24:103-111.
17. Holtenius K, Bjornhag G: The colonic separation mechanism in the guinea-pig (*Cavia porcellus*) and the chinchilla (*Chinchilla laniger*). Comp Biochem Physiol 1985; 82A:537-542.
18. Houston JW, Presturich JP: Chinchilla Care, 4th ed. Los Angeles, Borden Publishing, 1962.
19. Jenkins J: Husbandry and common diseases of the chinchilla (*Chinchilla laniger*). J Small Exotic Anim Med 1992; 2:15-17.
20. Jilge B: The gastrointestinal transit time in the guinea-pig. Z Versuchstierk 1980; 22:204-210.
21. Manning PJ, Wagner JE, Harkness JE: Biology and diseases of guinea pigs. *In* Fox JG, Cohen BJ, Loew FM, eds. Laboratory Animal Medicine. Orlando, Academic Press, 1984, pp 149-177.
22. Merry CJ: An introduction to chinchillas. Vet Tech 1990; 11:315-322.
23. Mitruka BM, Rawnsley HM: Clinical Biochemical and Hematological Reference Values in Normal Experimental Animals and Normal Humans, 2nd ed. Chicago, Year Book Medical Publishers, 1981, pp 70-73, 166-177.
24. Mösslacher E: Breeding and Caring for Chinchillas. Neptune City, NJ, T.F.H. Publications, 1986.
25. Navia JM, Hunt CE: Nutrition, nutritional diseases, and nutrition research applications. *In* Wagner JE, Manning PJ, eds. The Biology of the Guinea Pig. New York, Academic Press, 1976, pp 235-261.
26. Peiffer RL, Johnson PT: Clinical ocular findings in a colony of chinchillas (*Chinchilla laniger*). Lab Anim 1980; 14:331-335.
27. Popesko P, Rajtová V, Horák J: A Colour Atlas of Anatomy in Small Laboratory Animals. Vol. 1: Rabbit, Guinea Pig. London, Wolfe Publishing, 1992, pp 148-240.
28. Reuter RE: Venipuncture in the guinea pig. Lab Anim Sci 1987; 37:245-246.
29. Richardson VCG: Diseases of Domestic Guinea Pigs, 2nd ed. London, Blackwell Scientific, 2000.
30. Ritchey L: The Joy of Chinchillas. Menlo Park, CA (published privately), 1995.
31. Sisk DB: Physiology. *In* Wagner JE, Manning PJ, eds. The Biology of the Guinea Pig. New York, Academic Press, 1976, pp 63-92.
32. Timm KI, Jahn SE, Sedgwick CJ: The palatal ostium of the guinea pig. Lab Anim Sci 1987; 37:801-802.
33. Voss R: Male accessory glands and the evolution of copulatory plugs in rodents. Occasional Papers of the Museum of Zoology, No. 689. Ann Arbor, University of Michigan, 1979.
34. Walker EP: Mammals of the World, 3rd ed, Vol. II. Baltimore, Johns Hopkins University Press, 1975.
35. Webb R: Chinchillas. *In* Beynon PH, Cooper JE, eds. Manual of Exotic Pets. Ames, Iowa State University Press, 1991, pp 15-22.
36. Weir BJ: Chinchilla. *In* Hafez ESE, ed. Reproduction and Breeding Techniques for Laboratory Animals. Philadelphia, Lea & Febiger, 1970, pp 209-223.
37. Weir BJ: Notes on the origin of the domestic guinea-pig. Symp Zool Soc Lond 1974; 34:437-446.
38. Weir BJ: Reproductive characteristics of hystricomorph rodents. Symp Zool Soc Lond 1974; 34:265-301.
39. White EJ, Lang CM: The guinea pig. *In* Loeb WF, Quimby FW, eds. The Clinical Chemistry of Laboratory Animals. New York, Pergamon Press, 1989, pp 27-30.
40. Williams CSF: Practical Guide to Laboratory Animals. St Louis, CV Mosby, 1976, pp 3-11.

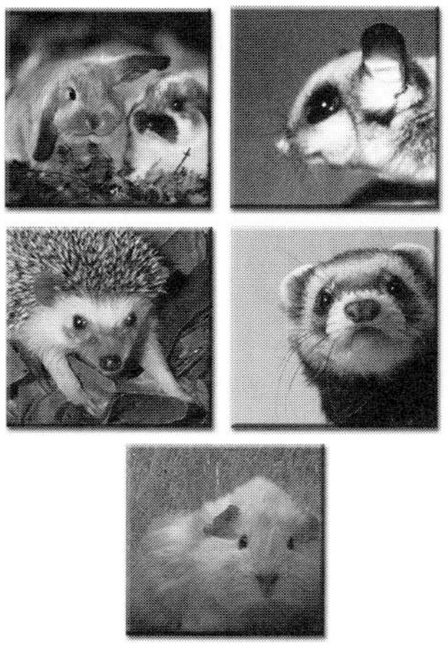

CHAPTER 24

Disease Problems of Guinea Pigs

Dorcas P. O'Rourke, DVM, MS, Diplomate ACLAM

Guinea pigs are New World, montane, hystricomorph rodents that are frequently kept as pets. Although superficially similar to mice and rats, guinea pigs have several anatomic and physiologic differences that can predispose them to unique disease conditions. This chapter deals with the diagnosis and treatment of guinea pig diseases.

GASTROINTESTINAL DISEASES

Antibiotic-Associated Enterotoxemia

Guinea pigs possess a predominantly gram-positive gastrointestinal flora and are exquisitely sensitive to antibiotics, which eradicate that flora. Drugs such as penicillin, ampicillin, chlortetracycline, clindamycin, erythromycin, and lincomycin will destroy the most susceptible gram-positive organisms, permitting overgrowth of *Clostridium difficile* and elaboration of its toxin.[10,35] Toxin production causes hyperactivity of secretomotor neurons, resulting in secretory diarrhea and hemorrhagic typhlitis.[59] Clinically, the guinea pig has diarrhea and is anorectic, dehydrated, and hypothermic.[35] Diagnosis is usually based on history, clinical signs, and lesions, because *C. difficile* is difficult to isolate. Antibiotic-associated enterotoxemia is treated symptomatically. Supportive therapy includes placing the animal in an incubator or putting its cage on a recirculating water blanket to correct hypothermia. Lactated Ringer's solution or other crystalline fluids should be administered intravenously, intraperitoneally, or subcutaneously to restore hydration. A daily maintenance dose of 10 mL/100 g should be administered to a dehydrated animal until it is drinking normally. Intestinal microflora can be reestablished by administration of a commercial *Lactobacillus* product. Alternatively, live-culture yogurt can be given orally at a dosage of approximately 5 mL/day. Although refaunation with rodent fecal slurry has been performed, transfaunation with healthy guinea pig flora has proven to be more successful. Chloramphenicol administered at 50 mg/kg q8h PO may be effective in suppressing further clostridial overgrowth.[10]

Antibiotic-associated enterotoxemia is prevented by treating guinea pigs with appropriate antibiotics. Trimethoprim-sulfa (30 mg/kg SC, IM, or PO q12h × 7 days), chloramphenicol (50 mg/kg PO q12h × 7 days), and enrofloxacin (10 mg/kg PO q12h) are effective and safe in guinea pigs. Sodium ampicillin (6 mg/kg SC q8h × 5 days) is well tolerated; however, it is toxic at

8 mg/kg.[60] Cefazolin at 50 mg/kg IM, SC is well tolerated; however, to be effective against *Bordetella* (a common guinea pig pathogen) at this dose, it would need to be administered every 30 minutes. Higher doses of cefazolin cause irritation at the injection site and death.[19] Whenever antibiotics are used to treat a guinea pig, the animal should also receive a *Lactobacillus* supplement during treatment and for 5 days beyond termination of antibiotic administration.[10]

Bacterial Enteritis

Salmonella typhimurium and *Salmonella enteritidis* are the most common causes of bacterial enteritis in guinea pigs. Transmission is by fecal contamination of feed. Animals that are stressed, particularly weanlings, pregnant sows, aged animals, and those with nutritional deficiencies, are particularly susceptible.[26] Signs include scruffy hair coat, weight loss, weakness, conjunctivitis, and abortion. Diarrhea may or may not be present. At necropsy, the spleen and liver are enlarged, and yellow necrotic foci may be present in the viscera.[10] Diagnosis is made by culture and sensitivity testing of a fecal sample. Treatment includes appropriate antibiotic and fluid therapy, keeping in mind that the affected animal could become an asymptomatic carrier. The disease can be prevented by keeping the environment clean, storing food in airtight containers, and thoroughly washing all fresh fruits and vegetables that are offered to guinea pigs. Salmonellosis is a zoonotic disease.

Other causes of bacterial diarrhea in guinea pigs include *Yersinia pseudotuberculosis, Clostridium perfringens, Escherichia coli, Pseudomonas aeruginosa,* and *Listeria monocytogenes*. Like *Salmonella*, these are contracted through fecal contamination of food. *Y. pseudotuberculosis* can cause abscesses of the intestine and of regional lymph nodes. *E. coli* causes wasting, depression, and death in weanlings. Intestines may contain yellow fluid.[27] Antibiotic treatment is based on culture and sensitivity analysis. Supportive therapy is also indicated. Tyzzer's disease, caused by *Clostridium piliforme* (formerly *Bacillus piliformis*), has been reported in guinea pigs. The organism is transmitted by the fecal-oral route, and young, stressed animals are particularly affected. Signs of Tyzzer's disease include diarrhea, an unthrifty appearance, and acute death.[35] In one case, dependent subcutaneous edema and excessive serous fluid were reported.[54] Lesions observed at necropsy include intestinal inflammation and focal hepatic necrosis. Because *C. piliforme* is an intracellular bacterium, it will not grow on routine culture media. Definitive diagnosis is made at necropsy by identification of the organisms on hematoxylin and eosin– or silver-stained sections of intestine or liver. Treatment has been unrewarding. This disease can be prevented by good husbandry practices and stress reduction, particularly at weaning.

Parasitic Diarrhea

Protozoal diarrhea in guinea pigs is caused by *Cryptosporidium wrairi*, which affects the small intestine. Transmission is by the fecal-oral route. Weanlings and immunosuppressed animals are most susceptible,[26] although immunocompetent adults can be affected.[9] Signs include failure to gain weight, weight loss, diarrhea, and death.[23] Immunocompetent guinea pigs recover within 4 weeks and are resistant to reinfection.[49] The organisms can be seen on fecal examination or identified histopathologically on the brush border of mucosal epithelial cells. No treatment has proved effective. Oocysts of *C. wrairi* can be destroyed in the environment with a 5% ammonia solution, freezing to below 32°F (0°C), or heating to above 149°F (65°C).[26] Cryptosporidiosis is a potentially zoonotic disease.

Guinea pigs are hosts to *Eimeria caviae, Balantidium caviae* (a protozoan), and *Paraspidodera uncinata* (a roundworm). In rare cases, *E. caviae* causes diarrhea, and *P. uncinata* can cause bronchoalveolar eosinophilia[11]; otherwise, these organisms cause no clinical disease.

Viral Diarrhea

There has been one report of a wasting syndrome involving diarrhea, anorexia, rapid weight loss, and acute death in weanling guinea pigs. Coronavirus-like particles were identified in the feces with the use of transmission electron microscopy; no other organisms were isolated.[28]

Malocclusion

Guinea pigs have hypsodontic (open-rooted) incisors, premolars, and molars that grow continuously; therefore, overgrowth of any of these teeth is possible. Although there is a strong genetic predisposition to malocclusion, diet, trauma, or infection may also play a role.[26] Maxillary premolars and molars overgrow laterally, abrading the cheeks, and mandibular teeth overgrow medially, abrading the tongue and occluding the oropharynx.[10] Overgrown incisors can be identified on physical examination (Fig. 24-1). Because premolar malocclusion usually goes unnoticed until the animal appears anorectic, prehends but cannot swallow food, and loses weight, an evaluation of cheek teeth should always be an integral component of a physical examination. Excess salivation *(slobbers)*, wetting of chin and forepaws, and secondary moist dermatitis are also signs of malocclusion.[26]

Malocclusion can be diagnosed by careful oral examination. Because the oral cavity of the guinea pig is narrow and large buccal folds are present, this examination is facilitated by first anesthetizing the animal with isoflurane. Gauze strips looped over the incisors can be used to open the mouth, and a vaginal

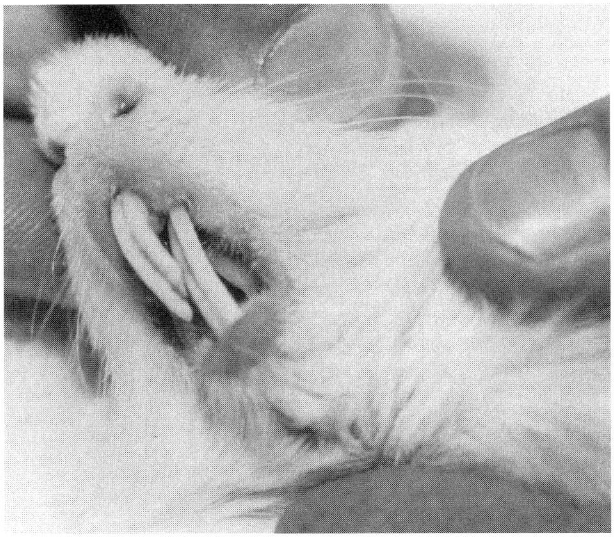

Figure 24-1 Malocclusion of incisors in a guinea pig.

speculum or otoscope can be used to carefully check the premolars and molars. The teeth can be trimmed with a dental drill, pediatric rongeurs, or a specially designed file. Use care if rongeurs are used to avoid splitting the teeth. Trimming needs to be repeated routinely (usually every 4 to 6 weeks) for the remainder of the animal's life. Vitamin C can be added to the diet of guinea pigs at 15 to 25 mg/day to prevent decreased collagen formation and subsequent tooth movement in the socket.[10] The disease can be prevented by not breeding affected animals and by feeding a proper diet (see Chapter 34).

RESPIRATORY DISEASES

Bacterial Pneumonia

Pneumonia is probably the most significant disease in guinea pigs, particularly in damp or humid environments. Guinea pigs are very susceptible to respiratory disease caused by *Bordetella bronchiseptica* and *Streptococcus pneumoniae. Bordetella*, a gram-negative rod, is commonly carried by rabbits, dogs, and nonhuman primates. Rabbits and guinea pigs are mutual sources of infection of *Bordetella*.[8] *Streptococcus*, a gram-positive coccus, is also transmitted by asymptomatic carriers of many species. Stress increases susceptibility to disease, and young guinea pigs are most often affected. The organisms are transmitted by direct contact, by aerosolization, and on fomites.[26] Signs include inappetence, nasal and ocular discharge, and dyspnea. *Bordetella* causes a purulent bronchopneumonia with consolidation of lung lobes and exudate in the tympanic bullae. Metritis and abortions have also been described. *Streptococcus* causes a fibrinopurulent pleuritis and pericarditis in addition to bronchopneumonia.[26] Torticollis and abortions may also occur with *Streptococcus*. The combination of *S. pneumoniae* infection and vitamin C deficiency has resulted in septic arthritis.[57]

Diagnosis of bacterial pneumonia is made by culture and sensitivity analysis of exudate. *Bordetella* antibodies can be detected by enzyme-linked immunosorbent assay (ELISA) or by indirect immunofluorescence; however, culture and sensitivity studies should be used to confirm active cases.[58] Radiographs may reveal consolidated lung lobes or an opacity in the tympanic bullae. Antibiotics commonly used to treat bacterial pneumonia in guinea pigs are chloramphenicol palmitate (30-50 mg/kg PO q12h × 7-21 days) and trimethoprim-sulfa (30-50 mg/kg PO q12h × 7 days), and enrofloxacin (5-10 mg/kg q12h × 7-21 days). A combination therapy using enrofloxacin and doxycycline (2.5 mg/kg PO q12h) for 7-21 days has also been effective. Long-term therapy (4-6 weeks) with any of these antimicrobial agents may be necessary. Trovafloxacin, a new quinolone, is effective against *S. pneumoniae* and was used successfully to treat experimentally induced Legionnaires' disease in guinea pigs.[40] *Lactobacillus* should be given during antibiotic treatment and for approximately 5 days afterward. Supportive care, such as lactated Ringer's solution, oxygen therapy, and vitamin C, can also be given. Good husbandry, avoidance of stress, and separation of guinea pigs from dogs and rabbits will help control pneumonia.

Other bacteria of clinical significance include *Haemophilus* species and *Streptobacillus moniliformis*. *Haemophilus* has been recovered from the respiratory tract of guinea pigs and rabbits; it can cause subcutaneous abscesses and is easily transmitted to rats.[7] *S. moniliformis* is usually implicated in cervical lymphadenitis and has caused granulomatous pneumonia in guinea pigs.[31]

Viral Pneumonia

A necrotizing bronchopneumonia has been described in guinea pigs. The incubation period is 5 to 10 days, and stressed animals are predisposed to developing disease. Morbidity is low, but mortality is high, and affected animals usually die acutely. Lesions include necrotizing, exfoliative bronchiolitis. Sloughed epithelium contains large, round to ovoid, basophilic intranuclear inclusions. An adenovirus is thought to be responsible for this disease.[15,17,25,32]

Pulmonary Neoplasia

Bronchogenic pulmonary adenoma is a common tumor found in guinea pigs. In one study, it occurred in approximately 30% of animals older than 3 years. This condition is sometimes misdiagnosed as pneumonia.

UROGENITAL DISEASES

Urinary Calculi

Urinary tract calculi are common in guinea pigs. In aged boars, congealed ejaculum can form proteinaceous urethral obstructions, resulting in urethritis. Females older than 3 years of age appear to be predisposed to cystitis and cystic calculi.[41] In one report, calcium oxalate uroliths were diagnosed in a number of guinea pigs with *Streptococcus pyogenes* cystitis. The bacteria formed nidi around which calcium was deposited, resulting in stone formation.[39] Signs of urolithiasis include anorexia, hematuria, dysuria, and a huddled, hunched posture.[48] Lesions include hemorrhage or congestion of bladder mucosa, hemorrhagic exudate within the bladder, and calculi adherent to the bladder wall.[41] *S. pyogenes* causes hyperemia of bladder mucosa and yellowish-gray deposits within the lumen.[39] Uroliths can sometimes be palpated; however, definitive diagnosis is most often made by radiography. Urinary acidifiers usually are not indicated because guinea pigs cannot easily remove an acid load.[26] Although potassium citrate is sometimes used to help prevent the formation of calculi, the efficacy of this drug has not been proven. In guinea pigs with urethral calculi, retrograde flushing might relieve the obstruction. If this procedure fails or if cystic or ureteral calculi are present, surgery should be considered. Isoflurane or sevoflurane is the anesthetic of choice for guinea pigs. Supportive care for urinary calculi includes antibiotic and fluid therapy.

Chronic Interstitial Nephritis

Chronic interstitial nephritis is commonly found at necropsy in guinea pigs older than 3 years of age. It has also been reported in guinea pigs with diabetes mellitus and hyperglycemia. Animals affected by staphylococcal pododermatitis may develop chronic renal amyloidosis and nephritis as sequelae.[26] Secondary interstitial nephritis can be prevented by proper diet, caging, and good sanitation, which reduce susceptibility to pododermatitis.

Renal Parasitism

Guinea pigs may harbor *Klossiella cobayae*, a renal coccidian. The organism lives in the epithelial cells lining the renal tubules. Sporocysts are shed in the urine. No clinical disease results from infection, and treatment is generally not recommended.[35] Sulfadimethoxine or trimethoprim-sulfa may be effective in treating renal parasitism.

Ovarian Cysts

Cystic rete ovarii have been identified in 76% of female guinea pigs between 18 months and 5 years of age, most commonly in animals age 2 to 4 years.[30] Cysts develop spontaneously, range in diameter from 0.5 to 7 cm, and increase in size as the animal ages. They may be single or multilocular, and they are usually filled with clear fluid (Fig. 24-2). In most cases, both ovaries are affected; however, if a single ovary is affected, it is usually the right one.[30] Testosterone can stimulate ovarian epithelial cell growth, resulting in cyst formation.[47] Affected animals present with abdominal distention, and occasionally with anorexia, fatigue, and depression.[6,30] If cysts are functional, bilateral symmetric hair loss can be seen in the flank region (Fig. 24-3). The most consistent sign of cysts in breeding sows is a decline in fertility after 15 months of age.

Diagnosis of an ovarian cyst is made by ultrasonography. A 6- or 10-MHz mechanical sector transducer oriented in the sagittal plane yields diagnostic real-time images. Treatment consists of ovariohysterectomy.[6] Other problems associated with cystic rete ovarii include leiomyomas,[16] cystic endometrial hyperplasia, and endometritis.[30] Ovarian and uterine neoplasms can be induced by exposure to estradiol, diethylstilbestrol, or testosterone.[43,46]

Vaginitis and Scrotal Plugs

Wet, soiled bedding combined with inguinal sebaceous secretions can become adhered to the penis, scrotum, or vulva, resulting in secondary infection or obstruction of urination and defecation. The condition can be corrected by gently soaking the affected part in a dilute chlorhexidine solution and carefully removing the debris. If indicated, systemic antibiotics can be given. This condition is easily prevented by appropriate sanitation and good husbandry practices.

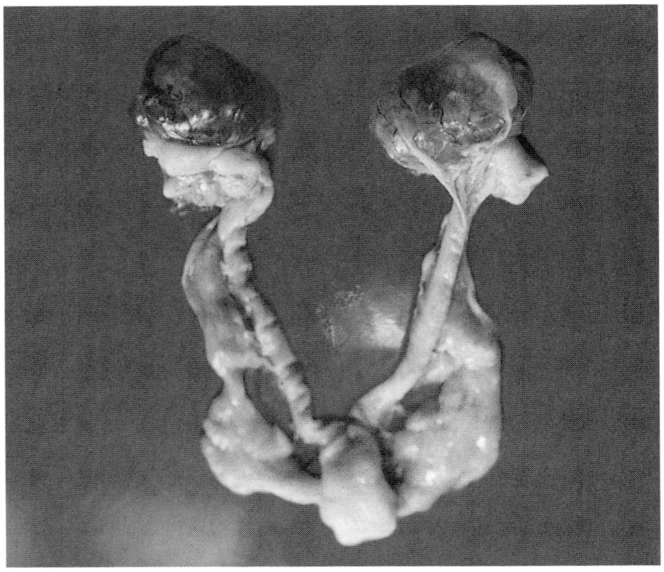

Figure 24-2 Ovarian cysts in a guinea pig. Ovarian cysts can develop in up to 76% of female guinea pigs and usually occur in both ovaries. *(Courtesy K. Rosenthal, DVM.)*

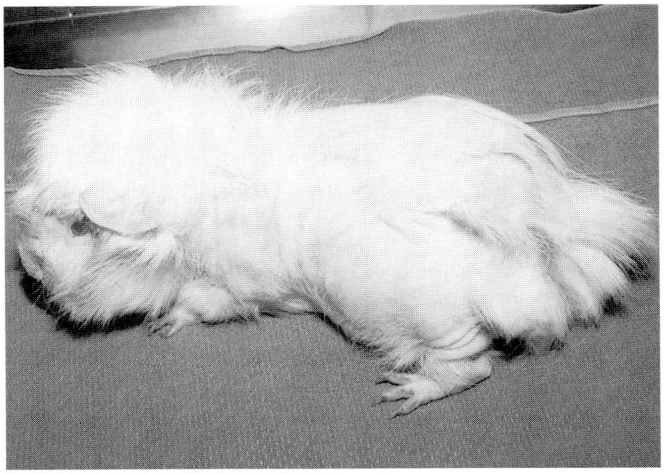

Figure 24-3 Alopecia secondary to ovarian cysts in a female guinea pig. *(Courtesy Elizabeth V. Hillyer, DVM.)*

Pregnancy Toxemia

Pregnancy toxemia (pregnancy ketosis) is most commonly seen in primiparous, obese sows during the final 2 weeks of gestation and the first week after delivery. Although pregnancy is a contributing factor, toxemia is not limited to females; boars are also susceptible to this disorder. Obesity and fasting are the most critical predisposing conditions. Dietary alterations, environmental changes, and other stressors also play a role in precipitating this disease.[18,35] Onset of signs is abrupt. The guinea pig becomes anorectic, quits drinking, and within 24 hours is prostrate and dyspneic. Convulsions and death can occur within 2 to 5 days. Clinically, the animal is hypoglycemic (less than 60 mg/dL), ketonemic, proteinuric, and aciduric (pH 5-6; normal pH = 9). The liver is enlarged and fatty, and the stomach is empty. In pregnant sows, the heavy, gravid uterus may compress its own vascular supply, resulting in ischemia, thromboplastin release, and disseminated intravascular coagulopathy.[26,35] Treatment of pregnancy toxemia is usually unrewarding. Keep the guinea pig warm, give fluids intravenously or, if necessary, intraperitoneally, and administer glucose intravenously or by mouth. If the animal is in shock, it also can be treated with corticosteroids and calcium gluconate. Stress of treatment, combined with anorexia and an empty stomach, may lead to a fatal enteritis.[26] The prognosis for recovery from pregnancy toxemia is guarded to grave.

Prevention is the preferred method of dealing with pregnancy toxemia. All guinea pigs should be kept on a good-quality diet, and care should be taken to prevent obesity. Feeding fresh vegetables will condition animals to a varied diet and lessen the chance of refusal when new foods are offered. Fresh water should always be available ad libitum, and environmental, physical, and social stresses should be avoided, particularly during late pregnancy.

Dystocia

Dystocia is common in guinea pigs. In female guinea pigs, during the last week of pregnancy, relaxin (a hormone released from the pituitary and endometrium) causes the fibrocartilage of the pubic symphysis to disintegrate, resulting in a 3-cm separation.[10,24] If a sow is not bred for the first time before she reaches 7 to 8 months of age, her pelvic symphysis will permanently fuse in close apposition, preventing passage of the fetuses during parturition (Fig. 24-4). Obesity, large fetuses, and uterine inertia can also cause dystocia.

In guinea pigs, pups are normally delivered within a 30-minute period, with a resting period of approximately 5 minutes between pups. Signs of dystocia include unproductive contractions and straining. Animals may present with depression and may have a bloody or greenish-brown vulvar discharge. Diagnosis is based on history and signs. If the pelvic symphysis is wide enough and the problem is uterine inertia, 0.2 to 3 IU/kg of oxytocin can be given intramuscularly to stimulate contractions.[18] If pups are manually extracted, the fetal membranes must be rapidly removed.[10] If oxytocin fails to stimulate contractions, or if the pubic symphysis is less than 20 to 25 mm dilated, immediate cesarean section is indicated.[18] The female can be given buprenorphine (0.05 mg/kg SC q8-12h), followed by isoflurane or sevoflurane via mask induction and maintenance. A standard ventral midline approach is used. The uterus is exteriorized and incised longitudinally. Once the pups are removed, they should be cleaned off and stimulated to breathe immediately. The uterus is closed with an inverted suture pattern. The linea is closed with absorbable suture and the skin with nonabsorbable suture, using a simple interrupted pattern for both closure locations (see Chapter 27). Guinea pigs do not tolerate the stress of anesthesia and surgery well; prognosis is guarded to poor.[18] Dystocia is best prevented by breeding guinea pigs before 6 months of age and by preventing obesity.

Mastitis

Mastitis in guinea pigs is caused by *E. coli* or *Pasteurella, Klebsiella, Staphylococcus, Streptococcus,* and *Pseudomonas* species. Wet, dirty cages and trauma caused by nursing pups predispose sows to infection. Organisms enter via the teat canal or through bite wounds on the teats. Clinically, the glands are initially swollen, red, and warm; later, they can become cool and cyanotic. The milk is often bloody. Infection can spread systemically and result in the death of both mother and pups. Guinea pigs with mastitis can be treated with systemic antibiotics, particularly chloramphenicol palmitate, trimethoprim-sulfa, and enrofloxacin. Hot packs can be applied to the affected glands. The environment should be cleaned, and the pups may be weaned early. If necessary, the mammary glands can be resected.[26]

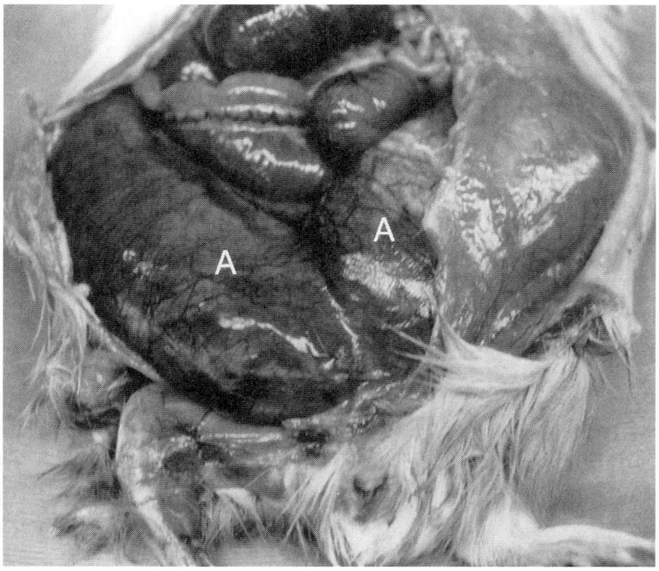

Figure 24-4 Postmortem examination of a guinea pig that died during a dystocia. Note the two large sacs (fetal membranes, *A*), each containing a fetus.

Mammary Gland Tumors

Most mammary gland tumors guinea pigs are benign fibroadenomas. Approximately 30% are adenocarcinomas, which are locally invasive but rarely metastasize.[10,35] If tumors are excised, make a wide excision that includes a large amount of normal tissue. Local lymph nodes should also be removed.

DERMATOLOGIC DISEASES

Dermatophytosis

Guinea pigs are susceptible to ringworm. Young animals are more susceptible because of their incompletely developed immune systems and lower amounts of fungistatic fatty acids in their sebum.[51] The dermatophyte most frequently isolated is *Trichophyton mentagrophytes,* although *Microsporum canis* has also been identified. Animals may be asymptomatic carriers; disease usually occurs secondary to overcrowding, poor husbandry, and other stressors. The organism is easily transmitted by direct contact and fomites. Lesions in the guinea pig are pruritic and consist of focal circular areas of alopecia with crusts. Lesions are usually seen first on the face, forehead, and ears and later spread over the back and down the limbs.[10]

Diagnosis is made by plucking or scraping hairs and crusts from the periphery of the lesion and placing these on dermatophyte test medium (DTM) or another appropriate culture medium. Ringworm can be treated topically with miconazole (q24h × 2-4 weeks).[26] Butenafine has been used effectively as a 1% cream applied topically (q24h × 10-20 days).[1] Fluconazole can be administered at 16 mg/kg PO q24h × 14 days.[37] Griseofulvin pediatric solution (25 mg/100 g PO q10 days × three treatments) has proved effective,[10] but griseofulvin is more commonly given at 25 mg/kg PO q24h × 14-28 days. Because it is teratogenic, this drug should not be given to pregnant animals.[10] Ringworm is a potentially zoonotic disease.

Ectoparasites

Guinea pigs are susceptible to infestation by mites (*Trixacarus caviae, Chirodiscoides caviae*), lice (*Gliricola porcelli, Gyropus ovalis*), and fleas (*Ctenocephalides felis*). Of these, *Trixacarus*, the sarcoptid mite, is the most significant pathogen (Fig. 24-5). *Trixacarus* is a burrowing mite that can also transiently infest humans. Signs of *Trixacarus* infestation include intense pruritus with excoriations and secondary infection. In some animals, pruritus is so severe that it may cause seizures. Lesions are seen on the thighs and back and can extend over the shoulders and neck.[50] Yellowish crusts can cover the affected skin. Microscopically, orthokeratotic hyperkeratosis, eosinophilic microabscesses, and necrotic areas can be seen. Cross-sections of mites may be present in the

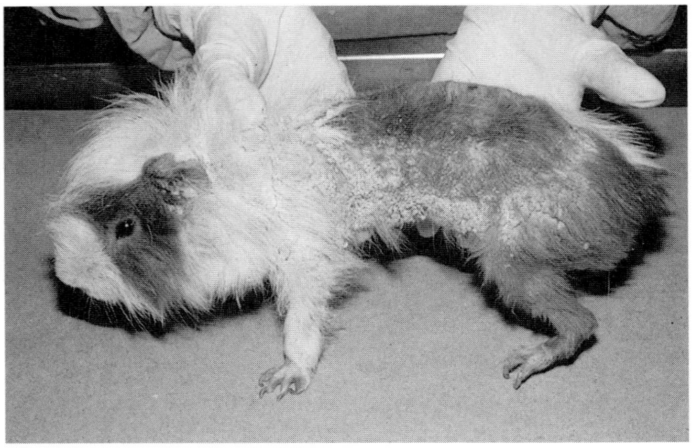

Figure 24-5 Sarcoptic mange in a guinea pig caused by *Trixacarus caviae.*

stratum corneum.[20] Hematologic changes associated with *Trixacarus* infestation are leukocytosis, monocytosis, eosinophilia, and basophilia.[44] *Chirodiscoides* is a nonburrowing fur mite that is much less of a problem than *Trixacarus*. *Chirodiscoides* can cause lesions on the perineal and hip area, but infestation is usually asymptomatic. *Gliricola* and *Gyropus* are debris-feeding lice that attach to the hair shafts (both adults and eggs). Alopecia, crusts, and a rough hair coat are seen with lice infestations.[50] All of these parasites are transmitted by direct contact.

Diagnosis of an ectoparasitic infection is made by skin scraping (mites), by plucking or combing hairs to look for eggs and adults (lice), or by visual identification (fleas). Potassium hydroxide digestion of skin scrapings may be necessary to visualize *Trixacarus*.[20]

Trixacarus is effectively treated with ivermectin (0.5-0.8 mg/kg SC, repeat in 7 days). Lice and *Chirodiscoides* also are treated with ivermectin (0.3 mg/kg SC, PO, repeat in 10 days).[50] Fleas can be treated with pyrethrin-based cat flea powder. Selamectin (6 mg/kg; Revolution, Pfizer, Exton, PA) is a topical parasiticide that has also been effective in guinea pigs. Treatment of any ectoparasite should be accompanied by thorough and repeated cleaning of the environment to prevent reinfestation.

Cervical Lymphadenitis

Cervical lymphadenitis *(lumps)* is a disease that commonly affects guinea pigs (Fig. 24-6). It is caused predominantly by *Streptococcus zooepidemicus,* Lancefield's group C, a gram-positive coccus. Occasionally, *S. moniliformis* is also involved.[35] *S. zooepidemicus* is normally present in the conjunctiva and nasal cavity of guinea pigs. If the animal's oral mucosa becomes abraded from malocclusion, dietary roughage (hay stems), or biting, bacteria invade the cervical lymph nodes and cause abscessation. Animals with intact nasal and conjunctival mucosa can also develop disease.[36] Stress increases susceptibility to infection.[26] Clinically, the guinea pig presents with pus-filled ventral cervical masses. Occasionally, bacteria spread systemically, resulting in septicemia or necrotizing bronchopneumonia.[31] Diagnosis is based on clinical signs and results of impression smears, Gram stains of the pus, and culture and sensitivity testing. Treatment consists of surgically excising the abscess (preferably) or draining of the abscess and copious flushing of the wound. A systemic antibiotic should be administered. This condition can be prevented by keeping the guinea pig on a good diet and in a clean, stress-free environment. *S. moniliformis* is a potentially zoonotic disease.[31]

Bite Wounds

Although guinea pigs are social animals, group housing can lead to bite wounds that occasionally abscess. Treatment consists of draining and irrigating the wound with saline solution[2] and administering appropriate systemic antibiotics, based on results of sensitivity testing.

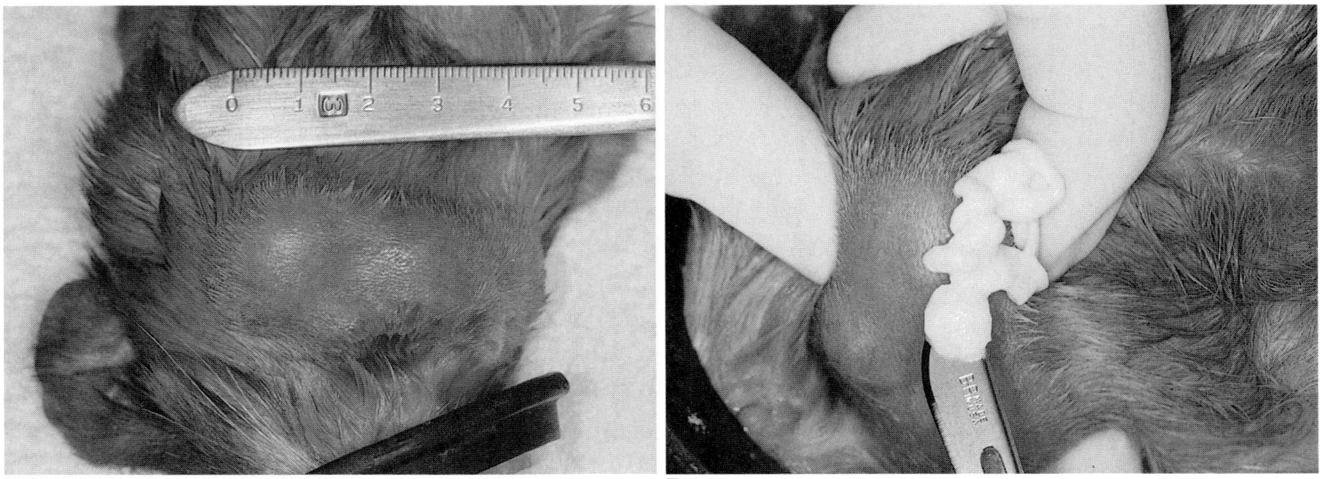

A B

Figure 24-6 Cervical lymphadenitis (also referred to as lumps) in a guinea pig. Infection is usually caused by *Streptococcus zooepidemicus* and occurs in the ventral cervical lymph nodes (**A**). Nodes are enlarged and filled with a thick, purulent exudate (**B**).

Pododermatitis

Pododermatitis (bumblefoot) is commonly seen in guinea pigs. Typically, the disease is found in obese animals that are housed on wire-bottom cages or with abrasive bedding. Areas of hyperkeratosis develop on the palmar and plantar surfaces of the feet. These ulcerate, permitting secondary invasion by *Staphylococcus aureus*.[35] Infection can extend deep into the tissues of the feet, traveling up tendons and into bone, resulting in osteomyelitis. Guinea pigs with pododermatitis are in significant pain, vocalize frequently, and are reluctant to walk. Diagnosis is based on clinical signs and identification of lesions. Radiography may be useful in identifying osteomyelitis. Treatment consists of appropriate systemic antibiotics, surgical debridement of lesions, chlorhexidine foot soaks, wound bandaging, and appropriate analgesic therapy. As with pododermatitis in most species, the prognosis is guarded. The disease is best prevented by keeping the environment clean dry; housing the animals on soft, nonabrasive bedding; and avoiding obesity.

Tumors

The most common skin tumor in guinea pigs is the trichofolliculoma, a benign basal cell epithelioma. Trichofolliculomas appear as solid or cystic masses, most commonly over the lumbosacral area (Figs. 24-7 and 24-8).[10,35] They are easily removed surgically.

Alopecia

Alopecia resulting from noninfectious causes is quite common in guinea pigs. Included in this group are barbering, endocrine alopecias, and vitamin deficiencies. Barbering is recognized by close examination of the area of hair loss. In barbering, broken hair shafts are present, and the underlying skin is not inflamed or pruritic.[35] Alopecia over the flank areas indicates self-barbering, which can occur secondary to boredom. Providing hay, other roughage, or chew toys may alleviate this problem. In group-housed guinea pigs, the dominant animal often barbers subordinates. Guinea pig sows in late

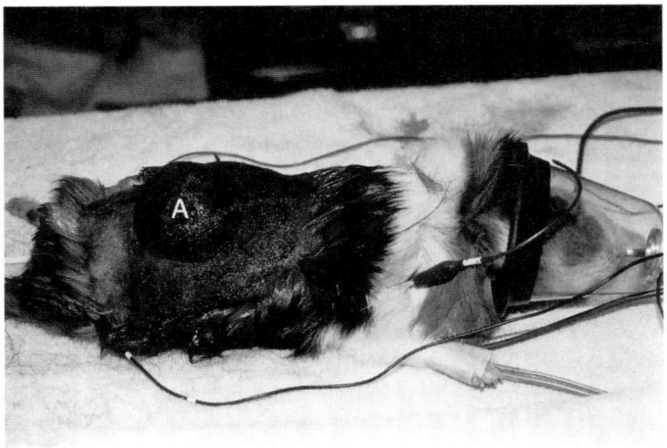

Figure 24-7 Guinea pig surgically prepared for removal of a trichofolliculoma *(A)*, a benign basal cell epithelioma, located over the lumbosacral area (see Figure 24-8).

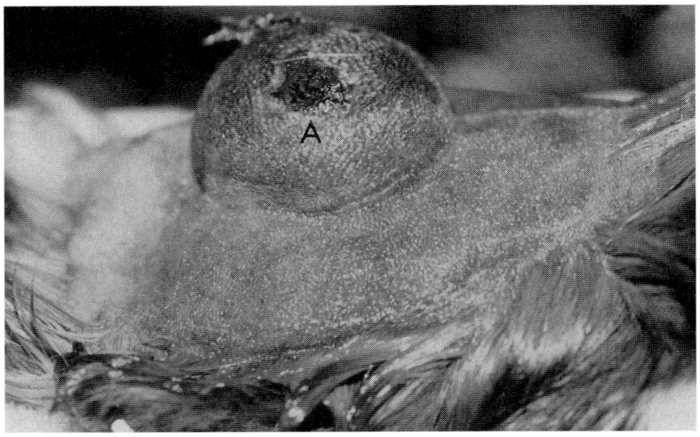

Figure 24-8 Close-up of the trichofolliculoma *(A)* in Figure 24-7.

gestation can experience transient endocrine alopecia.[22] Partial alopecia has been documented in weanlings.[35] Supplementation of the diet with hay has been demonstrated to reduce trichophagia.[22]

MUSCULOSKELETAL DISEASES

Scurvy

Guinea pigs possess a mutated gene for L-gulono-γ-lactone oxidase and cannot produce this enzyme. Therefore, they cannot convert glucose to ascorbic acid and are incapable of endogenous synthesis of vitamin C.[38] For this reason, guinea pigs require 15 to 25 mg/day vitamin C added to their diet; pregnant animals require 30 mg/day.[26] Ascorbic acid is necessary for collagen synthesis; lack of dietary vitamin C results in defective type IV collagen, laminin, and elastin, which compromises blood vessel integrity and results in joint and gingival hemorrhages.[34] Collagen also is necessary to anchor teeth tightly in their sockets; without it, teeth loosen and malocclusion occurs. In addition, vitamin C is necessary for appropriate retention of vitamin E.[33]

Signs of vitamin C deficiency include rough hair coat, anorexia, diarrhea, teeth grinding, vocalizing from pain, delayed wound healing, lameness, and increased susceptibility to bacterial infections.[35] Radiographically, long bone epiphyses and costochondral junctions of the ribs are enlarged. Pathologic fractures may also be evident. Young, growing animals are more susceptible to scurvy, and clinical disease can develop after as little as 2 weeks of ascorbic acid deprivation.[10]

Diagnosis of vitamin C deficiency is based on history, clinical signs, and radiographic lesions. Serum ascorbic acid levels can be used to confirm the diagnosis. Treatment should be initiated with parenteral ascorbic acid at a dose of 50 mg/day IP, IM, or SC. Once response is noted, vitamin C may be administered orally at the same dosage. After recovery, vitamin C should be supplemented daily in the diet. Fresh, good-quality guinea pig (not rabbit) chow provides adequate vitamin C if used within 90 days of the milling date (see Chapter 23). Fresh cabbage, kale, and oranges also provide a source of vitamin C: 100 g of kale contains 125 mg vitamin C, and 50 g of cabbage contains 30 mg vitamin C.[26] Vitamin C tablets can be added to the drinking water at a concentration of 200 to 400 mg/L[35]; medicated water should be replaced daily.

Osteoarthritis and Osteoarthrosis

Spontaneous osteoarthritis has been described in guinea pigs. Osteoarthritis of the knee in guinea pigs mimics the disease in humans both morphologically and epidemiologically. Obesity is a predisposing factor.[4]

Spontaneous cartilage degeneration and osteoarthrosis of the femorotibial joint of young guinea pigs has been described.[5] No cause has been identified, and the disease does not appear to be widespread.

Iatrogenic Muscle Necrosis

A combination of fentanyl and droperidol has been documented to cause muscle necrosis at the injection site in guinea pigs.[26] Ketamine and diazepam have also been implicated in nerve damage and self-mutilation distal to the injection site in guinea pigs.

NEUROLOGIC DISEASES

Lymphocytic Choriomeningitis Virus

Lymphocytic choriomeningitis virus (LCMV) is an arenavirus that causes meningitis and hind limb paralysis in guinea pigs, although it is more commonly reported in mice and hamsters. Lesions include lymphocytic infiltrates in the choroid plexus, ependyma, and meninges.[35] The virus is transmitted through inhalation, ingestion, or direct contact with contaminated urine, saliva, and feces. Biting insects can transmit LCMV, and transplacental transmission also occurs. LCMV can be transmitted to humans. Signs of LCMV infection in humans include headache, vomiting, and fever; fatalities are rare (See Chapter 40).

OPHTHALMOLOGIC DISEASES

Inclusion Body Conjunctivitis of Guinea Pigs

Conjunctivitis due to *Chlamydophila psittaci* has been described in guinea pigs.[13] Animals age 1 to 3 weeks are most commonly affected. The mode of transmission is unknown. Signs include conjunctival reddening and serous ocular discharge. Diagnosis is made by the identification of intracytoplasmic inclusions in conjunctival scrapings.[35] Because the disease resolves spontaneously in 2 to 3 weeks, no treatment is recommended. Although *C. psittaci* is a zoonotic pathogen, no documented cases of transmission from guinea pig to human exist.

MISCELLANEOUS DISEASES

Ototoxicity

Ototoxicity has been reported in guinea pigs after administration of various drugs. Gentamicin can be ototoxic when applied topically.[12] Cortisporin otic suspension (Glaxo Wellcome, Research Triangle Park, NC), which contains neomycin and polymyxin B, is also ototoxic to guinea pigs.[42] Cisplatin administered at 7.5 mg/kg IM twice within 5 days induced ototoxicity in guinea pigs.[45]

Diabetes Mellitus

Spontaneous diabetes mellitus has been described in adult male Abyssinian-Hartley guinea pigs. The diabetes is noninsulin-dependent and is similar to adult-onset diabetes in humans. Affected animals develop bladder hypertrophy and voiding dysfunction and have a life span of about 5 years.[3] An adult female guinea pig was diagnosed with diabetes mellitus after the animal presented with cystitis and urination of small, frequent amounts. The guinea pig responded to NPH insulin[53]; Caninsulin (Intervet Canada, Whitby, Ontario) worked best.[52] Diabetes mellitus may be transient, and a correct, low-fat, high-fiber diet is important in treatment and prevention.[29,52]

Adrenal Tumors

Adrenal tumors have been documented in guinea pigs. One case report described an adult male guinea pig that presented with obesity, bilateral alopecia, hepatomegaly, and depression. An adrenal tumor and ureterolith were diagnosed by ultrasound. Both were removed surgically, but the guinea pig died from surgical complications.[21]

Heat Stress

Guinea pigs are susceptible to heat stress. Guinea pigs housed outdoors can develop heat stress in ambient temperatures as low as 70° to 75°F (21° to 24°C). Guinea pigs suffering from heat stress will salivate profusely in an attempt to thermoregulate. They exhibit shallow, rapid respiration, pale mucous membranes, and elevated rectal temperature. These signs may be followed by coma and death. Treatment is supportive and includes cool water baths and administering corticosteroids and parenteral fluids. Prognosis is very guarded.

Metastatic Mineralization

Metastatic mineralization in guinea pigs is normally an incidental finding at necropsy. The etiology is unclear and is possibly related to subclinical mineral imbalances and dehydration or oversupplementation of dietary vitamin D_3 or minerals. Although the disease is usually clinically unapparent, it can manifest as muscle stiffness and renal dysfunction.[35] Lesions are seen in animals older than 1 year of age and include mineralization of kidneys, heart, vessels, stomach, and colon. There is no treatment.

Cavian Leukemia

Lymphosarcoma is the most common tumor of guinea pigs. The disease is caused by a type C retrovirus. Animals present with a scruffy coat and lymphadenopathy. Hepatomegaly, splenomegaly, and mediastinal masses are occasionally seen. Diagnosis is based on the results of a complete blood count and cytologic examination of aspirates of enlarged nodes or abdominal or pleural fluids. Leukemic animals have a total white blood cell count of 25,000 to 500,000 cells/mm^3.[10] At necropsy, lymph nodes and visceral organs may be enlarged, with infiltration by proliferating lymphoblasts. The course of the disease is 2 to 5 weeks. Prognosis is poor, although some animals have responded initially to chemotherapy.[35]

REFERENCES

1. Arika T, Tokoo M, Hase T, et al: Effects of butenafine hydrochloride, a new benzylamine derivative, on experimental dermatophytosis in guinea pigs. Antimicrob Agents Chemother 1990; 34:2250-2253.
2. Badia JM, Torres JM, Tur C, et al: Saline wound irrigation reduces the postoperative infection rate in guinea pigs. J Surg Res 1996; 63:457-459.
3. Belis JA, Curley RM, Lang CM: Bladder dysfunction in the spontaneously diabetic male Abyssinian-Hartley guinea pig. Pharmacology 1996; 53:66-70.
4. Bendele A, McComb J, Gould T, et al: Animal models of arthritis: relevance to human disease. Toxicol Pathol 1999; 27:134-142.
5. Bendele AM, White SL, Hulman JF: Osteoarthritis in guinea pigs: histopathologic and scanning electron microscopic features. Lab Anim Sci 1989; 39:115-121.
6. Beregi A, Zorn S, Felkai F: Ultrasonic diagnosis of ovarian cysts in ten guinea pigs. Vet Radiol Ultrasound 1999; 40:74-76.
7. Boot R, Thuis HCW, Veenema JL: Serological relationship of some V-factor dependent Pasteurellaceae (*Haemophilus* sp.) from guinea pigs and rabbits. Lab Anim 1999; 33:91-94.
8. Boot R, Thuis H, Wieten G: Multifactorial analysis of antibiotic sensitivity of *Bordetella bronchiseptica* isolates from guinea pigs, rabbits and rats. Lab Anim 1995; 29:45-49.
9. Chrisp CE, Suckow MA, Fayer R, et al: Comparison of the host ranges and antigenicity of *Cryptosporidium parvum* and *Cryptosporidium wrairi* from guinea pigs. J Protozool 1992; 39:406-409.
10. Collins B: Common diseases and medical management of rodents and lagomorphs. *In* Jacobson ER, Kollias GV, eds. Exotic Animals. New York, Churchill Livingstone, 1988, pp 261-316.
11. Conder GA, Richards IM, Jen L-W: Bronchoalveolar eosinophilia in guinea pigs harboring inapparent infections of *Paraspidodera uncinata*. J Parasitol 1989; 75:144-146.
12. Conlon BJ, McSwain SD, Smith DW: Topical gentamicin and ethacrynic acid: effects on cochlear function. Laryngoscope 1998; 108:1087-1089.
13. Deeb BJ, DiGiacomo RF, Wang S-P: Guinea pig inclusion conjunctivitis (GPIC) in a commercial colony. Lab Anim 1989; 23:103.
14. Earnest-Koons KA, Griffith JW, Lang CM: Incidence and classification of thyroid lesions in 210 guinea pigs. Lab Anim Sci 1988; 38:514.
15. Feldman SH, Richardson JA, Clubb FJ Jr: Necrotizing viral bronchopneumonia in guinea pigs. Lab Anim Sci 1990; 40:82-83.
16. Field KJ, Griffith JW, Lang CM: Spontaneous reproductive tract leiomyomas in aged guinea-pigs. J Comp Pathol 1989; 101:287-294.
17. Finnie JW, Noonan DE, Swift JG: Adenovirus pneumonia of guinea pigs. Aust Vet J 1999; 77:191-192.
18. Fish RE, Besch-Williford C: Reproductive disorders in the rabbit and guinea pig. *In* Kirk RW, Bonagura JD, eds. Kirk's Current Veterinary Therapy, Vol. 11. Philadelphia, WB Saunders, 1992, pp 1175-1179.
19. Fritz PE, Hurst WJ, White WJ, et al: Pharmacokinetics of cefazolin in guinea pigs. Lab Anim Sci 1987; 37:646-651.
20. Fuentealba C, Hanna P: Mange induced by *Trixacarus caviae* in a guinea pig. Can Vet J 1996; 37:749-750.
21. Gaschien L, Ketz C, Lang J, et al: Ultrasonographic detection of adrenal gland tumor and ureterolithiasis in a guinea pig. Vet Radiol Ultrasound 1998; 39:43-46.
22. Gerold S, Huisinga E, Iglauer F, et al: Influence of feeding hay on the alopecia of breeding guinea pigs. J Vet Med 1997; 44:341-348.
23. Gibson SV, Wagner JE: Cryptosporidiosis in guinea pigs: a retrospective study. J Am Vet Med Assoc 1986; 189:1033-1034.
24. Goldsmith LT, Weiss G, Steinetz BG: Relaxin and its role in pregnancy. Endo Disorders Preg 1995; 24:171-186.
25. Griffith JW, Brasky KM, Lang CM: Experimental pneumonia virus of mice infection of guinea pigs spontaneously infected with *Bordetella bronchiseptica*. Lab Anim 1997; 31:52-57.
26. Harkness JE, Wagner JE: The Biology and Medicine of Rabbits and Rodents, 3rd ed. Philadelphia, Lea and Febiger, 1989.
27. Hurley RJ, Murphy JC, Lipman NS: Diagnostic exercise: depression and anorexia in recently shipped guinea pigs. Lab Anim Sci 1995; 45:305-308.
28. Jaax GP, Jaax NK, Petrali JP, et al: Coronavirus-like virions associated with a wasting syndrome in guinea pigs. Lab Anim Sci 1990; 40:375-378.
29. Johnson-Delaney CA: Small mammal endocrinology. Proc Annu Conf Assoc Avian Vet, Small Mammal and Reptile Program, 1998, pp 99-111.
30. Keller LSF, Griffith JW, Lang CM: Reproductive failure associated with cystic rete ovarii in guinea pigs. J Vet Pathol 1987; 24:335-339.
31. Kirchner BK, Lake SG, Wightman SR: Isolation of *Streptobacillus moniliformis* from a guinea pig with granulomatous pneumonia. Lab Anim Sci 1992; 42:519-521.
32. Kunstyr I, Maess J, Naumann S, et al: Adenovirus pneumonia in guinea pigs: an experimental reproduction of the disease. Lab Anim 1984; 18:55-60.
33. Liu JF, Lee YW: Vitamin C supplementation restores the impaired vitamin E status of guinea pigs fed oxidized frying oil. J Nutr 1998; 128:116-122.
34. Mahmoodian F, Peterkofsky B: Vitamin C deficiency in guinea pigs differentially affects the expression of type IV collagen, laminin, and elastin in blood vessels. J Nutr 1999; 129:83-91.
35. Manning PJ, Wagner JE, Harkness JE: Biology and diseases of guinea pigs. *In* Fox JG, Cohen BJ, Loew FM, eds. Laboratory Animal Medicine. Orlando, Academic Press, 1984, pp 149-181.
36. Murphy JC, Ackerman JI, Marini RP, et al: Cervical lymphadenitis in guinea pigs: infection via intact ocular and nasal mucosa by *Streptococcus zooepidemicus*. Lab Anim Sci 1991; 41:251-254.
37. Nagino K, Shimohira H, Ogawa M, et al: Comparison of the therapeutic efficacy of oral doses of fluconazole and griseofulvin in a guinea pig model of dermatophytosis. J Antibiotics (Tokyo) 2000; 53:207-210.
38. Nishikimi M, Kawai T, Yagi K: Guinea pigs possess a highly mutated gene for L-gulono-γ-lactone oxidase, the key enzyme for L-ascorbic acid biosynthesis missing in this species. J Biol Chem 1992; 267:21967-21972.
39. Okewole PA, Odeyemi PS, Oladummade MA, et al: An outbreak of *Streptococcus pyogenes* infection associated with calcium oxalate urolithiasis in guinea pigs (*Cavia porcellus*). Lab Anim 1991; 25:184-186.
40. Pechere JC, Gootz TD: Bacteriological activity of trovafloxacin, a new quinolone, against respiratory tract pathogens. Eur J Clin Microbiol Infect Dis 1998; 17:405-412.
41. Peng X, Griffith JW, Lang CM: Cystitis and cystic calculi in aged guinea pigs. Lab Anim Sci 1987; 34:527.
42. Perry BP, Smith DW: Effect of Cortisporin otic suspension on cochlear function and efferent activity in the guinea pig. Laryngoscope 1996; 106:1557-1561.
43. Porter KB, Tsibris JCM, Porter GW, et al: Use of endoscopic and ultrasound techniques in the guinea pig leiomyoma model. Lab Anim Sci 1997; 47:537-539.
44. Rothwell TLW, Pope SE, Rajczyk ZK, et al: Haematological and pathological responses to experimental *Trixacarus caviae* infection in guinea pigs. J Comp Pathol 1991; 104:179-185.

45. Saito T, Zhang ZJ, Yamada T, et al: Similar pharmacokinetics and differential ototoxicity after administration with cisplatin and transplatin in guinea pigs. Acta Otolaryngol (Stockh) 1997; 117:61-65.
46. Silva EG, Tornos C, Deavers M, et al: Induction of epithelial neoplasms in the ovaries of guinea pigs by estrogenic stimulation. Gynecol Oncol 1998; 71:240-246.
47. Silva EG, Tornos C, Fritsche HA, et al: The induction of benign epithelial neoplasms of the ovaries of guinea pigs by testosterone stimulation: a potential animal model. Mod Pathol 1997; 10:879-883.
48. Spink RR: Urolithiasis in a guinea pig. Vet Med Small Anim Clin 1978; 73:501-502.
49. Suckow MA, Chrisp CE, Rush HG: Cryptosporidiosis in immunocompetent guinea pigs. Lab Anim Sci 1989; 39:470.
50. Timm KI: Pruritus in rabbits, rodents, and ferrets. Vet Clin North Am Small Anim Pract 1988; 18:1077-1091.
51. Vangeel I, Pasmans F, Vanrobaeys M, et al: Prevalence of dermatophytes in asymptomatic guinea pigs and rabbits. Vet Rec 2000; 146:440-441.
52. Vannevel J: Diabetes in the guinea pig: not uncommon. Can Vet J 1998; 40:613.
53. Vannevel J: Diabetes mellitus in a 3-year-old, intact, female guinea pig. Can Vet J 1998; 39:503-504.
54. Waggie KS, Wagner JE, Kelley ST: Naturally occurring *Bacillus piliformis* infection (Tyzzer's disease) in guinea pigs. Lab Anim Sci 1986; 36:504.
55. Wallach JD, Boever WJ: Diseases of Exotic Animals. Philadelphia, WB Saunders, 1983, pp 135-195.
56. Williams CSF: Practical Guide to Laboratory Animals. St Louis, CV Mosby, 1976, pp 3-11.
57. Witt WM, Hubbard GB, Fanton JW: *Streptococcus pneumoniae* arthritis and osteomyelitis with vitamin C deficiency in guinea pigs. Lab Anim Sci 1988; 38:192-194.
58. Wullenweber M, Boot R: Interlaboratory comparison of enzyme-linked immunosorbent assay (ELISA) and indirect immunofluorescence (IIF) for detection of *Bordetella bronchiseptica* antibodies in guinea pigs. Lab Anim 1994; 28:335-339.
59. Xia Y, Hu HZ, Liu S, et al: *Clostridium difficile* toxin A excites enteric neurons and suppresses sympathetic neurotransmission in the guinea pig. Gut 2000; 46:481-486.
60. Young JD, Hurst WJ, White WJ, et al: An evaluation of ampicillin pharmacokinetics and toxicity in guinea pigs. Lab Anim Sci 1987; 37:652-656.

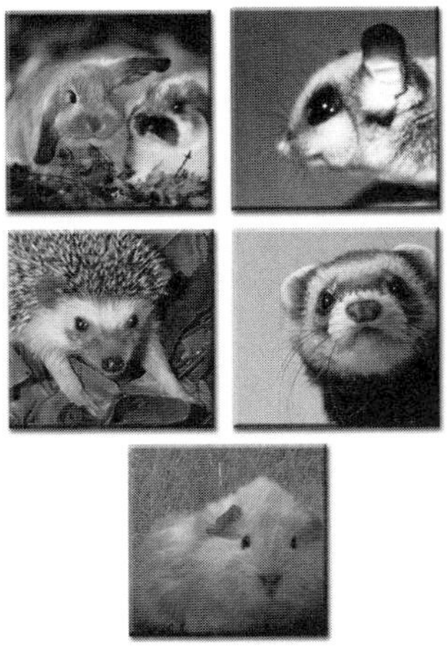

CHAPTER 25

Disease Problems of Chinchillas

Thomas M. Donnelly, BVSc, Diplomate ACLAM

Because of the paucity of information from clinical settings, acquiring knowledge about the diseases, diagnosis, and treatment of pet chinchillas differs from procuring similar information about other exotic rodents. The vast majority of the early literature on diseases of chinchillas has come from the fur industry. Although their small size and ease of handling make them suitable experimental animals, chinchillas have been used almost exclusively in hearing research. They have an auditory sensitivity remarkably similar to that of humans and large bullae surrounded by thin bone, which allows easy surgical access to the middle ear. Little information on spontaneous diseases in chinchillas has come from the laboratory animal field.

Most papers in English that describe diseases in chinchillas were written in the 1950s and early 1960s and cover conditions observed in fur-ranched animals. In contrast, most papers written after 1980 are in non-English European languages, often without an English summary. There were approximately three clinical reports per decade for the 1970s, 1980s, and 1990s.

Although there were numerous publications over the past 50 years on chinchilla diseases, most were printed in fur-trade periodicals and newsletters and not in clinical or scientific journals. The situation is further complicated by the misidentification of non-English trade publications such as *Deutsche Pelztierzuchter (German Fur-Animal Breeder)* as scientific journals and their use as references in clinical reports.

I have emphasized this state of the body of knowledge on chinchilla diseases because many readers may find two aspects of this chapter unusual: (1) I cite referenced information that is not necessarily current but may seem new, and (2) although I describe the same diseases as are covered in recent, brief reviews, I place far greater emphasis on diseases associated with poor husbandry. I consider these problems to be more frequent reasons that an owner of a pet chinchilla seeks veterinary consultation.

GENERAL COMMENTS ON DISEASE PROBLEMS OF CHINCHILLAS

Diseases Likely to Be Seen in Practice

Husbandry and feeding mistakes are the most common causes of disease seen in practice; therefore, asking about the husbandry conditions before attempting a diagnosis is essential. Chinchillas hide signs of disease as a survival mechanism.

Unless the owner is well informed, the pet will be brought to the veterinarian at a much later stage of disease than a dog or cat. Owners often follow the recommendations of the pet store before seeking veterinary help, which is another reason a chinchilla is often seen in a late stage of disease.

DISEASES ASSOCIATED WITH POOR HUSBANDRY

Disorders of the Digestive System

When a problem arises in chinchillas, it is usually gastrointestinal. In my experience, disorders of the digestive tract not associated with infectious disease remain the most frequent problem seen in clinical practice. Inappetence and lethargy are common presenting signs. However, because these signs are also associated with infectious and metabolic diseases, I always recommend a thorough diagnostic workup.

Malocclusion of the teeth and slobbers Chinchillas frequently develop cheek teeth abnormalities related to tooth elongation (Figs. 25-1 and 25-2; see also Chapter 34). Crossley[8] detected dental abnormalities in 35% of apparently healthy chinchillas presented for clinical examination and incisor abnormalities in 55% of those presented because of clinical illness. Chinchillas with malocclusion have a history of intermittent or chronic dysphagia, altered chewing pattern, changed food preferences, and weight loss. Clinically, chinchillas may have epiphora, serous nasal discharge, excess salivation and wet chin (slobbers), and detectable swellings on the ventrolateral borders of the mandible. Clinical examination of the oral cavity under anesthesia, as in rabbits and guinea pigs, is unreliable in assessing the extent of dental problems, and radiology or computed tomography is required to evaluate disease.[9] Treatment involves removing spikes, reducing crown height, and equilibrating occlusal surfaces. Providing a diet with physical properties that more closely matches that of wild chinchillas generally improves the dental health of pet chinchillas. Such foods include hay, straw, green feed, and pressed mixed feeds with long chewable and gnawable ingredients. Owners should avoid diets that consist predominantly of pellets with a small amount of hay.

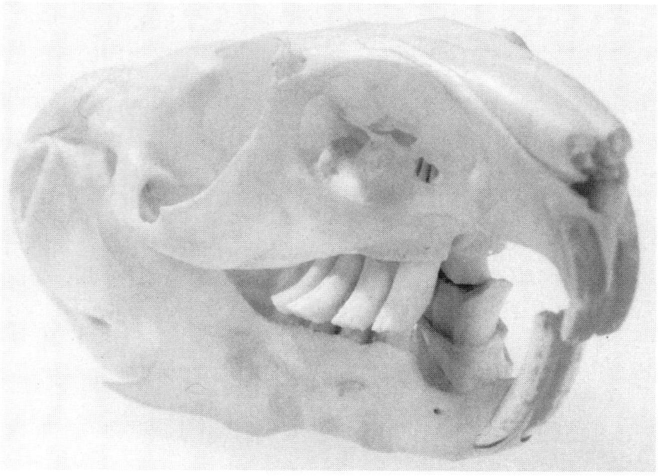

Figure 25-1 Skull of a chinchilla with severe molar malocclusion. Notice that the upper molars curve outward (see Figure 25-2 to see mandible).

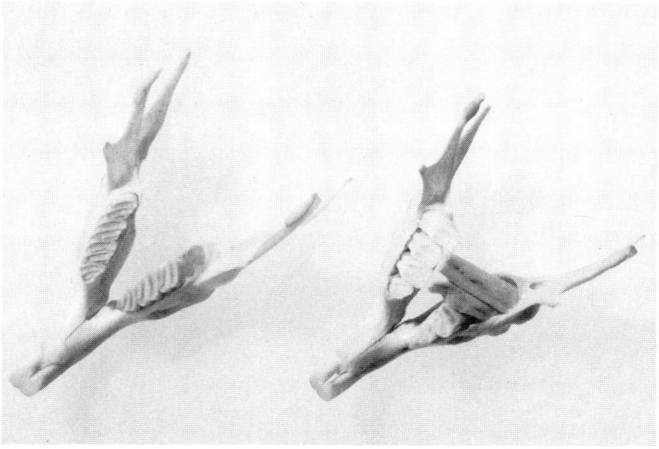

Figure 25-2 Two chinchilla mandibles. The mandible on the left shows normal molar occlusion. The mandible on the right is from the skull of the chinchilla in Fig. 25-1. Notice that the lower molars curve inward, in contrast to the upper molars, which curve outward. This is a severe case in which the molars no longer occluded and continued to grow, leading to trauma to the oral mucosa and tongue.

Choke and bloat Like rabbits and rats, chinchillas cannot vomit, and esophageal choke has been described in chinchillas of all ages.[7] Clinical signs include drooling, retching, dyspnea, and anorexia. Choke is more common in animals that are offered tidbits such as raisins, fruits, and nuts; in animals that eat their bedding; and in postparturient females that eat their placentas. Bloat or gastric tympany is another problem of lactating females and is associated with overeating of hay rich in clover, sudden food changes (especially the addition of fresh greens and fruits), and gastrointestinal inflammation. Affected animals are swollen, lie on their sides, hesitate to stir, and are dyspneic. Treat bloat by decompressing the stomach, either by passing a gastric tube or by transabdominally inserting a needle or trocar.

Gastric trichobezoars are often associated with fur-chewing. Clinical signs, including anorexia and lethargy, are similar to those in rabbits. Although their efficacy is questionable, the proteolytic enzymes in pineapple juice or papaya tablets are claimed to help break down fur in the stomach. However, pineapple juice and papaya tablets are sweet, and chinchillas may readily lap or eat them as a tasty treat. This treatment may not be efficacious, but is unlikely to cause harm. Treat dehydrated and anorectic animals with suspected trichobezoars with supplemental fluids, gastric motility stimulants, and force-feeding of a high-fiber food supplement—therapy similar to that used in rabbits.

Constipation In chinchillas, constipation has been described as a more common clinical problem than diarrhea.[29] Veterinarians easily overlook constipation because owners do not always recognize their pet's normal droppings. Healthy fecal pellets are plentiful and odorless, shaped like large grains of rice, either brown or black, and soft and plump when fresh.[7] Chinchillas with constipation strain to defecate, and the few pellets they pass are thin, short, hard, and occasionally blood-stained. The usual cause of constipation is feeding too much concentrated diet, which is high in energy and protein, without supplying sufficient roughage or fiber.[7] Therapeutically changing the diet by simply increasing the fiber is possible. Carefully adding small amounts of fresh food such as apples, carrots, or lettuce and omitting treats such as grains or raisins often achieves the desired results. If the constipation does not improve, laxatives such as those used in cats can be used. If there is no intestinal blockage, cisapride (0.5 mg/kg PO q8h) may be useful to enhance intestinal motility. Some breeders give vegetable oil or sweet butter on a spoon to avoid this problem. Other causes of constipation include obesity, lack of exercise, intestinal obstruction, and intestinal compression secondary to large fetuses.[28]

Diarrhea Diarrhea is another frequent reason for consultation. The most common cause of diarrhea in pet chinchillas is inappropriate feeding. This includes overfeeding of fresh green foods and offering damp hay that may be moldy or hay that is too young. Stress and sudden changes of food also seem to predispose chinchillas to diarrhea. The owner may first notice that feces are smeared on the resting board in the cage and fur around the anus is matted with feces. The diarrhea is acute, and usually the chinchilla does not appear sick. Hartmann[29] recommended withholding food for the first day and adding a palatable oral electrolyte replacement solution to the drinking water. A well-dried, high-quality hay that is older than half a year is offered on the second day, and an electrolyte solution is administered subcutaneously if the animal is dehydrated.

Bacterial and parasitic infections also cause diarrhea (see later section), but usually the owner describes signs of diarrhea that have been present for a few days. These chinchillas are often lethargic and have dry and dull fur. Because an animal may camouflage diarrhea by cleaning itself, fecal staining of the fur is not always apparent. Breeding females and young chinchillas up to 4 months of age are most susceptible to infectious diarrhea.[28]

Intestinal torsion and impaction Intestinal torsion, intussusception, or impaction of the cecum or colonic flexure can occur in chinchillas with chronic cases of constipation or gastroenteritis.[3,55] Ileus can be diagnosed radiographically by the presence of severely distended and gas-filled intestinal loops.[77] Animals may sit hunched, stretch out, or roll in an attempt to relieve pain. If the cause of these symptoms is impaction, a warm, soapy water or mineral oil enema can be carefully administered; intussusception or torsion requires surgery.

Rectal prolapse Rectal prolapse may also occur in chinchillas with severe constipation or diarrhea.[58] If diagnosed and treated quickly, the prolapse can be replaced and retained by a purse-string suture. If the tissue is edematous, gently soak it in a concentrated sugar solution, which sometimes reduces the swelling. Address the causative factors of the prolapse to prevent recurrence. Provide a bland, soft diet of baby food and cereals, except rice cereal, for 10 days after a prolapse has occurred. Gradually return the animal to a normal diet after the sutures are removed.

Reproductive Disorders

Fur-ring and paraphimosis Male chinchillas that groom excessively, strain to urinate, frequently produce small amounts of urine, or repeatedly clean their penis may have a fur-ring.[91,92] This is a ring of hair around the penis and under the prepuce that eventually stops the penis from retracting into the prepuce. In severe cases, an engorged penis is seen protruding 4 to 5 cm from the prepuce, resulting in paraphimosis.[36] The condition is not only painful but also may cause urethral constriction and acute urinary retention. Chronic paraphimosis can culminate in infection and severe damage to the penis, affecting the animal's breeding ability.

To remove the fur-ring, apply a sterile lubricant and cut or gently roll the fur-ring off the penis. In some chinchillas, sedation or anesthesia may be required to remove the fur-ring.[91,92]

Fur-ring is thought to result from the acquisition of fur from a female during copulation. However, because the condition is also seen in group-housed and single-housed males not exposed to females, fur may come from other males or from the same animal. Veterinarians should examine nonbreeding males for fur-rings at least four times a year and active studs every few days. In some chinchillas, the penis hangs out of the prepuce and is not engorged.[92] This is not associated with fur-ring but results from overexcitement brought on by separating a chinchilla from its mate or from overexhaustion because of too many females in the same cage.

Fetal resorption and dystocia Chinchillas have a high incidence of fetal resorption during pregnancy.[91] The normal gestation period for a chinchilla is 111 days, and the young are born fully furred. Chinchillas usually give birth to two kits early in the morning (before 8 AM) and only rarely late at night.[92] A chinchilla with dystocia is recognized by its extreme restlessness, frequent crying, and constant attention to its genital region. Dystocia is usually associated with the presentation of a single oversized fetus or malpresentation of one or more kits.[7] Uterine inertia has also been reported as a cause of dystocia.[72] In an uncomplicated dystocia, gentle traction of the fetus with feline obstetric forceps may correct the condition. However, if the chinchilla is in labor for longer than 4 hours, surgical intervention is indicated (see Chapter 27). Pet chinchillas respond well to cesarean section.[5,38,72,84,87]

Ectopic pregnancy and pulmonary trophoblastic emboli Gitlin and Adler[20] described a case of ectopic pregnancy in a chinchilla that died close to term. It was not determined whether the ectopic pregnancy was primary or secondary (i.e., due to rupture of a uterine horn during pregnancy). However, the chinchilla ovary is in free communication on its ventral aspect with the peritoneal cavity, in contrast to other rodents, in which an ovarian bursa surrounds the ovary.

Pulmonary trophoblastic emboli can occur in late gestation and after parturition.[35,88] In chinchillas, the fine structure of the interhemal membrane of the placental labyrinth is hemomonochorial, consisting of a single layer of syncytial trophoblasts, and is similar to that of guinea pigs. Trophoblastic pulmonary emboli also occur in pregnant women. In chinchillas and humans, this condition is considered an incidental finding, although it has occasionally caused death in women. In reported cases, ages of affected chinchillas varied from 14 months to 6 years, and one chinchilla also had trophoblastic infiltration of the myometrium.[35]

Traumatic Disorders

Conjunctivitis Irritation of the eyes that results in conjunctivitis without clinical signs of upper respiratory tract infection is often caused by excessive dust bathing. Dirty or poor-quality bedding and inadequate cage ventilation also can cause conjunctivitis. Treatment involves restricting dust bath access to 15-30 minutes per day, changing the type of dusting powder (see Chapter 23), and applying a protective ophthalmic preparation such as artificial tears or petrolatum ointment. If the condition does not respond rapidly, additional ophthalmic evaluation is recommended.

Fur slip Chinchillas possess a predator avoidance mechanism known as fur slip. When an animal is fighting or is being handled roughly, it can release a large patch of fur, thus enabling it to escape. A clean, smooth area of skin is left; hair may require several months to regrow.

Bite wounds Bite wounds that abscess often develop in group-housed animals, especially during breeding. Female chinchillas are larger than males and, like female hamsters, are more aggressive; older females may kill a young male housed in the same cage. Female chinchillas are highly selective in their choice of mates and will keep "unsuitable" males at bay by urinating, kicking, and biting.[92] In addition to causing abscesses, bite wounds sometimes result in the loss of parts of ears or toes. Culture of the abscesses often yields *Staphylococcus* species. Jenkins[37] found that surgical removal of the abscess was more successful than incision and curettage. Treatment with appropriate systemic antibiotics is also indicated.

Fractures Traumatic fractures of the tibia are commonly seen. The tibia is a long, straight bone with little soft tissue covering. It is longer than the femur, and the fibula is virtually nonexistent (Fig. 25-3). Tibial fractures are usually either transverse or short spiral fractures, and they usually are associated with bony fragments. Fractures commonly occur when a chinchilla is grabbed by its hind limb or catches its leg in a cage bar.

Like the bones of rabbits, those of chinchillas are thin and fragile, and surgical repair can be difficult (see Chapter 35). Soft, padded bandages and lateral splints usually do not provide adequate stability for fractures to heal.[31] Although intramedullary fixation has been used,[71] the effect of the pin on the thin cortices and narrow lumen can result in microstructural damage that leads to excessive bone resorption and premature pin loosening. For best results, surgically repair the fracture with either wire or external fixators (type II Kirschner-Ehmer apparatus) and then stabilize it with bandages.[47]

Chinchillas are active animals, and limiting mobility by placing the animal in a small cage is essential for fracture healing. Unfortunately, frequent visits to the veterinarian to reset the fracture are common. Advise owners that nonunion is a possible outcome and will result in a crooked leg. Should a limb need to be amputated, chinchillas usually adapt extremely well.

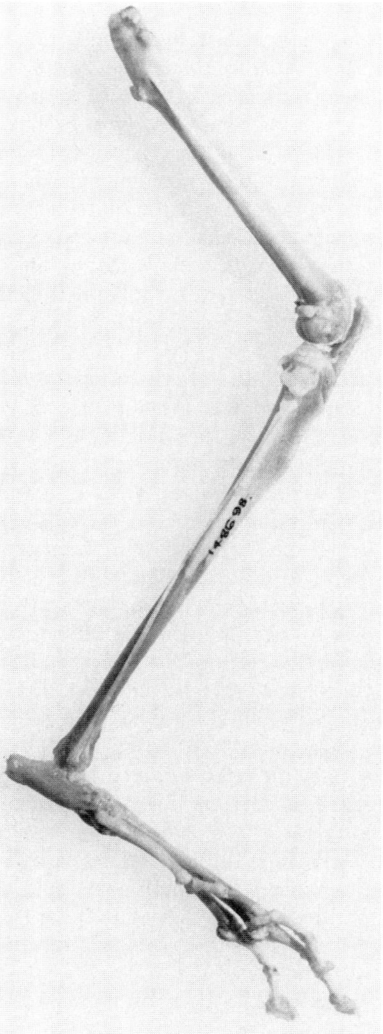

Figure 25-3 Hindlimb skeleton of an adult chinchilla. Notice the length of the tibia compared with the femur. The fibula is virtually nonexistent. Most traumatic fractures involve the tibia, and the fragile nature of the bone shows how challenging surgical fixation can be.

Dermatologic Disorders

Matted fur Chinchillas develop matted fur if they are kept in a warm (greater than 80°F [26.7°C]), humid environment or if they are deprived of a dust bath (see Chapter 23). Dust baths should be provided for approximately 30 minutes per day. Although the dust bath could be left with the chinchilla for longer periods, doing so could result in excessive bathing and subsequent conjunctivitis.

Alopecia and ringworm Dermatophytosis is uncommon in chinchillas. Although *Microsporum canis* and *Microsporum gypseum* have been incriminated in outbreaks of spontaneously occurring dermatophytosis, *Trichophyton mentagrophytes* is the dermatophyte most commonly isolated.[12] In infected chinchillas, small, scaly patches of alopecia on the nose, behind the ears, or on the forefeet are seen. Lesions may appear on any part of the body; in advanced cases, a large circumscribed area of inflammation with scab formation is not unusual. Although most mycologic studies of chinchillas are based on animals with clinical signs, *T. mentagrophytes* has been cultured from 5% of fur-ranched chinchillas with normal skin and 30% of those with fur damage.[12]

Because *T. mentagrophytes* does not fluoresce, ultraviolet light is not useful for diagnosis. Diagnosis requires microscopic examination of hair and skin samples and dermatophyte culture. For topical therapy, 2% chlorhexidine/2% miconazole shampoo or 0.2% enilconazole rinse is effective. Topical treatment removes spores from hair shafts, and systemic treatment acts at hair follicles. Systemic drugs that can be used are griseofulvin (microsized form: 50-100 mg/kg PO q24h divided into two to three doses), ketoconazole (10-15 mg/kg PO q24h), itraconazole (5-10 mg/kg PO q24h), and terbinafine (8-20 mg/kg PO q24h).

Captan mixed with a dust bath at 1 teaspoon per 2 cups of dust may help control the spread of infection.[94]

Fur-chewing Alopecia is usually associated with fur chewing in chinchillas. Chinchillas chew each other's fur, resulting in a coat with a moth-eaten appearance.

Eidmann[15] contrasted the histologic appearance of selected organs of 39 fur-chewers with those of 19 healthy chinchillas. The animals were of both sexes and various ages. Skin and fur samples were cultured for bacteria and fungi, feces were examined for parasites, and the numbers and types of intestinal bacteria were determined. Hematologic tests consisting of a complete blood count and selected serum enzyme measurements were done in all animals. The author concluded that an infectious cause of fur-chewing was unlikely and suggested that affected animals suffer from malnutrition and chew their fur for dietary requirements. The diagnosis of malnutrition was based on histologic and enzymatic evidence of mild fatty degeneration of the liver and lower numbers of cecal bacteria in fur-chewers. However, Eidmann[15] also suggested that multiple food factors (e.g., palatability, digestibility, fiber length and size of particles, amount of chewing or gnawing needed) are possibly involved in this type of malnutrition and that further dietary studies are required. Of particular interest was her correlation of thyroid hyperplasia to the size of chewed fur over the body. This was interpreted as a reactive response of the thyroid to the loss of insulation after fur loss. Both fur-chewers and control animals were found to have large numbers of *Giardia* parasites, but histologic examination of the intestines was not done.

Although a cause of fur-chewing could not be established, the conclusions of this study discredited popular theories supported by scant experimental evidence. Among these is the theory that a fungus is the cause of fur breakage,[81] on the basis of which some chinchilla fur ranchers regularly add fungicide to the dust bath. Another theory suggests that fur-chewers might have abnormal endocrine activity, because they have increased thyroid and adrenocortical activity.[89]

A current popular theory suggests that fur-chewing is a behavioral disorder. The vice is often transmitted from mother to offspring. Furthermore, the higher incidence of fur-chewing in commercial herds is often suggested as evidence for maladapted displacement behavior. There have been no documented attempts to treat fur-chewers with antidepressants such as fluoxetine hydrochloride (Prozac, Dista Products Co, Indianapolis, IN), despite success with its use in the treatment of tail chasing and lick granulomas of dogs. Based on rabbit and rodent dosages,[75] a dosage of 5 to 10 mg/kg PO q24h of fluoxetine hydrochloride is suggested for chinchillas.

Neurologic Disorders

Encephalitis Several disorders result in convulsions or other neurologic signs. In addition to the more common husbandry-associated conditions that are described here, encephalitis caused by listeriosis, lymphocytic choriomeningitis, or cerebrospinal nematodiasis should also be considered in the diagnostic workup (see later discussion).

Lead poisoning Two cases of lead toxicosis in pet chinchillas have been described. A retrospective study described a chinchilla that had seizures similar to those in dogs and cats.[60] Although the blood lead concentration was high (660 μg/dL), the authors did not observe nucleated red blood cells or basophilic stippling of the red blood cells in this chinchilla's blood smear. Blood lead concentrations of 25 μg/dL or higher are indicative of lead poisoning; however, concentrations of 15 μg/dL or higher are suspect. The affected chinchilla was treated successfully with calcium disodium edetate diluted to a 1% solution with 5% dextrose water (25 mg/kg SC, q6h × 5 days).[61] Hoefer[30] reported lead poisoning in a New York apartment-dwelling chinchilla that was presented with acute convulsions and blindness. The blood lead concentration was 340 μg/dL. This animal was treated successfully with calcium disodium edetate at 30 mg/kg SC q12h for 5 days. Both of these reports described chinchillas with lead toxicosis from cities with poor urban neighborhoods. Morgan et al.[61] demonstrated a positive correlation of lead poisoning in small companion animals with urban neighborhoods in which a high percentage of people live in poverty.

Heatstroke The ambient temperature range to which chinchillas are adapted is 65° to 80°F (18.3° to 26.7°C). Exposure to higher ambient temperatures, especially in the presence of high humidity, can result in heatstroke. A good rule of thumb is to add the unit values of the temperature (Fahrenheit) and humidity, and consider any value greater than 150 dangerous. For example, 85°F + 65% humidity = 150.

Affected animals lie down and exhibit rapid breathing; bright red mucous membranes; thick, stringy saliva; and, sometimes, bloody diarrhea. Owners often describe animals with engorged ear veins and bright pink or red ears and mucous membranes. Rectal temperature is usually greater than 103°F (39.4°C). Treatment is straightforward—cooling the animal by immersing it in tepid water baths and, if the animal is in shock, administering intravenous fluids. Do not place a chinchilla in an ice-cold water bath, because this can cause seizures. Advise owners not to position chinchilla cages near sunny windows or radiators.

Renal Disorders

Goudas and Lusis[23] described spontaneous calcium oxalate crystal precipitation in the renal tubules of six adult female chinchillas. Two of the chinchillas had a history of progressive weakness before death. The other cases were identified retrospectively by examination of microscopic sections of kidneys received by their laboratory during a 2-year period. Oxalate nephrocalcinosis is commonly seen in pets that ingest ethylene glycol (antifreeze). However, these chinchillas did not have access to antifreeze. Possible causes were feedstuffs made up of plants containing oxalic acid, moldy feed, and vitamin B_6 deficiency.

Male chinchillas can develop urinary calculi and urolithiasis.[39,63,86] The calculi are composed of calcium carbonate. Affected animals are presented with hematuria, dysuria, or anuria. Abdominal radiographs show radiodense calculi in the bladder or urethra. Ultrasound examination reveals a hyperechoic, smooth interface casting a shadow in the bladder. Treatment consists of surgical removal of the calculi and postoperative antibiotic therapy.

REPORTED INFECTIOUS DISEASES OF CHINCHILLAS

Table 25-1 summarizes all significant reports over the past 55 years of infectious diseases in chinchillas. There are two striking observations: (1) almost all of the reports come from

TABLE 25-1
Reports of Infectious Diseases in Chinchillas over the Past 60 Years

Organism	Groups of Fur-Ranched Chinchillas	Individual Pet or Laboratory Chinchillas
Yersinia	Hubbert (1972)	
	Langford (1972)	
	Kageruka, Mortelmans et al. (1976)	
	Gueraud (1988)	
	Emirsajllow, Furowicz et al. (1996)	
	Furowicz and Czernomysy (1999)	
Listeria	MacKay, Kennedy et al. (1949)	
	Shalkop (1950)	
	Smith (1953)	
	Leader and Holte (1955)	
	Cavill (1967)	
	Nilsson and Soderlind (1974)	
	Finley and Long (1977)	
	Novak, Ruttkay et al. (1994)	
	Wilkerson, Melendy et al. (1997)	
	Sabocanec, Culjak et al. (2000)	
Pseudomonas	Newberne (1953)	
	Larrivee and Elvehjem (1954)	
	Lusis and Soltys (1971)	
	Menchaca, Moras et al. (1980)	
	Lazzari, Vargas et al. (2001)	
Proteus	Larrivee and Elvehjem (1954)	Doerning, Brammer et al. (1993)
	Menchaca, Martin et al. (1978)	
Klebsiella	Bartoszcze, Matras et al. (1990)	
Clostridium	Moore and Greenlee (1975)	
	Bartoszcze, Nowakowska et al. (1990)	
	Nowakowska, Matras et al. (1991)	
Salmonella	Holm (1940)	Mountain (1989)
	Keagy and Keagy (1951)	Yamagishi, Watanabe et al. (1997)
	Gorham (1955)	
Giardia	Newberne (1953)	
	Shelton (1954)	
	Poole (1960)	
Toxoplasma	Keagy (1949)	Meingassner and Burtscher (1977)
Frenkellia		Dubey et al. (2000)
Cryptosporidium		Yamini and Raju (1986)
Sarcocystis		Rakich, Dubey et al. (1992)
Histoplasma		Burtscher and Otte (1962)
		Owens, Menges et al. (1975)
Baylisascaris	Sanford (1991)	

colonies of chinchillas raised for fur and involve bacterial diseases, and (2) most of the reports of bacterial disease in colonies were published 20 or more years ago. The two reports of infectious disease in pet chinchillas both involved protozoa or fungi.

Recent reviews of the diseases of chinchillas propagate the impression that these animals are very susceptible to infectious disease. However, my impression is that pet chinchillas are about as susceptible as dogs or cats to infectious disease.

Viral Infections

Chinchillas are susceptible to human herpesvirus 1 and may play a role as a temporary reservoir for human infections.

Goudas and Giltoy[22] described a spontaneous, herpeslike viral infection in a female chinchilla. Wohlsein et al.[95] reported a 1-year-old male chinchilla with a 2-week history of conjunctivitis that subsequently showed neurologic signs of seizures, disorientation, recumbency, and apathy. In this chinchilla, a nonsuppurative meningitis and polioencephalitis with neuronal necrosis and intranuclear inclusion bodies was found on histologic examination. Both eyes displayed ulcerative keratitis, uveitis, retinitis and retinal degeneration, and optical neuritis. The clinical signs, the distribution of the lesions, and the viral antigen suggested a primary ocular infection with subsequent spread to the central nervous system.

Bacterial Infections

Opportunistic infections caused by normal bacterial flora of chinchillas can cause frank disease, either localized to one organ (e.g., *Streptococcus* and *Pseudomonas* species, *Escherichia coli*) or as septicemia. Affected animals usually are immunocompromised by age, nutritional status, or husbandry-related stress.

Historically, *Pseudomonas aeruginosa* infections, yersiniosis, and listeriosis occurred frequently among fur-ranched chinchillas in Canada, the United States, and the United Kingdom. Estimates of fur-ranched chinchilla numbers in the United States in 1954 were greater than 100,000 animals. By the mid-1960s, these numbers were reduced significantly to only a few thousand. Reports since 1980 of yersiniosis and listeriosis in chinchillas come almost exclusively from fur-ranched chinchillas in Hungary, Poland, Slovakia, and Croatia.[44] These four European countries supply almost 50% of the annual 200,000 chinchilla pelts produced worldwide.

Several reports have described opportunistic systemic infections caused by *P. aeruginosa* in fur-ranched chinchillas.[41,45,50,57] Doerning et al.[10] described a case of *P. aeruginosa* infection in a laboratory chinchilla. The affected animal displayed a variety of clinical signs, including scrotal swelling, conjunctivitis, anorexia, weight loss, and corneal and oral ulcerations. The animal was treated with chloramphenicol therapeutically and with butorphanol for analgesia, and it developed unusual intradermal pustules 8 days after recovery from the infection. A vaccine against *P. aeruginosa* has been developed for attempted immunization and is used in fur-ranched chinchillas.[49,54]

The causative agents of yersiniosis, *Yersinia pseudotuberculosis* (formerly *Pasteurella pseudotuberculosis*) and *Yersinia enterocolitica*, occur worldwide in areas of moderate and subtropical climate, and outbreaks in chinchillas are commonly described.* *Y. enterocolitica* is the species most frequently isolated from chinchillas. Yersiniosis is an enteric disease that damages epithelium of the ileum, cecum, and colon, resulting in mucosal hemorrhage and ulceration. Lymphoid infiltration results in hypertrophy of Peyer's patches and mesenteric lymph nodes and necrotizing granulomas. Systemic spread results in granulomatous lesions in the lungs, spleen, and liver and death. A "chinchilla-type" strain of *Y. enterocolitica* (biovar 3, antigens or serovar 1, 2a, 3) appears to persist enzootically among chinchilla stock worldwide.[96] The pathogenicity of enteric *Yersinia* appears to depend on a plasmid that is essential for expressing virulence. Plasmid-mediated pathogenic functions are survival in serum, resistance to phagocytosis, cell adhesion, and cytotoxicity.[11,73] However, bacterial endocytosis in intestinal epithelial cells seems not to be encoded by a plasmid.

*References 16, 19, 25, 34, 43, 54, 73, 96.

Listeriosis in chinchillas was first reported by MacKay et al. in 1949.[52] It was and still is common in fur-ranched chinchillas but not in laboratory or pet chinchillas.* Although Gray and Killinger[24] claimed that chinchillas appear to be the animal most susceptible to infection with *Listeria monocytogenes*, this has not been proved. Case reports of listeriosis in chinchillas describe fur-ranched animals in high northern latitudes (e.g., Canada, Washington, the United Kingdom, Croatia, Hungary, Slovakia) that are fed silage or substitute roughage in pellets such as beet pulp during the winter.† Knowledge of *L. monocytogenes* and the various forms of disease that it causes has been limited until recently, but advances in taxonomy, isolation methods, bacterial typing, molecular biology, and cell biology have extended understanding of this organism.[48,76] *L. monocytogenes* is a highly adaptable environmental bacterium that can exist as both an animal pathogen and a plant saprophyte; it is also part of the normal microbial flora in healthy ruminants and is found in environmental sources such as decaying vegetation.

Most animal and human cases of listeriosis arise from the ingestion of contaminated food; the disease is common in animals fed on silage.[48] Unlike most foodborne pathogens that primarily cause gastrointestinal disease, *L. monocytogenes* causes several easily recognized invasive syndromes, such as encephalitis, abortion, and septicemia. However, the epidemiologic aspects and pathogenesis of infection remain poorly understood. In chinchillas, listeriosis is a cecal disease with bloodborne dissemination. The main target organ is the liver, where the bacteria multiply inside hepatocytes. Early recruitment of polymorphonuclear cells leads to lysis of hepatocytes, bacterial release, septicemia, and, in surviving hosts, the development of lung, brain, spleen, lymph node, and liver abscesses. The invasion of peripheral nerve cells and rapid entry into the brain, which causes the classic histopathologic lesion of monocytic perivascular cuffing, is believed to be a unique characteristic of its virulence.

Other recorded infections in chinchillas include clostridial enterotoxemia, salmonellosis, and *Klebsiella* infection. Bartoszcze et al.[2] described an outbreak of *Klebsiella pneumoniae* infection in fur-ranched chinchillas in Poland. Affected animals displayed loss of appetite, respiratory distress, and diarrhea and died 5 days after onset of clinical signs. At necropsy, the primary lesions were suppurative pneumonia and renal tubular necrosis. Affected animals were treated with gentamicin (2 mg/kg IM/SC q12h q5days); half the treated animals recovered.

Moore and Greenlee[59] described an enterotoxemia associated with *Clostridium* species in chinchillas; Nowakowska et al.[69] described enterotoxemia caused by *Clostridium perfringens* enterotoxin; and Bartoszcze et al.[1] described chinchilla deaths due to *C. perfringens* A enterotoxemia.

There are two case reports of *Salmonella* infection in companion chinchillas. Mountain[62] reported a case of *Salmonella arizona* septicemia in a chinchilla in the United Kingdom, and Yamagishi et al.[97] reported a case of septic infection in a companion chinchilla with *Salmonella enteritidis* in Japan. In the 1940s and 1950s, veterinarians described salmonella epizootics

*References 18, 26, 46, 51, 66, 68, 78, 80, 85, 90, 93.

†References 6, 18, 26, 68, 78, 93.

characterized by gastroenteritis and abortion in fur-ranched chinchillas in the United States.[21,33,41]

Systemic Fungal Infections

There are two case reports of *Histoplasma capsulatum* infection in chinchillas. Burtscher and Otto[4] described histoplasmosis in a chinchilla imported from the United States to Switzerland. Owens et al.[70] diagnosed histoplasmosis in a female chinchilla that originated from a commercial chinchilla ranch in central Missouri. At necropsy, pulmonary lesions included multiple hemorrhagic foci, alveolar consolidation, and bronchopneumonia, and the organism was present in numerous giant cells. Multifocal pyogranulomatous splenitis and hepatitis, with *H. capsulatum* in giant cells, also was noted. *H. capsulatum* was subsequently cultured from timothy hay used for food.

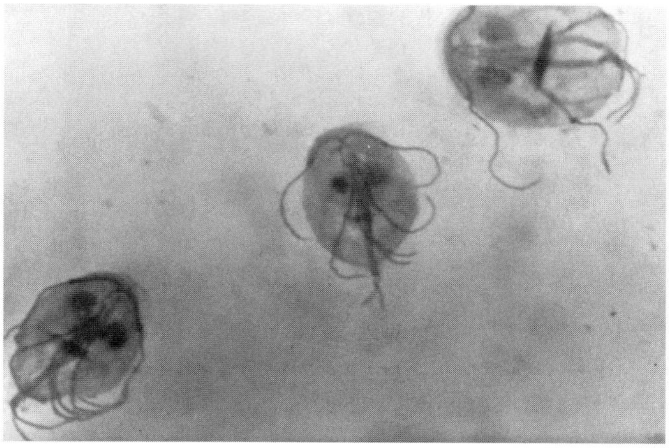

Figure 25-4 Wet mount of a fresh fecal sample showing motile trophozoites of *Giardia* species. Notice the prominent pair of nuclei containing a single karyosome of condensed chromatin, flagella running longitudinally between the nuclei, and a pair of curved median bodies. The arrangement of the organelles resembles a wide-eyed face.

Parasitic Diseases

Protozoal infections Although toxoplasmosis was commonly found in fur-ranched chinchillas in the past, it is now rarely seen.[40] At necropsy, lesions include enlarged spleens and mesenteric lymph nodes and hemorrhagic lungs. Meingassner and Burtscher[56] described two chinchillas with focal necrotic meningoencephalitis caused by *Toxoplasma gondii.* Several lobulated *Frenkelia* cysts up to 0.6 mm in diameter were found in the brains of the two animals, independent of and remote from the toxoplasmal inflammatory reaction. The authors considered that chinchillas may be susceptible to a *Frenkelia* species occurring in other free-living species. Dubey et al.[13] found tissue cysts of *Frenkelia microti* in the brain of a chinchilla bred in Minnesota and used for biomedical research. This was the first report of *Frenkelia* infection in chinchillas in the United States.

In the past, group-housed chinchillas in fur ranches and research colonies often had a high prevalence of giardiasis.[64,82] We now know that chinchillas normally harbor *Giardia* organisms in low numbers.[15] Stress and poor husbandry are believed to cause an increase in parasite numbers, resulting in severe diarrhea and death. However, the role of *Giardia* species in causing disease in pet chinchillas is difficult to establish, because these organisms are seen in both healthy and sick animals. *Giardia* can be identified on a fresh fecal smear (Fig. 25-4). Reports of giardiasis in pet chinchillas in the United States are more frequent on the West Coast than on the East Coast. Signs of giardiasis in pet chinchillas include a cyclic sequence of appetite loss and diarrhea associated with a declining body and fur condition. Until further research on chinchillas is done, the pathogenicity of *Giardia* species and its association with disease remain controversial. If giardiasis is suspected, treat with metronidazole, albendazole, or fenbendazole (see Metronidazole Toxicity).

Rakich et al.[74] described a case of acute hepatic sarcocystosis in a pet female chinchilla. The source of infection was unknown. The owners had housed and fed it with six other chinchillas that remained healthy. Yamini and Raju[98] described gastroenteritis associated with *Cryptosporidium* species in a pet chinchilla. The 8-month-old chinchilla came from a pet shop and developed severe diarrhea. Despite extensive antibiotic treatment and administration of intravenous fluids, the chinchilla died.

Nematode and cestode infections Disease outbreaks of cerebral nematodiasis caused by the raccoon ascarid *Baylisascaris procyonis* have been reported in chinchillas from western Canada.[79] Affected chinchillas showed ataxia, torticollis, paralysis, incoordination, and tumbling. Outbreaks of fatal central nervous system disease were linked to use of hay contaminated by raccoon feces. Raccoons infected with *B. procyonis* are more common in northern temperate regions of North America, especially the midwestern and northeastern United States.

Chinchillas can serve as an intermediate host for cestodes including *Taenia serialis, Taenia pisiformis, Echinococcus granulosus,* and *Hymenolepis nana.*[21] In the 1950s, infections were seen when chinchillas were given feed accidentally contaminated with infected dog feces. A recent report described more than 600 cysts of *Taenia crassiceps* found in the abdominal cavity of a pet chinchilla imported from The Netherlands into Japan.[42]

MISCELLANEOUS DISEASE PROBLEMS

Cardiomyopathy

Based on anecdotal reports of cardiomyopathy in two young black velvet females, breeders in the United States have suggested that cardiac problems may exist in chinchillas. Heart murmurs ranging from mild to moderate are described in chinchillas, and murmurs are often auscultated in young chinchillas presented for routine examination.[32] However, to date there have been no reports of cardiac disease in chinchillas, and the relationship of murmurs to cardiac disease is not understood at this time. The exception was a 2-year-old male chinchilla in which a heart murmur was detected as an incidental finding on physical examination.[32] Cardiac ultrasonography and electrocardiography revealed a ventricular septal defect and tricuspid regurgitation. (Ultrasound examination of two other animals, one with a murmur and one without, did not reveal abnormalities.) The animal died suddenly, 16 months after initial presentation, with no clinical signs. At necropsy, a marked papillary muscle dysplasia, mitral valve malformation, and a ventricular septal defect were noted. (The half-brother of this chinchilla, which also had a heart murmur, had died suddenly 1 week earlier, but a necropsy was not done.) Until this problem is further investigated, ultrasound examination and echocardiography are probably warranted for any animals in which murmurs are detected. At present, clinical management is empiric.

Metronidazole Toxicity

Administration of metronidazole has been anecdotally associated with liver failure in chinchillas. It is not known whether this association was related to toxicity of the drug or to a preexisting condition. Since the first edition of this book, I am not aware of any reports of metronidazole toxicity in chinchillas treated with the drug.

To treat chinchillas with giardiasis, I recommend anthelmintic benzimidazoles (e.g., albendazole). The nitroimidazole drugs, such as metronidazole, that are commonly prescribed to treat protozoal infections are not well tolerated in humans and are associated with poor compliance in children compared with adults.[83] Furthermore, recent reports have shown albendazole to be as effective as metronidazole in the treatment of giardial infections in children, with fewer adverse effects.[14,27] However, veterinarians consider albendazole to have more risks (i.e., teratogenicity and toxicity). Treat with albendazole at a dosage of 25 mg/kg PO q12h for 2 days or fenbendazole 50 mg/kg PO q24h for 3 days.

Diabetes Mellitus

A single case of diabetes mellitus was reported in a 5-year-old obese female chinchilla.[53] The animal had a 3-week history of poor appetite, lethargy, and weight loss. Physical assessment of the chinchilla showed polydipsia, polyuria, and bilateral cataracts. The blood glucose concentration was greater than 400 mg/dL, and urinalysis showed significant glucosuria and ketonuria. Daily treatment with 2 IU insulin was begun and then was increased to 12 IU. The ketonuria and polydipsia resolved, and after 10 days the blood glucose concentration dropped to 216 mg/dL. However, the animal's condition was difficult to stabilize, and hyperglycemia (greater than 400 mg/dL) returned after 2 weeks of therapy. The chinchilla was euthanatized, and microscopic examination of pancreatic islets showed prominent vacuolation, consistent with diabetes mellitus. Treatment of diabetes mellitus in rodents is difficult. However, regulation of the diet may arrest the disease. Feed that is high in protein, low in fat, and high in complex carbohydrates and contains 50 μg of chromium per kilogram of diet is suggested.[17]

Neoplasia

Despite the long life span of chinchillas (reported to be up to 20 years) compared with other rodents, references to neoplasia in chinchillas have been rare. Tumors such as neuroblastoma, carcinoma, lipoma, and hemangioma were listed in the *Annual Reports of the San Diego County Livestock Department* during the 1950s. One report in 1953 described a malignant lymphoma in a chinchilla,[65] and another in 1963 described an hepatic carcinoma.[67] The striking absence of reports of neoplasia up to the present probably reflects the emphasis on chinchillas as fur-producers or research animals.

A 5-year retrospective review of chinchillas presented to the Animal Medical Center in New York revealed only one case of a neoplasm, which was an incidental finding at necropsy. A 1-year-old female chinchilla presented for acute onset of neurologic signs caused by chronic otitis media and died shortly after presentation. Necropsy results showed a uterine leiomyosarcoma, and there were no associated metastases. With increasing ownership of pet chinchillas and the increased number of animals being presented for geriatric problems, it is likely that case reports of tumors will be described.

REFERENCES

1. Bartoszcze M, Nowakowska M, Roszkowski J, et al: Chinchilla deaths due to *Clostridium perfringens* A enterotoxin (letter). Vet Rec 1990; 126:341-342.
2. Bartoszcze M, Matras J, Palec S, et al: *Klebsiella pneumoniae* infection in chinchillas [letter]. Vet Rec 1990; 127:119.
3. Bowden RST: Diseases of chinchillas. Vet Rec 1959; 71:1033-1039.
4. Burtscher H, Otte E: [Histoplasma in the chinchilla.] (German.) DTW Dtsch Tierarztl Wochenschr 1962; 69:303-307.
5. Caspari EL: Caesarean section in a chinchilla [letter; comment]. Vet Rec 1990; 126:490.
6. Cavill JP: Listeriosis in chinchillas (*Chinchilla laniger*). Vet Rec 1967; 80:592-594.
7. Cousens PJ: The chinchilla in veterinary practice. J Small Anim Pract 1963; 4:199-205.
8. Crossley DA: Dental disease in chinchillas in the UK. J Small Anim Pract 2001; 42:12-19.
9. Crossley DA, Jackson A, Yates J, et al: Use of computed tomography to investigate cheek tooth abnormalities in chinchillas (*Chinchilla laniger*). J Small Anim Pract 1998; 39:385-389.
10. Doerning BJ, Brammer DW, Rush HG: *Pseudomonas aeruginosa* infection in a *Chinchilla laniger*. Lab Anim 1993; 27:131-133.
11. Donnelly TM, Quimby FW: Biology and diseases of other rodents. *In* Fox JG, Anderson LC, Loew FM, et al, eds. Laboratory Animal Medicine, 2nd ed. London, Academic Press, 2002, pp 248-307.
12. Donnelly TM, Rush EM, Lackner PA: Ringworm in small exotic pets. Semin Avian Exotic Pet Med 2000; 9:82-93.
13. Dubey JP, Clark TR, Yantis D: *Frenkelia microti* infection in a chinchilla (*Chinchilla laniger*) in the United States. J Parasitol 2000; 86:1149-1150.
14. Dutta AK, Phadke MA, Bagade AC, et al: A randomised multicentre study to compare the safety and efficacy of albendazole and metronidazole in the treatment of giardiasis in children. Indian J Pediatr 1994; 61:689-693.
15. Eidmann S: [Studies on the etiology and pathogenesis of fur damage in the chinchilla.] (German.) Hannover, Germany, Tierarztliche Hochschule, 1992, p 163.
16. Emirsajllow-Zalewska W, Furowicz AJ, Aleksic S, et al: Evaluation of pathogenicity determinants of *Yersinia pseudotuberculosis* strains isolated from chinchillas from the Western Pomerania area. Adv Agric Sci 1996; 5:19-24.
17. Ewringmann A, Gobel T: [Diabetes mellitus in rabbits, guinea-pigs and chinchillas.] (German.) Kleintierpraxis 1998; 43:337, 348.
18. Finley GG, Long JR: An epizootic of listeriosis in chinchillas. Can Vet J 1977; 18:164-167.
19. Furowicz AJ, Czernomysy-Furowicz D: [Eradication of *Yersinia pseudotuberculosis* infection from a chinchilla farm.] (Polish.) Magazyn Weterynaryjny 1999; 8:130-132.
20. Gitlin G, Adler JH: Coexisting intrauterine and abdominal (intraperitoneal) pregnancy with possible superfoetation (superfecundation) and with adhesion of placenta to foetus in a chinchilla (*Chinchilla laniger*). Acta Zool Pathol Antverp 1969; 49:65-76.
21. Gorham JR, Farrell K: Diseases and parasites of chinchillas. *In* Proceedings of 92nd Annual Meeting of the American Veterinary Medical Association, Minneapolis, 1955, pp 228-234.

22. Goudas P, Giltoy JS: Spontaneous herpes-like viral infection in a chinchilla (*Chinchilla laniger*). Wildl Dis 1970; 6:175-179.
23. Goudas P, Lusis P: Oxalate nephrosis in a chinchilla (*Chinchilla laniger*). Can Vet J 1970; 11:256-257.
24. Gray ML, Killinger AH: *Listeria monocytogenes* and listeric infections. Bacteriol Rev 1966; 30:309-382.
25. Gueraud JM: [Threat of an epidemic of yersiniosis in chinchillas.] (French.) Bull Acad Vet France 1988; 61:95-98.
26. Hajtos I, Ralovich B: [New data on the occurrence and epidemiology of the listeriosis in Hungary.] (Hungarian.) Magyar Allatorvosok Lapja 1994; 49:7.
27. Hall A, Nahar Q: Albendazole as a treatment for infections with *Giardia duodenalis* in children in Bangladesh. Trans R Soc Trop Med Hyg 1993; 87:84-86.
28. Harkness JE: A practitioner's guide to domestic rodents. Denver, American Animal Hospital Association, 1993.
29. Hartmann K: [Husbandry-related diseases in the chinchilla.] (German.) Tierarztliche Praxis 1993; 21:574-580.
30. Hoefer HL: Chinchillas. Vet Clin North Am Small Anim Pract 1994; 24:103-111.
31. Hoefer HL: Chinchillas. *In* Proceedings of the North American Veterinary Conference, 1995. Orlando, pp 672–673.
32. Hoefer HL, Crossley DA: Chinchillas. *In* Meredith A, Redrobe S, eds. BSAVA Manual of Exotic Pets, 4th ed. Quedgeley, Gloucester, British Small Animal Veterinary Association, 2002, pp 65-75.
33. Holm GC, Graves PH: Paratyphoid in chinchilla. Vet Med 1940; 35:501.
34. Hubbert WT: Yersiniosis in mammals and birds in the United States: case reports and review. Am J Trop Med Hyg 1972; 21:458-463.
35. Ilha MR da S, Bezerra Junior PS, Sanches AWD, et al: [Trophoblastic pulmonary embolism in chinchillas (*Chinchilla laniger*).] (Portuguese.) Ciencia Rural 2000; 30:903-904.
36. Ivey ES, Hoefer HL: Pollakiuria in a chinchilla. Lab Anim 1998; 8:21-22.
37. Jenkins JR: Husbandry and common diseases of the chinchilla (*Chinchilla laniger*). J Small Exotic Anim Med 1992; 2:15-17.
38. Jones AK: Caesarean section in a chinchilla [letter; comment]. Vet Rec 1990; 126:441.
39. Jones RJ, Stephenson R, Fountain D, et al: Urolithiasis in a chinchilla [letter]. Vet Rec 1995; 136:400.
40. Keagy HF: Toxoplasma in the chinchilla. J Am Vet Med Assoc 1949; 94:15.
41. Keagy HF, Keagy EH: Epizootic gastroenteritis in chinchillas. J Am Vet Med Assoc 1951; 118:35-37.
42. Kugi G, Nonaka N, Ganzorig S, et al: [*Taenia crassiceps* larvae in a chinchilla (*Chinchilla brevicaudata*).] (Japanese.) J Vet Med Jpn 1999; 52:449-452.
43. Langford EV: *Pasteurella pseudotuberculosis* infections in western Canada. Can Vet J 1972; 13:85-87.
44. Lanszki J, Demeter-Pedery T, Mayer-Farkas B: [Hungary is an important producer of chinchillas: possibilities of development in the future.] (Hungarian.) Allattenyesztes Es Takarmanyozas 1999; 48:869-871.
45. Lazzari AM, Vargas AC, Dutra V, et al: [Infectious agents isolated from *Chinchilla laniger*.] (Portuguese.) Ciencia Rural 2001; 31:337-340.
46. Leader RW, Holte RJA: Three outbreaks of listeriosis in chinchillas. Cornell Vet 1955; 45:78-83.
47. Lorinson D, Gressl H, Immler R: [Treatment of fractures in dwarf rabbits, guinea-pigs and chinchillas, particularly by external fixation.] (German.) Wiener Tierarztliche Monatsschrift 1996; 83:232-237.
48. Low JC, Donachie W: A review of *Listeria monocytogenes* and listeriosis. Vet J 1997; 153:9-29.
49. Lusis PI, Soltys MA: Immunization of mice and chinchillas against *Pseudomonas aeruginosa*. Can J Comp Med Vet Sci 1971; 35:60-66.
50. Lusis PI, Soltys MA: *Pseudomonas* infections in man and animals. J Am Vet Med Assoc 1971; 159:416.
51. MacDonald DW, Wilton GS, Howell J, et al: *Listeria monocytogenes* isolations in Alberta 1951-1970. Can Vet J 1972; 13:69-71.
52. MacKay KA, Kennedy AH, Smith DLT, et al: *Listeria monocytogenes* infection in chinchillas. Annual Report Ontario Veterinary College, Guelph, 1949, pp 137-145.
53. Marlow C: Diabetes in a chinchilla [letter]. Vet Rec 1995; 136:595-596.
54. Matthes S: [Vaccination of rabbits and fur animals.] (German.) Tierarztliche Praxis 1985; 13:107-112.
55. McGreevy PD, Carn VM: Intestinal torsion in a chinchilla (letter). Vet Rec 1988; 122:287.
56. Meingassner JG, Burtscher H: [Double infection of the brain with *Frenkelia* species and *Toxoplasma gondii* in *Chinchilla laniger*.] (German.) Vet Pathol 1977; 14:146-153.
57. Menchaca ES, Moras EV, Martin AM, et al: [Infectious diseases of the chinchilla: IV. *Pseudomonas aeruginosa*.] (Spanish.) Gaceta Veterinaria 1980; 42:96-102.
58. Misirlioglu D, Ozmen O, Cangul IT, et al: A case of rectum prolapsus and intestinal invagination in a male chinchilla. Veteriner Cerrahi Dergisi 2000; 6:51-53.
59. Moore RW, Greenlee HH: Enterotoxaemia in chinchillas. Lab Anim 1975; 9:153-154.
60. Morgan RV, Moore FM, Pearce LK, et al: Clinical and laboratory findings in small companion animals with lead poisoning: 347 cases (1977-1986). J Am Vet Med Assoc 1991; 199:93-97.
61. Morgan RV, Pearce LK, Moore FM, et al: Demographic data and treatment of small companion animals with lead poisoning: 347 cases (1977-1986). J Am Vet Med Assoc 1991; 199:98-102.
62. Mountain A: *Salmonella arizona* in a chinchilla [letter]. Vet Rec 1989; 125:25.
63. Newberne PM: Urinary calculus in a chinchilla. North Am Vet 1952; 33:334.
64. Newberne PM: An outbreak of bacterial gastro-enteritis in the South American chinchilla. North Am Vet 1953; 34:187-188, 191.
65. Newberne PM, Seibold HR: Malignant lymphoma in a chinchilla. Vet Med 1953; 48:428-429.
66. Nilsson O, Soderlind O: [*Listeria monocytogenes* isolated from animals in Sweden during 1958-1972.] (Swedish.) Nordisk Veterinaermedicin 1974; 26:248-255.
67. Nobel TA, Neumann F: Carcinoma of the liver in a nutria (*Myocaster coypus*) and a chinchilla (*Chinchilla laniger*). Refuah Veterinarith 1963; 20:161-162.
68. Novak S, Ruttkay D, Solar I: [Results of screening for bacterial diseases on large-scale chinchilla (*Chinchilla laniger*) farms.] (Slovakian.) Slovensky Veterinarsky Casopis 1994; 19:19-21.
69. Nowakowska M, Matras J, Bartoszcze M, et al: [*Clostridium perfringens* enterotoxaemia in chinchillas.] (Polish.) Medycyna Weterynaryjna 1991; 47:156-157.
70. Owens DR, Menges RW, Sprouse RF, et al: Naturally occurring histoplasmosis in the chinchilla (*Chinchilla laniger*). J Clin Microbiol 1975; 1:486-488.
71. Price DA, Juliff WF: Intramedullary fixation of the chinchilla tibia. J Am Vet Med Assoc 1957; 131:56.
72. Prior JE: Caesarian section in the chinchilla. Vet Rec 1986; 119:408.
73. Raevuori M, Harvey SM, Pickett MJ: *Yersinia enterocolitica*: experimental pathogenicity for chinchilla. Acta Vet Scand 1979; 20:82-91.
74. Rakich PM, Dubey JP, Contarino JK: Acute hepatic sarcocystosis in a chinchilla. J Vet Diagn Invest 1992; 4:484-486.

75. Rossoff IS: Handbook of Veterinary Drugs and Chemicals: A Compendium for Research and Clinical Use, 2nd ed. Taylorville, IL, Pharmatox Publishing, 1994.
76. Rouquette C, Berche P: The pathogenesis of infection by *Listeria monocytogenes*. Microbiologia 1996; 12:245-258.
77. Rübel GA, Isenbügel E, Wolvekamp P: Atlas of Diagnostic Radiology of Exotic Pets. Philadelphia, WB Saunders, 1991.
78. Sabocanec R, Culjak K, Ramadan K, et al: Incidence of listeriosis in farm chinchillas (*Chinchilla laniger*) in Croatia. Veterinarski Arhiv 2000; 70:159-167.
79. Sanford SE: Cerebrospinal nematodiasis caused by *Baylisascaris procyonis* in chinchillas. J Vet Diagn Invest 1991; 3:77-79.
80. Shalkop WT: *Listeria monocytogenes* isolated from chinchillas. J Am Vet Med Assoc 1950; 116:447-448.
81. Shaull EM: Fur quality and fur breakage in the chinchilla. Chinchilla World 1988; 37:9.
82. Shelton GC: Giardiasis in the chinchilla: II. Incidence of the disease and results of experimental infections. Am J Vet Res 1954; 15:75-78.
83. Shepherd RW, Boreham PF: Recent advances in the diagnosis and management of giardiasis. Scand J Gastroenterol Suppl 1989; 169:60-64.
84. Sims E: Caesarean section in a chinchilla [letter, comment]. Vet Rec 1990; 126:490.
85. Smith HC: Isolation of *Listeria monocytogenes* from chinchillas. Vet Med 1953; 48:294-295.
86. Spence S, Skae K: Urolithiasis in a chinchilla [letter]. Vet Rec 1995; 136:524.
87. Stephenson RS: Caesarean section in a chinchilla [letter]. Vet Rec 1990; 126:370.
88. Tvedten HW, Langham RF: Trophoblastic emboli in a chinchilla. J Am Vet Med Assoc 1974; 165:828-829.
89. Vanjonack WJ, Johnson HD: Relationship of thyroid and adrenal function to "fur-chewing" in the chinchilla. Comp Biochem Physiol A 1973; 45:115-120.
90. Vazquez-Boland JA, Gamallo JA, Ripio MT, et al: [Listeriosis in domestic animals: a short review of epidemiology, diagnosis and public health implications and description of prevalence in Spain] (Spanish). Medicina Veterinaria 1996; 13:333-344.
91. Weir BJ: Aspects of reproduction in chinchillas. J Reprod Fertil 1966; 12:410-411.
92. Weir BJ: Chinchilla. *In* Hafez ESE, ed. Reproduction and Breeding Techniques for Laboratory Animals. Philadelphia, Lea and Febiger, 1970, pp 209-323.
93. Wilkerson MJ, Melendy A, Stauber E: An outbreak of listeriosis in a breeding colony of chinchillas. J Vet Diagn Invest 1997; 9:320-323.
94. Williams CSF: Practical Guide to Laboratory Animals. St Louis, CV Mosby, 1976.
95. Wohlsein P, Thiele A, Fehr M, et al: Spontaneous human herpesvirus type 1 infection in a chinchilla (*Chinchilla laniger* f. dom.). Acta Neuropathol 2002; 104:674-678.
96. Wuthe HH, Aleksic S: *Yersinia enterocolitica* serovar 1, 2a, 3 biovar 3 in chinchillas. Zentralbl Bakteriol 1992; 277:403-405.
97. Yamagishi S, Watanabe Y, Tomura H, et al: [Septic infection of a companion chinchilla with *Salmonella enteritidis*.] (Japanese.) J Jpn Vet Med Assoc 1997; 50:345-348.
98. Yamini B, Raju NR: Gastroenteritis associated with a *Cryptosporidium* sp in a chinchilla. J Am Vet Med Assoc 1986; 189:1158-1159.

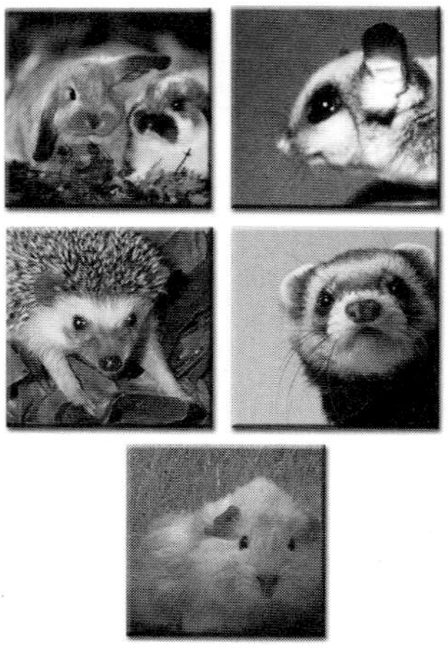

CHAPTER 26

Medical Management of Prairie Dogs

Richard S. Funk, MA, DVM

Until recently, prairie dogs were becoming increasingly popular as pets. However, because of the 2003 monkeypox zoonotic outbreak in the United States, the U.S. Department of Health and Human Services issued a nationwide ban on the sale of prairie dogs. Although they are arguably not suitable pets for most people, prairie dogs are nonetheless being presented to veterinarians for diagnosis and treatment of a variety of problems. This chapter reviews the basic biology of prairie dogs and discusses frequently encountered medical problems associated with their keeping. Prairie dogs are, of course, not dogs, but ground-dwelling and burrowing, diurnal, highly social squirrels. They are called prairie dogs because of their association with prairies and grasslands and because of their barking calls, which are somewhat reminiscent of small dogs.

BIOLOGY AND HUSBANDRY

Classification

Prairie dogs are members of the order Rodentia, whose dentition is characterized by four incisors that grow throughout life and a diastema between the incisors and the cheek teeth. They are in the family Sciuridae, which also contains squirrels, chipmunks, marmots, and woodchucks. Prairie dogs are generally classified into one genus, *Cynomys* (from the Greek, "a dog-like mouse"), with five species, as follows[12]:

1. *Cynomys ludovicianus*—Black-tailed prairie dog; occupies the Great Plains from southern Saskatchewan to northern Mexico
2. *Cynomys leucurus*—White-tailed prairie dog; occurs in Wyoming, Montana, Colorado, and Utah
3. *Cynomys parvidens*—Utah prairie dog; occurs in Utah; threatened U.S. Department of Interior (USDI)
4. *Cynomys gunnisoni*—Gunnison's prairie dog; occurs in New Mexico, Arizona, Utah, and Colorado
5. *Cynomys mexicanus*—Mexican prairie dog; occurs in northeastern Mexico; listed as "endangered" by both the USDI and the International Union for Conservation of Nature and Natural Resources (IUCN)

Virtually all of the prairie dogs in the pet trade today are black-tailed prairie dogs, and this chapter is based on that species, unless otherwise noted. The black-tailed prairie dogs seen as pets currently were legally captured as youngsters, mainly in Texas (R. Sands Jr., personal communication, 1999). Thousands of juveniles were collected each spring and supplied to a steadily increasing market both in the United States and abroad, including Japan. However, Japan recently banned the importation of prairie dogs because of the potential zoonotic diseases that they could carry. Prairie dog ownership is regulated in some areas; for example, they cannot be possessed as pets in Arizona. If properly cared for, prairie dogs may live for 8 to 10 years, although far too many fail to reach this potential, primarily because of husbandry-related problems. Books for prairie dog owners are available.[15,16]

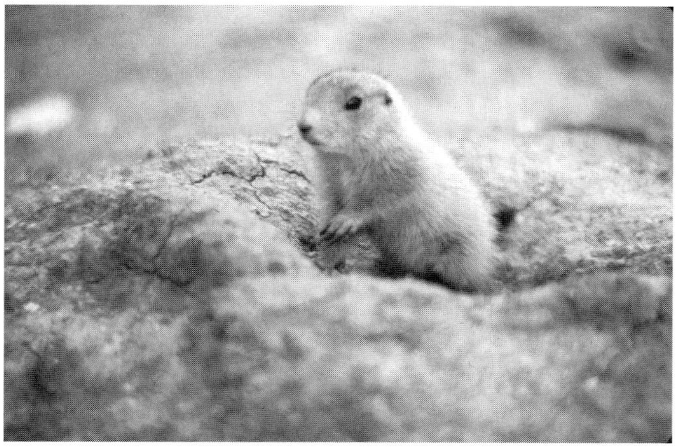

Figure 26-1 Prairie dogs are adapted to a terrestrial and burrowing mode of life. *(Courtesy Sunset zoo, Manhattan, Kansas).*

Anatomy

Prairie dogs (Fig. 26-1) are adapted to a terrestrial and burrowing mode of life. Black-tailed prairie dogs have a robust body and a stout head with tiny pinnae, relatively large eyes, and a neck scarcely narrower than the head. The tail is of medium length with a black terminal portion; hence these animals have been given the vernacular name of the "black-tailed" prairie dog. There are five digits on the rear feet and four on the front; each digit ends with a sharp nail. Fur coloration is pale to darker brown or tan, less frequently gray or reddish brown, and occasionally white. The color is lighter ventrally, and youngsters are paler than adults. The body length is about 12 to 16.5 inches with a 3- to 4-inch tail, and males are larger than females. The weight of wild-caught adults ranges from 0.7 to 1.4 kg, but obese captives can weigh up to 2.3 kg. The radius and ulna are separate, and the forearm is quite flexible about the elbow. The tibia and fibula are not fused. Prairie dogs are hindgut fermenters. The anal gland may be protruded as a triad of papillae; owners may refer to this as "the flower" (Fig. 26-2).

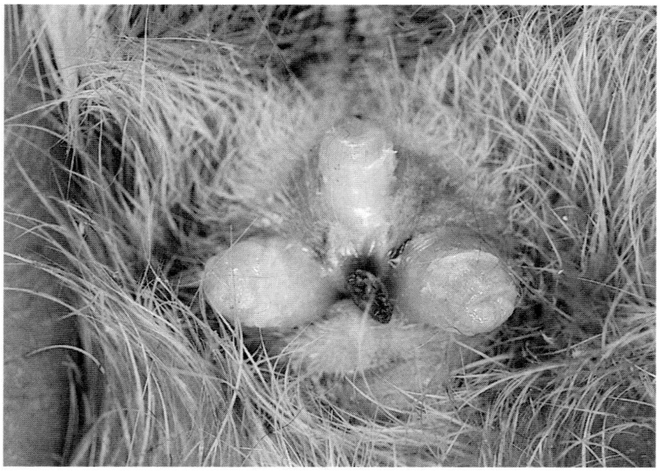

Figure 26-2 Anal glands of a male black-tailed prairie dog.

As is typical of rodents, prairie dogs possess four incisors, two in the upper jaw and two in the lower jaw. The incisors grow continuously and have no innervation. Prairie dogs lack canine teeth. The open-rooted cheek teeth are used for grinding. Cheek teeth have a series of ridges and cusps and are made mainly of soft dentin, with an outer harder enamel.[12] Malocclusion of the incisors can be caused by injury, disease, or diet. Individuals often grind their incisors together as normal behavior, and teeth are commonly broken when animals chew on the wire mesh or bars of cages.

Biology

Basic biological data are summarized in Table 26-1. Female prairie dogs are monoestrous and produce one litter annually, between April and June, beginning usually after 2 years of age. The females within a coterie exhibit synchronous breeding. During the breeding season, territorial defensiveness is heightened in both sexes. In my experience, females in heat tend to give off a peculiar, slightly sweet odor for 2 to 3 weeks, during which time the vulva may slightly enlarge. Gestation is 34 to 37 days, and the litter size is 2 to 10 pups, which are born naked and blind. Growth is rapid. The pups are furred and crawling by day 27, open their eyes between days 33 and 37, and are weaned by 49 days after birth. Pups may exit the burrows and begin foraging during the sixth week of life.

Pregnant and lactating females nest in isolated, grass-lined nests. They exhibit hostility to other prairie dogs during this time and typically seek out and kill the offspring of other females.[12] Some intact males become less tractable during the mating season, and others become extremely aggressive. It is rare for private owners to successfully breed prairie dogs; in captivity, a female that has been bred should be isolated from other prairie dogs until her brood is weaned.

Social Organization

The basic social unit of a prairie dog is termed a coterie.[12] Among black-tailed prairie dogs, a typical coterie consists of 8 to 10 animals with 1 adult male, 3 to 4 adult females, and several yearlings and juveniles. Females tend to stay within the coteries in which they were born and therefore are closely related to each other. Juvenile males typically disperse. Black-tailed prairie dogs

TABLE 26-1
Biological Data for Black-Tailed Prairie Dogs

Parameter	Range
Life span (yr)	8-10
Adult weight (kg)	0.7-2.3 (males heavier)
Body temperature	95.7°-102.3°F (35.3°-39.0°C)
Resting heart rate (beats/min)	83-318
Sexual maturity (yr)	2-3
Estrous cycle (wk)	2-3 (January through April)
Gestation (days)	34-37
Litter size (no. of pups)	2-10
Litters per year	1
Weaning age (wk)	6-7

Data from references 7, 10, 12, and 17.

may become dormant during the winter, but they do not truly hibernate.

In nature, the social organization of prairie dogs is intense and complex. The members of each coterie defend their burrow against outsiders. Many such coteries make up a prairie dog town, which can often spread over 10,000 acres. In the 1980s, South Dakota eliminated the largest remaining prairie dog town, which occupied 450,000 acres.[3] Historically, there were even larger towns. A wild prairie dog spends almost all of its time with other prairie dogs, a point to be kept in mind when dealing with solitary pets. The burrows are up to 34 m long and 5 m deep, and they are used by a wide variety of other animals, including vertebrates; prairie dog towns form the basis of a vanishing ecosystem.[10]

Vocalizations are quite complex, and a variety of sounds are used for different situations. Some researchers are investigating the calls of prairie dogs, which seem to communicate more information than we have yet deciphered.[10] Many owners recognize 6 to 10 distinctive vocalizations. Pets often greet their owners, and owners can learn to tell when the calls indicate excitement, irritation, aggression, and so on.

Being highly social animals, prairie dogs require frequent attention and interaction, and they welcome the company of their owners. Owners who let the novelty of their prairie dog wear off and stop interacting with it will see their pet become less tame and more prone to bite. A common complaint of prairie dog owners is that their 2- or 3-year-old pet is becoming more irascible. On questioning, these owners usually admit that they are now spending less time with their prairie dog.

Housing

Prairie dogs prefer temperatures of 68° to 72°F (20° to 22°C) and a relative humidity of 30% to 70%,[7,8] but they actually can do well at greater extremes. A prairie dog cage should allow plenty of room for normal activity and some exercise. Because prairie dogs do not climb well, climbing shelves and ladders are not recommended. Wood should not be used in the cage, because prairie dogs will chew it; in addition, wood cannot be adequately cleaned. Wire and stainless steel cages are usually adequate. Digging behavior will result in some bedding, hay, and food being flung or pushed out of the cage; a mat or tray underneath the cage to catch this material is advisable. An entirely enclosed, solid-sided cage restricts ventilation, leading to respiratory disease and problems with regulation of temperature and humidity; therefore, at least one side of the cage should be open and well ventilated. The cage should be escape-proof and free of hazards such as sharp edges or wire projections.

The floor of the cage can be either solid or wire. With appropriate bedding, solid-floored cages can be more esthetically pleasing, and deep bedding can provide the pet prairie dog with an opportunity to burrow. Wire mesh flooring is easier to maintain, but foot and hock injuries and infections are possible. If wire flooring is not frequently cleaned, it can become soiled with feces and can lead to pododermatitis.

Bedding materials should be clean, nontoxic, relatively dust-free, absorbent, and easily serviced; wood shavings, commercial pellets, and shredded or processed paper bedding products are suitable. Cedar shavings may be irritating or toxic. Sand and soil are generally unsuitable for a caged environment. A nest box or tunnel can provide some feeling of security by simulating a burrow system. Most prairie dogs cannot be trained to use a litter box.

Prairie dogs need a dry cool environment with good ventilation but without constant drafts. Avoid cold, damp sites (e.g., basements) and hot sites (e.g., next to a window). High traffic or noisy areas (e.g., next to a home entertainment center) should also be avoided. Pet prairie dogs are calmer when kept in a relatively stress-free environment. A regular photoperiod of 10 to 12 hours of light should be provided; if the ambient lighting is dim and decreases during the winter, the pet prairie dog may become sluggish or dormant if it also experiences a concomitant decrease in ambient temperature.

Clients who live in dry climates may keep their prairie dogs outdoors successfully if the enclosure is escape-proof, vermin-proof, vandal-proof, and hazard-proof, and if the prairie dog's desire to dig is taken into account. Areas with high rainfall and high humidity (e.g., Florida) may not be suitable for outdoor housing.

Nutrition

In nature, prairie dogs mainly graze on grasses. They also eat a variety of leaves, herbs, and flowering plants, occasionally some invertebrates, and rarely carrion. In captivity, prairie dogs generally get little exercise and are fed inappropriate diets, which often results in health problems. Obesity is almost the rule for captive prairie dogs older than 1 year of age. Diets that are high in fruits, nuts, raisins, carbohydrates, animal protein, dog food and treats, and table food predispose prairie dogs to obesity. Hepatic lipidosis and dental problems commonly accompany obesity.

Recommended diets for captive prairie dogs should take into account their natural diet. Grasses and timothy or mixed grass hay should be offered daily. Rabbit pellets can be given at 20 to 40 g/kg of body weight per day,[17] or a combination of rabbit pellets and rodent blocks can be fed at 15 to 30 g/day.[11] This amount should be reduced at maturity. A small amount of good-quality greens and vegetables can also be provided, as well as a very tiny amount of fruits and grains. As yet, no thorough research has documented the "best" diet for captive prairie dogs. Exercise should be given out of the cage on a daily basis, and clients should be encouraged to weigh their prairie dogs regularly. Fresh, clean water should always be available, preferably from a sipper tube that is cleaned regularly (prairie dogs may fill a water bowl with hay or food). Hospitalized prairie dogs may become inappetent because of the changes in environment and the food offered.

Handling and Restraint

The best procedure for picking up a tame prairie dog is to support the hind quarters with one hand, using the other hand to wrap around and support the chest. Scruffing is difficult because of the lack of loose neck skin, and prairie dogs usually resist this procedure. Even a tame prairie dog may not act very tame toward a veterinarian. A prairie dog that is not tame or is upset may bite or scratch with its sharp nails; in such cases, leather gloves or a towel may facilitate handling. Prairie dogs can inflict deep, painful bites. Two persons are often required to physically examine a prairie dog.

CLINICAL PATHOLOGY

For unanesthetized prairie dogs, small amounts of blood can be obtained from the cephalic or lateral saphenous veins.

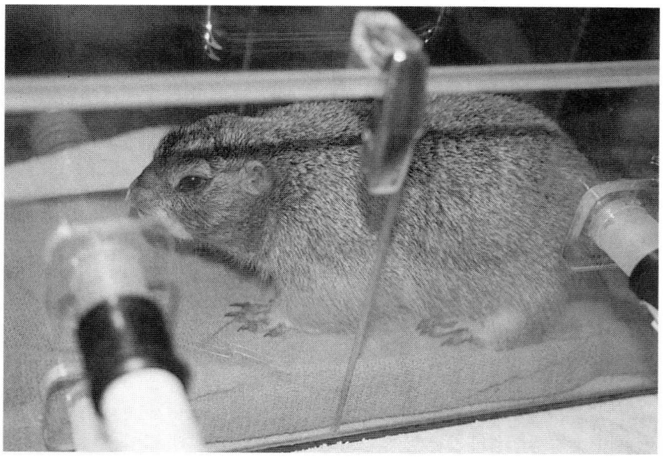

Figure 26-3 Anesthesia of a black-tailed prairie dog with isoflurane administered by chamber induction.

However, most prairie dogs resist restraint for venipuncture, and sedation facilitates this procedure. For larger samples, the jugular vein is the preferred venipuncture site. Table 26-2 lists normal hematologyic and blood biochemical values for the black-tailed prairie dog.

ANESTHESIA

Any sedated or anesthetized prairie dog should be placed on a heating pad and monitored for hypothermia. Obesity in a prairie dog complicates the response to injectable anesthetics. Use of a small chamber (Fig. 26-3) or face mask for induction, a mask for maintenance, a non-rebreathing circuit, and isoflurane anesthesia is preferred for all procedures requiring sedation or deeper anesthesia. Induction at 4% to 5% and maintenance at 1.75% to 2.5% isoflurane are usually satisfactory. Preanesthetic doses of glycopyrrolate (0.01 mg/kg IM, SC) or atropine (0.04 mg/kg IM, SC) may be given. Doses for injectable tranquilization or anesthetic agents are listed in Chapter 41. Analgesia may be provided with butorphanol (0.1-0.4 mg/kg IM, SC q8h) or ketoprofen (3-5 mg/kg IM, SC q12-24h).

SURGERY

Aside from castration and treatment for odontomas, there are no surgical procedures that are unique to prairie dogs. Procedures such as lacerations, abscesses, dental extractions, fracture repairs, biopsies, laparotomies, enterotomies, and amputations are managed in precisely the same fashion as in other rodents.

Reproductive surgeries are commonly requested. Although some reports suggest that such procedures performed at certain seasons (i.e., during fall and winter) may result in the patient's death, this information lacks merit. I have performed ovariohysterectomies and castrations during all months of the year without any adverse effects on the patients, and I have not observed any seasonal differences in their responses to anesthesia or surgery.[4] Surgical approaches for ovariohysterectomy, castration, and treatment of odontomas are described in Chapters 27 and 34.

TABLE 26-2
Normal Hematologic and Serum Biochemical Values in Captive Black-Tailed Prairie Dogs

Parameter*	Average	Range
Packed cell volume (%)	44	36-54
Red blood cell count ($\times 10^6/\mu L$)	7.7	5.9-9.4
Mean corpuscular conccentration (MHC) (pg)	21	18-24
Mean corpuscular hemoglobin concentration (MCHC) (g/dL)	35	32-39
Mean corpuscular volume (MCV) (fL)	59	54-71
Hemoglobin (g/dL)	16	13-20
White blood cell count ($\times 10^3/\mu L$)	5.5	1.9-10.1
Neutrophils ($\times 10^3/\mu L$)	3.8	0.9-7.1
Neutrophils (%)	69	43-87
Bands ($\times 10^3/\mu L$)	0	0
Lymphocytes ($\times 10^3/\mu L$)	1.4	0.3-3.5
Lymphocytes (%)	25	8-54
Monocytes ($\times 10^3/\mu L$)	0.2	0-0.7
Monocytes (%)	4	0-12
Eosinophils ($\times 10^3/\mu L$)	0.1	0-0.6
Eosinophils (%)	2	0-10
Basophils ($\times 10^3/\mu L$)	0.02	0-0.13
Basophils (%)	0.2	0-2
Alanine aminotransferase (ALT) (IU/L)	44	26-91
Alkaline phosphatase (IU/L)	47	25-64
Aspartate aminotransferase (AST) (IU/L)	25	16-53
Bilirubin, total (mg/dL)	0.2	0.1-0.3
Calcium (mg/dL)	9.7	8.3-10.8
Creatinine (mg/dL)	1.7	0.8-2.3
Fibrinogen (mg/dL)	273	100-600
Glucose (mg/dL)	157	120-209
Phosphorus (mg/dL)	7.6	3.6-10.0
Potassium (mEq/L)	4.6	4.0-5.7
Protein, total (g/dL)	7.0	5.8-8.1
Albumin (g/dL)	3.2	2.4-3.9
Sodium (mEq/L)	157	144-175
Solids, total (g/dL)	7.5	6.9-8.0
Urea nitrogen (mg/dL)	32	21-44

From Tell LA: Medical management of prairie dogs. Proc North Am Vet Conf 1995; 9:721-724.

*N = 30 for hematology counts; N = 29 for total protein; and N = 13-14 for total solids and the biochemical values.

PARASITIC DISEASES

Endoparasites

A coccidian protozoan, *Eimeria ludoviciani,* has been reported in the black-tailed prairie dog and oocysts may be identified in the feces.[14] Although some infected prairie dogs may have softer stools than normal, the animals are generally active and alert and often are just adjusting to their new diet in captivity. Coccidiosis can be treated with sulfadimethoxine in conjunction with good husbandry.

Trichomonads have been seen in several newly acquired prairie dogs, as well as in animals that have been in captivity for varying periods. In one pet shop (which also sold reptiles), most of the prairie dogs were found to have flagellates within 10 days after arrival at the store. Treatment with metronidazole (40 mg/kg PO q24h × 5-7 days) was successful at eliminating these infections. Water bowls must be changed during treatment. Giardiasis has been seen in a few captive prairie dogs; metronidazole is an effective treatment.

Tapeworms have been reported in wild prairie dogs, but only rarely in captive animals. Prairie dogs with tapeworm infestation can be treated with praziquantel (8 mg/kg IM, SC; repeat in 3 weeks).

The pulmonary mite, *Pneumocoptes penrosei,* was found in the lungs of a prairie dog that died acutely with bronchiectasis and emphysema.[1] Little is known about the incidence of infection with these mites; ivermectin has been suggested as a possible treatment.[1]

Nematode ova have only rarely been found in fecal examinations of recently captured prairie dogs. Prairie dogs with these parasites can be treated with anthelmintics, including pyrantel pamoate and fenbendazole (see Chapter 41). The raccoon ascarid, *Balisascaris procyonis,* was found in a research colony of prairie dogs housed temporarily in cages that previously had housed raccoons.[2] The affected prairie dogs exhibited neurologic signs including ataxia, head tilt, and stumbling. No treatment appears to be very effective against this potentially zoonotic infection (see Chapter 21).

Ectoparasites

Fleas are common on wild prairie dogs, but captured animals are usually treated with a malathion dip before entering the pet trade (R. Sands Jr., personal communication, 1999). Captive animals may acquire fleas either in a pet shop or in the home environment. Pyrethrin-based sprays and shampoos or fipronil applied topically have proved successful for flea control in captive prairie dogs. As with flea control in dogs and cats, environmental control is critical; both an adulticide and larval hormone regulators should be used. A concern with fleas in prairie dogs is the possibility of bubonic plague (see Bacterial Diseases). Ticks and lice also may be encountered on wild prairie dogs, but they are killed by the malathion dips. Ticks can be removed manually or killed with injectable ivermectin (0.2 mg/kg IM, SC). Pyrethrins and carbaryl will kill lice. The sucking louse, *Linognathoides cynomyis,* is host-specific for black-tailed prairie dogs. Several clinicians have encountered sarcoptiform mites in captive prairie dogs with alopecia, and treatment with ivermectin proved effective; these mites were not specifically identified. On two occasions, I have manually removed a bot fly larva (presumably *Cuterebra* species) from solitary skin lesions on the neck of black-tailed prairie dogs kept in outdoor cages in Florida by different owners; the wounds healed after manual removal of the bots and treatment with topical antibiotic ointment.

BACTERIAL DISEASES

Yersinia pestis, a gram-negative, nonmotile, pleomorphic bacillus that occurs as several strains of varying virulence and can produce endotoxins,[5] causes bubonic plague. This disease is enzootic in prairie dog towns and can kill prairie dogs; it is also an important zoonotic disease. A concern with recently captured prairie dogs is that any fleas infesting the animal at the time of capture could potentially carry the plague bacterium. Because fleas can harbor the plague bacterium for more than a year,[5] these parasites can serve both as vectors and as a means for perpetuation of the disease in nature. Ticks and lice can also harbor the plague bacterium.[1] Outbreaks of plague occasionally occur throughout the range of prairie dogs. Nonspecific signs of plague in prairie dogs include lethargy, anorexia, and death. Hepatic, splenic, or lymphatic lesions may be observed at necropsy, but diagnosis is based on laboratory cultures of the bacterial pathogen. The disease is reportable and quarantinable, and extreme caution should be used if such a diagnosis is suspected. Bubonic plague was unknown in the United States until 1900, and some researchers believe that it was introduced by shipborne rats and their fleas.

Yersinia pseudotuberculosis can cause yersiniosis in wild prairie dogs but has not yet been reported in pets. Transmission is usually fecal-oral, and nonspecific signs in infected prairie dogs may include lethargy, anorexia, and weight loss. Hepatic, splenic, or lymphatic lesions may be observed at necropsy. Treatment with chloramphenicol or tetracycline may be effective.[1]

Salmonellosis, characterized by diarrhea and listlessness, has occurred in captive prairie dogs. Some animals have become septic and died. Treatment consists of broad-spectrum antibiotics, fluid therapy, and gavage feeding, if indicated. *Salmonella* infection is potentially zoonotic.

Pasteurella multocida has been isolated from subcutaneous abscesses and from some prairie dogs with respiratory disease.[7] Abscesses should be surgically removed if possible. Abscesses also respond to lancing, draining, or curettage and flushing and to treatment with systemic antibiotics based on results from culture and sensitivity testing. If respiratory pasteurellosis is complicated by other factors such as obesity or dental disease, it may be refractory to treatment.

DERMATOLOGIC DISEASE

Dermatophytosis

There have been a few reports in prairie dogs of dermatophytosis (ringworm) caused by *Microsporum gypseum*[13] and *Trichophyton mentagrophytes.*[7] Affected animals exhibited alopecia, hyperpigmentation, and hyperkeratosis. Treatment consisted of bathing the animal with selenium sulfide shampoo (Selsun Blue, Chattem Consumer Products, Chattanooga, TN) or a combination of 2% miconazole shampoo (Miconazole Shampoo, EVSCO Pharmaceuticals, Buena, NJ) and selenium sulfide shampoo (q72h × 3 weeks). In addition, topical tolnaftate ointment (q24h × 2 weeks) and griseofulvin (Fulvicin-UF, Schering-Plough Animal Health Corp., Union, NJ) (250 mg/kg q24h, duration unspecified) are given on crushed carrots.

Necropsy data collected over several years from prairie dogs in a zoo indicated that dermatitis was present in 5 of 16 animals, and two prairie dogs had unidentified fungal mycelia in the skin.[6]

Barbering

Barbering (i.e., chewing of the hair by either a cagemate or the affected animal) can occur and can lead to pelage lesions. As in other rodents, a barbering site appears as if the hair were cut short *(mowed)* over the involved area; the underlying skin is usually normal. Treatment involves separating the pet from its cage mates, increasing the number and length of social interactions between the pet and its owner, and otherwise manipulating the environment. The differential diagnosis should include mites and dermatophytes.

Miscellaneous Skin Conditions

Skin abscesses and cellulitis can result from bite wounds[7] or other penetrating wounds (e.g., from exposed cage wiring). Unidentified nematodes were found in a prairie dog with dermatitis.[7] Fleas may contribute to a pruritic dermatitis. A commonly observed alopecia occurs on either side of the tip of the nose, and represents sites where the hair has been rubbed off as the prairie dog sticks its nose through the cage wire spaces. Pododermatitis associated with *Staphylococcus aureus* has also been reported in prairie dogs.[7]

RESPIRATORY DISEASE

Prairie dogs are frequently presented for evaluation and treatment of respiratory disease. Prairie dogs with respiratory disease may exhibit dyspnea, cyanosis, a nasal or ocular discharge, lethargy, and anorexia. Obesity, poor ventilation, high humidity, and a high dust content in the cage can all predispose prairie dogs to respiratory distress. In some cases, correction of the inappropriate environmental conditions resolves the problem. It may be difficult to determine whether an obese prairie dog actually has a respiratory infection or whether the signs are attributable to its obesity.

Infections with bacteria (including *Escherichia coli, Klebsiella, Pasteurella, Pseudomonas, Salmonella)*, mycoplasma, and fungi (*Aspergillus)* have been reported in prairie dogs with pneumonia. As yet, no bacterial or fungal respiratory pathogens peculiar to prairie dogs have been identified. Diagnostic regimens are similar to those used for other rodent species and may include radiography and tracheal washes (both performed with the animal under sedation). As in other rodents, treatment consists of appropriate antimicrobial agents, especially when determined by culture and sensitivity assays, and supportive care. Nebulization, bronchodilation with an appropriate agent, or use of an oxygen cage (being careful not to induce hyperthermia) may be helpful. Mycoplasma infections can be difficult to diagnose, but they may be responsive to fluoroquinolone therapy.

Prairie dogs with cardiomyopathy, intrathoracic masses, odontomas, or intraoral masses (see Dental Disease) may also be presented in respiratory distress. For example, a prairie dog that was examined for respiratory distress at our clinic had a piece of a plastic toy wedged horizontally between the posterior upper dental arcades; its removal resolved the clinical signs.

In general, prairie dogs with dyspnea have a relatively poor prognosis for long-term survival unless the problem is caught relatively early.

CARDIAC DISEASE

Dilated cardiomyopathy is frequently seen in captive prairie dogs older than 3 to 4 years of age.[8,9] Affected animals usually have dyspnea at presentation and may be inactive and inappetent. The condition may be mistaken for a primary respiratory disease. Diagnosis is based on radiographic findings (Fig. 26-4) and results of an echocardiogram. I have treated dilated car-

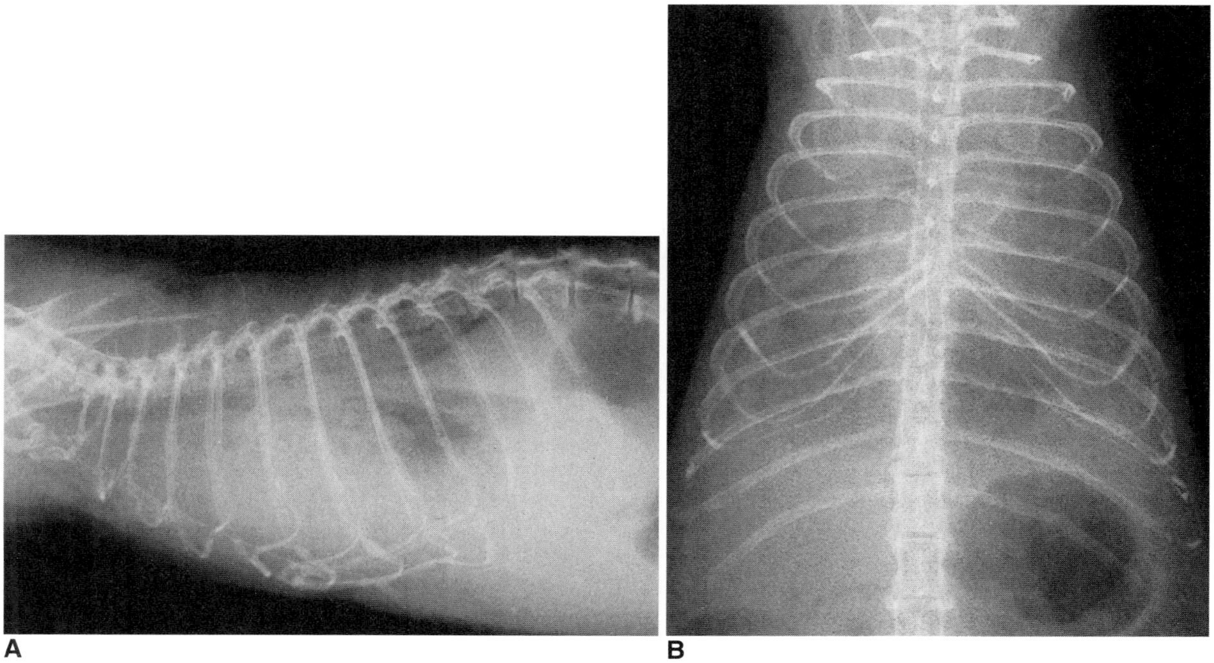

Figure 26-4 A, Lateral and B, ventrodorsal radiographs of an adult male black-tailed prairie dog with dilated cardiomyopathy; the fractional shortening was only 18%.

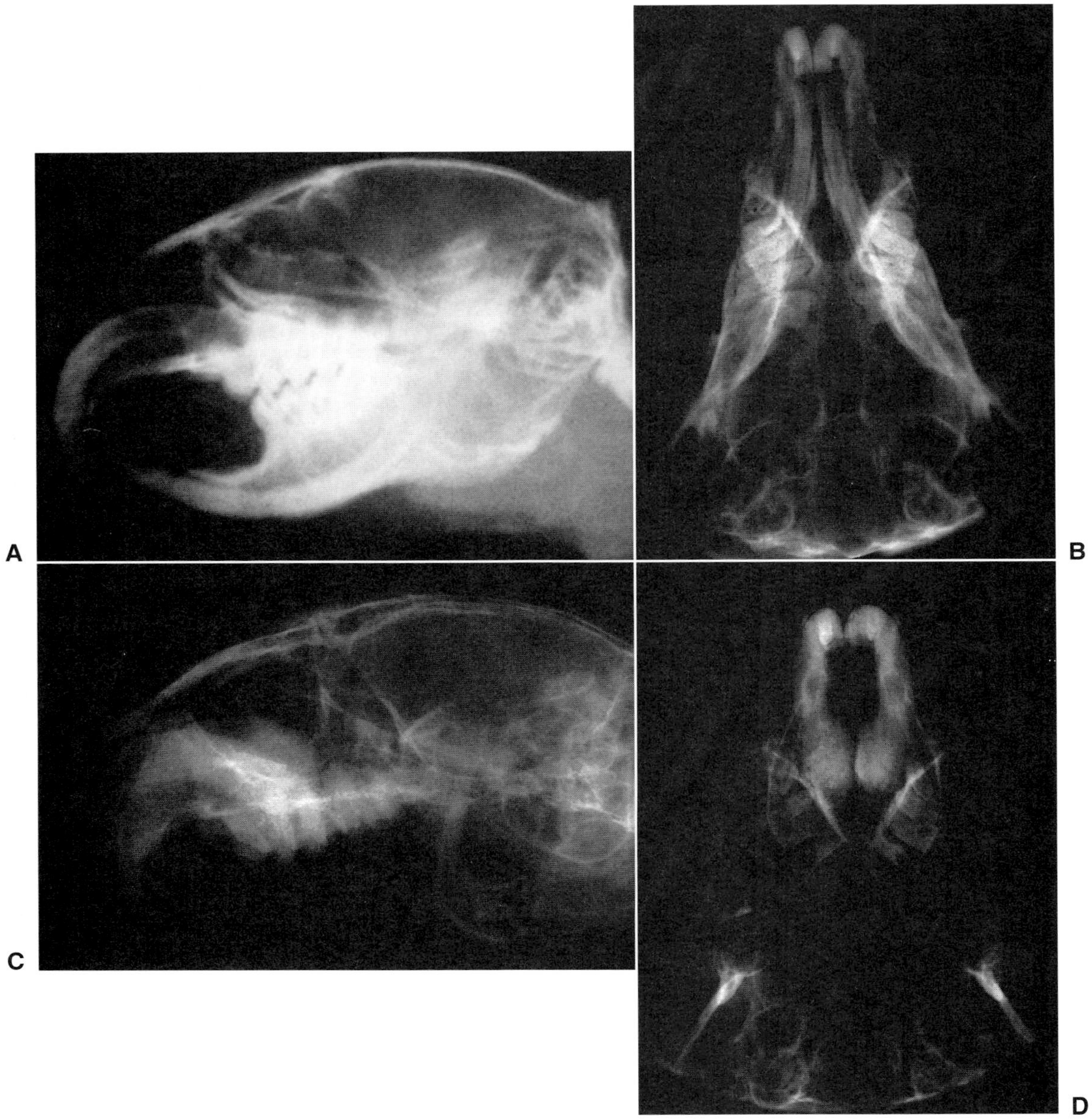

Figure 26-5 Skull radiographs of odontomas in a black-tailed prairie dog. **A**, Lateral and **B**, ventrodorsal views of a normal animal with uniform width of incisors in apical segments that are symmetrical and elongated. **C**, Lateral and **D**, ventrodorsal views of an animal with odontomas showing bilateral tumor causing bullous radiopacity and asymmetric enlargement in apical half of incisors. *(From Wagner RA, et al: Exotic DVM 1999; 1:7-10.)*

diomyopathy with enalapril maleate (compounded into a palatable suspension and administered PO q12h). However, the response to this therapy has been disappointing, partly because the condition is usually quite advanced when first diagnosed. A nutritional deficiency has been suspected to play a role, but this has not yet been confirmed.[8]

DENTAL DISEASE

Malocclusion may occur in either the incisors or the cheek teeth (see Chapter 34). Owners may see incisor malocclusion, but anorexia and hypersalivation are also clinical signs of malocclusion. Incisors may be damaged by trauma as in a fall, or by the prairie dog's constant chewing and rattling of the cage bars or wire. Cheek teeth malocclusions are more common in prairie dogs that are given a higher percentage of soft, low-fiber food than is recommended. As in other rodents and lagomorphs, clinical access to the cheek teeth is difficult even with sedation. Once the animal is sedated, the mouth can be opened to allow better visualization of the teeth and to facilitate filing, clipping, or grinding with a dental drill. Rabbit cheek spreaders, oral specula, and dental elevators work well with prairie dogs. As in other species, dental radiographs are essential for assessing the tooth roots and jaws. Maloccluded teeth that are trimmed need to be rechecked at 6- to 8-week intervals because malocclusions can be lifelong. If a dental drill is used, it should be operated at a low speed; higher velocities may actually worsen malocclusions by further damaging the open roots of the affected teeth. Untreated malocclusions can lead to malnutrition, starvation, and death. Abscessed teeth need to be extracted; the dental arcades then need to be monitored at least three to four times yearly for complications.

Odontomas appear to be relatively common in prairie dogs and may be associated with maloccluded incisors and nodular hard palate lesions.[18] Prairie dogs with odontomas exhibit dyspnea, open-mouthed breathing, incisor malocclusion, obstruction of nasal air flow, and occasionally nasal discharge. Radiographs reveal a bullous radiopacity in the apical half of the incisors with asymmetrical enlargement and encroachment of the roots on the midline (Fig. 26-5). In one study,[18] medical management with antibiotics, decongestants, and steroids was palliative; surgical extraction of the affected incisors resulted in incisor fracture and incomplete removal and failed to eliminate the clinical signs. Surgical placement of a hard plastic catheter via a rhinotomy site, coursing past the odontoma into the anterior nasopharynx, eliminated the respiratory signs. The cause of these odontomas is unknown, but it appears that constant incisor damage from the pet's behavior (e.g., repetitive cage wire rattling) contributes to the development of an odontoma. Nutritional factors may also play a role (see Chapter 34).

Dental problems can also result from traumatic tooth fractures, jaw fractures, and neoplasia of the oral cavity.

NEOPLASIA

Few neoplasms have been reported in prairie dogs. In one report, neoplasms were found in three captive males at necropsy; these tumors included a stomach adenocarcinoma with liver metastasis, a kidney adenocarcinoma, and an oral squamous cell carcinoma with kidney metastasis.[6] Adenocarcinoma of the stomach and adenoma of the kidney have also been found in wild prairie dogs.[17] Hepatocellular carcinomas have been reported in captive prairie dogs and resembled a similar disease in woodchucks, suggesting a viral etiology.[19]

FORMULARY

Chapter 41 contains a formulary for prairie dogs that is derived from the cited references and my own clinical experience. Prairie dogs are hindgut fermenters and have a gram-positive gastrointestinal flora. Therefore, it may be prudent to avoid certain antibiotics which in similar rodents can cause enterotoxemia, including the macrolides (erythromycin, tylosin, and spiramycin), the lincosamides (clindamycin and vancomycin), and perhaps the β-lactams (although published doses exist for amoxicillin). No thorough investigation of the pharmacologic effects of various medications in prairie dogs has been published.

Several veterinarians vaccinate prairie dogs against rabies using a killed vaccine, but this use is extralabel and raises a number of questions, including legal issues. Rabies has been reported rarely in wild prairie dogs, but I am unaware of its diagnosis in a pet. Vaccinations are not recommended.

ACKNOWLEDGMENTS

I thank R. Sands, Jr., for freely sharing information about prairie dogs and their capture for the pet trade; L. Philips, for much technical assistance in the clinic; and L. B. Funk, for her support of this project.

REFERENCES

1. Collins BR: Common diseases and medical management of rodents and lagomorphs. *In* Jacobson ER, Kollias GV Jr, eds. Contemporary Issues in Small Animal Practice: Exotic Animals. New York, Churchill Livingstone, 1988, pp 261-316.
2. Dixon D, Reinhard G, Kazacos K, et al: Cerebrospinal nematodiasis in prairie dogs from a research facility. J Am Vet Med Assoc 1988; 193:251-252.
3. Dold C: Making room for prairie dogs. Smithsonian 1998; 28:61-68.
4. Funk RS: Prairie dog reproductive surgeries. Proc North Am Vet Conf 2000; 14:1002.
5. Gasper PW, Watson RP: Plague and yersiniosis. *In* Williams ES, Barker IK, eds. Infectious Diseases of Wild Animals, 3rd ed. Ames, Iowa State University Press, 2001, pp 313-329.
6. Griner LA: Pathology of Zoo Animals. San Diego, Zoological Society of San Diego, 1983, pp 388-391.
7. Johnson-Delaney CA: Exotic Companion Medicine Handbook for Veterinarians. Lake Worth, Wingers Publishing, 1996, pp 17-23.
8. Lightfoot TL: Clinical examination of chinchillas, hedgehogs, prairie dogs, and sugar gliders. Vet Clin North Am Exotic Anim Pract 1999; 2:447-469.
9. Lightfoot TL: Therapeutics of African pygmy hedgehogs and prairie dogs. Vet Clin North Am Exotic Anim Pract 2000; 3:155-172.
10. Long ME: The vanishing prairie dog. Natl Geog 1998; 193:116-131.
11. Ness RD: Prairie dog tips. Proc North Am Vet Conf 1998; 12:851-852.
12. Nowak RM: Walker's Mammals of the World, 6th ed., Vol. 2. Baltimore, Johns Hopkins University Press, 1999, pp 1258-1260.
13. Porter SL: *Microsporum gypseum* infection in three Mexican prairie dogs. Vet Med 1979; 74:71.
14. Seville RS: *Eimeria* spp. from black- and white-tailed prairie dogs (*Cynomys ludovicianus* and *Cynomys leucurus*) in central and southeast Wyoming. J Parasitol 1997; 83:1.
15. Stoica K, Callis B, Watson L: Bringing a Prairie Dog Pup Into Your Home. Canton, Ohio, K. Stoica, 2001.
16. Storer P: Prairie Dog Pets. Columbus, TX, Country Storer Enterprises, 1995.
17. Tell LA: Medical management of prairie dogs. Proc North Am Vet Conf 1995; 9:721-724.
18. Wagner RA, Garman RH, Collins BM: Diagnosing odontomas in prairie dogs. Exotic DVM 1999; 1:7-10.
19. Woolf A, King J, Tennant B: Primary hepatocellular carcinoma in a black-tailed prairie dog, *Cynomys ludovicianus.* J Wildl Dis 1982; 18:517.

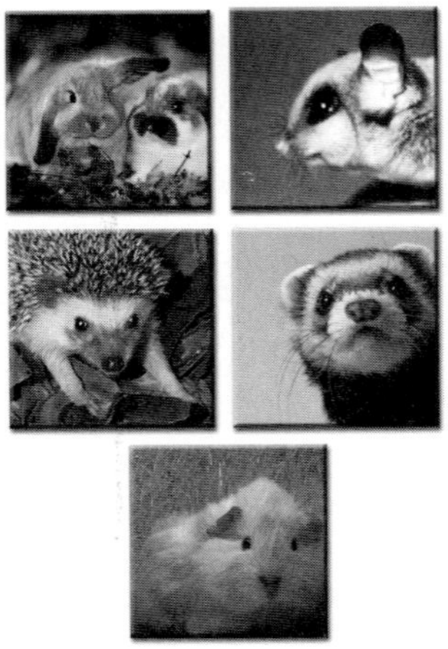

CHAPTER 27

Soft Tissue Surgery

R. Avery Bennett, DVM, MS, Diplomate ACVS, and Holly S. Mullen, DVM, Diplomate ACVS

Little information has been published on surgery in pet guinea pigs and even less on surgery in chinchillas. Both species are hystricomorph members of the order Rodentia and have similar biology, anatomy, physiology, disease susceptibility, and surgical conditions. In recent years, prairie dogs have been kept as companion animals. Prairie dogs are also rodents, but they are more closely related to squirrels (family Sciuridae) than to the hystricomorph rodents.

The natural history of rodents has a significant impact on their ability to survive surgical procedures. Rodents are shy and fearful prey species. With fear, pain, and stress, they lose the will to live and may die for no apparent reason. They may appear to recover from anesthesia and surgery, only to die at home 2 or 3 days later. This seems to be especially true of guinea pigs. It appears that the more human contact the pet is used to receiving, the better they bear the stresses of illness and surgery; those that are frequently held, played with, and coddled are more likely to survive than those that spend all their time in a cage. It is important to bear this fact in mind when discussing options and prognosis with owners.

Pet rodents that are stressed may stop eating to the point of starvation. Histricomorph rodents ferment cellulose in their cecum; if they become anorectic, life-threatening complications can occur. Some patients struggle violently, injuring themselves. Some become so frightened that their levels of circulating catecholamines become very high, which can negatively affect anesthesia, and some die acutely from these high levels of catecholamines. This concern underscores the need for appropriate preoperative and postoperative analgesic, antianxiety, and tranquilizing agents. If a patient seems to be stressed by the hospital environment and surgery is not urgent, it may be best to hospitalize the animal for a day or two, allowing it to acclimate to the new environment before surgery. In some cases, it may be best to perform multiple short procedures rather than several procedures with a long anesthetic time.

Because these herbivorous rodents eat frequently, a short fast of 1 to 2 hours is generally recommended, only to allow them to clear their mouth of food material. They are physiologically unable to vomit, so the risk of aspiration pneumonia is negligible. Because gastrointestinal function is vital to recovery, a long fast is not recommended. It has been shown that small mammals with a negative energy balance have a greater chance of having postoperative complications.[8]

Parenteral fluid administration is recommended for most procedures, as it is in other animals. Vascular access can be difficult to obtain in these small patients; however, obtaining vascular access through an intravenous catheter or an intraosseous cannula allows for the administration of fluids during anesthesia and also provides a means by which emergency drugs can be administered if necessary. If it is possible to maintain vascular access postoperatively, continue administering fluids at a maintenance level until the patient is eating and drinking normally.

The reported total blood volume of small mammals is 57 mL/kg body weight.[4,8] With loss of 15% to 20% of the total blood volume, most mammals experience hypovolemic shock and release high levels of catecholamines. Life-threatening consequences usually occur with loss of 20% to 30% of the total blood volume.[4,8] This would be equivalent to only 4.5 to 6.8 mL of blood in a 400-g guinea pig. Crystalloid, colloid, whole blood from a conspecific, or a blood substitute can be used in patients experiencing serious blood loss.

When selecting suture material for use in a pet rodent, keep in mind the propensity of these animals to develop a caseous, suppurative response to foreign materials such as sutures. Absorbable materials that are degraded by hydrolysis rather than proteolysis are recommended (e.g., polyglactin 910, polyglycolic acid, polydioxanone, poliglecaprone). Catgut is degraded by proteolysis and should not be used in rodents because of its reactive nature. Many surgeons recommend stainless steel for cutaneous sutures; however, this material is very stiff and the cut ends often cause serious irritation, actually stimulating rather than preventing self-mutilation. Soft, absorbable, braided materials (e.g., polyglycolic acid, polyglactin 910) are rapidly absorbed and are better tolerated than stiffer materials such as monofilament absorbable sutures (e.g., polydioxanone, poliglecaprone).

Many rodents chew out even steel skin sutures. Skin closure is best accomplished with an intradermal or subcuticular technique. This can be time-consuming if the surgeon is not adept. Skin staples are quickly applied, and most rodents will not bother them because there are no ends to poke and irritate the adjacent skin. Guinea pigs and chinchillas are less likely to bother surgical incisions than are other species of rodents; this is not the case with prairie dogs, however. If the patient demonstrates a tendency toward self-mutilation, midazolam (1-2 mg/kg IM, SC q4-6h) may help modulate the behavior, allowing appropriate recovery and healing. This treatment may be needed for only a day or two, until the patient becomes accustomed to having a surgical wound. Most patients that have proper postoperative analgesia do not bother their surgical wound initially, though they may begin to pay attention to it during later stages of healing if it becomes pruritic.

Small suture size and use of a small-gauge needle are also important. Suture sizes 4-0 to 7-0 are most commonly used in these species of pet rodents. Hemostatic clips are valuable for controlling hemorrhage, especially because of the small size of these patients and because the vessels are often in inaccessible locations.

Guinea pig skin is relatively thicker than that of chinchillas. Chinchilla skin is fragile and can easily be damaged during clipping for aseptic surgery. To help minimize the risk of tearing, flatten the skin in front of the clipper blade, move slowly over the skin, and frequently clean and lubricate the clipper blades. Tearing of the skin is not a significant problem in guinea pigs or prairie dogs. For skin preparation, a standard surgical scrub is recommended, alternating with warm saline solution–soaked gauze (instead of alcohol) to minimize evaporative cooling, because these species are prone to hypothermia. The soaked sponges can be warmed in a microwave before use, being careful not to overheat them.

Intraoperatively, monitor the patient's body temperature closely and provide supplemental heat with a circulating warm-water blanket, a forced warm-air blanket, a radiant heat lamp, or some combination of these.

GUINEA PIGS AND CHINCHILLAS

Ovariohysterectomy

Indications for ovariohysterectomy in hystricomorph and sciurimorph rodents include dystocia, uterine prolapse, pyometra, masses, and, potentially, behavior alteration. Ovariohysterectomy of young female rodents may decrease the incidence of mammary neoplasia; however, this has not been documented in hystricomorph rodents.

The ovaries are located caudolateral to the kidneys and are approximately 8 mm in length and 5 mm in width.[8,18] The uterus is bicornuate in rodents. The oviduct lies in close proximity to the dorsal aspect of the ovary, encircling it before joining the uterine horn.[14] The uterine horns join to form a uterine body, which is divided internally by a well-developed intercornual ligament. Caudally, the horns join to form a single cervical os. The mesovarium, mesometrium, and broad ligaments are sites of fat storage in guinea pigs and chinchillas, adding to the difficulty of the procedure.

Once the patient is anesthetized, clip the abdomen and prepare it for aseptic surgery. Place the patient in dorsal recumbency and drape appropriately. Make a 2- to 3-cm incision centered midway between the umbilicus and pubis. There is usually little subcutaneous tissue, and the linea alba is broad, making it easy to identify. Immediately dorsal (deep) to the body wall is the thin-walled cecum, and the bladder (also thin-walled) is just caudal to the cecum. It is vital to avoid iatrogenic injury to these structures, especially the cecum. Leakage of cecal contents can cause life-threatening complications. In addition, because the cecal wall is so thin, it is difficult to achieve adequate closure of a typhlotomy. Because of the potential for damage to these organs, a spay hook is not recommended for ovariohysterectomy in guinea pigs or chinchillas.

Locate the uterus between the bladder and the colon. Use a blunt instrument or a finger to move the cecum and bladder to the side on which the surgeon is standing, allowing visualization of the uterine horn on the opposite side. Grasp the uterus gently with forceps, and exteriorize it. Trace it cranially to locate the ovary on that side. The ovaries are supported by a short mesovarium that originates in the area of the caudal pole of the kidney. The mesovarium is short, and the ovaries are more difficult to exteriorize than in carnivores. It may be necessary to extend the incision cranially to avoid accidental tearing of the friable, fat-filled ovarian ligament. The broad ligaments also contain a large amount of fat, which can make identification of the ovarian vessels difficult. A single artery and vein run medial to each ovary and uterine horn.[3] Identify the vessels supplying the ovary within the mesovarium, and by using gentle blunt dissection, create an opening in the mesovarium to allow placement of two hemostatic clips or two ligatures of an absorbable synthetic suture. Transect the suspensory ligament, mesovarium, and vessels distal to the ligatures. It is important to remove the entire oviduct that encircles the ovary. Remnants of oviduct can develop into cystic masses within the abdomen.[8]

Repeat the procedure on the contralateral side, and bluntly dissect the broad ligament on each side to the level of the uterine body. Strip the broad ligament on each side caudally to the uterine vessels and uterine body. Ligate the vessels with the uterine body unless they appear particularly large, in which case ligate them separately. The uterus may be ligated with an encircling ligature or with a transfixation ligature. It has been recommended that the uterus be ligated cranial to the cervix to prevent spillage of urine into the abdomen when the uterus is transected.[8] The ovaries and uterus are removed as a unit.

Closure of the abdomen is routine. Use 4-0 monofilament absorbable suture for the linea alba and 5-0 absorbable suture for the subcutaneous/subcuticular closure. If necessary, use 4-0 or 5-0 nonabsorbable suture or skin staples to close the skin.

Pyometra

Pyometra is infrequently reported in guinea pigs and chinchillas.[19] Possible pathogens include *Escherichia coli*,

Corynebacterium pyogenes, and *Staphylococcus* and *Streptococcus* species. Affected animals are usually presented for vaginal discharge and may be lethargic and anorectic. Some guinea pig owners report polydipsia and decreased appetite. Radiographic and abdominal ultrasound examinations are valuable in obtaining a diagnosis and in ruling out dystocia and abdominal masses. Vaginal cytology, along with culture and sensitivity testing, confirms the tentative diagnosis.

Stabilize the patient and perform a complete blood cell count and plasma biochemical panel before surgery. Vascular access is required, because these patients are usually dehydrated and may have other metabolic abnormalities. It allows for administration of intravenous antibiotics. An appropriate antibiotic is administered after cultures are obtained intraoperatively.

Definitive treatment of pyometra is ovariohysterectomy, which is performed as soon as the patient is stable enough to undergo general anesthesia and surgery. Take care not to spill uterine contents into the abdomen during removal of the uterus. Irrigate the abdomen with warm saline solution before routine closure. Fluid therapy is continued postoperatively until the patient is eating and drinking normally. Recovery is usually uneventful.

Uterine Torsion

Uterine torsion is uncommon in most domestic pets but has been reported in gravid guinea pigs after 30 days of gestation and in gravid chinchillas.[19] Signs are the same as those for dystocia, but usually signs of circulatory shock and acute collapse are also present. The mortality rate is high, and the diagnosis is usually made at necropsy. This is an emergency situation. Stabilize the patient metabolically as much as possible before performing an emergency ovariohysterectomy. Vascular access and a minimum database are vital before surgery is performed.

Dystocia

Dystocia is relatively common in guinea pigs and chinchillas because of the relatively large size of the fetuses in these animals.[12,19] Guinea pigs should be bred before they are 6 months of age because bony fusion of the pubic symphysis occurs between 6 and 9 months of age and fat accumulates in the pelvic canal. If the pubic symphysis fuses before the first litter is delivered, dystocia results.[12] If a guinea pig delivers a litter before bony fusion of the pubic symphysis has occurred, cartilaginous fusion is preserved and future litters are possible without dystocia. Female guinea pigs are sexually mature at 28 to 35 days of age. Weaning typically occurs at 14 to 28 days of age.[5] In female chinchillas, fusion of the pubic symphysis is normal and does not cause dystocia. Male and female chinchillas reach sexual maturity at 4 to 12 months of age, much later than guinea pigs.[12] Chinchillas are seasonally polyestrous and age at puberty is a function of when they were born. Those born in the late summer do not reach maturity until the next fall breeding season.[7]

Gestation is approximately 59 to 72 days (usually 63 to 68 days) in guinea pigs and 111 days in chinchillas.[5,8] Average litter size is three to four in guinea pigs and chinchillas (range, one to six). In guinea pigs, approximately 10 days before parturition, the pubic symphysis begins to spread. Once the gap is 15 mm, parturition should occur within 48 hours[5]; at parturition, the symphysis is about 22 mm wide. This gap can be palpated externally and is a sign of impending parturition.[12] If the symphysis is open or if the sow has had a previous litter without intervention, and the sow has been in unproductive labor for longer than 30 to 60 minutes, give 0.5 to 1 U of oxytocin intramuscularly. If no young are delivered after 15 minutes, surgical intervention is considered necessary.[13]

Dystocia in guinea pigs and chinchillas can be surgically treated by either cesarean section or ovariohysterectomy of the intact gravid uterus. Cesarean section is performed to obtain viable fetuses or to preserve the reproductive viability of the sow for future breeding if the fetuses are not viable. For either procedure, make a routine ventral midline abdominal incision and exteriorize the gravid uterus. For a cesarean section, isolate the uterus with saline solution–moistened sponges, and make a transverse or longitudinal incision in the dorsal or ventral uterine body. A longitudinal, ventral incision is usually easiest. Deliver the neonates to an assistant, and close the incision with a single interrupted or continuous layer of 4-0 or 5-0 monofilament absorbable suture material. Irrigate the abdomen with warm saline solution before closing. If a cesarean section is performed to retrieve viable young but the sow will not be used for breeding in the future, ovariohysterectomy is performed routinely after removal of the fetuses, without closure of the hysterotomy incision. If the sow's pubic symphysis has fused, ovariohysterectomy should be performed.

Ovariohysterectomy of the intact gravid uterus can be performed to retrieve the offspring and prevent future pregnancy. The technique is similar to that used for routine ovariohysterectomy. After ligating and dividing the ovarian pedicles, clamp the uterine vessels and uterine body. Transect and remove the gravid uterus, passing it to an assistant. The assistant opens the uterus and removes and revives the neonates while the surgeon ligates the uterine vessels and uterine stump. It is often necessary to ligate the uterine vessels separately and transfix the uterus, because these structures are enlarged during pregnancy. Clamping of the uterine vessels occludes the blood supply to the fetuses, so the work must proceed quickly. The viability of the neonates is not affected by removing them with the uterus en bloc.

Contamination of the abdomen by uterine contents should be avoided. If the uterus is exceptionally large or engorged with blood and the sow is anemic, the en bloc technique is not recommended. If ovariohysterectomy is indicated, a cesarean section is performed first and the uterus is allowed to involute before removal so that some of the blood in the uterus returns to the patient's circulation. An intravenous or intramuscular dose of oxytocin speeds this process. Alternatively, oxytocin can be injected directly into a uterine artery, delivering the hormone directly to the involuting uterus.

Guinea pig and chinchilla young are precocious at birth. Their eyes are open, they ambulate well, and they can eat solid foods; however, they should be allowed to nurse as soon as the sow has recovered from anesthesia. Guinea pigs that are orphaned at less than 1 week of age have a high mortality rate, indicating they do need to have sow's milk.[5]

Uterine Prolapse

Uterine prolapse in guinea pigs and chinchillas is usually associated with parturition. In most cases, the sow has a tissue mass protruding from the vulva after delivery of young (Fig. 27-1). Most often, the owner discovers live young at the same

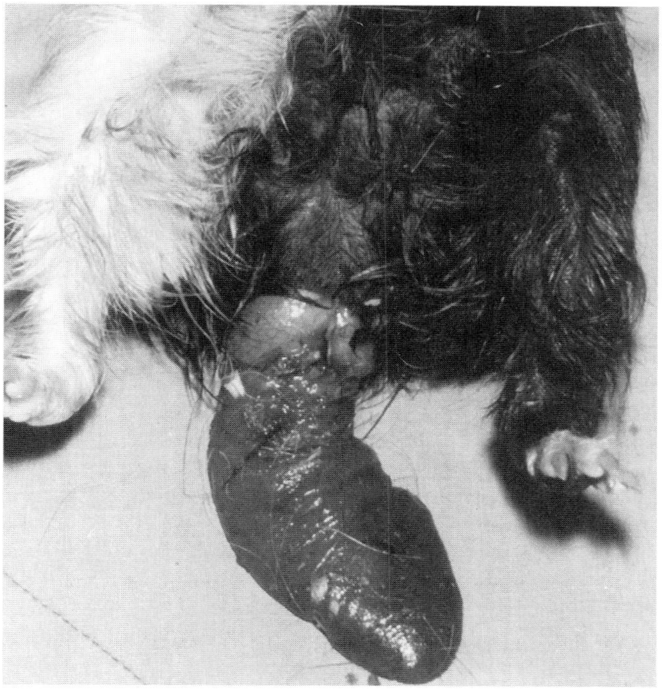

Figure 27-1 This guinea pig was presented for uterine prolapse the morning after farrowing. She was treated by ovariohysterectomy.

time the prolapse is noticed. The sow may be stable at presentation or may be debilitated, depending on how long the uterus has been prolapsed. The patient is stabilized medically before anesthesia is administered. Epidural anesthesia should be considered for patients that are not stable enough to undergo general anesthesia. With the patient under general anesthesia, clean and assess the prolapsed tissue. The prolapsed uterus is usually contaminated by the housing substrate. If it appears to be viable, reduce the prolapse. A concentrated sugar solution or 50% dextrose applied topically to the prolapsed tissue usually helps to reduce edema.

If the reproductive viability of the sow is to be preserved, make sure to reduce the prolapsed uterine horn into its proper location in the abdomen. If the horn is not replaced appropriately, it is likely to prolapse again after the retaining sutures are removed. An appropriately sized blunt probang is used to gently push the horn to approximately midabdomen. After the horn is reduced, monitor the sow closely for reprolapse. If this occurs, emergency ovariohysterectomy is indicated. Use of a pursestring suture is not recommended because the prolapsed uterus can remain in the vagina and cause urinary obstruction.

In most cases, ovariohysterectomy should be recommended. If the uterine tissue is not viable, ovariohysterectomy must be performed after the patient has been adequately stabilized. Prognosis depends on the stability of the patient at presentation. If the patient is alert and active, a fair to good prognosis is offered.

Mammary Gland Neoplasia

Mammary gland neoplasia is uncommon in older guinea pigs and is even more rare in animals younger than 3 years of age.[13] There are no published reports of mammary neoplasia in chinchillas, but one case has been diagnosed (D. Reavill, personal communication, 2003). Both male and female guinea pigs have mammary glands located inguinally as a single pair.[18] Chinchillas have two pairs of mammary glands. Neoplasias of the glands, both benign and malignant, have been reported to occur in guinea pigs of both sexes; about 70% are benign fibroadenomas, and 30% are mammary adenocarcinomas.[1] Liposarcoma, adenoma, papillary cystadenoma, and carcinosarcoma have also been reported.[16]

Because of the possibility of malignant neoplasia, do a preoperative biopsy or fine-needle aspiration and cytological examination of the mass. If the mass is malignant, metastasis may occur, making it important to stage the disease, by using radiographs and abdominal ultrasound findings, before surgery. Malignant tumors usually metastasize to regional lymph nodes, abdominal viscera, or lungs. If possible, biopsy or excise regional lymph nodes during surgical removal of malignant mammary tumors to stage the disease.

The left and right inguinal mammary glands do not have a common blood or lymphatic supply.[11] If a malignant mammary gland tumor is detected in one gland, mastectomy of that gland with removal and biopsy of the gland and its associated inguinal lymph node is recommended. Information regarding the incidence of bilateral disease or of a neoplasm developing in the second gland after one is excised is lacking; however, this appears to be uncommon based on clinical experience. Excision should include all mammary tissue on that side; however, plan carefully to allow for adequate closure because tissue is not abundant in this area. If the tumor is benign, be more conservative with the excision, leaving adequate skin and subcutaneous tissue for a simple, tension-free closure.

Make a fusiform incision around the affected gland, and dissect the gland and its associated deep, subcutaneous tissue. If the tumor is ulcerated or known to be malignant, the skin overlying it is also removed. Usually, there are several blood vessels in the subcutaneous tissue supplying the tumor that may be large and may need to be ligated. Bluntly dissect around the mass, ligating or clipping vessels as they are encountered. Use electrosurgical dissection and coagulation of vessels for tumor removal. Locate and ligate the caudal superficial epigastric artery and vein exiting the inguinal ring where they enter the tissue to be excised. Locate and remove the inguinal lymph node. Close the surgical defect in two layers. Close the subcutaneous tissue separate from the skin; this decreases tension on the skin edges, promoting proper healing. Drains are not usually needed, and "tacking" the skin to deeper structures is discouraged. Tacking seems to cause irritation and stimulates the patient to chew at the incision postoperatively. Close the skin with 4-0 or 5-0 nonabsorbable suture or skin staples.

If bilateral mammary tumors are present (these have been rare in our experience), two unilateral mastectomies are staged 2 to 4 weeks apart, allowing one side to heal and the skin to stretch before the other gland is removed. If staging is not possible and a bilateral mastectomy must be done, a rotation flap or advancement flap can be used to close the considerable defect. Use tension-relieving suture techniques such as walking sutures and far-near-near-far skin sutures to minimize tension on the incision and facilitate healing.

Castration

Castration is primarily used to control reproduction in guinea pigs and chinchillas. It is easier than performing an ovariohysterectomy and is associated with less morbidity and mortality. It may also be indicated to decrease aggression and for medical reasons (e.g., testicular tumor). If a boar guinea pig is to be housed with a female that has a fused pubic symphysis, castration is recommended to prevent the sow from getting pregnant, which would likely result in dystocia. The testicles of most rodents are comparatively large and descend during the first week or two of life.[3] This is not the case with prairie dogs. The inguinal canals remain open, and a functional cremaster muscle allows the testicles to migrate into and out of the abdominal cavity.[6] Hystricomorph rodents do not have a well-developed scrotum, and the testicles are located lateral to the penis in the inguinal region on each side (Figs. 27-2 and 27-3).

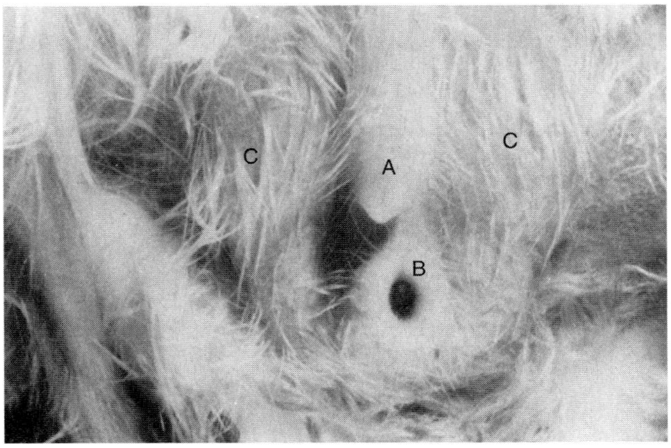

Figure 27-2 The genitalia of a male chinchilla. The penis *(A)* is directed caudally and almost touches the anus *(B)*, and the testicles *(C)* are located lateral to the penis.

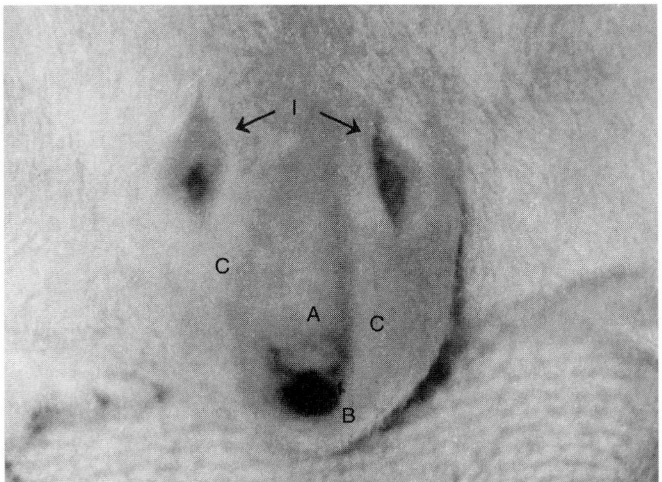

Figure 27-3 The genitalia of a male guinea pig. Incisions have been made in the location where they are made for castration. *A,* Penis; *B,* anus; *C,* testicles; *I,* incisions.

Rodents have a large epididymal fat pad within the vaginal tunic that helps prevent intestinal herniation. The large seminal vesicles also partially occlude the internal inguinal ring, preventing herniation. Most rodents have large fat bodies in the abdominal cavity on each side, through which the spermatic cord passes into the inguinal canal (Fig. 27-4).[14] Because of the anatomy, inguinal hernias are very rare in these rodents and visceral herniation after castration has not been reported. Although herniation frequently is reported as a major concern in castration of rodents, the concern may be only theoretical. In most mammals that have a large inguinal canal without these anatomic protective mechanisms, herniation of viscera into the scrotum is a significant concern. Some surgeons believe that guinea pigs are more likely to herniate their large seminal vesicles through the inguinal ring and recommend closure of the inguinal ring for that reason. One of us (H.S.M.) has observed this in one guinea pig, but there are no reports in the literature. It may not be necessary to close the inguinal canal during castration of rodents.

Castration of guinea pigs and chinchillas may be performed by a closed or an open technique. With the patient in dorsal recumbency, clip the fur around the scrotum, penis, and the inner thighs, and prepare the area for aseptic surgery. Three methods of castration are commonly used: closed, open with closure of the inguinal rings, and open with preservation of the epididymal fat pad. Because of the anatomy described earlier, it is not likely that the inguinal canal needs to be closed. One of us (R.A.B.) has used a standard open technique without any complications such as visceral herniation. If the surgeon is unsure, a closed technique requires the least amount of

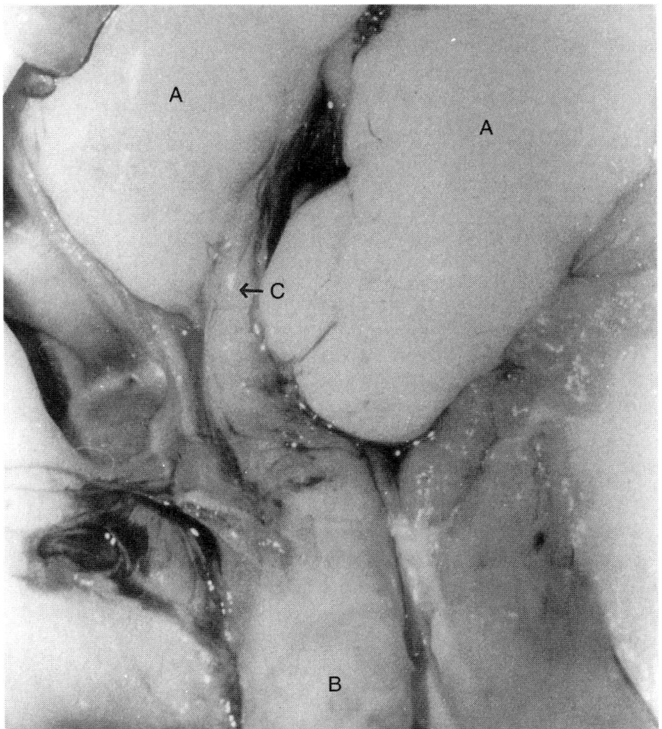

Figure 27-4 Large fat bodies *(A)* in the abdomen of rodents prevent visceral herniation into the scrotum but allow the testicles *(B)* to move into the abdomen. *C,* Spermatic cord.

exposure, and it is impossible for viscera to herniate into the scrotum because the tunic is tied off.

Palpate both testes, being careful not to confuse the body of the penis with a testicle. The penis can feel similar to a testicle under the skin, especially if one testicle is retracted into the abdomen. The testes are wider and rounder than the body of the penis, and the penis, which is located on the midline, cannot be pushed back into the abdomen as the testicles can. If one testicle is in the abdomen, gentle caudoventral pressure results in its return into the scrotum. For the closed technique, holding one testicle between the thumb and forefinger, make a 1.0- to 1.5-cm incision through the scrotum parallel to the penis on each side, about in the middle of the scrotum (see Fig. 27-3). The incision should not penetrate the tunica vaginalis.

Grasp the tunic and remove the testicle from the scrotum with the tunic intact. The tunic is tightly adhered to subcutaneous tissues. Carefully and gently dissect the tunic from its attachments circumferentially. The tunic is also tightly adhered to the end of the scrotum by the ligament of the tail of the epididymis. Break down this ligament to allow the testicle to be exteriorized. Once the testicle is removed from the scrotum, apply caudal traction to it and strip the fascial attachments, using a dry gauze sponge, until the narrow portion of the cord is exposed. Remember, you only need to remove the testicle; pulling the cord far out is of no added benefit and may damage the ipsilateral ureter. Be careful to avoid tearing the vaginal tunic during this dissection. Once the testicle has been exteriorized adequately, ligate the cord using a two- or three-clamp technique. Crushing the tissue with the clamps before placing the ligatures is helpful with the closed technique because the tissue cord is thicker since the vaginal tunic is incorporated. This ensures a more secure ligature, but it can also cause the tunic to tear. It is important that the goal is only to remove the testicle; the epididymal fat pad need not be removed, and leaving it in place may help prevent hernias. With the closed technique, herniation into the scrotum is not possible unless the ligature fails or the tunic tears; however, at least in theory, the intestine could pass into the inguinal canal until it is stopped by the ligature around the vaginal tunic.

A second technique commonly used includes open castration and closing of the inguinal ring to prevent inguinal hernia formation. Make the incisions as described previously, and incise the vaginal tunic to allow exteriorization of the testicle, the ductus deferens, their vascular supply, and the epididymal fat pad. Once the tunic is incised, the testicles are easily exteriorized because they are not attached to the internal (parietal) surface of the vaginal tunic. The ligament of the tail of the epididymis must be broken down to free the testicle from its caudal attachment to the vaginal tunic. With the open technique, the testicle can be exteriorized farther and the cord to be ligated is of a smaller diameter than with the closed technique. Double-ligate the spermatic cord proximal to the epididymal fat pad, and transect it distal to the ligatures. Remove the testicle and trace the vascular pedicle craniad until the inguinal canal, through which the cord passes, is identified. It may be necessary to extend the skin incision cranially to reach the inguinal ring. Place a single, interrupted suture across the inguinal canal, being careful not to damage or occlude the external pudendal artery and vein, which pass through the canal.

The third technique involves an open castration, being careful to remove only the testicle and leaving the epididymal fat pad intact to prevent visceral herniation. The procedure is the same as that described for an open technique, but only the testicle is removed; the entire epididymal fat pad is left in place. The vaginal tunic may be closed primarily or left unsutured. The theory is that the epididymal fat will prevent viscera from herniating into the scrotum.

Primary closure of the skin with an intradermal pattern is recommended. Guinea pigs and chinchillas seem particularly prone to the development of scrotal abscesses after castration. If this occurs, it is much more likely that visceral herniation will follow. The infection causes tissue necrosis in the area of the inguinal canal, widening the opening and allowing intestine to herniate. It is currently unknown why this occurs more commonly in histricomorph rodents. One theory is that the location of the incisions and the way the animal stands favor contamination of the incisions. Owners should be warned of this potential complication before surgery is performed. Aseptic technique must be strictly adhered to. Gentle tissue handling is critical, because traumatic manipulations can cause tissue necrosis and predispose to infection. Applying a layer of cyanoacrylate tissue adhesive over the incision may help prevent bacterial invasion from the bedding into the incision. Clean paper bedding is used until the incisions have healed (approximately 2 weeks). Perioperative or prophylactic antibiotic therapy should be considered as well.

Cystotomy

Cystic calculi are relatively common in guinea pigs and are the primary differential diagnosis for hematuria.[6] Clinical signs include hematuria, stranguria, dysuria, incontinence, anorexia, and pain. Urinary tract obstruction because of calculi is uncommon. Most commonly, urinary tract obstruction occurs in male guinea pigs because of plugs of sperm and seminal fluid.[18] If calculi cause obstruction, they should be removed. Calculi may lodge in the urethra, bladder, ureters, or renal pelves. Ureteral calculi are usually located at the caudal bend of a ureter as it enters the bladder. If a calculus is obstructing all or part of the ureteral lumen, it should be removed if possible. This requires magnification and microsurgery because of the small diameter of the ureter, even if it is dilated because of the obstruction. Perform an excretory urogram to assess the viability of the kidneys preoperatively. If the kidney on the affected side is nonfunctional or severely hydronephrotic, it may be necessary to perform a nephrectomy to remove the nidus for further urinary tract infection. In other species, end-stage kidneys have been associated with systemic hypertension.[15]

Make a ventral midline laparotomy approach just cranial to the pubis. Exteriorize the bladder, and examine the urinary tract carefully. Isolate the bladder with saline solution–moistened gauze sponges. If possible, place an indwelling urinary catheter in males with multiple small cystic calculi to prevent stones from migrating into the urethra during surgery. Often, a small (24-gauge) Teflon intravenous catheter can be passed into the penile urethra. Magnification is very helpful for this procedure. Make a 5- to 10-mm cystotomy incision along the ventral aspect of the bladder, beginning at the apex. A urachal diverticulum may be present at the apex. If so, it should be excised because it can harbor bacteria, predisposing to recurrent cystitis. Remove the stones and irrigate the bladder to make sure all stones are gone. Use a small intravenous catheter passed from the neck of the bladder into the urethra to confirm the patency of the urethra before closure.

Submit the calculi for stone analysis and culture and sensitivity testing.

If a distal ureteral stone is present, gently manipulate it toward the bladder and remove it through a cystotomy, if possible. Ureterotomy should not be done unless the surgeon is experienced in microsurgical techniques. Ureterotomy may be done if the ureter is sufficiently dilated by the presence of the obstructing calculus to allow primary ureteral closure with 7-0 or 8-0 absorbable suture. In our experience, the ureter is not usually dilated, and the calculus cannot usually be moved from its position in the ureter by gentle palpation. In such cases, the ureteral calculus is left within the ureter. If the kidney is not producing urine based on the excretory urogram, perform a nephrectomy. Unfortunately, if one kidney is removed and a calculus occurs in the other, the resulting obstruction may be fatal.

Before closing the cystotomy, trim about 1 mm of mucosa from one side of the cystotomy incision. Submit this section of bladder for culture. A positive mucosal culture confirms a bacterial cystitis. Close the cystotomy in a single-layer, simple interrupted pattern with a 4-0 or 5-0 monofilament absorbable material. Irrigate the abdomen with warm saline solution and close routinely. Appropriate antibiotic therapy is instituted initially with a safe, broad-spectrum antibiotic, which may be extended or changed based on the results of the culture and sensitivity testing. The patient is maintained on fluid therapy for 36 to 48 hours postoperatively. Hematuria may persist for several days postoperatively. Dietary management includes limiting access to alfalfa hay products and is discussed further in Chapters 13 and 15.

If the calculi are not causing urinary tract obstruction, surgery may not be necessary. The patient should be closely monitored for clinical signs that would indicate obstruction. Anemia is seen in guinea pigs with chronic hematuria due to urinary calculi. If anemia occurs, surgery is also indicated.

Not all of the factors that predispose individual rodents to the development of cystic calculi have been determined. It is difficult to cure this condition in guinea pigs, and recurrence is common.[3] Cultures of the bladder wall and the calculus should be obtained during the procedure to rule out bacterial cystitis as the cause of the calculi formation.

Cutaneous Dermal Masses

Skin and subcutaneous tumors are the second most frequently reported neoplasms in guinea pigs.[2,16] Frequently, they grow to a large size before the animal is presented for treatment. Most are benign trichofolliculomas, trichoepitheliomas, or sebaceous adenomas, all of which are typically cystic (Fig. 27-5). These cysts may contain sebum, hair, and keratin debris. They can grow quite large without causing clinical problems. Other neoplasms reported to occur in and under the skin include fibroma, fibrosarcoma, fibrolipoma, lipoma, sarcoma, and adenocarcinoma.[16] Aspiration of sebaceous debris from a cutaneous mass suggests the presence of one of the benign cystic neoplasms listed. If this type of sebaceous debris is not present cytologically, submit an aspirate or biopsy to determine the type of tumor present.

Excision of the mass and definitive biopsy are recommended, even if a benign cyst is suspected. Benign cystic masses can become infected. If surgery is delayed and the cyst becomes infected, the guinea pig will probably also be ill, complicating anesthesia and surgery. Guinea pigs have a moderate amount of loose skin over the dorsum, but excision of very large masses may require undermining adjacent skin to achieve closure or skin flaps, and creative closure of the defect may be necessary.

Cervical Lymphadenitis

Cervical lymphadenitis, a condition known as *lumps* in guinea pigs, is a streptococcal infection of the cervical lymph nodes. It is believed to occur secondary to oral mucous membrane trauma and usually results in lymph node abscessation (Fig. 27-6).[13] Isolate affected guinea pigs from other guinea pigs until the condition has resolved. The optimal treatment is complete surgical excision of any involved lymph nodes. Provide supportive care and antibiotic therapy based on the results of culture and sensitivity testing of samples taken at surgery. If the abscesses are small, this approach may result in a cure; however, even with total excision of all grossly infected tissue, the condition can recur shortly after surgery in adjacent tissues. It is important to perform surgery as early as possible, while the abscesses are small.

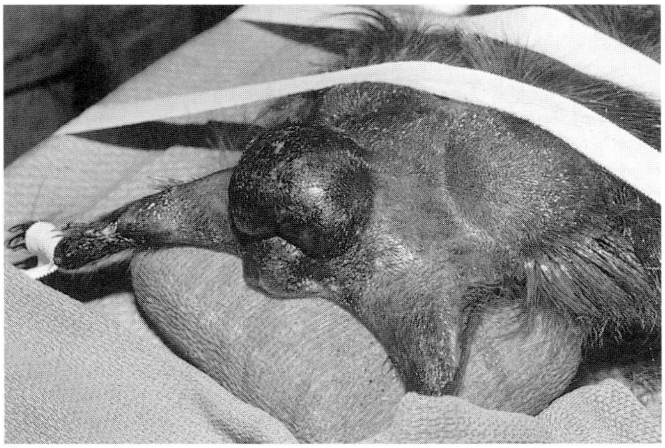
A

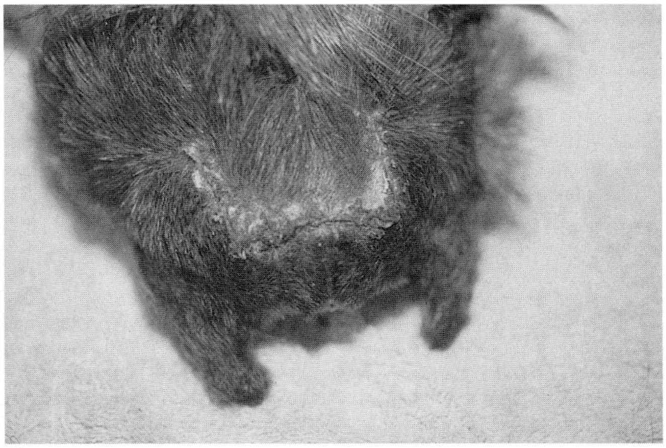
B

Figure 27-5 A, A large sebaceous cyst on the rump of a guinea pig positioned and prepared for surgical removal. **B,** The same guinea pig 2 weeks after surgery.

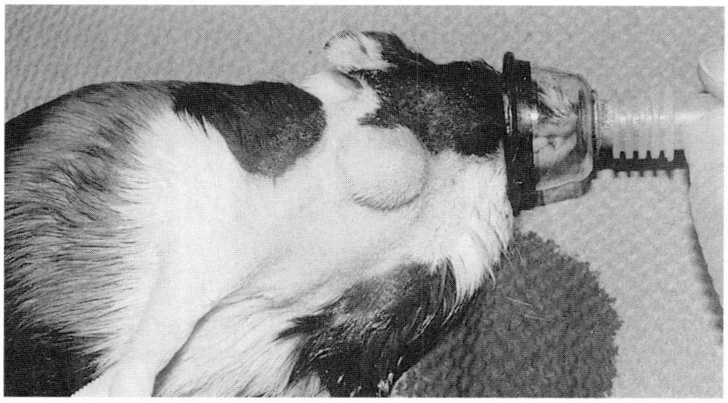

Figure 27-6 Cervical lymphadenitis in a guinea pig.

If excision is not possible, it has been recommended that the abscess be lanced, drained, and flushed, leaving the wound open for granulation. Wound irrigation and topical as well as systemic antibiotic therapy may resolve the abscesses; however, recurrence is very common. Persistent, nonhealing abscesses can be cauterized with silver nitrate.[11] The silver nitrate is caustic and kills bacteria within the cauterized tissue. Unfortunately, it also causes necrosis of healthy tissue.

More recently, antibiotic-impregnated polymethylmethacrylate (AIPMMA) beads have been used to control microscopic disease after excision of these abscesses. Excise the abscesses and place AIPMMA beads in the dead space created by tissue removal. Loosely pack the site with beads. Close the subcutaneous tissues and skin over the beads routinely. The beads release antibiotic into the local tissue for an extended period and do not need to be removed (see Chapter 34).

Thoracotomy

Thoracotomy is challenging in guinea pigs and chinchillas because endotracheal intubation is difficult. Various techniques for intubating guinea pigs have been described.[9,17] If thoracotomy is indicated and the patient cannot be intubated per os, a temporary tracheostomy can be performed to establish an airway, allowing for ventilation of the patient during surgery. Make a 1.0- to 1.5-cm skin incision on the ventral cervical midline. Bluntly dissect through the subcutaneous tissues and identify the sternocephalicus muscles. Separate these muscles along the midline, being careful not to damage the thyroid vein. Identify the trachea, and bluntly dissect the peritracheal tissues off the cartilage, preserving the recurrent laryngeal nerves. Place a 3-0 nylon suture around the cartilage ring cranial to the proposed tracheotomy site and another caudal to the proposed site. Tie these sutures to create a large loop of suture with long suture tails, which are used to pull the trachea to the surface, facilitating tracheostomy tube placement. Make a transverse incision in the trachea approximately one third of the diameter of the trachea. Insert a sterile endotracheal tube (1.5-2.0 mm) into the aborad segment of the trachea. After the procedure is completed and the patient is awake, remove the tracheostomy tube and allow the surgical site to heal by second intention.

The primary indications for thoracotomy in guinea pigs and chinchillas are pulmonary abscesses and neoplasms.[10] Pulmonary tumors are the most common neoplasm observed in guinea pigs.[16] Most are benign, bronchogenic, papillary adenomas, but alveolar and bronchogenic carcinomas are also reported. Most pulmonary tumors are slow growing, and clinical signs do not occur until late in the course of the disease.

If the mass is small enough, it can be removed through a lateral thoracotomy at the sixth to eighth intercostal space, depending on the location of the tumor. A standard approach is made. Magnification is very important for this type of procedure. The lung lobe containing the tumor is exteriorized, and the hilus is identified. The pulmonary artery and vein are identified, isolated, and double-ligated. The bronchus is closed with a transfixation ligature, and the lobe is removed by transection of the bronchus distal to the transfixation ligature and between the vascular ligatures. Alternatively, hemostatic clips can be used instead of ligatures. Closure is routine and includes placing a thoracostomy tube to maintain negative intrapleural pressure during recovery. A 3.5-Fr or 5-Fr red rubber catheter serves this purpose well. Once negative pressure has been maintained for 24 hours, remove the tube. The tube within the thoracic cavity stimulates production of 1 to 2 mL of effusion per kilogram body weight per day.

For large masses and cranial mediastinal masses, a median sternotomy is preferred. Place the patient in dorsal recumbency and do a ventral midline approach. The approach is analogous to that used for larger animals with one exception. Because the sternebrae are very narrow, it is not feasible to split them longitudinally. Instead, cut the ribs on one side at their attachments to the sternebrae. After removal of the mass, close with figure-of-eight sutures of monofilament absorbable material encircling the sternebrae at each rib. A second layer, apposing the muscles ventrally, provides additional stability. Subcutaneous tissues and skin are closed routinely. Place a chest tube to allow control of the pleural space postoperatively.

Pulmonary abscesses are also treated by pulmonary lobectomy; however, patients with abscesses are usually more systemically ill. Additionally, during manipulation of the lung lobe, purulent material can flow from the affected lobe into the bronchus and then into other lobes. These factors make the prognosis guarded to poor for guinea pigs and chinchillas with pulmonary abscesses undergoing surgical removal. Long-term antibiotic therapy can be considered as an alternative; however, because of the caseous nature of the pus, medical management often is not successful in resolving the infection.

Miscellaneous Procedures

Exploratory laparotomy for abdominal masses in guinea pigs and chinchillas is indicated for hepatic cysts or neoplasms, uterine neoplasms (Fig. 27-7), ovarian cysts or neoplasms, and gastrointestinal obstruction.

Ovarian cysts occur in middle-aged to older sows. Bilaterally symmetrical, nonpruritic alopecia along the back, flanks, and rump is often present and is usually the reason for presentation. A fluctuant abdominal mass may be palpable. Ultrasonography aids in differentiation of a cyst from an ovarian tumor. Administration of 100 IU (1000 USP units) of human chorionic gonadotropin administered intramuscularly in two doses given 2 weeks apart may temporarily resolve the clinical signs.[6] Ovariohysterectomy is the treatment of choice. It is helpful to drain the fluid from the cyst before the ovaries are removed.

Ovarian tumors, most commonly teratomas, occur in sows older than 3 years of age.[2] Some teratomas may be as large as 10 cm in diameter.[16] They are usually unilateral and rarely

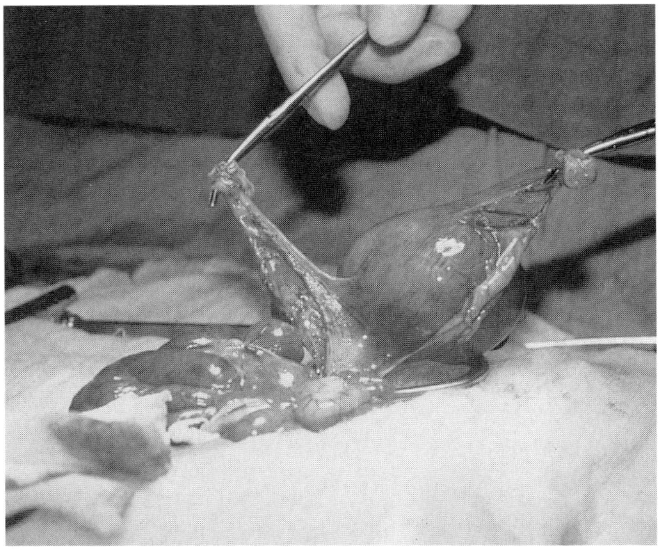

Figure 27-7 A right uterine horn leiomyoma in a 4-year-old guinea pig with a palpable abdominal mass.

metastasize. Affected sows present for depression, weakness, or collapse due to spontaneous intraabdominal hemorrhage from the tumor. Acute death from blood loss can occur. Ovariohysterectomy is the treatment of choice for sows with these tumors.

The etiology and management of pododermatitis are discussed in Chapters 19 and 20. These fibrous granulomas of the plantar surface of the feet are usually seen in guinea pigs kept on wire floors. The prognosis for cure is guarded. Many lesions recur after treatment. It is imperative to change the husbandry conditions. Surgery should not be attempted unless the owners are willing and able to house the patient on a soft bedding and can keep the bedding clean by changing it daily. This must be done for the rest of the animal's life. Aggressive excision of the lesions, followed by bandaging and open-wound management (allowing the surgical wounds to granulate and epithelialize), has met with some success. The patient is also given appropriate systemic antibiotic therapy.

Alternatively, debridement and placement of AIPMMA beads has resulted in a cure in some cases. Debride the infected areas of purulent material and infected tissue. Place small AIPMMA beads in the defect, and suture the skin together over the beads, across the defect, to hold them in place. Pad and bandage the feet. Change the bandages every day initially and then every 2 to 3 days. One of us (R.A.B.) has left beads in the feet permanently, and they have not appeared to cause lameness.

PRAIRIE DOGS

Black-tailed prairie dogs (*Cynomys ludovicianus*) belong to the order Rodentia and the family Sciuridae (squirrel-like rodents). Surgery in prairie dogs is analogous to that performed in other species of rodents. When presented with a unique situation requiring surgery in a prairie dog, the surgeon should rely on experiences with other rodents and other mammals to extrapolate for prairie dogs. There are some unique characteristics of performing ovariohysterectomy and castration in prairie dogs that are reviewed here.

Prairie dogs hibernate in the winter. In the fall, they eat more and accumulate fat, on which they survive during their hibernation. Because this excess fat accumulation can make spaying and castration more challenging, it is often recommended that these procedures be performed in the spring, when there is potentially less fat. However, obesity is a serious problem in captive prairie dogs regardless of the season. Young prairie dogs are less likely to be obese. Therefore the ideal time to castrate or spay a prairie dog is in the spring of its first year of life. These procedures can be performed at any age or any season, recognizing that fat accumulation may make surgery more challenging.

Another consideration in castration of prairie dogs is the late age at which the testicles descend. Spring is the breeding season for prairie dogs. In mature prairie dogs, in breeding season, the testicles are easily identified in the scrotum, lateral to the penis. However, in immature prairie dogs they are located in the abdomen. As in other species, it is generally recommended that prairie dogs be castrated before puberty to prevent the development of aggressive behaviors. It is likely that castration of adults will also reduce their aggressive behaviors.

Ovariohysterectomy

Female prairie dogs, like other rodents, store fat in the mesovarium and mesometrium. This makes ovariohysterectomy somewhat more challenging. They also have a large cecum, which can be damaged iatrogenically during efforts to locate the uterus. In obese immature females, the uterus is quite small and embedded in fat, making it difficult to locate. Until the practitioner is familiar with the procedure, it is recommended that adequate exposure be obtained by making a somewhat large incision. Once the technique has been perfected, smaller initial incisions can be used.

Make an incision from just caudal to the umbilicus to just cranial to the pubis. Because many prairie dogs are obese, there is usually a thick layer of subcutaneous fat that must be incised to allow the linea alba to be identified. Incise the linea alba with a standard technique, being careful not to damage the underlying cecum. In many cases, the fat in the mesometrium displaces the uterus toward midline, making it easy to identify. Use only a blunt instrument or a finger to identify and exteriorize the uterus to avoid iatrogenic damage to the cecum. Keep in mind that, especially in young animals, the uterus will be only a thin tubular tissue along the edge of the fat-filled mesometrium.

Depending on the amount of fat, it may be difficult to identify the ovarian vessels. Gently crush the fat dorsal to the ovary between the thumb and first finger. This will break away the fat but not tear the vessels, allowing them to be more accurately identified. Double-ligate or clip the ovarian vessels and transect them to free up the ovary. The vessels within the fat of the mesometrium are usually small. Break down the mesometrium in a cranial-to-caudal direction, using blunt dissection, until the entire horn is exteriorized and the uterine body is identified. Trace along the uterine body cranially to the opposite side until the other ovary is located. Repeat the procedure to allow excision of the contralateral ovary and uterine horn. Ligate the uterine body using a standard technique. Close the body wall with 4-0 monofilament absorbable suture and the subcutaneous tissue with a soft, braided absorbable material. Subcuticular

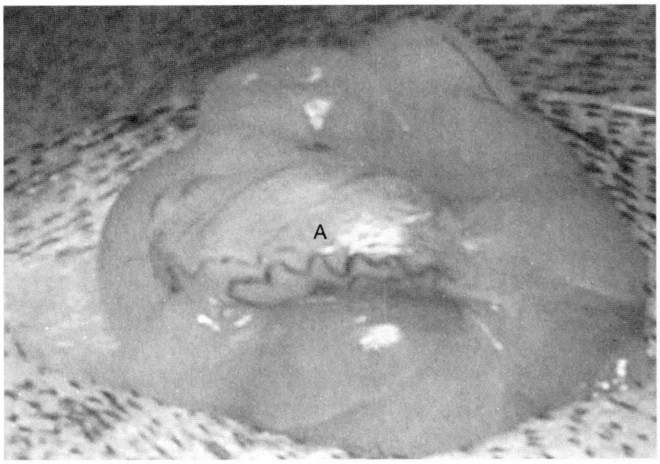

Figure 27-8 When the abdominal approach is used for castration of prairie dogs, the fat that is easily exteriorized usually contains the testicle. *A*, Testicle.

closure is preferred because prairie dogs are likely to chew out even skin staples.

Castration

In mature males, the testicles are easily palpated in the scrotum. The anatomy is very similar to that of guinea pigs and chinchillas, with the scrotal sacs located bilaterally and adjacent to the penis. Castration in adults is analogous to that described for guinea pigs and chinchillas.

In immature males, the testicles are located within the abdomen. An abdominal approach is recommended. This approach can be used for any rodent or rabbit because the inguinal canal is large enough that the testicles can be brought into the abdomen for removal. The vasa deferentia lay in a position analogous to that of the uterus in females—dorsal to the neck of the bladder (similar to where the uterine body would be located)—and extend laterally to the testicles.

Make a 3-cm ventral midline incision in the caudal abdomen approximately 1 to 2 cm cranial to the prepuce. Be sure to avoid the cranial flexure of the penis. Dissect through the subcutaneous fat, which may be abundant depending on the prairie dog's nutritional status, and identify the body wall. The linea alba is difficult to identify in the caudal abdomen. Make a midline body wall incision to enter the abdominal cavity. The vas deferens is located along the abdominal fat body on each side. Insert a forceps or hemostat into the abdominal cavity and retrieve either the vas deferens or the fat body. If you retrieve the fat, the testicle will usually come out with it (Fig. 27-8). Pull on the vas deferens to exteriorize the testicle. If fat is exteriorized and the testicle is not found, replace the fat and repeat the procedure until the testicle is exteriorized.

The testicle has two attachments. At the caudal aspect, the gubernaculum testis is adhered to the epididymis and must be broken down. The gubernaculum, which becomes the ligament of the tail of the epididymis, can be clamped and torn off the epididymis, or it can be ligated and transected, freeing the caudal aspect of the testicle. The cranial attachment is the testicular artery and vein. Identify these vessels and ligate them by using a two- or three-clamp technique. Transect the vessels and remove

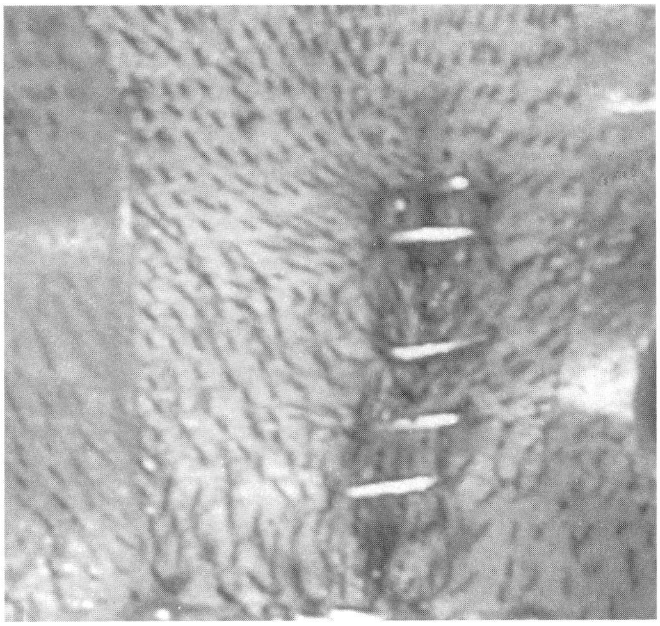

Figure 27-9 The abdominal incision for castration of prairie dogs is made just cranial to the pubis. It can be closed with skin staples.

the testicle. Repeat the procedure on the other side. Close the body wall with 4-0 monofilament absorbable suture. Close the subcutaneous fat and skin routinely. Soft, braided absorbable suture is preferred for the fat and intradermal closure. Alternatively, skin staples can be used (Fig. 27-9).

REFERENCES

1. Collins BR: Common disease and medical management of rodents and lagomorphs. *In* Jacobson ER, Kollias GV, eds. Exotic Animals. New York, Churchill Livingstone, 1988, pp 261-316.
2. Cooper JE: Tips on tumors. Proc North Am Vet Conf 1994; pp 897-898.
3. Harkness JE: A Practitioners Guide to Domestic Rodents. Denver, American Animal Hospital Association, 1993.
4. Harkness JE, Wagner JE: Biology and Medicine of Rabbits and Rodents, 3rd ed. Philadelphia, Lea & Febiger, 1989, p 62.
5. Harkness JE, Wagner JE: Biology and Medicine of Rabbits and Rodents, 3rd ed. Philadelphia, Lea & Febiger, 1989, pp 161-166.
6. Hillyer EV: Common clinical maladies of pet rodents. Proc North Am Vet Conf 1994; pp 909-910.
7. Hoeffer HL: Chinchillas. Vet Clin North Am Small Anim Pract 1994; 24:103-111.
8. Jenkins JR: Surgical sterilization in small mammals, spay and castration. Vet Clin North Am Exotic Anim Pract 2000; 3:617-645.
9. Kramer K, Grimbergen JA, van Iperen DJ, et al: Oral endotracheal intubation of guinea pigs. Lab Anim 1998; 32:162-164.
10. Mullen HS: Section Three: Guinea pigs and chinchillas. Soft tissue surgery. *In* Hillyer EV, Quesenberry KE, eds. Ferrets, Rabbits, and Rodents: Clinical Medicine and Surgery. Philadelphia, WB Saunders, 1997, pp 329-336.
11. Mullen HS: Nonreproductive surgery in small mammals. Vet Clin North Am Exotic Anim Pract 2000; 3:629-645.
12. Peters LJ: The guinea pig: an overview. Part I. Compend Contin Educ Pract Vet 1991; 4:15-19.
13. Peters LJ: The guinea pig: an overview. Part II. Compend Contin Educ Pract Vet 1991; 5:20-27.

14. Popesko P, Rajtova V, Horak J: Atlas of the Anatomy of Small Laboratory Animals, Vol. 1. Rabbit and Guinea Pig. London, Wolfe Publishing, 1992, pp 148-240.
15. Syme HM, Barber PJ, Markwell PJ, et al: Prevalence of systolic hypertension in cats with chronic renal failure at initial evaluation. J Am Vet Med Assoc 2002; 220:1799-1804.
16. Toft JD: Commonly observed spontaneous neoplasms in rabbits, rats, guinea pigs, hamsters and gerbils. Semin Avian Exotic Pet Med 1991; 1:80-92.
17. Turner MA, Thomas P, Sheridan DJ: An improved method for direct laryngeal intubation in the guinea pig. Lab Anim 1992; 26:25-28.
18. Wagner JE, Manning PJ: The Biology of the Guinea Pig. New York, Academic Press, 1976.
19. Wallach JD, Boever WJ: Diseases of Exotic Animals: Medical and Surgical Management. Philadelphia, WB Saunders, 1983.

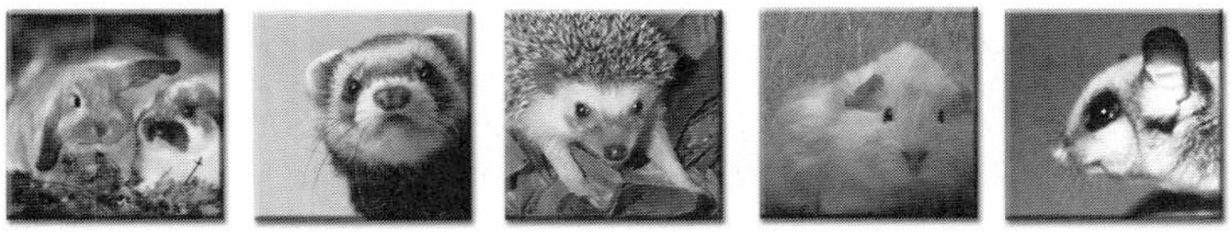

SECTION FOUR

SMALL RODENTS

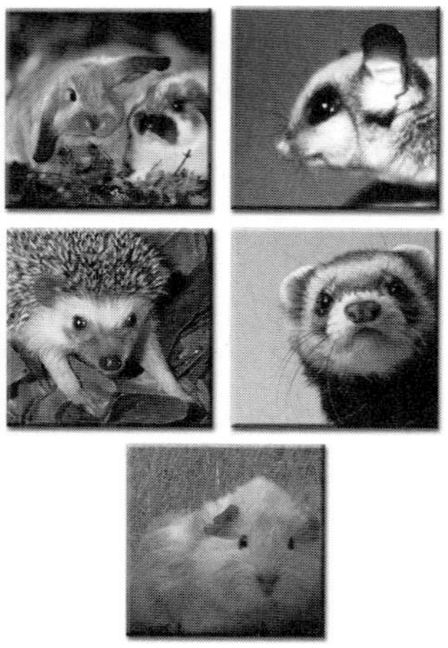

CHAPTER 28

Basic Anatomy, Physiology, Husbandry, and Clinical Techniques

Craig Bihun, DVM, DVSc, and Louise Bauck, DVM, MVSc

The traditional small pet rodents such as the golden hamster (*Mesocricetus auratus*), the white mouse (*Mus musculus*), the gerbil (*Meriones unguiculatus*), and the rat (*Rattus norvegicus*) all continue to remain popular but have been supplemented by color and coat varieties not formerly available and by species such as the Siberian or dwarf hamster (*Phodopus sungorus*) (Fig. 28-1), the Chinese hamster (*Cricetus griseus*), the spiny mouse (*Heteromys* species), the spiny rat (*Proechimys* species), the degu (*Octodon* species), the chinchilla (*Chinchilla laniger*), the jerboa (*Jaculus jaculus*), and the African pygmy mouse (*Baiomys* species). Although very little specific husbandry and medical information about the newly introduced exotic species is available, nutritional requirements and husbandry details are similar for many of these small rodents. Degus and chinchillas are actually hystricomorph rodents related to guinea pigs. Spiny rats and mice have a buff-colored coat with a coarse or spiny appearance, are medium-sized (150-200 g), and are characterized by large, attractive ears. Pygmy mice are among the smallest of mammals (each weighing approximately 10 g). They have a rich brown dorsal surface and white abdomen. They scamper very quickly and for this reason are difficult to catch and handle.

GENERAL CHARACTERISTICS

Gerbils

Gerbils are excellent pets for older children. They tend to scamper and may slough their tail skin if picked up incorrectly; therefore, they are unsuitable for most children younger than 10 years of age. They are more active than hamsters, and their agility in climbing and burrowing makes providing living quarters for them interesting. They are usually gentle when handled correctly. Gerbils are available in white, black, buff, gray, and spotted varieties. Gerbils are territorial in nature and are best kept singly (cannibalism can result from attempting to keep incompatible pairs or males together). Gerbils are more disease resistant than hamsters, although older gerbils may develop a variety of neoplastic and degenerative conditions. Epilepsy has been reported in gerbils but is uncommon in many pet strains.

Hamsters

The most common hamster kept as a pet is the golden hamster. Hamsters are the least hardy of the small rodents when newly purchased, and stress-related diseases such as proliferative ileitis are common. Hamsters are usually large and slow enough for children to hold. They are nocturnal, but if they are scooped up gently with two hands, they usually awaken without attempting to bite. Touching a hamster's back with a finger in an attempt to rouse it is likely to provoke a start or a threat response. Excited hamsters often jump from hands or tables, so appropriate caution should be used when they are handled. Hamsters are available in many color varieties and in a long-haired ("teddy bear") breed. All hamsters are well known for their ability to escape; most chewing can be attributed to this behavior. Chewed or damaged cage parts should be replaced immediately; if a hamster is cared for by a child, then an adult should regularly check the pet's cage for signs of wear. Hamsters may be stressed

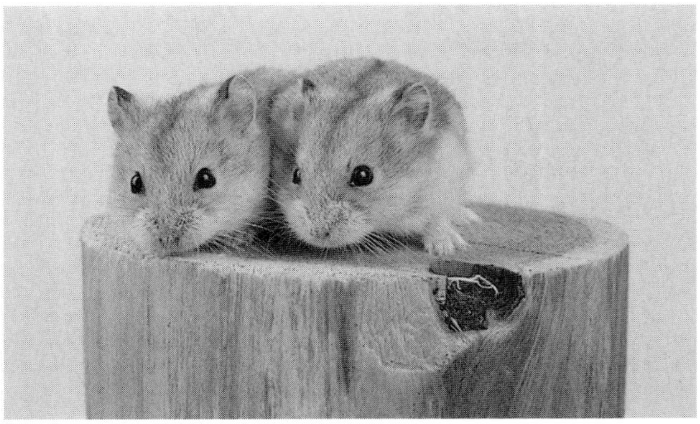

Figure 28-1 A pair of dwarf hamsters (*Phodopus* species).

by hot and humid environments; an effort should be made to keep hamsters in a cool area of the house during the summer months. The noise of an exercise wheel may annoy some adults. Plastic exercise wheels that are almost noise free are available, although some hamsters may chew on them if other materials, such as soft wood blocks, are not available.

Dwarf hamsters (usually Siberian dwarfs) are mouse-sized and have a furred short tail, white underparts, and a grayish dorsal surface. They are excitable and more difficult to restrain than other hamsters. Many dwarf hamsters do not hesitate to bite when restrained. Also, they are subject to stress-related enteropathies.

All pet hamsters should be kept singly. Male hamsters fight each other; female hamsters also fight with males and with other females, particularly once they are pregnant.

Mice

Standard laboratory mice are usually white but also are available in pet varieties, including satin (shining hair coat), long-haired, pied (spotted) (Fig. 28-2), and various solid colors. An adult mouse weighs approximately 30 g. Most mice make good pets for older children (10 years of age and up). Mice rarely bite but may scamper quickly, so younger children may not be able to handle them. Mice are largely nocturnal but are easily roused. Female mice are much recommended over males because they are less odorous. Mice are hardy pets and rarely suffer from infectious disease; however, mite infestations are common and are difficult to treat. Mammary tumors may plague older animals. Male mice are aggressive toward each other, but female mice often get along well.

Rats

Rats are most popular in the pet market in hooded color varieties, in which the coat color is present only over the head and shoulders. Rats are hardy as young animals but may suffer from obesity, chronic respiratory disease, and mammary tumors when older. Rats are large enough to be easily grasped by children, and they rarely bite. Some may be excitable and run when removed from their cages; however, rats have been known to return to their cage after an "escape."[1] Male and female rats get along well, and males may be present while females are raising a litter. Rats are relatively intelligent and seem interested in humans; they can be trained to come when called for a treat.

HUSBANDRY

Housing and Equipment

One of the most important requirements for any cage to house pets is that it is easy to clean. Poor husbandry and hygiene frequently result if the cage is heavy or awkward to disassemble. This is particularly true if children are assigned the sole responsibility for cage cleaning (a practice that is not recommended). Easy-to-clean cages have lightweight plastic bottoms, preferably with sides deep enough to contain bedding (Fig. 28-3). Aquariums are excellent for containing bedding, but they may be poorly ventilated and are often too heavy to be easily cleaned. However, their large screen tops are easily removed and

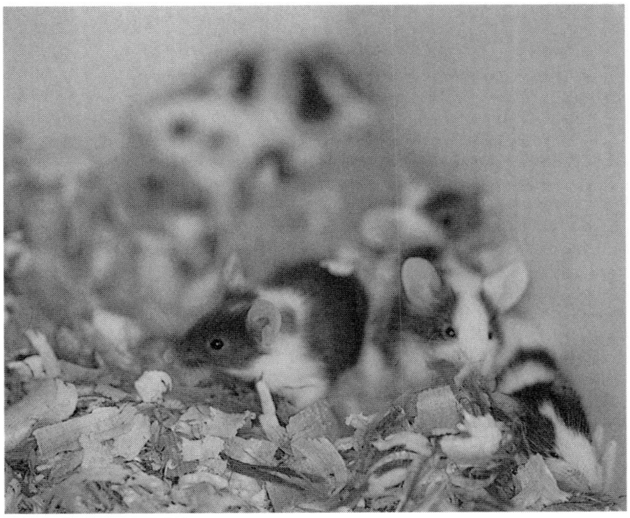

Figure 28-2 A group of pied mice.

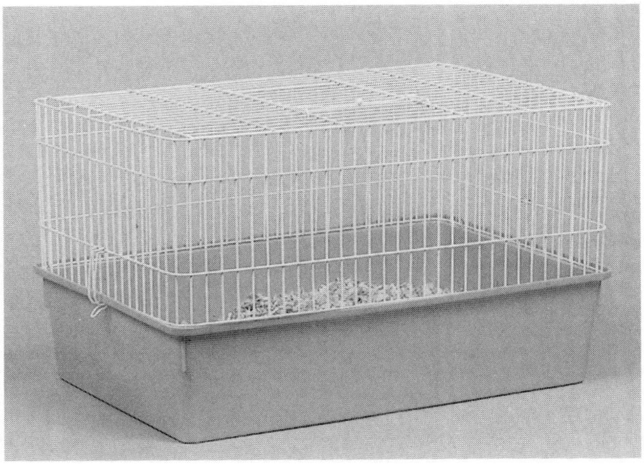

Figure 28-3 A cage appropriate for large rodents. It has a lightweight plastic bottom and sides that can contain bedding material.

do allow easy access to the pet. Conventional cages should have a large door (or doors) to facilitate easy removal of the animal. Screen tops for aquariums should be fitted with a locking mechanism. Solid plastic cages featuring plastic connector tunnels (S.A.M., Pennplax Inc., Garden City, NY; and Habitrail, Hagen Inc., Mansfield, MA) provide an interesting environment for the animal but must be cleaned regularly as ventilation in them may be less than in cages constructed principally of wire.

Commercial laboratories often use overhead hoppers to provide access to large food pellets or "blocks." This prevents the hoarding and soiling of food with feces. Although hoarding is a natural and probably desirable behavior for such pets as hamsters, it makes it difficult to judge the amount of food that is available to the pet. Hoppers are not widely available for pet rodents, and most owners use small, heavy plastic dishes or crocks.

Water bottles can easily be mounted on or in most conventional cages with the necessary adaptors or fittings. Accidental or negligent water deprivation is a common problem in pet rodents. Although water bottles may look full, sipper tubes can occasionally become blocked by air bubbles, or leaks may lead to the quick emptying out of all the water. Leaks can occur if the rubber fittings are old or if a foreign body such as a wood shaving is present in the sipper tube. Patency of the water bottle should be checked after every installation, and water should be changed *daily* with fresh water so that accidental water deprivation is avoided.

Exercise wheels have been used with most of the small rodent species, including pygmy mice and rats. However, hamsters are the best known for use of the wheel. Some female hamsters are capable of running up to 10 km in a single night.[1] When providing an exercise wheel for a long-haired hamster, keep its hair trimmed so that it does not become entangled in the wheel. Check metal wheels for sharp projections. Spherical exercise balls also are popular for use with pet hamsters, although owners should be cautioned that stairwells, direct sunshine, small children, and other pets may be hazardous to pets using these exercise devices. Despite the possible dangers that these plastic spheres present, it is uncommon for hamsters to actually sustain any injuries.

Exercise balls and related devices can play a valid role in environmental enrichment and exercise and may contribute to the bond between human and pet. Quality-of-life factors for pet rodents depend on human interactions. Many children quickly lose interest in a newly purchased pet rodent that is largely nocturnal. Possible sequelae are failure to keep the cage hygienic, failure to provide food and water, or, ultimately, failure to keep the animal as a pet. Devices such as exercise balls, commercial mazes, and tunnel constructs can be used to reverse this loss of interest, promoting interaction and bonding. Obviously, parental supervision is desirable if pets are owned by young children, especially during the pet's exercise and out-of-cage activities.

Bedding

Many different beddings are popular for use with pet rodents, including newer beddings such as recycled paper products, compressed wheat straw, citrus litter, aspen or oak beddings, and a variety of corncob by-products.

Pine shavings remain the most commonly used bedding for small pet rodents in many parts of North America. Corncob products and recycled paper products are excellent for certain rodents such as gerbils and dwarf hamsters. Cedar shavings also are popular, but their use remains controversial. Cedar has been shown to affect microsomal oxidative liver enzymes in rats and mice. Although enzymatic changes can affect factors such as drug metabolism, no clinical signs associated with these changes have been documented.[23] Because the changes may interfere with certain aspects of medical research, laboratory rodents are rarely housed on cedar shavings.

There are anecdotal reports of respiratory and skin effects in pet species, but little is known about the exact mechanism of these effects or which species might be sensitive. Cedar shavings were originally thought to have allergenic effects in gerbils (excoriations and ulcers affecting the muzzle and face). However, this was largely disproved when the harderian gland of affected gerbils was found to be involved (abnormal grooming procedures failed to distribute the secretions normally).[8,19] The housing of gerbils on shavings is indirectly involved in the development of facial lesions. Sand or dust normally present in the natural environment is absent in cages with shavings, and dust bathing is thought to be part of gerbils' normal grooming procedure. Sandboxes can be provided for gerbils in much the same way that they are for chinchillas. White, yellow, and red cedar shavings contain one or more aromatic oils and terpenes that may be irritating to animals when present in sufficient quantities. These aromatic oils are reputed to repel insects and other pests; thus, they could conceivably have beneficial effects in certain circumstances. Very aromatic batches of cedar might not be recommended for use with certain species such as dwarf hamsters; there have been anecdotal reports of hair loss and respiratory disease in this species when cedar shavings are used.

Feeding

Seed diets are commonly given to pet rodents, and the constant refilling of the feed dish allows the animals to select very palatable seeds such as sunflower seeds. These high-fat, low-calcium seeds can be offered as a treat food but should not be fed in excess, particularly to rats and hamsters. Rats are prone to obesity, and hamsters are prone to osteoporosis; a seed diet may exacerbate these problems. Certain seed diets are composed of hulled seeds with added vitamins and minerals. These diets differ slightly from the traditional diet of vitamins and minerals in a pelleted vehicle (similar in appearance to a rabbit pellet) that is mixed with a variety of seeds. Unfortunately, most pet rodents simply ignore these pellets when they are mixed with seeds.

More uniform nutrition can be provided with the use of formulated diets, in the form of blocks (Fig. 28-4) or pellets. These formulated diets are now packaged specially for the pet industry (e.g., Nutri-block, Hagen Inc., Rodent Maintenance and Rodent Performance, Oxbow Pet Products, Murdock, NE). Although hoppers are not widely available, blocks and pellets are easy to feed and check and are more visible than hoarded seeds. Conversion to this type of diet is usually simple, because most rodents find pellets and blocks very palatable. Rats might be an exception: they undoubtedly find them palatable, but, much like pet birds, they often avoid new foods. A gradual introduction is recommended instead of a sudden change.

Most of the small rodents have similar nutritional requirements, although minor differences in protein requirements have been noted for gerbils.[8] A typical formulated diet suitable for pet

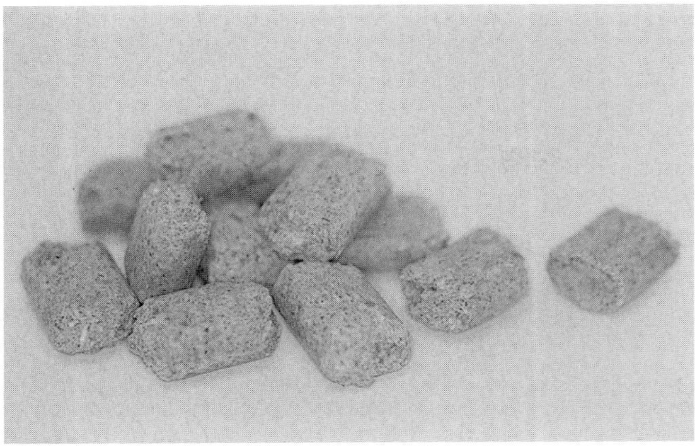

Figure 28-4 An example of a block-style rodent diet. This diet prevents preferential selection of seeds from a mix.

mice, rats, gerbils, and hamsters should have a minimum protein content of 16% and a fat content of 4% to 5%. The analysis for a seed mix is basically meaningless, because seed hulls and other discarded items are included in the analysis. Also, pet rodents select certain items from mixes, so that it is impossible to assess the nutritional value of a mixed seed diet. High-protein snacks or treats may occasionally be given to pet rodents, but fatty treats should be avoided. Offer treats in very small amounts to pets that are unfamiliar with new items. Reproduction in certain species such as gerbils and rats may require dietary protein levels of 20% or higher.[8]

ANATOMIC AND PHYSIOLOGIC FEATURES

General

Gerbils, hamsters, mice, and rats belong to the largest mammalian order, Rodentia. The word *rodent* is derived from the Latin verb *rōdere*, which means "to gnaw." These particular species have a common dental formula of $2(I\frac{1}{1}\ C\frac{0}{0}P\frac{0}{0}\ M\frac{3}{3})$. The four prominent, orange-colored incisors are open rooted and therefore grow continuously; in contrast, the molars are fixed rooted. In general, a crown/length ratio for the upper to lower incisors is approximately 1:3. Clinicians sometimes mistake the longer length of the lower incisors as overgrowth and clip the teeth; this is to be avoided. The chisel-like occlusal surface of the incisors is the result of differential wearing. The outer, convex surface of the incisors is covered by hard enamel, whereas the inner surface is lined only by cementum and dentin. The prominent space between the incisors and the molars is referred to as the *diastema* and is occupied by cheek tissue.

The small rodents have bulging, somewhat exophthalmic eyes; this presumably accounts for their frequent blinking. An important structure located behind the eyeball is the harderian gland. This gland produces lipid- and porphyrin-rich secretions that appear to play a role in ocular lubrication and pheromone-mediated behavior. The porphyrins impart a red tinge to the tears; under ultraviolet light, they fluoresce. Normally, the lacrimal secretions are spread over the pelage during daily grooming. However, in stressful situations and in certain disease conditions, there may be an overflow of tears; this can be inaccurately diagnosed as bleeding from the eyes and nose.

Hamsters, mice, and rats have four front toes and five hind toes; the opposite is true in gerbils. The small rodents all have tails, although the length and hair cover of the tails vary. Gerbils, mice, and rats have tails that are longer than their bodies. Hamsters have short, haired tails; the dwarf hamster's tail is slightly longer and almost prehensile in function. Gerbils' tails are well furred and have a tufted end. Rats' tails are thick, rasplike, and virtually hairless. The tails of mice also are covered only by sparse, fine hair.

Rodents do not possess sweat glands and are unable to pant. Mice salivate in response to warm temperatures. Otherwise, the ears and tails of rodents are responsible for their limited ability to dissipate heat. For these reasons, rodents are prone to heat stress and should not be exposed to extremely high temperatures.

Gerbils, hamsters, mice, and rats have, respectively, 4, 6 to 7, 5, and 6 pairs of nipples. Mammary gland tissue may extend over the shoulders and as far caudad as the perianal region. This is an important anatomic characteristic to remember when a list of differential diagnoses for skin masses is being considered. Mammary tumors or infections can be present anywhere along this tract.

Rodents are monogastric and are usually herbivorous or omnivorous. They are also, to varying degrees, coprophagic; fecal pellets often constitute a significant proportion of what they consume. The fecal pellets presumably provide nutrients, such as B vitamins, that are produced by the colonic bacteria. Regurgitation is difficult in these species because of the presence of a limiting ridge at the junction of the esophagus and the stomach. For this reason and because these small creatures have such a high metabolic rate, preoperative fasting is not required or recommended.

Normal physiologic, biochemical, hematologic, and urologic reference values are provided in Tables 28-1 through 28-4, respectively.

The small rodents are polyestrous and are spontaneous ovulators. Reproductive problems are not common. Rodents are usually efficient, prolific breeders, and pet owners often become acutely aware of overpopulation problems associated with the housing together of animals of the opposite sex. Vaginal cytologic analysis can be used to determine fairly accurately the stage of the estrous cycle. A small pipette can be used to instill and recover a small volume of normal saline from the vagina. A smear is then prepared with the recovered fluid. In general, proestrus is characterized by the presence of nucleated cells only, estrus by the presence of cornified cells only, metestrus by the presence of cornified cells and leukocytes, and diestrus by the presence of epithelial cells and leukocytes. Mating is confirmed by the presence of a "copulatory plug" within the vagina or on the cage floor. The copulatory plug is a straw-colored, gelatinous substance formed by secretions from the accessory sex glands of the male. The presence of sperm in a vaginal smear also is predictive of normal female and male fertility and, indeed, of pregnancy.

Other pertinent reproductive values are presented in Table 28-5.

Gerbils

Gerbils are adapted to a desert environment. They require very little water and produce only a small volume of concentrated urine. In their natural habitat, they can obtain most, if not

TABLE 28-1
Normal Physiologic Reference Values for Gerbils, Hamsters, Mice, and Rats*

Value	Gerbil	Hamster	Mouse	Rat
Average life span (mo)	24-39	18-36	12-36	26-40
Maximum reported life span (mo)	60	36	48	56
Average adult weight (g), male	46-131	87-130	20-40	267-500
Average adult weight (g), female	50-55	95-130	22-63	225-325
Heart rate (beats/min)	260-600	310-471	427-697	313-493
Respiratory rate (breaths/min)	85-160	38-110	91-216	71-146
Tidal volume (mL)	NA	0.8	0.15	0.6-1.2
Minute volume (mL)	NA	64	24	220
Rectal temperature (°C)	38.2	37.6	37.1	37.7
Approximate daily diet consumption of adult (g)	5-7	10-15	3-5	15-20
Approximate daily water consumption of adult (mL)	4	9-12	5-8	22-33
Approximate daily fecal production (g)	1.5-2.5	2-2.5	1-1.5	9-15
Recommended environmental temperature (°C)	18-22	21-24	24-25	21-24
Recommended environmental relative humidity (%)	45-55	40-60	45-55	45-55

NA, not available.
*Average reference values from data given in references 1, 3, 4, 6, 12 and 13.
Note that reference values may not represent the mean or range for certain populations or strains of animals; for this reason, the values should be interpreted as approximations.

TABLE 28-2
Serum Biochemical Reference Values for Gerbils, Hamsters, Mice, and Rats*

Value	Gerbil	Hamster	Mouse	Rat
Total protein (g/dL)	4.6-14.7	5.5-7.2	59-103	5.9-7.8
Albumin (g/dL)	1.8-5.8	2.0-4.2	2.5-4.8	3.3-4.6
Globulin (g/dL)	0.8-10.0	2.5-4.9	0.6	2.2-3.5
Glucose (mg/dL)	47-137	60-160	73-183	74-163
Cholesterol (mg/dL)	90-141	65-148	59-103	44-138
Urea nitrogen (mg/dL)	17-30	14-27	18-31	12-22
Creatinine (mg/dL)	NA	0.4-1.0	0.48-1.1	0.38-0.8
Creatine kinase (IU/L)	NA	366-776	155	111-334
Aspartate aminotransferase (IU/L)	NA	43-134	101-214	54-192
Alanine aminotransferase (IU/L)	NA	22-63	44-87	52-144
Alkaline phosphatase (IU/L)	NA	6-14.2	43-71	40-191
Lactate dehydrogenase (IU/L)	NA	134-360	366	225-275
Total bilirubin (mg/dL)	0.8-1.6	0.24-0.72	0.3-0.8	0.23-0.48
Sodium (mEq/L)	143-147	124-147	143-164	142-150
Potassium (mEq/L)	3.6-5.9	3.9-6.8	6.3-8.0	4.3-6.3
Chioride (mEq/L)	93-118	92-103	105-118	100-109
Phosphorus (mg/dL)	3.7-11.2	4.0-8.2	5.2-9.4	5.3-8.4
Calcium (mg/dL)	3.7-6.1	8.4-12.3	4.6-9.6	7.6-12.6
Magnesium (mg/dL)	NA	1.9-2.9	1.4-3.1	2.6-3.2

NA, Not available.
*Average reference values from data given in references 2, 4, 8, 9, 10 and 13. Note that the ranges should be considered as guides; values are likely to vary between groups of animals according to such variables as strain, age, sex, fasted, and methodology.

TABLE 28-3
Hematologic Reference Values for Gerbils, Hamsters, Mice, and Rats*

Value	Gerbil	Hamster	Mouse	Rat
Red blood cells (×10⁶/µL)	7.0-10.0	5.0-9.2	7.9-10.1	5.4-8.5
Hemoglobin (g/dL)	12.1-16.9	14.6-20.0	11.0-14.5	11.5-16.0
Hematocrit (%)	41-52	46-52	37-46	37-49
Platelets (×10³/µL)	400-600	300-570	600-1200	450-885
White blood cells (×10³/µL)	4.3-21.6	5.0-10.0	5.0-13.7	4.0-10.2
Neutrophils (%)	5-34	10-42	10-40	6-17
Lymphocyes (%)	60-95	50-95	55-95	9-34
Eosinophils (%)	0-4	0-4.5	0-4	0-6
Monocytes (%)	0-3	0-3	0.1-3.5	0-5
Basophils (%)	0-1	0-1	0-0.3	0-1.5
Total blood volume (mL/kg)	60-85	65-80	70-80	50-65

*Average reference values from data given in references 2, 4, 6, and 10.
Note that reference values may not represent the range for certain populations or strains of animals; for this reason, the values should be interpreted as approximations.

TABLE 28-4
Urinalysis Reference Values for Gerbils, Hamsters, Mice, and Rats*

Value	Gerbil	Hamster	Mouse	Rat
Urine volume (mL/24 hr)	A few drops–4	5.1-8.4	0.5-2.5	13-23
Specific gravity	NA	1.060	1.034	1.022-1.050
Average pH	NA	8.5	5.01	5-7
Protein (mg/dL)	NA	NA	Males proteinuric	<30

NA, not available.
*Average reference values from data given in references 2, 4, 9, and 13. Note that the ranges should be considered as guides; values are likely to vary between groups of animals according to such variables as strain, age, sex, fasting, and methodology.

all, of their water requirements from metabolic processes and from any available fruit or vegetable matter. Despite this remarkable natural ability, pet gerbils should always have access to fresh water.

The gerbil red blood cell has a life span of approximately 10 days. The rapid turnover of red blood cells is reflected on a stained blood smear as a pronounced basophilic stippling in a high percentage of these cells. Gerbil blood is normally hypercholesterolemic; this characteristic is probably a reflection of their high-fat diet and their love of food such as sunflower seeds.

Gerbils of both sexes have a distinct, orange-tan, oval area of alopecia on the midventral region that is referred to as the *ventral marking gland* or *pad*. This structure is composed of large sebaceous glands that are under the control of gonadal hormones. In the pubescent male, the gland starts to enlarge and produces an oily, musk-scented secretion. Gerbils can often be seen rubbing their abdomen on objects; this is thought to be a form of territorial marking.

Hamsters

Hamsters are short-tailed, stocky rodents that are known for their abundance of loose skin. They have large, potentially reversible cheek pouches that are paired muscular sacs extending as far back as the scapula. The pouches are evaginations of the oral mucosa and are used for transporting food, bedding material, and occasionally young. Hamsters also have a distinct forestomach that, similar to a rumen, has a high pH and contains microorganisms.

Hamsters have distinctive hip or flank glands that should not be misdiagnosed as skin tumors. These dark brown patches are found bilaterally along the costovertebral region. They are poorly developed in the female, but in the mature male they are prominent and become wet and matted during sexual excitement. Djungarian hamsters (*Phodopus* species) have a midventral sebaceous gland, similar to that of gerbils. Secretions from this sebaceous gland play a role in territorial marking and mating behavior.

Female hamsters are typically larger than the males. Female hamsters are unique in that they produce a copious vaginal discharge, normally just after ovulation (day 2 of the estrous cycle). These secretions should not be misinterpreted as indicating a bacterial infection of the genital tract. Female hamsters also have paired vaginal pouches that collect exfoliated cells and leukocytes. For this reason, it is difficult to use vaginal cytologic examination to determine the stage of estrus.

Hamsters are permissive hibernators. Low environmental temperatures stimulate them to gather food. At temperatures of about 41°F (5°C), they may curl up and enter a deep sleep. This state should not be confused with death.

TABLE 28-5
Normal Reproduction and Growth Reference Values for Gerbils, Hamsters, Mice, and Rat*

Value	Gerbil	Hamster	Mouse	Rat
Estrogen cycle length (days)	4-7	4-5	4-5	4-5
Estrus (heat) duration (hr)	12-18	8-26	9-20	9-20
Length of gestation (days)	23-26	15-18	19-21	21-23
Pups per litter	3-8	5-10	7-11	6-13
Weight at birth (g)	2.5-3.5	1.5-3	1-1.5	4-6
Eyes open (days)	16-21	12-14	12-14	12-15
Ears open (days)	5	4-5	10	2.5-3.5
Hair coat starts (days)	6	9	10	7-10
Start to eat dry food (days)	16	7-10	12	14
Optimal weaning age (days)	21-28	19-21	18-21	21
Age of maturation of male (wk)	9-18	8	6	4-5
Age of maturation of female (wk)	9-12	6	6	4-5
Recommended minimum breeding age (wk)	10-14	8	8	9
Chromosome number (diploid)	44	44	40	42

*Average reference values from data given in references 1, 2, 3, 4, 6, 7, 12, 13.
Note that the reference values may not represent the mean or range for certain populations or strains of animals; as a result, the values should be interpreted as approximations.

Mice

Male mice are typically twice the size of female mice. Like most other male rodents, they have open inguinal canals, an os penis, and a complex urogenital system that contains several prominent accessory glands. Intermale aggression is a common problem, particularly if the males were not raised together or if they are housed in a confined space with mature females. Male mice produce a characteristic, musty odor. Pheromones play an important role in mouse behavior and are mediated through tissues such as the vomeronasal (Jacobson's) organ, which is located in the floor of the nasal cavity. Estrus is suppressed in female mice that are housed in large groups (the Whitten effect). Recently bred mice that are exposed to a strange male may have impaired implantation (the Bruce effect).

Rats

Because of the popularity of rats in the biomedical research community, an extensive amount of information is available on rat anatomy, physiology, behavior, and diseases. Readers are encouraged to consult any of the references listed at the end of this chapter for more detailed information. In general, rats are typical rodents, many of the pertinent features of which have already been covered. Several other points are useful to remember. Albino strain rats, compared with their pigmented peers, have poor eyesight and rely heavily on their vibrissae for spatial orientation. Rats do not have gallbladders. The white hair coat of rats often yellows with age, and the tail becomes more dry and scaly. Aged male rats develop brown, granular sebaceous secretions at the base of their hair shafts, which some owners may mistake as an ectoparasite.

SEXING

In general, measuring the distance between the anus and the genital papilla is a reliable method of determining the sex of young animals. The anogenital distance is greater in males than in females. In addition, the genital papilla is usually more prominent and has a round opening in the male. Elevating an animal's front end or applying gentle pressure to the abdomen often forces the testicles into the scrotum, further assisting sex determination. Grossly observable nipples are found only on the females of these species. They are noticeable at about 10 days of age in female mice and rat pups (Fig. 28-5).

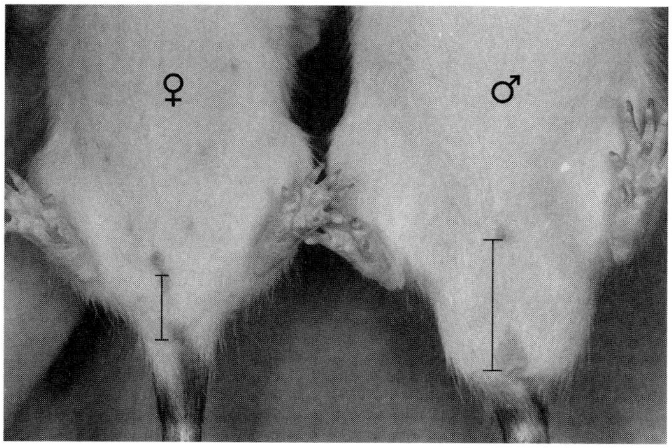

Figure 28-5 A male juvenile rat *(right)* and a female juvenile rat *(left)*. Note the greater anogenital distance, the prominent presence of the scrotum, and the absence of nipples in the male.

Other, more species-specific criteria also can be used. In gerbils, weanling males have a darkly pigmented scrotum, and in sexually mature males the midventral abdominal gland is large. The flank gland in hamsters is androgen sensitive and therefore appreciably larger in mature males than in females. Viewed from above, male hamsters have a rounded perineal profile because of the presence of inguinal canal fat pads that tend to keep the testes in the scrotum. Female hamsters have a flat profile that culminates in a point at the tail.

CLINICAL TECHNIQUES

Handling and Restraint

When handling a small rodent, the goal is to avoid stressing or physically harming the small patient while at the same time minimizing the risk of being bitten. In general, the key to successful handling is being gentle yet firm and decisive in your actions. Knowledge of the animal's behavior also is helpful, because each species reacts somewhat differently, yet predictably, to restraint.

Gerbils are docile in nature and are very amenable to being picked up and loosely held in a cupped hand. An excited or threatened gerbil often exhibits a rhythmic thumping of the hind limb; this should be taken into consideration when you approach the animal, because it is at this time that it is more likely to bite. For fully restraining a gerbil, the over-the-back grip or the scruff-of-the-neck technique is recommended. The animal may be caught initially by grabbing the base of the tail; however, use caution, because the skin can tear, resulting in a serious "degloving" injury. Damage is especially apt to occur in young animals or when the more distal segments of the tail are grasped. Allow the forefeet to grasp the edge of the cage or examining table so that the animal directs its efforts toward moving away from the restrainer. Approaching the animal from behind, place your forefinger and index finger on either side of the neck and exert pressure on the body of the mandible to immobilize the head. Hold the rest of the animal against the palm of your hand with your remaining fingers.

The scruff-of-the-neck technique involves grasping the loose fold of skin along the neck and back (Fig. 28-6). While holding the animal by the tail, use the forefinger and thumb to gently pin down the head; this prevents the animal from turning and biting. Using the same fingers, grasp a sufficient amount of loose skin over the neck. Holding the tail with the little finger of the same hand provides additional support. Both methods of restraint result in good exposure of the head and ventral abdomen and facilitate physical examination and the administration of parenteral or oral drug therapy. Also, restriction of the animal's breathing is minimal as long as the skin is not held too tautly and compression of the chest cavity is avoided.

Hamsters have a dubious reputation for being biters. They do not tolerate excessive or prolonged restraint as well as some other rodents do. If suddenly awakened from a deep sleep, they usually exhibit typical threatening behavior, such as rolling on their backs or standing on their hind limbs and vocalizing. However, if you avoid startling these animals, they can be quite receptive to being scooped up in the palm of your hand. When full restraint is required, a modification of the scruff grip is used. Because the hamster has an abundance of loose skin over the back and shoulders, a full-handed grip is required to achieve complete immobilization. To do this, grasp the skin between the tips of all four fingers and the base of thumb and lower palm of your hand.

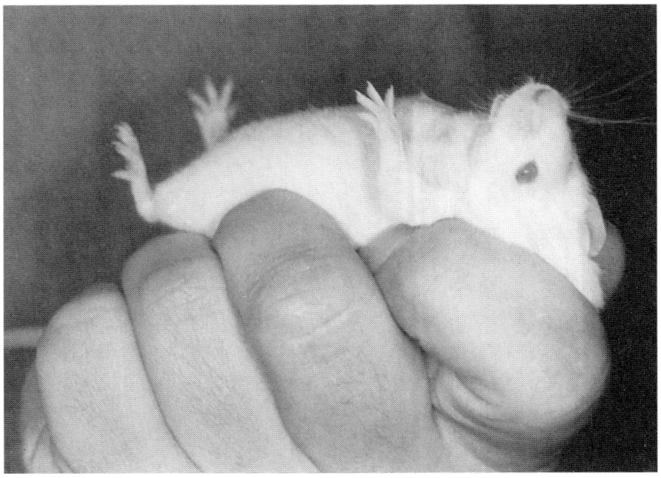

Figure 28-6 Scruff-of-the-neck handling technique in a mouse.

Mice are very active and are quick to jump away from a person handling them. Take precautions to ensure that, if the animal does escape, it will not injure itself and can be easily recaptured. Mice often bite when being handled, emphasizing the need for proper restraint of this species. Handle mice as you would gerbils. Initially, grab them by the base of the tail; then, use the scruff-of-the-neck method of restraint (see Fig. 28-6).

Most pet rats are very friendly and do not object to being picked up and gently manipulated. They rarely bite unless they are agitated or hurt. Pick up a rat by grabbing it over the neck and shoulders. Position your forefinger just below the mandible on one side of the head and your thumb on the opposite side, either above or below the forelimb (Fig. 28-7). Provide additional support by holding the tail and hind limbs with the opposite hand. The base of the tail may be used to temporarily catch an animal if it is not receptive to the direct approach; however, if the animal appears to be stressed by the procedure, it is probably best to take a short break and try again later.

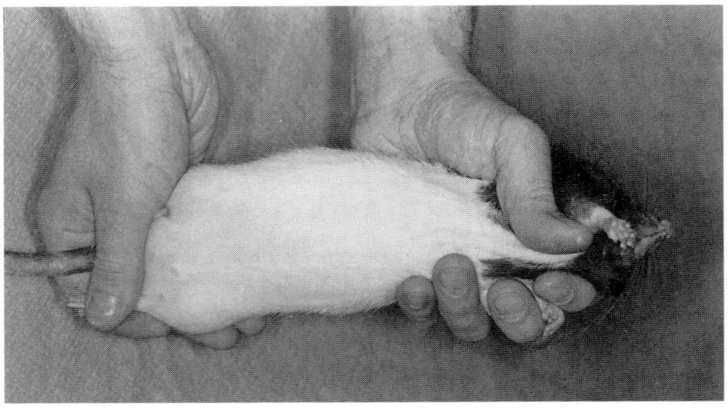

Figure 28-7 Over-the-back method of rat restraint.

Restraint devices for rodents of all sizes can be purchased commercially (Fig. 28-8, *A*) or custom-made with materials in the clinic. Animals may simply be placed in stockinet or wrapped in a thin cloth or soft paper towel (the "burrito" technique). The advantage of a paper towel is the ability to tear away a small section to expose a specific area for detailed examination, treatment, or drug administration. Syringe cases can be modified so that the animal contained within the case can breathe through a hole cut in the narrow end. Cone-shaped polyethylene bags that have had the tip removed also are designed for this purpose (Fig. 28-8, *B*); alternatively, you can modify a clear plastic bag by cutting off one of the corners. This last approach is advantageous because it allows the clinician to observe an animal and, at the same time, permits parenteral drug administration through the plastic.

In situations in which the animal obviously is not tame, the animal is very distressed, or a painful manipulation is planned, use of a soft leather, Kevlar, or wire mesh glove may be considered. However, the use of any foreign device is likely to be in itself distressing to the animal. In addition, the physical barrier of the glove material makes it more difficult for the handler to gauge the exact amount of force needed for adequate restraint. Caution must be used to avoid overrestraint, which can impair respiration or otherwise harm the patient.

Blood Collection

The exact technique chosen to collect blood depends on factors such as the species, the volume of blood required, the skill of the technician, and the clinical situation. Certainly, when dealing with individual pet animals, emphasis is placed on using the safest, least stressful, and least traumatic method. To avoid unduly compromising the animal, keep the volume of blood collected near the minimum required to run the desired tests. The general guideline for sampling blood is to remove no more than 10% of the total blood volume. Removal of this volume of blood should have no obvious effect on a healthy subject and can be repeated in 3 to 4 weeks. When collecting samples from clinically ill animals, use discretion and perhaps reduce the volume appropriately. Approximate total blood volumes are provided in Table 28-3. In general, try not to collect more than 0.3, 0.65, 0.14, and 1.3 mL of blood from the adult gerbil, hamster, mouse, and rat, respectively.

An excellent article describing blood sampling from the lateral saphenous vein of the gerbil, hamster, mouse, and rat was published in 1998.[9] This technique is advantageous in that it is minimally invasive, does not require anesthesia, can be performed by a single person when combined with the appropriate restraint, and can be repeated at the same location multiple times. The procedure does require some skill and is normally appropriate when relatively small quantities of blood are required, although volumes of 300 to 400 μL from a mouse can be obtained. Readers are encouraged to read the full article. Briefly, the patient is first immobilized. A mouse, for example, may be placed head first in a 50-mL syringe case that has been modified by placing one or more small breathing holes in the tip (Fig. 28-9). Extend an exposed hind limb by firmly grasping the skin just in front or just behind the knee, the exact "grip" depending on the leg being bled and the hand being used. Shave the hair over the lateral tarsal area, by carefully using a scalpel blade or with a small, quiet clipper (i.e., rechargeable personal trimmer), to better expose the superficially located vein. The vein is best exposed by wetting down the area with alcohol or silicon grease, or both. The grease alone is particularly useful in reducing the risk of clotting when blood contacts the skin, and it is less irritating than alcohol to the animal. Puncture the vessel at a 90-degree angle to the skin with a needle of appropriate size (a 25-gauge needle is usually sufficient in the mouse). A drop of blood immediately appears and can be collected with the use of standard microcapillary tubes or a microtube container. After the required volume is obtained, release the skin. This usually is sufficient to stop the bleeding; if it is not, apply gentle pressure to the puncture site. If necessary, the animal can be bled again at the same site after the scab that forms over the initial wound is gently rubbed off.

In gerbils, mice, and rats, the lateral tail veins can be used to collect small to moderate volumes of blood. The veins are located on either side of the tail and are quite superficial; in young albino mice and rats, they can easily be seen. General anesthesia is not required for this technique, but the animal must be properly restrained. Commercially available or custom-made restrainers that suitably immobilize the animal but provide access to the tail assist in making this a one-person procedure. Dilate the tail vessels by placing the tail in warm water or under a heat lamp (i.e., 25-30 cm away from a 60-W heating lamp). Incubation of the animal at a temperature of 104 °F (40 °C)

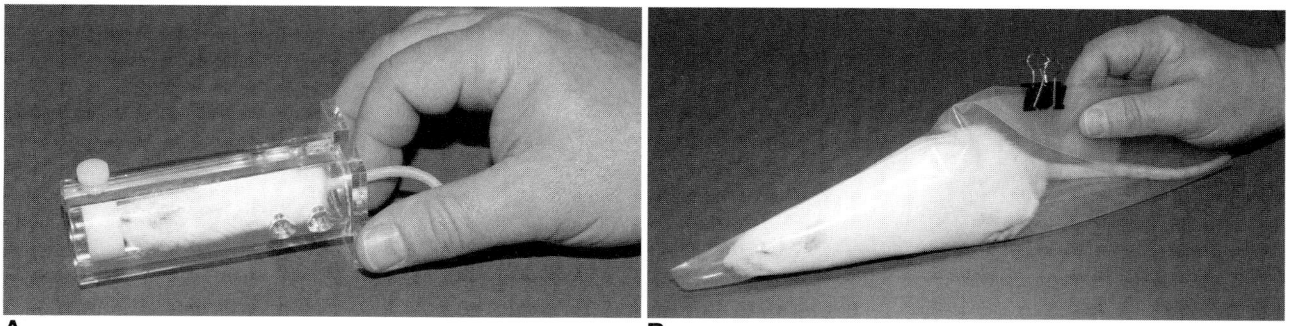

A B

Figure 28-8 Rat and mouse restrainers. **A,** Mouse in a commercial mouse restrainer (Broome Restraints, Plas-Labs, Lansing, MI). **B,** Rat in a plastic film tube (Decapicone, Braintree Scientific, Inc., Braintree, MA).

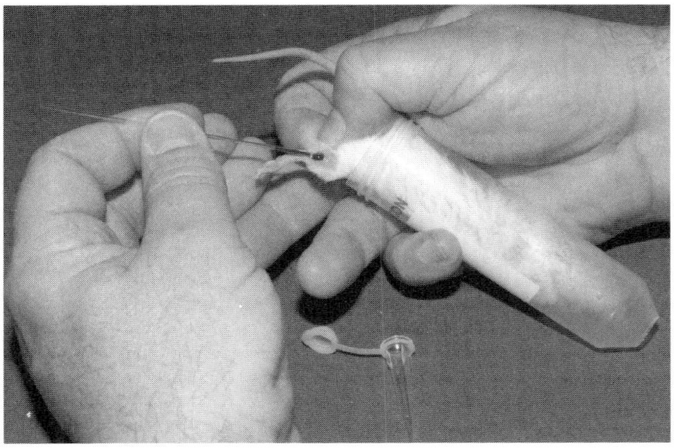

Figure 28-9 Blood collection from the lateral saphenous vein in a mouse.

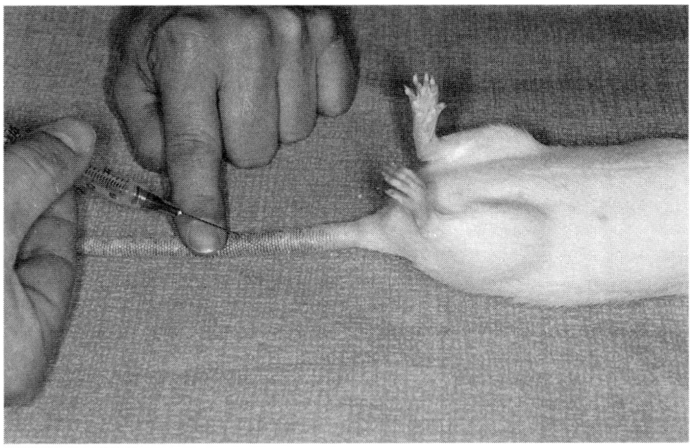

Figure 28-10 Obtaining a blood sample from a ray by venipuncture of the tail artery.

for 10 to 15 minutes before blood collection also is effective. Occlude the veins by placing a tourniquet around the base of the tail; a rubber band and mosquito hemostat are suitable for this purpose. With a needle of appropriate gauge for the species, enter the skin at a shallow angle, at a point approximately one third down the length of the tail. If the initial attempt at collection is unsuccessful, try again at a site closer to the base of the tail. To avoid collapsing the vessel, use a small-volume syringe to withdraw the sample, or collect the blood into a microhematocrit tube as it flows freely from the needle hub. A modified butterfly catheter (i.e., with all but the proximal 5 mm of tubing removed) also may be used. For repeated intravenous injections or blood sampling in the rat, use a 24-gauge pediatric over-the-needle catheter to catheterize the vessel. After the sample has been collected, remove the needle or catheter and apply gentle pressure to the puncture site until hemostasis is achieved.

The ventral tail artery in the rat is another very accessible vessel from which several milliliters of blood may easily be collected. The artery courses along the ventromedial aspect of the tail, although it is not as superficial as the lateral tail veins. Anesthesia is required for this technique, preferably with an anesthetic agent that maintains the animal's blood pressure. Place the lightly anesthetized animal in dorsal recumbency. Use a 22-gauge needle and a 3-mL syringe from which the plunger has been removed. Alternatively, some practitioners prefer to use a 23-gauge butterfly needle with a short tubing connected to a 3-mL syringe. Make the first puncture attempt at a point one third down the tail's length. Enter the skin at a 20- to 30-degree angle to the tail, with the bevel of the needle facing upward (Fig. 28-10). A perceptible "pop" usually indicates that the artery has been entered; this is quickly followed by filling of the syringe (or butterfly tubing) with blood. The high blood pressure in this vessel negates the need for the negative pressure produced by withdrawal of the plunger. Indeed, the presence of the plunger within the syringe case impairs recognition of correct penetration of the vessel. After the required volume of blood has been collected, withdraw the needle and apply pressure to the puncture site. Note that more time is required to stop the bleeding from the tail artery than from the tail vein.

Although blood collection from the orbital venous plexus or sinuses of small pet rodents was described in the previous edition of this text, it is no longer recommended because of the risk of injury to the eye and surrounding structures.

Cardiac puncture is useful for obtaining large volumes of blood. This procedure must be reserved for blood collection in animals that will be euthanatized because of the inherent risk of lacerating a lung lobe or a coronary vessel. General anesthesia is always required. Place the animal in dorsal recumbency; with the thumb and fingers of one hand, lightly compress the chest to locate and isolate the heart. Insert the needle at a 30-degree angle from the horizontal, at a location just underneath but slightly to the left of the manubrium. Successful entry into one of the chambers of the heart is signaled by a reduced resistance to insertion and the presence of blood in the needle hub.

Urine Collection

Although rodents do not produce a large amount of urine, small volumes are easy to obtain for testing with the commonly available urine reagent strips. The easiest and least traumatic approach is to gently restrain the animal over a clean, solid surface such as a stainless steel examining table. When the animal is faced with a foreign environment and under some restraint, the normal reflex is to urinate. Although midstream collection of single drops is preferred, a table-top collection is often sufficient for the tests of interest.

Drug Administration

The administration of drugs to small rodents poses some unique challenges to veterinary clinicians. Most drugs are not licensed for use in these animals, and therefore their use must be considered extralabel. In addition, most drug formulations are concentrated. To administer an accurate dose and to avoid causing tissue damage, drugs must be suitably diluted for parenteral use, and a tuberculin or insulin syringe should be used to ensure delivery of accurate volumes. Ideally, the diluent selected should be the same one in which the drug is currently formulated. Otherwise, an isotonic solution, such as sterile physiologic saline (0.9% sodium chloride), is acceptable for most water-soluble compounds.

Table 28-6 summarizes the recommended anatomic sites, maximum volumes to be administered, and needle gauges to be used for the conventional routes of drug administration. As a general rule, select the smallest-gauge needle that is compatible with the viscosity of the compound that is being injected; this helps minimize any discomfort to the animal.

Subcutaneous injections are preferred for drug administration because they are easy to give, pose the least risk to the animal, and allow the delivery of relatively large volumes. With the animal restrained by the scruff of the neck, make the injection into the tented fold of skin that is held between the thumb and forefinger (Fig. 28-11). If an assistant is restraining the animal, use a fold of skin along the back, flank, or abdomen. Aspirate before injection to ensure that the needle has not entered a blood vessel or passed through the skin.

Intraperitoneal (IP) injection is an easy means of drug or fluid administration. Because relatively large volumes can be delivered, potentially irritating solutions can be generously diluted. In addition, the large surface area of the abdominal cavity and its abundant blood supply facilitate rapid absorption. However, there are several drawbacks associated with this method. Administered compounds must first pass through the portal circulation; therefore, some metabolism or biotransformation may take place before the drug reaches the general circulation. Administration is also not 100% reliable. Some reports suggest that 10% to 20% of IP injections are not actually delivered intraperitoneally but instead are deposited, to some extent subcutaneously or intramuscularly; within the lumen of the intestine, uterus, or urinary bladder; or within a retroperitoneal space. There is also some discussion as to the optimal location for injection. The lower left abdominal quadrant, lower right abdominal

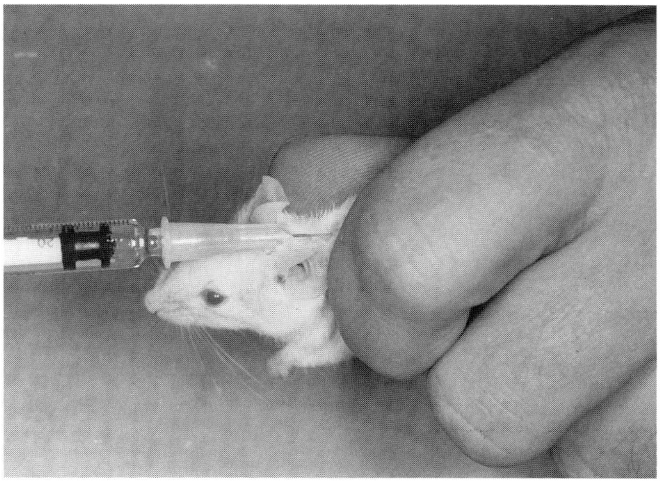

Figure 28-11 Subcutaneous injection in the neck skin fold of a restrained mouse.

TABLE 28-6
Recommended Routes for Drug Administration for Gerbils, Hamsters, Mice, and Rats

Route	Gerbil	Hamster	Mouse	Rat
Intramuscular				
Site	Quadriceps, gluteals	Quadriceps, gluteals	Quadriceps	Quadriceps, gluteals, triceps
Maximum volume (mL)	0.1 per site	0.1 per site	0.03 per site	0.2-0.3 per site
Needle gauge	23-26	23-26	23-26	22-26
Intraperitoneal				
Site	Lower right quadrant of abdomen	Lower right quadrant of abdomen	Lower right quadrant of abdomen	Lower right quadrant of abdomen
Maximum volume (mL)	2-3	3-4	1-3	10
Needle gauge	22-26	22-26	22-26	22-26
Intravenous				
Site	Lateral tail veins	Not recommended	Lateral tail veins	Lateral tail or saphenous veins
Maximum volume (mL)	0.2-0.3	—	0.2-0.3	0.5-3 slowly
Needle gauge	23-26	—	23-26	22-26
Intragastric				
Site	Stomach	Stomach	Stomach	Stomach
Maximum volume (mL)	NA	NA	5-10 mL/kg	5-10 mL/kg
Needle gauge	18-22, 3-4 cm long Bulbed feeding needle	18, 4-4.5 cm long Bulbed feeding needle	18-22, 2-3 cm long Bulbed feeding needle	15-18, 6-8 cm long Bulbed feeding needle or 8-Fr flexible catheter
Subcutaneous				
Site	Neck, back	Neck, back, abdomen	Neck, back, abdomen	Neck, back, abdomen
Maximum volume (mL)	2-3	3-5	2-3	5-10
Needle gauge	21-26	21-26	22-26	21-26

quadrant, and lower midline just above the urinary bladder have all been recommended. If the main concern is to avoid the spleen and cecum, then probably it is best to direct any injection into the lower right side. Tilting the animal downward while injecting has also been suggested; however, this does little to actually move internal organs out of harm's way. Finally, the practice of withdrawing the syringe plunger once the needle is inserted is of limited value; if the needle has penetrated the intestinal tract, the viscosity of intestinal contents usually precludes aspiration.

The fact that muscle masses in these animals are small restricts the number of practical injection sites and the volume of drug that can safely be given by the intramuscular route. If this route must be used, the recommended locations are the quadriceps muscle group, which covers the anterior aspect of the thigh, and the gluteal muscles of the hip (Fig. 28-12). Avoid the posterior thigh muscles, because the sciatic nerve courses along the back of the femur. Irritating substances that are inadvertently injected in close proximity to this nerve may result in lameness or in the animal's self-mutilation of the affected limb.

Many intravenous injection routes have been described; however, most require some degree of technical skill or the use of anesthesia. Consequently, this route often is not practical in pet rodents. If intravenous therapy is imperative, then accessing the lateral tail veins is recommended (see Blood Collection). Alternatively, an intraosseous catheter can be placed in the proximal femur of larger rodents. A small (24- to 26-gauge) needle can be used as a catheter. Except for very depressed animals, anesthesia is required for this procedure.

Achieving therapeutic blood levels of drugs through the use of medicated food or water is difficult, because sick animals usually reduce their food and water consumption. The palatability of medicated food or water often is affected, and too may result in altered food and water intake. If medication is to be given orally in the hospital setting, then intragastric gavage is recommended. Intragastric gavage is easy to perform on the conscious animal if a bulbed metal feeding needle or a flexible feeding tube is used (Fig. 28-13). A bulb-ended tube is particularly advantageous in that it helps limit the possibility of the tubes inadvertently entering the trachea. Before intubation, determine the approximate length of stomach tube that must be inserted by externally measuring the distance from the nares to the last rib. Lubricate the tube with water or a drop of glycerin to facilitate easy passage. Restrain the animal with its neck extended. Insert the tube at the level of the diastema (interdental space), and slowly advance it toward the back of the mouth. In the conscious animal, the tube should pass around the epiglottis and enter the esophagus. Smooth advancement of the tube indicates correct placement; incorrect placement is accompanied by violent struggling and dysphagia. With a flexible catheter, the use of a mouth gag is prudent to prevent the animal from biting through the tube.

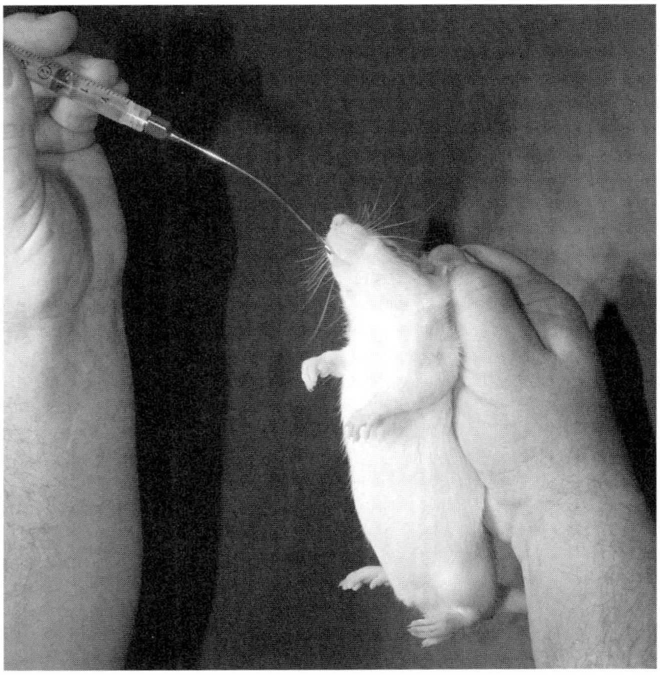

Figure 28-13 Intragastric drug administration in a rat. A 16-gauge, 3-inch metal feeding needle with a curved bulb end is passed gently down the esophagus into the stomach.

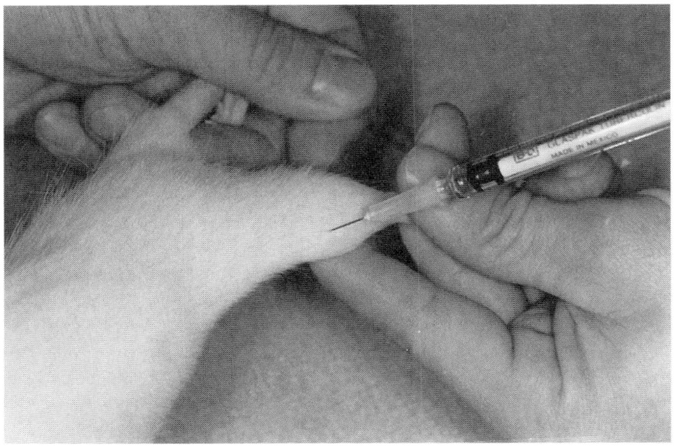

Figure 28-12 Intramuscular injection into the anterior muscle mass of the hind limb of a rat.

Compounding pharmacists can easily prepare oral medications in suitable concentrations for the treatment of pet rodents at home. Most drugs can be compounded into very dilute concentrations in a flavored syrup base. To administer a drug, restrain the rodent as previously described and insert the tip of a small dosing syringe into the lateral cheek pouch. Most rodents readily accept oral medications that taste sweet. Occasionally, a hamster reaches with its front paws in an attempt to push the syringe away. Always show the client how to administer an oral medication to a pet rodent before prescribing a drug, to ensure that the client is comfortable performing the procedure.

REFERENCES

1. Baker HJ, Lindsey JR, Weisbroth SH: The Laboratory Rat. Volume 1: Biology and Diseases. New York, Academic Press, 1979.
2. Bober R: Technical review: drawing blood from the tail artery of a rat. Lab Anim 1988; 17:33–34.
3. Boorman GA, Eutis SL, Elwell MR, eds. Pathology of the Fischer Rat: Reference and Atlas. San Diego, Academic Press, 1990.

4. Field KJ, Sibold AL: The Laboratory Hamster and Gerbil. New York, CRC Press, 1999.
5. Flecknell PA: Laboratory Anesthesia: A Practical Introduction for Research Workers and Technicians, 2nd ed. London, Academic Press, 1996.
6. Foster HL, Small JD, Fox JG, eds. The Mouse in Biomedical Research. Vol. III: Normative Biology, Immunology, and Husbandry. New York, Academic Press, 1983.
7. Fox JG, Cohen BJ, Loew FM, eds. Laboratory Animal Medicine. Orlando, Academic Press, 1984.
8. Harkness JE, Wagner JE: The Biology and Medicine of Rabbits and Rodents, 4th ed. Baltimore, Williams & Wilkins, 1995.
9. Hem A, Smith AJ, Solberg P: Saphenous vein puncture for blood sampling of the mouse, rat, hamster, gerbil, guinea pig, ferret, and mink. Lab Anim 1998; 32:364-368.
10. Hoffman RA, Robinson PF, Magalhaes H, eds. The Golden Hamster: Its Biology and Use in Medical Research. Ames, Iowa State University Press, 1968.
11. Hrapkiewicz K, Medina L, Holmes DD: Clinical Laboratory Animal Medicine: An Introduction, 2nd ed. Ames, Iowa State Press, 1998.
12. Kohn DF, Wixson SK, White WJ, et al., eds. Anesthesia and Analgesia in Laboratory Animals. New York, Academic Press, 1997.
13. Laber-Laird K, Swindle MM, Flecknell P, eds. Handbook of Rodent and Rabbit Medicine. Oxford, UK, Elsevier Science, 1996.
14. Loeb WF, Quimby FW, eds. The Clinical Chemistry of Laboratory Animals, 2nd ed. Philadelphia, Taylor & Francis, 1999.
15. Merck Veterinary Manual, 8th ed. Whitehouse Station, NJ, Merck & Co, 1998.
16. Olfert ED, Cross BM, McWilliam AA, eds. Canadian Council on Animal Care: Guide to the Care and Use of Experimental Animals, 2nd ed, Vol. 1. Ottawa, Canadian Council on Animal Care, 1993.
17. Percy DH, Barthold SW: Pathology of Laboratory Rodent and Rabbits. Ames, Iowa State University Press, 2001.
18. Siegel HI, ed. The Hamster Reproduction and Behaviour. New York, Plenum Press, 1985.
19. Thiessan D, Pendergrass M: Harderian gland involvement in facial lesions in the Mongolian gerbil. J Am Vet Med Assoc 1982; 181:1375-1377.
20. Thiessen D, Yahr P: The Gerbil in Behavioral Investigations. Austin, University of Texas Press, 1977.
21. Van Hoosier GL, McPherson CW, eds. Laboratory Hamsters. Orlando, Academic Press, 1987.
22. Waynforth HB, Flecknell PA: Experimental and Surgical Techniques in the Rat, 2nd ed. London, Academic Press, 1992.
23. Weichbrod RH, Cisar CF, Miller JG, et al: Effects of cage beddings on microsomal oxidative enzymes in rat liver. Lab Anim Sci 1988; 38:296-298.

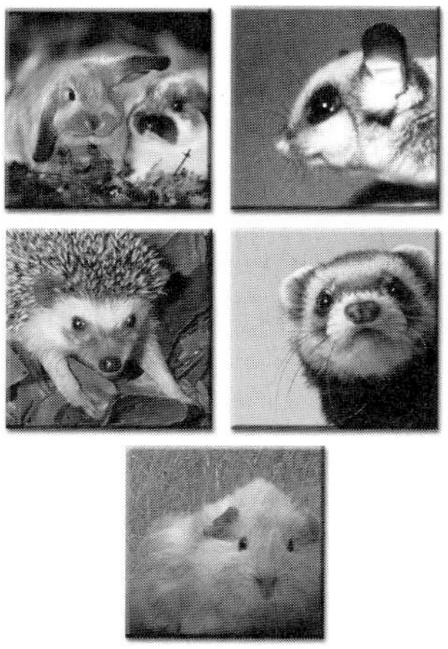

CHAPTER 29

Disease Problems of Small Rodents

Thomas M. Donnelly, BVSc, Diplomate ACLAM

The most challenging medical diagnoses are those made in areas of discovery. All too often, the animal and its condition are familiar, and the diagnosis and treatment are routine. However, some cases involve original investigation in emerging fields of veterinary medicine.

The treatment of rodents as pets is one of these emerging fields, presenting a terrain bristling with complexities for many veterinarians. First among these is the common perception of rodents. Most people do not consider them pets, and they usually are called "vermin." Moreover, almost all scientists consider rodents experimental tools. Veterinarians are not immune to such prejudices, and some may feel reluctant to examine a fully grown, red-eyed, wheezing rat. Owners of pet rodents often feel the same aversion for unsympathetic veterinarians and as a result travel long distances to see one who understands their needs. A second area of concern is the unfamiliarity of clinical veterinarians with rodent biology. Although much information has been accumulated on wild and laboratory rodents, very little of this information pertains to pet rodents. Geriatric diseases, the pharmacokinetics of common drugs, and the beneficial and harmful effects of human handling, contact, and care are a few of the phantom areas in this field. Yet the spectrum of problems affecting rodents does not differ greatly from that of dogs and cats.

One intent of this chapter is to describe the common diseases of pet rodents seen in practice so that their relative novelty becomes a challenge and not a stumbling block. Another is to inform clinicians about reasonable methods to diagnose common diseases of rodents accurately.

THE DIAGNOSTIC CHALLENGE

Pet Rodent Etiquette

Establishing and familiarizing the veterinary staff with a few simple rules of so-called pet rodent etiquette can make the physical examination a positive and fruitful experience. This preparation leaves the clinician confident and free of undue anxiety that can arise when he or she is presented with a concerned, overprotective owner. The veterinarian should be ready to apply his or her acumen and therapeutic skills toward treating the patient. Establishing clear communication between clinician and owner greatly facilitates the rodent's treatment and recovery.

Scheduling an Appointment

Rats and hamsters are essentially nocturnal animals and are only occasionally active during the day.[55] In contrast, gerbils and mice are active during both the night and day.[50] Healthy rodents are generally active during the awake part of their normal circadian cycle. When a sleep-deprived, drowsy, and irritable animal is brought to the clinician, subtle signs of diseases may be overlooked. This is especially true with hamsters. When possible, receptionists should schedule appointments for rats and hamsters during early evening hours. Appointment times are not as critical for gerbils and mice. Taking the time to explain the reasoning behind appointment scheduling to clients who are unwilling to make an evening appointment often not only changes their minds but also sets the veterinarian-client relationship off to a good start.

Instruct the client to bring the rodent to the hospital in its own cage. Husbandry and sanitation are essential to taking a good clinical history. Only by seeing the cage, water supply, feed containers, bedding, and food can the clinician understand the environment in which the rodent lives. Clients should be tactfully instructed not to clean the rodent's housing before the appointment because, by doing so, they may inadvertently destroy information important for diagnosis and treatment.

Reception Area

The waiting area for owners with pet rodents should be quiet. Receptionists should avoid planning appointments for natural predators, such as outdoor cats or hunting dogs, when a pet rodent is scheduled for an examination.

The rodent's sense of smell is well developed, and its world is rich in olfactory stimuli and pheromonal cues. Rodents are more sensitive to the effects of heat than cold. Even though wild golden hamsters and gerbils are desert-dwelling animals, their main method of thermoregulation involves escape from the heat by burrowing or seeking cool places. Mice in particular are very sensitive to the effects of heat. Waiting areas for rodents should be kept relatively cool. The dry-bulb temperature range of 64.4° to 78.8°F (18°-26°C), recommended by the National Institutes of Health, is ideal for housing rodents. Also, the opportunity for a habituated rodent to nestle next to the familiar smell of its owner can only be afforded in a quiet and safe waiting area.

Educating clients and receptionists about ways to make a trip to the clinic less stressful is well worth the time investment that it requires. If proper attention is devoted to education, then the veterinarian is likely to see a rodent amenable to examination instead of one ready to fight, flee, or cringe.

Medical History

In reaching a correct diagnosis, facts about the history and nature of a rodent's problem are generally more useful than the clinical history for a companion animal. Skill is required to extract a reliable, unbiased history of a pet's disease. Some owners are good at noticing changes and can provide important information, but others are not.

Find out what owners know about rodents. Have they had rodents as pets before? Where did they obtain their information on caring for their pet? Was it from the Internet, a book, a pet store, or first-hand experience? Books about rodents for owners of all ages are listed in the Suggested Reading section at the end of this chapter. Although these books are generally available, most veterinarians have not seen them. Many of these books are informative about husbandry requirements; however, many provide incorrect or misleading descriptions of diseases. For this reason, the sections on diseases must be carefully evaluated. Knowing your clients' sources of information further helps you assess their ability to provide an accurate history.

Do not become unsettled if an owner appears to know more than you do. Such a client can be very informative, enthusiastic, and willing to take an active role in treatment. When discussing a pet's problem with the owner, communicate on a level commensurate with his or her aptitude and background. Parents often present a sick rodent that belongs to their child, who is often the family member most knowledgeable about the pet's habits and behavior. When obtaining a medical history in these cases, the young owner's presence is invaluable.

Ask neutral questions that do not bias responses. For example, "Tell me about your rat's drinking habits." Try to avoid direct or leading questions such as, "Have you noticed that your rat is drinking more water?" because they may influence the response. Posing general questions such as, "Anything else?", "What do you mean?", or "Tell me more about that" helps encourage the owner to elaborate on his or her responses. Do not be afraid to say, "I'm not sure what you mean," and never belittle owners' opinions of their pets' illness. Try to obtain answers to the following specific questions:

- Where did the pet come from? A pet store? A laboratory?
- How long has the owner had the pet?
- Are there other pets in the household? If so, are they the same species or another species?
- What food does the owner give the pet? Where is the food purchased?
- What food does the pet prefer and what does it actually eat?
- Where is the food stored and for how long?
- Who is responsible for feeding and cleaning? How routinely are these tasks performed?
- How long have the signs of illness been apparent? Who first noticed them and why?
- Has the pet's condition deteriorated, improved, or remained stable?

Pets isolated from other rodents and household animals and those acquired from a private breeder or laboratory are less likely to have infectious disease than are animals obtained from a pet store.

Many diseases are the result of poor or inappropriate diets. Pet rodents often selectively eat only one ingredient (e.g., sunflower seeds) when offered mixed-seed, vegetable, and fruit diets. In households with children, a regular feeding routine may not occur, and pets are inappropriately fed by doting children. Owners are often ignorant of the availability of specially formulated diets for laboratory rodents. These diets, which are pelleted, are convenient and nutritionally balanced sources of nourishment. However, most diets are only available in 50-lb bags and can only be purchased from wholesale feed distributors. A list of these diets and the feed manufacturers (and their web sites) can be found in the annual Buyer's Guide issue of *Lab Animal* (see Suggested Reading and Resources).

Presently, two feed manufacturers, Oxbow Pet Products (Murdock, NE; www.oxbowhay.com) and Mazuri (St Louis, MO; www.mazuri.com) have developed pelleted diets for pet rodents and rabbits. The diets are available in 2-, 5-, 10-, and 50-lb bags by direct order or from selected retail locations. Oxbow has also developed Critical Care, a product used specifically for force-feeding rodents and rabbits that are anorexic because of illness or recovery from surgery.

Clinical Examination

Seeing how a pet rodent is maintained provides information that is helpful in reaching a diagnosis or a reasonable prognosis. Information obtained from a physical examination is limited because of a rodent's size. However, the significance of the rodent's history and husbandry can only be evaluated after thoroughly examining the animal. With appropriate handling and a few specialized but simple pieces of equipment, the major organ systems can be thoroughly reviewed. If the same procedure is followed consistently, it eventually requires less and less time to perform.

Observe the pet rodent in its cage for activity, condition of grooming, and the presence of a head tilt or any discharge. If the rodent is dyspneic or depressed, be extremely careful when handling the animal because it is probably very sick and could die from the stress of a physical examination. Also warn the owner of your guarded prognosis.

Pet rodents that have been frequently and gently handled usually require minimal restraint. Less cooperative patients need to be more firmly restrained, and the use of a towel or even heavy gloves may be required (see Chapter 28). Although pet rodents do not often bite, their nips can be painful and may elicit an unfortunate reflex response from the handler that results in the pet being pitched onto the floor or at a wall. In addition to the potential for traumatic injury that this circumstance entails, the rodent may escape and become harmed.

In general, the first component of the physical examination that I perform is to accurately measure the patient's weight. Weight measurement is essential for calculating appropriate dosages of medications and provides an opportunity for gauging the rodent's temperament before the actual physical examination begins. Rodents are easily weighed in metal or plastic containers placed on a small digital scale or a triple-beam balance.

A binocular loupe and an otoscope are useful to evaluate physical signs. Start at the head, examining first the ears, eyes, and nose for discharge and the oral cavity for dentition. In most rodents except mice, the otoscope allows careful examination of the mouth and ears. Lymph nodes and glands of the head can be observed for size and palpated for consistency. Assessing the head is probably the most time-consuming part of the examination.

Palpate the abdomen for consistency and the presence of unusual masses. However, do not squeeze the animal too hard because overzealous palpation can result in visceral rupture. Examine the anogenital region for discharges and staining of the fur or skin. When a rodent is picked up, it generally urinates and defecates. Have a dipstick ready to perform an immediate urinalysis; feces can be caught in a small tube and examined later, if required. Observe the condition of the fur and assess the body condition in general. Palpate the limbs for tenderness or fractures and pay special attention to the paws, observing the length of the nails and the state of the footpads.

Respiration and heart rates are difficult to measure in rodents because rates are very rapid. Instead, look for signs of dyspnea. A sensitive pediatric stethoscope is useful to auscultate large rodents. Some respiratory infections, such as mycoplasmosis, are clinically silent. These diseases can be better heard than seen; abnormal sounds called "snuffling" in rats and "chattering" in mice are noticeable without a stethoscope.

The value of determining rectal temperature is questionable. A rodent is stressed by the examination, and as a result its body temperature increases. Furthermore, it is easy to cause rectal damage and prolapse in these animals because of their small size. Finally, most thermometers are too big to use in pet rodents. However, rectal temperatures can be measured safely by using small, semiflexible temperature probes connected to a digital clinical thermometer. These probes are reusable; are available in polyvinyl chloride, nylon, and Teflon; and range in size from 1 to 3 mm in diameter. They are ideal for monitoring body temperature when performing surgery on pet rodents. A list of manufacturers can be found in the annual Buyer's Guide issue of the journal *Lab Animal* (see Supplemental Reading and Resources) listed under "Research/Animal Research Equipment/Temperature Probes."

The clinician can obtain a small amount of blood for a smear and microhematocrit from a hind-limb skin stab, nail-clip, or nick of the tip of the tail (see Chapter 28). Obtaining larger amounts of blood for a complete blood count and biochemical analysis may not be practical because of the quantity and quality of blood required. Rats often have chronic renal disease; a blood urea nitrogen concentration can be estimated by using a blood dipstick, and proteinuria can be detected by urine dipstick analysis.

Technologic advances have made possible electrocardiography and accurate and sensitive recordings of heart rate, respiratory rate, and blood pressure. However, the cost of this equipment may prohibit its use in most small exotic animal practices. Advances in high-resolution film screen combinations that require relatively low radiographic exposures and developments in ultrasound have allowed diagnostic imaging to become a useful, ancillary examination. A 1993 review describes the limitations of diagnostic imaging in small pets.[67] The *Atlas of Diagnostic Radiology of Exotic Pets* contains many excellent radiographs of the anatomy of rodents in health and disease.[61]

DISEASES

General Comments

Diseases of small rodents seen in practice The prevalence and type of small rodent diseases seen in practice are quite different from those seen in a research setting. Although this may seem rather obvious, much of the literature describing the maladies of pet rodents has been indiscriminately inferred from conditions seen in laboratory rodents. The diagnosis and treatment of pet rodents involve evaluation and care of an individual animal in a household, not the health management of rodents from a research colony. Derangements likely to be seen in practice include trauma-induced injuries, infectious diseases, and problems related to nutrition and aging; genetic disorders are uncommon. Natural infections that would be considered rare in a laboratory animal colony often are transmitted to rodent pets by other pets and by children; for example, pet animals other than rodents are a major reservoir of dermatophytes,[24] and human beings are the main natural host of *Streptococcus pneumoniae* and *Streptococcus pyogenes*.[41] Rodents used for research are maintained in tightly controlled environments designed to reduce the impact of unwanted variables in animal experiments.[18] However, pet rodents generally are exposed to temperature, humidity, and light-cycle changes; a broad range of foods; numerous microorganisms borne by animals and human beings; and various types of handling. As a result, pet rodents exhibit a wider range of physiologic and pathologic responses than do rodents used for research. Consequently, the disease presentation of many pet rodents does not conform to the classic description of the disease.

Veterinarians must be discerning in selecting information about rodents. Research-oriented scientific publications can be more confusing than helpful for small pet practice. Many research articles treat rodents as part of a herd or as experimental tools, and disease is diagnosed at necropsy. Successful diagnosis and resolution of disease are not addressed, and it is in this area that our understanding must be broadened. Fortunately, exceptions to this are now becoming more numerous. Clinical case reports and columns such as "What's Your Diagnosis?" in laboratory animal journals are more numerous and clinically oriented, and several newer publications specifically address problems seen in pet rodents. Some suggested sources of information for veterinarians are listed under Suggested Reading and Resources.

Significant diseases and life spans Pet mice, rats, gerbils, hamsters, and degus are subject to a limited number of naturally occurring medical problems. The most common, spontaneous outbreaks of disease are caused, or at least stimulated, by shortcomings in feeding and management. Some of these problems, unique to each species, are listed and grouped by the primary organ system affected in Table 29-1. The average life span of each species is also given. Most problems in these species are dermatopathies, enteropathies, or pneumonia. Certain problems such as malnutrition, hypothermia, and trauma, which are also commonly seen in small exotic animal practice but are not necessarily unique to a species, are not presented.

Prophylaxis for small rodents Prevention of disease in rodents is far more successful than treatment. Disease prevention is primarily based on common-sense husbandry practices, such as purchasing healthy, genetically sound animals; supplying balanced fresh food appropriate in protein and caloric content; providing clean, fresh water; furnishing adequate shelter that includes shade from direct sunlight; avoiding drafts and excessive temperature or humidity changes; keeping cages clean by preventing the accumulation of excess feces and urine; isolating sick animals from a group for treatment; and protecting vulnerable animals from more aggressive members of their group (e.g., young animals from older animals and male hamsters from female hamsters) or from natural predators living in the same household (e.g., mice from cats). Other sound husbandry practices include housing different species separately to prevent interspecies disease transmission (e.g., rats carry *Streptobacillus moniliformis* in their nasopharyngeal cavity, which causes septicemia in mice) and reducing obesity by limiting food intake and providing cage accessories that allow play and exploration (e.g., exercise wheels, tunnels, and ramps).

Unlike larger companion animals, pet rodents are not vaccinated. The introduction of ivermectin, although not approved for use in any rodent species, has allowed routine systemic treatment of pet rodents with pinworms and mites.

Dental problems are seen in pet rodents because of their continually erupting teeth. Overgrown incisors are seen most

TABLE 29-1
Common Problems of Small Rodents Seen in Clinical Practice

	SPECIES (AVERAGE LIFE SPAN)				
Organ System	**Mice (1.5-2.5 years)**	**Rats (2-3 years)**	**Hamsters (1.5-2 years)**	**Gerbils (3-4 years)**	**Degus (7-10 years)**
Integumentary and mammary gland	Alopecia, bite wounds, ectoparasites, mammary neoplasia	Ulcerative dermatitis, mammary gland neoplasia	Bite wounds, scent gland tumors, cutaneous lymphoma	Nasal dermatitis, ventral gland, lesions, tail-slip	
Digestive	Neonatal enteritis, endoparasites	Salivary gland inflammation, incisor overgrowth	Diarrhea, enterotoxemia, weight loss	Enteritis	
Respiratory	Chronic respiratory disease	Chronic respiratory disease, pneumonia	Pneumonia		Pneumonia
Urinary	Urinary obstruction	Chronic renal disease			
Reproductive			Vaginal discharge, maternal cannibalism		
Ocular		Red tears	Exophthalmos		Cataracts
Cardiovascular			Atrial thrombosis, congestive heart failure		
Endocrine			Hyperadrenocorticism		Diabetes mellitus
Nervous					Epileptic seizures

frequently in rats and mice. Specially designed cheek dilators, mouth specula, rongeurs, and filing rasps for treating dental problems are now commonly available (see Chapter 34).

Clinical Signs and Treatment

Mice

Integumentary system and mammary glands Most of the problems seen in pet mice are associated with the skin. A survey from a large research animal diagnostic laboratory indicated skin disease in mice represents 25% of all cases (for all species) submitted for diagnosis.[37] I categorize four groups of skin problems in mice: behavioral disorders, husbandry-related problems, microbiologic and parasitic infections, and idiopathic conditions. Behavioral, husbandry-related, and infectious causes of skin disease are relatively straightforward to diagnose and treat. However, many skin diseases characterized by chronic or ulcerated skin (often secondarily colonized by bacteria) are diagnosed as idiopathic. This group is commonly unresponsive to either topical or systemic treatment, and affected individuals are often euthanatized.

Mice exhibit well-studied social and sexual behavior. Social dominance, a form of behavior relating to the social rank and dominance status of an individual mouse in a group, is manifested as barbering and fighting. Barbering is a unique condition seen in group-housed mice in which the dominant mouse nibbles off the whiskers and hair around the muzzle and eyes of cagemates (Fig. 29-1). There are no other lesions, and only one mouse (the dominant one) retains all its fur. Removing the dominant mouse stops barbering; frequently, however, another mouse assumes the dominant role. Barbering is often seen in female mice caged together. Male mice, except littermates raised together from birth, are more likely to fight, often very savagely, and inflict severe bite wounds on one another, especially over the rump, tail, and shoulders.

Mechanical abrasion resulting from self-trauma on cage equipment is a form of husbandry-related alopecia. Small patches of alopecia appear on the lateral surfaces of the muzzle. These result from metal feeders that chafe, poorly constructed watering device openings, and metal cage tops. Unlike barbering, dermatitis may also be associated with the alopecic area. Treatment consists of replacing the poorly constructed equipment with nonabrasive equipment.

Individually housed mice can display aberrant stereotypic behavior such as polydipsia and bar chewing that results in mechanical abrasion and alopecia. In this situation, replacing the cage equipment does not help. Instead, provide environmental enrichment toys such as running wheels or hollow tubes. Nursing mice often have ventral abdominal and thoracic alopecia; this is normal and is nearly always associated with the extensive distribution of mammary glands. Absorbent cotton or cotton-wool may wrap around the legs of suckling mice and cause necrosis and sloughing of limb extremities.[58]

Most infectious causes of alopecia and dermatitis are associated with fur mites. Generalized thinning of the hair, especially on difficult-to-groom areas such as the head and trunk, is seen (Fig. 29-2). The coat often appears greasy and, in cases of heavy infestation, mice are noticeably pruritic with self-inflicted

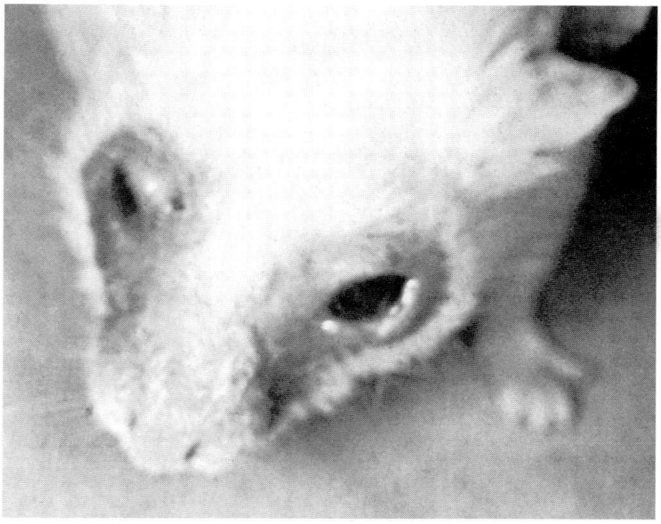

Figure 29-1 Barbering in a mouse. Barbering is often seen in mice housed in groups, in which the dominant male chews the facial hair and whiskers of his cagemates.

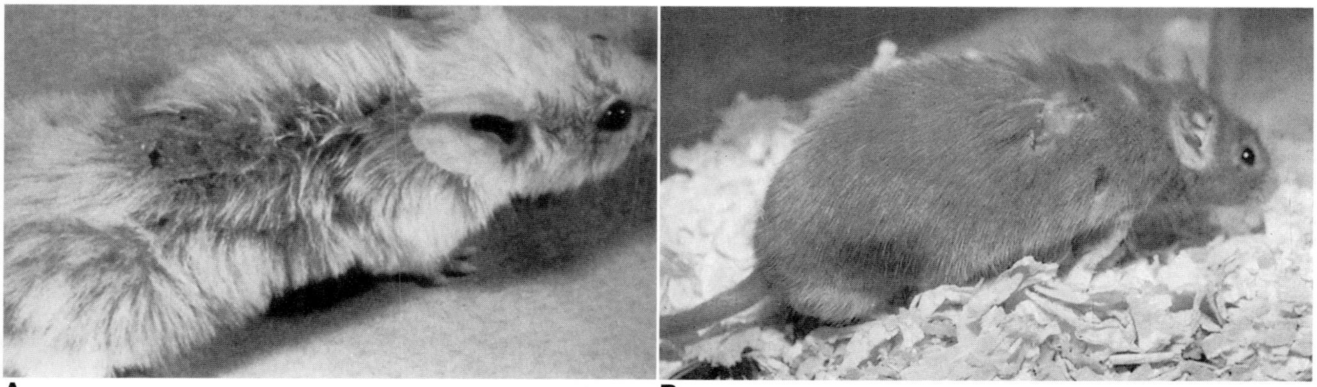

A **B**

Figure 29-2 A, Alopecia is commonly associated with mite infestation in mice. B, Noticeable pruritus and self-inflicted dermal ulceration may be observed. Three mite species are commonly seen: *Myobia musculi*, *Mycoptes musculinus*, and *Rhadfordia affinis*.

dermal ulcers. Three mite species are commonly seen: *Myobia musculi, Myocoptes musculinus,* and *Radfordia affinis*. The most clinically significant species is *M. musculi*, but infestations are usually caused by more than one species. Mites are spread by direct contact with infected mice or infested bedding. Diagnosis is based on identifying adult mites, nymphs, or eggs on hair shafts with a hand lens or a stereoscopic microscope. Adults and nymphs appear pearly white and elongate (being about twice as long as they are wide); eggs are oval and seen attached to the base of hairs or inside mature females.

Treat mice with mite infestations with ivermectin (0.2 mg/kg SC or PO) twice at 10-day intervals. Alternatively, place a few drops of ivermectin solution (diluted to 1:100 in equal parts of water and propylene glycol for three treatments) on the mouse's head to allow spread by grooming and ingestion.[6] Fragrant wood chips such as cedar and pine are high in volatile hydrocarbons and have long been known to have ectoparasiticidal properties. However, the hydrocarbons also induce cytochrome P-450 enzymes in the liver, which increase the metabolism of many common anesthetics and drugs (e.g., the sleep time of pentobarbital is decreased). Fragrant wood chips may also be associated with skin hypersensitivity, so I recommend replacing this type of bedding with paper or recycled paper litter.

Sometimes an owner presents a single pet mouse with clinical signs of mite infestation but with no evidence of mites or known history of recent exposure to other animals. Biopsy samples may be useful in these cases to distinguish active acariasis from dermal hypersensitivity to mites or other allergens such as wood chip bedding. Dermal hypersensitivity to *M. musculi* is well described in certain inbred strains of mice (B6 and NC) and is characterized by severe pruritus, the presence of fine dandruff all over the body, and occasionally ulcerative dermatitis.[23] The prevalence of dermal hypersensitivity in outbred pet mice strains is unknown. In these cases, treat the mouse with ivermectin as if it had clinical acariasis and monitor treatment response. If unresponsive, categorize these mice into the idiopathic group and offer the owner additional diagnostic tests and treatments.

Ringworm is uncommon in pet mice but can be caused by *Trichophyton mentagrophytes*. Lesions, when present, are most common on the face, head, neck, and tail. The lesions appear scruffy with patchy areas of alopecia and variable degrees of erythema and crusting. Pruritus is usually minimal to absent, and the lesions do not fluoresce under a Wood's lamp.[19]

Skin swellings are usually tumors or abscesses. Results of fine-needle aspirate often reveal the nature of the contents and allow diagnosis. Three bacterial species, *Staphylococcus aureus, Pasteurella pneumotropica,* and *S. pyogenes*, have been isolated as the causes in various well-described cases.[15] All are considered opportunistic pathogens and can cause abscesses in other organs (e.g., *P. pneumotropica* is sometimes associated with conjunctivitis, panophthalmitis, and swollen eye abscesses). Antibiotic therapy with penicillins or cephalosporins, concurrent with drainage and debridement of the abscess, is effective.

Idiopathic skin disease in mice is characterized by ulcerative dermatitis with pruritus. In affected mice, test results for primary ectoparasitic, bacterial, or mycotic infections are negative. Histopathologic and immunofluorescent microscopic examination of selected inbred strains of mice have revealed an underlying vasculitis attributed to immune complex deposits in dermal vessels. In these mice, dietary factors and dysregulated fatty acid metabolism have been implicated in the pathogenesis. Two treatments appear to alleviate or resolve lesions. Gavaging affected mice with 0.1 mL/day of liquid from Derm Caps (DVM Pharmaceuticals, IVAX Corporation, Miami, FL), an essential fatty acid supplement containing omega-3 fatty acids, regressed lesions and resolved pruritus in 10 of 10 affected mice.[42] In another report, persimmon leaf extract administered daily for 4 weeks significantly decreased skin lesions, serum immunoglobulin E levels, and scratching behavior in affected mice.[48]

The most common spontaneous tumors associated with the skin are mammary adenocarcinomas, followed by fibrosarcomas. The incidence of mammary tumors varies according to the mouse strain and the presence or absence of mouse mammary tumor viruses; in some strains, the incidence is as high as 70%.[70] In wild and outbred mice, the incidence of fibrosarcoma ranges from 1% to 6%.[30] By the time a diagnosis is made, subcutaneous tumors are nearly always malignant and often have ulcerated. Although tumors can be treated by surgical excision, the chance of recurrence is high and the prognosis is poor. Attempts to treat tumors in mice by radiation or chemotherapy have not been reported.

Digestive system Endoparasites are relatively common in mice. However, only two parasites regularly seen in the digestive tract, the protozoan parasites *Spironucleus muris* and *Giardia muris*, are considered pathogenic, even though they are not associated with clinical signs in immunocompetent hosts. A diagnosis is made by demonstrating characteristic trophozoites in wet mounts of fresh intestinal contents or feces. Treatment is metronidazole added to the drinking water (0.04%- 0.10% for 14 days), but it does not completely eliminate the infection.[31] In individual pet animals, metronidazole can be compounded into a fruit-flavored suspension and given at dosages used in other rodents.

Pinworms are ubiquitous and considered nonpathogenic. Two are commonly encountered in mice: *Syphacia obvelata* and *Aspicularis tetraptera*. The only indication of pinworm infestation often is rectal prolapse from straining. To establish a diagnosis of *S. obvelata* infestation, make a clear cellophane tape impression of the perianal skin. Adult *S. obvelata* females deposit ova around the anus. *A. tetraptera* does not deposit its ova in this area, and fecal smear or flotation is required to confirm a diagnosis. Ivermectin (2 mg/kg PO given twice at a 10-day interval) eliminates pinworms from mice. Ivermectin 1% is diluted 1:9 in vegetable oil to establish a concentration of 1.0 mg/mL; affected mice are dosed with a volume of 0.2 mL/100 g PO.[21] The recommended package label dose for mice with ectoparasites (0.2 mg/kg given twice at a 10-day interval) does not eliminate pinworms.[34]

Diarrhea is not usually seen in adult mice. Digestive disease in adult mice is usually caused by a varying combination of pathogenic and opportunistic infectious agents. Fecal flotation and fresh wet mounts of feces usually yield positive results and do not necessarily give a definitive diagnosis. However, these techniques are sometimes helpful in identifying heavy endoparasite infections. Treatment is generally directed at clinical signs and consists of the judicious use of antimicrobials.

Respiratory system Diseases of the upper and lower respiratory tracts are common in pet mice and rats. Animals may display sniffling, sneezing, chattering, and labored breathing. If dyspnea is suspected, do not overhandle the animal during clinical examination because it may die. Collecting tracheal and nasal secretions is not recommended; swabbing is highly traumatic, and the disease is generally caused by a mixed viral, mycoplasmal, and bacterial infection. Antibiotic treatment is helpful but usually does not eliminate the disease.

The two most common causes of clinical respiratory disease in mice are Sendai virus and *Mycoplasma pulmonis*. Sendai virus is associated with an acute respiratory infection in which mice display chattering and mild respiratory distress. Neonates and weanlings may die. Adults generally recover within 2 months. When the disease expression exceeds this pattern, the cause is most likely concurrent mycoplasmal infection. *M. pulmonis* causes chronic pneumonia, suppurative rhinitis, and occasionally otitis media. Purulent exudate accumulates in inflamed and thickened nasal passages, causing chattering and dyspnea. Survivors develop chronic bronchopneumonia, bronchiectasis, and occasionally pulmonary abscesses (this does not happen in rats). Antibiotic therapy may alleviate clinical signs but does not eliminate the infection. For treatment, enrofloxacin (10 mg/kg) in combination with doxycycline hyclate (5 mg/kg) given every 12 hours PO for 7 days is sometimes helpful.

Urinary system Urethral obstruction in male mice has been described as a result of infection of the preputial glands with *S. aureus* and of the bulbourethral glands with *P. pneumotropica*. Accessory sex gland secretions and, rarely, urolithiasis have also been implicated. Mice often are presented to the veterinarian because they mutilate their penis as a result of these conditions. In addition, occasional injury of the penis is seen in young males from aggressive breeding activity and abrasion on the cage. Treatment involves isolating the affected mouse, cleaning and debriding the affected areas, and treating with antibiotics.

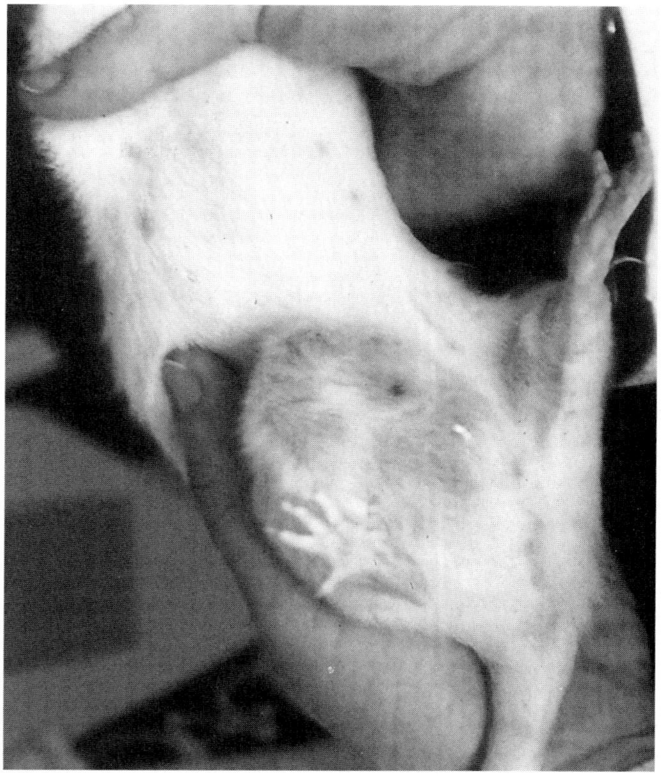

Figure 29-3 Mammary fibroadenoma in the inguinal region of a female rat.

Rats

Integumentary system and mammary glands Ulcerative dermatitis caused by *S. aureus* infection results from self-trauma associated with fur mite infestation or, more commonly, scratching of the skin over an inflamed salivary gland. Rats have a remarkable ability to resist infection with *S. aureus*.[18] Treatment consists of clipping the toenails of the hindpaws, cleaning the ulcerated skin, and applying a topical antibiotic. Systemic treatment is rarely necessary.

The most common subcutaneous tumor in rats is fibroadenoma of the mammary glands. The distribution of mammary tissue is extensive, and the tumors can occur anywhere from the neck to the inguinal region (Fig. 29-3). Tumors can reach 8 to 10 cm in diameter and develop in both males and females. The surgical technique for tumor removal is straightforward (see Chapter 30), and survival after mastectomy is good if the tumor is benign.[32] Adenocarcinomas represent fewer than 10% of mammary tumors in rats. The prevalence of mammary tumors, as well as that of pituitary tumors, is significantly lower in ovariectomized rats than in sexually intact Sprague-Dawley rats.[32] However, recurrence of fibroadenomas is common in uninvolved mammary tissue, and often several surgeries are needed. In contrast, mammary tumors in mice are nearly always malignant and often are not amenable to surgical removal.

Ectoparasitic infestation is less common in rats than in mice. Occasionally, the fur mite *Radfordia ensifera* is seen. Although *R. ensifera* infestation produces few ill effects, heavy infestation may lead to self-trauma and ulcerative dermatitis. Other mites, including *Demodex* species, have been described in rats maintained in laboratories[75]; however, they are seldom seen, and no reports of infestations in pet rats appear in recent literature. Diagnosis and treatment are the same as those for mice.

Avascular necrosis of the tail, or ringtail, is a highly photogenic lesion of rats and probably for this reason is always described in textbooks and articles on diseases of rats. It occurs primarily in young laboratory rats in low-humidity environments and often in rats housed in hanging cages; it is rarely seen in pet animals. If ringtail is diagnosed, treatment involves amputating the tail below the necrotic annular constriction.

Digestive system Inflammation and edema of the cervical salivary glands is caused by sialodacryoadenitis virus, a coronavirus. Owners of infected rats often describe their pets as having mumps. Sialodacryoadenitis virus infection is highly contagious. It initially causes rhinitis followed by epithelial necrosis and inflammatory swelling of the salivary and lacrimal glands. Cervical lymph nodes also become enlarged. There is no treatment for this disease. Glandular healing follows within 7 to 10 days, and clinical signs subside within 30 days, with minimal residual lesions remaining. During acute inflammation, affected rats are at high risk for anesthesia-related death because of the decreased diameter of the upper respiratory tract lumen; also, ocular lesions such as conjunctivitis, keratitis, corneal ulcers, synechiae, and hyphema can develop from lacrimal dysfunction. The eye lesions usually resolve but occasionally progress to chronic keratitis and megaglobus.

Overgrowth of the incisors is common in rats, and their teeth can grow into the nasal cavity (Fig. 29-4). See Chapter 34 for further discussion of this problem.

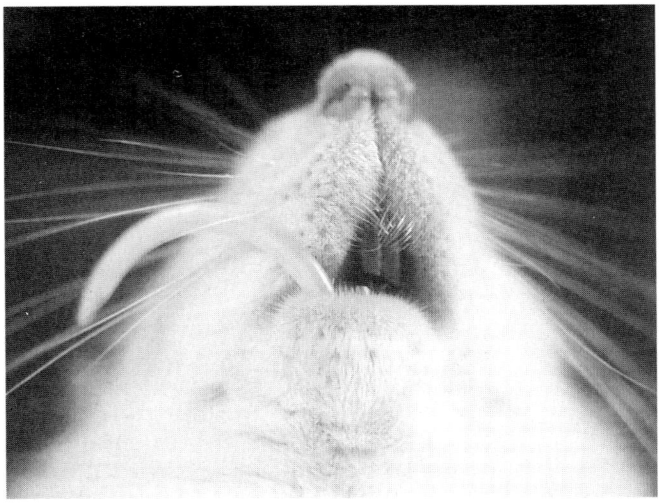

Figure 29-4 Overgrown incisors in a rat. Overgrown teeth can be cut with a high-speed drill.

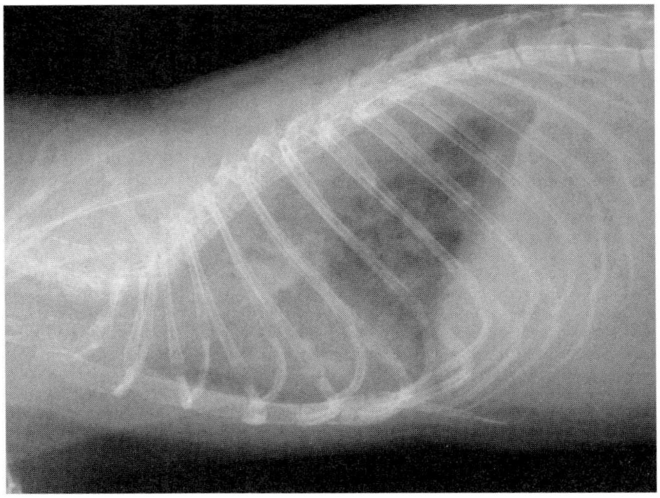

Figure 29-5 Lateral radiographic view of a 1.5-year-old male rat with chronic respiratory disease. The lungs have multifocal areas of pulmonary infiltrate. The cause of disease is usually multifactorial, involving concurrent infection with *Mycoplasma pulmonis*, Sendai or other viruses, and cilia-associated respiratory bacillus, as well as management and genetic factors.

Respiratory system Respiratory disease caused by infectious agents is the most common health problem in rats. Three major respiratory pathogens cause overt clinical disease: *M. pulmonis*, *S. pneumoniae*, and *Corynebacterium kutscheri*. Other organisms such as Sendai virus (a parainfluenza virus), pneumonia virus of mice (a paramyxovirus), rat respiratory virus (a hantavirus),[46] cilia-associated respiratory (CAR) bacillus, and *Haemophilus* species are minor respiratory pathogens that by themselves rarely cause overt clinical disease. However, these minor respiratory pathogens interact synergistically as copathogens with the major respiratory pathogens to produce two major clinical syndromes: chronic respiratory disease (CRD) and bacterial pneumonia.

CRD is the best understood multifactorial respiratory infection in rats. *M. pulmonis* is the major component of CRD, also known as murine respiratory mycoplasmosis. Rats may live 2 to 3 years with CRD. Clinical signs are highly variable, and initial infection develops without any clinical signs. Early signs involve both the upper and the lower respiratory tracts and may include snuffling, nasal discharge, polypnea, weight loss, hunched posture, ruffled coat, head tilt, and red tears.[15,35] Thoracic radiographs may be helpful in the diagnosis of CRD (Fig 29-5). The most important aspect of CRD for clinicians is that respiratory mycoplasmosis varies greatly in disease expression because of environmental, host, and organismal factors that influence the host-pathogen relationship. Examples of such factors include intracage ammonia levels; concurrent Sendai virus, coronavirus (sialodacryoadenitis virus), pneumonia virus of mice, rat respiratory virus, or CAR bacillus infection; the genetic susceptibility of the host; the virulence of the *Mycoplasma* strain; and vitamin A or E deficiency.[15] For many years, the standard treatment for laboratory rats was to add tetracycline to sweetened water. However, this treatment is ineffective in rats because blood antibiotic concentrations are below minimum inhibitory concentrations, and pulmonary tissue concentration of tetracycline is noninhibitory. Instead, administer enrofloxacin (10 mg/kg PO q12h for 7 days) in combination with doxycycline hyclate (5 mg/kg PO q12h for 7 days). Although mycoplasma and CAR bacillus are susceptible to this antibiotic therapy, the respiratory viruses are not. In addition, certain strains of rats have a heightened cellular immune response to mycoplasma that aggravates respiratory damage. Therefore, warn owners that antibiotic treatment will not cure CRD but may alleviate clinical signs. Reducing ammonia levels in cages by removing bedding and using clean paper daily may also help. Despite developing high antibody titers to mycoplasma and high antibiotic tissue levels, affected animals typically have persistent *M. pulmonis* infection. Chronic signs of infection often include middle ear infection (by way of the eustachian tube); ciliostasis and subsequent buildup of lysozyme-rich inflammatory exudate in airways; and, eventually, bronchiectasis and bronchiolectasis from inflammatory damage to the bronchiolar membranes. Abscesses may develop in scattered areas of one or both lungs. In these animals with advanced CRD, reducing ammonia levels in cages and administering bronchodilators and low levels of short-acting corticosteroids are also sometimes helpful in reducing clinical signs.

Bacterial pneumonia is nearly always caused by *S. pneumoniae* (Fig. 29-6) but seldom develops in the absence of some combination involving *M. pulmonis*, Sendai virus, or CAR bacillus. Infection with *C. kutscheri* (Fig. 29-7) also results in pneumonia but only in debilitated or immunosuppressed animals. In pet rats, immunosuppression can result from diabetes, neoplasia, or dietary deficiencies. *C. kutscheri* pneumonia is rare in pet rats. Pneumonia caused by *S. pneumoniae* can be of sudden onset. Young rats are more severely affected than are older ones, and often the only sign they exhibit is sudden death. Mature rats may demonstrate dyspnea, snuffling, and abdominal breathing. A purulent exudate may be seen around the nares and on the front paws (from wiping of the nostrils). A tentative diagnosis can be based on identifying numerous gram-positive diplococci on a Gram stain of the exudate or in a sample submitted for cytologic examination (Fig. 29-8). Severe bacteremia is an important consequence of advanced disease and results in multiorgan abscesses and infarction. Treatment must be aggressive, and the use of beta-lactamase–resistant penicillins such as cloxacillin, oxacillin, and dicloxacillin (all of which can be administered orally) is recommended. There are no published dosages of these drugs for rats, and the dosage is empirical.

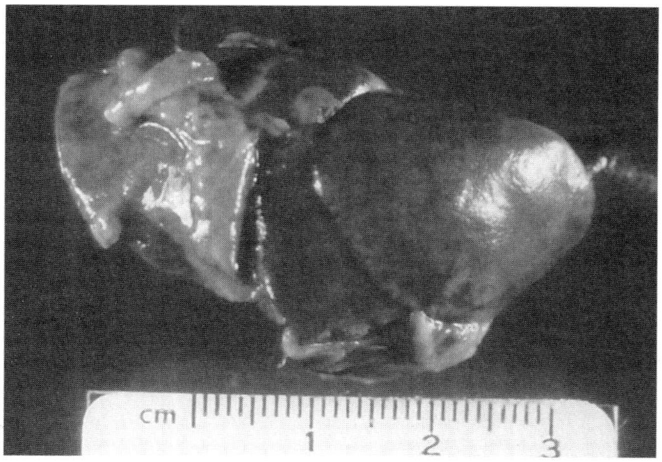

Figure 29-6 Fibrinopurulent pneumonia in a rat caused by *Streptococcus pneumoniae.*

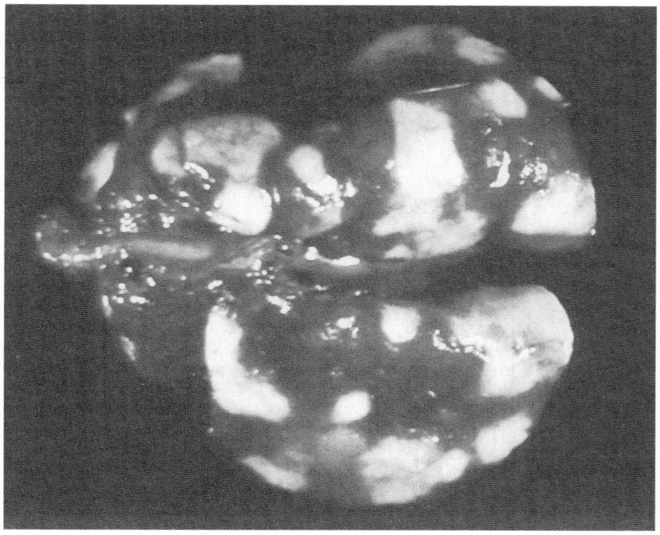

Figure 29-7 Gross appearance of the lungs in a diabetic rat with pneumonia caused by *Corynebacterium kutscheri* infection. Lobular pneumonia is the result of the hematogenous spread of the organism. Compare the appearance of these lungs with that of the lungs in Fig. 29-6.

Urinary system Chronic progressive nephrosis (CPN) is the best-known age-related disease of rats. In CPN, the kidneys are enlarged and pale and have a pitted, mottled surface that often contains pinpoint cysts (Fig. 29-9). Lesions consist of a progressive glomerulosclerosis and myriad tubulointerstitial disease primarily involving the convoluted proximal tubule (Fig. 29-10).[27] The most striking change in renal function is a proteinuria level exceeding 10 mg/day that progressively increases in severity with age. The features of CPN are qualitatively similar among different strains of laboratory rats, but the onset, incidence, and severity of the disease vary considerably. The disease occurs earlier and is of greater severity in males than in females; urinary protein excretion averaging 137 mg/day has been documented in

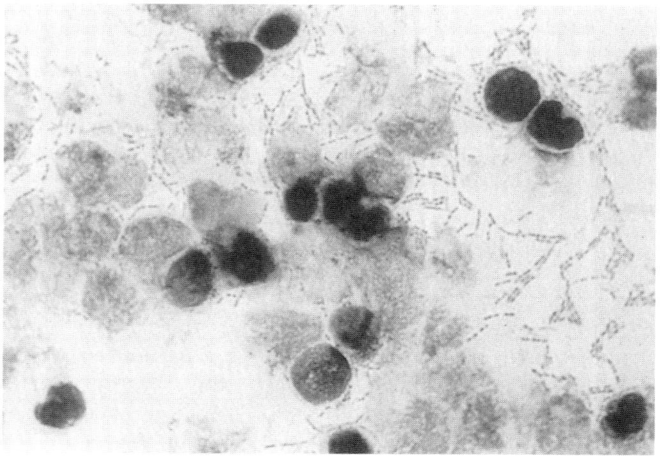

Figure 29-8 Photomicrograph of a Giemsa-stained smear from a rat with a nasal exudate. Multiple diplococci characteristic of *Streptococcus pneumoniae* are visible. The polymorphonuclear cells characteristic of purulent exudate are clearly evident.

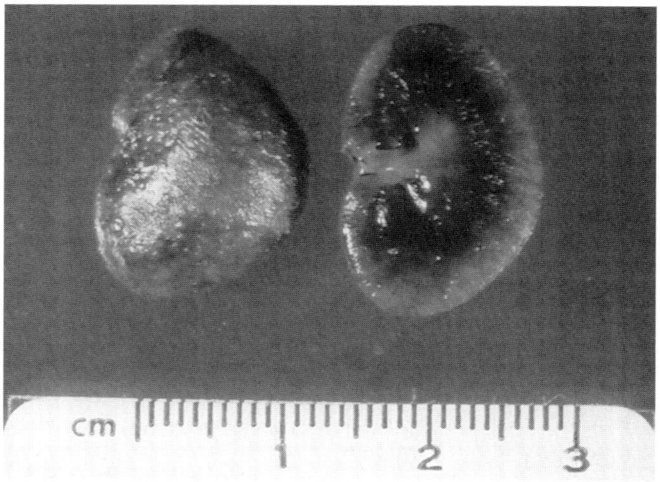

Figure 29-9 Enlarged, pale kidneys from a rat with chronic progressive nephrosis. Note the pitted, mottled surface containing pinpoint cysts.

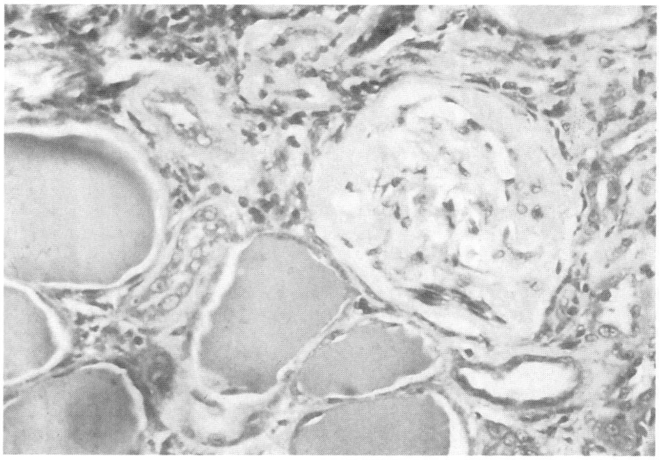

Figure 29-10 Photomicrograph of severe glomerulosclerosis in a rat. The proximal tubules are dilated and contain copious amounts of a protein-rich material; this finding indicates the deterioration of glomeruli that fail to filter and retain plasma protein.

18-month-old male Sprague-Dawley rats, whereas excretion averaging 76 mg/day was reported in female rats of the same age.[65] Dietary factors appear to have an important role in the progression of CPN. Restricting calories, feeding diets low in protein (4%-7%), and limiting the source of dietary protein reduce the incidence and severity of CPN. Feeding soy protein (as opposed to casein) and substantially restricting calories reduce the incidence and severity of CPN; feeding low-calorie diets that contain high protein levels does not. Exposure to drugs and chemicals also exacerbates CPN. Treatment is supportive and involves feeding a low-protein diet and administering anabolic steroids.

Ocular system The harderian glands of rats are located behind the eyes. They secrete various porphyrins that give the tears a reddish color. Harderian gland secretion increases in response to stress and disease, and the tears dry around the eyes and external nares (the nasolacrimal duct drains into the nasal cavity), resembling crusts of blood (Fig. 29-11). Owners commonly report bleeding from the eyes and nose of their pet rats. The porphyrins fluoresce under ultraviolet light and can be readily differentiated from blood with a Wood's lamp. The condition is known as chromodacryorrhea or red tears, and although it is not pathologic, it is a consequence of acute-onset stress such as that caused by pain, illness, or restraint. Red tears often indicate a chronic underlying disease, and their presence warrants a thorough evaluation of the affected pet rat.

Hamsters Although many types of hamsters live in the wild, only a few types are kept as pets. The most common is the golden or Syrian hamster (*Mesocricetus auratus*), which has been kept as a pet since the 1940s. Although two other species of hamsters, the common or European hamster (*Cricetus cricetus*) and the ratlike Chinese hamster (*Cricetulus griseus*) are used in research, they do not make good pets because of their aggressive nature. However, dwarf hamsters such as the Djungarian (*Phodopus sungorus*) and Roborovski (*Phodopus roborovskii*) are being seen increasingly as pets because they have a docile disposition, do not attempt to bite or run away, and do well in captivity. Very few reports of spontaneous diseases in these animals have been published; Cantrell and Padovan have prepared the most complete review to date on this subject.[11] The description of diseases refers to Syrian hamsters.

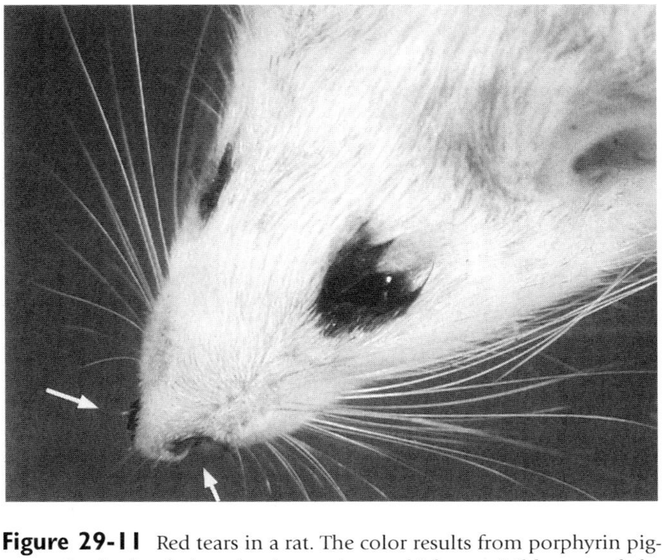

Figure 29-11 Red tears in a rat. The color results from porphyrin pigments in the harderian gland secretions, which are visible around the nares (*arrows*).

Integumentary system and marking glands The most common skin problem seen in hamsters is haircoat roughness. This is a nonspecific sign of fighting, aging, and a variety of diseases. Female hamsters are heavier than males and generally are more aggressive, not only toward other hamsters, but also their owners. They can inflict severe bite wounds on cagemates, and nonestrous females can be especially aggressive toward young males and may kill them.

Hamsters have distensible cheek pouches that may be mistaken for lesions by the owner.[9] Sometimes the cheek pouches become impacted, and the material must be removed from the pouches with fine forceps. A radiograph of the head often shows the extent of the impaction.[61] Predisposing causes of impaction, such as malocclusion of incisors or molars, should be investigated. Male hamsters have large, pendulous testes and pigmented sebaceous flank glands, which clients may mistake for tumors.

Digestive system The most common problems seen in pet hamsters are enteropathies. Diarrhea may occur in hamsters of any age and is known as *wet-tail*, although this euphemism is frequently used to describe the disease in young hamsters. Proliferative ileitis is the most significant intestinal disease of 3-to10-week-old hamsters and results in a high mortality rate. It is caused by the intracellular bacterium *Lawsonia intracellularis*, which is also responsible for proliferative enteropathy in pigs and ferrets.[43,57] Treatment must be aggressive and involves correcting any life-threatening electrolyte imbalance, administering antibiotics, and force-feeding. Several antibiotic treatments are recommended, including tetracycline hydrochloride (400 mg/L of drinking water for 10 days), tetracycline (10 mg/kg PO q12h for 5-7 days), enrofloxacin (10 mg/kg PO or IM q12h for 5-7 days), and trimethoprim-sulfa combination (30 mg/kg PO q12h for 5-7 days). Symptomatic treatment with bismuth subsalicylate may be given if diarrhea persists. Give replacement electrolyte and glucose solutions orally, and administer electrolyte replacement fluids such as saline or lactated Ringer's solution at a dose of 20 mL/100 g q24h. Offer liquid food such as pureed baby spinach, apples, carrots, and lettuce mixed in equal parts with a slurry made from rodent pellets, or offer a nutritional supplement such as Critical Care (Oxbow Pet Products). Adding 1 tablespoon of honey to the feed mixture may make it more palatable. If the hamster does not eat, force-feed small amounts of liquid feed. Potential sequelae to proliferative ileitis in surviving hamsters are obstruction, intussusception, or rectal prolapse (see Chapter 30).[16]

Diarrhea in adult hamsters is associated with enterotoxemia caused by *Clostridium difficile* and may develop 3 to 5 days after treatment with antibiotics such as penicillin, lincomycin, or bacitracin. Bovine antibodies against toxigenic *C. difficile* administered orally will protect hamsters against experimental antibiotic-associated enterotoxemia.[47]

Tyzzer's disease (*Clostridium piliforme*, previously known as *Bacillus piliformis*) was described in hamsters and gerbils obtained from a pet store supplier.[51] In this outbreak, hamsters and gerbils had a high mortality rate but the rats and mice did not. Affected rodents were depressed and dehydrated and had scruffy coats and diarrhea; many animals had no clinical signs before death. The authors concluded that the clinical outbreak was precipitated by severe stress, including that caused by overcrowding, high environmental temperature and humidity, heavy internal and external parasite load, and nutritionally inadequate diets, despite the prophylactic treatment of drinking water with oxytetracycline. Tyzzer's disease, first recognized in 1917 in a colony of Japanese waltzing mice by Tyzzer at Harvard,[72] is frequently listed in laboratory animal textbooks as an intestinal disease of rodents and other animals. However, the actual prevalence of the infection in rodents is unknown. The report concerning the pet store illustrates the opportunistic nature of *C. piliforme* in immunosuppressed animals. The disease is not seen in healthy immunocompetent animals.

Weight loss is seen in aged hamsters and is often associated with hepatic and renal amyloidosis. One research report described amyloidosis in 88% of hamsters older than 18 months of age.[26] In long-term research studies, amyloidosis is described as the principal cause of death in laboratory hamsters, with a higher incidence, increased severity, and earlier age of onset in female hamsters than in male hamsters.[62] Social stress induced by crowding correlates with the incidence of disease.[25] In pet hamsters, the incidence and clinical signs of amyloidosis have not been described and, because overcrowding is usually not a problem, the incidence may be low. However, if the condition is present, clinicians should expect edema and ascites caused by hypoproteinemia of hepatic and renal origin. If amyloidosis is diagnosed in a pet hamster, the prognosis is poor and treatment supportive.

Respiratory system In one survey, 6 of 14 laboratories in the United States reported pneumonia as the second most common clinical condition in hamsters after diarrhea.[60] An earlier survey conducted in Germany noted respiratory infections in 8% of all clinical conditions in hamsters.[45] Histologic evidence of bronchopneumonia resembling bacterial pneumonia and of interstitial pneumonia resembling viral pneumonia has been described, but there are no reports of observed clinical cases. Consequently, other authors have stated that respiratory disease is uncommon in hamsters.[28] The true prevalence remains to be established.

Purulent rhinitis associated with pneumonia and sticky eyelids has been described in hamsters and is associated with a poor prognosis.[38] Bacterial pneumonias, especially those caused by *Streptococcus* species, may be inadvertently transmitted by children to pet hamsters. Rapid diagnosis can be made by identifying the characteristic gram-positive diplococci on a Gram stain of a sample of nasal and ocular discharges. Follow-up culture and treatment with chloramphenicol (chloramphenicol palmitate, 50 mg/kg PO q8h; chloramphenicol succinate, 30 mg/kg IV or IM q8h) are recommended until antibiotic sensitivity results are available.[2]

Reproductive system Female hamsters have a 4-day estrous cycle that ends with a copious postovulatory discharge. The discharge is creamy white and has a distinctive odor; it fills the vagina and usually extrudes through the vaginal orifice (female hamsters have three orifices: urinary, genital, and anal). Its stringy nature is distinctive, and if touched it can be drawn out as a thread of about 4 to 6 inches in length. Owners often describe the discharge as pus and mistakenly believe it to be abnormal.

Pyometra has been observed clinically, although rarely, in pet hamsters. A tentative diagnosis is made by ultrasound examination of the abdomen, and ovariohysterectomy is the treatment of choice.

In group-housed laboratory female hamsters, cannibalism of young accounts for about 95% of all preweaning mortality.[60] Other factors such as cold ambient temperatures (<50 °F [10 °C]), lean diets, and low body weight (especially during pregnancy) appear to increase cannibalism.[63,64] Instruct the owners of pet hamsters to give the mother ample food and water and to leave her alone in a quiet, warm place for at least 1 or preferably 2 weeks. Disturbing the mother by handling the young or nest and not providing adequate nesting material, warmth, food, or water often results in litter desertion and cannibalism.

Cardiovascular system Atrial thrombosis has been described in aging research hamsters,[33] and in certain strains the incidence is high (up to 73%).[12] Most thromboses develop in the left atrium from heart failure and lead to a consumptive coagulopathy (Fig. 29-12). Although the incidence does not differ between the sexes in aged hamsters, atrial thrombosis occurs on average at a younger age in females (13.5 months) than in males (21.5 months).[12] Aged pet hamsters have clinical signs of cardiomyopathy such as hyperpnea, tachycardia, and cyanosis. Untreated hamsters typically die within 1 week after these signs are evident. The endocrine status of the animal and especially the amount of circulating androgens influence the incidence of atrial thrombosis. Thus castration of male hamsters is linked to an increase in the prevalence of atrial thrombosis.[66]

Cardiomyopathy should be suspected in aged pet hamsters (older than 1.5 years) that present clinically with signs of tachypnea, lethargy, anorexia, and cold extremities. Diagnosis is based on clinical signs and results of radiography and ultrasonography of the heart. Treatment of heart disease is symptomatic and involves empirical use of digoxin, diuretics, angiotensin-converting enzyme inhibitors, and prophylactic anticoagulants. Recommended dosages for hamsters are available for some of these drugs; otherwise, extrapolate dosages from those used in ferrets and closely monitor the response. Verapamil, a calcium antagonist, administered at a dose increasing from 0.25 mg to 0.50 mg SC q8h over a 4-week period, prevented severe myocardial lesions in untreated 2-month-old inbred female myopathic hamsters.[39]

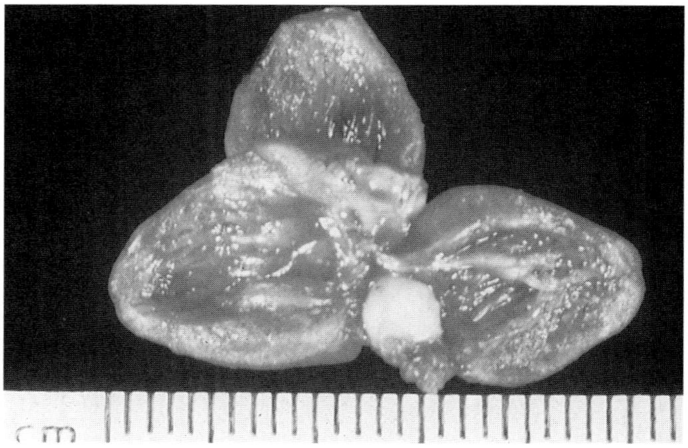

Figure 29-12 Thrombosis in the atria of the heart of a hamster caused by cardiomyopathy. (Courtesy Heidi L. Hoefer, DVM.)

Endocrine system Surveys of spontaneous lesions in laboratory hamsters describe a high incidence of adrenocortical hyperplasia and adenoma.[62] However, despite extensive histopathologic study, there has been only one clinical report of hyperadrenocorticism, or Cushing's disease, in three hamsters, with high serum cortisol concentrations documented in only one of the three animals.[5] Hamsters with clinical signs resembling those of Cushing's disease are occasionally seen in practice (Fig. 29-13). Diagnosis is based on documenting classic signs seen in dogs, such as a history of polydipsia, polyuria, and polyphagia; clinical signs of alopecia and hyperpigmentation; and high concentrations of plasma cortisol and serum alkaline phosphatase. Reference values of cortisol concentrations are low compared with those of other species and range from 0.5 to 1.0 μg/dL in normal males and females.[76] Hamsters may secrete both cortisol and corticosterone[56]; therefore, at present, meaningful measurement of plasma cortisol concentrations in hamsters is empirical. If hyperadrenocorticism is suspected, the cause, such as hypersecretion by a functional tumor, primary adrenal hyperplasia, or excess adrenocorticotropic hormone production, often is more difficult to determine. Hamsters respond to exogenous adrenocorticotropic hormone stimulation.[76] In the clinical report of the three hamsters, one hamster that was treated with metyrapone (8 mg PO q24h for 1 month) responded well; another hamster treated with o,p′-DDD (mitotane) (5 mg PO q24h for 1 month) did not improve and was then given a similar dose of metyrapone, also without success.[4] Further research needs to be done on this syndrome.

Ocular system Exophthalmos is common in hamsters. It is usually a result of ocular infection or trauma to the periorbital area, or it occurs iatrogenically during restraint. Hamsters with sialodacryoadenitis (caused by cytomegalovirus infection) may develop keratoconjunctivitis sicca, exophthalmos, and subsequent proptosis. Occasionally, a hamster's eye is displaced forward if the caregiver restrains the animal too tightly by holding the skin at the back of the neck. If the hamster is treated soon after the exophthalmos occurs, then the prognosis for saving the eye is good. Cleanse the ocular area gently with an ophthalmic wash, and lubricate the eye with sterile ophthalmic lubricant. Gently retract the lid margins around the globe until the eye returns to its normal position. Treat the eye with an antibiotic ophthalmic ointment for a minimum of 7 to 10 days. Occasionally, tarsorrhaphy is needed to prevent recurrence. Enucleation may be necessary if the eye cannot be replaced or if it has been severely traumatized.

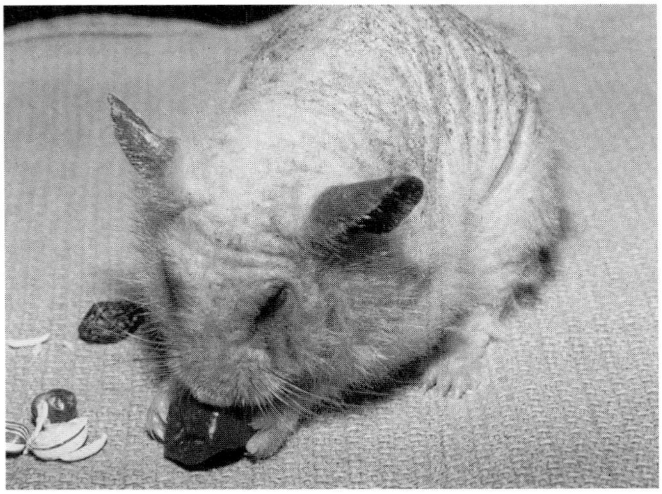

Figure 29-13 Generalized alopecia associated with adrenocortical hyperplasia in a hamster.

Neoplasia Lymphoma is the most common neoplasm in Syrian hamsters. Clinicians see three variations. In older hamsters, lymphoma is the most frequently observed neoplasm of the hematopoietic system.[71] These tumors are often multicentric, involving the thymus, thoracic lymph nodes, mesenteric lymph nodes, superficial lymph nodes, spleen, liver, and other sites. Cytology of the tumors is variable. A second variation, cutaneous lymphoma, which resembles mycosis fungoides, an epidermotropic T-cell lymphoma in humans, is seen in adult hamsters.[29] Lethargy, anorexia, weight loss, patchy alopecia, and exfoliative erythroderma have been described in affected animals. Pathologists have noted dense infiltrates of neoplastic lymphocytes in the dermis, with extension into the epidermis. The third variation is an epizootic of lymphoma in young hamsters. The causative agent is hamster polyomavirus (HaPV).[4] When HaPV is first introduced into a naive population of breeding hamsters, an epizootic of lymphoma, with an incidence as high as 80%, can result. Once enzootic in a hamster population, the occurrence of lymphoma declines to a much lower level. Enzootically infected hamsters develop HaPV skin tumors rather than lymphoma. Hamsters with HaPV lymphoma appear thin, often with palpable abdominal masses. Tumors often arise in the mesentery but can arise in the axillary and cervical lymph nodes. The tumors are often lymphoid, but erythroblastic, reticulosarcomatous, and myeloid types occur. Anecdotal reports of chemotherapy in hamsters have been based on protocols using drugs that can be administered subcutaneously, orally, or intraperitoneally at dosages used in other small animals.

Gerbils

Integumentary system and marking glands Facial eczema, sore nose, and nasal dermatitis all describe a common skin condition seen in gerbils. Clinical lesions adjacent to the external nares appear erythematous initially; these lesions progress to localized alopecia and then to an extensive moist dermatitis (Fig. 29-14). The cause is believed to be an increase in the secretion of porphyrins by the harderian gland (as in chromodacryorrhea in rats), which act as a primary skin irritant. Various staphylococcal species (*S. aureus* and *S. xylosus*) may act synergistically to produce the dermatitis.[10,68] Stress may cause excessive harderian gland secretion. Two examples of stress are overcrowding and exposure to an environmental humidity of greater than 50% (in this case, the coat stands out and appears matted instead of lying sleekly against the body). Gerbils require sandbathing to keep their coats from becoming oily. Keeping the gerbil in a dry environment, cleaning its face, and providing soft clay or sand bedding instead of abrasive wood chip bedding usually alleviate the problem. Use topical or parenteral antibiotics (except streptomycin) in gerbils with severe dermatitis.

The tail of gerbils is covered by thin skin. Unlike rats or mice, if a gerbil is picked up by the tip of its tail, the skin often slips off, leaving a raw, exposed tail that eventually becomes necrotic and sheds (Fig. 29-15). If the tail skin is lost, surgically amputate the bare tail where the skin ends. The tail usually sloughs if it is left untreated. When picking up a gerbil, avoid grasping the

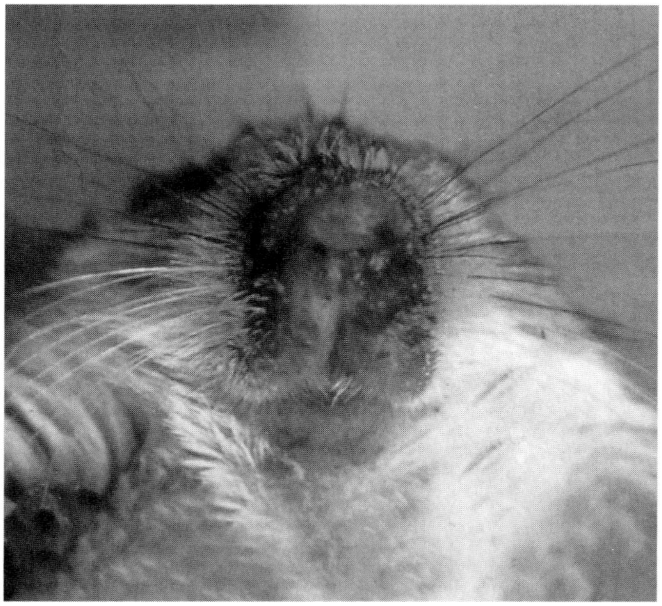

Figure 29-14 Sore nose (facial eczema, nasal dermatitis) in a gerbil. This condition may result from an increase in harderian gland secretion complicated by infection with *Staphylococcus* species.

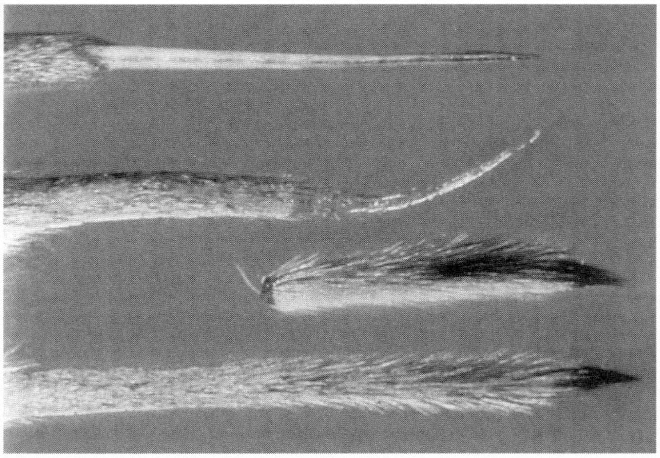

Figure 29-15 One normal *(bottom)* and two *(top)* gerbil tails with varying degrees of tail-slip. Tail-slip can result from the restraint of a gerbil by its tail.

tail unless it is gently held at the base. The best holding technique involves placing the palm of the hand over the gerbil's back and encircling the body with thumb and fingers. Gerbils bite if they are not handled securely, despite the claim in many reviews that they rarely bite human handlers regardless of provocation.

Gerbils have large, ventral, abdominal marking glands that are androgen dependent (Fig. 29-16). Owners may mistake this normal ventral gland for a tumor. In aged animals, the gland may become infected or neoplastic. Local debridement and topical antibiotic ointments are indicated for treatment of infected glands. Do a wide excisional biopsy if you suspect a tumor such as adenocarcinoma.

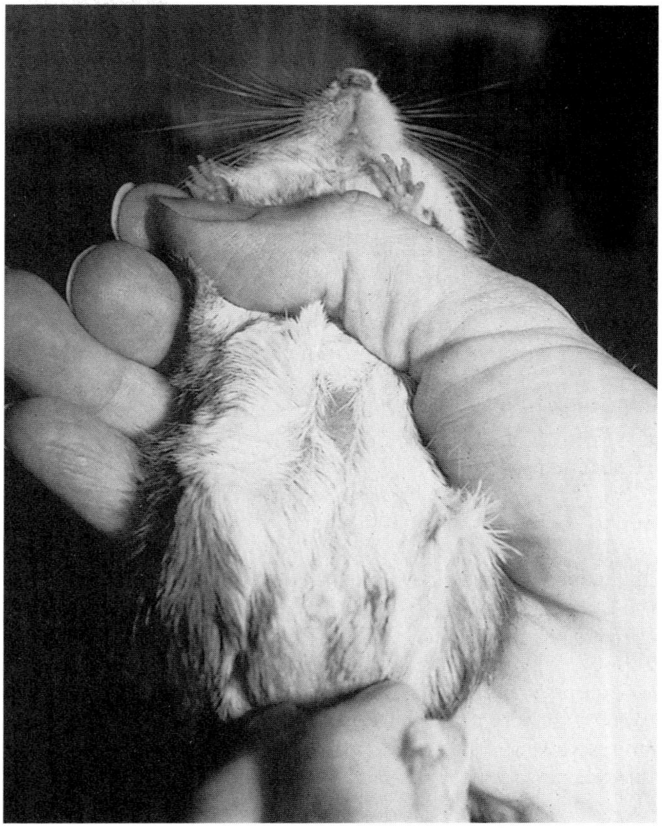

Figure 29-16 Ventral marking glands on a male gerbil.

Digestive system Naturally occurring Tyzzer's disease is the most frequently described fatal infectious disease of gerbils.[13,36,51,59,77] In reported cases, common findings were sudden death or death after a short illness and the presence of multiple foci of hepatic necrosis. Diarrhea and gross and microscopic lesions in the intestinal tract were variably present. Experimentally induced Tyzzer's disease in gerbils has confirmed that these animals are extremely susceptible to infection[74]; the probable route of infection is oral. Gerbils exposed to infected bedding contract the disease.

Gerbils will develop spontaneous, insidious periodontal disease if fed a standard rat or mouse diet for more than 6 months.[73] On the same diet, approximately 10% of animals become obese, and some may even develop diabetes. Various pelleted commercial diets are available that are suitable for rats, mice, hamsters, and gerbils.

Central nervous system Approximately 20% to 40% of gerbils develop reflex, stereotypic, epileptiform (clonic-tonic) seizures beginning at 2 months of age. The susceptibility is inherited, seen in selectively bred lines, and is caused by a deficiency in cerebral glutamine synthetase.[40] There is no treatment. Most animals outgrow the behavior with time. The seizures generally pass in a few minutes; they may be mild or severe and have no lasting effects.

Reproductive system Cystic ovaries are reported to occur frequently in laboratory Mongolian gerbils.[54] Removal of the affected ovary is recommended.

Tumors and aging After 2 to 3 years of age, approximately 25% to 40% of gerbils develop neoplasia.[49,73] Squamous cell carcinoma of the sebaceous ventral marking gland in males and ovarian granulosa cell tumor in females account for 80% of tumors seen in animals older than 3 years. Besides neoplasia, older gerbils have a high incidence of chronic interstitial nephritis.[8] Aged gerbils have a remarkable propensity for the development of aural cholesteatoma, a nonneoplastic keratinizing epithelial mass that occurs in the middle ear and mastoid region, erodes bone, and invades the labyrinth and the cranial cavity.[14]

Degus Degus, or trumpet-tail rats, are native to Chile. Taxonomically, they are in the same diverse order as guinea pigs and chinchillas. Degus have been used as laboratory animals for 20 years, but there are very few reports on naturally occurring diseases. One report describes a 3-month-old pet degu with a tibial fracture that was repaired by medullary fixation.[7] Like chinchillas, captive degus must be provided with a dust bath twice a week.[1] Although degus do not drink much water, owners should change water bottles regularly to prevent bacterial overgrowth. The testicles of male degus are intraabdominal and the method of castration is by laparotomy.[20]

Integumentary system Clinicians should not hold degus by the tail because they will spin like a top, leaving the veterinarian holding only the skin. Degus familiar with their owners do not show this behavior and tail shedding is uncommon.[1]

Endocrine and ocular system Degus develop spontaneous diabetes mellitus caused by amyloidosis of Langerhans islets. Cellular infiltration of Langerhans islets induced by cytomegalovirus, alpha cell crystals with the presence of a herpes-type virus, and foods such as guinea pig chow or fresh fruit that increase blood glucose concentrations are also associated with the development of diabetes in degus.[22,53,69] Owners should feed degus a commercial rodent diet supplemented with vegetables. Like prairie dogs, it is easy to overfeed degus and obesity is likely to occur. No treatments have been described for diabetic degus.

Degus can develop cataracts within 4 weeks of the onset of diabetes.[17] A congenital cataract unrelated to diabetes has also been described.[78]

Neoplasms Various neoplasms have been described in degus. Hepatocellular carcinoma is the most frequently described; however, there have been only four reported cases in animals 5 to 6 years of age.[50,52] Other reported tumors include bronchioloalveolar carcinoma,[3] reticulum cell sarcoma,[52] splenic hemangioma,[52] lipoma,[52] rhabdomyosarcoma,[50] and transitional cell carcinoma.[44]

MEDICATION AND ANTIBIOTIC THERAPY IN PET RODENTS

Because of the small size of pet rodents, even pediatric-strength medications often must be diluted for use in these species. Knowing the precise weight of the animal, diluting medications, and administering medications with a tuberculin or insulin syringe will increase dosing accuracy. Medication often is given by mixing it into feed or water. However, rats do not drink if they find the taste of their water objectionable. Ball-ended dosing needles are ideal for gavage, but always carefully calculate the volume of the dose and depth of penetration when using the dosing needle to prevent gastric rupture. Intravenous injections are difficult to administer; intraperitoneal injection (for anesthetics), intramuscular, or subcutaneous injections are commonly substituted.

Exercise caution when administering antibiotics to rodents. Streptomycin and procaine are toxic in mice; nitrofurantoin causes neuropathologic lesions in rats; and gerbils cannot tolerate dihydrostreptomycin and streptomycin. Hamsters are similar to guinea pigs in their susceptibility to clostridial enterotoxemia when they are given penicillins, erythromycin, or lincomycin. Many antibiotics are added to the drinking water of pet rodents, but the water must contain high concentrations and fresh solutions must be prepared daily to achieve therapeutic levels. As an example, tetracycline is often added to the drinking water of rats and mice at a dose of 5 mg/mL for the treatment of respiratory mycoplasmosis. Rats often do not drink the medicated water because of its unpleasant taste. Some researchers add sugar to the water to encourage drinking, but such supplementation is controversial.

Antibiotics that are apparently safe to use in rodents (especially guinea pigs and hamsters) include enrofloxacin, ciprofloxacin, trimethoprim-sulfa combinations, and chloramphenicol. Other sulfonamides, tetracycline, and piperacillin should be used sparingly in hamsters, and ampicillin and amoxicillin should be avoided (see Chapter 28). Many compounding pharmacies can now prepare medications in flavored syrups or treats that are palatable to rodents.

CLIENT EDUCATION

Most clients purchase books on pet rodents in pet stores and often rely on the recommendations of the pet store owner before asking for advice from a veterinarian. Unfortunately, many of the available owner's manuals are not familiar to veterinarians. Having some knowledge about pet rodents from these handbooks, clients often raise questions about what they have read, and clinicians may not appear well informed from the client's perspective if they are unfamiliar with their references. The rodent owners then often return to the pet store owner for guidance; unless their animals are very sick, the owners do not return to the veterinarians for advice on husbandry and diseases. At this point, the prognosis for very ill pets is poor.

Familiarity with the pet hobbyist literature breaks the cycle of mistrust and ignorance. Many hobby books on pet rodents are highly entertaining and informative about the husbandry and biology of the animals. However, the medical information in these books should be carefully reviewed by the veterinarian. Purchasing some of these books and then recommending them to pet rodent owners is an effective method of educating clients and establishing a good rapport with them. The books are generally less expensive than veterinary textbooks and are written for a range of age groups (e.g., children and parents) and levels of interest. Barron's Educational Series and Dorling Kindersley are two reputable publishers of readily available books. TFH Publications, another reputable publisher, no longer publishes. Access www.tfh.com for availability of titles.

REFERENCES

1. Altmann D, Schwendenwein I, Wagner K: Zu biologie, haltung, ernahrung und erkrankungen des degus (*Octodon degus*). Erkrankungen Der Zootiere 1994; 36:277-292.
2. Anderson NL: Pet rodents. *In* Birchard SJ, Sherding RG, eds. Saunders Manual of Small Animal Practice, 2nd ed. Philadelphia, WB Saunders, 1999, pp 1512-1538.
3. Anderson WI, Steinberg H, King JM: Bronchioloalveolar carcinoma with renal and hepatic metastases in a degu (*Octodon degus*). J Wildlife Dis 1990; 26:129-131.
4. Barthold SW, Bhatt PN, Johnson EA: Further evidence for papovavirus as the probable etiology of transmissible lymphoma of Syrian hamsters. Lab Anim Sci 1987; 37:283-288.
5. Bauck L, Orr JP, Lawrence KH: Hyperadrenocorticism in three teddy bear hamsters. Can Vet J 1984; 25:247-250.
6. Baumans V, Havenaar R, van Herck H, et al: The effectiveness of Ivomec and Neguvon in the control of murine mites. Lab Anim 1988; 22:243-245.
7. Beregi A, Felkai F, Seregi J, et al: Medullary fixation of a tibial fracture in a three-month-old degu (*Octogon degus*). Vet Rec 1994; 134:652-653.
8. Bingel SA: Pathologic findings in an aging Mongolian gerbil (*Meriones unguiculatus*) colony. Lab Anim Sci 1995; 45: 597-600.
9. Bivin WS, Olsen GH, Murray KA: Morphophysiology. *In* Van Hoosier GL, McPherson CW, eds. Laboratory Hamsters. Orlando, Academic Press, 1987, pp 9-41.
10. Bresnahan JF, Smith GD, Lentsch RH, et al: Nasal dermatitis in the Mongolian gerbil. Lab Anim Sci 1983; 33:258-263.
11. Cantrell CA, Padovan D: Biology, care, and use in research. *In* Van Hoosier GL, McPherson CW, eds. Laboratory Hamsters. Orlando, Academic Press, 1987, pp 369-387.
12. Carlton WW: Spontaneous cardiac lesions. *In* Proceedings of the ILSI Histopathology Seminar on the Cardiovascular System of Laboratory Animals. Orlando, International Life Sciences Institute, 1991.
13. Carter GR, Whitenack DL, Julius LA: Natural Tyzzer's disease in Mongolian gerbils (*Meriones unguiculatus*). Lab Anim Care 1969; 19:648-651.
14. Chole RA, Henry KR, McGinn MD: Cholesteatoma: spontaneous occurrence in the Mongolian gerbil *Meriones unguiculatis*. Am J Otol 1981; 2:204-210.
15. Committee on Infectious Diseases of Mice and Rats, Commission on Life Sciences, National Research Council: Infectious Diseases of Mice and Rats. Washington, DC, National Academy Press, 1991.
16. Cunnane SC, Bloom SR: Intussusception in the Syrian golden hamster. Br J Nutr 1990; 63:231-237.
17. Datiles MBD, Fukui H: Cataract prevention in diabetic *Octodon degus* with Pfizer's sorbinil. Curr Eye Res 1989; 8:233-237.
18. Donnelly TM, Rush EM, Lackner PA: Ringworm in small exotic pets. Semin Avian Exotic Pet Med 2000; 9:82-93.
19. Donnelly TM, Stark DM: Susceptibility of laboratory rats, hamsters, and mice to wound infection with *Staphylococcus aureus*. Am J Vet Res 1985; 46:2634-2638.
20. Fehr M, Schanen H, Grof D, et al: Anatomical basics and description of a method of castration in the degus [in German]. Kleintierpraxis 1994; 39:837-840.
21. Flynn BM, Brown PA, Eckstein JM, et al: Treatment of *Syphacia obvelata* in mice using ivermectin. Lab Anim Sci 1989; 39:461-463.
22. Fox JG, Murphy JC: Cytomegalic virus-associated insulitis in diabetic *Octodon degus*. Vet Pathol 1979; 16:625-628.
23. Friedman S, Weisbroth SH: The parasitic ecology of the rodent mite, *Myobia musculi*. IV. Life cycle. Lab Anim Sci 1977; 27:34-37.
24. Georg LK: Animal ringworm in public health. Washington, DC, US Department of Health, Education, and Welfare, 1960, Report No 727.
25. Germann PG, Kohler M, Ernst H, et al: The relation of amyloidosis to social stress induced by crowding in the Syrian hamster (*Mesocricetus auratus*). Zeitschrift fur Versuchstierkunde 1990; 33:271-275.
26. Gleiser CA, Van Hoosier GL, Sheldon WG, et al: Amyloidosis and renal paramyloid in a closed hamster colony. Lab Anim Sci 1971; 21:197-202.
27. Gray JE: Chronic progressive nephrosis, rat. *In* Jones TC, Mohr U, Hunt RD, eds. Urinary System. Berlin, Springer-Verlag, 1986, pp 174-178.
28. Harkness JE: A practitioner's guide to domestic rodents. Denver, American Animal Hospital Association, 1993.
29. Harvey RG, Whitbread TJ, Ferrer L, et al: Epidermotropic cutaneous T-cell lymphoma (*Mycosis fungoides*) in Syrian hamsters (*Mesocricetus auratus*). A report of six cases and the demonstration of T-cell specificity. Vet Derm 1992; 3:13-19.
30. Heider K, Eustis SL: Tumors of the soft tissues. *In* Turusov VS, Mohr U, eds. Tumours of the mouse, 2nd ed. Lyon, International Agency for Research on Cancer, 1994, pp 611-631.
31. Herweg C, Kunstyr I: Effect of intestinal flagellate *Spironucleus [Hexamita] muris* and of dimetridazole on intestinal microflora in thymus-deficient (nude) mice. Zentralblatt fur Bakteriologie, Parasitenkunde, Infektionskrankheiten and Hygiene, Abteilung, 1, Originale A 1979; 245:262-269.
32. Hotchkiss CE: Effect of surgical removal of subcutaneous tumors on survival of rats. J Am Vet Med Assoc 1995; 206:1575-1579.
33. Hubbard GB, Schmidt RE: Noninfectious diseases. *In* Van Hoosier GL, McPherson CW, eds. Laboratory Hamsters. Orlando, Academic Press, 1987, pp 169-178.
34. Huerkamp MJ: Correspondence [letter]. Lab Anim Sci 1990; 40:5.
35. Kohn DF, Barthold SW: Biology and diseases of rats. *In* Fox JG, Cohen JB, Loew FM, eds. Laboratory Animal Medicine. Orlando, Academic Press, 1984, pp 91-122.
36. Koopman JP, Mullink JW, Kennis HM, et al: An outbreak of Tyzzer's disease in Mongolian gerbils (*Meriones unguiculatus*). Z Versuchstierkd 1980; 22:336-341.
37. Krogstad AP, Franklin CL, Besch-Williford CL: An epidemiological and diagnostic approach to murine skin lesions [abstract]. Proceedings of the 52nd American Association for Laboratory Animal Science National Meeting, Baltimore, 2001, p 94.
38. Kuntze A: Diseases of guinea-pigs and golden hamsters important in practice. [German.] Monatshefte fur Veterinarmedizin 1992; 47:143-147.
39. Kuo TH, Ho KL, Wiener J: The role of alkaline protease in the development of cardiac lesions in myopathic hamsters: effect of verapamil treatment. Biochem Med 1984; 32:207-215.
40. Laming PR, Cosby SL, O'Neill JK: Seizures in the Mongolian gerbil are related to a deficiency in cerebral glutamine synthetase. Comp Biochem Physiol C 1989; 94:399-404.
41. Lancefield RC: Group A streptococcal infections in animals—natural and experimental. *In* Wannamaker LW, Matsen JM, eds. Streptococci and Streptococcal Diseases. New York, Academic Press, 1972, pp 313-326.
42. Lawson GA, Sato A, Schwiebert RS, et al: The efficacy of Derm Caps in the treatment of ulcerative dermatitis in C57BL/6 mice and related strains [abstract]. *In* Proceedings of the 52nd American Association for Laboratory Animal Science National Meeting, Baltimore, 2001, p 78.
43. Lawson GHK, Gebhart CJ: Proliferative enteropathy. J Comp Pathol 2000; 122:77-100.
44. Lester PA, Rush HG, Sigler RE: Renal transitional cell carcinoma and choristoma in a degu (*Octodon degu*). *In* Proceedings of the 52nd American Association for Laboratory Animal Science National Meeting, Baltimore, 2001, p 99.

45. Lindt VS: Uber krankheiten des syrischen goldhamsters (*Mesocricetus auratus*). Schweizer Archiv fur Tierheilkunde 1958; 100:86-97.
46. Livingston RS, Simmons JH, Purdy GA, et al: Serologic diagnosis of rat respiratory virus (RRV) infection [abstract]. *In* Proceedings of 52nd American Association for Laboratory Animal Science National Meeting Baltimore, 2001, p 70.
47. Lyerly DM, Bostwick EF, Binion SB, et al: Passive immunization of hamsters against disease caused by *Clostridium difficile* by use of bovine immunoglobulin G concentrate. Infect Immun 1991; 59:2215-2218.
48. Matsumoto M, Kotani M, Fujita A, et al: Therapeutic effects of persimmon leaf extract on atopic eczema in NC/Nga mice. [Japanese.] Nippon Eiyo Shokuryo Gakkaishi [J Jap Soc Nutrition Food Sci] 2001; 54:3-7.
49. Matsuoka K, Suzuki J: Spontaneous tumors in the Mongolian gerbil (*Meriones unguiculatus*). [Japanese.] Exp Anim 1995; 43:755-760.
50. Montali RJ: An overview of tumors in zoo animals. *In* Montali RJ, Migaki G, eds. The Comparative Pathology of Zoo Animals. Washington, DC, Smithsonian Institution Press, 1980, pp 531-542.
51. Motzel SL, Gibson SV: Tyzzer disease in hamsters and gerbils from a pet store supplier. J Am Vet Med Assoc 1990; 197:1176-1178.
52. Murphy JC, Crowell TP, Hewes KM, et al: Spontaneous lesions in the degu (*Rodentia, Hystricomorpha: Octodon degus*). *In* Montali RJ, Migaki G, eds. The Comparative Pathology of Zoo Animals. Washington, DC, Smithsonian Institution Press, 1980, pp 437-444.
53. Najecki D, Tate B: Husbandry and management of the degu. Lab Anim 1999; 28:54-62.
54. Norris ML, Adams CE: Incidence of cystic ovaries and reproductive performance in the Mongolian gerbil, *Meriones unguiculatus*. Lab Anim 1972; 6:337-342.
55. Nowak RM: Walker's Mammals of the World, 6th ed. Baltimore, The Johns Hopkins University Press, 1999.
56. Ottenweller JE, Tapp WN, Burke JM, et al: Plasma cortisol and corticosterone concentrations in the golden hamster (*Mesocricetus auratus*). Life Sci 1985; 37:1551-1558.
57. Peace TA, Brock KV, Stills HF Jr: Comparative analysis of the 16S rRNA gene sequence of the putative agent of proliferative ileitis of hamsters. Int J Syst Bacteriol 1994; 44:832-835.
58. Percy DH, Greenwood JD, Blake B, et al: Diagnostic exercise: sloughing of limb extremities in immunocompromised suckling mice. Contemp Top Lab Anim Sci 1994; 33:66-67.
59. Port CD, Richter WR, Moise SM: Tyzzer's disease in the gerbil (*Meriones unguiculatus*). Lab Anim Care 1970; 20:109-111.
60. Renshaw HW, Van Hoosier GL Jr, Amend NK: A survey of naturally occurring diseases of the Syrian hamster. Lab Anim 1975; 9:179-191.
61. Rübel GA, Isenbügel E, Wolvekamp P: Atlas of Diagnostic Radiology of Exotic Pets. Philadelphia, WB Saunders, 1991.
62. Schmidt RE, Eason RL, Hubbard GB: Pathology of Aging Syrian Hamsters. Boca Raton, CRC Press, 1983.
63. Schneider JE, Wade GN: Effects of maternal diet, body weight and body composition on infanticide in Syrian hamsters. Physiol Behavior 1989; 46:815-821.
64. Schneider JE, Wade GN: Effect of ambient temperature and body fat content on maternal litter reduction in Syrian hamsters. Physiol Behavior 1991; 49:135-139.
65. Short BG, Goldstein RS: Nonneoplastic lesions in the kidney. *In* Mohr U, Dungworth DL, Capen CC, eds. Pathobiology of the Aging Rat. Washington, DC, International Life Sciences Institute Press, 1992, pp 211-225.
66. Sichuk G, Bettigole RE, Der BK, et al: Influence of sex hormones on thrombosis of the left atrium in Syrian (golden) hamsters. Am J Physiol 1965; 208:465-470.
67. Silverman S: Diagnostic imaging of exotic pets. Vet Clin North Am Small Anim Pract 1993; 23:1287-1299.
68. Solomon HF, Dixon DM, Pouch W: A survey of staphylococci isolated from the laboratory gerbil. Lab Anim Sci 1990; 40:316-318.
69. Spear GS, Caple MV, Sutherland LR: The pancreas in the degu. Exp Mol Pathol 1984; 40:295-310.
70. Squartini F, Pingitore R: Tumours of the mammary gland. *In* Turusov VS, Mohr U, eds. Tumours of the Mouse, 2nd ed. Lyon, International Agency for Research on Cancer, 1994, pp 47-100.
71. Strauli P, Mettler J: Tumours of the haematopoietic system. *In* Tursusov VS, ed. Tumours of the Hamster. International Agency for Research on Cancer, 1982.
72. Tyzzer EE: A fatal disease of the Japanese waltzing-mouse caused by a spore-bearing bacillus (*Bacillus piliformis* N. sp.). J Med Res 1917; 37:307-338.
73. Vincent AL, Rodrick GE, Sodeman WA Jr: The pathology of the Mongolian gerbil (*Meriones unguiculatus*): a review. Lab Anim Sci 1979; 29:645-651.
74. Waggie KS, Ganaway JR, Wagner JE, et al: Experimentally induced Tyzzer's disease in Mongolian gerbils (*Meriones unguiculatus*). Lab Anim Sci 1984; 34:53-57.
75. Walberg JA, Stark DM, Desch C, et al: Demodicidosis in laboratory rats (*Rattus norvegicus*). Lab Anim Sci 1981; 31:60-62.
76. Wardrop KJ, Van Hoosier GL: The hamster. *In* Loeb WF, Quimby FW, eds. The Clinical Chemistry of Laboratory Animals. New York, Pergamon Press, 1989, pp 31–39.
77. White DJ, Waldron MM: Naturally-occurring Tyzzer's disease in the gerbil. Vet Rec 1969; 85:111-114.
78. Worgul BV, Rothstein H: Congenital cataracts associated with disorganized meridional rows in a new laboratory animal the degu (*Octodon degus*). Biomedi Express 1975; 23:1-4.

SUGGESTED READING AND RESOURCES

Children

Step by Step Series: Chinchillas; Gerbils; Guinea Pigs; Hamsters; Dwarf Rabbits; Rabbits. TFH Publications (www.tfh.com), paperback, 64 pp.

Barron's Young Pet Owners Guides: Taking Care of Your Gerbils; Guinea Pig; Hamster; Rabbit. Barron's Educational Guides, Hauppauge, NY, paperback, 32 pp.

Dorling-ASPCA Pet Care Guides for Kids: Guinea Pigs; Hamster; Rabbit. Houghton Mifflin, Boston, hardback, 32 pp.

Adults

Complete Introduction (KW) Series: Chinchillas; Gerbils; Guinea Pigs; Hamsters; Rabbits. TFH Publications (www.tfh.com), hardback, 128 pp.

Proper Care Series: Gerbils; Guinea Pigs; Dwarf Rabbits; Fancy Rats. TFH Publications (www.tfh.com), hardback, 256 pp.

Barron's Complete Pet Owners Manuals: Chinchillas; Degus; Dwarf Hamsters; Gerbils; Guinea Pigs; Hamsters; Mice; Prairie Dogs; Rats; Fancy Rats; Rabbits; Dwarf Rabbits. Barron's Educational Guides, Hauppauge, NY, paperback, 64-104 pp. Since 1999, all publications in the Complete Pet Owners Manuals are written by experienced veterinarians. These books have good husbandry and basic disease sections and are the best value for their price.

Veterinary Resources

Exotic DVM
Zoological Education Network
PO Box 541749
Lake Worth, FL 33454-1749
800-946-4782
www.exoticdvm.com

Lab Animal
345 Park Ave South, 10th floor
New York, NY 10010-1707
www.labanimal.com
This site has an online subscription form for the United States. For subscriptions to other parts of the world go to: www.agenda-rm.co.uk/subscription_form.pdf

Association of Exotic Mammal Veterinarians (AEMV)
PO Box 396
Weare, NH 03287-0396
www.aemv.org

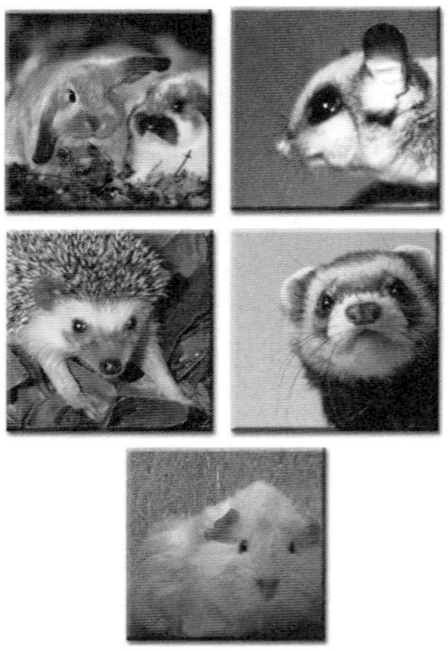

CHAPTER 30

Soft Tissue Surgery

R. Avery Bennett, DVM, MS, Diplomate ACVS, and
Holly S. Mullen, DVM, Diplomate ACVS

Small rodents such as hamsters, gerbils, rats, and mice are popular pets. Despite their small size and relatively low purchase price, their owners are frequently as emotionally attached to them as they would be to a dog or a cat. This attachment often leads owners to request surgical and medical treatments that have costs much greater than the replacement value of the pet.

As members of the myomorph group of rodents, hamsters, gerbils, rats, and mice share a similar anatomy. Rats and mice are murid rodents, whereas gerbils and hamsters are cricetid rodents. All are monogastric, have a bicornuate uterus, and have testicles that are usually descended into a large, well-developed scrotum, but that can be easily retracted into the abdomen through open inguinal canals. The female reproductive tract is more like that of dogs and cats than rabbits and hystricomorph rodents. The mesovarium and uterine body are relatively short. There is a single cervical os and the oviduct encircles the ovary as it does in other rodents. This group of rodents is sexually mature at 40 to 60 days of age.[19] Rats and mice have a long, hairless tail; gerbils have a long, haired tail; and hamsters have a short, lightly haired tail. Hamsters have large cheek pouches in which they store food.

PRESURGICAL CONSIDERATIONS

Patient Support

Most surgeries in small rodents are analogous to those performed in dogs and cats. The small size of the patient makes it more challenging for several reasons. As surgical patients, rodents are especially prone to complications such as hypovolemia from blood loss, hypothermia, and renal and respiratory compromise.[5,32] Rodents are species that serve as a food source for predator species. As such, they have evolved to "give up and die" when that will spare them a slower, more painful death. Therefore fear, pain, and stress have profound effects on their survival during and after surgical procedures. It is believed that catecholamine release is responsible for such a stress-related death. This catecholamine release can have effects on anesthesia as well. Efforts should be made to minimize pain, fear, and stress during the hospitalization period. Providing analgesia is a vital component of a successful outcome.

Because they are especially prone to asymptomatic renal and respiratory disease, a preoperative database should include a complete blood count, plasma biochemical analysis, urinalysis, and whole-body radiographs, especially to evaluate the lungs. Rats and mice frequently have subclinical *Mycoplasma* pneumonia. Renal disease is common in older rodents. It can be difficult to obtain urine in a small rodent; however, they urinate frequently. Put the rodent in a clean, dry, plastic or glass container. Usually, within a few minutes, a few drops of urine can be collected from the container, which is all that is required to evaluate the urine by dipstick and determine the specific gravity. Proteinuria and dilute urine indicate underlying renal disease. At the very least, a preoperative database should include a packed cell volume, total protein, urine specific gravity, and a blood urea nitrogen (BUN) estimate by an azotemia test strip. These tests require only a few drops of blood and urine.

Rodents are physiologically unable to vomit, so a prolonged fast is not necessary.[25] They also have relatively low hepatic glycogen stores.[13,25] A short fast of 1 hour will allow the animal to clear food material from its mouth. Administration of fluids containing dextrose (SC, IV, or IO) will help combat loss of energy stores.

Rodents have a large body surface area/volume ratio, predisposing to the development of hypothermia during long anesthetic and surgical procedures. A temperature monitor probe is ideal for continuous evaluation of core body temperature. The body temperature of a rat can drop 18°F (10°C) after 20 minutes of anesthesia.[14] Hypothermia decreases the metabolism and excretion of many anesthetic drugs.[26] A short operative time accomplished by having all the necessary equipment ready and accessible will help minimize the development of hypothermia. Alcohol should be avoided for skin preparation because the evaporative cooling will potentiate the development of hypothermia. A circulating warm water blanket under the patient should be set at 104°F (40°C) because these patients have a higher resting body temperature than dogs and cats. A heat lamp should be placed above the patient to augment the water blanket. Forced warm air blankets also seem useful in combating hypothermia. Other sources of supplemental heat are also available, including hot water bottles or examination gloves filled with warm water. Closely monitor all heat supplement devices to prevent accidentally burning the patient. The patient should be draped as quickly as possible because the drape will help hold in heat.

Relatively small amounts of hemorrhage can be disastrous in such small patients. It is best to have blood from a conspecific available for transfusion when significant blood loss is anticipated. Strict attention to hemostasis is vital. The average cotton-tipped applicator holds approximately 0.1 mL of blood when completely soaked. Loss of 10% to 15% of the total blood volume (approximately 1% of body weight) is usually safe. Loss of more than 5 cotton-tipped applicators full of blood (0.5 mL, or 10 drops) in a 50-g mouse is equivalent to more than 20% of the blood volume and is potentially dangerous.[13] Approximately 1.2, 1.4, and 4.0 mL of blood is equivalent to more than 20% of the blood volume (a potentially dangerous amount to lose) in the average-sized gerbil, hamster, and rat, respectively.[13] Intravascular fluid volume may also be supported with the aid of crystalloid fluids such as lactated Ringer's solution with or without dextrose. Intraosseous cannulas such as spinal needles are easily inserted in a normograde fashion into the proximal femur or proximal tibia of pet rodents. This will provide access to the vascular system for fluid support and emergency drug therapy, if needed. Fluids may also be administered subcutaneously or intraperitoneally with slower absorption. This route is not acceptable for treating animals in shock or with hypovolemia. A dose of 10 mL/kg SC of 4% dextrose has been recommended.[25]

The thoracic cavity of many small rodents is relatively small. Placing the patient in dorsal recumbency can compromise respiration because of the pressure of the viscera on the diaphragm. Tilting the patient such that the viscera displace caudally may be beneficial for the respiratory system of the anesthetized patient.[25]

The subcutis in small rodents is relatively thick and holds subcuticular sutures well. Rodents are fastidious groomers and do not tolerate skin sutures well. They also seem prone to self-mutilation of surgical wounds. Gentle tissue handling, strict attention to aseptic technique, and closing with no external sutures will help minimize the risks of this. Chromic catgut should be avoided because of its reactive nature, which might stimulate the patient to chew at the incision postoperatively. We prefer 5-0 to 7-0 absorbable suture in a subcuticular or intradermal closure to avoid the use of skin sutures. If necessary, tissue glue may also be used to facilitate skin closure. Small incisions can be opposed with only tissue adhesive. Rodents tend to chew at skin sutures and can chew out wire sutures as well as nylon ones. Steel skin staples appear to be more resistant to being chewed out.

Instrumentation

Microsurgical instruments are constructed so that only the tips are miniaturized.[4] The handles should be of normal length (5.5 to 7 inches) to help provide stability to the tips, diminishing the effects of tremors. The handles should be round to facilitate the required rolling action between the thumb and first two fingers. This is most important for the needle holders, where a curved needle must be rolled through the tissue. Many prefer needle holders without a clasp or box-lock because the motion that occurs when the lock is set and released may be enough to cause the needle to tear tissues. In general, ophthalmic instruments are not well suited to small mammals. The short length makes it difficult to manipulate tissues within a body cavity.

A microsurgical pack should consist minimally of a microsurgical needle holder (Micro Surgery Needle Holder, straight, T/C without lock, 8 inches; Micro Surgery Needle Holder, curved, without lock, 7.125 inches, pencil-style grip), microsurgical scissors (Tew-Barraquer Scissor, curved, 7 inches), and a microsurgical thumb forceps (Micro Surgical Forceps, straight, 7 inches, pencil-style grip) (all RICA Surgical Products, Inc., Chicago, IL). Many microsurgeons prefer jeweler's forceps to microsurgical forceps (Long Jeweler's Forceps No. 3, RICA Surgical Products, Inc.). These are significantly less expensive and serve their purpose adequately but are not ideal. Heiss Self Retaining Retractors (RICA Surgical Products, Inc.) work well as abdominal and tissue retractors. Hemostatic clips are also very useful and are available in four sizes, with small and medium (Hemoclips, stainless steel, 200 clips/box and Samuels Hemoclip Applier, 6.25 inches, RICA Surgical Products, Inc.) being most applicable for pet rodent surgery. Such a surgical pack can be put together for approximately $1000. After gaining experience, other microsurgical instruments such as micro mosquito hemostats may be added to the pack.

Small gauze pads (2 × 2 inches) can be cut from the standard 4 × 4-inch sponges. Sterile cotton-tipped applicators should also be available. These are useful for absorption of fluids as well as gentle tissue dissection and manipulation. Absorbable gelatin sponge (Gelfoam, Pharmacia & Upjohn Co., Kalamazoo, MI) and other absorbable hemostatic agents are valuable for controlling hemorrhage. Surgicel (Ethicon, Inc., Johnson & Johnson, Sommerville, NJ) is oxidized regenerated cellulose resembling cloth. It is a hemostatic aid that adheres nicely to internal tissues but is not capable of absorbing much fluid. Topical thrombin (Thrombin-JMI, GenTrac, Middleton, WI) is available in various size vials. Thrombin stimulates clot formation, and this product is a liquid. Either Gelfoam or Surgicel can be soaked in topical thrombin before placing it over the hemorrhaging structure to aid in hemostasis.

Magnification

Some form of magnification is recommended for surgery in rodent patients. The dexterity and manipulation required of fingers and hands are far greater than can be achieved with unaided vision. Small amounts of hemorrhage appear more significant under magnification and individual vessels are much more easily identified for coagulation, minimizing the degree of hemorrhage associated with a procedure. Binocular loupes are available in various styles, with the hobby loupe being the least expensive and simplest. Hobby loupes have several disadvantages, including a set focal distance, no focal light source, and the inability to look around the lenses when magnification is not required.

A modification of the hobby loupe is marketed with interchangeable lenses and a cool halogen focal light source (MDS, Inc., Brandon, FL). These allow the surgeon to change the degree of magnification to that appropriate to the size of the patient and to be able to illuminate inside body cavities. This type of loupe still has a set focal length and the surgeon is committed to looking through the lenses.

SurgiTel (General Scientific Corp., Ann Arbor, MI) eliminates most of the problems associated with the hobby loupes. It has a focal halogen light source, lenses do not cover the entire visual field so the surgeon is not committed to looking through the lenses, and lenses also have a focal range, rather than a set focal distance, which allows the entire patient to be in focus during surgery.

Electrosurgery

Electrosurgery uses high-frequency alternating current to generate energy. There are two electrodes (an active electrode and an indifferent electrode) with concentration of current density at the tip of the smaller (active) electrode. Burns can result if the ground plate contacts only a small area. The Surgitron (Ellman International, Inc., Hewlett, NY) uses radiofrequency current that is received, with the indifferent electrode acting as an antenna. The area of contact between the patient and the indifferent electrode is irrelevant. If only a small area of the patient is over the electrode it will not burn the patient, which is especially advantageous when working with small mammal patients. The bipolar forceps are most useful for hemostasis within body cavities because the current passes between the tips of the electrodes, coagulating the tissue. Ellman has created an adaptor switch that allows the surgeon to switch from monopolar (used for cutting the skin) to bipolar (used for coagulating within a body cavity) and back without having to unplug electrodes.

The Surgitron Dual Frequency 120 (Ellman International, Inc.) radiowave energy is emitted at 4.0 MHz, providing control of absorption depth in tissue and resulting in minimal cellular damage and heat conduction (Fig. 30-1). This unit features a unique isolated circuitry system that maintains a constant frequency of 4.0 MHz. With other units there is variation in the frequency output. With this constant frequency, there are only 15 μm of lateral heat damage compared with 90 μm from the older Surgitron units and more than 100 μm with a carbon dioxide laser. The standard electrosurgical units generally produce more than 750 μm of lateral heat damage.

Another unique feature of this machine is the three-button finger switch. The finger switch has a button for cutting, another for coagulating, and a third for bipolar cautery. Everything is incorporated into the unit, thereby keeping it all in the sterile field. A technician is not required to switch from bipolar to monopolar, as is required with the other electrosurgical units.

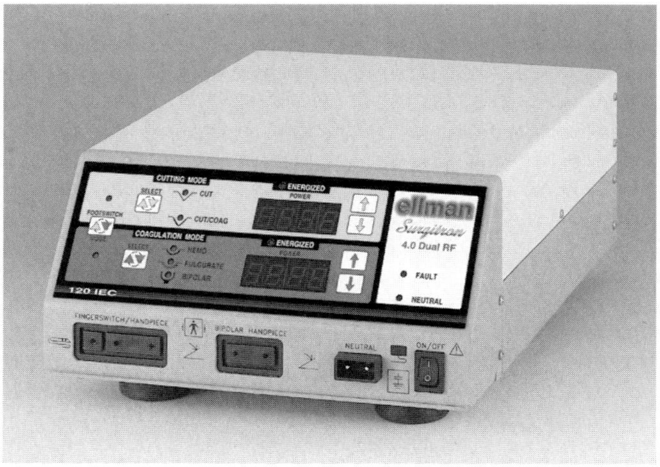

Figure 30-1 The Surgitron Dual Frequency 120 radiosurgical unit is small and has both monopolar and bipolar capabilities. It operates with radiofrequency electromagnetic waves, with the ground plate acting as an antenna.

Carbon Dioxide Laser

The carbon dioxide (CO_2) laser (AccuVet CO_2, Lumenis, Norwood, MA) has recently gained popularity in small exotic animal surgery.[23] It produces a beam of light energy at a wavelength of 10,600 nm. This wavelength of energy is highly absorbed by water molecules, making it ideal for cutting with a focal beam or vaporizing tissue when used with a diffused beam. The CO_2 laser seals vessels less than 0.6 mm in diameter, so that many of the incisions made with this unit are bloodless and result in less postoperative swelling because the lymphatic vessels are also sealed. Incisions made with the CO_2 laser are reportedly less painful than those made with a blade or electrosurgical or radiosurgical units because the energy beam seals nerve endings as well. When used appropriately, the amount of lateral heat damage is said to be less with a laser than with other modalities[23]; however, when used incorrectly, lasers can cause significant lateral thermal damage.

A diode laser (Sharplan 810 and 980, Lumenis) is also available and produces a beam of energy in the 635-nm to 980-nm range. The main advantage of this type of laser in surgery of rodents is that it can be used through an endoscope or in a fluid-filled medium. It has deeper tissue penetration but is less precise than the CO_2 laser. The diode laser can be used for photodynamic cancer therapy, chromophore-enhanced tissue ablation, or coagulation of blood.[23]

Lasers can cause injury to the operator or assistant as well as to the other tissues of the patient. Proper safety training for all personnel, therefore, is important when using lasers in surgery.

Patient Preparation

Standard aseptic technique is essential with pet rodent patients. Rodents are susceptible to infections and their cages often require them to be in close proximity to their urine and feces. Care must be taken to avoid damaging the skin during preparation for surgery. The area clipped should be minimized to help control heat loss. Clear plastic drapes allow respiration to be monitored during the procedure. A plastic drape with a 3.5 × 5-inch adhesive center and an overall size of 40 × 54 inches is commercially available (Veterinary Transparent Surgical Drape, Veterinary Specialty Products, Inc., Boca Raton, FL). This allows the surgeon to maintain a sterile field over the entire table and still be able to monitor the patient. A smaller drape is also available (24 × 24 inches) for minor procedures but is not large enough to create a sterile field on a surgical table. These drapes may also hold heat in better than cloth or paper drapes.

CASTRATION

The indications for castration of rodents are to prevent breeding (it is easier to castrate males than ovariectomize females), prevent or treat aggression (castration is recommended before puberty), and decrease urine marking behaviors (it is best to castrate an animal before it develops these behaviors). Testicular tumors occur in rodents, especially rats. They are usually Leydig cell tumors, which are considered benign but can get quite large.[30] The incidence varies with strain of rat and increases with age. Testicular tumors are usually bilateral and multilobulated. If unilateral, the affected side is very large and the unaffected testis is small because of atrophy. Prostatic and testicular tumors are also reported in gerbils.[30]

The procedure for castration of rats, mice, hamsters, and gerbils is basically the same.[8] The testicles are located caudoventrally in the inguinal area and are readily retracted into the abdomen. They can be easily propulsed back into the scrotum with a gentle rolling pressure on the caudal abdomen, in a caudal direction just cranial to the pubis. The testicles are relatively large and are contained in a well-defined scrotal sac. The epididymal fat is responsible for preventing intestinal herniation.[19] It is difficult to remove the testicle without removing the fat. Performing a closed castration avoids the risk of intestinal herniation or evisceration; however, the risk of this occurring has not been clearly documented. Alternatively, the tunic can be ligated after an open castration.

After routine clipping and surgical preparation of the scrotum, an open or closed technique may be used. A single transverse or midline 0.5- to 1.0-cm incision is made at the distal (caudal) tip of the scrotum. Alternatively, two incisions can be made, one in each side of the scrotum. It is best to place the incision as far dorsally as possible to minimize incisional contamination by the cage substrate. Another method involves cutting off the tip of the scrotum to allow both testicles to be exteriorized and removed (Fig. 30-2).

The closed technique is analogous to that described for guinea pigs and chinchillas (see Chapter 27). For the open technique, extend the incision through the tunic on each side of midline to allow exteriorization of each testicle. Manually break the ligament of the tail of the epididymis, and apply caudal retraction to the testicle to expose the spermatic cord. Ligate or clip the cord and transect it distal to the ligature. The tunic may be left open or closed using a 4-0 to 6-0 synthetic, absorbable material. The skin incision may be left open to heal by second intention or may be closed with a tissue adhesive or staples. The substrate must be kept clean and changed frequently. Generally, sexual activity should cease in 1 to 2 weeks after castration; however, in rodents that have had sexual experiences before castration, mounting and intromission usually persist for several weeks after castration.[14] Complications associated with castration include hematoma formation, self-trauma, excess activity, and infection.[25]

Some surgeons prefer an abdominal approach for castration of rodents.[14,17] The technique is analogous to that described in Chapter 27 in prairie dogs.

OVARIOHYSTERECTOMY AND OVARIECTOMY

Indications for ovariohysterectomy in rodents include dystocia, pyometra, masses, and, potentially, behavior alteration. Ovariectomy of young female rodents has been shown to significantly decrease the potential for the development of mammary neoplasia.[16] Ovariectomized female rats also had a significantly lower incidence of pituitary tumors and had a higher rate of survival to day 630. Ovariectomy, however, also predisposes rats to osteopenia.[16,20] Pyometra is rare in small rodents but can occur in any species. Female hamsters have an odorous, mucoid vaginal discharge at estrus, and this discharge should not be mistaken for

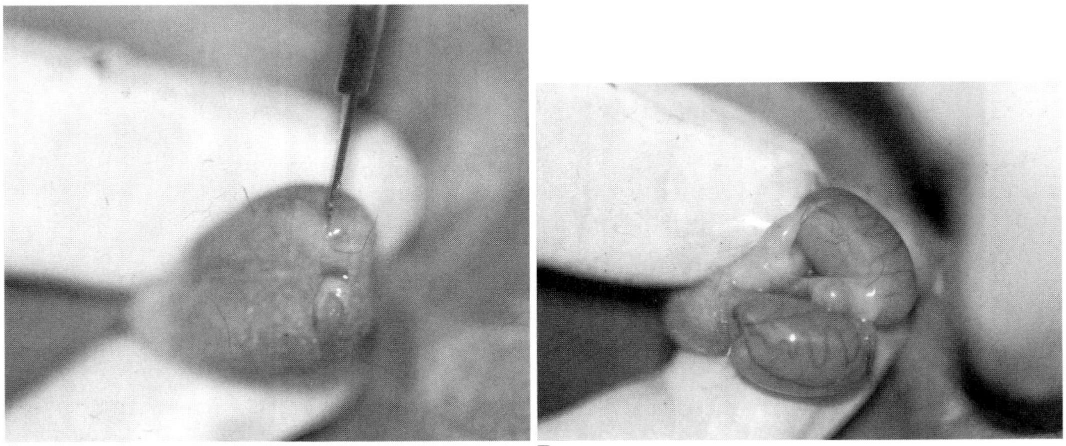

A B

Figure 30-2 A, One technique for castrating small rodents, such as this rat, is to cut off the end of the scrotum B, The testicles are exposed, allowing ligation and transection of the spermatic cord.

pyometra.[15] Ovariohysterectomy is used to treat cysts as well as ovarian and uterine tumors of small rodents. Benign and malignant tumors of the uterus and ovaries have been reported.[30] Benign endometrial stromal tumors occur in up to 66% of some strains of rats more than 21 months old. These are more common in virgin rats than in breeding females. Ovarian tumors tend to be benign in hamsters and gerbils. Uterine tumors tend to be benign in rats and malignant in hamsters and gerbils.

The ovaries are located at the caudal pole of the kidneys within a rather large fat pad (Fig. 30-3). The oviduct wraps around the ovary, encircling it cranially. The suspensory ligaments are long and the ovaries can be exteriorized without breaking the ligament. There are a single artery and vein that run medial to each ovary and the ipsilateral uterine horn.[13]

Place the patient in dorsal recumbency and prepare it for aseptic surgery. Make a 1- to 2-cm ventral midline celiotomy incision midway between the umbilical scar and the pubis. In rodents the incision is relatively large to be able to access the ovarian vessels. Gerbils of both sexes have a sebaceous gland located midventrally on the abdomen near the umbilicus.[15] If this interferes with the abdominal incision, divert the incision to one side and undermine the skin to expose the linea alba. The uterine horns are identified dorsal to the apex of the bladder. Grasp one horn and exteriorize it through the incision. Identify the vessels within the mesovarium supplying the ovary and create an opening in the mesovarium to allow placement of hemostatic clips or an absorbable synthetic suture ligature. Monofilament absorbable synthetic suture of size 4-0 or 5-0 is suitable. Transect the suspensory ligament, mesovarium, and vessels distal to the ligatures. Repeat the procedure on the contralateral side, and bluntly dissect the broad ligament on each side to the level of the uterine body. It has been recommended that the uterus be ligated cranial to the cervix to prevent urine from spilling into the abdomen when the uterus is transected. This appears to be of little concern clinically. Care must be taken to avoid damaging the urinary bladder, which lies immediately dorsal to the uterus. Gentle tissue handling and avoiding manipulation of the gastrointestinal tract are important because rodents, especially hamsters, are prone to the development of adhesions.[25] A three-layer closure is recommended to close the body wall, subcutaneous tissue, and skin or subcutis as separate layers. The substrate should be changed at least twice daily to minimize incisional contamination.

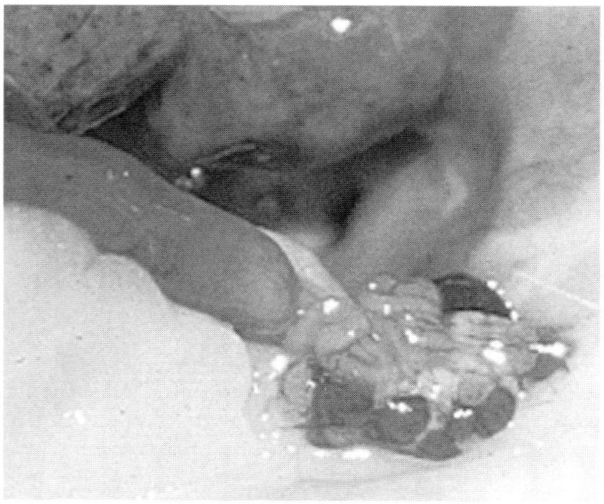

Figure 30-3 As in other rodents, the ovaries of rats are located at the caudal pole of the kidney surrounded by fat. The oviduct encircles the ovary.

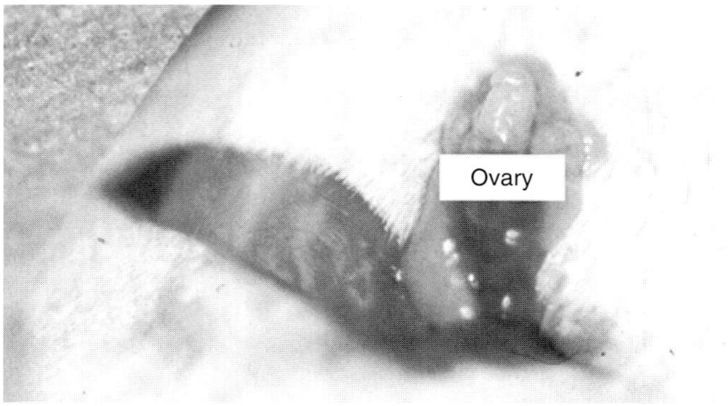

Figure 30-4 For ovariectomy in rodents, a transverse incision is made dorsally at approximately the level of the third lumbar vertebra. The ovary is easily exteriorized through blunt dissection caudal to the last rib.

Ovariectomy is performed routinely in laboratory rodents.[13,19,25] The risk of pyometra after ovariectomy appears to be negligible. The procedure is easier to perform than ovariohysterectomy, with minimal morbidity (Fig. 30-4). The dorsal skin incision can be made longitudinally or transversely so that the skin can be slid from one side to the other, allowing removal of both ovaries through one incision, or separate incisions can be made to approach each ovary. Approximately 1 cm ventral to the dorsal spinous processes of the third lumbar vertebra, immediately caudal to the last rib, bluntly dissect through the body wall with a mosquito hemostat. Pressure on the abdomen will cause the ovary to be extruded through the incision, allowing its removal. If it does not exteriorize, insert a forceps or hemostat and retrieve the ovary located just caudal to the kidney on that side. In a laboratory animal facility, the ovaries are removed by blunt dissection with no ligation because hemorrhage is generally minimal. Clinically, a ligature or clip on the ovarian vessels will help prevent hemorrhage. Transect the pedicle distal to the ligature and remove the ovary. The oviduct, which encircles the ovary, is also removed. If incompletely removed the lining produces fluid and a cyst can develop.[19] The muscle can be opposed with 4-0 or 6-0 synthetic, absorbable suture, but this is not usually necessary. The skin is moved to the other side and the procedure is repeated. Close the skin with a subcuticular suture or tissue adhesive.

Cesarean section has been reported in a gerbil.[24] In rodent species the patient should be tilted to allow the viscera and gravid uterus to fall away from the thoracic cavity. When making the skin incision, avoid the enlarged mammary glands and associated blood vessels. The uterus is vascular when gravid and the incision in the uterus is made carefully in a relatively avascular area. The uterus is closed in a simple continuous pattern oversewn with an inverting pattern. Oxytocin can be administered after removal of the fetuses to aid with uterine involution.

MAMMARY GLAND NEOPLASIA

Mammary gland neoplasia is the most common spontaneous neoplasm of mice and rats.[7,30] Although reported, it appears to be rare in gerbils and hamsters. Most mammary tumors in rats and hamsters are benign, whereas in mice and gerbils they are malignant.[7,30] In mice, they are rapidly metastatic, invasive, and much more difficult to remove.[6,13] Mouse mammary tumor virus predisposes to the development of mammary adenocarcinoma and is passed transplacentally and through milk.

Rat mammary gland tumors are known to be sensitive to hormone stimuli,[30] and Sprague-Dawley rats ovariectomized at 90 days of age had a significantly lower incidence of mammary tumors (4%) than intact rats (47%).[16] These ovariectomized rats also had a significantly lower incidence of pituitary chromophobe adenomas (4% compared with 66%). Estrogen does not seem to be the major factor in tumor development because exogenous estrogen did not increase the incidence of tumor development.[16] It is theorized that high levels of prolactin from pituitary tumors actually cause tumor development. However, estrogen may contribute to the development of pituitary tumors. Ovariectomy also improved survival to 630 days of age (89% compared with 59% of intact rats). It has been reported that tumor removal prolongs survival to 630 days[12]; however, a study by Hotchkiss[16] that compared data from other studies with rats in which tumors were not removed failed to confirm this. Clinically it appears that ovariohysterectomy in conjunction with mammary tumor removal helps prevent the formation of new tumors and tumor recurrence (Michael Weisse, personal communication, 2002).

In rats, mammary gland tumors are usually benign mammary fibroadenomas (50%-90%, depending on the strain)[1,21] and are uncommon in rats younger than 1 year of age.[16] Fewer than 10% of mammary tumors are malignant.[1,13,33] Mammary tumors are usually single, large, firm, not attached to deeper structures, and well tolerated by the animal. They do not metastasize to distant locations and clinical problems are generally associated with the large size, sometimes being larger than the patient (Fig. 30-5).[1,28] It has been reported that 16% of aged male rats develop mammary fibroadenomas.[10]

Mammary gland tissue is extensive in rats and mice, extending from the cervical to the inguinal region ventrally and as high as the shoulders and flanks laterally (Fig. 30-6). Mammary gland tumors can be found anywhere in these areas and grow rapidly to large sizes. Mammary tissue is confined to the ventral thorax and abdomen of hamsters and gerbils.

Treatment of mammary tumors in all small rodents consists of excising the tumor and associated mammary gland, in conjunction with an ovariohysterectomy in some cases. If ulcerated or suspected to be malignant, the skin overlying the tumor should be removed. Generally there are several blood vessels that may be very large in the subcutaneous tissue supplying the tumor that need to be ligated. Bluntly dissect around the mass, ligating or clipping vessels as they are encountered. With large tumors, ligate arteries before veins to allow some blood to drain from the tumor into the patient circulation. Speed and hemostasis are vital for a successful outcome. Electrosurgical or laser dissection and coagulation of vessels are applicable to tumor removal. Close the surgical wound in one or two layers. If possible, close the subcutaneous tissue separately from the skin. Drains are not usually needed and "tacking" the skin to deeper structures is discouraged. Tacking causes irritation and stimulates the patient to chew at the incision postoperatively. It is best to remove excess skin after tumor removal so the amount needed to close can more accurately be determined. If time is critical, only the skin is closed with staples, which are rapidly applied.

OTHER CUTANEOUS MASSES

A variety of cutaneous neoplasms have been reported in rodents.[30] These include fibromas, fibrosarcomas, lipomas, undifferentiated sarcomas, squamous cell carcinomas, and hemangiosarcomas. Fibromas tend to be small, firm, and well circumscribed, whereas fibrosarcomas are usually large, locally invasive, and early to metastasize. Hamsters and gerbils have scent marking glands. It is important to know the normal location and appearance of these glands so as not to confuse them with a pathologic process. Hamsters have a bald spot near each hip that is the location of the gland, and Djungarian hamsters have a midventral sebaceous gland. Gerbils have a similar single gland on the ventral abdomen.

A review of the literature in one report documented that 8 of 34 tumors reported in gerbils were associated with the scent

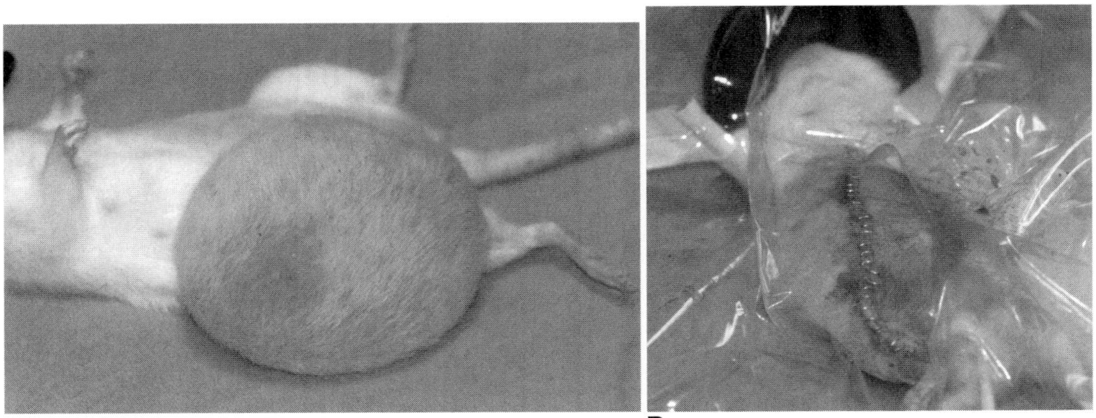

A B

Figure 30-5 A, Rat mammary fibroadenomas can grow quite large. This tumor weighed more that the rat did after tumor removal. B, Because speed is important in removing large mammary tumors, a single-layer closure with skin staples is usually adequate.

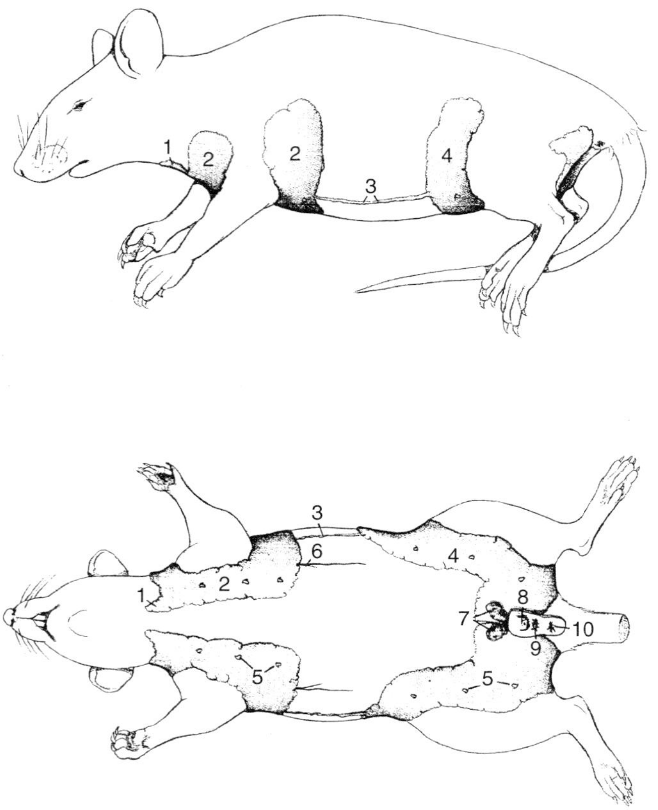

Figure 30-6 Mammary tissue is extensive in rats and tumors occur in any location. *1-4,* Mammary glands; *1,* cervical gland; *2,* thoracic gland; *3,* abdominal gland; *4,* inguinal gland; *5,* mammae papillae; *6,* superficial cranial epigastric vein (subcutaneous abdominal vein); *7,* preputial gland; *8,* prepuce; *9,* opening of vagina; *10,* anus. (From Popesko P, Rajtová V, Horák J: Atlas of the Anatomy of Small Laboratory Animals. Vol. I: Rabbit and Guinea Pig; Vol. 2: Rat, Mouse and Golden Hamster. Bratislava, Príroda Publishing, 1990 [Czechoslovak edition]).

gland, including three squamous cell carcinomas, a sebaceous adenoma, three sebaceous adenocarcinomas, and a papilloma.[30] Wide excision is recommended because the neoplasm is locally invasive.[18] Of the 34 cutaneous tumors reported in gerbils, 12 were squamous cell carcinomas, eight were melanomas, five were sebaceous adenomas, three were fibrosarcomas, and two were mammary adenocarcinomas.

Rats have a specialized sebaceous gland around the external ear canal called Zymbal's gland. Malignancy of this gland presents as a large, ulcerated swelling or mass within or ventral to the ear canal.[1,29] Squamous cell carcinoma is the most common histologic diagnosis. These tumors are locally aggressive but late to metastasize to the lymph nodes and lungs. Surgical removal can be curative if adequate surgical margins can be obtained.

Rats of both sexes also have bilateral preputial glands (Fig. 30-6). Although inflammation is most commonly reported, malignancy can occur. These are modified sebaceous glands as well and one or both can be affected. Carcinomas of these glands are typically invasive and can metastasize. Early detection and removal with adequate surgical margins can effect a cure. It is important to protect the urethral papilla during resection.

MISCELLANEOUS ABDOMINAL PROCEDURES

Exploratory laparotomy is indicated in pet rodents for a variety of reasons. The procedure is similar to that used in larger mammalian species. Some rodents, especially hamsters, are prone to the development of adhesions, which can cause clinical problems postoperatively.[25] Gentle tissue handling, minimizing handling of viscera, and avoiding the use of reactive suture material, such as chromic catgut, are important in preventing adhesion formation. Verapamil (200 μg/kg PO q8h for 3 days), a calcium channel blocker, has been shown to reduce the formation of adhesions in hamsters after laparotomy.[9]

Cystotomy

Cystotomy is generally performed for removal of cystic calculi, which are relatively uncommon but do occur in small rodents.[3,22] Clinical signs include hematuria, stranguria, dysuria, incontinence, anorexia, and expression of pain. All the factors predisposing individual rodents to the development of cystic calculi have not been determined. It is difficult to cure this condition in rodents and recurrence is common.[14] Cultures of the bladder wall and the calculus should be obtained during the procedure.

Cystotomy is performed as for other species, except that the suture material and needle must be small and delicate tissue handling is required. Midline skin and body wall incisions are made just cranial to the pubis, allowing the bladder to be exteriorized. Identify the bladder and isolate it with moist 2 × 2-inch gauze sponges. Make an incision on the ventral surface of the bladder, thus avoiding the trigone. After removing the calculus and collecting samples for culture, irrigate the bladder and flush the urethra with an intravenous catheter before closure of the cystotomy. The bladder wall of rodents is relatively thin. It is closed with 6-0 to 8-0 monofilament, synthetic, absorbable suture material on a small, atraumatic, and swaged-on needle with a simple interrupted pattern. Irrigate the abdominal cavity before closure of the celiotomy. Calculi are usually calcium based and may respond to dietary management. If the patient is not urinating postoperatively, catheterize the urethra with an appropriate-sized intravenous catheter that is left in place for 2 to 3 days to allow tissue swelling to subside.[25]

Abdominal Masses

Abdominal masses can arise from any organ. Hamsters are prone to polycystic disease. The cysts can become quite large and are most often found in the liver and kidneys. Hamsters are also prone to the development of lymphosarcoma. In addition to involvement of the peripheral lymph nodes, tumors may be found in the liver, kidney, spleen, and bowel.[30]

Gerbils have a high incidence of spontaneously occurring neoplasia, especially if they are older than 2 years. Tumors of the reproductive tract, liver, pancreas, and spleen have all been described.[30]

Renal tumors have been reported in rats. Nephroblastomas are seen most often in young rats; older rats with renal neoplasia usually have renal tubular adenoma or adenocarcinoma. These tumors are often bilateral.[7,30]

Adrenal tumors occur commonly in older rodents but are usually found incidentally at necropsy. There are at least 15 reports of adrenal tumors in gerbils.[30] Adrenal tumors also occur commonly in older rats and are typically adrenocortical in origin. They may be malignant or benign (pheochromocytomas). The incidence varies with the strain of rat, and metastasis has been reported.[30] In hamsters, adrenal adenomas are commonly reported benign tumors, occurring more often in males.[30] Affected hamsters are generally 2 to 3 years old.

Cystic Ovarian Disease

Cystic ovaries have been reported in all the small rodents, but most often in hamsters and gerbils. The incidence of thecomas in hamsters is approximately 2%.[30] These cysts may become very large without causing significant signs of discomfort (Fig. 30-7). They can become large enough to compress abdominal organs and compromise function. They can also make it difficult for the hamster to take in adequate amounts of nutrition. Before surgical removal, it is recommended to drain the cyst to improve the patient's ability to ventilate and the surgeon's exposure to the reproductive tract. In gerbils, 29 of 37 tumors of the female reproductive tract were ovarian in origin and the other 8 were uterine.[30] Uterine adenocarcinoma is common in Syrian hamsters. These tumors have been documented to metastasize and to be spread by implantation of malignant cells during surgery.[30]

PULMONARY LOBECTOMY

A technique has been described for pulmonary lobectomy for rats in a laboratory setting.[27] The rats are maintained under anesthesia with a face mask. The mask fits tightly around the muzzle

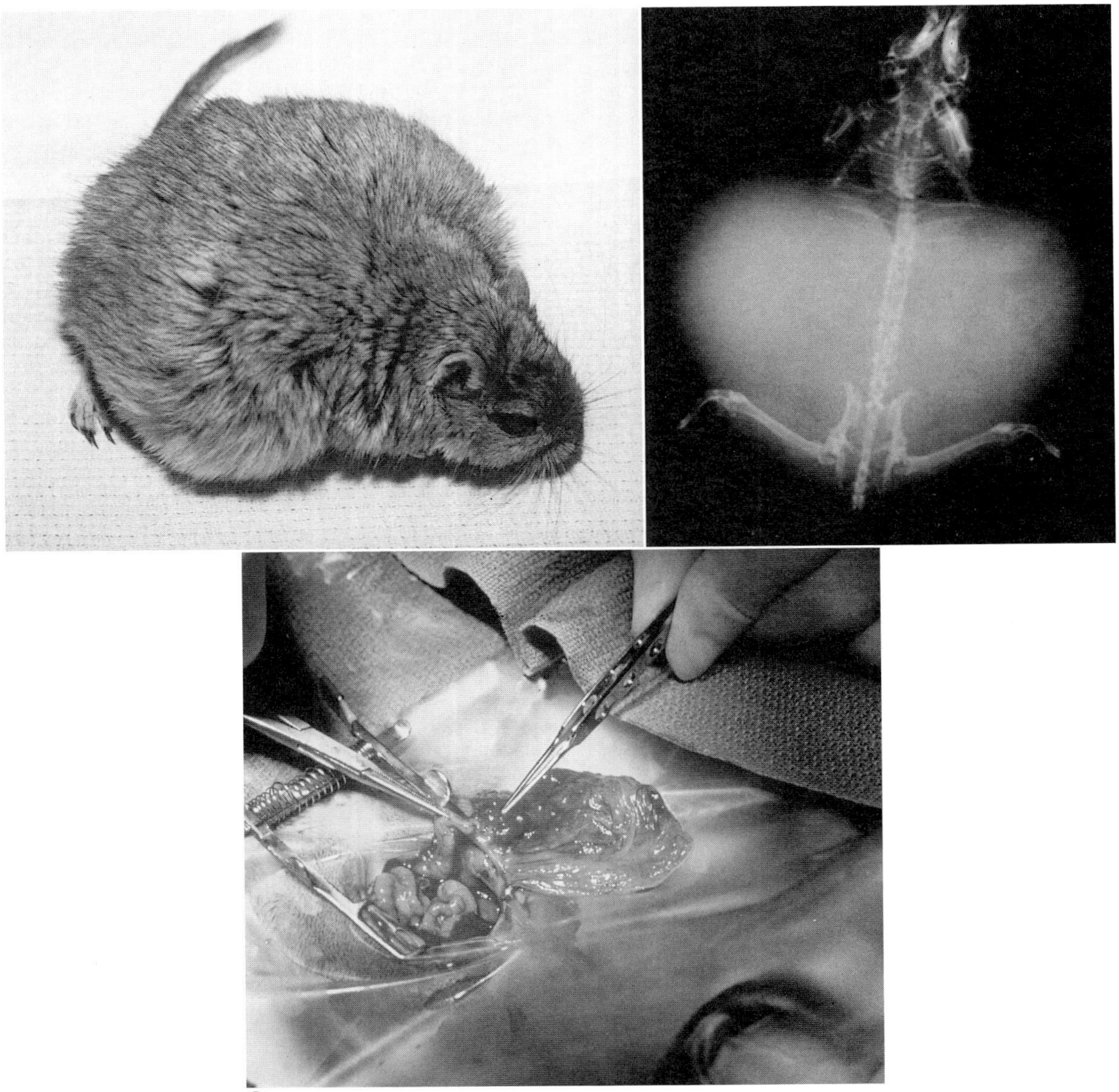

A B

C

Figure 30-7 **A,** A 2-year-old female gerbil with abdominal distention caused by a large right ovarian cyst. **B,** Ventrodorsal radiograph of the same hamster. **C,** Intraoperative view of the drained cyst before ovariohysterectomy.

and allows the patient to be ventilated. Ventilation is supported during thoracotomy at 20 beats/min and the lungs are directly visualized to evaluate for sufficient expansion. An intercostal approach is used. An incision is made over the lateral thoracic wall and muscles are divided, paying attention to hemostasis. The thoracic cavity is entered by using a hemostat to penetrate between ribs into the thoracic cavity at the fourth intercostal space. The hemostat is then spread to open the intercostal space, avoiding vessels. A Heiss retractor is used to maintain exposure while the lung is exteriorized. The hilus is clipped with a medium-sized Hemoclip and the tissue transected distal to the clip. Two sutures of 3-0 nylon are used to oppose the ribs. Before tying the second, a catheter is inserted into the chest to allow air and fluid to be evacuated. Muscle layers are closed appropriately along with the subcutis and skin. The chest tube can be maintained if needed or removed after evacuation of the chest cavity. This procedure takes less than 10 minutes to perform and the chest is generally open for less than 3 minutes.[27] Of the 54 rats on which this procedure was performed, 51 survived. The fatalities occurred early in the study and were related to hemorrhage.

ABSCESSES

Subcutaneous Abscesses

Abscesses are not uncommon in small rodents, particularly hamsters, and they usually occur because of a bite wound or other trauma. Some affected animals are asymptomatic except for having an abnormal swelling. Others are systemically ill and are administered supportive care as necessary. Radiographs are indicated when abscesses are on the face or feet to evaluate for the presence of bone involvement.

Abscesses are easily diagnosed by finding pus on cytologic examination of a fine-needle aspirate. Implantation of antibiotic-impregnated polymethylmethacrylate beads is indicated in most cases. If it is not feasible to excise the entire abscess, remove as much of the abscess as possible, including the fibrous capsule. Submit a section of the wall for culture and sensitivity testing as well as histopathologic evaluation. Fill the resulting defect loosely with antibiotic-impregnated polymethylmethacrylate beads and close the subcutis and skin routinely. Administer a broad-spectrum antibiotic systemically pending culture and sensitivity results.

Dental Abscesses in Hamsters

Hamsters are very prone to periodontal disease and dental caries.[2,31] Their incisors grow continuously but their cheek teeth do not. Once a cheek tooth is removed, no new tooth will grow to replace it. A facial abscess located ventral or rostral to the eye may be caused by a tooth root abscess. These facial abscesses need to be irrigated and drained; however, they will recur if the underlying cause, the abscessed tooth root, is not addressed.

As in most rodents, the roots of the incisor teeth are long and deeply seated in the skull. By the time a facial abscess has formed, the tooth root is usually so loosened by decay that extraction is not difficult. Remove the tooth by elevating the periodontal membrane while alternately and steadily retracting the exposed tooth. Close the defect in the gingiva with a single absorbable suture. Clean the facial abscess area several times daily until the wound has granulated closed.

ENUCLEATION

Rodents have a large venous orbital sinus that surrounds the muscles and harderian gland caudal to the globe. This is the site used for blood collection with a capillary tube in a laboratory setting. If this is damaged during enucleation, significant hemorrhage occurs. Indications for enucleation are those that cause end-stage ocular disease. These murid rodents do not have a third eyelid. Proptosis is somewhat common in small rodents, especially hamsters. If left untreated even a few hours, it may not be possible to save the eye.

Two techniques are described for enucleation of rodents.[25] The transconjunctival approach involves dissecting tissues off the globe, staying as close to the globe as possible with the dissection, thus avoiding the sinus. This will leave tissue in the orbit, which will help prevent the sunken appearance common after enucleation. If the tissue is infected, a transpalpebral approach is recommended. This approach involves dissecting tissues as close to the bony orbit as possible, again avoiding the venous sinus. By using this technique, no tissue is left in the orbit. An antibiotic-impregnated polymethylmethacrylate prosthetic globe can be made to help control infection and prevent the sunken appearance.

CHEEK POUCH EVERSION IN HAMSTERS

Hamsters have well-developed cheek pouches bilaterally that are lined by a thin epithelial membrane.[2,15,31] These pouches are used to store extra food. One or both pouches can spontaneously evert and, if so, they will need to be replaced. The cause is unknown and recurrence is common unless the pouch is sutured in place.

Sedate the hamster and gently replace the everted pouch with a cotton-tipped applicator or a 1 mL syringe case. Place a single, full-thickness, percutaneous suture into the cheek pouch with 4-0 or 5-0 monofilament, nonabsorbable suture material and a small needle (Fig. 30-8). If using a cotton-tipped applicator, be careful not to include cotton in the tissue bite. A stent is not necessary because the suture is not tightened enough to cause necrosis. Recovery is uneventful, and the hamster is able to eat right away. Remove the suture in 14 days. There are no reports of recurrence after this procedure.

PROLAPSED BOWEL IN HAMSTERS

Hamsters are prone to proliferative ileitis ("wet tail," or regional enteritis), a disease characterized by excessive glandular proliferation in the epithelium of the ileum.[31] Signs seen with this disease include diarrhea (sometimes containing blood) and tenesmus. Intestinal neoplasia of the colon and small intestine can cause similar signs and must be differentiated from proliferative ileitis. Prolapse of the small intestine, colon, or rectum can result from the excessive straining seen with both these conditions. Other conditions causing tenesmus, such as parasitism and diet-induced diarrhea, can also lead to prolapse.

Hamsters with bowel prolapse are usually sick and should receive necessary medical treatment that includes the administration of fluids, dextrose, and antibiotics before they undergo emergency surgery. It is very important to ascertain what segment of bowel is prolapsed before surgery. A nonnecrotic rectal pro-

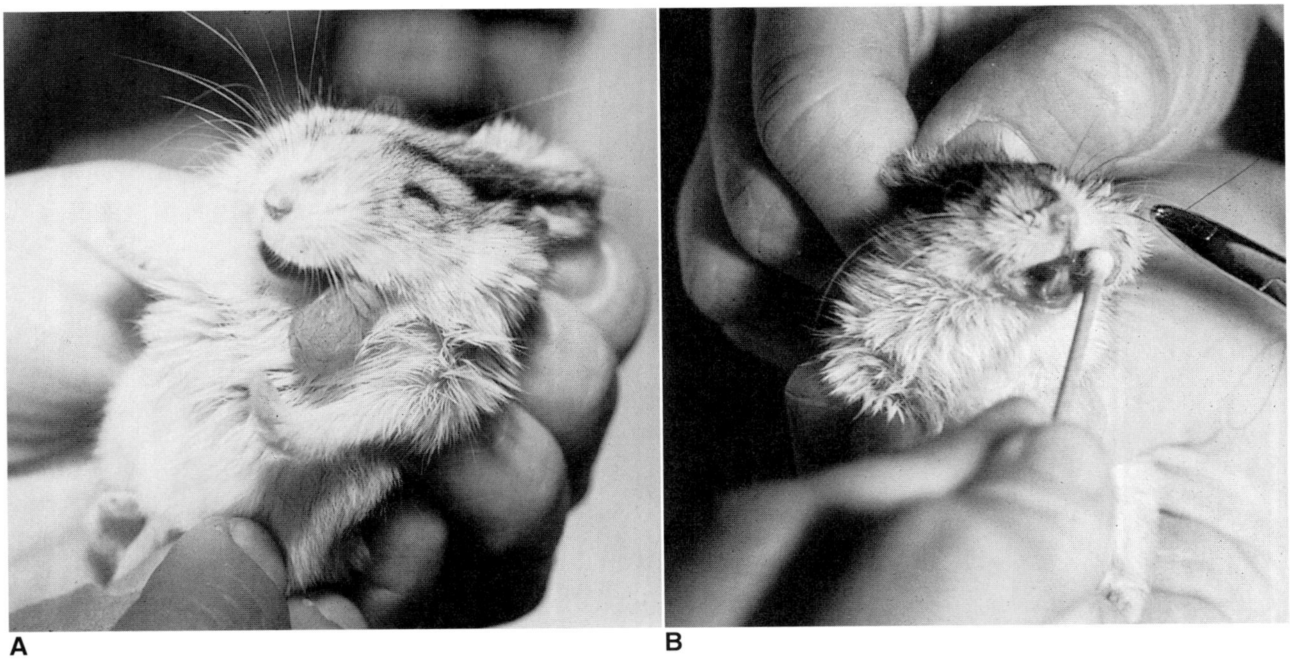

Figure 30-8 A, An everted cheek pouch in a dwarf hamster (*Phodopus sungoris*). B, Surgical repair. A cotton-tipped applicator swab is used for holding the cheek pouch in position while a full-thickness, percutaneous suture is placed.

lapse can be replaced and maintained in reduction with a purse-string suture. A necrotic rectal prolapse must be amputated and sutured, whereas a small intestinal or colonic prolapse (intussusception) requires abdominal exploration. All these conditions are considered surgical emergencies.

Determine what has prolapsed by carefully examining the tissue. If there is an orifice at the end of the tissue, it is a section of bowel. If the tissue is solid, it may be a rectal mass or polyp that has extruded on a stalk. Once you have determined that the bowel has prolapsed, gently pass a small, blunt-ended probe (e.g., a tomcat catheter or cotton-tipped miniapplicator) on each side of the prolapsed tissue. If this probe passes easily along the side of the prolapsed tissue for a distance greater than 1 cm, it is an intestinal or colonic prolapse (Fig. 30-9).

Lubricate a simple, nonnecrotic rectal prolapse and gently replace it with a cotton-tipped miniapplicator or a soft urinary catheter. Purse-string suture the anus with 5-0 nonabsorbable suture material so that the anus is snug, but not tight, over a 5-Fr catheter. The purse-string suture can be removed in 3 to 5 days; meanwhile, treat the medical condition causing the prolapse.

Amputate a necrotic rectal prolapse by using a full-thickness incision through the prolapse at its healthy junction with the remaining rectum, 180 degrees around the prolapse. Suture healthy rectum to healthy anus with a 6-0 monofilament, synthetic absorbable suture in a simple interrupted pattern. Amputate the remaining prolapsed tissue and close the second half of the anastomosis in the same manner. A purse-string suture is not needed (Fig. 30-10).

Hamsters with intussuscepted, prolapsed bowel have a poor prognosis for survival because they usually present in a debilitated condition because of a primary disease that caused the straining and the prolapse.

To surgically treat a prolapsed intestine, do a routine ventral midline abdominal exploratory examination. Identify the intussuscepted segment and gently reduce it if possible. Resect the necrotic portion of the intussusceptum, preserving the blood supply to the viable bowel. If it is not possible to reduce the intussusception, amputate it internally and have an assistant withdraw it externally by applying traction on the segment protruding from the anus. Do an end-to-end anastomosis of the healthy bowel with 6-0 or 7-0 monofilament, absorbable suture material. Six to eight simple interrupted sutures are usually needed to close the anastomosis. Test the site for leaks by gently milking intestinal contents past it. Close the defect in the mesentery with 6-0 absorbable suture material. Intestinal plication is no longer recommended because it takes a lot of time and is associated with more postoperative complications than not plicating.

Follow proper technique for enteric surgery, which includes changing gloves and instruments after completing the anastomosis, followed by irrigating the abdomen and subcutaneous tissues during routine closure.

TAIL AMPUTATION

Degloving injury to the tail of rodents is common. It occurs more often in gerbils because the skin on the tail is more loosely attached than in other rodents. The skin over the tail is thin and easily pulled off during restraint or if it becomes caught. A gerbil's tail can be mutilated by a cage mate if the animals do not get along. The exposed, skinless tail will eventually slough off, but may be painful or, if denervated, the affected rodent may chew on it until it sloughs. It is unlikely that sepsis would occur from this type of injury but infection is a risk in these animals. These factors favor a recommendation of amputation.

The procedure is simple. Place the animal in ventral recumbency and suspend the tail with tape away from the

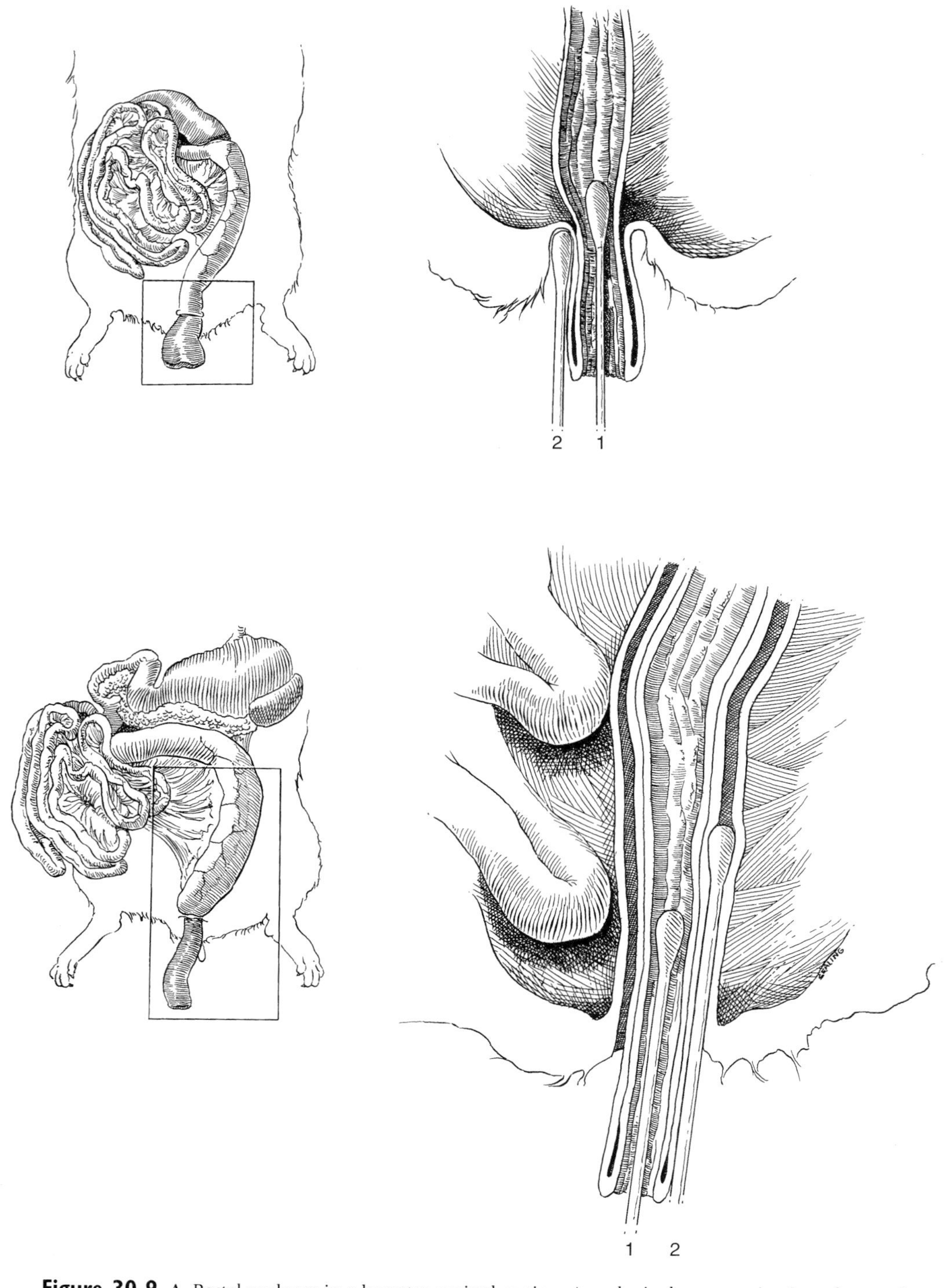

Figure 30-9 **A,** Rectal prolapse in a hamster, sagittal section. A probe is shown passing into the rectal lumen (*1*) but not on either side of the prolapse (*2*). **B,** Intestinal prolapse. The probe is shown passing into the intestinal lumen (*1*) as well as to either side of the prolapse (*2*).

body while the site is prepared for aseptic surgery. Incise the healthy skin several millimeters proximal to the edge of the degloving to create fresh skin edges for suturing. Retract the skin proximally as far as possible and disarticulate the tail between the two most cranial coccygeal vertebrae exposed. This will allow adequate soft tissue coverage over the vertebral bone. Bleeding from the coccygeal vessels is generally easy to control with cautery or a ligature. Close the subcutis with 5-0 or 6-0 absorbable suture and close the skin with suture or tissue adhesive. Sensation to the tail stump can be blocked by injecting 0.01 mL of bupivacaine or lidocaine several millimeters proximal to the site. Self-trauma to the amputation site is rare if gentle tissue handling and minimal cautery are used.

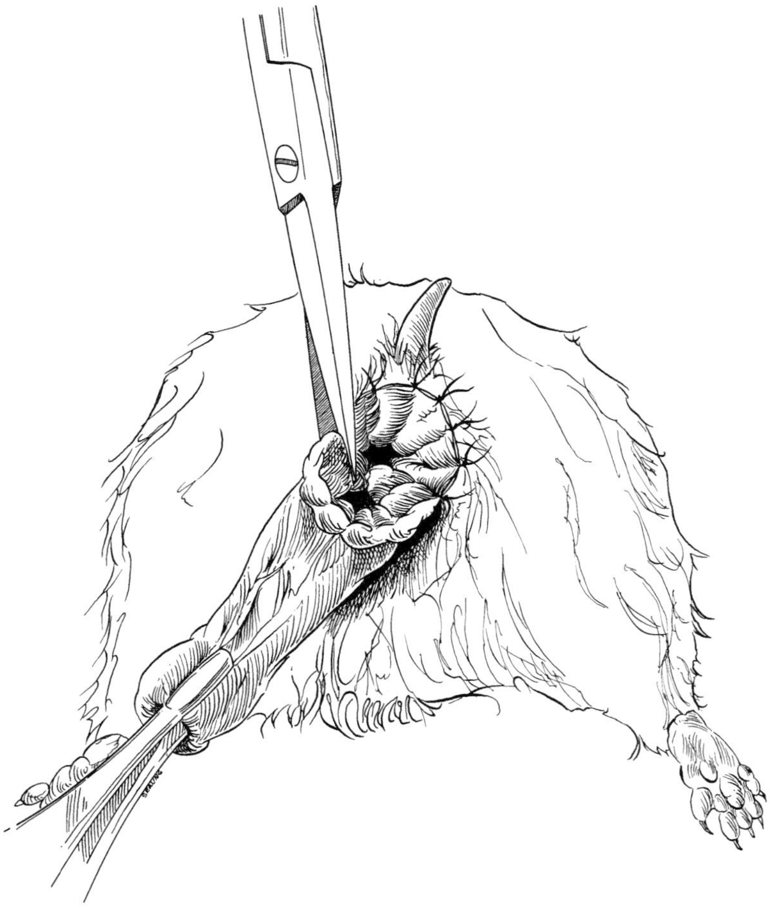

Figure 30-10 Amputation of a necrotic rectal prolapse in a hamster. Almost half of the rectocutaneous closure has been completed.

RECOVERY

During the recovery period, every attempt should be made to prevent energy loss. Hypothermia decreases the patient's metabolic rate and the rate of excretion of drugs prolonging the recovery period.[26] During the recovery period, the patient should be placed in a well-ventilated, oxygen-enriched, warm, quiet environment. Incubators are ideal for this purpose. They allow for proper temperature control, administration of oxygen, and adequate humidity. If an incubator is not available, circulating warm water heating blankets, heating lights, and warm water bottles may be used for thermal support. The patient is turned every 30 to 60 minutes to minimize the risk of hypostatic pulmonary congestion during recovery. The patient is placed in a cage lined with clean paper towels to keep the incision clean as the scab forms. It is best to keep the paztient alone so that other animals do not traumatize the surgical wound. Also, other animals, including conspecifics, often unexpectedly attack any animal they perceive to be injured.

The use of bandages should be minimized because they are not well tolerated by rodents. A paste made from metronidazole tablets applied to the wound will often discourage self-trauma because of its bitter taste. Analgesia is also very helpful at preventing self-trauma. A yoke can be fashioned to help prevent the patient from chewing at its wound. The technique for construction and application of such a yoke has been previously described.[17] Observe the patient carefully to make sure it is eating and drinking before discharge. The incision is evaluated and sutures removed if adequately healed in 10 to 14 days. Providing appropriate analgesia also helps prevent self-trauma during recovery.

Analgesia

Although often ignored, providing intraoperative and postoperative analgesia is important in small rodents.[25] Signs of pain in rodents include an increased heart rate, increased respiratory rate, decreased appetite, trembling, and bruxism. Many agents have been given with good success and appear to be effective in providing the recovering patient with pain relief.[11] Butorphanol (0.1-0.5 mg/kg IM, SC q4-6h for mice, and 2 mg/kg IM, SC q4-6h for rats) can be given intraoperatively and postoperatively. The dose should be repeated as necessary every 4 to 6 hours. Other analgesics include buprenorphine (0.05-0.10 mg/kg SC q8-12h in mice, and 0.01-0.05 mg/kg SC q8-12h in rats), which has a longer analgesic effect than butorphanol. Morphine (2-5 mg/kg SC q2-4h in mice and rats) is recommended. The veterinarian should consider the species variation in the dosage being used and the lasting analgesic effect. Morphine is not suitable as an analgesic agent in hamsters because this species shows high resistance to its effects. Nonsteroidal anti-inflammatory medications are gaining popularity as postoperative analgesics. Carprofen (4 mg/kg SC, PO q12h for rats and mice) has been recommended. Meloxicam (0.2-0.3 mg/kg PO q12h) has shown great efficacy as an analgesic in a clinical setting.

REFERENCES

1. Altman NH, Goodman DG: Neoplastic diseases. *In* Baker HJ, Lindsey JR, Weisbroth SH, eds. The Laboratory Rat. Vol I. Biology and Diseases. Orlando, Academic Press, 1979, pp 333-337.
2. Battles AH: The biology, care, and diseases of the Syrian hamster. Compend Contin Educ Pract Vet 1985; 7:815-824.
3. Bauck LA, Hagan RJ: Cystotomy for treatment of urolithiasis in a hamster. J Am Vet Med Assoc 1984; 184:99-100.
4. Bennett RA: Preparation and equipment useful for surgery in small exotic pets. Vet Clin North Am Exotic Anim Pract 2000; 3:563-585.
5. Castro JE: Surgical procedures in small laboratory animals. J Immunol Meth 1974; 4:213-216.
6. Collins BR: Common diseases and medical management of rodents and lagomorphs. *In* Jacobson ER, Kollias GV, eds. Exotic Animals. New York, Churchill Livingstone, 1988, pp 261-316.
7. Cooper JE: Tips on tumors. Proc North Am Vet Conf, 1994, pp 897-898.
8. Dulisch ML: A castration procedure for the rabbit, rat, hamster, and guinea pig. J Zoo Anim Med 1976; 7:8-11.
9. Dunn RC, Steinleitner AJ, Lambert H: Synergistic effect of intraperitoneally administered calcium channel blockade and recombinant tissue plasminogen activator to prevent adhesion formation in an animal model. Am J Obstet Gynecol 1991; 164:1327-1330.
10. Flecknell PA: Laboratory Animal Anesthesia. London, Academic Press, 1987.
11. Flecknell PA: Post-operative analgesia in rabbits and rodents. Lab Anim 1991; 20:34-37.
12. Goya RG, Lu JK, Meites J: Gonadal function in aging rats and its relation to pituitary and mammary pathology. Mech Aging Dev 1990; 56:77-88.
13. Harkness JE: Anesthesia, surgery. *In* Harkness JE, ed. A Practitioner's Guide to Domestic Rodents. Denver, American Animal Hospital Association, 1993, pp 37-50.
14. Harkness JE,Wagner JE: Biology and Medicine of Rabbits and Rodents, 3rd ed. Philadelphia, Lea & Febiger, 1989.
15. Hillyer EV: Common clinical maladies of pet rodents. Proc North Am Vet Conf, 1994, pp 909-912.
16. Hotchkiss CE: Effects of surgical removal of subcutaneous tumors on survival of rats. J Am Vet Med Assoc 1995; 206:1575-1579.
17. Hoyt RF Jr: Abdominal surgery of pet rabbits. *In* Bojrab MJ, ed. Current Techniques in Small Animal Surgery, 4th ed. Baltimore, Williams & Wilkins, 1998, pp 777-790.
18. Jackson TA, Heath LA, Hulin MS, et al: Squamous cell carcinoma of the midventral pad in three gerbils. J Am Vet Med Assoc 1996; 209:789-791.
19. Jenkins JR: Surgical sterilization of small mammals. Spay and castration. Vet Clin North Am Exotic Anim Pract 2000; 3:617-627.
20. Krohn B, Erben RG, Weiser H, et al: Osteopenia caused by ovariectomy in young female rats and prophylactic effects of 1,25-dihydroxyvitamin D_3. Zentralbl Veterinarmed A 1991; 38:54-60.
21. Krohn DE, Barthold SW: Biology and diseases of rats. *In* Fox JG, Cohen BJ, Loew FM, eds. Laboratory Animal Medicine. Orlando, Academic Press, 1984, pp 116-122.
22. Lidderdale JA, St Pierre SJ: Cystotomy for treatment of urolithiasis in a hamster. Vet Rec 1990; 127:364.
23. Mader DM: Use of laser in exotic animal medicine. Vet Pract News 2000; 12:1.
24. Mighell JS, Baker AE: Caesarean section in a gerbil. Vet Rec 1990; 126:441.
25. Redrobe S: Soft tissue surgery of rabbits and rodents. Semin Avian Exotic Pet Med 2002; 11:231-245.
26. Robinson WR, Peters RH, Zimmerman J: The effects of body size and temperature on metabolic rate of organisms. Can J Zool 1983; 61:281-288.
27. Roman CD, Hanley GA, Beauchamp RD: Operative technique for safe pulmonary lobectomy in Sprague-Dawley rats. Contemp Top Lab Anim Sci 2002; 41:28-30.
28. Squire RA, Goodman DG, Valerio MG, et al: Tumors. *In* Benirschke K, Garner FM, Jones TC, eds. Pathology of Laboratory Animals. Vol II. Orlando, Academic Press, 1978, pp 1051-1283.
29. Strandberg JD: Neoplastic diseases. *In* Van Hoosier GL Jr, McPherson CW, eds. Laboratory Hamsters. Orlando, Academic Press, 1987, pp 157-168.
30. Toft JD: Commonly observed spontaneous neoplasms in rabbits, rats, guinea pigs, hamsters, and gerbils. Semin Avian Exotic Pet Med 1991; 1:80-92.
31. Van Hoosier GL Jr, McPherson CW: Laboratory Hamsters. Orlando, Academic Press, 1987.
32. White WJ, Field KJ: Anesthesia and surgery of laboratory animals. *In* Harkness JE, ed. Vet Clin North Am Small Anim Pract 1987; 17:989-1017.
33. Young S, Hallowes RC: Tumours of the mammary gland. *In* Turusov VS, ed. Pathology of Tumours in Laboratory Animals. IARC Sci Publ No 5, Vol 1, Part 1. Lyon, France, IARC, 1973, pp 31-74.

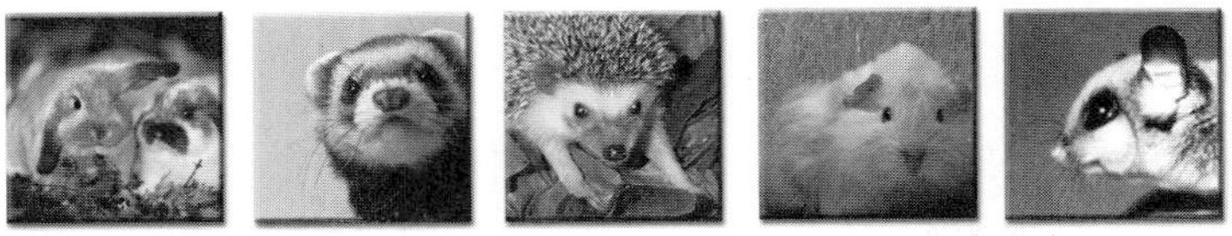

SECTION

FIVE

OTHER SMALL MAMMALS

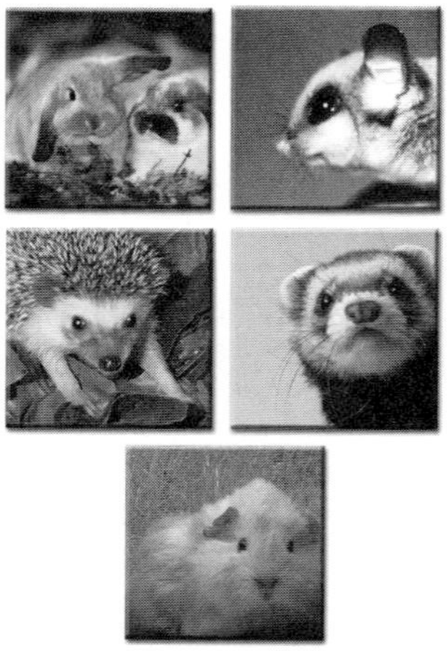

CHAPTER 31

Sugar Gliders

Robert D. Ness, DVM, and Rosie Booth, BVSc

BIOLOGY

Natural History

Sugar gliders (*Petaurus breviceps*) are small, nocturnal arboreal marsupials that are native to New Guinea and the eastern coast of Australia.[4] They inhabit open areas in tropical or coastal forests and dry, inland, sclerophyll tropical forests. They are social animals, with colonies of 6 to 10 animals occupying a territory of up to 1 hectare. Dominant males mark territory and other group members with scent gland secretions. Animals in a group nest communally in leaf-lined tree holes. During periods of extreme cold or food scarcity, sugar gliders conserve energy by going into torpor for as many as 16 hours per day.[3]

Anatomy and Physiology

Marsupials: General Marsupials are best known for possessing a pouch in which the female raises her young (Fig. 31-1). The degree of pouch enclosure is dependent on the species. The pouch is absent in all males and in female South American short-tailed opossums, which are considered to be more primitive marsupials. The female sugar glider has a pouch, containing four teats, in which she raises one or two young.

Epipubic bones (ossa marsupialia or eupubic bones) are unique to certain marsupials, but they are diminished or absent in gliders. These small bones are thought to provide an attachment for muscles that support the pouch. Their absence may be an adaptation to gliding that reduces skeletal weight.

The metabolism of marsupials is approximately two thirds that of placental (eutherian) mammals. The normal heart rate of a sugar glider is 200 to 300 beats/min, and the respiratory rate is 16 to 40 breaths/min.[1] The cloaca is a common terminal opening of the rectum, urinary ducts, and genital ducts. Cloacal temperature is lower than the actual body temperature; the average cloacal temperature is 89.6°F (32°C).[8] True rectal temperature in marsupials can be measured by directing the thermometer dorsally into the rectum from within the cloaca. The rectal temperature is usually 97.3°F (36.3°C).[3] Measurement of the tympanic temperature is another means to determine core body temperature.

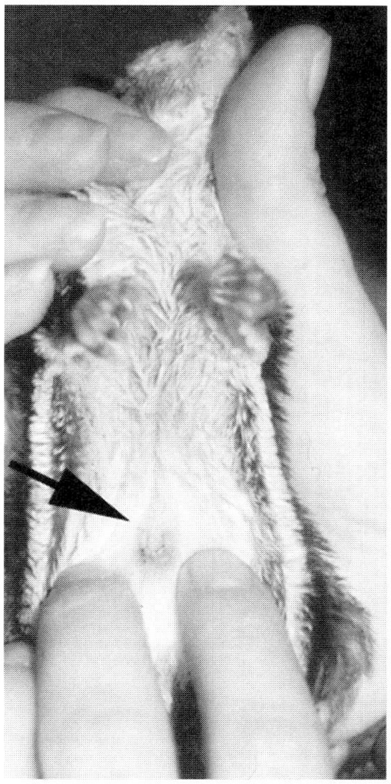

Figure 31-1 Female sugar gliders raise one or two young in their pouch *(arrow)*, which contains four teats.

Anatomic characteristics Sugar gliders have soft, velvety fur that is gray with a central black stripe dorsally and cream-colored ventrally. Similar to American flying squirrels, sugar gliders possess a patagium (gliding membrane) that stretches between their front and hind legs (Fig. 31-2). Adult males weigh between 100 and 160 g and females weigh between 80 and 130 g, although these ranges vary among subspecies. Body length ranges from 160 to 210 mm and tail length from 165 to 210 mm. Gliding distances are reported to be as long as 50 m.[16] Being a nocturnal prey species, sugar gliders have large, protruding, widely spaced eyes. They have five toes on their hind feet, with an opposable first digit and syndactyly of the second and third digits (Fig. 31-3). Dominant males mark territory and group members with secretions from androgen-sensitive frontal (forehead) (Fig. 31-4), gular (throat), and paracloacal scent glands.

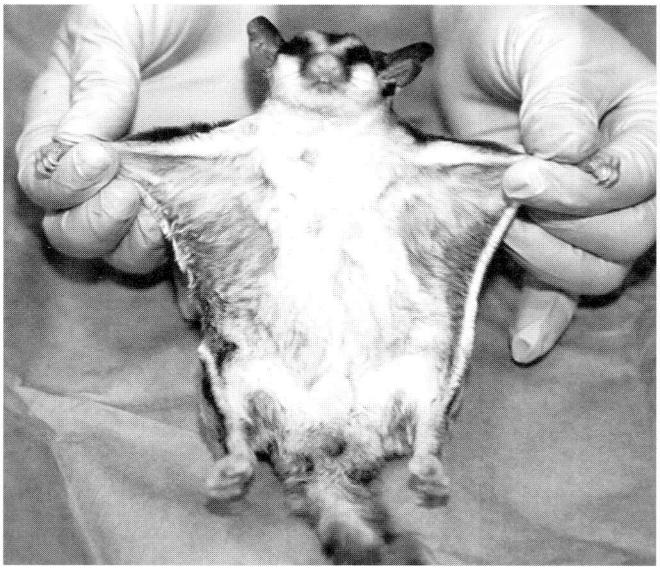

Figure 31-2 The patagium, or gliding membrane, of sugar gliders stretches between their front and hind legs.

Reproduction Sugar gliders are seasonally polyestrous, with the natural breeding season in Australia occurring between June and November. They are polygynous, with a dominant male that breeds with the mature females in the colony.[4] Young (joeys) are typically born in the spring, when insects are plentiful. Litter size is usually two (81%) or, less commonly, one (19%).[4] Two litters

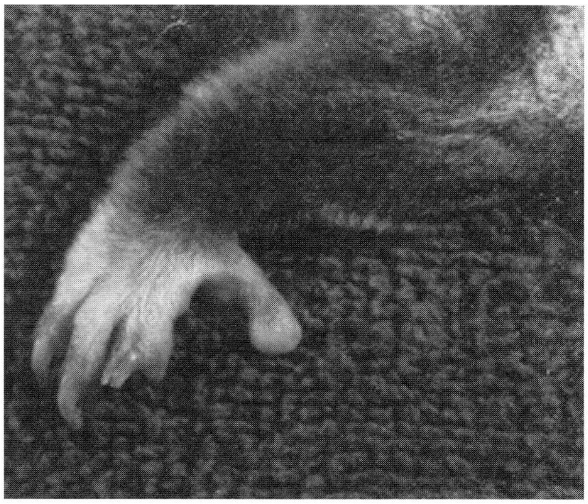

Figure 31-3 The hind foot of sugar gliders has five toes, with syndactyly of the second and third digits and an opposable first digit.

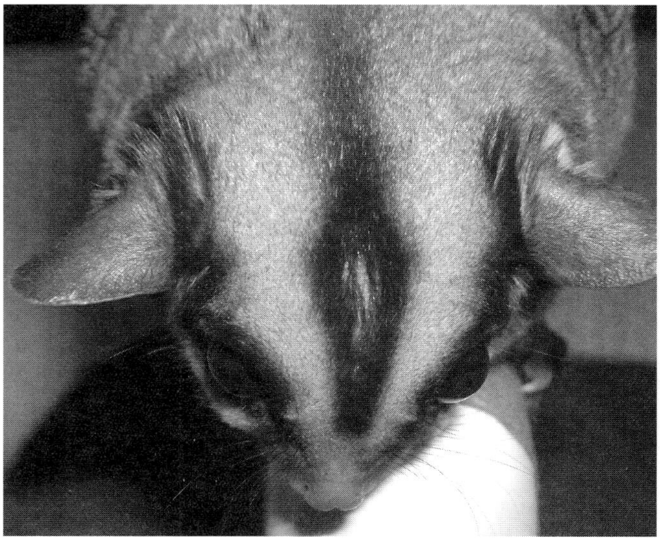

Figure 31-4 Male sugar gliders have a frontal scent gland on their head. Secretions from this gland are used to mark territory and group members.

in a single breeding season are common. The estrous cycle is 29 days in length, and gestation is 15 to 17 days.[17] Young weigh only 0.2 g at birth when they migrate to the pouch. They remain in the pouch for 70 to 74 days. After they outgrow the pouch, the young are left in the nest until they are weaned at 110 to 120 days of age. The young remain with the colony until they are forcibly dispersed, at 7 to 10 months of age.[1] Sexual maturity is reached at 8 to 12 months of age in females and at 12 to 15 months in males.[14]

The reproductive anatomy of sugar gliders is unique when compared with that of other mammals routinely treated in practice. Female sugar gliders have two uteri and two long, thin, lateral vaginas that open into a single cul-de-sac divided by a septum. Both sexes have paracloacal glands, which are more developed in the male.[15] Males have a large prostate with a constriction at the anterior third. They also have two pairs of Cowper's glands in addition to three paracloacal glands. The testes are located in a prepenile pendulous scrotum (Fig. 31-5), and the penis is bifid (Fig. 31-6). Males do not urinate from the forked end of the penis, but rather from the proximal portion. Therefore, the distal penis can be amputated in cases of penile trauma or paraphimosis.

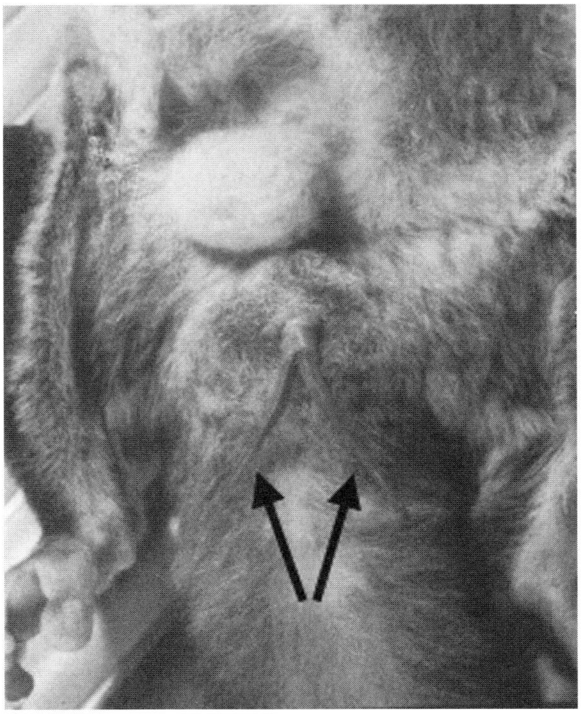

Figure 31-6 In male sugar gliders, the penis is bifid *(arrows)*. Males do not urinate from the tip of the forked penis, but from its base.

Behavior

Sugar gliders make good pets if they are given sufficient socialization and ample space. When hand-reared, they adapt well to captivity and develop a strong bond with their human companions. They are time-consuming pets, with recommended socialization periods of at least 2 hours per day. Basic handling for socialization and companionship is best achieved at night, when the animals are more interactive and playful. If awakened and handled during the day, sugar gliders become agitated and irritable.

Sugar gliders are most responsive to and trusting of individuals they know, but they respond well if approached with patience and gentle handling. They enjoy cuddling and curling up in shirt pockets or pouches, where they feel safe. They should not be allowed to crawl into tight-fitting clothes, such as pants pockets, because of the risk of injury.

Advantages of these pets include their small size, playfulness, and intelligence. The life span of sugar gliders is longer than that of other comparably sized pets; they can live from 10 to 12 years in captivity.[1] Disadvantages include their nocturnal nature, housing requirements, specific dietary needs, and musky odor.

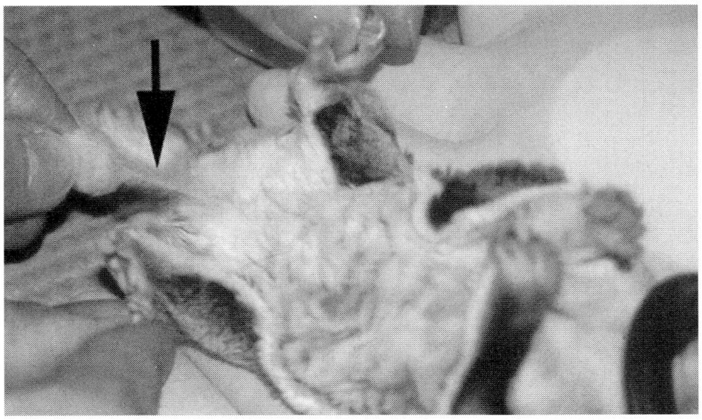

Figure 31-5 The prepenile scrotum of a male sugar glider is attached to the body wall by a long scrotal neck *(arrow)*.

Husbandry

Caging Because of their active nature, sugar gliders should have cages as large as possible. These animals need space to climb, run, and jump. Minimum cage size is 36 × 24 × 36 inches (91 × 61 × 91 cm), but larger is better. Cages should be made of wire for good ventilation, with wire spacing no more than 1.0 × 0.5 inch (2.5 × 1.3 cm) wide. Sugar gliders tolerate temperatures between 65° and 90° F (18° and 32° C), with an ideal range of 75° to 80° F (24° to 27° C).[10] The cage must have designated areas for food, water, shelter, and exercise. Several food and water dishes should be placed in various locations throughout the cage. A nest box or sleeping pouch positioned high in the cage gives the sugar glider a place to sleep during the day. Bedding in the nest site consisting of hardwood shavings, recycled paper substrate, or shredded paper is recommended. Branches, perches, and shelves can be placed at various levels of the cage to satisfy the natural behavior of climbing. Sugar gliders enjoy playing with bird toys, such as swings and chew toys. Plastic wheels without open rungs, such as a hamster wheel, are used for exercise. A variety of objects may be placed throughout the cage to stimulate and entertain these animals.

Sugar gliders need permanent access to a nest box for sleeping and hiding, with minimal daytime disturbances. Nest box size depends on colony size, but boxes should be at least 6 × 6 inches (13 × 13 cm) with a hinged lid and a circular opening on the front with a sliding closure.[4] Bird nest boxes or small hollow logs are suitable. Nesting material can consist of hardwood shavings, recycled paper products, shredded bark, dried leaves, coconut fibers, sea grass, or equivalent materials. Artificial wool, cloth strips, and similar materials are not suitable because fibers have been known to entrap an animal's limbs. Nest boxes need to be cleaned and bedding material changed regularly, at least every 1 to 2 weeks. If nest box closures are secure, the nest box can be relocated from an outdoor aviary into the house for interaction each evening and then returned to the aviary to allow for nocturnal activity.

Nutrition and feeding

Natural diet Sugar gliders are omnivorous. The diet of a wild sugar glider can include sap and gum from eucalyptus and acacia trees, nectar and pollen, manna and honeydew, and a wide variety of insects and arachnids.[4] Sugar gliders possess enlarged lower incisors for chewing into the bark of trees. The lengthened fourth digit on the manus aids in extracting insects from crevices. Sugar gliders also have an enlarged cecum, which functions principally in microbial fermentation of complex polysaccharides in gum.

The diet varies with the season. During the spring and summer months, these animals are primarily insectivorous. During the winter months, sugar gliders feed on gum from the eucalyptus and acacia trees, as well as on sap and sugar from the trees and sap-sucking insects.

Field energetics studies have demonstrated that wild sugar gliders consume 182 to 229 kilojoules (kJ)/day.[11] This is equivalent to approximately 17% of body weight in wet weight of food.[11] Captive gliders expend less energy in exercise and consume more easily assimilated foods than do those in the wild; therefore, the total energy offered to gliders in captivity should be less.

Captive diet Captive diets must satisfy the numerous specializations of these omnivores. The captive diet should include nectar, insects, and other protein sources, as well as limited amounts of fruits and vegetables.[10] Protein is a critical nutrient in the diet of sugar gliders. Various protein sources include insects (mealworms and crickets), eggs, newborn mice, lean meat, and commercial protein sources (high-quality cat food or monkey chow). Other natural dietary components are sap and nectar, which provide necessary carbohydrates. Sources include fresh nectar, maple syrup, honey, and artificial nectar products. Examples of commercial products include prepared lory diets and Gliderade (Avico, Fallbrook, CA). Various commercial diets for sugar gliders and insectivores are available and should be included as part (at least 24%) of the diet. Leafy green vegetables provide a source of fiber and some vitamins. Sugar gliders accept a wide variety of other foods, including fruits, vegetables, nuts, and seeds (sunflower and pumpkin). Fruit juices and strained baby food can be offered if they are free of preservatives. Because these foods are not a significant component of the natural diet, they should constitute less than 10% of the captive diet. Sprinkle a broad-spectrum vitamin and mineral supplement with a good calcium supply on the food daily.

Fruit-based diets are harmful to captive sugar gliders because they provide inadequate protein and calcium and predispose animals to osteoporosis and periodontal disease. Although sugar gliders readily accept fruits, nuts, and grains, these are not a substantial part of their natural diet. Contrary to the nutritional needs observed in the wild, much of the information found in lay publications lists fruits and vegetables as a major portion of the captive diet.

A simplified diet for captive sugar gliders has been proposed.[9] The diet consists of 50% insectivore/carnivore diet and 50% Leadbeater's mixture (an artificial nectar mix originally formulated for Leadbeater's possums [*Gymnobelideus leadbeateri*]), with a small amount of other foods as treats. Various insectivore/carnivore diets are marketed, with the choice depending on reliability of the company, availability to the owner, and acceptance by the pet. The Leadbeater's mixture consists of 150 mL water, 150 mL honey, one shelled hard-boiled egg, 25 g high-protein baby cereal, and one teaspoon vitamin and mineral mixture. This mixture is kept refrigerated until served, with unused portions discarded after 3 days. The mixture can be frozen for later use. Acceptable treat foods can include lean meats, diced fruit, bee pollen, and gut-loaded insects. Treats should constitute less than 5% of the diet.

Hand-rearing Orphaned marsupial-pouch young must be maintained at a stable temperature close to the body temperature of the mother, which may range from 86° to 93°F (30° to 34°C). The young depend less on artificial heat as their fur begins to grow. A snug artificial pouch can be made from a child's cotton sock to provide security and warmth. Place the pouch in a temperature-controlled box. By the time the pelage is thick and complete, the orphan has reached a homeothermic state and no longer requires an artificial heat source.

If the age of the orphaned young is not known, estimate the age from the body weight and stage of development (Table 31-1). Sugar glider pouch life is 70 to 74 days, and weaning occurs at 120 days.[17] From day 75 to day 100, the young are left in an insulated nest while the mother is foraging. When an orphan has reached this stage, a soft toy the size of an adult sugar glider is useful to provide security from the time of pouch exit to weaning. The artificial nest can be a fleecy cotton bag that is big enough to accommodate the animal and the toy; it should be placed in a box maintained at 77°F (25°C).

Feed unfurred young every 1 to 2 hours (including throughout the night), and feed just-furred young every 4 hours. Gradually reduce the frequency to twice daily, then once daily, until the young are weaned. Feed a low-lactose milk formula (e.g., puppy Esbilac [PetAg, Inc., Hampshire, IL]). Marsupial milk increases in energy at the time of pouch exit to provide for the young's increased energy demands of locomotion and thermoregulation. This change can be simulated by adding canola oil (rape seed oil) to the milk at the rate of 1 mL of oil per 20 mL of milk.

Juvenile sugar gliders usually lap readily from the tip of a syringe, or they can be taught to lap from a small plastic lid. At each feeding, measure and record milk intake. Measure body weight daily until the weight stabilizes, then weekly. Frequency of feeding and quantity of food can be adjusted to achieve a satisfactory growth rate. Start offering solids at about 100 days, at which time the young glider should weigh approximately 54 g, and wean at 130 days, when body weight is approximately 78 g. Pureed baby food with meat and vegetables or blended adult diet is suitable starter food.

CLINICAL TECHNIQUES

Handling and Restraint

Sugar gliders are rather easy to handle but can be difficult to restrain. As mentioned earlier, sugar gliders are very energetic

TABLE 31-1
Growth and Development of Young Sugar Gliders

Age (days)	Weight (g)	Milestones	Total Daily Intake (mL)
1	0.2	Birth	—
20	0.8	Ears free from head; papillae of whiskers visible	0.2
40	3.2	Ears pigmented; whiskers erupted; eye slits present	0.6
60	12	Intermittently detached from teat; dorsal stripe, fur, and gliding membrane developing	2.5
70	20	Left in nest; eyes open; fully furred	4
80-90	35-44	Fur lengthens	6-8
100	54	Emerging from nest, starting to eat solids	8-10
120-130	78	Weaning	Feed up to 20% of body weight in pureed solids
200	100	Subadult	Feed up to 20% of body weight in solids

Adapted from Booth RJ: General husbandry and medical care of sugar gliders. *In* Bonagura JD, ed. Kirk's Current Veterinary Therapy XIII. Philadelphia, WB Saunders, 2000, pp 1157-1163.

and hyperactive during the late evening hours, which makes them difficult to handle or restrain. Therefore, schedule clinical examinations early in the day, when the animals are normally less active.

Nest boxes make useful transport boxes if they are constructed with hinged lids and lockable slides over the circular entrance. If the hinged lid is partially opened, the glider can be captured with a hand protected by a small cotton bag, which is then inverted over the glider. Bag seams should be double sewn so that no frayed threads can become tangled around the sugar glider's appendages. Palpate the head through the bag, then grasp the glider firmly around the back of the head, behind the ears, as you cup its body in the rest of your hand. Peel the bag back to expose the face for examination or to apply a face mask to induce anesthesia.

Other methods of restraint include grasping the glider at the base of its tail or cupping the animal in the palm of your hand. The ventrum and hindquarters can be examined by lifting the animal by the base of its tail while allowing the glider to grasp a surface with its front feet. This method also permits palpation of the abdomen and examination of the pouch. To examine the head and chest, hold the sugar glider in a small towel with its head exposed. These animals do not tolerate being scruffed.

Full clinical examination or diagnostic sampling is best performed with the animal under isoflurane anesthesia. Do a complete head-to-toe examination, assessing the function of all major systems. Measure the temperature, pulse, and respiratory rate, and weigh the animal before it recovers from anesthesia. During recovery, place the sugar glider in a cotton bag or pouch and administer oxygen by face mask. Recovery is usually rapid. Assess locomotion before anesthesia or after full recovery, when the sugar glider is contained in a small cage with simple horizontal perches.

Blood Collection

Collecting a blood sample from a sugar glider can be difficult. Sedation or full anesthesia with an inhalant anesthetic (e.g., isoflurane) is required for diagnostic sampling. Use a 0.5-mL insulin syringe or a 1-mL tuberculin syringe with a 25- to 27-gauge needle to collect blood samples. Because of the small size of these animals, only small volumes of blood (up to 1% of body weight in grams) can be safely drawn.

Reliable venipuncture sites in sugar gliders are the jugular vein and the cranial vena cava.[12] These sites yield the greatest blood volume (up to 1 mL) from an adult sugar glider. For jugular venipuncture, insert the needle midway between the point of the shoulder and the ramus of the mandible on the ventral aspect of the neck, lateral to the trachea and esophagus. The cranial vena cava can be sampled at the thoracic inlet. The needle is directed caudally at a 30-degree angle off midline toward the opposite hind leg.

Small blood samples can be obtained from various peripheral veins. The medial tibial artery can be accessed to collect up to 0.5 mL of blood.[1] Although this vessel is readily visible, it is quite mobile. For venipuncture of the cephalic, lateral saphenous, femoral, or ventral coccygeal veins, use a 0.5-mL insulin syringe with a 27-gauge needle. These veins are superficial and easily collapse if too much negative pressure is applied. Up to 0.25 mL of blood can be drawn from these veins.

Hematologic and plasma biochemical values obtained from 11 captive sugar gliders are listed in Table 31-2. These values should be used as a guide as the sample size is too small to consider them as definitive reference ranges.

Treatment Techniques

Fluid therapy is administered by routes commonly used in other small animals and includes oral, subcutaneous, and intraosseous routes. Administer subcutaneous fluids along the dorsal midline of the thorax. Take care not to administer the fluids laterally into the patagium because fluids are more slowly absorbed from this area and can cause discomfort and distress in the patient. Administer intraosseous fluids in the proximal femur by using the same technique to place an intraosseous catheter as is used in other small mammals. Calculate the volume of fluids to be administered by estimating the percent dehydration in addition to the daily fluid requirements (comparable to methods used in similarly sized mammals). The choice of fluids depends on the animal's condition and diagnosis.

TABLE 31-2
Hematologic and Plasma Biochemical Reference Values for Captive Sugar Gliders*

Measurement	*n*	95% CI
Hemoglobin (g/dL)	2	13-15†
Hematocrit (%)	8	45-53
Red blood cell count (× $10^6/\mu L$)	9	5.1-17.8
Mean corpuscular hemoglobin concentration (g/dL)	3	31-33†
Mean cell volume (μm^3)	3	58-62†
Mean corpuscular hemoglobin (pg)	3	18-21†
Platelets (× $10^3/\mu L$)	7	105-220
White blood cell count, total (× $10^3/\mu L$)	10	5.0-12.2
Neutrophils (× $10^3/\mu L$)	10	1.5-3.0
Bands (× $10^3/\mu L$)	10	0
Lymphocytes (× $10^3/\mu L$)	10	2.8-9.2
Monocytes (× $10^3/\mu L$)	9	0.1-0.2
Eosinophils (× $10^3/\mu L$)	10	0-0.1
Basophils (× $10^3/\mu L$)	10	0
Sodium (mmol/L)	9	135-145
Potassium (mmol/L)	9	3.3-5.9
Blood urea nitrogen (mg/dL)	9	18-24
Creatinine (mg/dL)	11	0.3-0.5
Bilirubin, total (mg/dL)	11	0.4-0.8
Alanine aminotransferase (ALT) (IU/L)	10	50-106
Aspartate aminotransferase (AST) (IU/L)	9	46-179
Creatine phosphokinase (IU/L)	7	210-589
Protein, total (g/dL)	11	5.1-6.1
Albumin (g/dL)	10	3.5-4.3
Glucose (mg/dL)	11	130-183
Calcium (mg/dL)	9	6.9-8.4
Phosphorus (mg/dL)	5	3.8-4.4

CI, Confidence interval.
*Values shown are the 95% confidence intervals after outliers were removed. Statistically, 90% of the population should have values within these limits. Because the sample size is small, these values should be used as guidelines. Data were analyzed using SPS version 10.0.
†Sample size too small to calculate meaningful confidence intervals (actual range quoted).

Injections can be given in a variety of routes and sites. Give intramuscular injections in the epaxial muscles of the neck and upper thorax or in the muscle mass in the anterior thigh (biceps femoris). Subcutaneous injections are safely administered along the dorsal midline of the thorax. Intravenous injections are difficult and must be administered in the cephalic or lateral saphenous veins with the animal under general sedation.

Radiography

General anesthesia is required to position a sugar glider for diagnostic radiographs. If young are detached from the teat, remove them before radiography.

In very small animals, mammography film yields superb definition of both soft tissues and skeletal elements. Special cassettes with slightly slower screens are required, but otherwise standard radiographic equipment can be used. Because of the greater detail provided by this film and screen combination, greater exposure is required (preferably higher milliamperage). Some experimentation will be required to arrive at the best settings for each individual radiographic machine. A suitable starting point for a sugar glider is 60 kilovolts (kV) at 30 milliamperes (mA) for 0.2 to 0.3 sec (see also Chapter 37).

Drug Dosages

Various antimicrobial agents have been used successfully in captive sugar gliders, despite the absence of pharmacologic studies in this species. When using metabolic scaling, it should be remembered that the small body size is offset to some extent by the low metabolic rate of marsupials. Approximate drug dosages can be extrapolated from the low-end ranges for cats, ferrets, and hedgehogs.[7] Dosages provided in Table 31-3 have been extrapolated from dosages used in other species and have been used successfully in sugar gliders.[14]

DISEASES AND SYNDROMES

Gastrointestinal Disease

Malnutrition Because of the misinformation regarding their dietary requirements, sugar gliders in captivity commonly suffer from malnutrition. Common diet-related conditions in captive sugar gliders include hypoproteinemia, hypocalcemia, and anemia. Hypocalcemia is primarily caused by an imbalance of dietary calcium, phosphorus, and vitamin D. Lack of dietary protein is a cause of anemia and hypoproteinemia. With chronic malnutrition, hepatic and renal biochemical values are abnormal, because these organ systems become affected. Malnourished sugar gliders are weak, lethargic, and debilitated at presentation. These animals are usually thin and dehydrated; if they are severely hypocalcemic, seizures and pathologic fractures can develop. Pale mucous membranes, edema, and bruising may be present in anemic and hypoproteinemic patients, and secondary infections are common in debilitated animals. Treatment involves general supportive care and correction of the underlying dietary problems.

Obesity Captive sugar gliders easily become overweight when fed a diet that is too high in fat or protein. Lack of exercise also contributes to the problem. Obesity can lead to cardiac, hepatic, and pancreatic disease, as in other species.[10] Lipid deposits can form in the eyes of juvenile sugar gliders if the mother is fed a diet too high in fat. These deposits appear as small white spots within the eyes and can affect the animal's sight. Treatment of obesity includes modifying the diet and increasing exercise.

Nutritional osteodystrophy Nutritional osteodystrophy, also known as metabolic bone disease or nutritional secondary hyperparathyroidism, is a common cause of hind limb paresis and paralysis in pet sugar gliders. The condition resembles the syndrome seen in calcium-deficient captive reptiles. The importance of full-spectrum light, particularly ultraviolet light, is well established in reptiles; however, because sugar gliders are nocturnal, its importance in this species is unclear. The clinical presentation of nutritional osteodystrophy is sudden onset of hind limb paresis (Fig. 31-7); spinal trauma and general malnutrition are differential diagnoses. Radiographs may reveal long bone, pelvic, and vertebral osteoporosis. Hypocalcemia and hypopro-

TABLE 31-3
Drug Dosages for Sugar Gliders

Agent	Dosage and Administration	Comments
Antiparasitics		
Fenbendazole	20-50 mg/kg PO q24 h × 3 days	Roundworms, hookworms, whipworms, and tapeworms
Oxfendazole	5 mg/kg PO once	Roundworms and adult tapeworms
Ivermectin	0.2 mg/kg PO, SC, repeat at 14 days	Roundworms, hookworms, whipworms, and mites
Carbaryl 5% powder	Use topically or in nest box	Use sparingly for ectoparasites
Pyrethrin powder	Use topically	Ectoparasites
Antimicrobials		
Amoxicillin	30 mg/kg PO, IM q24h*	
Cephalexin	30 mg/kg SC q24h	Injectable form not available in United States
Enrofloxacin	5 mg/kg IM, PO q24h	Potential tissue necrosis when administered parenterally
Lincomycin	30 mg/kg IM, PO q24h*	
Metronidazole	80 mg/kg PO q24h*	
Trimethoprim/sulfa	15 mg/kg PO q12h	
Analgesics		
Butorphanol	0.5 mg/kg IM q8h	Analgesia
Flunixin meglumine	0.1 mg/kg IM q12h	Analgesia and antiinflammatory
Acepromazine and butorphanol	1.7 mg/kg (A) and 1.7 mg/kg (B) PO	Postoperative analgesia and sedation to prevent self-trauma to incision site
Acepromazine and ketamine	1 mg/kg (A) and 10 mg/kg (B) SC	Postoperative analgesia and sedation to prevent self-trauma to incision site
Anesthetics		
Isoflurane	1%-5 %	Anesthetic agent of choice
Sevoflurane	1%-5 %	
Tiletamine/zolazepam	8-12.4 mg/kg	Use with caution: reports of toxicity
Ketamine	20 mg/kg IM	Follow with isoflurane

Modified from Pye GW, Carpenter JW: A guide to medicine and surgery in sugar gliders. Vet Med 1999; 94:891-905.
*Daily dose can be divided.

teinemia are seen on plasma biochemical profiles. The clinical history often indicates a calcium-deficient diet comprising 75% fruit and 25% muscle meat.[1] Patients identified in the early stages may respond to cage rest, parenteral calcium, and vitamin D_3 with dietary correction.

Calcitonin-salmon (50 to 100 IU/kg; e.g., 200 IU/mL Miacalcin [Sandoz Ltd, Hanover, NJ]) can be used in more severely affected animals.[13] However, calcitonin should only be given when plasma calcium concentrations are within reference ranges. Calcitonin decreases calcium resorption from bone because it inhibits osteoclastic activity; however, because serum calcium and phosphorous concentrations also decrease, calcitonin must be used in conjunction with a calcium supplement. Until more is known about specific nutritional requirements of sugar gliders, diets should contain about 1% calcium, 0.5% phosphorus, and 1500 IU/kg vitamin D on a dry weight basis.[1] Insects should be gut-loaded with calcium before being fed to sugar gliders.

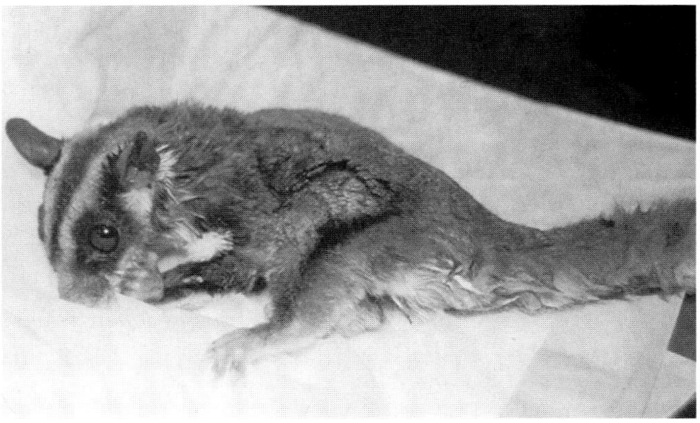

Figure 31-7 Sudden onset of hind limb paresis is the most common clinical sign of nutritional osteodystrophy, or metabolic bone disease. This syndrome is common in captive sugar gliders that are fed an inadequate diet.

Dental disease Periodontal disease and tartar buildup are common in sugar gliders fed soft, carbohydrate-rich diets.[1] Tartar can be scaled while the patient is anesthetized. Treat associated gingivitis with systemic antibiotics. Including insects with hard exoskeletons in the diet helps deter tartar buildup.

Advanced tooth decay or traumatic incisor fracture can lead to exposed root canals. The root canal is too small for filling, and extracting the lower incisor risks fracturing the mandibular symphysis. Therefore, diet modification is the best way to allow the patient to cope with the root exposure.[1]

Respiratory Disease

The differential diagnoses in sugar gliders that are presented with signs of tachypnea or dyspnea include trauma, bacterial pneumonia, cardiac failure, heat stress, and abdominal distention from various causes. Radiography with the animal anesthetized with isoflurane will assist with diagnosis and is usually safe, even in severely compromised animals.

Urogenital Disease

Failure to breed in females can be related to obesity or inappropriate social situations. In the closely related Leadbeater's possum, abscesses in both lateral vaginas were observed in an aged female. This animal presented with lethargy and abdominal distention, and the diagnosis was made by radiography and exploratory laparotomy.

Self-mutilation of the penis and scrotum is sometimes seen in stressed males (see later discussion). In animals with severe injuries, amputation of the penis may be necessary. Because males urinate from the base of the penis, amputation of the forked end of the penis will not interfere with urination.

Dermatologic and Musculoskeletal Diseases

Stress-related disorders Stress in sugar gliders can manifest in numerous ways. Self-mutilation of the tail, limbs, scrotum, and penis is common. Because sexual frustration may be a factor, castration is recommended for a pubescent male that mutilates his penis or scrotum.[10] Stressed sugar gliders can also present with coprophagy, hyperphagia, polydipsia, and pacing.[7] Some patients simply present with alopecia, presumably from increased adrenal activity caused by stress. Providing proper nutrition and hygiene, normal social grouping, appropriate nesting areas and cage accessories, and protection from potential predatory species can help reduce stress in captive sugar gliders.

Traumatic injuries Trauma is a common presentation in captive sugar gliders. Bite wounds from pet dogs, cats, and ferrets are potentially fatal to these little animals, not only because of the physical trauma but also because of the potential infection acquired from the wound. Sugar gliders can also be injured by household accidents, such as falling into toilet bowls, chewing on electrical cords, being shut in a door or window, or being stepped on by family members. Common injuries include cuts, punctures, and fractures.

Ophthalmic injuries occur frequently in sugar gliders because of their slightly protruding eyes. Corneal scratches with ulceration and conjunctivitis are most common.

Neurologic Disease

The most common neurologic condition of pet sugar gliders is paresis or paralysis secondary to nutritional spinal osteopathy. If a sugar glider presents with neurologic signs, differential diagnoses should include trauma and, less commonly, middle ear infection, bacterial meningitis, toxoplasmosis, and cryptococcosis.

Infectious Disease

Bacterial diseases Infectious diseases are not well documented in captive sugar gliders, but these animals are presumed to be susceptible to the same pathogens as are other marsupials in their family. Sugar gliders have died from infection with *Pasteurella multocida* contracted from rabbits kept in the same area.[14] The disease is characterized by generalized abscesses in various organs and subcutaneous areas and sudden death. *Clostridium piliforme* infection, giardiasis, and cryptosporidiosis have been diagnosed in captive sugar gliders.[8] Significant pathogens in related possum species include *Yersinia pseudotuberculosis, Salmonella* species, *Mycobacterium* species, *Cryptococcus neoformans*, and *Leptospira* species.[3]

Parasitic diseases Diseases caused by parasites have not been specifically reported in captive sugar gliders. Parasites are most often found in wild sugar gliders or in captive gliders kept outdoors. Various nematodes, trematodes, tapeworms, mites, lice, and fleas are all potential parasites of sugar gliders.[10] Specific parasites identified in sugar gliders include trematodes (*Athesmia* species) in the liver and nematodes (*Parastrongyloides, Paraustrostrongylus,* and *Paraustroxyuris* species) in the gut.[1] Ectoparasitic mites recovered from sugar gliders include trombiculid (*Guntheria kowanyam*), astigmatid (*Petauralges rackae*), and atopomelid mites.[1] Marsupials are susceptible to *Toxoplasma gondii,* which causes neurologic signs and sudden death.

Various anthelmintics have been used in gliders without apparent side effects, but pharmacologic studies have not been conducted. Dosages for several anthelmintics are provided in Table 31-3. Pyrethrin or carbaryl powder can be applied topically and in nest boxes to control mite infestation.[7]

Neoplasia

Neoplasia, in particular lymphoid neoplasia, is relatively common in captive gliders.[1] Cutaneous lymphosarcoma has been reported in a sugar glider.[6]

SURGERY AND ANESTHESIA

Anesthesia

Isoflurane and sevoflurane are the anesthetics of choice for sugar gliders. The use of either of these agents facilitates physical examination, venipuncture, and radiographic examination, as well as anesthesia for general surgery. Anesthesia can be induced with the use of a large face mask as an induction chamber to deliver 5% isoflurane. Transient apnea may occur during induction; therefore, monitor the heart rate closely. If the heart rate is stable, gentle pressure to the thorax usually stimulates breathing. Once anesthesia is induced, a small face mask or a 1-mm Cook endotracheal tube (Global Veterinary Products, New Buffalo, MI; www.globalvetproducts.com) can be used to deliver isoflurane at 2% to 3% for maintenance. Intubate gliders by using a stylet and fine-bladed laryngoscope.[1] While extending the glider's head to maximally lift the soft palate, extend its tongue and use the laryngoscope to see the larynx.

A mixture of tiletamine hydrochloride and zolazepam hydrochloride (Telazol, Fort Dodge Animal Health, Fort Dodge, IA) reportedly caused neurologic signs and death in apparently healthy sugar gliders when administered at 10 mg/kg.[5] Other reports suggest that Telazol can be used in sugar gliders at 8.4 to 12.8 mg/kg without problems.[2] Therefore, use this drug combination with caution in sugar gliders.

Soft Tissue Surgery

General surgical considerations Sugar gliders should be fasted for at least 4 hours before surgery.[14] For gastrointestinal surgery, a longer fasting period may be indicated. Administer subcutaneous fluids before surgery, or place an intraosseous catheter to administer fluids during the operation. Maintain the patient's body temperature during surgery with the use of a circulating hot-water pad or forced warm-air unit. Magnification with a binocular head loupe during surgery aids in identifying small structures and vessels. Minimize blood loss during surgery by using an electrosurgical unit, and ligate small vessels with fine nonreactive monofilament suture, such as 5-0 polydioxanone (PDS). Sugar gliders commonly chew at skin sutures; therefore, close the skin with subcutaneous sutures and apply tissue glue.

Sugar gliders typically recover smoothly from anesthesia. Administer analgesics after surgery to minimize self-trauma to the incision, and provide postoperative pain relief. Butorphanol (0.5 mg/kg IM) can be administered up to three times daily for postoperative pain.[14] Recommended dosages for other analgesic choices are listed in Table 31-3.[7] To maintain body temperature, allow the patient to recover from anesthesia in an incubator. Restricted activity and usual postoperative procedures are recommended as in other species.

Castration Induce and maintain general anesthesia with isoflurane administered by a small face mask. Clip and surgically prepare the area on and around the base of the scrotum on the ventral abdomen. Make a short, longitudinal skin incision in the neck of the scrotum near the body wall (see Fig. 31-5). Bluntly dissect to identify and isolate the vas deferens and blood vessels. Ligate these with 5-0 PDS and ablate the scrotum distal to the ligation. Close the remaining flap of skin from the scrotal neck over the ligated stump of the vas deferens with tissue glue.

Ovariohysterectomy Induce and maintain general anesthesia as described previously. Clip and surgically prepare the area around the pouch on the ventral abdomen. Make a 1- to 2-cm skin incision paramedial to the pouch, leaving enough skin along the edge of the pouch for closure.[14] Identify the linea alba by blunt dissection, then incise into the abdominal cavity. The bladder is visible as the abdominal cavity is entered in this area. Carefully exteriorize the bladder to bring the reproductive tract into view. The ovaries appear as small, red, granular structures. Identify and ligate the ovarian branch of the ovarian artery. Ligate and remove the uterus above the lateral vaginal canals. Close the linea alba; then close the skin routinely with subcutaneous sutures and tissue glue.

Patagium repair Small wounds (less than 5 mm) to the patagium may be left to heal by second intention, but they should be thoroughly clipped, debrided, and cleaned. Take particular care to remove hair from the wound edges with a scalpel blade. Larger wounds may require suturing, and care must be taken to correctly align the two skin layers. Magnification will assist this process. Fine (4-0 or 5-0) absorbable suture material with a swaged-on suture is recommended. If the gliding membrane is extensively damaged, it may need to be reshaped to remove any skin tags or flaps that could become snagged on wire enclosures. To discourage self-trauma, sutures must not be tight. Sugar gliders can reach almost all parts of their body, even with a fitted Elizabethan collar, so comfortable sutures are important.

REFERENCES

1. Booth RJ: General husbandry and medical care of sugar gliders. *In* Bonagura JD, ed. Kirk's Current Veterinary Therapy XIII. Philadelphia, WB Saunders, 2000, pp 1157-1163.
2. Bush MJ, Graves AM, O'Brien SJ, et al: Dissociative anesthesia in free-ranging male koalas and selected marsupials in captivity. Aust Vet J 1990; 67:449-451.
3. Fleming MR: Thermoregulation and torpor in the sugar glider *Petaurus breviceps* (Marsupilia: Petauridae). Aust J Zool 1980; 28:521.
4. Henry SR, Suckling GC: A review of the ecology of the sugar glider. *In* Smith PA, Hume ID, eds. Possums and Gliders. Sydney, Australian Mammal Society, 1984, pp 355-358.
5. Holz P: Immobilization of marsupials with tiletamine and zolazepam. J Zoo Wild Med 1992; 23:426-428.
6. Hough I, Reuter RE, Rahaley RS, et al: Cutaneous lymphosarcoma in a sugar glider. Aust Vet J 1992; 69:93-94.
7. Johnson-Delaney CA: Exotic Companion Medicine Handbook for Veterinarians (Supplement). Lake Worth, FL, Wingers Publishing, 1997, pp 1-23.
8. Johnson-Delaney C: Feeding sugar gliders. Exotic DVM 1998; 1:4.
9. Johnson-Delaney CA: The marsupial pet: sugar gliders, exotic possums, and wallabies. Proceedings of the North American Veterinary Conference, 1998, pp 329-339.
10. Nagy KA, Suckling GC: Field energetics and water balance of sugar gliders, *Petaurus breviceps* (Marsupialia: Petauridae). Aust J Zool 1985; 33:683.
11. Ness RD: Introduction to sugar gliders. Proceedings of the North American Veterinary Conference, 1998, pp 864-865.
12. Ness RD: Clinical pathology and sample collection of exotic small mammals. Vet Clin North Am Exotic Anim Pract 1999; 2:591-619.
13. Ness RD: Sugar glider *(Petaurus breviceps):* general husbandry and medicine. Exotic Small Mammal Medicine and Management Supplement, Proceedings of the Annual Conference of the Association of Avian Veterinarians, 2000, pp 99-107.
14. Pye GW, Carpenter JW: A guide to medicine and surgery in sugar gliders. Vet Med 1999; 94:891-905.
15. Smith MJ: The reproductive system and paracloacal glands of *Petaurus breviceps* and *Gymnobelideus leadbeateri* (Marsupialia: Petauridae). *In* Smith PA, Hume ID, eds. Possums and Gliders. Sydney, Australian Mammal Society, 1984, pp 321-330.
16. Suckling GC: Sugar glider. *In* Strahan R, ed. The Mammals of Australia. Chatswood, Australia, Reed Books, 1995, pp 229-231.
17. Tyndale-Biscoe H, Renfree M: Reproductive Physiology of Marsupials. Cambridge, Cambridge University Press, 1987, pp 18, 19, 22, 59, 123.

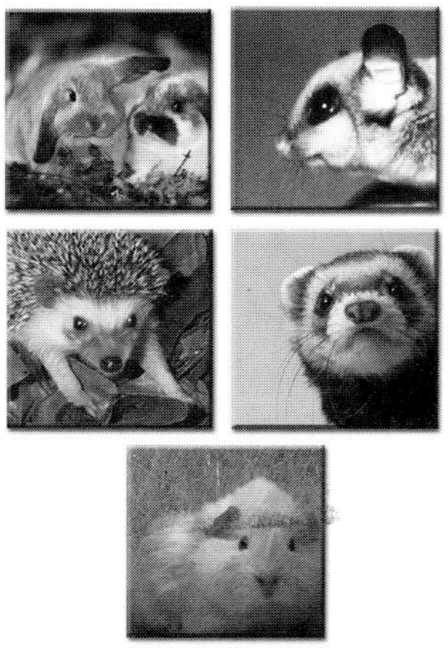

CHAPTER 32

African Hedgehogs

Evelyn Ivey, DVM, Diplomate ABVP, and
James W. Carpenter, MS, DVM, Diplomate ACZM

Because of their small size, spiny coat, and relatively recent appearance in the pet trade, African hedgehogs can be challenging patients. Hedgehogs are illegal in some states and municipalities; in other states, a permit is required. Anyone who breeds hedgehogs for sale or for-fee exhibition must be registered with the U.S. Department of Agriculture, although changing regulations may soon exclude breeders with three or fewer pairs from this requirement. In the past, enforcement of national and local regulations was inconsistent; however, a recent outbreak of foot-and-mouth disease in Europe has led to increased scrutiny of hedgehog owners in some areas. Hedgehog owners are advised to check with appropriate regulatory agencies.

BIOLOGY AND ANATOMY

Taxonomy and Natural History

Hedgehogs are members of the family Erinaceidae, within the order Insectivora. The two most familiar hedgehog species are the central African hedgehog *(Atelerix albiventris)* (Fig. 32-1) and the European hedgehog *(Erinaceus europaeus)*. The central African hedgehog, also known as the white-bellied, four-toed, or "African pygmy" hedgehog, is native to the savanna and steppe regions of central and eastern Africa.[40] Unless otherwise noted, the information in this chapter refers to pet African hedgehogs.

Wild African hedgehogs are nocturnal; they spend daylight hours hidden in burrows or other cavities. At night, they are very active invertebrate predators, jogging several miles in search of insects, earthworms, slugs, and snails.[40] Males and females are territorial and are solitary except during courtship and when raising young. Although all hedgehog species appear to be capable of entering a torpid state under cold conditions, the central African hedgehog probably does not normally experience cold temperatures in the wild, and torpor is considered to be undesirable in captives.[24,40] Excessively high temperatures can also induce a torpid state.[40]

Anatomy

Basic hedgehog anatomy is depicted in Figure 32-2. Hedgehogs are adept at climbing, digging, swimming, and constant jogging. The tibia and fibula are fused distally. The stance is plantigrade. The manus has five digits, the pes has four. Hedgehogs have brachydont (closed-rooted) teeth. The first incisor in each quadrant is large and projects forward. The mandibular first incisors occlude into a space between the maxillary first incisors, an arrangement that is suited to spearing insects. The stomach is simple, and a vomiting reflex is present. There is no cecum, and the colon is smooth.

The crown and dorsum are covered in a dense coat of several thousand smooth spines. Hair and sebaceous glands are absent in the spiny skin.[40] The epidermis in this area is thin, and there is a thick fibrous dermal layer that contains much fat and few blood vessels. Hedgehog spines are composed of keratin and have a complex internal structure that confers lightness, strength, and elasticity. Each spine has a round basal bulb that firmly

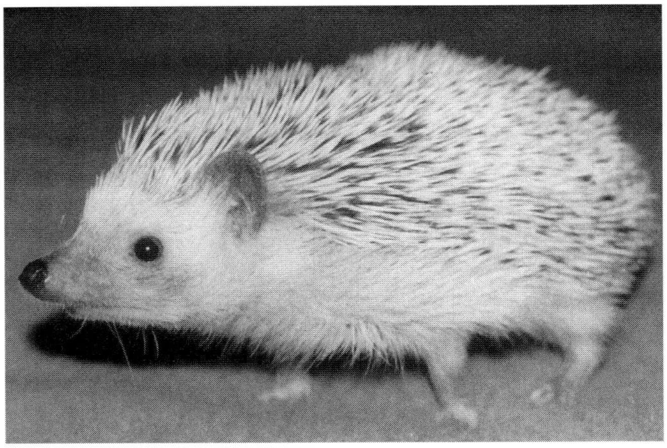

Figure 32-1 Healthy African hedgehog. Note that in normal ambulation, the ventrum is lifted well off the substrate.

attaches it within the follicle. Histologically, the spines are in anagen phase, and healthy spines are difficult or impossible to pull from the follicle without breakage. Spines may last up to 18 months and are replaced individually. Spines are absent from the midline of the crown. The haired skin and the soles of the feet are rich in sweat and sebaceous glands. The toenails are round in cross-section and are highly curved.

A wary hedgehog will raise the spines on its head and crouch. If a frightened hedgehog is touched, contraction of the panniculus muscle pulls the loose spiny skin over the entire body. Several muscles assist in pulling the panniculus over the body and tucking in the legs and rump. The panniculus is thickened at the rim to form the orbicularis muscle, a purse-string–like muscle that closes the loose skin over the animal. A hedgehog may remain rolled up for hours with relatively little muscular effort.

An unrolled hedgehog's gender is easily determined; the male has a conspicuous prepuce that opens on the mid-abdomen, whereas the female's urogenital opening is a few millimeters cranial to the anus (Fig. 32-3). There is no scrotal sac; the testes

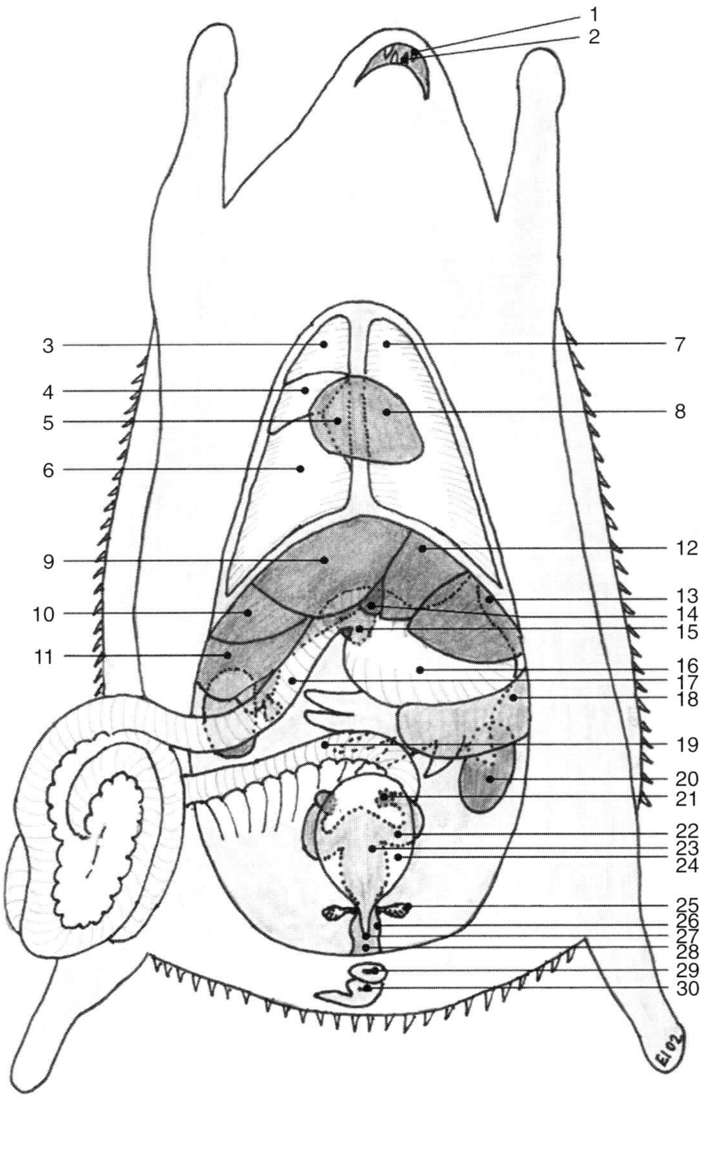

Figure 32-2 Anatomy of a female African hedgehog. The pelvis has been removed. *1,* Maxillary incisor; *2,* mandibular incisor; *3,* right cranial lung lobe; *4,* right middle lung lobe; *5,* accessory lung lobe; *6,* right caudal lung lobe; *7,* left lung lobe; *8,* heart; *9,* right medial liver lobe; *10,* right lateral liver lobe; *11,* caudate liver lobe; *12,* left medial liver lobe; *13,* left lateral liver lobe; *14,* gallbladder; *15,* quadrate liver lobe; *16,* stomach; *17,* duodenum; *18,* spleen; *19,* colon; *20,* left kidney; *21,* left ovary; *22,* left uterine horn; *23,* upper vagina; *24,* urinary bladder; *25,* Cowper's-like gland; *26,* midvaginal gland; *27,* urethral opening; *28,* urogenital sinus; *29,* vulva; *30,* anus.

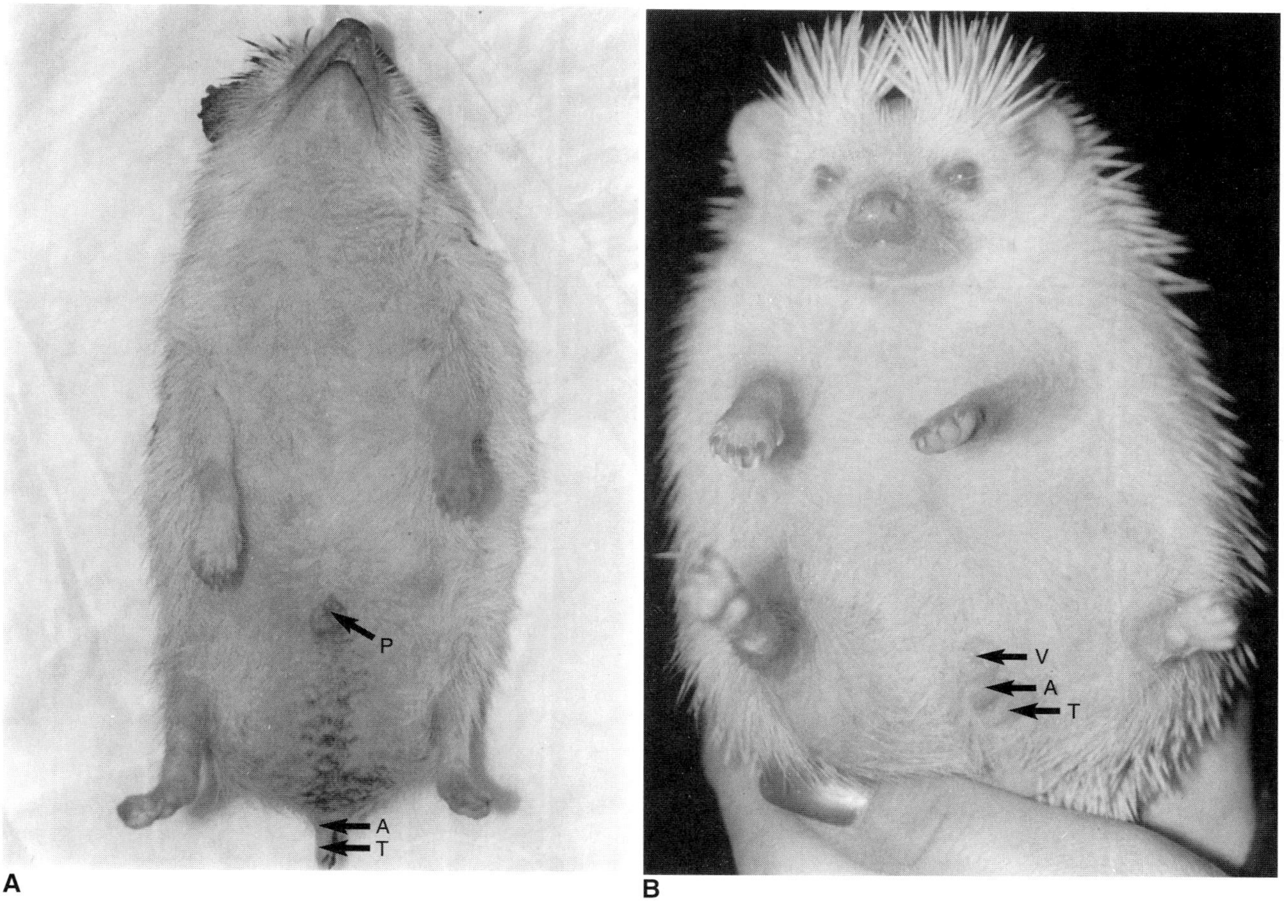

Figure 32-3 Gender determination: **A**, male and **B**, female. *A*, Anus; *P*, prepuce; *T*, tail; *V*, vulva.

are located in a para-anal recess[4] surrounded by fat and can be palpated in reproductively active males (Fig. 32-4). Male accessory glands include paired prostate glands, seminal vesicles, bulbourethral glands, and Cowper's-like glands.[40] The uterus is bicornate; there is no uterine body, but rather a continuous lumen over the cervix. There is a single cervix and a long vagina that is always patent. A fan-shaped gland, homologous to the Cowper's-like gland of the male, lies on each side of the vagina. The urethral opening is located in the distal vagina, several millimeters from the vulva. Both sexes have up to 10 nipples. Mammary glands, when fully developed, form two continuous strips of tissue.

African hedgehogs are polyestrous and breed throughout the year in captivity. The estrus cycle for *A. albiventris* empirically seems to be similar to that of other hedgehog species, for which the estrus cycle has been reported to be 3 to 17 days of estrus, followed by 1 to 5 days of diestrus.[40] There is some indirect evidence to suggest that ovulation is induced.[4,40] Sterile matings with pseudopregnancy may occur. Although the gestation period is 34 to 37 days, it is possible that delayed implantation may occur and extend the apparent gestation period to 40 days.[40] Hedgehogs are born hairless, with closed eyes and ears. At birth, the spines are buried within a layer of skin; within the first few hours, they are exposed by an inflating and subsequent deflating of the skin with fluid and removal of the covering by the

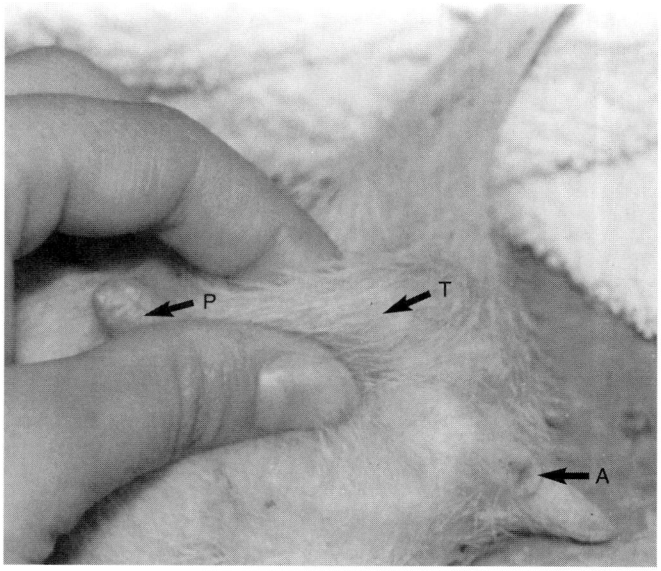

Figure 32-4 The testes *(T)* are located in a para-anal recess. *A*, Anus; *P*, prepuce.

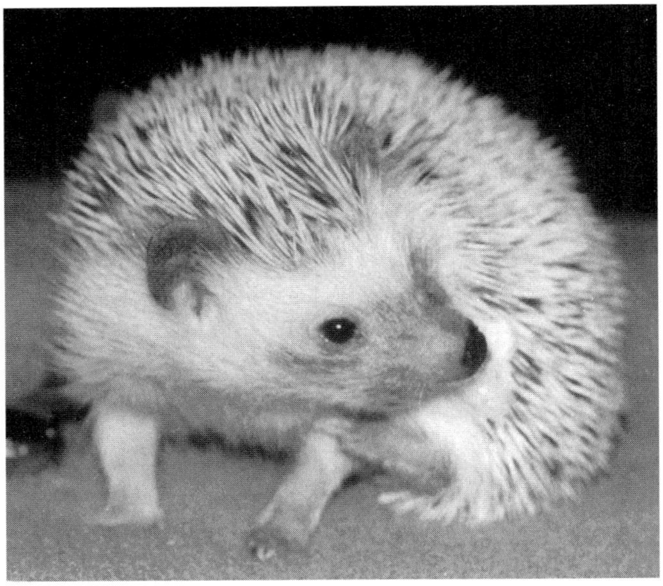

Figure 32-5 Anting. After chewing on the leather watchband, the hedgehog has applied frothy saliva to its spines.

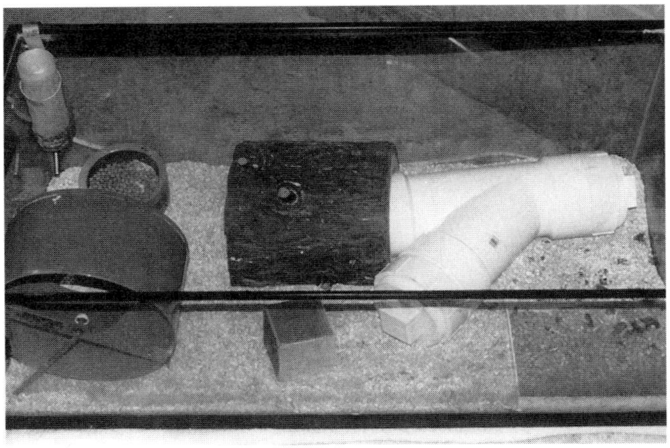

Figure 32-6 This 10-gallon tank is a small enclosure. Note that a hiding place, litter pan, hedgehog-safe wheel, soft substrate, and heating pad have been provided.

mother. These first spines are white, but they are replaced by darker spines over the first 3 days of life. Colostral transfer is believed to occur early in lactation.

Hedgehogs have very sensitive senses of smell and hearing, especially in the ultrasonic range. Their sense of vision is not as well developed and is essentially monochromatic. Frightened or agitated hedgehogs make a distinctive hissing sound. Other vocalizations include grunts, squeals, and snuffling, but these are uncommon except during courtship and between mothers and offspring. The cerebrum of hedgehogs is relatively small, and their learning capabilities seem to be less than those of rodents or carnivores.[40] They do demonstrate the ability to recognize their owners and with patient training may learn simple commands. Both genders of wild and captive hedgehogs demonstrate a unique behavior called self-anointing, or anting (Fig. 32-5). This behavior may be elicited by a variety of substances, particularly those with a strong or unusual odor, such as fish, wool, and various plants and vegetables. The hedgehog takes the material or object into the mouth, mixes it with frothy saliva, and applies the mixture to its spines with the tongue. Many speculations have been offered as to the purpose of this behavior, the most plausible of which seems to be one of imparting an individual odor to the animal and its home range.[40] With patient, gentle handling, most hedgehogs learn to accept and even enjoy handling. Although some owners may attempt to convert their pets to a diurnal schedule (reverse lighting schedules may help), most hedgehogs retain the nocturnal lifestyle of their wild counterparts.

HUSBANDRY

Housing

Hedgehogs are solitary in the wild; in captivity they are usually maintained in individual cages. Some fanciers successfully keep groups of females with or without a single male, or even groups of males, but this can lead to disproportionate feeding and injuries from fighting. Although young animals that are raised together may tolerate each other as adults, hedgehogs typically become aggressive toward cagemates when they reach sexual maturity. Healthy hedgehogs are very active, and as large a cage as possible should be provided; 2 × 3 feet (0.6 × 0.9 m) are minimal floor dimensions. Hedgehogs are able to climb and escape through small holes, so the cage must be secure and lidded. Glass tanks are suitable but are heavy when they are sufficiently large (Fig. 32-6). Hedgehog droppings can be soft and messy, making wood cages difficult to keep clean. Plastic-bottomed cages with wire walls are suitable, provided that the wire spacing is sufficiently close (1-inch square is acceptable). Widely spaced wires can lead to limb entrapment or death if the hedgehog puts its head between the wires and becomes ensnared by its spines. A hiding place, which may be a cardboard or wooden box, flowerpot, cloth bag, or polyvinyl chloride (PVC) tube, is an essential furnishing. The cage substrate should be soft and absorbent and will require frequent changing. Aspen or pine shavings work well, as do hay and recycled newspaper bedding. Wire, cedar, corncob, and dusty or scented substrates are not recommended. Any cloth in the cage should have a tight weave that will not allow nails to become entrapped.

Hedgehogs should be maintained at ambient temperatures between 72° and 90°F (23° and 32°C); 75° to 85°F (24° to 29°C) is optimal. African hedgehogs may go into torpor if they are too cool or too warm. A heating pad placed under part of the enclosure or a ceramic reptile heater may be used. Low humidity (less than 40%) is preferred. Hedgehogs avoid bright light; however, a day cycle of 10 to 14 hours of mild light should be provided. Hedgehog droppings are relatively soft and, depending on diet, can be quite messy. Although some hedgehogs use a litter tray, other hedgehogs deposit their droppings at random. Placing all of the droppings in the litter tray on a daily basis may facilitate litter training. Other litter training tips include providing a cardboard enclosure over the tray, placing the animal in the tray, after feeding, placing another hedgehog's feces in the tray, and placing the tray where the animal seems most inclined to eliminate. Natural plant litters used for cats make the best litter substrate. Clay, clumping-type litter, or sand may stick to the animal and should not be used. Many hedgehogs defecate in their hide boxes and exercise wheels and subsequently walk in their feces, and so daily spot cleaning of the cage is often necessary. Exercise wheels are highly recommended. The wheel needs to have a solid or fine plastic mesh for hedgehogs to run on because their legs tend to become entrapped by traditional wire rodent wheels (see Fig. 32-6). Hedgehogs should be let out into a large area on a daily basis for exercise. Cardboard tubes, straw, safe climbing structures, swimming tubs, and other toys provide interest. Dirty hedgehogs may be bathed with the use of a mild pet shampoo and a soft-bristle vegetable brush.

Diet

Wild African hedgehogs feed on a diversity of invertebrate prey as well as plant materials and occasional vertebrate prey.[40] Although many of the natural food items are known, the nutritional contents of invertebrates vary tremendously; this makes it very difficult to deduce nutrient requirements based on the wild diet. Insectivorous mammals are traditionally fed diets that are 30% to 50% protein and 10% to 20% fat (dry matter basis).[2] Hedgehogs seem to require a higher level of dietary fiber than carnivores do; this may be related to the large quantity of insect exoskeletons that make up the natural diet.

The bulk of the captive diet should consist of a commercially prepared hedgehog food. Scientific studies regarding hedgehog nutritional needs are lacking; however, commercial diets appear to be the most balanced staple that a pet owner can offer. If hedgehog food is not used, premium food for less active cats should form the basis of the diet. Ferret food is high in fat and is not recommended. With many individuals, food must be rationed to prevent obesity. Depending on the animal's weight and activity, 1 to 2 tablespoons of the main diet is typically fed daily. Growing animals and reproductively active females may be fed the usual diet *ad libitum,* and calcium-rich foods are recommended.

In addition to the main diet, approximately 1 to 2 teaspoons of varied moist foods (e.g., canned cat or dog food, cooked meat or egg, or low-fat cottage cheese) and about one-half teaspoon of fruit (e.g., banana, grape, apple, pear, berries) or vegetables (e.g., beans, cooked carrots, squash, peas, tomatoes, leafy greens) should also be provided daily. Acceptable treats include mealworms, earthworms, waxworms, crickets, and cat treats; these may be hidden in the bedding to promote foraging activity. Hedgehogs should not be fed raw meat or eggs, which may harbor *Salmonella.* Milk, although relished by many hedgehogs, can cause diarrhea. Nuts, seeds, and large items or hard foods such as raw carrots can become lodged in the roof of the mouth and should be avoided (Fig. 32-7). The need for vitamin or mineral supplementation, if any, is not known, but supplementation does not appear to be necessary for animals fed a commercial diet. Moist or perishable foods should be offered in the evenings. Hedgehogs may be slow to accept novel foods, and any diet changes must be made with care. Fresh water should be available at all times. Most, but not all, hedgehogs can learn to drink from water bottles.

Breeding

Although pet hedgehogs may become sexually mature at 2 months, females should be at least 6 months of age before breeding. There is anecdotal evidence that female hedgehogs may undergo fusion of the pelvic symphysis if not bred by 18 months of age; dystocia may occur if an older female is bred for the first time. Pregnancy is most easily determined by weighing the female every few days; a gain of 50 g or more within 2 to 3 weeks of being placed with a male is suggestive of pregnancy.[43] At 30 days, a general swelling of the abdomen or mammary enlargement may be detected. Infanticide, usually followed by cannibalism of the young, can occur. Novice hedgehog breeders should give the female strict privacy from other hedgehogs and humans from about 5 days before delivery through 5 to 14 days after delivery. Females that are conditioned to frequent handling are less likely to desert or kill their young in response to human contact.[43] Male hedgehogs must not be allowed near the neonates because cannibalism often results.

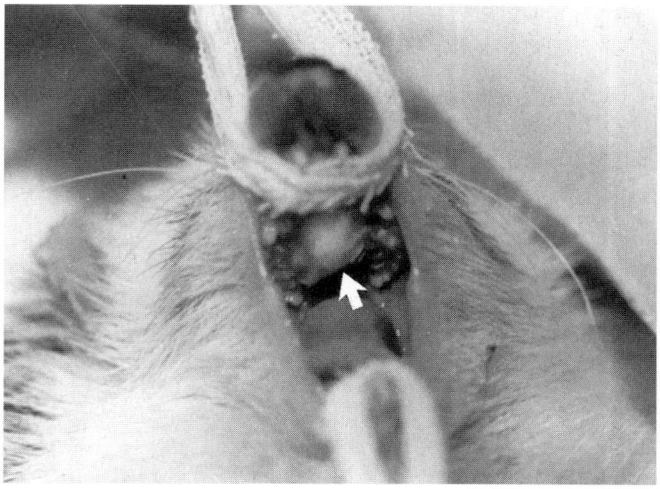

Figure 32-7 A peanut *(arrow)* has become lodged against the palate. Hard foods should be chopped into small pieces, because lodged items may lead to dysphagia and stomatitis. *(Courtesy Dr. Heidi Hoefer.)*

Neonatal Care

Normal pups (or "hoglets") stay close to their dam and littermates when resting. In cases of lactation failure or abandonment by the female, fostering of the pups to another dam with similarly aged pups is usually successful. If a surrogate dam is unavailable, a milk replacer may be fed through a dropper, feeding tube, or narrow-tipped syringe.[44] Based on the composition of European hedgehog milk, a canine milk replacer with added lactase (Lactaid, McNeil-PPC, Ft. Washington, PA) seems to be the most logical formula.[23,40,44] Hand-rearing of hedgehogs is often associated with high mortality. Neonates should be fed as much as they will consume every 2 to 4 hours for about 3 weeks. The ambient temperature should be maintained at 90° to 95°F (32° to 35°C) for the first few weeks.[43] Neonates should gain approximately 1 to 2 g/day during the first week, 3 to 4 g/day during the second week, 4 to 5 g/day during the third and fourth weeks, and 7 to 9 g/day until they are 60 days old.[40,43] Neonates should be stimulated to eliminate after each feeding by massaging the ventrum and perineal area with a cloth or swab moistened in warm water. At 4 to 6 weeks, parent- or hand-raised young should be weaned by offering canned dog or cat food, minced beef, or freshly molted mealworms. A slight weight loss may occur during weaning.[43]

BASIC PROCEDURES AND PREVENTATIVE MEDICINE

Restraint and Examination

Even very tame hedgehogs often roll up when an examination or other procedure is attempted. Hedgehogs do bite, but infrequently. Patience and a quiet room with subdued light may help calm wary hedgehogs. High-pitched sounds, such as the jingling of instruments, should be avoided. A small towel and light gloves may facilitate handing. Some hedgehogs may be induced to voluntarily uncurl if supported in normal standing position and gently rocked up and down in a "see-saw" fashion. When the snout pokes out, place a thumb firmly on the back of the neck to prevent the head from tucking in. Press the thumb of the other hand into the back so that it also uncurls.[40] Other techniques include holding the animal face-downward over a table, placing it on its back, or pushing it toward the edge of a table; these maneuvers may induce extension of the legs as the animal seeks, respectively, to reach the surface, right itself, or avoid falling. The hind legs are then grasped, and the hedgehog is held in a face-down position. Some hedgehogs uncurl if their rump spines are stroked slowly in a circular or backward motion for several minutes; the animal is then pinned against the table by grasping the spiny dorsal skin. Once uncurled, hedgehogs may be restrained by holding the spined skin as one would hold the scruff of other species (Fig. 32-8).

A superficial examination may be performed as the animal moves about within a transparent container, but a thorough examination usually requires chemical restraint. Healthy hedgehogs should be active and inquisitive, or curled up in a tight ball. Hydration may be assessed by eyelid turgor. Body temperature is lower than that of most mammals (Table 32-1). The eyes should be clear, and the pinnal margins should be free of crusting or ragged edges. The teeth should be white and the gingiva a uniform pink. Inspect the oral cavity and tongue for ulcers, foreign material, and masses. The nose is normally moist and active. Normal lymph nodes are difficult to palpate, but lymph nodes may become enlarged in cases of neoplasia or infection.[19,37] The heart should have a regular rhythm and no murmurs. Respiration is normally silent, except in the defensive or aggressive animal, in which forceful expulsion of air through the nose creates a loud hissing sound. The abdominal contour as the animal rests in the hand of the clinician should be flat. Palpate the abdomen for organomegaly, masses, and fluid. Check the prepuce or vulva for inflammation, discharge, or adherent debris. Testicles may be palpable in the paraanal area (see Fig. 32-3). Normal stools are very dark brown, and the consistency varies from very soft to pellet-like. Healthy, untroubled hedgehogs walk with the ventrum raised clear off the table (see Fig. 32-1), but weak or wary hedgehogs tend to crouch. Inspect the toes for encircling fibers and overgrown nails. The skin in the spiny areas may have a mildly dry or flaky appearance, but excessive flaking, quill loss, erythema, and crusting are abnormal.

TABLE 32-1
Biodata for African Hedgehogs

Average body weight (captive)	Female, 300-600 g; male, 400-600 g
Life span	Average, 4-6 yr*; may live to 8 yr
Temperature	95.7°-98.6°F (37.4°-36.0°C)
Adult dental formula	$2(I^3_2\ C^1_1\ P^3_2\ M^3_3) = 36$; variations have been noted
Gastrointestinal transit time	12-16 hr
Heart rate	180-280 beats/min*
Respiratory rate	25-50 breaths/min*
Age of sexual maturity	Female, 2-6 mo; male, 6-8 mo
Reproductive life span	Female, 2-3 yr; male, throughout life
Gestation	34–37 days
Milk composition	Protein, 16 g/100 g; carbohydrate, trace; fat, 25.5 g/100 g
Litter size	3-4 (range, 1-7)
Birth weight	10-18 g
Eyes open	14-18 days
Deciduous teeth eruption	Begins on day 18; all deciduous teeth erupted by 9 wk
Permanent teeth eruption	Begins at 7-9 wk
Age at weaning	4-6 wk (start eating solids at 3 wk)

Data from references 23, 28, 40, 43, 44, and 48.
*Evelyn Ivey, DVM, personal observation, 2002.

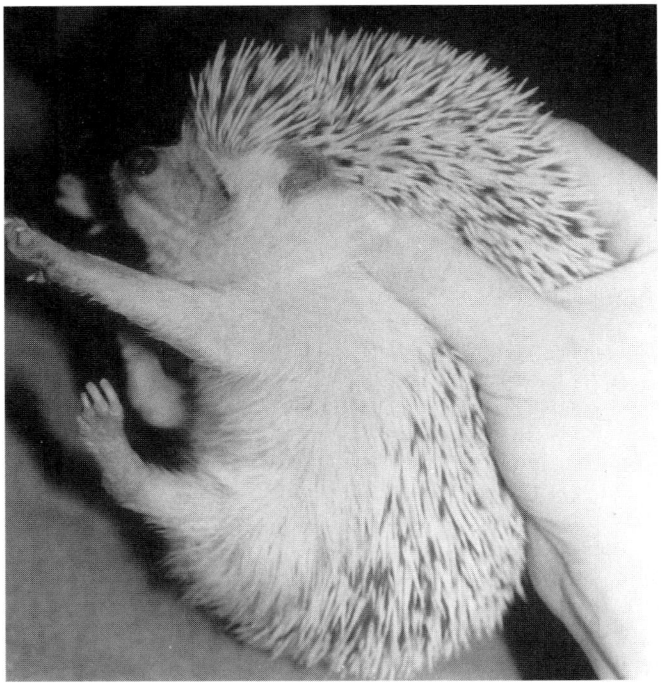

Figure 32-8 Some hedgehogs may be restrained by "scruffing" the dorsum.

Clinical Techniques

Isoflurane alone is commonly used for anesthetic induction and maintenance. Hypersalivation may occur, and premedication with atropine is advised.[26] Injectable agents, including ketamine, diazepam, midazolam, xylazine, tiletamine/zolazepam, and medetomidine, have also been used but may prolong recovery.[31,44] Tracheal intubation may be indicated for longer or oral procedures and is accomplished with a 1.0- to 1.5-mm endotracheal tube, a Teflon intravenous catheter, or a feeding tube.[5,44]

The jugular vein is usually used to collect blood samples. Although visualization of the vein may be difficult, its anatomic location is similar to that in other small mammals. Alternatively, the cranial vena cava may be used. The technique for caval venipuncture is similar to that used in ferrets, but there is a greater risk of cardiac puncture due to the relatively cranial position of the hedgehog heart. The femoral, lateral saphenous, or cephalic veins may be used for injections or to collect small samples (up to 0.5 mL). Retro-orbital blood collection has also been described,[17] but it is not recommended for use on companion animals. Maintaining an intravenous catheter in all but extremely weak hedgehogs is difficult. A femoral or tibial intraosseous catheter may be placed as a substitute for vascular access.[5,24]

Reference ranges for hematologic and serum biochemical values are presented in Table 32-2. A urine sample may be collected by cystocentesis or catheterization; however, reference values are not available.[5,44]

Subcutaneous injections can be given in the spiny or furred areas. The dermis under the spiny skin is poorly vascularized, so drugs or fluid given in this location may not be absorbed for several hours. Intramuscular injections may be given in the thigh. Oral medication may be difficult to impossible to administer to some animals. Some animals accept pleasant-tasting medications via a syringe. Many hedgehogs will consume mealworms that have been injected with medication; for those that do not, medications may be mixed with a favorite food. Topical medications are frequently ingested during the grooming process, although bandages can be used to cover medications placed on the extremities.[27] When weak or debilitated hedgehogs are hospitalized, cage temperatures of 80° to 85°F (27.7° to 29.4°C) should be provided. Anorectic animals should be fed a protein-rich, high-calorie canine or feline diet via syringe or tube.[44]

Radiographic detail is greatly diminished by the presence of the spines. Anesthesia usually is required for proper positioning unless the patient is too weak to roll up. Extend the legs and body for both the lateral and ventrodorsal views. For the lateral view, the elasticity of the dorsal skin makes it possible to pull the spines away from most of the chest and abdomen; a plastic kitchen clip (as is used to seal potato chip bags) is useful (Fig. 32-9).

Preventative Medicine

Because hedgehogs often hide signs of illness, annual or semiannual examinations are recommended. Hedgehogs are prone to a number of dental disorders, including periodontal disease. A palatable pet enzymatic dentifrice may be placed on a crunchy treat daily or several times per week to help prevent this. Tartar-control treats made for dogs and cats may also help loosen tartar. Although dry foods help prevent tartar accumulation, they may cause excessive wearing of the teeth. An accurate scale to monitor weight allows early detection of obesity or weight loss. Owners should be advised of the risks associated with cold temperatures, which include metabolic derangement and immunocompromise. Nails must be trimmed to prevent ingrowth. Currently, there are no vaccines for pet hedgehogs. Because hedgehogs are not typically maintained in mixed-gender groups, elective castration or ovariohysterectomy is not usually needed to prevent unwanted offspring. Animals may be identified with microchips or with nontoxic fabric paint applied to a few spines.[24]

Table 32-2
Hematologic and Serum Biochemical Reference Values of African Hedgehogs

Measurement	Normal Values*
Hematologic values	
Hematocrit (%)	36 ± 7 (22-64)
Red blood cell count (× $10^6/\mu L$)	6 ± 2 (3-16)
Hemoglobin (g/dL)	12.0 ± 2.8 (7.0-21.1)
Mean corpuscular volume (fL)	67 ± 9 (41-94)
Mean corpuscular hemoglobin (pg)	22 ± 4 (11-31)
Mean corpuscular hemoglobin concentration (g/dL)	34 ± 5 (17-48)
Platelets (× $10^3/\mu L$)	226 ± 108 (60-347)
White blood cell count (× $10^3/\mu L$)	11 ± 6 (3-43)
Neutrophils (× $10^3/\mu L$)	5.1 ± 5.2 (0.6-37.4)
Lymphocytes (× $10^3/\mu L$)	4.0 ± 2.2 (0.9-13.1)
Monocytes (× $10^3/\mu L$)	0.3 ± 0.3 (0.0-1.6)
Eosinophils (× $10^3/\mu L$)	1.2 ± 0.9 (0.0-5.1)
Basophils (× $10^3/\mu L$)	0.4 ± 0.3 (0.0-1.5)
Biochemical values	
Alkaline phosphatase (IU/L)	51 ± 21 (8-92)
Alanine aminotransferase (IU/L)	53 ± 24 (16-134)
Amylase (IU/L)	510 ± 170 (244-858)
Aspartate aminotransferase (IU/L)	34 ± 22 (8-137)
Bilirubin, total (mg/dL)	0.3 ± 0.3 (0.0-1.3)
Blood urea nitrogen (mg/dL)	27 ± 9 (13-54)
Calcium (mg/dL)	8.8 ± 1.4 (5.2-11.3)
Chloride (mEq/L)	109 ± 10 (92-128)
Cholesterol (mg/dL)	131 ± 25 (86-189)
Creatine kinase (IU/L)	863 ± 413 (333-1964)
Creatinine (mg/dL)	0.4 ± 0.2 (0.0-0.8)
Gamma-glutamyl transferase (IU/L)	4 ± 1 (0-12)
Glucose (mg/dL)	89 ± 30
Lactate dehydrogenase (IU/L)	441 ± 258 (57-820)
Phosphorus (mg/dL)	5.3 ± 1.9 (2.4-12.0)
Potassium (mEq/L)	4.9 ± 1.0 (3.2-7.2)
Protein, total (g/dL)	5.8 ± 0.7 (4.0-7.7)
Albumin (g/dL)	2.9 ± 0.4 (1.8-4.2)
Globulin (g/dL)	2.7 ± 0.5 (1.6-3.9)
Sodium (mEq/L)	141 ± 9 (120-165)
Triglycerides (mg/dL)	38 ± 22 (10-96)

From Physiological Data Reference Values: International Species Information System, Apple Valley, MN, 2002.
*Mean ± SD (range in parentheses).

COMMON DISEASES

Ocular, Otic, and Oral

Hedgehogs seem to be prone to corneal ulcers and other ocular injuries. Diagnosis and treatment is as for other species,

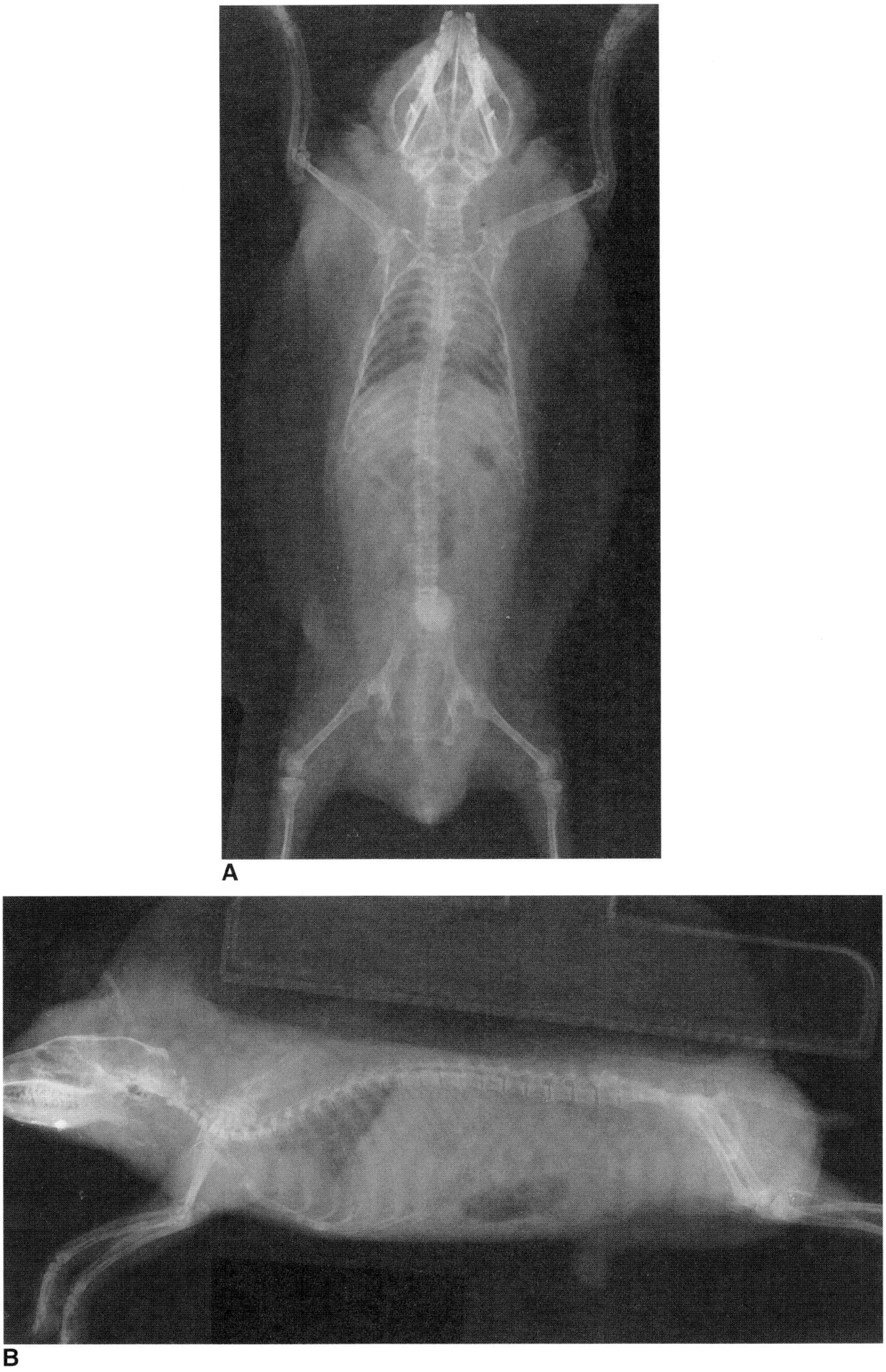

Figure 32-9 Radiographs of a healthy male hedgehog, showing ventrodorsal (A) and lateral (B) views. A large plastic clip was used to retract the dorsum in the lateral view.

although treatment may be difficult if owners are unable to administer topical medication. Blind hedgehogs seem to navigate their captive environments with minimal detriment to their quality of life. Ocular proptosis was a relatively common presenting complaint in one report.[47] The ocular sequelae to proptosis were severe and resulted in enucleation or euthanasia in all eight cases. Moderate to marked orbital inflammation was present in each case; sinusitis, neoplasia, and fungal elements were not observed. Two of the animals had concurrent neurologic disease that may have resulted in ocular trauma; no known trauma occurred in the other cases. Hedgehogs have a shallow orbit that may predispose them to proptosis, especially if excessive fat accumulation or orbital inflammation is present. In hedgehogs with a unilateral proptosis, tarsorrhaphy may be indicated as a prophylactic measure for the remaining eye.[47] Otitis externa has been seen; signs include purulent discharge, odor, and sensitivity of the face and ear.[44,48] Differential diagnoses include bacterial or yeast infection, which in some cases may be secondary to acariasis. Diagnosis and treatment is as for other small mammals.

Oral neoplasms, particularly squamous cell carcinomas, are relatively common (Fig. 32-10). Dental disease is also common; tartar, gingivitis, and periodontitis may occur. On examination, reddened and swollen gingiva, tartar, gingival recession, and loose teeth may be present. Signs include decreased appetite, ptyalism, halitosis, and pawing at the mouth. Tooth fractures and dental abscesses also occur. Dental radiographs, extractions, cleaning, and antibiotic administration should be performed as in other species. In cases in which advanced periodontal disease requires extraction of all the teeth, hedgehogs can be maintained on soft food.[44] Excessive tooth wear may occur with hard feeds, and animals with this condition should be fed a predominantly moist diet. Hedgehog teeth are not continuously growing and should not be trimmed or filed. Hedgehogs are susceptible to wedging of hard items (e.g., peanuts) against the palate (see Fig. 32-7); signs are similar to those seen with dental disease. Stomatitis may occur in males that bite their mates during copulation; treatment is with soft food and antibiotics.[24]

Respiratory

A case of fatal corynebacterial bronchopneumonia was reported in a pet African hedgehog.[39] Other bacteria such as *Bordetella bronchiseptica* and *Pasteurella multocida* can cause respiratory infections in European hedgehogs and are possibly important in *Atelerix* as well.[44] Predisposing factors for upper and lower respiratory tract infection include suboptimal environmental temperature, dusty or unsanitary bedding, malnutrition, concurrent disease, and other causes of immunocompromise. Signs include nasal discharge, increased respiratory noise, dyspnea, lethargy, inappetence, and sudden death. As in other species, diagnostic testing includes radiographs, hematologic testing, and culture of tracheal or lung lobe aspirates. Treatment includes antibiotics, nebulization, supportive care, and correction of husbandry problems. Additional differential diagnoses for dyspnea include pulmonary neoplasia and cardiac disease. Lungworms can also cause pneumonia, but this is unlikely in indoor pets.[19,44] The existence of cytomegalovirus in African hedgehogs has been questioned and is in any case highly unlikely in domestically raised pets.[7]

Cardiovascular and Hematologic

Dilated cardiomyopathy is common in pet hedgehogs, and necropsy findings from several cases have been described.[33] Affected hedgehogs are typically 3 years of age or older, although the disease may occur in animals as young as 1 year of age. Signs

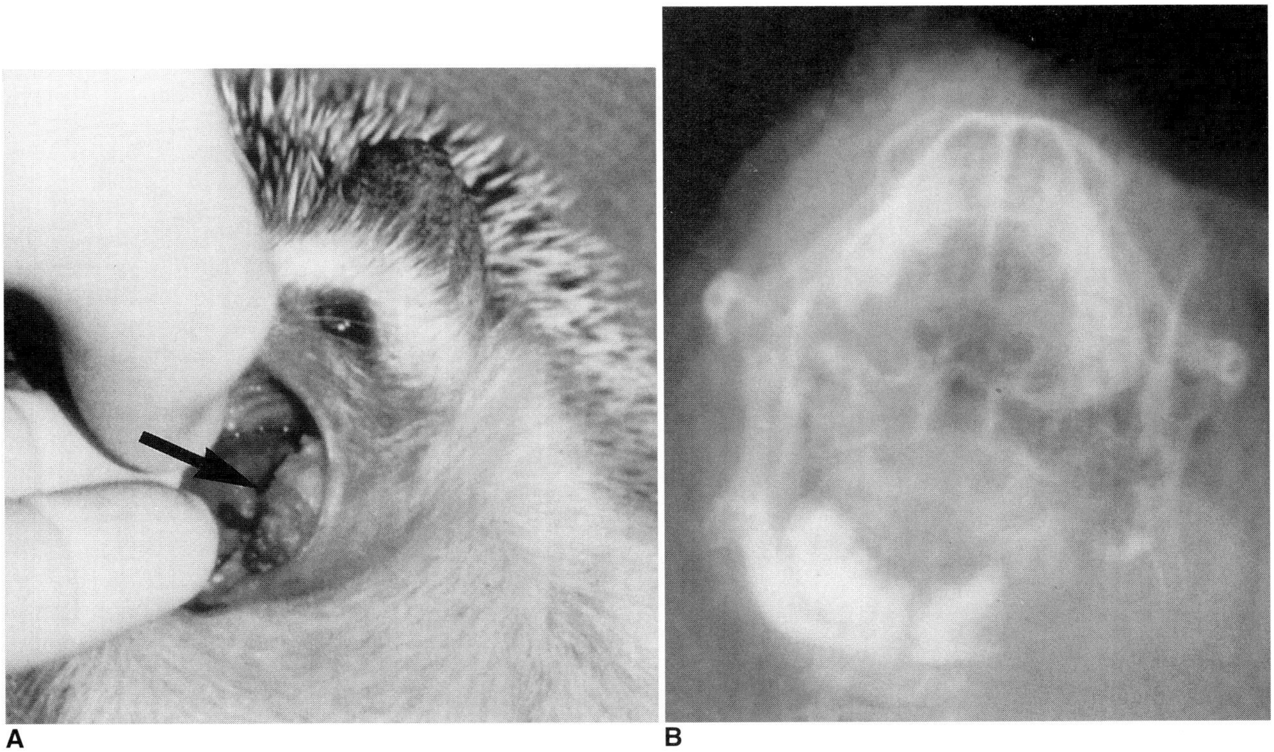

Figure 32-10 A, Oral mass *(arrow)*. B, Open-mouth rostrocaudal skull radiograph of the hedgehog depicted in A. Severe osteolysis of the left mandible is present along with the soft tissue swelling. Histopathologic examination demonstrated the mass to be a squamous cell carcinoma. *(B, Courtesy College of Veterinary Medicine, Kansas State University.)*

include dyspnea, decreased activity, weight loss, a heart murmur, ascites, and acute death. Radiographs typically demonstrate varying degrees of cardiac enlargement, pulmonary edema, pleural effusion, hepatic congestion, and abdominal fluid (Fig. 32-11). Reported histologic lesions of the myocardium have included fibrosis, edema, degeneration, and necrosis, with myofiber atrophy, hypertrophy, and disarray.[33] Histologic lesions may be confined to either ventricle (more commonly the left), but in some cases both ventricles are affected. Pulmonary and renal infarcts may occur in some affected animals. The etiology of cardiomyopathy in hedgehogs is not known, but there may be a genetic or dietary component.

If cardiac disease is suspected, obtain full-body radiographs and an echocardiogram. Normal echocardiographic measurements have not been published, but a subjective evaluation of wall motion and chamber size is often sufficient to confirm a diagnosis of cardiomyopathy. In our experience with a small number of healthy hedgehogs, fractional shortening should be at least 25%, and wall thickness should be at least 1.5 mm. A complete blood count and biochemical profile are useful to screen for concurrent problems and to serve as a reference for monitoring the effects of therapeutic agents. Therapy with digoxin, furosemide, and enalapril may be helpful initially, but the long-term prognosis for hedgehogs with congestive heart failure is poor. Splenic extramedullary hematopoiesis has been noted at necropsy in several hedgehogs with diverse diseases[37]; the clinical significance of this is not known.

Gastrointestinal and Hepatic

Enteritis may be caused by *Salmonella* or other bacteria. Salmonellosis in hedgehogs may be clinically silent or may cause diarrhea, weight loss, decreased appetite, dehydration, lethargy, and death. It must be emphasized that salmonella has been identified in pet African hedgehogs as well as European hedgehogs.[1,9] Diagnosis should be confirmed with fecal culture, using a *Salmonella*-enriching medium. Although treatment is indicated in animals with clinical signs of disease, owners should be advised of the zoonotic potential and the risks of creating antibiotic resistance. Alimentary candidiasis (*Candida albicans*) was suspected based on results of fecal cytology and culture in a hedgehog that was presented with weight loss, depression, and blood in the stool.[8] Fatal cryptosporidiosis of the ileum, jejunum, and colon was reported in a juvenile hedgehog.[15] Although numerous species of nematodes, cestodes, and protozoa have been identified in wild hedgehogs, their significance in pets appears to be minimal. Nevertheless, fecal examination by float and wet mount is indicated in newly acquired animals and in those with signs of enteritis.[5]

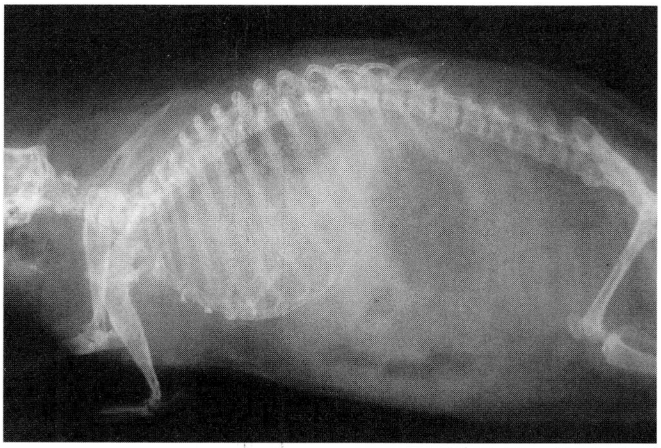

Figure 32-11 Lateral radiograph of a hedgehog with dilated cardiomyopathy. Loss of the cardiac border, dorsal elevation of the trachea, pleural effusion, and evidence of aerophagia are present. *(Courtesy Dr. Heidi Hoefer.)*

Pyloric and intestinal obstructions can occur and are most often caused by rubber, hair, or carpet fibers. Signs include acute anorexia, lethargy, and collapse. Vomiting may or may not be present. Presurgical diagnosis of acute gastrointestinal obstruction may be complicated by the fact that marked gaseous dilation of the gastrointestinal tract can be a nonspecific finding in ill hedgehogs. A fatal, 720-degree intestinal mesenteric torsion has also been reported.[11] Alimentary inflammation, including esophagitis, gastritis, enteritis, colitis, and gastric ulceration with perforation, has also been seen in African hedgehogs.[12] Most of these animals had nonspecific signs such as decreased appetite and weight loss; gastrointestinal signs such as vomiting and diarrhea were not observed.

Diarrhea can also be associated with some commercial diets or inappropriate foods such as milk. Changing the brand of pellets and eliminating inappropriate food items may resolve the condition. Gastrointestinal neoplasia, particularly lymphosarcoma, is relatively common.[36] Other differential diagnoses for gastrointestinal signs include dietary change, toxins, hepatic disease, and malnutrition. Hedgehogs do not rely on bacterial fermentation for digestion, and there is no evidence of antibiotic sensitivity as is seen in herbivorous mammals.[19]

Hepatic lipidosis is relatively common in hedgehogs. In one survey of common necropsy findings in 14 hedgehog cases, hepatic lipidosis was found in 50% of the animals.[37] Hepatic lipidosis may be caused by nutritional imbalances, starvation, obesity, toxicosis, and pregnancy, and it can also be a sequela to infectious or neoplastic disease. Signs include lethargy, inappetence, and icterus, particularly in the axillary region. Diarrhea or signs of hepatic encephalopathy may also be present. Treatment for hepatic lipidosis is similar to that in other species.

Other important causes of liver failure include primary and metastatic hepatic neoplasia.[26] Multifocal hepatic necrosis caused by human herpes simplex virus 1 was reported in a hedgehog that had been treated with dexamethasone.[3] This animal was found dead after a single day of anorexia; the dexamethasone was administered 2 weeks before death (the dose and duration of treatment were not specified). Transmission from the hedgehog's owners was suspected in this case.

Urinary

Cystitis and urolithiasis have been seen in pet hedgehogs.[6,21,22] Signs may include changes in urine color, stranguria, pollakiuria, inappetence, and lethargy. Composition of urinary tract calculi has not been reported, but a causal relationship with cat food diets has been anecdotally described.[22] Urinalysis with culture and radiographs should be obtained. Renal disease is also common and in many cases may be secondary to systemic disease. Nephritis, tubular necrosis, glomerulosclerosis, infarcts, and various glomerulonephropathies have been identified histologically.[11,37]

Reproductive

Posthitis caused by substrate entrapment in the prepuce is common. Hemorrhagic vulvar discharge is often caused by uterine neoplasia.[24] Pyometra and metritis have been reported.[11] Dystocia also occurs and is treated as in other small mammals.[43] Premature births occasionally occur, and the prognosis for young without a suckling reflex is poor.[43] Agalactia may be suspected if neonates lose condition within 72 hours after birth. Diagnosis may be confirmed by attempting to express the mammary glands[43]; however, this procedure usually requires anesthesia and may cause the dam to abandon or cannibalize her young. Possible causes of agalactia include malnutrition of the dam, stress, lack of oxytocin, inadequate mammary development in young females, and mastitis. Supportive care for weak neonates includes warming to normal body temperature over 1 to 3 hours, fluid support, and caloric support once normothermia has been achieved.[43]

Musculoskeletal

Myositis secondary to cellulitis has been reported.[11] Osteoarthritis and intervertebral disk diseases have also been observed.[3,11] Fractures most frequently occur when a limb becomes entrapped in a rodent wheel or wire cage. Splinting may be performed for distal limb fractures and requires anesthesia.[42] Surgical correction may also be performed, but any fixation device must be able to withstand the strong rolling-up mechanism.[20] Lameness may be caused by ingrown toenails, arthritis, nutritional deficiencies, pododermatitis, constriction of a foot or digit by fibrous foreign material, neurologic disease, or neoplasia.[5,22,26]

Neurologic

Ataxia may be caused by a state of torpor. Demyelination (discussed later), trauma, toxins, infarcts, malnutrition, and neoplasia are other possibilities. As in other species, head tilt or circling may be caused by otitis media or primary neurologic disease. Hypocalcemia may occur in cases of postpartum eclampsia, with malnutrition, or for unknown reasons and usually responds to calcium supplementation.[27] Intervertebral disk disease has been anecdotally reported.[3,11] Neurologic signs resulting from rabies, *Baylisascaris*, and polioencephalomyelitis are also possible.[27]

An emerging neurologic disease of pet hedgehogs is a degenerative syndrome sometimes referred to as progressive paresis/paralysis or *wobbly hedgehog syndrome*.[12,16,24,27] Clinical onset most commonly occurs at 2 to 3 years of age, although neonates and older animals have also been affected. The clinical course typically begins with hindlimb ataxia and paresis and progresses in an ascending fashion to tetraplegia with muscle atrophy (Fig. 32-12). Animals with initial signs of forelimb or generalized weakness have also been seen. Death usually occurs within 18 to 25 months after the onset of signs. The diagnosis is confirmed by necropsy. Gross lesions are not evident, but histopathologic lesions are usually seen in the spinal cord. The brain is commonly affected in advanced cases, and peripheral nerves may also be involved. Primary lesions include axonal swelling, degeneration of spinal cord ventral tracts, and axonal and myelin degeneration in brain white matter.[16] To date, there has been no histologic evidence of a viral or autoimmune cause. The etiology for this syndrome is unknown, but pedigree analyses for numerous animals throughout the country strongly suggest a genetic cause; diet may also play a role (D. Graesser, personal communication, 2001). There is no known treatment other than supportive care. A similar syndrome has been described in European hedgehogs[29]; signs included progressive ataxia and paresis. Histologic examination demonstrated vacuolation and demyelination in spinal cord and brain white matter. Focal meningitis with mixed inflammatory perivascular cuffing was also seen. A viral cause was suspected, but isolation attempts were not successful.

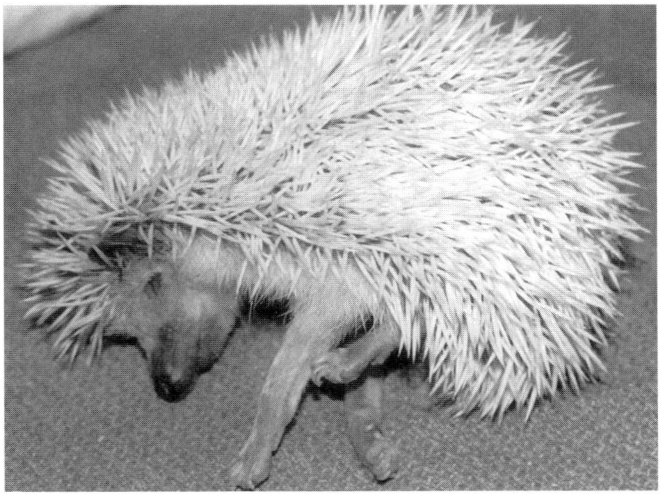

Figure 32-12 Progressive paresis/paralysis syndrome. This hedgehog was presented with a several-month history of ascending tetraparesis and muscle wasting. This syndrome has been associated with neuronal degeneration and demyelination.

Integumentary

Acariasis is very common. *Caparinia tripolis* is probably the most common mite that infests pet hedgehogs, whereas *Caparinia erinacei* may be more common in wild African hedgehogs.[40,45] Although *Chorioptes* species has been frequently implicated in pet hedgehog acariasis,* it is probable that the mites in these cases were misidentified *Caparinia*, which they closely resemble (J. H. Greve, personal communication, 2002). However, detailed descriptions of index specimens are lacking. In some cases, *Notoedres* mites may also infest pet hedgehogs.[22,40] Some hedgehogs have subclinical infestations, which may account for the high prevalence of mites in the pet population. Infested bedding or fomites from pet stores may be another source. Signs include seborrhea, quill loss, and white or brownish crusts (mite droppings) at the base of the quills and around the eyes (Fig. 32-13). Hedgehogs can scratch themselves with their hindlimbs or rub against stationary objects, but many individuals do not demonstrate obvious signs of pruritus. Acariasis also causes nonspecific signs such as lethargy and decreased appetite. Diagnosis is confirmed by a skin scraping. Treatment consists of three to five doses of ivermectin spaced 7 to 14 days apart. Amitraz and permethrin have also been reported to be

*References 13, 19, 24, 25, 27, 44.

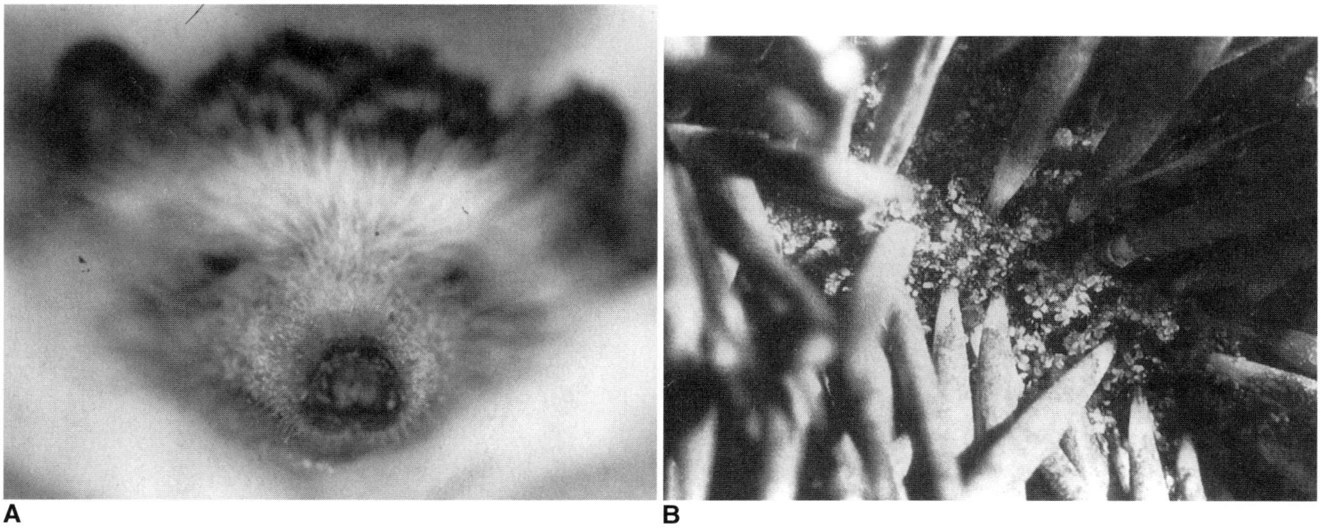

Figure 32-13 Acariasis in a hedgehog. **A,** Note the accumulation of brown mite droppings on the face. **B,** The mites in this case have left a large accumulation of white droppings at the base of the spines. In advanced cases, many spines will be missing. *(**A,** Courtesy Dr. Heidi Hoefer; **B,** courtesy Dr. R. Avery Bennett.)*

safe and are possibly more effective in some cases.[25,45] All bedding must be removed and cage furnishings disinfected or discarded. During the treatment period, the cage is lined with paper that is changed daily. All hedgehogs in the home should be treated concurrently.

Ear mites (*Notoedres cati*) are occasionally seen.[40,48] Signs include accumulation of waxy otic debris and otic pruritus. Diagnosis is confirmed by identifying mites in the ear or in swabbed material. Ear mites in hedgehogs may be treated as in cats. Pet hedgehogs may be infested with fleas; shampoo and powder products that are safe for kittens appear to be safe for hedgehogs. Ticks and fly larvae are uncommon in indoor hedgehogs and are removed individually.

Dermatophytes, usually *Trichophyton* species (especially *T. erinacei*), but also *Microsporum* species, can cause a crusting, usually nonpruritic dermatitis, especially around the face and pinnae. Some infections are secondary to other dermatopathies, such as acariasis or trauma.[44] Diagnosis is confirmed by fungal culture. Treatment consists of topical antifungal agents, with systemic griseofulvin or ketoconazole if needed. Lyme sulfur dips may also be used. Other hedgehogs in the home may be subclinically infected, and treatment of all animals may be indicated.[5] Contact dermatitis may result from unsanitary bedding.[5] Cellulitis has been linked to secondary myositis and sepsis; the primary cause in most of these cases was trauma.[11]

Suspected allergic dermatitis has been anecdotally described. One report described food allergy as a cause of erythema, especially on the ventrum. The offending feeds, if known, were not specified.[48] Cases of facial, axillary, and groin dermatitis with pruritus and histologic evidence of allergy of unknown source have also been reported.[13,27] Restricted antigen diets, antihistamines, and glucocorticoids may be helpful in such cases.[13]

A single case of pemphigus foliaceus has been reported.[46] Signs included generalized loss of spines; dry, flaking skin; moist erythema on the legs, anus, ears, and chin; and epidermal collarettes on the ventral abdomen and limbs. Dexamethasone injections were successful in resolving the condition; initially injections were given twice daily, but over 16 months this frequency was gradually reduced to once every 10 days.

Pinnal dermatitis occurs when skin secretions accumulate along the margins of the pinnae, causing a ragged-edged or crusty appearance. Dermatophytes are an important cause; other possibilities include localized acariasis, nutritional deficiencies, dry skin, and nonspecific seborrhea with hyperkeratosis.[19] Cutaneous and subcutaneous nodules may be seen. Differential diagnoses include papillomas, abscesses, mycobacteriosis, *Cuterebra* larvae, and neoplasia[19,38,42] (Fig. 32-14). Pruritus may occur with the development of new spines, as occurs in young hedgehogs.

Lacerations or other wounds are occasionally seen. Hedgehogs often bite cagemates below the spined skin on the hind legs. If spines in the area of a wound need to be removed, they must be clipped, because they cannot be pulled. Bandages and dilute chlorhexidine baths are well tolerated.[44] If the cutaneous muscle is damaged, it must be closed in a separate layer.[20] Contraction of the rolling-up musculature can cause wound dehiscence. Papillomas of suspected viral etiology have been reported, although histologic findings were not described; recurrence in other sites after excision is common.[5,42]

Neoplastic

Captive African hedgehogs have a remarkably high incidence of neoplasia; two separate institutions reported an incidence of at least 30% in their hedgehog necropsy cases.[12,37] Reported tumor types are diverse, and any body systems can be affected.[30,32,35] Metastasis was noted in several cases; sites included lung, lymph nodes, spleen, mesentery, and other tissues.[35] More than one tumor type occurs in as many as 8% of patients with neoplasia.[35,36] In one survey of 50 cases of neoplasia, the median age at time of tumor diagnosis was 3.5 years (range, 2 to 5.5 years), and incidence was statistically unrelated to gender.[36] More than 80% of the tumors in this survey were classified as malignant. Mammary gland and uterine tumors are common in females, and most are malignant.[34,35] Hemolymphatic

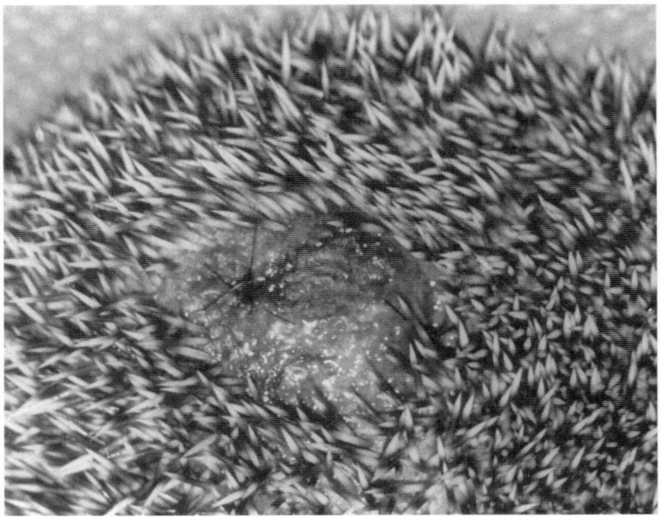

Figure 32-14 Cutaneous lymphosarcoma in a hedgehog. The indentation in the center of the mass corresponds to a biopsy site.

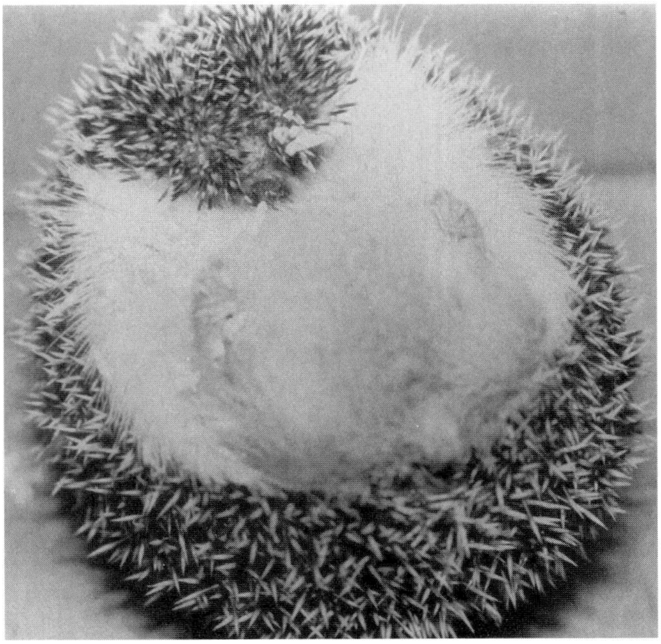

Figure 32-15 Obesity in a hedgehog. This hedgehog is so obese that it cannot roll up completely.

neoplasias are common, particularly alimentary lymphosarcoma, multicentric lymphosarcoma, and myelogenous leukemia. Neoplastic lymphocytes and eosinophilic granulocytes may be seen in peripheral blood.[18,22,35] Oral squamous cell carcinoma is another common tumor and is usually locally infiltrative[35] (see Fig. 32-10). An oncogenic retrovirus was suspected based on electron microscopy findings from two adult captive African hedgehogs with skeletal sarcomas.[30]

In addition to the presence of masses, clinical signs of neoplasia may include chronic weight loss, anorexia, lethargy, diarrhea, dyspnea, and ascites. Patients with oral squamous cell carcinoma may demonstrate swelling of the maxillary or mandibular gingiva, loose teeth, and gingivitis. As in other species, diagnosis of neoplasia is confirmed by results of cytologic or histologic examination. Radiography for evidence of invasion or metastasis, hematologic and biochemical testing, and abdominal ultrasonography may be useful in identifying concurrent problems as well as the location and extent of neoplastic tissue. Treatment usually includes surgical excision and supportive care, although other treatment modalities may be helpful.

Nutritional

Captive hedgehogs, particularly those whose diet consists mainly of cultured invertebrates, may have problems associated with calcium deficiency.[2] Vitamin excess or deficiency may also occur with unbalanced diets.[44] Obesity is common. Healthy hedgehogs should be able to roll up completely, without any fat deposits protruding. Obese hedgehogs may have large axillary fat deposits or a decreased ability to roll up (Fig. 32-15). Treatment includes eliminating high-fat foods, rationing the main diet, and increasing exercise. Weight reduction should be gradual to prevent hepatic lipidosis, and owners should monitor their pet's weight with an accurate scale.

The Lethargic, Weak, Anorectic Hedgehog

The nonspecific signs of lethargy, weakness, and anorexia frequently are the only historical and physical findings, even in hedgehogs with severe system-specific disease. Examples include advanced meningeal lymphoma without neurologic signs, debilitating acariasis without evident pruritus, severe gastric ulceration without gastrointestinal signs,[11] and extensive necrosuppurative pneumonia without respiratory signs.[39] Hedgehogs with advanced neoplasia, hepatic disease, or renal failure may have nonspecific signs at presentation. Other causes include suboptimal environmental temperature, inappropriate or novel foods, dental problems, and competition for food with cagemates. This frequent presentation of hedgehogs emphasizes the importance of diagnostic testing, even if anesthesia is required.

ZOONOSES AND SUITABILITY AS PETS

Several strains of *Salmonella* species occur in hedgehogs, and cases of transmission from pet African hedgehogs to humans have been documented.[1,9] Hedgehogs' messy droppings and propensity to walk in their feces may facilitate dissemination of salmonella in the household. As with reptiles, it should be assumed that all pet hedgehogs can carry and transmit this pathogen, and animals should be handled accordingly (e.g., wash hands after handling, do not allow animals or fomites to contact food or food preparation areas). Subclinically infected animals may shed intermittently, so cultures should not be used to rule out the carrier state. Treatment aimed at eliminating the carrier state is unlikely to be successful and should not be attempted, because resistance may result.[6] Several cases of human dermatophytosis transmitted from pet hedgehogs have been documented.[41] In addition, some people are extremely sensitive to contact with African hedgehog spines and develop a transient but markedly pruritic urticaria within minutes after handling a hedgehog.[14] One person reportedly developed a more persistent papular eruption after the urticaria. People with cat allergies may be predisposed to this sensitivity.

A single case of Chagas' disease (*Trypanosoma cruzi*) was reported in a captive African hedgehog that was housed outdoors in Texas.[10] Rabies has not been reported in captive hedgehogs, but the profuse salivation that occurs during self-anointing is occasionally mistaken as a sign of rabies. Tick-borne diseases including tularemia and Q-fever have been reported in wild African hedgehogs,[42] but these diseases have not been reported in captive-bred hedgehogs. Wild-caught African hedgehogs may be infected with foot-and-mouth disease. This virus can be transmitted to humans, but it presents a far greater threat to hoofed stock. To prevent introduction of this disease to the United States, importation of African hedgehogs was banned by the U.S. Department of Agriculture in 1991. The current trade in the United States consists entirely of captive-bred individuals.

Because hedgehogs are not particularly personable and have a relatively short life span, their suitability as pets has been questioned. In our experience, most hedgehogs are tame with their owners if handled consistently from an early age. As pets, hedgehogs have the advantages of being small, quiet, and solitary, and they have minimal odor. Unlike many other exotic species, their care is relatively straightforward and husbandry-related problems (other than obesity) are infrequent. Hedgehogs do not appear to suffer from boredom or stress in appropriate captive environments, and behavioral problems are rare. From a conservation perspective, the current U. S. pet hedgehog trade does not affect wild populations and has not led to the establishment of feral populations. Although some hedgehogs do resent handling as adults, they are nevertheless very active and interesting animals.

ACKNOWLEDGMENTS

We thank the following people for their assistance in preparing this manuscript: Connie George; Donnasue Graesser; Marc S. Kraus, DVM; and Pamela F. J. Powers.

REFERENCES

1. African pygmy hedgehog-associated salmonellosis—Washington, 1994. MMWR Morb Mortal Wkly Rep 1995; 44:462-463.
2. Allen ME: The nutrition of insectivorous mammals. Proc Joint Conf Am Assoc Zoo Vet/Am Assoc Wildl Vet, 1992, pp 113-115.
3. Allison N, Chang TC, Steele KE, et al: Fatal herpes simplex infection in a pygmy African hedgehog *(Atelerix albiventris)*. J Comp Pathol 2002; 126:76-78.
4. Bedford JM, Mock OB, Nagdas SK, et al: Reproductive characteristics of the African pygmy hedgehog, *Atelerix albiventris*. J Reprod Fertil 2000; 120:143-150.
5. Bennett RA: Husbandry and medicine of hedgehogs. Annu Proc Assoc Avian Vet, 2000, pp 109-114.
6. Brown SA: African hedgehogs: husbandry, restraint, and common problems. Annu Proc Midwest Exotic Pet Semin, 1996, pp 1-7.
7. Brunnert SR, Hensley GT, Citino SB, et al: Salivary gland oncocytes in African hedgehogs *(Atelerix albiventris)* mimicking cytomegalic inclusion disease. J Comp Pathol 1991; 105:83-91.
8. Campbell T: Intestinal candidiasis in an African hedgehog *(Atelerix albiventris)*. Exotic Pet Pract 1997; 2:79.
9. Craig C, Styliadis S, Woodward D: African pygmy hedgehog–associated *Salmonella tilene* in Canada. Can Commun Dis Rep 1997; 23:129-131; discussion, 131-132.
10. deMarr TW, Kassell NL, Blumer ES: Chagas' disease in an African hedgehog. Proc Am Assoc Zoo Vet, 1994, pp 151-153.
11. Done LB: What you don't know about hedgehog diseases. Proc North Am Vet Conf, 1999, pp 824-825.
12. Done LB, Dietze M, Cranfield M, et al: Necropsy lesions by body systems in African hedgehogs *(Atelerix albiventris)*: clues to clinical diagnosis. Proc Joint Conf Am Assoc Zoo Vet/Am Assoc Wildl Vet, 1992, pp 110-112.
13. Ellis C, Mori M: Skin diseases of rodents and small exotic mammals. Vet Clin North Am Exotic Anim Pract 2001; 4:493-542.
14. Fairley JA, Suchniak J, Paller AS: Hedgehog hives. Arch Dermatol 1999; 137:561-563.
15. Graczyk TK, Cranfield MR, Dunning C, et al: Fatal cryptosporidiosis in a juvenile captive African hedgehog *(Atelerix albiventris)*. J Parasitol 1998; 84:178-180.
16. Graesser D, Dressen P, Spraker T: Wobbly hedgehog syndrome. Proc Annu Conf Am Assoc Vet Lab Diagn, 2001, pp 82.
17. Hamlen H: Retro-orbital blood collection in the African hedgehog *(Atelerix albiventris)*. Lab Anim 1997; 26:34-37.
18. Helmer PJ: Abnormal hematologic findings in an African hedgehog *(Atelerix albiventris)* with gastrointestinal lymphosarcoma. Can Vet J 2000; 41:489-490.
19. Hoefer HL: Clinical approach to the African hedgehog. Proc North Am Vet Conf, 1999, pp 836-838.
20. Isenbügel E, Baumgartner RA: Diseases of the hedgehog. *In* Fowler ME, ed. Zoo and Wild Animal Medicine. Current Therapy 3. Philadelphia, WB Saunders, 1993, pp 294-302.
21. Johnson DH: Hedgehog with suspected bilateral renal calculi. Exotic DVM 2001; 3:5.
22. Johnson-Delaney CA: Other small mammals. *In* Meredith A, Redrobe S, eds. BSAVA Manual of Exotic Pets, 4th ed. Gloucester, UK, British Small Animal Veterinary Association, 2002, pp 102-115.
23. Landes E, Zentek J, Wolf P, et al: Investigations into the composition of hedgehog milk and development of hedgehog young. Kleintierpraxis 1997; 42:647-658.
24. Larsen RS, Carpenter JW: Husbandry and medical management of African hedgehogs. Vet Med 1999; 94:877-890.
25. Letcher JD: Amitraz as a treatment for acariasis in African hedgehogs *(Atelerix alibventris)*. J Zoo Anim Med 1988; 19:24-29.
26. Lightfoot TL: Clinical examination of chinchillas, hedgehogs, prairie dogs, and sugar gliders. Vet Clin North Am Exotic Anim Pract 1999; 2:447-469.
27. Lightfoot TL: Therapeutics of African pygmy hedgehogs and prairie dogs. Vet Clin North Am Exotic Anim Pract 2000; 3:155-172.
28. Morgan KR, Berg BM: Body temperature and energy metabolism in pygmy hedgehogs. Am Zool 1997; 5:150A.
29. Palmer AC, Blakemore WF, Franklin RJM, et al: Paralysis in hedgehogs *(Erinaceus europaeus)* associated with demyelination. Vet Rec 1998; 143:550-552.
30. Peauroi JR, Lowenstine LJ, Munn RJ, et al: Multicentric skeletal sarcomas associated with probable retrovirus particles in two African hedgehogs *(Atelerix albiventris)*. Vet Pathol 1994; 31:481-484.
31. Pye GW: Marsupial, insectivore, and chiropteran anesthesia. Vet Clin North Am Exotic Anim Pract 2001; 4:211-237.
32. Ramos-Vara JA: Soft tissue sarcomas in the African hedgehog *(Atelerix albiventris)*: microscopic and immunohistologic study of three cases. J Vet Diagn Invest 2001; 13:442-445.
33. Raymond JT, Garner MM: Cardiomyopathy in captive African hedgehogs *(Atelerix albiventris)*. J Vet Diagn Invest 2000; 12:468-472.

34. Raymond JT, Garner M: Mammary gland tumors in captive African hedgehogs. J Wildl Dis 2000; 36:405-408.
35. Raymond JT, Garner MM: Spontaneous tumors in captive African hedgehogs *(Atelerix albiventris)*: a retrospective study. J Comp Pathol 2001; 124:128-133.
36. Raymond JT, Garner MM: Spontaneous tumors in hedgehogs: a retrospective study of fifty cases. Proc Joint Conf Am Assoc Zoo Vet, Am Assoc Wildl Vet, Assoc Rept Amph Vet, Nat Assoc Zoo Wildl Vet, 2001, pp 326-327.
37. Raymond JT, White MR: Necropsy and histopathologic findings in 14 African hedgehogs *(Atelerix albiventris)*: a retrospective study. J Zoo Wildl Med 1999; 30:273-277.
38. Raymond JT, White MR, Janovitz EB: Malignant mast cell tumor in an African hedgehog *(Atelerix albiventris)*. J Wildl Dis 1997; 33:140-142.
39. Raymond JT, Williams C, Wu CC: Corynebacterial pneumonia in an African hedgehog. J Wildl Dis 1998; 34:397-399.
40. Reeve N: Hedgehogs. London, T & AD Poyser Ltd, 1994.
41. Rosen T: Hazardous hedgehogs. South Med J 2000; 93:936-938.
42. Smith AJ: Husbandry and medicine of African hedgehogs *(Atelerix albiventris)*. J Small Exotic Anim Med 1992; 2:21-28.
43. Smith AJ: Neonatology of the hedgehog *(Atelerix albiventris)*. J Small Exotic Anim Med 1995; 3:15-18.
44. Smith AJ: General husbandry and medical care of hedgehogs. *In* Smith AJ, ed. Kirk's Current Veterinary Therapy XIII Small Animal Practice. Philadelphia, WB Saunders, 2000, pp 1128-1133.
45. Staley EC, Staley EE, Behr MJ: Use of permethrin as a miticide in the African hedgehog *(Atelerix albiventris)*. Vet Hum Toxicol 1994; 36:138.
46. Wack R: Pemphigus foliaceus in an African hedgehog. Proc North Am Vet Conf, 2000, p 1023.
47. Wheler CL, Grahn BH, Pocknell AM: Unilateral proptosis and orbital cellulitis in eight African hedgehogs *(Atelerix albiventris)*. J Zoo Wildl Med 2001; 32:236-241.
48. Wrobel D, Brown SA: The Hedgehog: An Owner's Guide to a Happy, Healthy Pet. New York, Howell Book House, 1997.

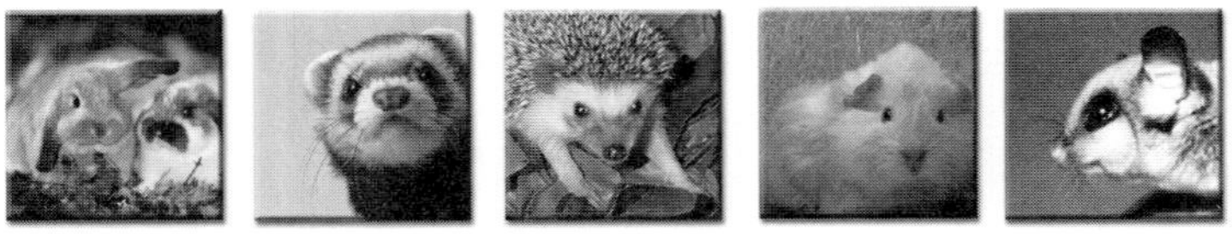

SECTION

SIX

GENERAL TOPICS

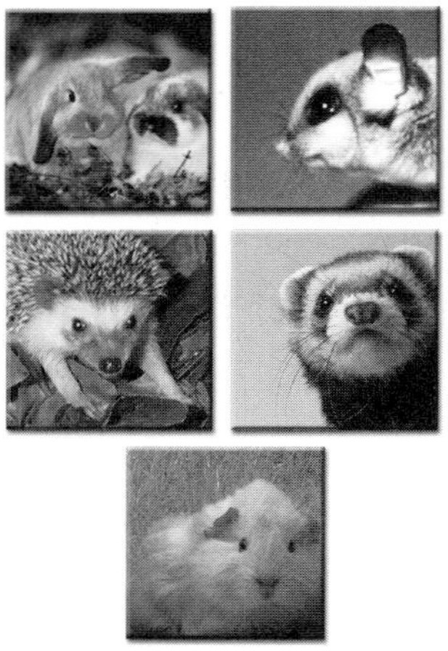

CHAPTER 33

Anesthesia, Analgesia, and Sedation of Small Mammals

Darryl J. Heard, BVMS, PhD, Diplomate ACZM

The following discussion emphasizes anesthetic regimens that I believe are appropriate for clinical practice, based on experience and available pharmacologic data. With sometimes a little modification, most of the same anesthetic drugs, equipment, and techniques used in small animal practice are suitable for ferrets, rabbits, and rodents. In the past decade, advances in monitoring and supportive care equipment have substantially improved the safe anesthetic management of small mammals. These include development of portable blood gas analyzers, pulse oximeters, accurate low-volume fluid infusors, and respiratory ventilators.

GENERAL PRINCIPLES

Most published small mammal anesthetic regimens were developed for research animals. Unfortunately, the objectives of research anesthesia are not always compatible with those of clinical practice. For example, parenteral anesthetic regimens were developed for prolonged invasive procedures from which animals were never recovered. Further, the only aim of some historical studies may have been to render the animal immobile (and hopefully analgesic), without consideration for physiologic consequences. These regimens also usually assumed that the animals were young and healthy. Great care must be taken to not use published drug dosages out of context. This is particularly true of formularies and review articles that simply collate anesthetic dosages without critical evaluation of clinical safety and efficacy. Conversely, because small mammal species are used as pharmacologic models, there are many excellent studies that describe the effects of anesthetics in these animals.

Small size has several physiologic consequences relevant to perianesthetic management. The smaller the animal, the higher the metabolic and tissue oxygen consumption rates, and the lower the tolerance to even brief hypoxemia. Small rodents begin to develop irreversible central nervous system injury within 30 seconds or less of respiratory arrest. Increased oxygen requirement is associated with increased alveolar ventilation and more rapid inhalant anesthetic uptake and excretion.

A high metabolic rate implies rapid metabolism and excretion of parenterally administered drugs. This is enhanced by the evolutionary adaptation of many herbivores (rabbits and rodents included) to detoxify ingested plant chemicals (e.g., the presence of circulating atropine esterases in many rabbit breeds). Consequently, injected drugs generally have a shorter duration of effect than do comparable doses in larger mammals; this explains, in part, the higher dose per kilogram that is required for many drugs.

High metabolic rate and small glycogen reserve predispose to hypoglycemia in the perianesthetic period. Small body size is also associated with a greater ratio of surface area to volume and, often, a higher body temperature. Convective heat loss is rapid, and therefore, hypothermia is assured unless supplemental heat is provided. Small body size implies small blood volume; relatively small amounts of blood loss are significant and may lead to hemorrhagic shock and death. For this reason, the use of electrocautery during surgery is recommended for hemostasis. Small body size also implies a small airway diameter. Because airway resistance is inversely related to radius,[4] slight changes in diameter (e.g., caused by edema and mucus accumulation) have a dramatic effect on respiratory work.

Despite improvements in expertise and equipment, morbidity and mortality are inversely related to anesthetic duration. Therefore, it is important to minimize anesthetic duration by inducing the animal only after the surgeon or diagnostician is prepared to begin the procedure.

Physical restraint is often an important part of the perianesthetic period and is discussed in other chapters. Physical restraint devices (e.g., rabbit squeezeboxes, cat bags) are a useful adjunct to anesthesia, particularly in the induction period. However, care must be taken to avoid excessive and inappropriate physical restraint in place of adequate analgesia and anesthesia.

PREANESTHETIC PREPARATION

Physical Examination

All animals should be physically examined and their medical history reviewed before induction. An accurate admission weight and subsequent daily weights are part of essential patient care. Assessment of cardiopulmonary function is emphasized, and baseline values for respiration rate, heart rate, and temperature are determined for reference during anesthesia. A good-quality pediatric stethoscope is highly recommended for cardiopulmonary auscultation.

Most small mammals are either primary or obligate nasal breathers, and upper respiratory tract disease is common (e.g., snuffles in rabbits, odontomas in prairie dogs). Consequently, assessment of the patency of one or both nares and the nasopharynx is essential, especially if a mask is to be used for inhalant anesthesia.

Minimum diagnostic testing might include blood collection for packed cell volume, total protein, glucose, and urea nitrogen (with or without urine specific gravity). These tests require a very small blood volume, and the information they can provide may be critical in determining the animal's "fitness" for anesthesia. Further diagnostic tests (e.g., hematology, plasma biochemical panel, radiographs) are performed as indicated (see the medicine chapters on specific species).

Fasting

For each patient, the advantages of fasting should be weighed against its disadvantages. There is little experimental evidence from which critical evaluation and recommendations can be made. Fasting is recommended to reduce the volume of the gastrointestinal tract and, consequently, mechanical compression of the diaphragm and lungs. This is particularly important in large-breed rabbits and in obese animals, which have small thoracic cavities relative to abdominal space. Fasting appears to reduce, but not eliminate, the predisposition to regurgitate in guinea pigs and ferrets.

Fasting exhausts glycogen stores, resulting in hypoglycemia, and may contribute to ileus in the perianesthetic period (e.g., rabbits, guinea pigs). Further contraindications to fasting include, but are not limited to, prolonged anorexia, insulinoma (i.e., ferrets), hepatic dysfunction, and late pregnancy. Unless it is contraindicated, I recommend that small mammals be fasted for 0 to 4 hours. Water is also removed up to 4 hours before induction.

Stabilization

Ideally, all patients are physiologically stable before anesthetic induction. If sufficient time is available, abnormalities such as dehydration, anemia, hypoglycemia, electrolyte imbalances, and acid-base disturbances are corrected (see the medicine chapters on specific species). Drugs (e.g., antibiotics) and blood products (i.e., transfusions, Oxyglobin [Biopure Corporation, Cambridge, MA]) that have the potential to produce anaphylactic or anaphylactoid reactions are also administered at this time. Vascular access is attained in unstable animals and in those undergoing prolonged procedures or procedures that are likely to produce significant hemorrhage (e.g., tumor removal, gravid ovariohysterectomy).

Premedication

Although a major aim is to minimize anesthetic and recovery time, the use of tranquilizers and sedatives in the perianesthetic period is valuable to reduce anxiety and smooth induction, maintenance, and recovery. Recommended premedication dosages are given in Table 33-1. An analgesic plan is also essential for any anesthetic regimen.

Parasympatholytics (antimuscarinics, anticholinergics) Parasympatholytics are used to reduce respiratory and salivary secretions that may obstruct respiration. However, it has been argued they may also enhance obstruction by making secretions more "tacky." Parasympatholytics also ameliorate or prevent vagally mediated bradyarrhythmias. Unlike rodents, many

TABLE 33-1
Table of Drug Doses (mg/kg) for Premedication and Sedation of Small Mammals*

Drug†	Ferret	Rabbit	Rat	Mouse	Gerbil	Hamster	Guinea Pig, Chinchilla
Acepromazine	0.1-0.3	0.25-1.0	0.5-2.5	0.5-2.5	—‡	0.5-5.0	0.5-1.5
Diazepam	2	1-5	3-5	3-5	3-5	3-5	1-5
Midazolam	1	1-2	1-2	1-2	1-2	1-2	1-2
Xylazine	1	1-5	10-15	10-15	5-10	5-10	5-10
Atropine	0.05	0.8-1.0	0.05	0.05	0.05	0.05	0.05
Glycopyrrolate	0.01	0.01-0.02	0.01-0.02	0.01-0.02	0.01-0.02	0.01-0.02	0.01-0.02

*Use lower end of dose range for debilitated, geriatric, or obese animals and for those that are relatively large for the species.
†Routes of administration are generally IM or SC.
‡Acepromazine is not recommended for use in gerbils because it may lower the seizure threshold.
Adapted, in part, from Mason DE: Anesthesia, analgesia, and sedation for small mammals. *In* Hillyer EV, Quesenberry KE, eds. Ferrets, Rabbits, and Rodents: Clinical Medicine and Surgery. Philadelphia, WB Saunders, 1997, pp 378-391.

rabbits have circulating levels of atropine esterases that make the efficacy of atropine unpredictable. Increasing the dosage increases the likelihood of inducing both a therapeutic effect and toxicosis.

In rabbits, atropine sulfate (0.2-2.0 mg/kg SC, IM) only briefly induces a moderate tachycardia, but glycopyrrolate (0.1 mg/kg SC, IM) elevates heart rate for longer than 50 minutes.[20] In rats, atropine sulfate (0.05 mg/kg SC, IM) and glycopyrrolate (0.5 mg/kg SC, IM) produce an increase in heart rate for 30 and 240 minutes, respectively.[20] Although both atropine and glycopyrrolate provide protection against bradycardia in rabbits and rodents anesthetized with ketamine/α_2-adrenergic agonist combinations, glycopyrrolate is more effective in maintaining heart rate within the normal range. Neither glycopyrrolate nor atropine influences respiratory rate, core body temperature, or systolic blood pressure when used alone or in combination with the injectable anesthetics mentioned.

Phenothiazines As with other phenothiazines, the peak effect of acepromazine may not be attained for 30 to 45 minutes, even when it is administered by intravascular injection. The tranquilization level attained is inversely related to the amount of environmental stimulation. Acepromazine blocks α_2-adrenergic receptors, producing arteriovenous dilation and subsequent hypotension. It also prolongs the duration of anesthesia and the time to recovery of postural reflexes. Acepromazine should be used only in healthy, hemodynamically stable animals.

Benzodiazepines The benzodiazepines are anxiolytics, sedatives, anticonvulsants, and central muscle relaxants that have minimal cardiopulmonary effects. However, because diazepam is solubilized in propylene glycol, it may produce marked hypotension in debilitated patients if it is administered by rapid intravenous injection. Diazepam is slightly less potent than midazolam, but it has a longer duration of effect. It is poorly absorbed from intramuscular injection sites but well absorbed orally. Midazolam is water soluble, miscible with ketamine solutions, and well absorbed after either intramuscular or oral administration.

Benzodiazepines provide good sedation and relaxation in most small mammals and are a useful adjunct to induction of debilitated patients because of their minimal cardiopulmonary effects. Benzodiazepines are frequently combined with dissociative anesthetics to improve muscle relaxation and duration of effect. The effects of benzodiazepines can be reversed with flumazenil.

α_2-Adrenergic agonists The sedative-hypnotic α_2-adrenergic agonists include xylazine, detomidine, and medetomidine. Xylazine is least potent; medetomidine is most potent and is selective for the receptor. Xylazine is often combined with ketamine to improve muscle relaxation, analgesia, and duration of effect. The α_2-adrenergic agonists produce respiratory depression and either hypertension or hypotension. Bradycardia can be marked and is caused by central and peripheral vagal effects, a response to the hypertension, or both. The analgesia produced appears to be additive to that of ketamine.

The effects of these sedative-hypnotics, when used alone, can be reversed given sufficient environmental stimulation. They can also be reversed by an α_2-adrenergic antagonist (i.e., yohimbine, tolazoline, or atipamezole). Tolazoline (10-50 mg/kg), when compared with yohimbine (1 mg/kg), appeared more effective and safer for the reversal of xylazine in xylazine/ketamine anesthesia in rats.[14] Yohimbine given to rats at a dose of 20 mg/kg IP produced a high mortality rate (22%).

ANALGESIA

The provision of analgesia in anesthetic regimens is mandatory for painful procedures. The principles and techniques for small mammal analgesia have been well reviewed by Robertson[21] and Flecknell.[8] The two main groups of analgesic premedicants used in small mammal anesthesia are opioids and nonsteroidal antiinflammatory drugs (NSAIDs). These can be combined or used alone. Opioids produce respiratory depression that may be additive to that of other drugs used in the perianesthetic period. Their effect on the cardiovascular system is variable, depending on the species. In ferrets and rats they tend to produce hypotension, whereas in mice and rabbits they are hypertensive. Ketamine, even at low doses,[21] may also provide analgesia and is worth including for this reason in some anesthetic regimens. Local and regional anesthesia (discussed later) also has the potential to further enhance analgesia. Recommended doses for analgesics are given in Table 33-2.

TABLE 33-2
Analgesic Drug Dosages (mg/kg) for Small Mammals

Analgesic	Ferret	Rabbit	Rat	Mouse, Gerbil, Hamster	Chinchilla, Guinea pig, Prairie dog
Buprenorphine	0.01-0.03 IM, SC, IV q6-12h	0.01-0.05 IM, SC, IV q6-12h	0.05 IM, SC q8-12h	0.1 SC q6-12h	0.05 IM, SC q6-12h
Butorphanol	0.4 IM, SC q4h	0.1-0.5 IM, SC q4h	2 IM, SC q2-4h	1-5 SC q4h	2 IM, SC q4h
Carprofen	4 IM, SC q24h	4 IM, SC q24h 1.5 PO q12h	5 IM, SC, PO q24h	5 SC q12h	4 IM, SC q24h
Flunixin	0.5-2 IM, SC q12-24h	1-2 IM, SC q12h	2.5 IM, SC q12h	2.5 SC q12h	2.5 IM, SC q12-24h
Ketoprofen	3 IM, SC q24h	3 IM, SC q24h	5 IM, SC, PO q24h	?	?
Meloxicam*	0.2 IM, SC 0.3 PO q24h	0.2 IM, SC 0.3 PO q24h	1-2 SC PO q12h	1-2 IM, SC, PO q24h	?
Meperidine	5-10 IM, SC q2-4h	10 IM, SC q2-3h	10-20 IM, SC q2-3h	10-20 SC q2-3h	10-20 IM, SC q2-4h
Morphine	0.5 IM, SC q4-6h	2-5 IM, SC q4h	2-5 IM, SC q4h	2-5 SC q4h	2-5 IM, SC q4h
Oxymorphone	0.05-0.2 IM, SC q8-12h	0.05-0.2 IM, SC q8-12h	0.2-0.5 IM, SC q6-12h	0.2-0.5 SC q6-12h	0.2-0.5 IM, SC q6-12h

Adapted from Flecknell[8] and Mason.[19]
*Only the oral form of meloxicam is currently available in the United States.
Adapted from Flecknell PA: Analgesia of small mammals. Vet Clin North Am Exotic Anim Pract 2001; 4:47-56 and Mason DE: Anesthesia, analgesia, and sedation for small mammals. *In* Hillyer EV, Quesenberry KE, eds. Ferrets, Rabbits, and Rodents: Clinical Medicine and Surgery. Philadelphia, WB Saunders, 1997, pp 378-391.

LOCAL AND REGIONAL ANESTHESIA

Many species of small mammals are amenable to local anesthesia for minor procedures and epidural anesthesia for major procedures (e.g., cesarean section). Guinea pigs and rabbits are used as research models for epidural and intrathecal administration of local anesthetics and analgesics.[7,13] Most local anesthetics have a low therapeutic index (particularly the long-acting drugs such as bupivacaine), and commercial preparations usually contain drug concentrations suitable for humans. Consequently, great care must be taken to calculate and prepare appropriate volumes of local anesthetic for infiltration. For example, if the toxic dose of lidocaine in a rabbit were 10 to 20 mg/kg, the equivalent volume of a 2% lidocaine solution would be 0.5 to 1.0 mL/kg.

PARENTERAL ANESTHESIA

Drug Administration

Injection routes for parenteral anesthetics in small mammals include subcutaneous (SC), intramuscular (IM), intraperitoneal (IP), intravenous (IV), and intraosseous (IO). Intraosseous catheterization sites are described in the chapters on species medicine. Although drugs are routinely administered by subcutaneous and intramuscular injection in cats and dogs, great care should be taken when using these routes in small mammals. Potentially irritant solutions (e.g., high or low pH solutions) should not be administered by these routes because of the risk of self-mutilation. Diluting the solution, avoiding large-volume injections, and injecting in the proximal muscles of the legs reduce the risk of this adverse effect. Alternatively, drugs are administered by intraperitoneal injection. Recommended drug doses for injectable anesthetics in small mammals are presented in Table 33-3.

Dissociative Anesthetics

The most commonly used dissociative anesthetics are ketamine and tiletamine. Dissociative anesthesia is so named because it produces dissociation between areas of the central nervous system rather than generalized suppression of neuronal function. Consequently, muscle relaxation is usually poor, and many reflexes such as swallowing and palpebral response are maintained even at high doses. Some small mammals (particularly guinea pigs) may retain some limb motion at dosages that would be expected to produce surgical anesthesia, making determination of anesthetic depth difficult.

Both ketamine and tiletamine increase central and peripheral sympathetic tone, resulting in hypertension and tachycardia. However, they also directly depress myocardial contractility, and this effect may be unmasked if the patient is hypovolemic or in shock. This may induce periods of apneustic breathing. That is, the animal intersperses periods of tachypnea with prolonged apnea. The respiratory depression may be additive to that caused by other drugs, including inhalant anesthetics. Ketamine decreases blood flow to the gravid uterus and should be avoided, if possible, in late pregnancy.

Dissociative anesthetics are administered by intramuscular, intraperitoneal, intravenous, or intraosseous injection. As discussed earlier, intramuscular injection of ketamine alone or in combination with xylazine in some small mammal species has been associated with self-mutilation.

Ketamine Ketamine alone in small mammals produces short-term immobilization with poor muscle relaxation. Large doses usually are required to produce prolonged immobility and surgical anesthesia. Ketamine in rabbits has a very short duration of action, apparently, in part, because of renal excretion.[4] Consequently, renal impairment markedly prolongs its duration of effect.

TABLE 33-3
Drug Dosages (mg/kg) for Injectable Anesthetics in Small Mammals*

Drug or Combination	Ferret	Rabbit	Rat	Mouse	Gerbil	Hamster	Guinea Pig, Chinchilla
Ketamine-acepromazine	*10-30:* 0.05-0.3 IM, IV	*25-40:* 0.25-1.0 IM, IV	*50-150:* 2.5-5.0 IP, IV	*50-150:* 2.5-5.0 IP	NA	*50-150:* 2.5-5.0 IP	*20-50:* 0.5-1.0 IP, IV
Ketamine-xylazine	*10-30:* 1-2 IM, IV	*20-40:* 3-5 IM, IV	*40-90:* 5 IP, IV	*50-200:* 5-10 IP	*50-70:* 2-3 IP	*50-150:* 5-10 IP	*20-40:* 3-5 IP, IV
Ketamine-diazepam	*10-30:* 1-2 IM, IV	*20-40:* 1-5 IM, IV	*40-100:* 3-5 IP, IV	*40-150:* 3-5 IP	*40-150:* 3-5 IP	*50-150:* 5 IP	*20-50:* 3-5 IP, IV
Tiletamine/zolazepam	22 IM, IV	5-25 IM, IV†	50-80 IP, IV	50-80 IP	50-80 IP	50-80 IP	20-40 IP, IV
Propofol	3-6 IV	3-6 IV	10 IV	NA	NA	NA	10 IV

IM, intramuscular; IP, intraperitoneal; IV, intravenous; NA, not applicable.
*Use lower end of dose range for IV injection; for debilitated, geriatric, or obese animals; and for animals that are relatively large for the species.
†Avoid use of higher dosages because of risk of renal injury.
Adapted, in part, from Mason DE: Anesthesia, analgesia, and sedation for small mammals. *In* Hillyer EV, Quesenberry KE, eds. Ferrets, Rabbits, and Rodents: Clinical Medicine and Surgery. Philadelphia, WB Saunders, 1997, pp 378-391.

Ketamine combinations Xylazine and other α_2-adrenergic agonists are frequently combined with ketamine for short-term immobilization and surgical anesthesia. Great care must be taken when using these combinations, particularly at the higher doses. They produce mild to severe dose-dependent hypotension, bradyarrhythmias, and respiratory depression, with associated hypercapnia, acidemia, and hypoxemia. As with all parenteral anesthetic regimens, some form of oxygen supplementation or assisted ventilation, or both, is recommended. Ketamine/benzodiazepine combinations appear to produce less cardiopulmonary depression and analgesia, but good muscle relaxation.

Multiple anesthetic episodes with ketamine (50 mg/kg)/xylazine (10 mg/kg) intramuscularly were incriminated in producing myocardial necrosis and fibrosis in Dutch belted rabbits.[18] Similarly, detomidine, alone and in combination with ketamine or diazepam, was associated with myocardial necrosis and fibrosis in New Zealand white rabbits.[9] The postulated mechanism for this effect was decreased coronary blood flow. However, other causes such as hypovitaminosis E, excessive anesthetic dose, and hypoxemia could not be ruled out. Acute reversible lens opacity in rats and mice was observed after administration of xylazine alone or in combination with ketamine.[6] These "cataracts" were associated to a varying degree with proptosis, obtunded blink response, corneal surface drying, and mydriasis.

Tiletamine/zolazepam Tiletamine and zolazepam are combined in equal amounts in a commercial preparation (Telazol [Fort Dodge Laboratories, Fort Dodge, IA]), and the dose is calculated based on the total dose of the two drugs. Tiletamine is two to three times as potent as ketamine and longer acting than ketamine. Although this combination produces a moderately effective anesthesia for minor surgical procedures when used alone in ferrets, rats, and gerbils, very high doses are required to produce even immobility in response to noxious stimuli in other species (i.e., rabbits, mice, hamsters, and guinea pigs). In rabbits, high doses of tiletamine/zolazepam produce dose-dependent renal tubular necrosis within 7 days after injection.[5] Another major disadvantage of tiletamine/zolazepam is prolonged recovery time. This is dose- and perhaps species-dependent. Differential metabolism of zolazepam and tiletamine within species may also result in unmasking of the adverse effects of tiletamine (i.e., struggling and disorientation) during recovery.

Propofol The alkylphenol propofol is a chemically unique, short- and rapid-acting, noncumulative parenteral anesthetic that is administered intravenously. It is used as an induction agent and for maintenance of anesthesia when administered as a continuous intravenous infusion or intermittent bolus. Propofol's rapid onset of action is a result of its rapid uptake into the central nervous system; its short duration of action is related to rapid redistribution and efficient elimination from the plasma by metabolic processes. Propofol produces dose-dependent decreases in cardiopulmonary function. A combination of arterial and venous dilation, together with a decrease in myocardial contractility, produces hypotension. Respiratory depression is caused by decreases in both respiratory rate and tidal volume. Apnea can occur and is related to the dose, rate of injection, and presence of other drugs.

The total dose of propofol required for anesthetic induction depends on the rate of administration. In rats, both fast (20 mg/kg per minute) and slow (2.5 mg/kg per minute) rates of administration result in larger induction doses than those attained at an intermediate rate (10 mg/kg per minute; induction dose = 13 mg/kg).[16] However, despite different induction dose requirements at different rates of administration, duration of anesthesia is not significantly different.

The effects of propofol in rabbits (and presumably in other small mammals) are similar to those described in domestic animals.[1,2] Propofol alone produces inadequate analgesia for painful procedures, and maintenance of anesthesia with infusions is not recommended unless respiratory and circulatory support are provided. Propofol is indicated for induction of healthy rabbits and other small mammals if vascular access can be attained before anesthesia. A slow infusion can also be used to produce sufficient sedation to facilitate mask induction. It is recommended that the animals be intubated and ventilated as soon as possible after induction.

INHALATION ANESTHESIA

Inhalation anesthesia is the primary component of most, if not all, clinical anesthetic regimens in small mammals. It allows rapid induction, recovery, and control of anesthetic depth, and the adverse physiologic effects are usually dose dependent and reversible.

Inhalant Anesthetics

The main inhalant anesthetic presently used in small mammal practice is isoflurane. Isoflurane is associated with rapid induction and recovery and rapid control of anesthetic depth. It produces a dose-dependent cardiopulmonary depression, does not sensitize the myocardium to catecholamine-induced arrhythmias, and is a poor analgesic.[10,11] Respiratory depression is slightly greater for isoflurane than for halothane, and there appears to be some species differences in magnitude of cardiopulmonary depression.

Sevoflurane has recently become commercially available and will probably supplant isoflurane as the inhalant of choice. Sevoflurane is similar to isoflurane, except that it produces even more rapid induction and recovery. This is because it is less soluble in tissue and blood than isoflurane. Sevoflurane requires an agent-specific vaporizer; it cannot be used in either a halothane or an isoflurane vaporizer because of its different vapor pressure. Sevoflurane is only half as potent as isoflurane (see later discussion), and at present it costs approximately twice as much per milliliter.

Inhalant Anesthetic Potency

Minimum anesthetic concentration (MAC) is a measure of inhalant anesthetic potency. MAC is defined as the anesthetic concentration (volume %) that produces immobility in 50% of an anesthetized population subjected to a noxious stimulus. Knowledge of the MAC value in one species is used to approximate vaporizer settings for surgical anesthesia in other species, because MAC is similar within and across animal classes. Vaporizer settings for maintenance of surgical anesthesia are approximately 25% higher than the MAC. For example, the MAC of isoflurane is usually between 1.5% and 2.0%, so the maintenance vaporizer settings for isoflurane range from 2.0% to 2.5%. Several factors must be accounted for when using MAC as a guide to vaporizer setting. Hypothermia decreases MAC, as does premedication with opioids and other premedicants.

MAC is not used to predict induction and recovery times because it is measured when inhalant anesthetic levels in the lower respiratory tract have equilibrated with those in the central nervous system. Inhalant anesthetic tissue and blood solubilities, ventilatory efficiency, and circulation time primarily determine the induction and recovery times. Rabbits often have shallow rapid respirations under inhalation anesthesia that may be associated with decreased alveolar ventilation and delayed attainment of maintenance alveolar anesthetic levels. This probably explains the need sometimes to "maintain" rabbits early in a procedure at isoflurane vaporizer settings of about 4% to 5%. Inclusion of premedication in the anesthetic regimen and use of intubation ameliorate this situation. Intubation allows for assisted ventilation, improved alveolar ventilation, and, therefore, better control of anesthesia.

Inhalant Anesthetic Induction

Inhalant anesthesia may be used either alone or as an adjunct to parenteral anesthesia for induction. The anesthetic is administered either into an induction chamber or through a mask (Fig. 33-1). The advantage of an induction chamber is that the animal does not have to be physically restrained during the involuntary excitement phase of induction. This reduces the risk of injury to both handler and patient. The disadvantages include greater potential for environmental contamination with inhalation anesthetic and difficulty in monitoring.

Mask induction of physically restrained animals without premedication and supplemental injectable anesthesia is not recommended. This is because most animals go through an involuntary excitement phase that may result in injury to either the handler or the animal. This is particularly true of rabbits and ferrets. Rabbits also have the propensity to suddenly kick out with their hindlimbs, sending them flying to the ground or fracturing their lumbar vertebrae. It is recommended that

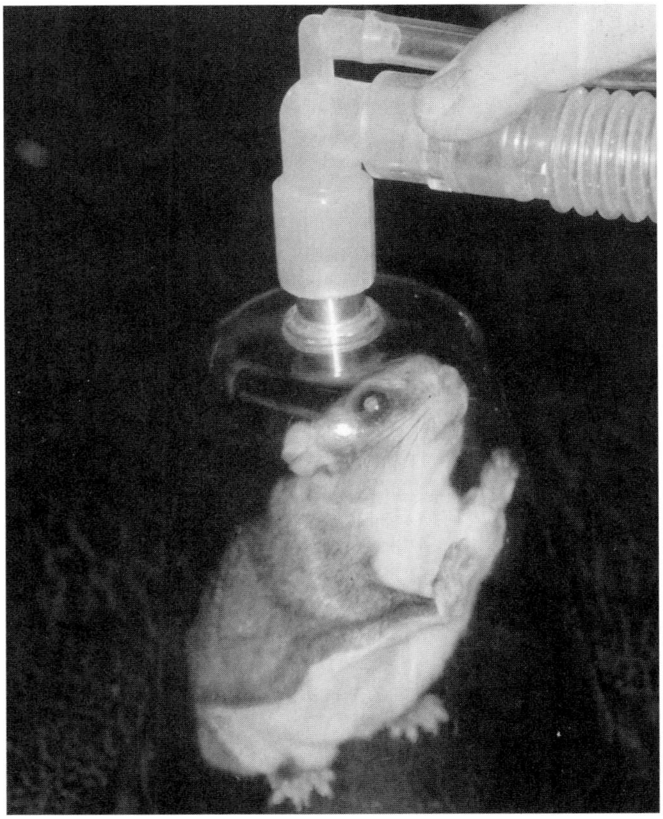

Figure 33-1 Small mammals may be induced with an inhalant anesthetic in oxygen administered into a translucent container such as this commercial dog mask containing a flying squirrel.

premedication be administered whenever an inhalant is used for induction.

Anesthetic chambers and masks are translucent to allow visibility of the patient (see Fig. 33-1). The top of the chamber should be secured to prevent the animal's forcibly opening it and escaping. For induction of an awake or lightly sedated animal, inhalant anesthetic is introduced into the container through one opening, and waste gas removed from another opening. The vaporizer is set at maximum concentration, and the oxygen flow rate set at 2 to 4 L/min, depending on the size of the container. It will take a period of time for the concentration in the induction chamber to equilibrate with the vaporizer setting. Once the animal loses its righting response (usually 5 to 10 minutes), it is removed from the chamber and a mask is placed over its nose and mouth. The chamber is removed outside or closed to allow waste gases to be safely voided to the atmosphere. The animal is then either maintained on anesthetic via the mask or intubated after it is sufficiently relaxed.

When maintaining anesthesia with a mask, it is important to place the animal's head and neck in extension to facilitate air movement. Assess respiratory pattern, rate, and noise to ensure minimum resistance to breathing. If the animal appears to be having respiratory difficulty, move the head and neck to see if the obstruction can be corrected. If not, use cotton-tipped applicators to clear the oropharynx and nares. If this fails to relieve the problem, either use intubation or awaken the animal and cancel the procedure. A pulse oximeter (discussed later) is invaluable for assessing the adequacy of arterial hemoglobin saturation.

Equipment

An animal's small size is an indication for the use of non-rebreathing systems (e.g., the Bain coaxial and other variations of the T-piece) for administration of inhalant anesthetics (Fig. 33-2).[17] These systems provide reduced respiratory resistance and mechanical dead space, and they are simple and inexpensive to construct. T-piece breathing systems are recommended for the smallest patients. Rebreathing bags can be constructed from small balloons to facilitate visualization of respiratory movement. Fresh gas flow rate for non-rebreathing systems is about 200 mL/kg per minute.

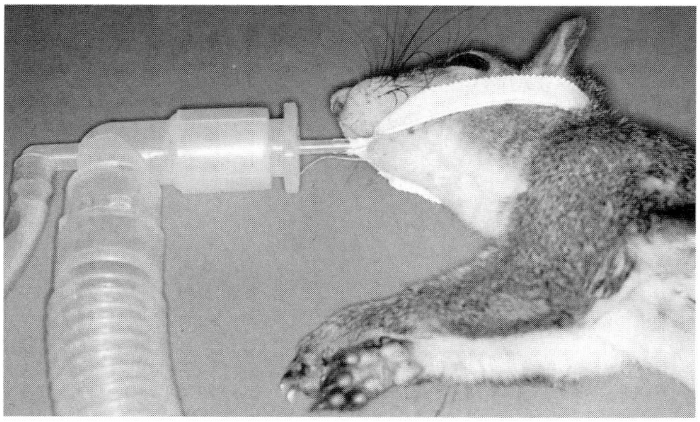

Figure 33-2 Non-rebreathing systems, such as this modified T-piece connected to an intubated squirrel, are commonly used for administration of inhalant anesthetics in small mammals.

Because intubation of some small mammals is very difficult (see later discussion), inhalation anesthesia is often maintained with the use of a mask connected to the breathing system. Systems have been developed for small rodents that allow concurrent scavenging of waste anesthetic gases. These usually include the fresh gas line entering the mask and an exit line for removal of waste gases.

Endotracheal Intubation

Endotracheal intubation is indicated for upper airway protection, administration of oxygen and inhalant anesthetics, and assisted ventilation. Respiratory obstruction and hypoventilation are common causes of morbidity and mortality of anesthetized small mammals and a major limitation to the performance of some diagnostic and surgical procedures. With a little practice and the use of appropriate technique and equipment, intubation of ferrets, rabbits, and some rodents can and should be a routine standard of care, especially for complex and prolonged procedures.

Endotracheal tubes Endotracheal tube size recommendations are provided in Table 33-4. A variety of commercially available endotracheal tubes are available; the smallest cuffed and uncuffed tubes have internal diameters (ID) of 3 and 1 mm, respectively. Unfortunately, the latter (Global Veterinary Products, Inc, New Buffalo, MI) is very flexible, easily occluded, and opaque. Endotracheal tubes are preferably clear, to allow visualization of condensation or occlusion with mucus or blood. Cole endotracheal tubes were originally developed for pediatric patients. They have a small-diameter portion that fits into the glottis and a wide portion that connects to the breathing system. This design decreases resistance to respiration. For the smallest patients (e.g., rats), endotracheal tubes are constructed from over-the-needle catheters or urinary catheters and attached to commercial endotracheal tube adapters.

Ferrets Endotracheal intubation in ferrets is relatively simple and is similar to that in cats. Jaw tone is often high even at moderate levels of anesthesia, and gauze placed around the upper and lower jaws is usually necessary to facilitate opening. The tongue is pulled forward to visualize the glottis (Fig. 33-3). Topical application of a small amount of local anesthetic reduces laryngospasm and facilitates intubation.

TABLE 33-4
Guidelines for Endotracheal Tube Size Selection for a Variety of Small Mammals

Species	Endotracheal Tube Internal Diameter (mm)
Ferret	2.0-3.5
Rabbit	2.0-3.5
Rat	16-18 gauge over-the-needle catheter
Guinea pig, chinchilla	14-16 gauge over-the-needle catheter, ≤2
Hamster	16 gauge over-the-needle catheter
Squirrel	≤2
Prairie dog	2.0-2.5
Hedgehog	14-16 gauge over-the-needle catheter, ≤2

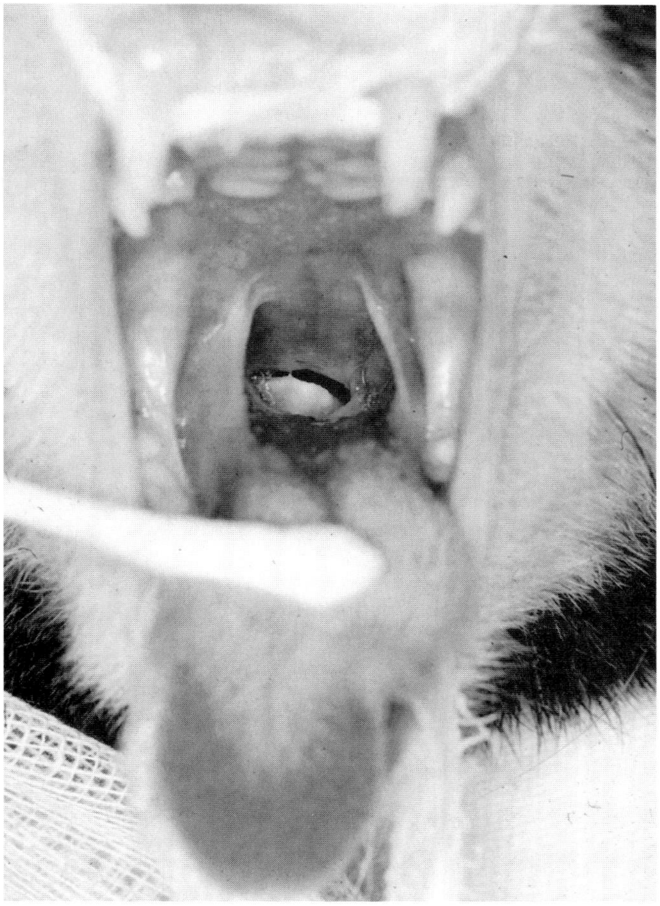

Figure 33-3 The ferret glottis is readily visualized by opening the animal's mouth with gauze placed around the upper and lower incisors. The tongue has been pulled forward to reveal the white epiglottis at its base.

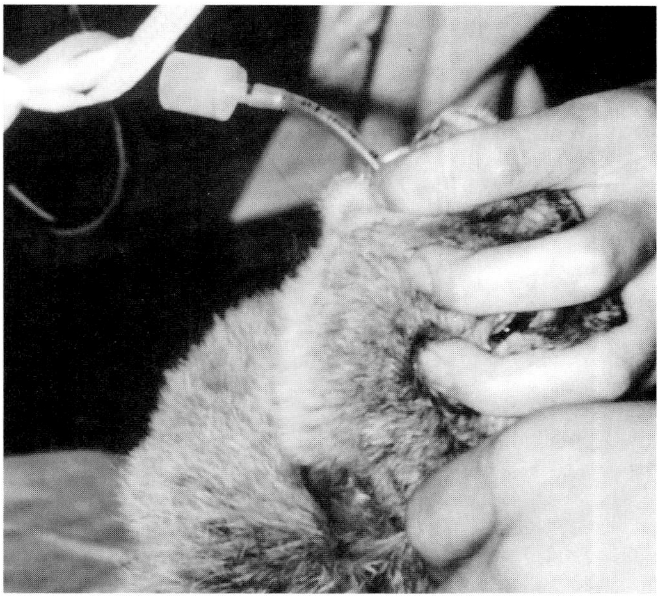

Figure 33-4 Endotracheal intubation of a rabbit requires that the head and neck be hyperextended to align the glottis with the oropharynx. The rabbit is placed in sternal recumbency, and the head grasped with one hand.

Rabbits In rabbits, it is essential that the animal's head and neck be hyperextended to align the larynx and trachea with the oropharynx (Fig. 33-4). Care is taken to prevent excessive hyperextension, which may result in spinal injury. Because rabbits are nasal breathers, the epiglottis must be displaced ventral to the soft palate for visualization of the glottis through the oropharynx. Regardless of technique, the animal should be adequately relaxed before intubation is attempted as indicated by the absence of a response to an ear or toe pinch.

Primarily two types of technique are used: blind and direct visualization. An additional technique, not recommended for routine clinical practice because of the potential for laryngeal trauma, uses retrograde placement of a guide wire or catheter through the larynx and out through the mouth. The endotracheal tube is then passed over the wire into the larynx.

I prefer the blind technique for routine intubation. However, this technique requires spontaneous respiration for accurate endotracheal tube placement, because it relies on respiratory noise. The relaxed rabbit is placed in sternal recumbency on a table at a height comfortable for the anesthetist. If you are right handed, stand on the right side of the animal and grasp the head with the left hand (see Fig. 33-4). Grasp the head from above and behind with the fingers under the lower jaw. Insert the endotracheal tube into the space between the incisors and the first premolar (Fig. 33-5) and pass it caudally over the base of the tongue. The anesthetist then lifts the head and neck into hyperextension and places his or her ear against the tube as it is passed toward the glottis (Fig. 33-6). The tube is advanced until maximum respiratory noise is detected. Sudden cessation of noise and gurgling sounds indicates that the tube is in the

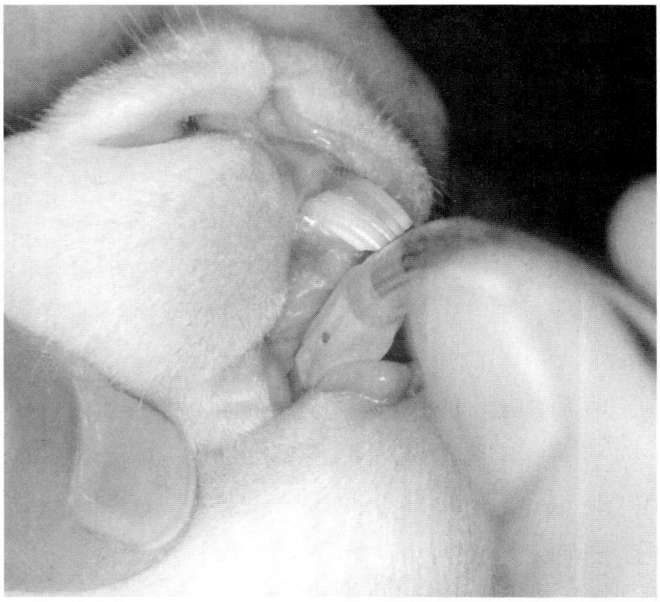

Figure 33-5 For the blind technique of endotracheal intubation in the rabbit, the endotracheal tube is inserted between the incisors and the premolars and passed back over the tongue.

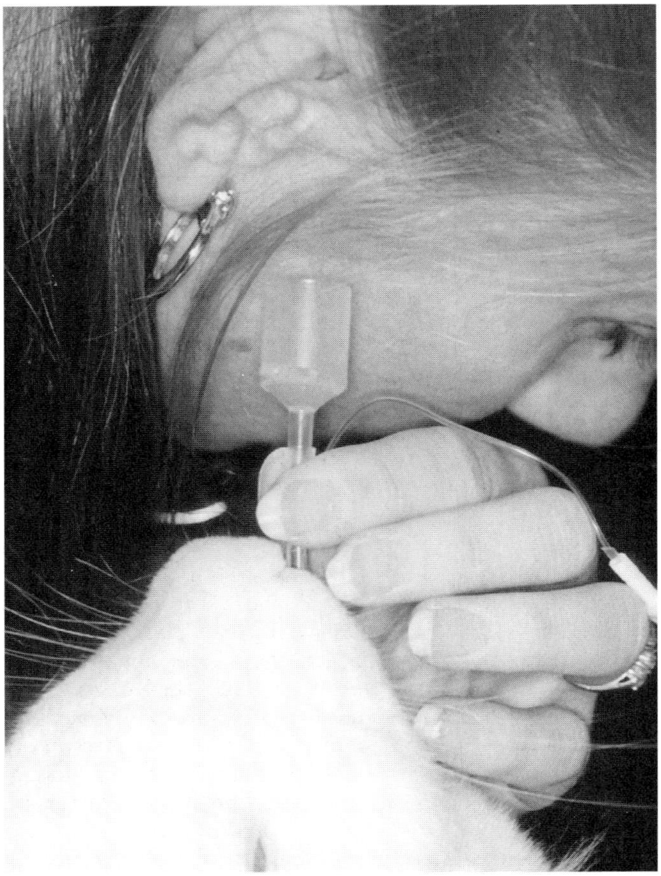

Figure 33-6 The blind technique for rabbit intubation relies on listening for respiratory noise through the endotracheal tube to identify its position relative to the glottis.

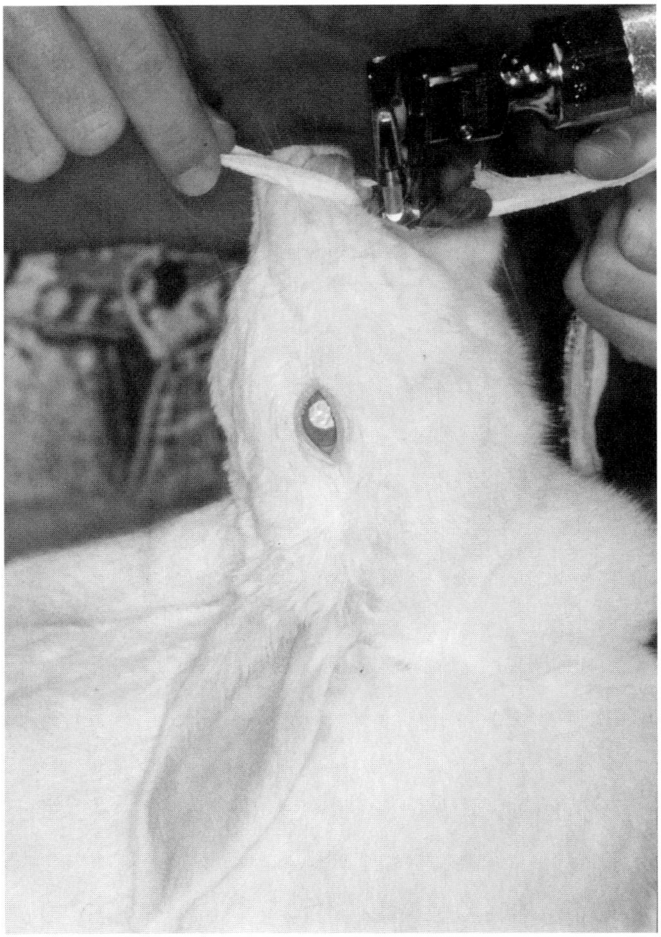

Figure 33-7 The direct visualization technique for endotracheal intubation in the rabbit requires that the mouth be opened with gauze placed around the upper and lower incisors. The head and neck are hyperextended, and a pediatric laryngoscope is used to visualize the glottis. Alternatively, the endotracheal tube is placed over a rigid 2.7-mm endoscope that is used for visualization of the glottis, or an otoendoscope can be used.

esophagus. Withdraw the tube until the normal respiratory noise is heard. The tube is then repetitively and gently advanced at the glottis until it enters the trachea. At the point of peak respiratory noise, it sometimes helps to rotate the endotracheal tube 180 degrees to displace the epiglottis. The use of a local anesthetic, either as a gel applied to the end of the tube or as a liquid poured down the tube, desensitizes the glottis and facilitates intubation. Be aware that the rabbit may forcefully cough the tube outward. Do not persist in intubation attempts for more than a few minutes or if there is evidence of either laryngeal edema or hemorrhage.

The direct visualization technique is similar to the blind technique. An assistant opens the animal's jaws using gauze tape placed around the upper and lower incisors (Fig. 33-7). The tongue is grasped by an additional gauze square and pulled up and to the side. A cotton-tipped applicator may assist in grasping the tongue. A laryngoscope with a pediatric straight blade (Miller No. 0 or 1) is then inserted into the oropharynx. Once again, to allow visualization of the glottis, the head and neck are hyperextended and the epiglottis is displaced. The endotracheal tube is then passed down the laryngoscope blade and through the glottis. Visualization of the glottis is usually lost as the endotracheal tube occludes the oropharynx. A small-diameter guide catheter may be placed instead, with the endotracheal tube passed over the catheter. Alternatively, the endotracheal tube may be placed over a rigid 2.9-mm endoscope that is used to visualize the glottis. Once the endoscope is in place, the tube is advanced into the glottis. However, this technique is often difficult because of obstruction of the scope by condensation and secretions. An otoendoscope can also be used to view the glottis, and the endotracheal tube is passed alongside the otoendoscope and inserted into the glottis (see Chapter 36). Placement of the rabbit in dorsal recumbency may facilitate visibility of the glottis.

Rodents Prairie dogs, chinchillas, squirrels, and other medium to moderately large rodents (e.g., African pouched rats, Patagonian cavies) can routinely be intubated for inhalation anesthesia by using a blind technique. The anesthetized rodent is placed in lateral recumbency, with the head and neck moderately extended. The tube is then passed in a manner similar to that described for the rabbit.

Although guinea pigs are commonly anesthetized, they present several obstacles to routine endotracheal intubation. They readily regurgitate if the oropharynx is stimulated, and their cheeks frequently contain stored food. They also produce profuse salivary secretions that can be controlled, in part, by glycopyrrolate. In addition, the soft palate is fused to the base of the tongue, and entry to the glottis requires passage through a small opening called the palatal ostium.[23] The palatal ostium is also present in chinchillas and capybaras, and probably in other hystericomorph rodents as well. The soft tissue at the base of the tongue is readily traumatized by a laryngoscope blade, resulting in profuse hemorrhage. The glottis is also very small relative to the size of the animal. For these reasons, I rarely intubate guinea pigs. However, other authors have described intubation of dorsally recumbent animals with the use of direct visualization techniques with modified pediatric No. 0 blades and 14-gauge over-the-needle catheters.[15]

Rat endotracheal intubation usually involves direct visualization of the glottis and requires some form of magnification and a focused light source (e.g., rigid endoscope). One technique describes transillumination with a high-intensity light source attached to the end of a flexible fiberoptic rod positioned so that it contacts the surface of the skin in front of the neck, near the pharyngoepiglottic region of the rat's neck.[26] For visualization of the glottis, I use either a rigid endoscope or an otoscope attached to a No. 2 ear speculum that has had the distal two thirds of the tip along the right side removed.[24] The rat is positioned in dorsal recumbency on a board. An elastic band is then affixed to the upper incisors and fastened to the board, to extend the head and neck. The tongue is pulled forward and to the side, and a cotton-tipped applicator is used to clear any secretions from around the glottis. Topical application of local anesthetic on the glottis reduces laryngospasm. A slight pressure exerted on the ventral surface of the neck may further facilitate visualization of the glottis. A blind technique, similar to that described previously for other rodents, has also been reported.[22]

Endotracheal tubes for rats are constructed from 14- to 16-gauge over-the-needle catheters. The needle stylette is cut to the same length as the catheter, and the end is then filed smooth so that the smoothed needle is approximately 1 mm shorter than the catheter.[22] Alternatively, a 70-mm length of malleable 20-gauge wire can be used as a stylet.[24] At 1.5 cm from the end of the catheter, the stylette is bent to a 30-degree angle. A surgical suture can be tied to the catheter at a point 4.5 cm from its end, to prevent excessive insertion of the catheter into the trachea. Mucous obstruction is common, and changing the tube may be necessary. This technique can also be used for hamsters.

Miscellaneous Hedgehogs are intubated with either a direct technique similar to that described for ferrets or a modification using a rigid endoscope. Sugar gliders are not routinely intubated, but, if needed, I would recommend the technique described for the rat.

Assessment of endotracheal tube placement If correct placement is in doubt, remove the endotracheal tube and reassess placement. The use of a pulse oximeter (see later discussion) is invaluable for determining potential oxygenation problems due to airway obstruction during intubation. Correct endotracheal tube placement is determined by (1) visualizing condensation on the inside of the endotracheal tube or on a metal surface placed at the end of the tube; (2) detecting air movement with a hair placed in front of the tube; (3) watching the non-rebreathing bag; (4) the response to intubation (e.g., coughing); or (5) the detection of exhaled carbon dioxide on a capnograph. To ensure the tube has not been placed into a single bronchus, premeasure the tube before use and auscultate both lung fields for respiratory sounds after intubation.

PERIOPERATIVE MONITORING

It is recommended that a trained person be assigned as anesthetist for each patient, regardless of the size or value of the animal. This approach facilitates monitoring, recording, and supportive care in the perianesthetic period and saves time when supportive intervention is required.

Anesthetic Depth

The presence of adequate muscle relaxation (i.e., immobilization) does not necessarily imply either unconsciousness or analgesia. Conversely, unconsciousness does not imply either adequate muscle relaxation or analgesia. Clinically, an assumption of unconsciousness is based on anesthetic dose and vaporizer setting, muscle relaxation, decreased reflex activity, and absence of limb and body movement.

In rabbits anesthetized with isoflurane, the eyelid aperture increases in a predictable dose-dependent manner[11]; this is true also in ferrets, but not rats.[10] This response is difficult to evaluate clinically, because either the cornea is protected with a lubricant or the eyelids are taped closed. The eyeball rotates medially, then either dorsally or ventrally at 0.8 MAC before becoming centrally fixed at greater than 1.5 MAC.[11] Palpebral and corneal reflexes are observed at 0.8 MAC but are abolished at greater than 2.0 MAC. In ferrets and rodents, the corneal reflex is a poor guide to anesthetic depth.[10] A fixed, dilated pupil that is unresponsive to light, and with no corneal reflex, is a cross-species indicator of excessive anesthetic depth and/or brain stem hypoperfusion/ischemia. Anal tone is usually retained until deep anesthetic levels, but this is difficult to assess in small rodents.

Evaluation of the physiologic and muscular response to a painful stimulus is used to assess pain and nociceptor response. The difficulty arises in providing a stimulus reflective of surgical pain that does not unintentionally traumatize tissues. This can be a pinch to toe, ear, or tail or a skin incision. Increasing depth toward a surgical plane of anesthesia is assumed when muscle tone (e.g., jaw muscle, anal sphincter) decreases, palpebral and corneal reflexes are obtunded, and the respiration pattern becomes regular and even. Sudden tachycardia, hypertension, or tachypnea in response to stimuli indicates inadequate anesthetic depth, inadequate analgesia, or both. Appropriate responses include stopping the painful stimulus, graded increases in anesthetic dose (e.g., increased vaporizer setting), or parenteral administration of an analgesic, usually an opioid, or ketamine. Although most inhalant anesthetics produce unconsciousness, they are poor analgesics. An exception is nitrous oxide, which is a good analgesic but does not produce unconsciousness alone.

Cardiovascular Monitoring

The heart rate in mammals is determined primarily by temperature, size, metabolism, respiratory state, and the presence or absence of painful stimuli. Heart rate is inversely related to body size. The resting heart rate (min^{-1}) for mammals is calculated from the allometric equation heart rate = $241 \times M_b^{-0.25}$, where M_b is the body weight in kilograms. A heart rate that is 20% faster or slower than the calculated rate for an individual animal is considered to be tachycardic or bradycardic, respectively.

Auscultation An esophageal stethoscope should be used in most small mammals during anesthetic procedures in which the patient is intubated. The esophageal stethoscope is not practical to use in small rodents, and it may induce regurgitation in guinea pigs. Alternatively, a quality pediatric stethoscope should be available for immediate use.

Electrocardiography The electrocardiograph should have a multichannel oscilloscope with nonfade tracing and freeze capabilities. Additionally, it must be able to record at speeds of 100 mm/sec and amplify the signal to at least 1 mV equal to 1 cm. Standard lead positions are used.

Doppler flow detection The Doppler flow detector uses a probe placed as close as possible to blood flow in either an artery or the heart. The probe contains a high-frequency sound transmitter as well as a receiver. There are three types of probe: human adult, human pediatric, and pencil. The pencil type has a small probe surface at the end of an elongated holder and is valuable for assessing blood flow in very small patients. Decreases in volume indicate either a decrease in blood flow or displacement of the probe. Always check the animal first when sound volume decreases or the Doppler probe appears not to be working. The Doppler may be used anywhere there are major arteries close to the skin. In small mammals, contact sites include the ventral aspect of the tail base; the carotid, femoral, and auricular arteries; and directly over the heart.

Arterial blood pressure measurement Sites for indirect blood pressure measurement include the legs, forearms, tail, and ears (rabbits). Indirect measurement is least accurate at low systemic pressures and when small arteries are used. It is important to have the appropriate cuff size; its width should be approximately 40% of the circumference of the limb. Cuffs that are too narrow or too wide give pressures that are erroneously high or low, respectively. Indirect blood pressure measurement techniques have been designed and validated for use in rats and rabbits.

Direct arterial blood pressure measurement is used less frequently than indirect measurement because it is technically difficult and requires an expensive monitor. It is most easily performed in rabbits because of the easily accessible auricular artery in the center of the pinna.

Respiratory Monitoring

The respiratory rate is inversely related to body weight and is determined by evaluating either thoracic wall or reservoir bag movement.

Auscultation As with cardiac auscultation, evaluation of the respiratory system in small patients requires a good-quality stethoscope with appropriate head and length of tubing, and an experienced ear. The esophageal stethoscope can be used to evaluate respiratory noise. However, there is more likely to be artifactual noise that must be distinguished from true respiratory noise.

Blood gas analysis Arterial blood gas analysis assesses the patient's oxygenation and acid-base status and adequacy of ventilation. Venous blood gas samples are more easily obtained, but interpretation is difficult. Arterial blood gas samples are obtained from any palpable artery. Collection sites include the femoral, metatarsal, and auricular (rabbit) arteries. Infiltration of the periarterial area with 1% lidocaine without epinephrine may prevent reflex vasoconstriction.

Pulse oximetry Pulse oximetry has been evaluated in both rabbits and rats, and it appears to be accurate at hemoglobin saturation levels greater than 85%.[25] Potential sites for placement of transmission pulse oximeter sensors include the ear, tongue, buccal mucosa, paw (Fig. 33-8), vulva, prepuce, and proximal tail. A reflectance pulse oximeter sensor is used in either the esophagus or the rectum or applied to the skin/fur surface on the ventral aspect of the neck, overlying the carotid artery (rat). In rabbits, the base of the tail and the paws appear more effective locations for pulse oximetry than the ears; this may be caused by excessive compression of the aural vasculature by the clamp holding the probe to the ear.

Pulse oximeters require adequate pulsations to allow them to distinguish arterial light adsorption. Therefore, they are inaccurate in the presence of decreased blood pressure, decreased pulse pressure, and vasoconstriction. The α_2-adrenergic agonists produce intense peripheral vasoconstriction and consequently make signal detection difficult. The oximeter measures a pulse but not peripheral perfusion; the presence or absence of a pulse is quickly detected, but the presence of a pulse does not ensure adequate blood flow.

Capnography Capnometry is the measurement of carbon dioxide concentrations in expired gases. Capnography refers to the display of these concentrations on an oscilloscope screen or recording chart, usually as a function of time. End-tidal carbon dioxide tension ($ETCO_2$) is used to provide a noninvasive estimate of the arterial partial pressure of carbon dioxide ($PaCO_2$). $ETCO_2$ is usually less than $PaCO_2$. Lung disease will increase this difference, as will sample errors. The most obvious sampling error is a system leak. Another sampling problem is related to the sampling rate and the minute ventilation of the patient. High sampling rates (e.g., 250 mL/min), when used in small patients, result in dilution with room air and, consequently, lower $ETCO_2$ values. In human pediatric patients, the sampling rate is set at 50 mL/min, but this rate is still too high in small exotic patients.

Thermoregulatory monitoring Body temperature measurement is a standard of care during all anesthetic procedures. Hypothermia is common in small anesthetic patients because of the large ratio of surface area to volume. Additionally, many

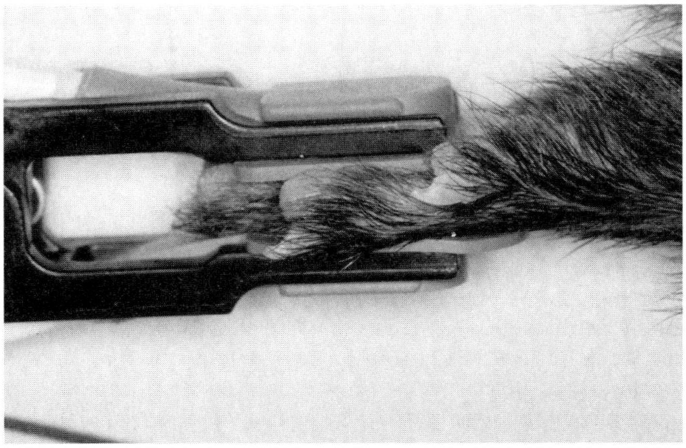

Figure 33-8 The paw of a small mammal is usually an effective site for placement of the pulse oximeter probe for monitoring hemoglobin saturation.

drugs used in the perianesthetic period suppress normal thermoregulatory mechanisms. Further, the anesthetic gases used during inhalation anesthesia are of low humidity and temperature. Body temperature is preferably measured continuously, and the thermometer should be sufficiently small to be used in small patients. For measurement of core body temperature, it is necessary to use a temperature probe attached to an esophageal stethoscope.

PERIOPERATIVE SUPPORTIVE CARE

Cardiovascular Care

Fluid therapy Vascular access is established in physiologically unstable patients and in those likely to decompensate from hemorrhage, endotoxemia, or other causes during the perianesthetic period. Small patient size makes venous and intraosseous catheterization difficult, but practice and attention to technique enable attainment of these essential skills for small mammal practice. Potential catheterization sites include the cephalic, saphenous, and auricular (rabbit) veins. Penetration of the skin before placement, with either a hypodermic needle or a scalpel blade, is done to prevent catheter buckling. Intraosseous catheter sites include the proximal femur, tibia, and humerus. Attaining vascular access is described in more detail in the species medicine chapters.

Subcutaneous administration of fluids is not an appropriate route for correction of deficits or replacement from hemorrhage in the perianesthetic period. Fluid absorption is minimal, because subcutaneous tissues are poorly vascularized and peripheral vasoconstriction is the usual response to dehydration and hypotension. Hypertonic dextrose solutions administered subcutaneously exacerbate dehydration and fluid deficits.

Selection of the appropriate fluid to infuse in the hemorrhaging patient depends on the severity and duration of hemorrhage, the initial hematocrit, the species, and the presence of underlying cardiopulmonary disease. The hematocrit and total protein do not acutely reflect hemorrhage severity. A general guideline to fluid selection is as follows: for 5% to 10% of blood volume lost, use balanced electrolyte solution at three times the volume of the estimated blood loss; for 10% to 20% loss, use plasma expanders (e.g., hetastarch [Hespan, B. Braun Medical Inc., Irving, CA], plasma); and for 20% to 30% loss, use whole blood transfusion.

Small-volume infusors are commercially available (e.g., Medfusion 3 2010i, Medexing, Duluth, GA), but they are expensive. However, they are essential for accurate fluid infusion in small anesthetized patients. Some infusors can be preprogrammed to flow rates for emergency and other drugs, so that all that is necessary for administration is to enter the body weight of the animal. They also allow a continuous infusion, which is preferable to bolus injection.

The rate of fluid infusion during anesthesia depends on the hydration status, daily fluid requirement, severity of hemorrhage, type of fluid to be infused, and presence or absence of underlying renal or cardiac disease. During most anesthetic episodes, the main goal of fluid therapy is to maintain vascular access and replace fluids lost (e.g., to dry anesthetic gases). I usually infuse a balanced electrolyte solution at 5 to 10 mL/kg per hour.

Drugs Pharmacologic manipulation of cardiovascular function is occasionally indicated in the anesthetized patient. The main difficulties are in early detection of instability and subsequent monitoring of drug effect. Positive inotropes, chronotropes, and vasoconstrictors (e.g., dopamine, dobutamine, ephedrine, epinephrine, norepinephrine) may be used. However, without arterial blood pressure measurement to adjust the infusion rates, these drugs may in themselves cause detrimental hypertension or arrhythmias, or both. The use of small-volume infusors, previously described, is essential for accurate administration of these drugs in small patients.

Respiratory Care

Ventilation General anesthetics usually produce a dose-dependent ventilatory depression. This effect may be either additive or synergistic with underlying disease, resulting in marked hypercapnia or ventilatory arrest. High inspired-oxygen concentrations also decrease the ventilatory drive. Ventilation is also affected by body position and by compression of the respiratory exchange tissues because of distended viscera or obesity. Inadvertent compression of the chest by surgeons is common in small exotic patients. Development of good hand position techniques, an attentive anesthetist, and the use of clear plastic drapes help prevent this cause of hypoventilation.

Ferrets, because of their very compliant chest walls, appear to be dependent on diaphragmatic movement for ventilation. Rabbits have very small chest cavities relative to body size and have a high prevalence of respiratory disease. Additionally, they often develop tachypnea under anesthesia with a normal to decreased alveolar ventilation. As discussed previously, guinea pigs have relatively small-diameter tracheas and are prone to airway obstruction because of regurgitation and profuse salivary secretions.

Adequacy of ventilation is most accurately assessed by measuring the $PaCO_2$. Capnography provides an indirect estimate of $PaCO_2$, but it is too inaccurate in most small exotic patients to be used for anything other than validation of successful endotracheal intubation. Visualization of chest wall movement is a deceptive guide to adequacy of ventilation. Consequently, I recommend either assisted or controlled ventilation of intubated patients under general anesthesia. Doxapram is not recommended for use in hypoventilating patients unless intubation and mechanical ventilation are impossible or contraindicated.

Ventilation is assisted or controlled by the application of positive pressure, either manually or mechanically. Many of the ventilators used in small animal anesthesia can be modified to ventilate very small patients. A commercially available ventilator and anesthetic-delivery machine (Anesthesia WorkStation, Halowell EMC, Pittsfield, MA) has been specifically designed for use in very small patients, primarily research rabbits and rodents. It is both a circle system for delivery of inhalant anesthetic and an optional ventilator with an adjustable pressure safety limit. Another ventilator for small animals (Vetronics, West LaFayette, IN), which uses a T-piece breathing system, is also commercially available. As an example of the ventilator settings required in a small mammal, rats were successfully ventilated at a frequency of 82 breaths per minute and a tidal volume of 1.5 mL/100 g body weight.[3]

The advantage of mechanical ventilation is that it frees the anesthetist to concentrate on other tasks. The disadvantages are that mechanical ventilators require a thorough theoretical and technical understanding for their safe use, they require endotracheal intubation, and they produce positive intrathoracic pressures that interfere with venous return to the heart and may cause lung trauma.

Manual ventilation provides the advantages, with a skilled anesthetist, of rapid adjustment of ventilatory pressures and volumes and responsiveness to the surgeon, who may require brief, irregular periods of ventilatory arrest to safely complete a procedure. Further research is necessary to evaluate the efficacy and appropriateness of ventilation techniques in small mammal practice. There may be situations in which some hypoventilation is preferable to the adverse effects of positive-pressure ventilation.

Oxygen support Administration of elevated inspired oxygen concentrations (greater than 40%) often is sufficient to overcome mild to moderate hypoxemia, assuming that no major pulmonary shunting is present. Although mammals are susceptible to pulmonary oxygen toxicity, this syndrome is unlikely to be observed in patients maintained on high inspired-oxygen concentrations for 24 hours.

Thermoregulatory Care

Measures to reduce hypothermia include minimizing anesthesia time, using warmed surgical preparation solutions, wrapping the body, increasing the room temperature, and using external heat sources (i.e., circulating warm-water blankets and forced-air warmers). Electric heat blankets are not used because they have the potential to cause severe burns. Similarly, heated fluid bags placed in contact with the skin can cause burns.

CARDIOPULMONARY RESUSCITATION

Cardiopulmonary resuscitation follows the same priorities as in other veterinary patients: airway (A), breathing (B), circulation (C), and drugs (D). As discussed earlier, the period of ischemia/hypoxia that can be tolerated by the brain before irreversible damage is incurred is indirectly related to metabolic rate and body temperature. Compared with cats and dogs, small mammals, because of their higher metabolic rates, have a shorter "window of time" during which resuscitation can be effective. To improve response time, emergency drug dosages are precalculated and drawn into labeled syringes in preparation for use. If endotracheal intubation is not possible, an indirect ventilation technique, using a bulb inflator placed over the nose, can be used in small rodents.[12]

RECOVERY

Recovery is a critical period during which the patient is placed in a warm, quiet environment and monitored. Supportive care established during anesthesia is continued into the recovery period until the patient is fully alert and physiologically stable. In particular, vascular access is maintained to allow emergency administration of drugs and fluids.

The anesthetic agents used, the duration of the procedure, and the magnitude of physiologic dysfunction incurred primarily determine the duration and quality of recovery. Prolonged recovery is usually caused by hypothermia, hypoglycemia, and anesthetic overdose or impaired drug elimination. Care must be taken when rewarming an animal that is possibly hypovolemic or hypoglycemic, as warming results in dilation of vasoconstricted peripheral vessels and increased metabolic demand for glucose. These phenomena may explain some of the sudden deaths that occur a few hours into recovery.

SPECIES ANESTHESIA

Drug doses for premedication, analgesia, and injectable anesthetics are given in Tables 33-1, 33-2, and 33-3, respectively. Induction and maintenance with isoflurane is acceptable for most nonpainful procedures. The addition of an analgesic is indicated for surgical and other painful procedures. Tranquilizers or sedatives may be used to facilitate the handling and induction of some animals. Techniques for endotracheal intubation were described previously, and guidelines for endotracheal tube size are given in Table 33-4. Anesthesia of sugar gliders and hedgehogs is similar to that of other small mammals of a similar size, and data should be extrapolated.

REFERENCES

1. Aeschbacher G, Webb AI: Propofol in rabbits: 1. Determination of an induction dose. Lab Anim Sci 1993; 43:324-327.
2. Aeschbacher G, Webb AI: Propofol in rabbits: 2. Long-term anesthesia. Lab Anim Sci 1993; 43:328-335.
3. Alpert M, Goldstein D, Triner L: Technique of endotracheal intubation in rats. Lab Anim Sci 1982; 32:78-79.
4. Bjorkman S, Redke F: Clearance of fentanyl, alfentanil, methohexitone, thiopentone and ketamine in relation to estimated hepatic blood flow in several animal species: application to prediction of clearance in man. J Pharm Pharmacol 2000; 52:1065-1074.
5. Brammer DW, Doerning BJ, Chrisp CE, et al: Anesthetic and nephrotoxic effects of Telazol in New Zealand white rabbits. Lab Anim Sci 1991; 41:432-435.
6. Calderone L, Grimes P, Shalev M: Acute reversible cataract formation induced by xylazine and by ketamine-xylazine anesthesia in rats and mice. Exp Eye Res 1986; 42:331-337.
7. Eisele P, Kaaekuahiwi MA, Canfield DR, et al: Epidural catheter placement for testing of obstetrical analgesics in female guinea pigs. Lab Anim Sci 1994; 44:486-490.
8. Flecknell PA: Analgesia of small mammals. Vet Clin North Am Exotic Anim Pract 2001; 4:47-56.
9. Hurley RJ, Marini RP, Avison DL, et al: Evaluation of detomidine anesthetic combinations in the rabbit. Lab Anim Sci 1994; 44:472-477.
10. Imai A, Steffey EP, Farver TB, et al: Assessment of isoflurane-induced anesthesia in ferrets and rats. Am J Vet Res 1999; 60:1577-1583.
11. Imai A, Steffey EP, Ilkiw JE, et al: Comparison of clinical signs and hemodynamic variables used to monitor rabbits during halothane- and isoflurane-induced anesthesia. Am J Vet Res 1999; 60:1189-1195.
12. Ingall JRF, Hasenpusch PH: A rat resuscitator. Lab Anim Care 1966; 16:82-83.
13. Kero P, Thomasson B, Soppi A-M: Spinal anaesthesia in the rabbit. Lab Anim 1981; 15:347-348.
14. Komulainen A, Olson ME: Antagonism of ketamine-xylazine anesthesia in rats by administration of yohimbine, tolazoline, or 4-aminopyridine. Am J Vet Res 1991; 52:585-588.
15. Kujime K, Natelson BH: A method for endotracheal intubation of guinea pigs (*Cavia porcellus*). Lab Anim Sci 1981; 31:715-716.
16. Larsson JE, Wahlström G: Optimum rate of administration of propofol for induction of anaesthesia in rats. Br J Anaesth 1994; 73:692-694.

17. Lerche P, Muir WW, Bednarski RM: Nonrebreathing anesthetic systems in small animal practice. J Am Vet Med Assoc 2000; 217:493-497.
18. Marini RP, Xiantang L, Harpster NK, et al: Cardiovascular pathology possibly associated with ketamine/xylazine anesthesia in Dutch belted rabbits. Lab Anim Sci 1999; 49:153-160.
19. Mason DE: Anesthesia, analgesia, and sedation for small mammals. *In* Hillyer EV, Quesenberry KE, eds. Ferrets, Rabbits and Rodents: Clinical Medicine and Surgery. Philadelphia, WB Saunders, 1997, pp 378-391.
20. Olson ME, Vizzutti D, Morck DW, et al: The parasympatholytic effects of atropine sulfate and glycopyrrolate in rats and rabbits. Can J Vet Res 1994; 58:254-258.
21. Robertson SA: Analgesia and analgesic techniques. Vet Clin North Am Exotic Anim Pract 2001; 4:1-18.
22. Stark RA, Nahrwold ML, Cohen PJ: Blind oral tracheal intubation of rats. J Appl Physiol 1981; 51:1355-1356.
23. Timm KI, Jahn SE, Sedgwick CJ: The palatal ostium of the guinea pig. Lab Anim Sci 1987; 37:801-802.
24. Tran DQ, Lawson D: Endotracheal intubation and manual ventilation of the rat. Lab Anim Sci 1986; 36:540-541.
25. Vegfors M, Sjoberg F, Lindberg L-G, et al: Basic studies of pulse oximetry in a rabbit model. Acta Anaesthesiol Scand 1991; 35:596-599.
26. Yasaki S, Dyck PJ: A simple method for rat endotracheal intubation. Lab Anim Sci 1991; 41:620-622.

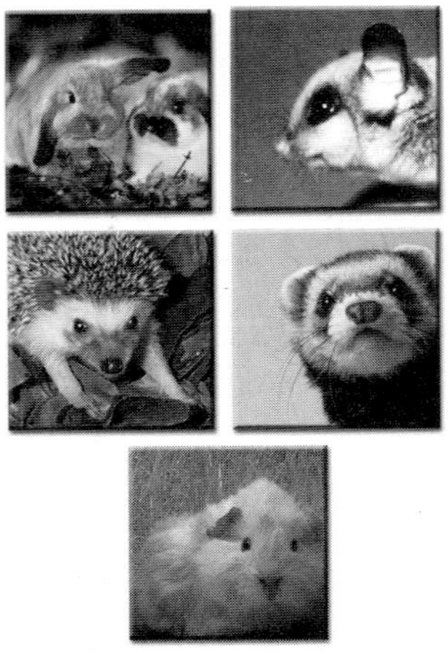

CHAPTER 34

Small Mammal Dentistry

PART I: David A. Crossley, BVetMed, MRCVS, FAVD, Diplomate EVDC
PART II: Sean Aiken, DVM, MS, Diplomate ACVS

PART I DENTAL ANATOMY AND DENTAL DISEASE

David A. Crossley, BVetMed, MRCVS, FAVD, Diplomate EVDC

Most animals seen by veterinarians have teeth. Where teeth are present, dental disease of one kind or another can and frequently does occur.

Until recently, most dental research has been intended to benefit mankind. However, these investigations, which used small carnivores, rats, mice, and hamsters, have also provided much useful species-specific information that is now being supplemented by veterinary research. Large-scale surveys have been undertaken to investigate dental disease in cats and dogs. Results consistently reveal a high incidence of periodontal disease of sufficient severity to require immediate professional treatment, with traumatic injury and other dental problems occurring much less frequently.[9,18] Also, periodontal disease and systemic disease have proved to be linked.[13] Clinical experience suggests that the pattern is similar for other commonly kept small carnivores, such as ferrets, and for insectivores, such as hedgehogs. Dental disease in other species is now beginning to receive attention,[7,11,12,16] but very little scientific information is available for many species. With these animals, careful extrapolation from related species, or those with similar dental anatomy, is necessary.

Treatment must be humane and appropriate for the species and the condition being treated. As more scientific data, veterinary dental training, and purpose-designed dental equipment become available, the continued use of outdated and often barbaric practices such as tooth clipping is no longer acceptable. It is the aim of this chapter to provide some background knowledge to veterinarians to guide them when dealing with dental problems in the lesser-known species.

Specialized dental equipment, including speculums, mouth gags, and long-shank dental burrs, are available for use in rabbits and rodents. Endoscopic equipment can also be used to examine the oral cavity and teeth (see Chapter 36).

BASIC DENTAL ANATOMY

What Is a Tooth?

Teeth are believed to have evolved from the circumoral dermal armor or skin scales of primitive fish.[28] During the evolution of land vertebrates, the teeth adapted for a wide range of functions primarily related to feeding: gathering food (prehension), cutting it into manageable portions, and crushing and grinding it to promote digestion. Teeth also developed other uses, such as tools for environmental manipulation (e.g., collection of bedding), for grooming, and as instruments of offense and defense. Teeth can be status symbols indicating health, rank, and sexual maturity. For example, in healthy rodents the facial surfaces of the incisors are typically deep orange or yellow because of iron pigments incorporated into the superficial layer of enamel (an exception is the guinea pig, which has white incisors). Abnormal incisor pigmentation indicates vitamin or mineral deficiency, local injury or infection, systemic illness, increased tooth eruption rate, or a combination of these factors.

With all the possible functions of teeth and the wide differences in the diets of different species, it is not surprising that tooth form varies considerably within and between species. The basic tooth form we are most aware of is that present in our own mouths (Fig. 34-1)—off-white, mineralized objects of reasonably consistent size with smooth, hard surfaces showing varying forms (incisors, canines, premolars, and molars) somewhat adapted for cutting, piercing, crushing, or grinding . In the center of each tooth is the dental pulp, composed of highly vascular, loose connective tissue surrounded by a single layer of odontoblasts, the cells that produce dentine. These have thin processes that extend through the dentine to its outer extremity. This makes the dentine a sensitive, living tissue. The tooth structure extends into the underlying jaw to form one or more tooth roots, which are somewhat longer than the crown. Around the roots is a sheet of tissue, the periodontal ligament, that contains a meshwork of collagen fibers extending from the cementum to surrounding alveolar bone, supporting the tooth. Many nerve endings are present in the periodontal ligament for proprioception and reflex control of complex chewing patterns. The jaw anatomy and dentition are adapted to accommodate a chewing pattern suitable for the natural diet of the animal. In most mammals, the upper and lower jaws are anisognathic, that is, of different sizes. Carnivores and most herbivores have lower jaws that are narrower and shorter than their upper jaws. However, rodent mandibles are wider, though still shorter, than their maxillas.

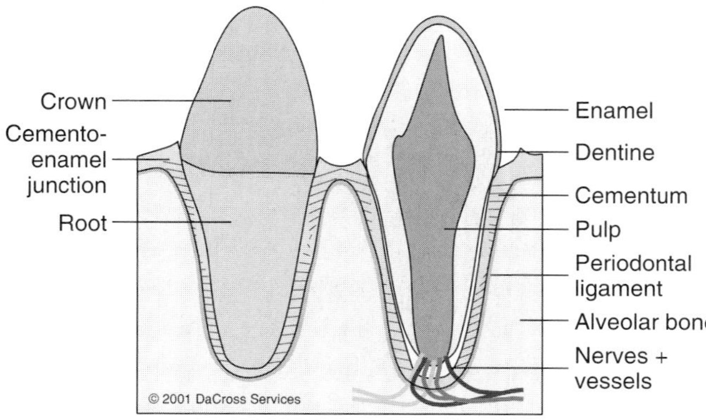

Figure 34-1 Basic mammalian tooth structure.

Dental Adaptations

Animals that manipulate the environment with their teeth and those that eat large volumes of abrasive, low-energy foods such as grass wear their teeth rapidly. This attrition can cause teeth to be completely worn away at an early age, severely reducing feeding efficiency and causing death by starvation. To avoid this, some species have developed complex folding of the tooth structure that both improves chewing efficiency and reduces the wear rate by increasing the proportion of the harder enamel exposed on the worn tooth surface. A further adaptation that occurs in horses and cattle involves elongation of the crowns until they extend nearly the full height of the jaws, with root formation delayed until maturity. These long-crowned (hypsodont) teeth continue to erupt until all the buried reserve crown has worn away, at which stage the animal is unable to chew and starves. Many species have gone a stage further, with teeth that remain immature, never forming anatomic roots (Fig. 34-2). As the tooth surface is worn away, reserve crown continues to erupt, with loss of tooth substance being compensated for by further apical growth. The lifelong growth and eruption of these aradicular hypsodont, or elodont, teeth permits increased longevity. As an additional benefit, with this form of dentition the size of the teeth can increase with growth.

Unlike our ancestors, modern human beings rarely have significant tooth wear. The teeth of hunter-gatherers are often worn down to gum level by what we consider to be middle age.[1,20] The reduction in tooth wear and current high incidence of malocclusion in humans have been caused by alterations in the diet associated with the development of agriculture and improvements in food processing technology. Modern diets need little effort or time for chewing, so there is less stimulus for jaw growth during development; the content is also refined, eliminating the abrasive components so the teeth are not worn

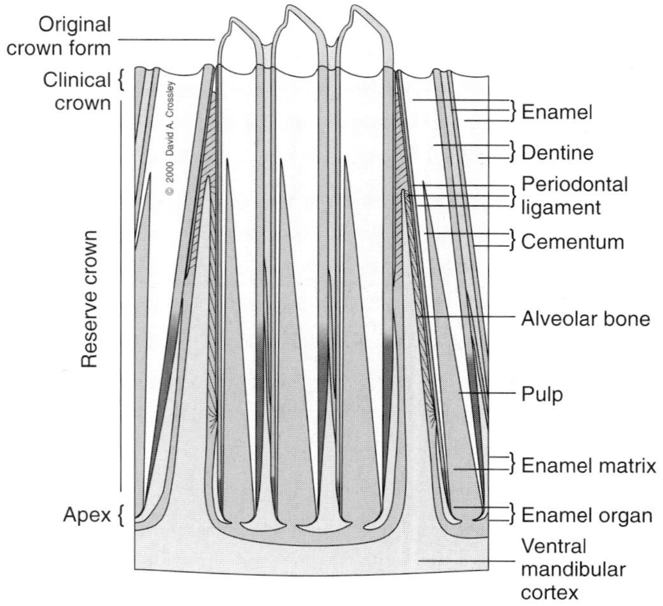

Figure 34-2 The complex tooth structure of continuously growing (elodont) cheek teeth in a young chinchilla. When the tooth first erupts, cusps are present on the surface. These are worn away to expose layers of enamel, dentine, and cementum.

away interproximally or occlusally. The resulting combination of smaller jaws with effectively larger teeth leaves insufficient space, causing crowding and displacement of the teeth. This has been seen within a single generation when native peoples have been introduced to modern diets.[10,36]

Those species that have adapted to accommodate greater tooth wear than seen in humans develop more severe problems when dietary changes reduce attrition rates. Horses fed on concentrate rations need their teeth "floated" at regular intervals to prevent occlusal irregularities such as spikes that form at the edges of the occlusal surfaces.[2,3] On a natural diet, equine cheek teeth erupt and wear approximately 3 mm per year. The problems affecting continuously growing teeth, such as the cheek teeth of rabbits, guinea pigs, and chinchillas, are potentially far more dramatic, with about 50 mm of growth and eruption in 1 year.[17]

Normal Occlusal Patterns

In species with relatively little tooth wear, such as carnivores and insectivores, the occlusal pattern largely depends on the apposing and interlocking of teeth in the opposing jaws. Although tooth positioning in herbivores is important, the pattern of tooth wear and jaw movement play an essential part.

Although each species has a typical dental formula (Table 34-1), individual variation is common. Missing, supernumerary, and abnormally shaped teeth are regularly seen. Examples include bilateral absence of "peg" teeth in rabbits, absence of third molars in chinchillas, and the presence of an extra incisor in each quadrant in ferrets.

CARNIVORES

In typical carnivores, the mandibular incisors occlude with their tips contacting the caudal surface of their maxillary counterparts. The mandibular canine slots into the gap, or diastema, between the maxillary third incisor and canine tooth and, with the mouth closed, its tip extends to the full height of the oral vestibule. Supereruption or suboptimal vestibular development results in the tips of these teeth penetrating the oral mucosa. Behind the canine teeth are the premolar and molar teeth. The more specialized the carnivore, the fewer of these teeth. Anatomically, the mesial (rostral) premolars and distal (caudal) molars are lost, accounting for the break in the sequence of tooth numbering in the modified Triadan tooth identification system (Fig. 34-3). The premolars, which are adapted for gripping or cutting, interdigitate, with each tooth ideally being opposite an interproximal space in the opposing jaw. Because the lower jaw is narrower than the upper, the mandibular premolars and molars fit medial to their maxillary counterparts. The lower first molar and upper fourth premolar are modified as large, cutting carnassial teeth. These teeth typically overlap as the mouth closes, producing a scissorlike slicing action as the intercuspal ridges of the lower tooth slide across those of the upper one. The temporomandibular joint has a hingelike function permitting this action, whereas the interlocking of the canine teeth further restricts lateral movement so the risk of direct cusp-on-cusp contact during function is minimal. In most true carnivores, the teeth caudal to the carnassials are small or absent.

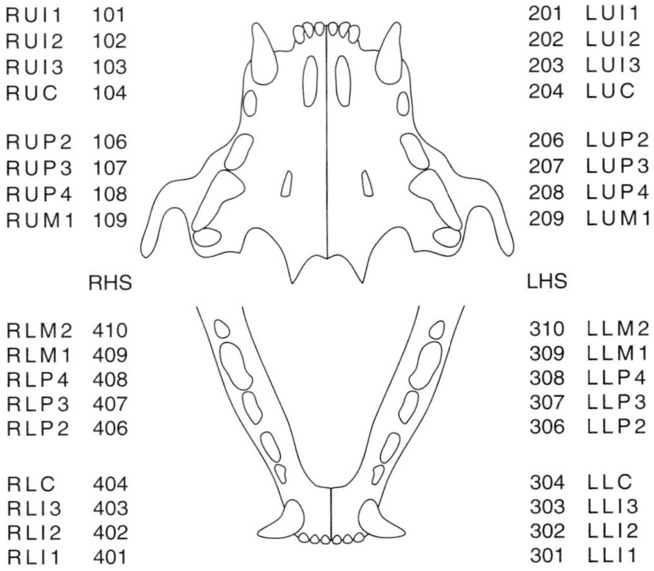

Figure 34-3 Anatomic abbreviation and modified Triadan tooth numbering for the ferret.

TABLE 34-1
Dental Formulas of Small Pet Mammals

Species	Dental Formula	Total Teeth
Ferret	$2 \times I\frac{3}{3}\ C\frac{1}{1}\ P\frac{3}{3}\ M\frac{1}{2}$	34
Rabbit	$2 \times I\frac{2}{1}\ C\frac{0}{0}\ P\frac{3}{2}\ M\frac{3}{3}$	28
Rat, mouse, hamster, gerbil	$2 \times I\frac{1}{1}\ C\frac{0}{0}\ P\frac{0}{0}\ M\frac{3}{3}$	16
Guinea pig, chinchilla	$2 \times I\frac{1}{1}\ C\frac{0}{0}\ P\frac{1}{1}\ M\frac{3}{3}$	20
Prairie dog	$2 \times I\frac{1}{1}\ C\frac{0}{0}\ P\frac{2}{1}\ M\frac{3}{3}$	22
Hedgehog	$2 \times I\frac{2}{2}\ C\frac{1}{1}\ P\frac{3}{2}\ M\frac{3}{3}$	34
Sugar glider	$2 \times I\frac{3}{2}\ C\frac{1}{0}\ P\frac{3}{3}\ M\frac{4}{4}$	40

I, Incisor; *C*, canine; *P*, premolar; *M*, molar.

RABBITS AND RODENTS

The teeth of rabbits and rodents are divided into two separate functional units, the incisors and the cheek teeth, that are separated by a long gap, the diastema (Figs. 34-4 and 34-5). Differential wear of the occlusal and interproximal surfaces of the teeth creates the typical occlusal pattern of mature animals. Rabbit and rodent incisors are strongly curved elodont teeth. Normal chewing activity, combined with active tooth-on-tooth grinding, produces the typical chisel-shaped wear pattern. In addition to wear caused by normal feeding, many rodents additionally require a suitable gnawing medium to maintain their incisors.

The cheek teeth are adapted to crushing or grinding the food. Grain eaters such as rats, mice, hamsters, and gerbils have 12 relatively small, short-crowned, rooted cheek teeth composed of three molars in each quadrant of the mouth. The occlusal surfaces have several small cusps that become worn to expose dentine as the animal ages. True herbivores tend to have more numerous or larger teeth with a large occlusal surface area adapted for grinding. The tooth structure is more complex, with

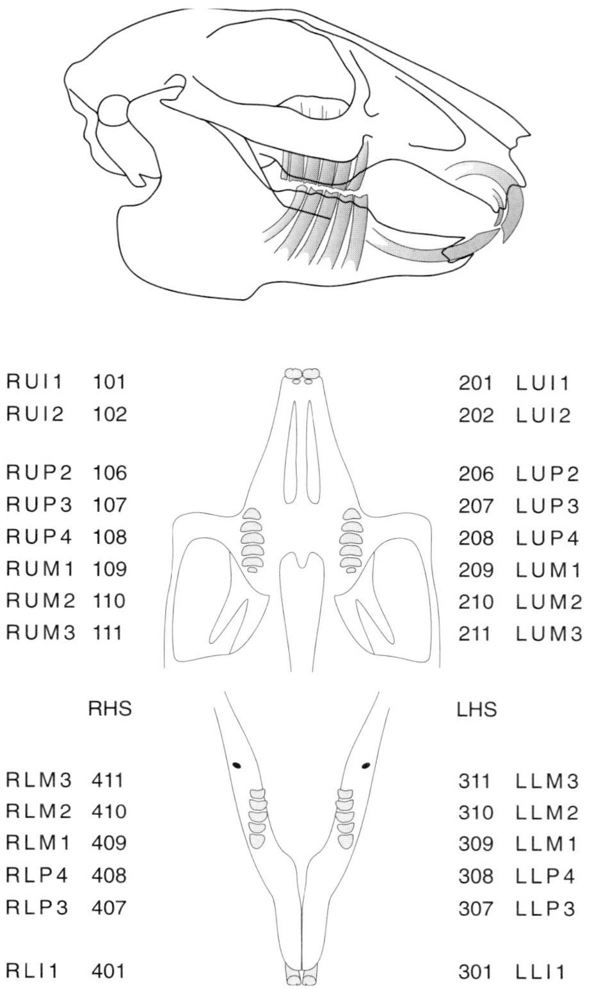

Figure 34-4 Resting jaw position and the arrangement of the teeth into two separate functional units, incisors and cheek teeth, in the rabbit. Note that the lower dental arcades are closer together than the upper ones. The anatomic abbreviation and corresponding modified Triadan tooth notation systems are shown.

a long crown and deep folds in the enamel. The cusps that are present when the teeth erupt are rapidly lost because of attrition of the occlusal surfaces, exposing the folded layers of cementum, dentine, and enamel that make up the tooth structure (Figs. 34-2 and 34-5). Some species, such as rabbits, chinchillas, and guinea pigs, have elodont cheek teeth.

Chewing in Rabbits

Rabbits use a largely vertical incisor action, the tips of the lower teeth sliding along the occlusal surface of the maxillary first incisors. Once the food is between the cheek teeth, the jaw is moved with a wide lateral chewing action (Fig. 34-6). To enable this, the mandible is retracted a little from its resting position, separating the incisors and bringing the cheek teeth into alignment. The temporomandibular joint only acts as a fulcrum on the working side, with different sections of the masseter and pterygoid muscles being used on either side of the mouth. When natural vegetation is consumed, the main power stroke approaches horizontal rather than vertical and occurs as the teeth near contact. With thicker and harder food, the power stroke becomes more vertical, starting during mouth closure. The folded cheek tooth structure wears to produce laterally orientated ridges on the occlusal surfaces of the cheek teeth. These interlock with those of the opposing teeth as the mouth closes, creating a very efficient cutting mechanism for reducing moist fibrous vegetation to short pieces. These are then ground to a digestible pulp that is moved into the pharynx and swallowed.

Chewing in Rodents

The incisors are primarily used with a rostrocaudal gnawing action from which rodents derived their name. However, they can also be used with a near vertical biting motion, such as during defensive or offensive behavior. The temporomandibular joint and masticatory muscles are highly adapted for rostrocaudal motion, with some rodents even having the ability to subluxate the joint. In most rodents, the cheek teeth occlude at rest. Because the diastema is shorter in the mandible than in the maxilla, this gives rodents their normal brachygnathic appearance (Fig. 34-5).

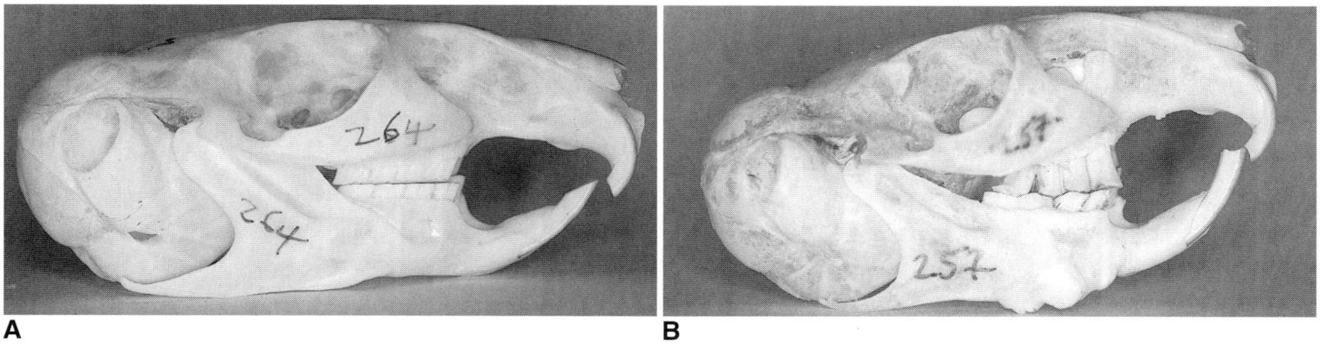

A B

Figure 34-5 A, Chinchilla skull with clinically healthy dentition. Note the shorter diastema in the lower jaw. Chinchillas are true herbivores. In a natural situation the cheek teeth wear about 1 mm every week; the incisors wear about three times as fast. B, The effects of cheek tooth elongation in the chinchilla. Note the bony changes at the cheek tooth apices.

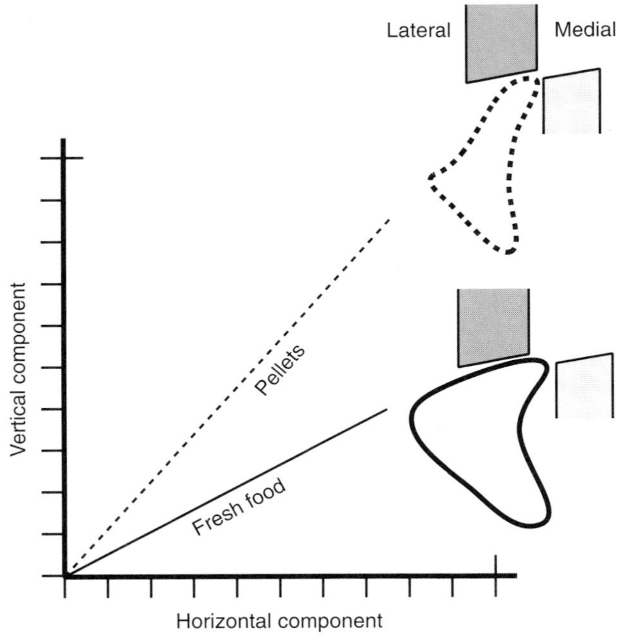

Figure 34-6 Jaw motion during chewing in the rabbit. The graph shows the relative angle and duration of the power strokes when chewing different types of food. *(Based on Morimoto T, Inoue T, Nakamura T, et al: Characteristics of rhythmic jaw movements of the rabbit. Arch Oral Biol 1985; 30:673–677.)*

Although the rat is generally described as a typical rodent, there are more than 1500 species of rodents, with many having considerably different dentition and feeding habits. In these species, it is only appropriate to extrapolate from the rat when the oral anatomy and function are similar. Rats naturally eat seeds and other high-energy foods, so they do not need highly specialized cheek teeth. These, like the incisors, are used with a largely rostrocaudal action. The cheek teeth of the lower jaw move forward along the line of the maxillary teeth during the power stroke, with chewing taking place on one or both sides. In those rodents with cheek teeth rows that converge rostrally, the chewing action is diagonal and on one side at a time. This chewing action is described as being propalineal.[14,40] Unlike rabbits, the folding of the cheek tooth structure in truly herbivorous rodents is not parallel between upper and lower teeth (see Fig. 34-5), so any enamel ridges that form during wear do not interlock. As the maxillary and mandibular arcades slide along each other, the angulation of the enamel ridges between arcades creates an efficient scissorlike cutting and grinding action.

HEDGEHOGS AND SUGAR GLIDERS

The teeth of hedgehogs are adapted for handling a wide range of invertebrate foods but are also capable of coping with other high-energy food items such as carrion, eggs, and fruit. The incisors and canines are short and, with the prominently cusped premolars, are used to grip and penetrate food items. The molars, having somewhat flattened crowns with multiple cusps, are more suitable for crushing. The diet eaten by sugar gliders is almost reverse that of hedgehogs, with fruit and tree sap being the main components, supplemented with protein from insects and other small animals. Sugar gliders have prominent sharp lower first incisors, the rest being small, as are the canines. The premolars are also small with the molars being somewhat larger.[24]

DENTAL DISEASE IN FERRETS

The range of dental disease seen in ferrets compares with that seen in dogs and cats, so texts on those species are recommended for detailed information on causes and treatment methods. As in these species, dental disease in ferrets is usually severe before it causes obvious clinical signs.

The inquisitive nature of ferrets results in many traumatic dental injuries. Surface wear and small chips in the tooth surface rarely cause oral discomfort. When oral pain is suspected, a thorough examination is essential to rule out the possibility of other causes, such as inflammation, a foreign body, or soft tissue injury. Areas of exposed dentine can be treated to reduce the sensitivity by applying fluoride or an unfilled resin (dental bonding agent) in the anesthetized patient. If related to dentine sensitivity, clinical signs will resolve rapidly after treatment. More severe dental trauma is likely to result in a complicated tooth fracture, that is, one that exposes the pulp. The treatment options in this case are endodontic therapy or extraction. Whichever is chosen, perform an intraoral, bisecting angle radiograph before surgery to assess the anatomy and to check for other pathologic lesions such as a jaw fracture. Because the periodontal support of damaged teeth is usually intact, an open surgical extraction is indicated for tooth removal. This approach also permits primary closure of the extraction site with the gingivomucoperiosteal flap that is raised for access.

Periodontal disease is common in ferrets. Accumulated plaque elicits a marked inflammatory response from the adjacent soft tissues. The problem can be reduced by providing food in a natural form to encourage prolonged chewing. To prevent plaque, tooth brushing can be done at least once daily with a small, soft-bristled toothbrush and either a pet dentifrice or an oral antiseptic gel that contains chlorhexidine. If significant gingivitis or periodontal disease is present, then professional periodontal debridement is indicated. Multirooted teeth that are affected where the roots divide (furcation involvement) and any teeth that have lost more than one third of their periodontal support are best extracted, as it is unlikely that plaque control will adequately prevent further progression of disease.

DENTAL DISEASE IN RABBITS

Rabbits are highly susceptible to anything that reduces chewing efficiency and food intake. As a result, one of the earliest indicators of a dental problem is weight loss. Owners can therefore best assess both dental and general health by measuring food intake and weighing their animals regularly.

Periodontal Disease

Because the exposed crowns are short and the tooth surface for plaque accumulation is minimal, conventional periodontal disease is rare in rabbits fed an appropriate diet (grass and hay). The minimal accumulated plaque and rapid tooth wear also mean that caries normally cannot become established. However, when tooth wear is reduced, the risk of both caries and periodontal disease increases. Periodontitis is accelerated by sharp fragments of food and other debris that impact into the periodontal space. Once a periodontal pocket is established, impacted debris increases and infection progresses rapidly toward the apex with risk of lateral or apical abscessation. Unfortunately, this is often difficult to detect both clinically and radiographically.

When early periodontal lesions are detected, conventional periodontal therapy, supragingival and subgingival scaling with extraction of compromised teeth, may be effective. However, undetected and recurrent lesions are common. Cleaned periodontal pockets can be packed with a perioceutic gel containing bioabsorbable doxycycline to help eliminate residual infection and provide some protection from further food impaction. Extraction results in iatrogenic malocclusion that requires lifelong management.

Trauma

Accidental incisor trauma is relatively common, usually resulting in fracture of one or more teeth. After more serious concurrent injuries are ruled out, assess the teeth and associated tissues both visually and radiographically. Dental radiographic films positioned intraorally allow detailed imaging of the incisor teeth. If significant alveolar damage or pulp exposure is evident, then analgesics are indicated. Treat the injuries appropriately, then smooth fractured tooth surfaces to prevent soft tissue irritation. Pulp exposure is painful and leads to pulpitis, which may progress to pulp necrosis and apical abscessation. When recognized early, aseptic partial pulpectomy and pulp capping with a setting calcium hydroxide cement, as both a dressing and a temporary restoration, often permit healing. Do not use conventional filling materials because they prevent normal tooth wear. Monitor the teeth over the next few weeks, trimming opposing teeth intermittently if necessary, until the fractured teeth have regrown and are wearing normally. If the incisors fail to regrow, reassess the area radiographically. Apical deformity or necrosis may be present and requires surgical intervention. Because trauma commonly results in apical damage, regrowing teeth may become deformed and fail to occlude. The choice is then between frequent trimming with a dental bur or extraction. Trimming permits rapid eruption with elongation of the pulp cavity, so pulp exposure becomes more likely with repeated treatment.

Luxation of the temporomandibular articulation is a very rare accidental injury in rabbits and is most frequently iatrogenic, caused by excessive opening of screw-operated mouth gags. Because luxation is usually accompanied by severe soft tissue damage, the prognosis is very poor. Separation of the mandibular symphysis, seen alone or as a complication of incisor fracture, is more common. If the teeth are undamaged, the symphysis can be stabilized easily by applying a bonded composite splint to the facial surfaces of the teeth, but restoring the normal alignment of the mandibles is difficult. Remove the splint after 2 weeks, otherwise it interferes with tooth wear. Cerclage wiring is less successful because the rostral mandible is tapered and the wire compresses the fibrous symphysis significantly, altering the occlusion. Even minor changes in occlusal angulation result in abnormal jaw function, malocclusion, and uneven tooth wear, although this may not become apparent for several months.

Malocclusion

Malocclusion most commonly results from pathologic tooth elongation. This affects a high proportion of adult domestic rabbits independent of breed. Trauma-induced malocclusions are rare. Primary skeletal malocclusions are seen in very young animals but are largely restricted to the extreme dwarf and lop breeds. In adults, malocclusion is accompanied by acquired tooth elongation. When rabbits are fed high-energy and compounded foods, the exposed crowns elongate because they are not worn adequately. The combination of incomplete wear and the consistent curvature of the cheek teeth results in "spike" formation on the edges of the occlusal surfaces (Fig. 34-9). As the teeth elongate, they come into contact with their counterparts in the opposing jaw, forcing the mouth open at rest until resting jaw tone prevents further eruption. Tooth growth slows down but does not stop as eruption is arrested, so the apices start intruding. If remodeling of surrounding tissues occurs fast enough, the tooth form remains normal. However, proximity to supporting bone or penetration into an abnormal environment upsets the germinal tissues, resulting in dysplastic changes to the newly formed dental tissues. In its mildest form, this is recognized as an increased curvature of the teeth, which further enhances spike formation.

Incisor malocclusions are occasionally skeletal in origin or the result of previous injury, in which case incisor extraction is the best, if only palliative, treatment. Repeated trimming with a bur in either a high- or low-speed dental handpiece is also possible. More often, the problem is caused by coronal elongation of the cheek teeth, which forces the mouth open, and treatment requires concurrent correction of the underlying elongation. Coronal reduction and occlusal equilibration (eliminating occlusal irregularities) is necessary to restore the occlusal surfaces of both the incisors and cheek teeth to a normal level and angle (Fig. 34-7). This must be performed without causing additional injury and is only effective when the curvature of the teeth has not changed and no teeth have tipped in their sockets. Coronal adjustments can only be done effectively by using dental power equipment such as a straight, low-speed, dental handpiece with an appropriate bur. Clipping and rasping are unacceptable because they result in tooth fracture, and the energy transmitted into the teeth damages the periodontal and periapical tissues.

The amount of tooth substance that requires removal can be difficult to judge. Preoperative radiography is essential for diagnosis, prognosis, and treatment planning. A lateral skull view is most useful because it shows how much the gingiva and alveolar bone have elongated with the crowns of the teeth, masking the overgrowth on visual inspection. The elongated gingiva sometimes has to be ground down along with the teeth to permit removal of sufficient tooth substance. Luckily, gingiva is not particularly sensitive, unlike oral mucosa, and it heals very rapidly so that analgesia is rarely required by 48 hours after treatment.

It takes several weeks after coronal reduction for the jaw muscles to fully adapt back to their normal contraction pattern. This, combined with the abnormal occlusal surfaces (lacking the normal ridging), means that chewing is very inefficient immediately after treatment and supportive feeding is necessary. However, discontinue supportive feeding as soon as possible and introduce a natural diet to promote normal chewing. Fresh growing grass is best, but freshly cut long grass and other natural vegetation (but not lawn clippings!) along with hay are acceptable. The food must be in its natural form to encourage a normal

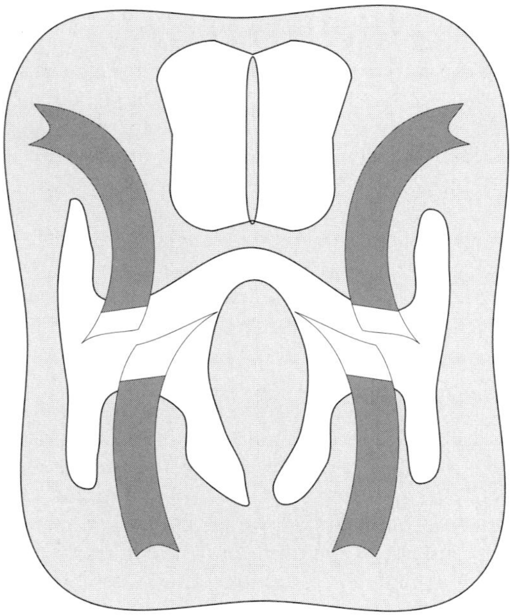

Figure 34-7 Diagram showing the typical pattern of coronal elongation in the rabbit with spike formation on the occlusal surfaces, medially in the lower cheek teeth and laterally in the upper. This can be effectively corrected by reducing the crown length to the level of the gingiva.

chewing pattern and promote tooth wear. Coronal reduction usually needs repeating several times at 4- to 6-week intervals before any significant improvement is seen. Unfortunately, in many rabbits coronal abnormalities are severe before they are diagnosed, in which case euthanasia may be preferable to the need for lifelong palliative treatment.

Apical (root) elongation of the first maxillary incisor teeth is commonly associated with malocclusion. Interference with apical growth leads to folding of the forming dental tissue, which appears as horizontal ridging as the affected part erupts into view. Apical intrusion frequently obstructs the lacrimal ducts as they pass around the incisor apices[6]; therefore rabbits with lacrimal discharge need dental examinations. If the incisors are extracted, the apical changes may resolve, correcting the problem if it is just lacrimal overflow. However, if obstruction is chronic or secondary infection is present, lesions usually persist. In rabbits with apical elongation, treating lacrimal overflow or discharge by catheterizing the lacrimal duct and flushing is likely to burst the duct above the obstruction, creating a new opening into the nasal cavity and bypassing the obstruction. Apical elongation of the mandibular cheek teeth results in palpable distortion of the normally smooth ventral border of the mandible, a useful diagnostic indicator. In the maxilla, the apices intrude into the orbit, preventing retraction (or manual retropulsion) of the eyes, with proptosis occurring in advanced cases.

More commonly, proptosis is caused by retrobulbar inflammation or an abscess of dental or other origin. External facial abscesses may be of dental origin, but external injury, a foreign body, or hematogenous spread from another site is likely. Mandibular abscesses are most frequently of dental origin. Endodontic abscesses of the incisors and periodontal abscesses of the cheek teeth all appear in and beneath the body of the mandible, and identifying their origin can be difficult. Treatment of dental abscesses involves removing the offending teeth and surgically debriding the area extensively for any chance of success (see Part II).

Some dental problems of rabbits in the United Kingdom have been linked to inadequate intake of dietary calcium and vitamin D.[19] This is attributed to selective feeding when excessive quantities of mixed-type foods are offered. These and most other dental diseases can be prevented by feeding rabbits what they originally evolved to eat: grasses and other low-growing herbage in their natural form.

DENTAL DISEASE IN RODENTS

Incisor Problems

The continuously growing incisor teeth of rodents are susceptible to injury, insufficient wear, and interference with eruption. Fractured teeth need to be checked for evidence of pulp exposure. If this has occurred, perform an aseptic partial pulpectomy and pulp capping (with a setting calcium hydroxide cement without additional restoration, as already described for rabbits) to protect the remaining pulp. Smooth the fractured tooth to prevent soft tissue irritation and monitor the animal weekly for regrowth. Trim the opposing teeth with a dental bur if necessary to maintain a normal occlusal relation. Once the tooth has regrown, continue to monitor it because injury transmitted to the periodontal and periapical tissues often results in deformity of the newly formed dental tissue. This causes a secondary malocclusion because the abnormal part eventually erupts into the mouth. Teeth that continue to grow unopposed are best extracted to eliminate the need for frequent trimming.

Rodents require material to gnaw to maintain normal occlusion of their incisors. Excessive attrition is very rare, but insufficient wear is common, resulting in an abnormal occlusal wear pattern and rapid tooth elongation. Unopposed, continuously growing incisors can erupt up to 1 mm per day, so these teeth require frequent trimming. Alternatively, the malocclusion may interfere with the eruption of the teeth, when apical growth continues until interference from surrounding structures deforms the germinal tissues. This results in folding of the newly formed tooth substance, if eruption is still occurring, or more severe apical deformity if eruption has ceased. When the maxillary incisors are affected (particularly those of squirrels and prairie dogs), this progresses to formation of a pseudo-odontoma, that is, a dysplastic malformation growing at a normal or reduced rate (these are not neoplastic lesions; Fig. 34-8). Experimentally, hypophysectomy[4,5,31] and hypomagnesemia[22,37] may also cause apical folding, whereas hypovitaminosis A causes a similar apical dysplasia.[8,26,30,39] However, these effects are only seen when the teeth are exposed to significant occlusal pressure.[22,37] Clinically, obstructed eruption combined with hypovitaminosis A appear to be the most significant factors, with hyperadrenocorticism as a likely additional factor. If the problem is recognized before a bulbous mass develops at the apex, then trimming the incisors and providing suitably abrasive food with an adequate vitamin A content, such as growing grass, as well as gnawing materials will correct the problem. Conversely, oversupplementing with vitamin A promotes an increase in apical growth that, in the case of a pseudo-odontoma, potentially causes rapid enlargement.

Unfortunately, once there is dramatic folding or a mass at the apex, eruption of affected teeth is arrested and the problem becomes one of a slowly expanding, space-occupying lesion. In

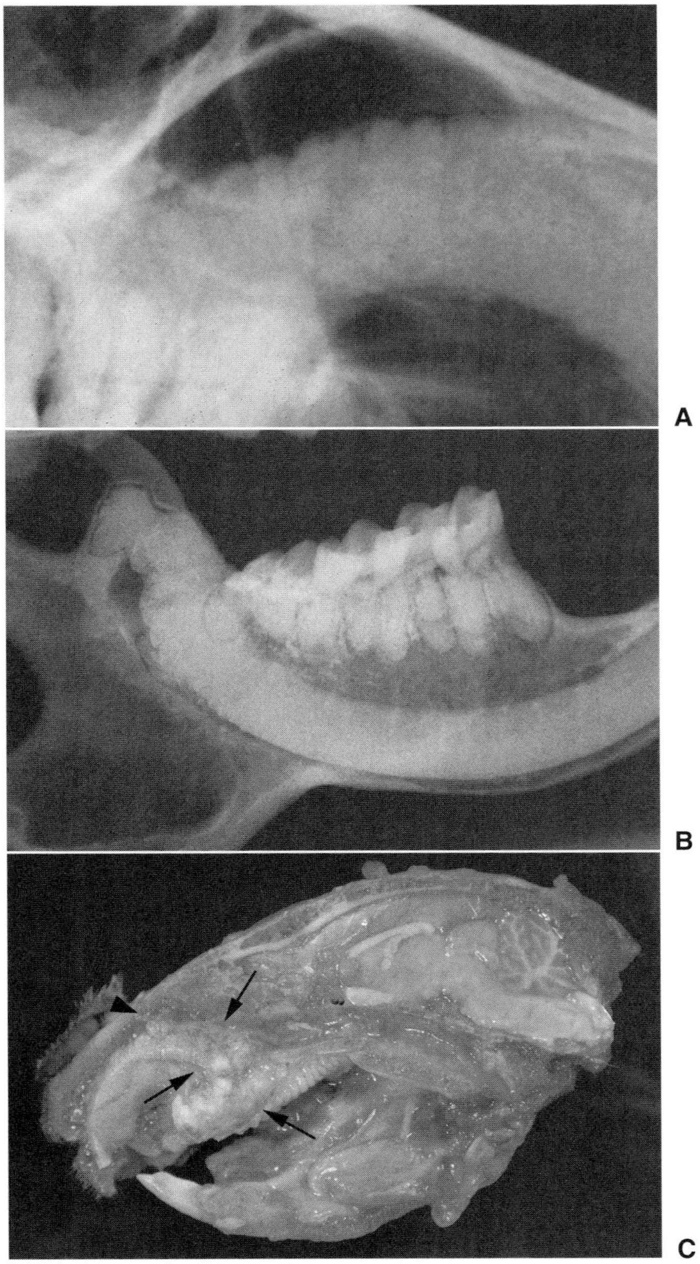

Figure 34-8 Pseudo-odontoma in a praire dog. **A,** Radiograph of the maxilla. **B,** Radiograph of the mandible of a prairie dog with arrested eruption of the incisors. A pseudo-odontoma is present at the apex of the maxillary incisor; however, it is masked by the cheek teeth. Note the short crowned, rooted cheek teeth. The elongated apices are grossly deformed. **C,** Head of a prairie dog with a pseudo-odontoma *(arrows)* at necropsy. The nasal passage is almost completely obstructed by the proliferative tissue *(arrowhead)*.

the mandible, this is rarely serious (see Fig. 34-11), but in the maxilla, there is a risk of nasal obstruction. If an intranasal mass is small, then an extraoral, lateral surgical approach permits extraction of the tooth and the accompanying mass. Because both sides are usually affected, bilateral surgery is necessary. With large masses that obstruct nasal air flow, the lateral approach is less practical. An accessory nostril can be surgically created dorsally at the level of, or slightly rostral to, the medial canthus.[35] If this is done, remove the caudal margins of the nasal bones without extending the incision further caudally (otherwise there is a risk of exposing the olfactory bulb). Incise the nasal epithelium, then trim both the skin and nasal epithelium, leaving just enough to suture them together around the margin of the new opening. However, this measure is only temporary because the intranasal mass will continue to grow. Complete resection of the mass is preferable. This may be attempted either by rhinotomy or by a transpalatal approach. Neither approach is easy, so rhinotomy with the aim of debulking of the mass and creating an accessory nostril is probably the most practical option.

Cheek Teeth Problems

Rooted cheek teeth are prone to developing typical plaque-associated periodontal disease, a common problem in pet rats. Scaling followed by tooth brushing will control early disease, but extraction is indicated with more advanced disease. This is performed by severing the periodontal ligament around each of the multiple tooth roots and carefully luxating the tooth. Caries are not common in wild rodents because they rarely carry cariogenic bacteria. However, in pet rodents, the combination of a diet containing refined carbohydrates and occasional items of human food that the owner has bitten into and inoculated with cariogenic bacteria increases the likelihood of disease. While restoring some caries lesions is technically possible, extraction is generally the preferred treatment.

Rodents with elodont cheek teeth have problems similar to those already described for rabbits. Elongation and altered curvature of the crowns of the cheek teeth tend to separate the occlusal surfaces, enhancing impaction of food and debris, formation of deep periodontal pockets, and periodontal abscessation. This is very common in chinchillas and usually causes obvious disease.

Spike formation is less common in chinchillas and guinea pigs than it is in rabbits; however, gross coronal elongation is more common. This condition forces the mouth open, creating a secondary incisor malocclusion with little effect on chewing function initially. In guinea pigs, the steeply angulated occlusal surfaces of the converging dental arcades force the mandible rostrally and the mouth open. This prevents adequate wear of the maxillary third molars and mandibular premolars, with the latter tending to elongate into or over the tongue, entrapping it. When the mouth is forced open beyond a certain degree, the tongue has difficulty compressing boluses of food into the pharynx, making swallowing difficult.

Treatment of cheek teeth overgrowth involves reducing the crown length and restoring the occlusal surface to a normal height and angulation. With the patient anesthetized, use a guarded flat or taper fissure bur in a straight, low-speed dental handpiece to remove excess coronal tissue. Some gingiva and bone may need to be removed from the alveolar crest as well because these often elongate with the teeth. As in rabbits, the jaw muscles require time before they return to normal function. Supportive feeding is initially required; however, place the animal on a diet of naturally abrasive vegetation as soon as possible. Although I have had some success in treating chinchillas and guinea pigs in the short term, the long-term prognosis is poor. The oral and dental anatomy makes treatment difficult and, in chinchillas, apical changes are usually advanced, preventing a return to normal. In guinea pigs, short-term use of an elastic jaw sling to support the mandible in normal occlusion appears to increase the success rate after occlusal correction (L. Legendre, personal communication, 2001). In chinchillas, elongated apices of the maxillary premolar and first molar encroach on the bony nasolacrimal canal and may obliterate the lacrimal ducts, causing persistent tear overflow. Although pathologic changes involving the incisors may obstruct the lacrimal ducts in rabbits, this has not been recognized in chinchillas.[12] Because the lacrimal punctae are very small, catheterizing the ducts is rarely possible, so perforating into the nasal cavity above the obstruction, either accidentally or deliberately, is not useful as treatment.

Extraction of Continuously Growing Teeth

Indications and case selection Although the possible reasons for extracting continuously growing teeth vary widely, the main indications are recurrent elongation or untreatable malocclusion. Although any tooth may be a candidate for extraction, removing the incisors is most common. In general, extracting all the incisors is best because removing only one usually results in secondary problems with the others. The exceptions to this are extracting the peg teeth in rabbits (although this is rarely indicated as a stand-alone procedure) and removing a single mandibular incisor in rodents. Most rodents will use both maxillary incisors with a single remaining mandibular tooth, although such cases need monitoring because maxillary incisors sometimes elongate or develop oblique wear patterns. Because of poor access, extracting elodont cheek teeth is more difficult than extracting incisors, particularly when they are elongated or deformed. There are also serious consequences for the opposing arcade. In rabbits, chinchillas, and guinea pigs, if more than two cheek teeth are extracted in one session, the trauma is often fatal. If a large number of teeth that are not already loose need extracting, stage the procedure, only removing one to three teeth at a time.

Extraction is a surgical procedure and should be performed aseptically whenever possible. Take radiographs immediately before the procedure to assess the dental anatomy and pathologic changes because the shape of continuously growing teeth can alter dramatically over a short time. If root deformity is minimal, a closed extraction technique is appropriate (Table 34-2). Otherwise an open surgical approach is required, with removal of overlying bone to access and remove the deformed tissues.

Because the typical reason to extract the incisors is that the teeth are nonfunctional, most patients have already adapted to

TABLE 34-2
Procedure for Closed Extraction of Continuously Growing Teeth

Step	Procedure
1	Shorten the teeth to approximately normal length to improve access to the mouth. Leave sufficient crown to manipulate teeth during extraction and to retain a mouth gag for intraoral examination and treatment.
2	Perform any intraoral treatment and obtain radiographs before extracting incisor teeth.
3	Disinfect the operating field by using a mucosal disinfectant such as 0.2% chlorhexidine aqueous solution (not a surgical scrub).
4	Separate the gingival epithelial attachment within the gingival sulcus around each tooth to be extracted, extending the incision into the periodontal ligaments.
5	Insert a purpose-designed luxator matched to the tooth anatomy into the periodontal space lateral to the first tooth, holding the instrument under gentle longitudinal pressure for 20 seconds. This cuts the periodontal ligament to the depth reached by the luxator, and the taper of the instrument wedges the tooth and alveolar bone in opposite directions.
6	Insert the instrument medially and hold it under tension. Lateral movement of the tooth now tears the periodontal attachment on the other surfaces of the tooth.
7	Work in turn on the other teeth that are being extracted before returning to the first one and repeating the process.
8	After repeating the luxation process 3 to 4 times, the teeth should become reasonably mobile. Once this stage is reached, the teeth can be intruded into their sockets to tear the remaining periodontal attachment.
9	Once fully loose, rock the teeth in their sockets while applying intrusive force. This damages the apical germinal tissues, reducing the risk of continued growth of the tooth after extraction.
10	Remove the teeth by rotating them out of their sockets along their paths of growth and eruption. Long cheek teeth may need to be removed in short sections (as performed in oral extraction in horses).
11	Check that the pulp has been removed intact with the teeth. If not, curette the apical region of the socket with a sterile instrument, removing remaining pulp tissue.
12	Flush sockets thoroughly with isotonic saline or lactated Ringer's solution to remove debris. Packing sockets with doxycycline perioceutic gel provides a slow release depot of antibiotic and reduces the risk of food impaction during healing.
13	Gently squeeze each alveolus to compress the stretched gingiva and loosen bone plates back into position. Maintain pressure with a damp swab to control any hemorrhage. Significant bleeding is very rare.
14	If the gingiva has been cut or torn, suture with fine, synthetic, rapidly absorbable material with a swaged-on cutting needle.
15	Obtain postoperative radiographs.
16	Give the owner detailed dietary advice and care instructions. Arrange follow-up examinations (postoperative, short-term, and long-term).

eating without using them. Therefore minimal postoperative care is required if this is the only treatment given. When occlusal adjustments are made to the cheek teeth, it may take several days for the animal to adapt to the changes, so assisted feeding of a special diet may be needed at first.

Potential complications Extraction and other jaw surgery in rabbits and rodents require a gentle technique to avoid tooth or jaw fracture. Iatrogenic folding fractures of the mandibular ramus are difficult to detect but easily treated, whereas gross fractures of the mandibular body are usually obvious but difficult to stabilize. Any fracture is serious because even a minute change in alignment results in cheek tooth malocclusion.

When discussing cases before treatment, advise clients that tooth fracture is common during extraction and that, if it happens, a second procedure may be necessary later. If a continuously growing tooth does fracture during extraction, the remaining portion is likely to continue growing. The small peg teeth in rabbits are the ones most likely to break. But unlike any remaining portions of the strongly curved larger first incisors, the roots of peg teeth are easy to extract. In the case of broken incisor roots, either extract them surgically or, if the fragments are not contaminated or infected, leave the apical fragment and observe for regrowth, extracting the regrown tooth later. If tooth regrowth is not visible after 2 months, take radiographs of the jaw because continued growth may not be externally apparent.

Providing that proper technique is used to destroy the apical germinal tissues during extraction (see Table 34-2), completely extracted teeth should not regrow. However, if a very gentle technique is used and the pulp remains in the socket, anything from a perfectly normal tooth to an amorphous mass of dentine can reappear after a few weeks to months.[32]

A common complication after cheek tooth extraction is tipping of the adjacent teeth toward the extraction site. Currently, there is no effective way of preventing this problem. Because the opposing teeth will not wear evenly, regular follow-up examinations are required after extracting cheek teeth. Occasional occlusal adjustment is needed to prevent malocclusion from progressing. If cheek teeth are extracted for treatment of a mandibular abscess, a further complication is formation of a fistula from the mouth to the skin under the jaw. This can be managed by daily cleansing of the affected skin and syringing a small quantity of water through the fistula to flush accumulated debris into the mouth.

Alternatives to extraction In animals with persistent problems with elongated cheek teeth, an alternative to extraction is to arrest the growth of the teeth. Without apical growth, either the affected tooth continues to erupt until it has insufficient periodontal support and is shed or, less often, it stops erupting. Several methods have been used to arrest tooth growth. Because the extent of the necrosis caused by cytotoxic materials cannot be controlled, endodontic methods that use these materials are inappropriate. Apical cryotherapy has been used experimentally, but again, controlling the area of necrosis is difficult, with the risk of extensive jaw necrosis. Surgical apicoectomy (root resection) is currently the most effective method. Access to the apices of the mandibular cheek teeth is practical. However, although access to the maxillary cheek tooth apices is technically possible, the extremely high risk of severe iatrogenic injury makes it impractical. For apicoectomy, remove the apical tissues, along with the dental pulp if possible, and close the surgical access site without any root filling. If asepsis has been maintained, no antibiotic treatment is necessary.

PART II SURGICAL TREATMENT OF DENTAL ABSCESSES IN RABBITS

Sean Aiken, DVM, MS, Diplomate ACVS

HISTORY AND DIAGNOSTIC WORKUP

Dental abscesses are common in rabbits. A rabbit with an abscess is usually brought to the veterinarian because it is anorexic or the owner has observed a facial swelling or purulent material in the rabbit's mouth. Abscesses may involve the mandibular or maxillary teeth, but mandibular abscesses are diagnosed more frequently. The abscesses may develop as a result of oral injury from malocclusion or overgrown teeth, food impaction between teeth, or fracture of a longitudinal tooth that extends below the gum line. Odontogenic abscesses may involve multiple adjacent teeth or be multicentric, involving multiple locations in the mandible or maxilla. In a recent study, the most common bacterial species isolated from dental abscesses in rabbits were similar to those isolated from other mammalian species and humans with periodontal infections. These included a mixture of anaerobic gram-negative rods, such as *Fusobacterium nucleatum*; anaerobic gram-positive non–spore-forming rods, predominantly *Actinomyces* species; and aerobic gram-positive cocci of the *Streptococcus milleri* group.[34] Other reported pathogens include *Pasteurella* and *Staphylococcus* species.[21]

The diagnosis of a mandibular or maxillary abscess is based on a good oral examination and skull or dental radiographs taken while the rabbit is sedated or anesthetized. Ventrodorsal, lateral, and oblique radiographic projections are needed to visualize all the tooth roots. When reading skull radiographs, compare the symmetry of the skull to identify abnormalities in the dental arcade and to locate abscess pockets. Displaced or deviated tooth roots and lysis of the surrounding alveolar bone, with or without evidence of surrounding periosteal new bone formation, will be visible (Fig. 34-9).

TREATMENT

Surgical Techniques

Treatment should be aimed at aggressive surgical debridement and appropriate antibiotic therapy. Dental abscesses originate at the tooth root and continue to enlarge until the fibrous wall that surrounds the abscess can no longer contain the expansion. The purulent material then breaks out of the capsule to form a new adjacent abscess pocket that is joined to the previous pocket by a small isthmus. Locating and removing the entire extent of the abscess can therefore be very difficult, especially in the maxilla (Fig. 34-10). After anesthetizing the rabbit, begin surgical debridement by incising the skin over the abscess and bluntly dissecting around the abscess wall. Isolate all involved

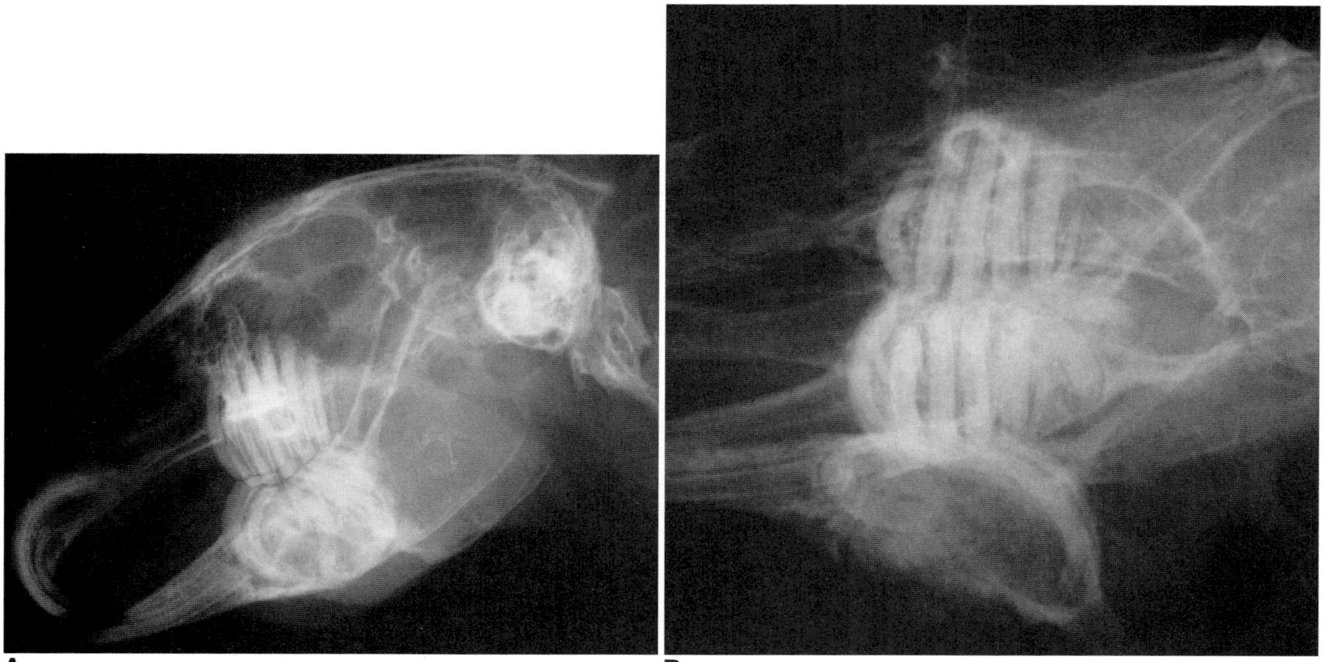

A B

Figure 34-9 A, Lateral radiographic projection of the skull of a rabbit with a mandibular abscess. The roots of the teeth are deviated. All the involved teeth must be extracted. **B,** Oblique radiographic projection of the skull demonstrating a mandibular abscess and a grossly malformed tooth.

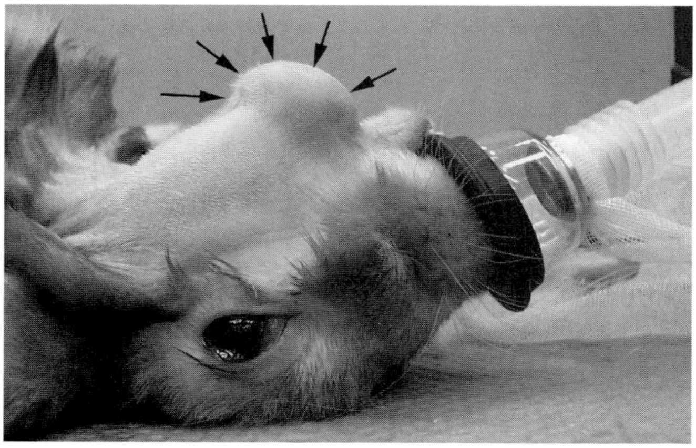

Figure 34-10 Lateral view of a rabbit positioned for surgical debridement of a left mandibular abscess. *Arrows* outline the extent of the soft tissue component of the abscess. The abscess may be much more extensive than is suggested by the soft tissue mass.

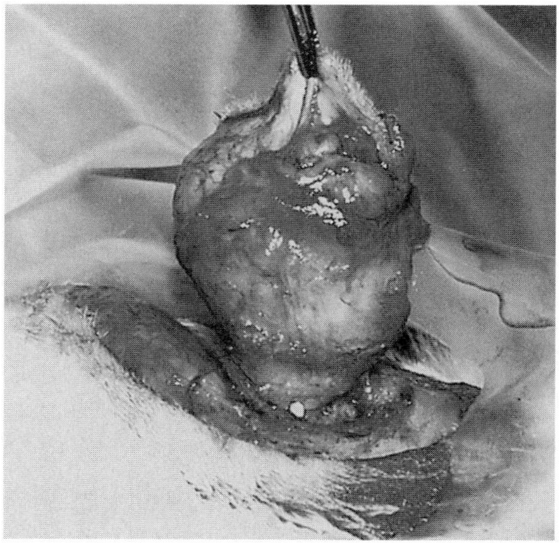

Figure 34-11 The soft tissue component of the mandibular abscess of a rabbit has been dissected to the level of the bone. The base of this mass should next be resected from the bone. Purulent material will be released that should be isolated from the surrounding soft tissues.

tissue from the healthy tissue to the level of the bone (Fig. 34-11). Take care not to penetrate the abscess until the entire extent of the fibrous capsule is exposed. Use cautery and fine absorbable suture material to achieve hemostasis. Cut the fibrous capsule from the underlying bone with a scalpel blade or Mayo scissors. This will release the purulent material, which then can be removed with suction or a bone curette. Collect samples of the fibrous capsule for both aerobic and anaerobic bacterial culture and sensitivity testing. With a large bone curette and bone rongeurs, expose the entire abscess pocket, which can be extensive (Fig. 34-12). Locate the involved tooth roots and remove all involved teeth through the abscess pocket. Because the bone may be weakened by the extensive abscess pockets, be very careful not to fracture the mandible while removing the involved teeth. Small root elevators, bone curettes, and bone rongeurs can be used for tooth extraction. Remove all inflam-

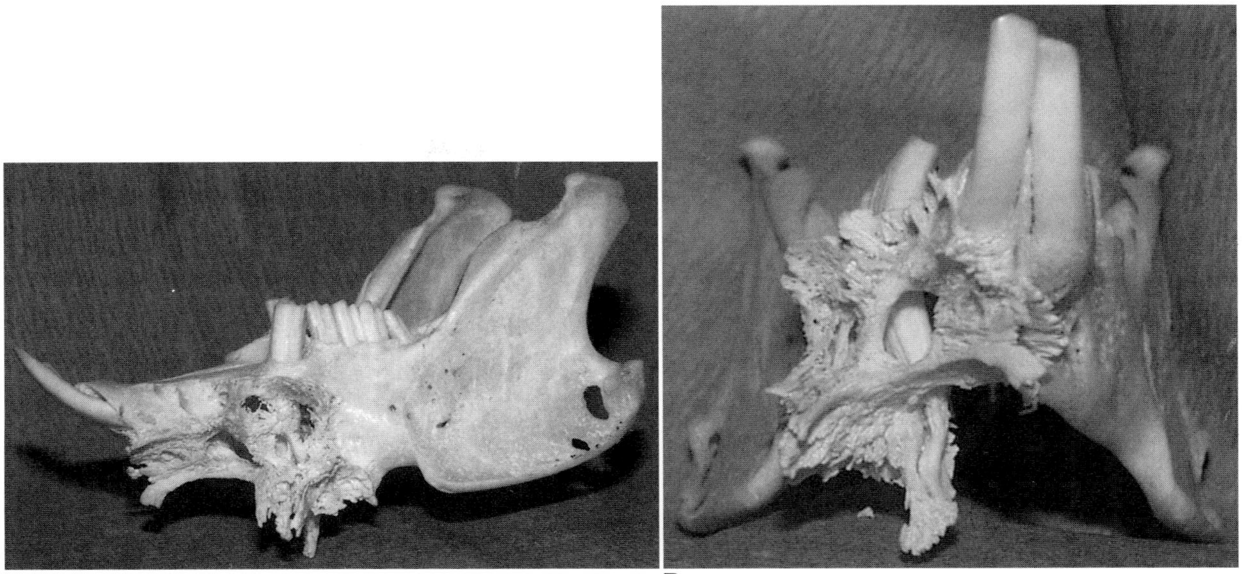

A B

Figure 34-12 A, Lateral view of a dissected skull from a rabbit with an extensive mandibular abscess. Note the abscess pocket and the extensive new bone formation involving the mandible. B, The frontal view illustrates the extensive bone loss around the tooth root, which makes fracture of the mandible during surgical debridement and tooth extraction a concern.

matory tissue from the bone defect with a bone curette, and lavage the site with sterile saline solution, taking care not to flood the oral cavity through the mucosal defects that result from tooth extractions.

After all the purulent material, fibrous lining, and involved teeth are removed, further treatment is aimed at preventing abscess recurrence. Many different treatment protocols have been used with varying degrees of success. One report suggested the use of calcium hydroxide in the bony defect, which is then removed after 1 week.[5] The high pH of the calcium hydroxide (pH = 12) is considered bactericidal. However, because severe soft tissue reactions and skin sloughing can develop if calcium hydroxide contacts the surrounding tissues, this treatment is not currently recommended.

Antibiotic-impregnated polymethylmethacrylate beads (AIPMMA) can be placed in the abscess pocket after debridement. The beads act as a local antibiotic delivery system, releasing a high concentration of antibiotic to the local tissues while maintaining very low systemic levels and toxicity. A variety of antibiotics, including cefazolin, ceftiofur, and gentamicin, can be used to make the beads. Although most of the antibiotic is released from the beads in the first 24 hours, antibiotic levels above the minimum inhibitory concentration continue to be released for 7 to 30 days, depending on the antibiotic and dose used.[15,38] To make the beads, aseptically mix 1 g cefazolin, ceftiofur, or gentamicin with a 20-g dose of polymethylmethacrylate powder, then add the liquid monomer.[15,38] Before it polymerizes, roll the mixture into 5-mm spheres or pour it into a bead mold, if available. Placing the beads on nylon suture material will help control the beads during implantation and aids in locating the beads at removal. The beads may be produced at the time of surgery or prepared in advance and gas sterilized. The beads are neither bioabsorbable nor bioactive, so ideally they should be removed when the antibiotic levels decrease below the minimum inhibitory concentration. Some authors suggest leaving the beads in place to avoid a second surgical procedure.

Ideally, the material used to fill the bone defect will eliminate dead space, be bactericidal, and promote bony healing. Bioactive ceramics will attach to soft tissue and bone, filling dead space, and have the added advantage of being osteoconductive, helping to eventually fill the defect with bone. Although these materials may have antibacterial properties, they also can be loaded with antibiotics for local release.[6,23,33] Currently, I treat bony abscesses in rabbits by aggressive surgical debridement, then by filling the defect with Consil (Bioglass, Nutramax Laboratories, Baltimore, MD), being careful to keep the material out of the surrounding soft tissues. With concurrent therapy with injectable penicillin (see below), the addition of antibiotics to Consil is not usually necessary unless a resistant organism has been identified by culture and sensitivity testing of a sample from the abscess before surgery. After the bone defect is filled with Consil, remove any excess skin and close the subcutaneous tissue and subcuticular skin with fine absorbable suture material.

Antibiotic Therapy

After surgery, maintain the rabbit on appropriate systemic antibiotic therapy for at least 2 to 4 weeks. Until results of the bacterial culture and sensitivity testing are known, choose an antibiotic combination that provides broad-spectrum coverage against both aerobic and anaerobic species. A recent unpublished report suggests good results with the long-term use of benzathine penicillin/procaine penicillin G (rabbits <2.5 kg, 75,000 U/rabbit q48h SC; for rabbits >2.5 kg, 150,000 U/rabbit q48h SC) for treatment of dental abscesses.[29] With the findings of a high proportion of anaerobic bacteria within these abscesses, the use of penicillin in combination with a broad-spectrum antibiotic effective against aerobic bacteria seems logical.

Mandibular and maxillary abscesses in rabbits are difficult problems to resolve, but with aggressive surgical debridement, control of dead space, and appropriate antibiotic therapy, some animals can be treated successfully. However, owners must be warned that multiple surgical procedures may be required and that even with aggressive therapy, treatment may not be successful.

REFERENCES

1. Andrews P, Martin L: Hominoid dietary evolution. Philosophical Transactions of the Royal Society of London. Series B: Biological Sciences 1991; 1270:199-209.
2. Baker GJ: A study of dental disease in the horse [thesis]. Glasgow, Scotland, University of Glasgow, 1979.
3. Baker GJ, Easley J: Equine Dentistry. London, WB Saunders, 1999.
4. Baum LJ, Becks H, Ray JC, et al: Hormonal control of tooth eruption. II. The effects of hypophysectomy on the upper rat incisor following progressively longer intervals. J Dent Res 1954; 33:91-103.
5. Becks H, Collins DA, Simpson ME, et al: Changes in the central incisors of hypophysectomised female rats after different periods. Arch Path 1946; 41:457-475.
6. Bellantone M, Coleman NJ, Hench LL: Bacteriostatic action of a novel four-component bioactive glass. J Biomed Material Res 2000; 51:484-490.
7. Burling K, Murphy CJ, da Silva Curiel J, et al: Anatomy of the rabbit nasolacrimal duct and its clinical implications. Prog Vet Comp Ophthalmol 1991; 1:33-40.
8. Burn CG, Orten AU, Smith AH: Changes in the structure of the developing tooth in rats maintained on a diet deficient in vitamin A. Yale J Biol Med 1941; 13:817-830.
9. Colmery B, Frost P: Periodontal disease: etiology and pathogenesis. Vet Clin North Am Small Anim Pract 1986; 16:817-833.
10. Corruccini RS, Lee GTR: Occlusal variation in Chinese immigrants to the United Kingdom and their offspring. Arch Oral Biol 1984; 29:779-782.
11. Crossley DA: Results of a preliminary study of tooth enamel thickness in the mature dentition of domestic dogs and cats. J Vet Dent 1995; 12:111-113.
12. Crossley DA: Dental disease in chinchillas in the UK. J Small Anim Pract 2001; 42:12-19.
13. Debowes LJ, Mosier D, Logan E, et al: Association of periodontal disease and histologic lesions in multiple organs from 45 dogs. J Vet Dent 1996; 13:57-60.
14. De Vree F: Mastication in guinea pigs, *Cavia porcellus*. Am Soc Zoo 1977; 17:886.
15. Ethell MT, Bennett RA, Brown MP, et al: In vitro elution of gentamicin, amikacin, and ceftiofur from polymethylmethacrylate and hydroxyapatite cement. Vet Surg 2000; 29:375-382.
16. Fairham J, Harcourt-Brown FM: Preliminary investigation of the vitamin D status of pet rabbits. Vet Rec 1999; 145:452-454.
17. Fish EW, Harris LJ: The effects of vitamin C deficiency on tooth structure in guinea pigs. Brit Dent J 1935; 58:3-20.
18. Golden AL, Stoller N, Harvey CE: A survey of oral and dental diseases in dogs anesthetised at a veterinary hospital. J Am Anim Hosp Assoc 1982; 18:881-889.
19. Harcourt-Brown FM: Calcium deficiency, diet and dental disease in pet rabbits. Vet Rec 1996; 139:567-571.
20. Hillson S: Teeth. Cambridge, Cambridge University Press, 1986.
21. Jenkins JR: Skin disorders of the rabbit. Vet Clin North Am Exotic Anim Pract 2001; 4:552-554.
22. Kusner W, Michaeli Y, Weinreb MM: Role of attrition and occlusal contact in the physiology of the rat incisor: V. Impeded and unimpeded eruption in hypophysectomised and magnesium deficient rats. J Dent Res 1973; 52:65-73.
23. Kwanabe K, Okada Y, Matsusue Y, et al: Treatment of osteomyelitis with antibiotic-soaked porous glass ceramic. J Bone Joint Surg Br 1998; 80:527-530.
24. McKay GM: Family *Petauridae*. *In* Walton DW, Richardson BJ, eds. Fauna of Australia. Mammalia. Vol 1B. Canberra, Australian Publishing Service, 1989, pp 665-678.
25. Morimoto T, Inoue T, Nakamura T, et al: Characteristics of rhythmic jaw movements of the rabbit. Arch Oral Biol 1985; 30:673-677.
26. Orten AU, Burn CG, Smith AH: Effects of prolonged chronic vitamin A deficiency in the rat with special reference to odontomas. Proc Soc Exp Biol Med 1937; 36:82-84.
27. Remeeus PGK, Verbeek M: The use of calcium hydroxide in the treatment of abscesses in the cheek of the rabbit resulting from a dental periapical disorder. J Vet Dentistry 1995; 12:19-22.
28. Romer AS: The Vertebrate Body, 4th ed. Philadelphia, WB Saunders, 1970.
29. Rosenfield ME: Successful eradication of severe abscesses in rabbits with long-term administration of penicillin G benzathine/penicillin G procaine. Available at: http://moorelab.sbs.umass.edu/-mrosenfield/bicillin/. Accessed Nov 2002.
30. Schour I, Hoffman MM, Smith MC: Changes in the incisor teeth of albino rats with vitamin A deficiency and the effects of replacement therapy. Am J Pathol 1941; 17:529-561.
31. Schour I, van Dyke HB: Changes in the teeth following hypophysectomy. 1. Changes in the incisor of the white rat. Am J Anat 1932; 50:397-433.
32. Steenkamp G, Crossley DA: Incisor tooth regrowth in a rabbit following complete extraction. Vet Rec 1999; 145:585-586.
33. Stoor P, Soderling E, Salonen JI: Antibacterial effects of a bioactive glass paste on oral microorganisms. Acta Odontol Scand 1998; 56:161-165.
34. Tyrrell KL, Citron DM, Jenkins JR, et al: Peridontal bacteria in rabbit mandibular and maxillary abscesses. J Clin Microbiol 2002; 40:1044-1047.
35. Wagner RA, Garman RH, Collins BM: Diagnosing odontomas in prairie dogs. Exotic DVM 1999; 1:7-10.
36. Waugh LM: Influence of diet on the jaws and face of the American Eskimo. J Am Dent Assoc Dent Cosmos 1937; 24:1640-1647.
37. Weinreb MM, Kusner W, Michaeli Y: Role of attrition and occlusal contact in the physiology of the rat incisor. VII. Formation of impeded and unimpeded incisors in magnesium deficient rats. J Dent Res 1973; 52:498-503.
38. Weisman DL, Olmstead ML, Kowalski JJ: In vitro evaluation of antibiotic elution from polymethylmethacrylate (PMMA) and mechanical assessment of antibiotic-PMMA composites. Vet Surg 2000; 29:245-251.
39. Wolbach SB, Howe PR: The incisor teeth of albino rats and guinea pigs in vitamin A deficiency and repair. Am J Pathol 1933; IX:275-293, plates 38-50.
40. Woods CA: How hystrichomorph rodents chew. Am Zoo Soc 1976; 16:215.

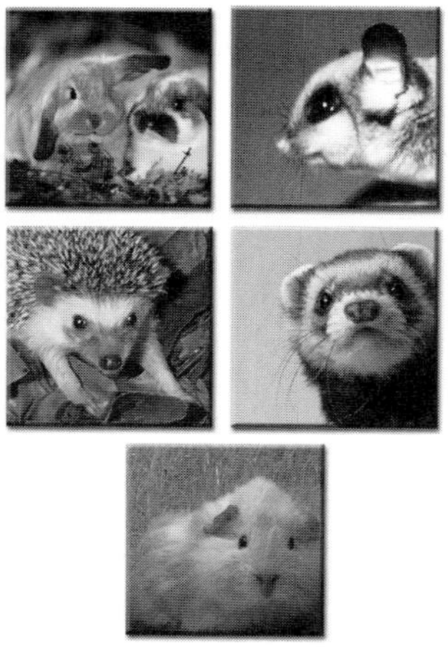

CHAPTER 35

Orthopedics in Small Mammals

Amy Kapatkin, DVM, Diplomate, ACVS

Orthopedic problems in rabbits, ferrets, and small rodents can be successfully managed by a surgeon who adheres to basic orthopedic principles and who understands the considerations unique to each species and how they resemble and differ from those that apply to dogs and cats.

FRACTURE MANAGEMENT AND FIRST AID

Orthopedic trauma in small mammals often results from household accidents, including injury from a falling object, a closing door, or an owner stepping on an animal. Also common is the trapping of a limb, which results from poor cage design or inappropriately sized wire mesh flooring. In cities with tall apartment buildings, "high-rise syndrome" is common, with injuries in ferrets similar to those of cats that have fallen from great heights. However, survival rates of ferrets with high-rise syndrome tend to be between those of cats and dogs.[13,17,41]

With any of these injuries, the first consideration is to assess the animal as a trauma patient. Shock, respiratory compromise, abdominal emergencies, and bleeding disorders need immediate attention. Once these life-threatening complications have been controlled, perform a thorough orthopedic and neurologic examination. Orthopedic trauma is never a medical emergency unless the patient has a spinal fracture, which results in paralysis if surgery is not performed immediately. If this is the case, the veterinarian and owner must consider the importance of anesthetic safety against that of neurologic competence.

After a patient has been treated for shock, its open fractures need immediate attention. *Closed fractures* are those that do not communicate with the external environment; *open fractures* are those that do. Open fractures are further divided into three subgroups based on the severity of the soft tissue injury:[3,7]

Grade I fractures result from the penetration of bone fragment to the external environment. If soft tissue trauma is minimal and can be surgically debrided, these fractures can be managed like closed fractures.

Grade II fractures result from external trauma to the soft tissues and are associated with significantly more damage to the soft tissues.

Grade III fractures result from external trauma and are characterized by a high degree of bone contamination and soft tissue destruction. Both grade II and grade III open fractures must be surgically managed as open fractures, even after surgical debridement.

In many small mammal species, fractures below the elbow and stifle are commonly open fractures because there is minimal soft tissue to protect the bone from breaking through the skin. Grade I open fractures are more common than those of other grades except in ferrets with high-rise syndrome, which often have more severe limb trauma. Rabbits with open fractures are difficult to manage. The very fine underfur around the fracture site must be clipped carefully to avoid tearing the delicate skin. A surgical clipper is the best tool for removing rabbit fur. Be patient and take care not to further complicate the wound.

When handling all open fractures, wear sterile gloves and use aseptic technique, even if the wounds are grossly contaminated. Ideally, take swab samples from the fracture site for aerobic and anaerobic cultures. Then, start broad-spectrum antibiotic therapy. Carefully debride the wound and lavage the area copiously with sterile saline. If definitive fracture repair is not planned at this time, place a sterile bandage and splint. If the fracture is above the elbow or stifle, placing a splint is not advisable unless it is a spica splint (over the shoulder or hip). However, because of the size and body conformation of most small mammals, spica splints are difficult to place. Rabbits with open fractures often do poorly because they tend to develop osteomyelitis, which is extremely difficult to cure in this species (see below).

Keep the patient comfortable and quiet, and give analgesics until definitive orthopedic treatment is safe. Most small mammals must be heavily sedated or anesthetized before a radiograph can be taken; thus, imaging is often postponed until an animal becomes stable (e.g., after 24-48 hours). Regardless of the fracture type, schedule fracture fixation as soon as anesthesia is safe for the patient. Definitive fixation maximizes the patient's comfort and improves the bone's ability to heal properly. Fracture stabilization allows the blood supply to aid in healing and increases the resistance of the bone to infection.[3]

The approach to orthopedic surgery in rabbits, ferrets, and other small mammals is distinct from that in dogs and cats in several ways. Although confining these animals after surgery is easy, preventing them from being active in their cages is not. Assume that rabbits and small rodents will chew at their skin sutures; thus the use of subcuticular sutures and perhaps tissue glue is preferred. Skin sutures should be avoided because of the difficulty involved in maintaining a collar on these animals to prevent chewing. However, if needed, collars for small rodents are commercially available from laboratory animal supply companies. When considering a splint or other external fixation, keep in mind that most animals will chew on the apparatus and can destroy it or cause self-injury. Many of the surgical implants that veterinarians are accustomed to using are too large for these small species. Even the smallest bone plates available from AO/ASIF (Association for the Study of Internal Fixation) can be too large. The smallest positive profile pins that are available may be more than 20% of the bone diameter and therefore inappropriate for use.[11,36]

The expense of each possible surgical repair must be considered. This includes the cost of the initial surgery and that of subsequent implant removals or bandage changes.

METHODS OF FIXATION

Choose the method of fixation for fracture repair in small mammals according to the basic rules outlined below. No one fixation method or approach can be used in every situation. An orthopedic surgeon must be knowledgeable about many different techniques and have the appropriate equipment. An investment in small instruments is worthwhile if you anticipate working often with exotic small mammals.

External Coaptation

External coaptation in small mammals can often be used quite effectively as a definitive orthopedic treatment for closed fractures. It works best for simple fractures affected by bending and rotational forces that cause bone ends to interdigitate with manipulation and to remain reduced. Fractures affected by compressive or shear forces, such as short oblique fractures, are poorly immobilized with external coaptation.[9]

While trying to reduce a fracture in these small animals, take care not to damage soft tissues and the blood supply. Palpation is often sufficient to determine if reduction has been achieved; however, radiography is still recommended to detect potential rotational or angular deformity. Apply standard splinting principles: maintain the affected limb in normal position, immobilize the joint above and below the fracture, and achieve at least 50% cortical contact in the reduced fracture in two radiographic views.[9]

Standard materials used for splints and casts in dogs and cats can be applied in managing fractures of rabbits, ferrets, and other small mammals. Rabbits are occasionally large enough to tolerate an aluminum rod with a light modified Robert Jones bandage. Otherwise, several products work well for splinting small mammals, such as Orthoplast (Johnson & Johnson, New Brunswick, NJ), and Vet-lite (Runlite SA, Micheroux, Belgium; see www.runlite.com for distributors). These are castlike materials that are very lightweight, thin, easy to use, and biomechanically strong. They are prepared in boiling water and conform to any shape when molded and allowed to cool. These products work best when used for a half cast with a light modified Robert Jones bandage, avoiding excessive pressure on the limb (Fig. 35-1). Although these materials cost more than routine casting materials, the final cost is reasonable because only a small piece of material is usually required. Vet-lite can be layered so that splint thickness and stiffness can be increased if desired. These products are very resistant to chewing by the animal and will not cause oral trauma or break apart and cause a gastrointestinal obstruction.

Monitor animals with splints and casts weekly to prevent complications. Common complications include soiling, which leads to the formation of pressure sores or local skin infections, and swelling, which results from excessive activity or from the splint being too tight. Joint laxity and stiffness from the coaptation are also commonly seen.[19,35]

Intramedullary Pinning

Intramedullary pinning in small mammals is a technique that is available to most practice situations. The implants and equipment are relatively inexpensive. Intramedullary pinning is a biomechanically sound technique in these species because the implant shares the load with the bone instead of bearing all the load. In research studies, healing is delayed beyond 12 weeks if the implant does all the load bearing.[24,28] Biodegradable pins made of polydioxanone materials are under investigation. These pins are biomechanically stiff enough to allow fracture healing, yet they resorb gradually by 24 weeks, when the bone is remodeling and no longer needs the support. This allows the forces to transfer from the implant to the bone without the need for a second surgery to remove the implant.[4,24,28]

Standard principles for intramedullary pinning are used in small mammals. The pin diameter should occupy at least 60% to 70% of the medullary cavity.[3] In these small species, anything larger than Kirschner wires, which come in diameters of 0.028, 0.035, 0.045, and 0.062 inches, can rarely be used. Use only smooth intramedullary pins to avoid breakage at the thread interface.[28]

Use the pins to obtain good axial alignment and to limit bending and rotational forces. Multiple pins used in a cross-pin fashion are probably best in supracondylar femoral or humeral fractures (Fig. 35-2). Antegrade placement of the pin is advantageous to avoid penetrating the joints and to enable custom direction of the pin.[28]

Bone Plating

Bone plating has limited clinical use in rabbits, ferrets, and small mammals. Extensive research has been done in rabbits with bone osteotomies repaired with rigid plate fixation. The purpose of these studies was to determine the ideal fracture

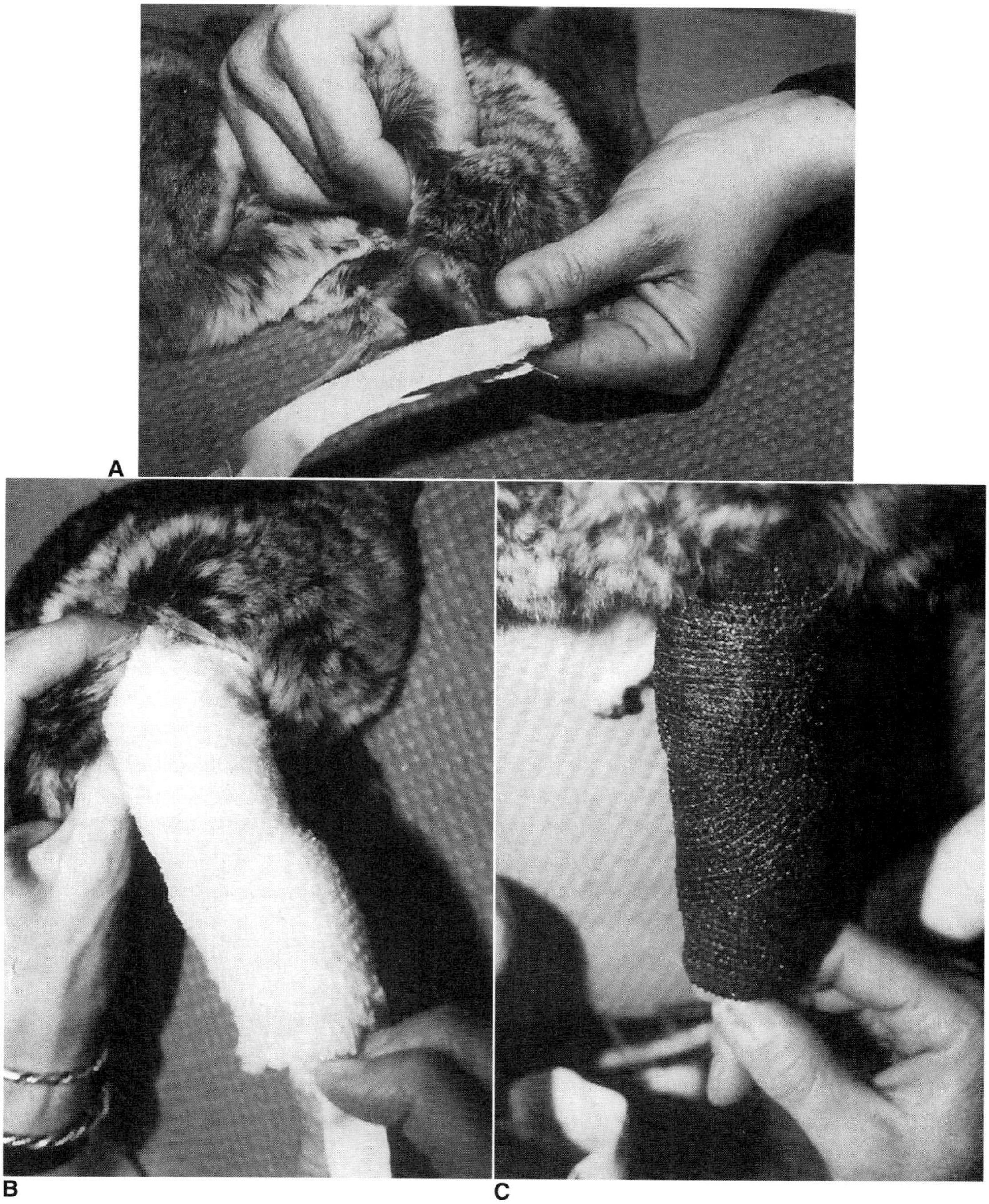

Figure 35-1 Splinting of a fractured tibia/fibula in a chinchilla. **A,** Tape stirrups placed on the fractured limb. **B,** Padding complete. **C,** Completed splint.

fixation, the type of bone healing, and the point in time at which the stiffness advantage of the plate becomes a disadvantage regarding load sharing of the bone. In studies of rabbits with transverse bone osteotomies, results have shown that bone heals faster than was previously thought. In dogs and cats, it has been assumed that the remodeling stage of bone healing lasts 8 to 12 months and plate implants should not be removed before that time. In rabbits, the optimal time for plate removal has been shown to be 6 to 8 weeks after surgery. However, this conclusion was based on studies of osteotomy repair in which the blood supply to the bone was not damaged and fractures were not comminuted. In a clinical situation, optimal plate removal is probably 3 to 4 months after fixation.[18,23,30,32]

In certain situations, the use of a plate is appropriate for fracture repair in a rabbit or ferret. Because of the conformation of these species, an open fracture of the humerus or femur can be difficult to manage with an external fixator. The soft tissue coverage over the femur and the humerus is considerable and

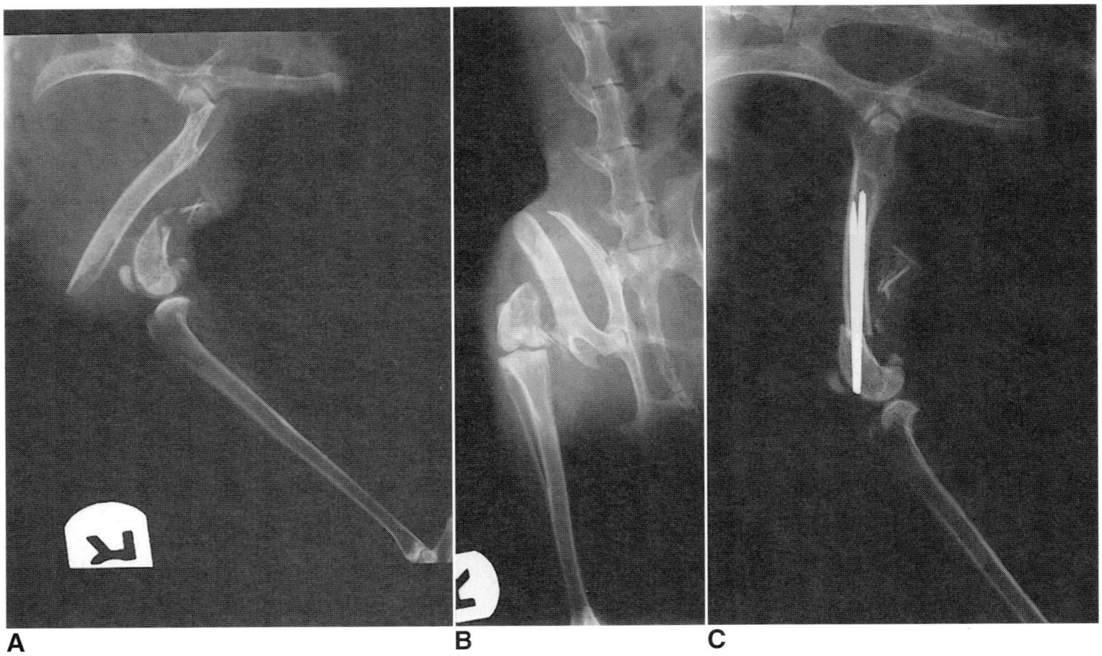

Figure 35-2 A and B, Radiographs of a supracondylar femoral fracture in a rabbit. C, Dynamic cross-pin repair of the fracture.

external skeletal fixation can be uncomfortable when used here. Because grade II or III open fractures should be repaired by either plating or external fixators, plating is sometimes the best choice. If plating is chosen, the implants commonly used are 1.5-mm and 2.0-mm cuttable plates (Synthes, Ltd., Wayne, PA). The cuttable plates offer the surgeon flexibility in choosing the appropriate length and stiffness of the plate. The standard size AO plates are too large and stiff for use in these small species. The principles of the application of AO bone plates are covered in other texts.[6,10]

The use of plating in these species presents some specific problems. The bones of rabbits have extremely thin cortices that make screw placement difficult without stripping the cortex. I have experienced complete collapse of the bone while trying to place a screw. In a clinical setting, rabbit fractures are rarely without comminution. The blood supply to the bone is already compromised, predisposing the rabbit to osteomyelitis and nonunion. Placing a bone plate with removal of the remaining periosteum and soft tissues only worsens this problem. Plating often overprotects a fracture, preventing load sharing and causing subsequent delayed healing or nonunion. If a plate is used, the animal will require staged plate removal, which is costly and unpopular with owners. Another disadvantage is the high cost of equipment and implants.

As for pins, biodegradable plates and screws have been evaluated, and their successful application looks promising. These implants degrade over time; thus they do not protect the bone from stress and do not need to be removed.[34]

External Skeletal Fixation

External skeletal fixation is probably the most common method of repairing fractures in small mammals. External fixators provide rigid stability, can be adapted for use in these small species, and cause minimal soft tissue damage.

The nomenclature of external fixators is outlined in Table 35-1. Type Ia fixators are useful for counteracting rotational forces but are subject to bending. Type Ib fixators are useful for counteracting craniocaudal bending forces. Double connecting bars can be added to limit compressive forces, but this is never needed in these small species.[11,36] Type II fixators are resistant to compressive and rotational forces. Their use is limited to bones below the elbow and stifle.[11,36] The type III configuration is very stiff and resists all forces. Its use is rarely indicated in rabbits, ferrets, and small rodents.[11,36]

Basic principles for applying external fixators are similar in all species. The pins should be inserted with low rotational speed (150 rpm). Manual insertion causes wobble and leads to premature loosening of the pins. High-speed drilling can cause

TABLE 35-1
Nomenclature for External Fixators

Type I	Unilateral connecting bar(s) with fixation pins penetrating one skin edge and two bone cortices
	Type Ia, uniplanar
	Type Ib, biplanar
Type II	Uniplanar with bilateral connecting bars and fixation pins that pass through two skin surfaces and two bone cortices
Type III	Combination of types I and II, namely, bilateral and biplanar

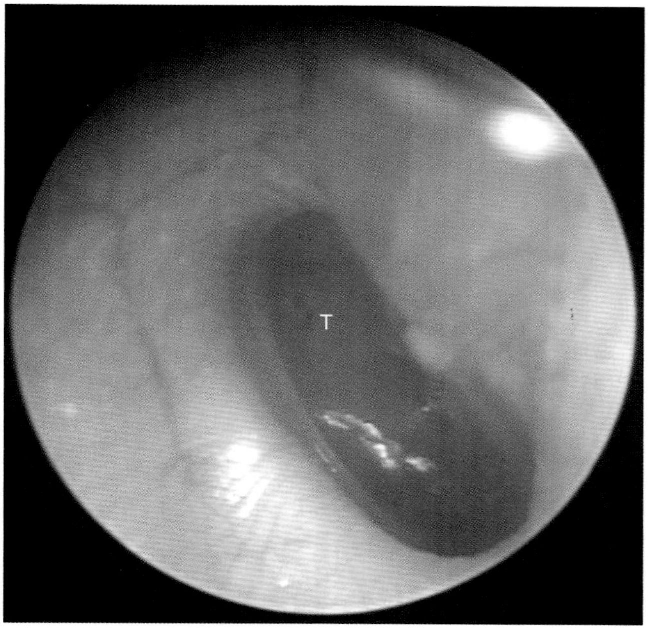

Plate 1 Endoscopic view of the horizontal ear canal and the normal tympanum *(T)* of a rabbit. *(Courtesy Stephen Hernandez-Divers, Ithaca, New York, and Michael Murray, Monterey, California.)*

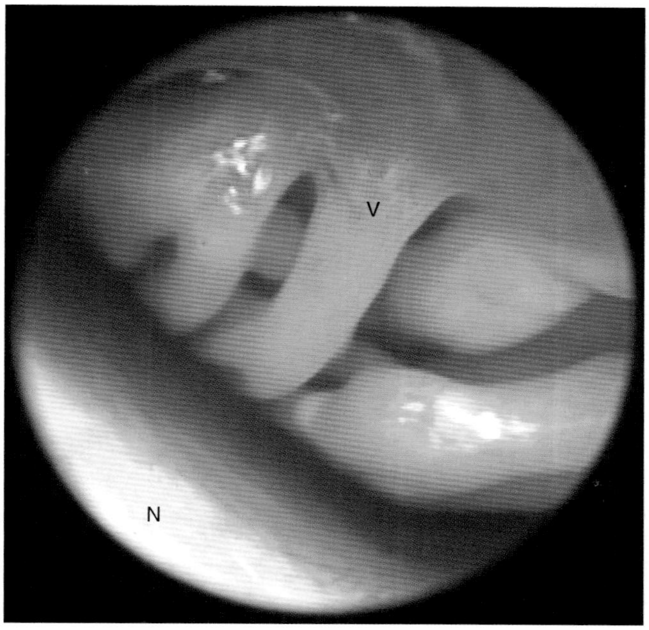

Plate 2 Endoscopic view of the ventral nasal concha *(V)* and the nasal septum *(N)* as seen from the common nasal meatus of a rabbit. *(Courtesy Stephen Hernandez-Divers, Ithaca, New York, and Michael Murray, Monterey, California.)*

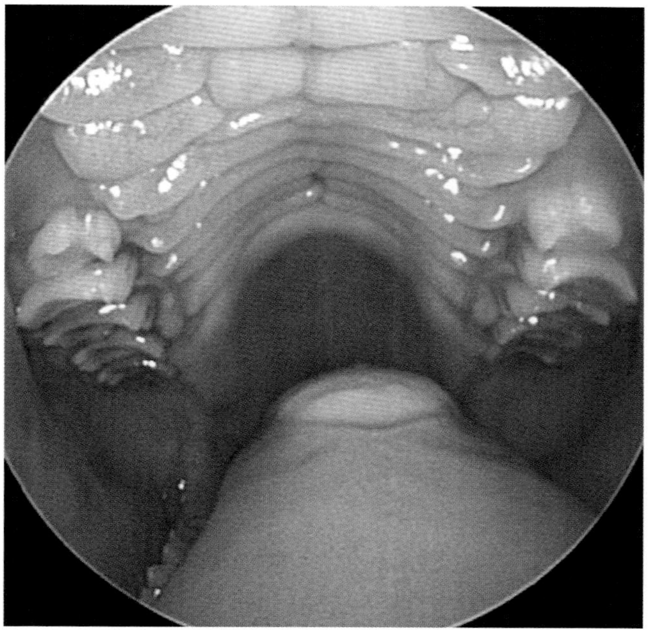

Plate 3 Typical wide-angle view into the oral cavity as provided by the rigid endoscope. Rotating the scope 180 degrees downward provides a view of the lower arcade. Closer, magnified view of individual teeth is made possible by advancing the telescope toward the tooth. *(Courtesy Stephen Hernandez-Divers, Ithaca, New York, and Michael Murray, Monterey, California.)*

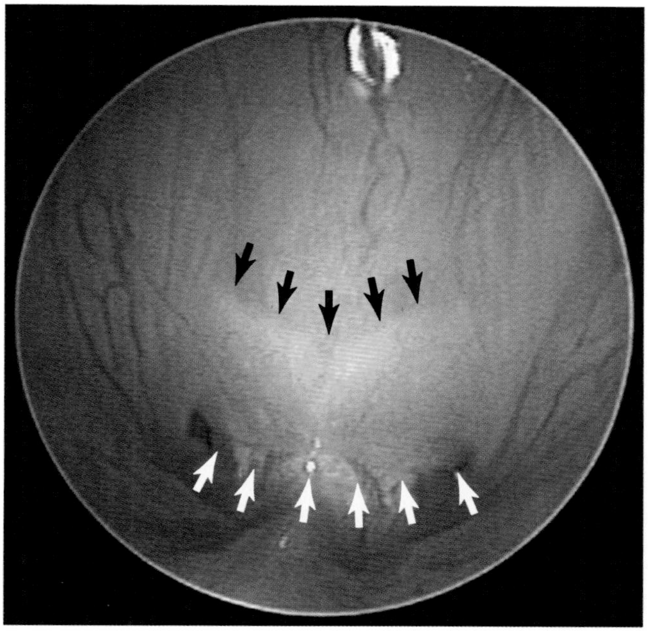

Plate 4 Nasal breathing in rabbits is facilitated by the entrapment of the epiglottis dorsal to the soft palate. The butterfly-shaped epiglottis *(black arrows)* is clearly visible through the relatively transparent caudal soft palate *(white arrows)*. The vascular pattern depicted here is typical for a rabbit. *(Courtesy Stephen Hernandez-Divers, Ithaca, New York, and Michael Murray, Monterey, California.)*

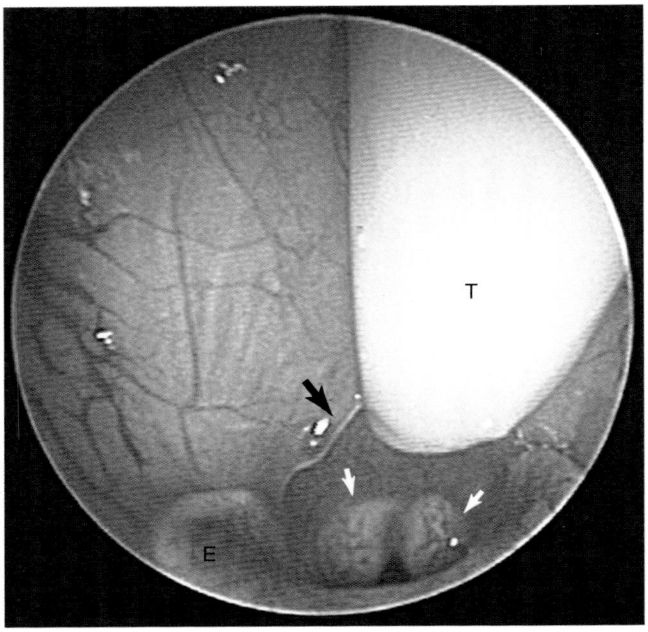

Plate 5 Gentle pressure on the soft palate *(black arrow)* frees the epiglottis *(E)* and allows the endotracheal tube *(T)* to be advanced and inserted between the arytenoid cartilages *(white arrows)*. *(Courtesy Stephen Hernandez-Divers, Ithaca, New York, and Michael Murray, Monterey, California.)*

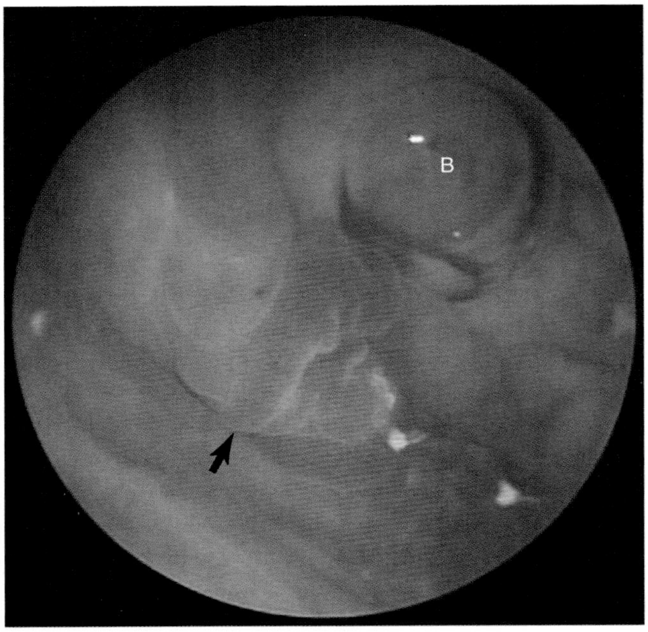

Plate 6 Cystoscopic view of the mucosal surface of the rabbit urinary bladder. Note the air bubble *(B)*. This rabbit had hematuria; a space-occupying mass *(arrow)* was outlined by the positive contrast of the urine within the bladder. Histologic diagnosis of epithelial hyperplasia was made from a biopsy sample. *(Courtesy Stephen Hernandez-Divers, Ithaca, New York, and Michael Murray, Monterey, California.)*

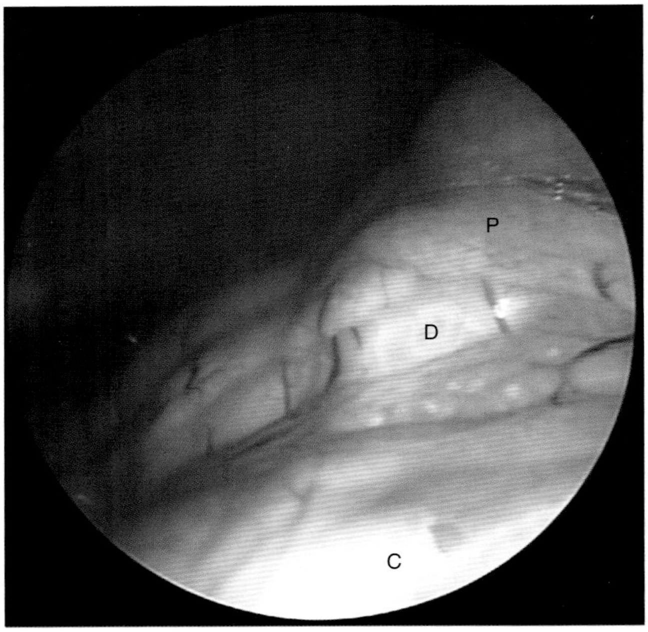

Plate 7 Laparoscopic (left cranial flank) view of the duodenum *(D)*, pancreas *(P)*, and cecum *(C)* of a rabbit. *(Courtesy Stephen Hernandez-Divers, Ithaca, New York, and Michael Murray, Monterey, California.)*

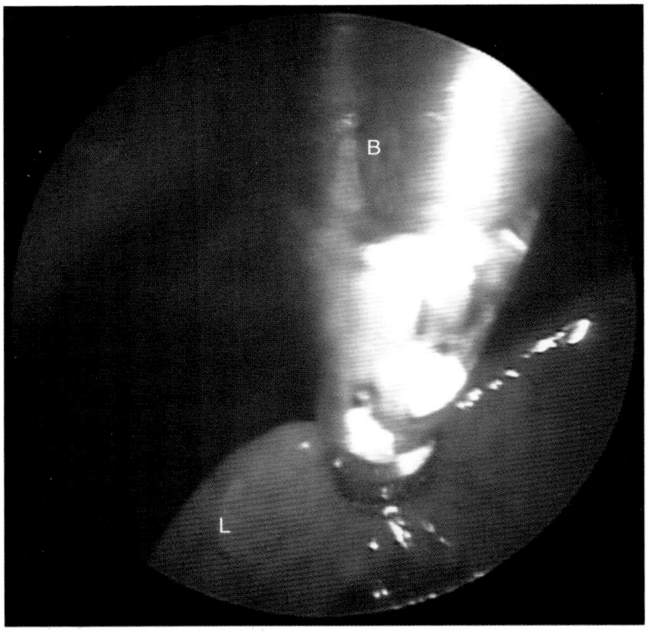

Plate 8 Endoscopic biopsy of the liver of a rabbit. The biopsy forceps *(B)* are used to take a tissue sample from the caudal edge of the liver *(L)*. *(Courtesy Stephen Hernandez-Divers, Ithaca, New York, and Michael Murray, Monterey, California.)*

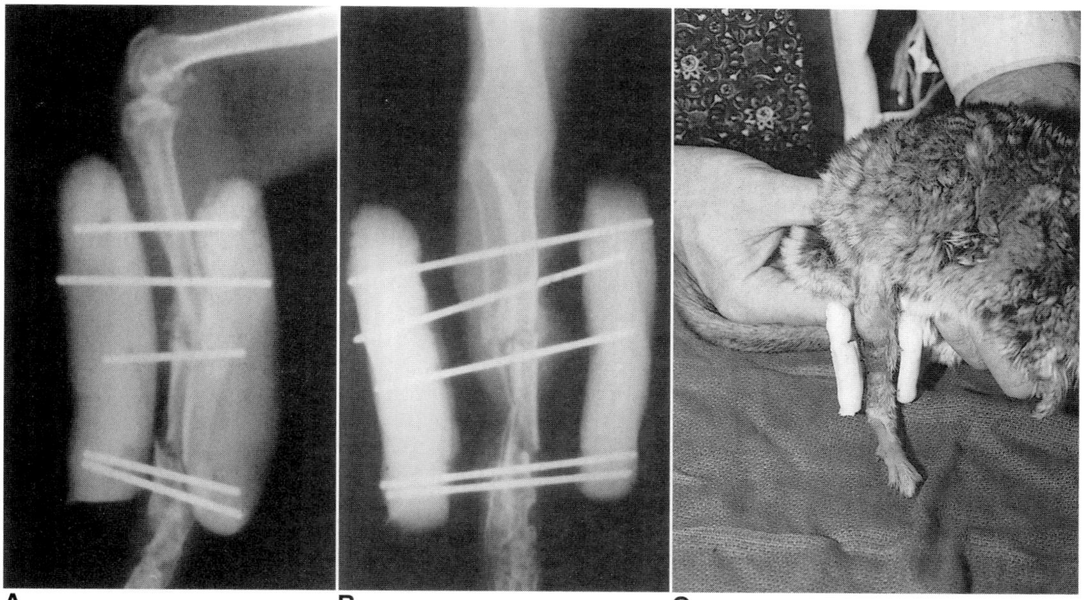

A B C

Figure 35-3 A and B, Postoperative radiographs of a tibia/fibula fracture with an external skeletal fixator in a chincilla. C, Example of polymethylmethacrylate bar fixation in a chinchilla.

bone necrosis, which also leads to the premature loosening of pins. Predrilling with a drill bit is an acceptable technique if smooth pins are used and is the correct method for inserting threaded (positive profile) pins. However, threaded pins are difficult to use in small mammals because of their small bone size and the size of pins that are available. When smooth pins are used, angle the pins at about 70 degrees to the longitudinal axis of the bone so that pullout of the pins is prevented. Try to place the pins in the center of the bone so that bone-pin interface stability is increased.[11,36]

Before repairing a fracture with an external fixator, decide whether a limited open approach or closed placement of the pins is best. In species with limited soft tissue covering the bone, it is advantageous not to destroy the tissues by opening the fracture. Therefore, in simple fractures, place the external fixator with a closed technique. With highly comminuted or open fractures that need a debridement, use a limited open technique to reduce the fracture and place the pins.

Rabbits, ferrets, and small rodents are usually too small to connect the pins with external fixator clamps and bars. Instead, use bone cement and acrylics as fixator bars. Biomechanically, these materials are as rigid as the metal bars and clamps (if used at an appropriate thickness) and are resistant to chewing by the animals.

Place the fixator pins approximately 1 cm away from the fracture line. Four pins per bone segment is ideal for maximum stiffness. Additional pins increase stiffness insignificantly. In these small species, four pins may provide too much stiffness; therefore I usually use three pins per segment. The fixator pin diameter should not exceed 20% of the bone diameter, so Kirschner wires are typically used. Position the connecting bar approximately 1 cm away from the skin. Placing the bar too far away from the skin decreases the stiffness and strength of the external fixators. Remember to allow for swelling when placing the bars. Spread out the pins evenly across the fracture segment to achieve maximum strength. Also remember to place the pins through a separate stab skin incision and not through the fracture opening or original incision (Fig. 35-3).[11,36]

Bone healing in rabbits with fractures stabilized by external fixation has been well studied. The current belief in external fixation is to stage the removal of the apparatus so that bone is allowed to take over load bearing at a fairly early stage of fixation. This process has been termed *dynamization*.[11,36] In studies of rabbits with tibial osteotomies used as the model, the ideal time to remove external fixators was 6 weeks. The strength and stiffness of the bone were greater if the fixator was removed at 6 weeks than if it was left in place for 12 weeks.[31,33] Clinically, many factors affect optimal removal time of a fixator, such as the age of the animal, the type of fracture, and the degree of vascular structure disruption.[11,36] Therefore the key is to examine these patients every 2 to 3 weeks after surgery and to stage removal when there are indications that the fracture has regained normal stiffness, even though strength may not be normal.[31] Experimentally, removing the fixator at 4 weeks causes some loss of reduction and is probably not advisable, even in perfectly reduced fractures.[31]

FRACTURE HEALING AND POSTOPERATIVE MANAGEMENT

Bone healing in rabbits, ferrets, and small rodents is the same as it is in other mammals. There are two major categories of bone healing: direct and indirect. Direct bone healing takes place if no periosteal or endosteal callus is present. This occurs when there is anatomic reduction and rigid stability of the fracture. Direct healing takes place by either contact healing or gap healing. With contact healing, bone union and haversian remodeling occur together. Gap healing takes place when a gap smaller than 800 μm is present. Layers of bone are laid down on two surfaces of the fracture. This transverse lamellar bone is then remodeled longitudinally through osteons and haversian remodeling.[14,24] Indirect bone healing is "classic" bone healing. For further details on bone healing, refer to other texts.[8,15,25,27]

Postoperative management of small mammals includes confinement, good husbandry, and frequent monitoring and maintenance of the fixation apparatus. Animals with closed fractures only need perioperative antibiotics (a dose given intravenously every 2 hours during surgery), but open fractures require extended antibiotic therapy. Ideally, the antibiotic is chosen according to the sensitivity pattern of the bacterial culture taken initially.

Some of the techniques used in managing open fractures in dogs and cats are not feasible in exotic small mammals. Placing drainage systems or treating open wounds daily with sterile flushes and bandages is extremely difficult. Animals chew excessively at bandages or reach the wound unless a hard splint made of one of the previously discussed casting materials has been placed on the limb. In some species, daily flushes can only be managed with heavy tranquilization or anesthesia. This is expensive and stressful, especially for rodent species. Therefore wound management should be definitive at the time of surgery, if at all possible.

Instruct the owner to keep the pet confined and quiet and how to force feed the pet if necessary. Good husbandry is extremely important for the pet experiencing the added stress of recovery.

If a splint is used, review bandage care with the owner. He or she needs to check the toes for swelling or discharge. These species often chew at splints even if they appear comfortable. Extreme discomfort in these animals often manifests as quietness and anorexia. Recheck the splints at least every 2 weeks, with the first recheck scheduled within a few days of splint placement.

Evaluate the fracture radiographically every 3 to 4 weeks. In these species, this usually requires heavy sedation or anesthesia. Because radiographic findings often lag behind clinical healing, good palpation of the fracture is also important. Depending on the type of fixation, changes can be made in the apparatus as healing becomes evident on radiography.

COMPLICATIONS

The ultimate goal in fracture repair is bony union. Unfortunately, this does not always occur despite our use of sophisticated techniques. A delayed union, nonunion, or malunion can result.

Delayed Union

Fractures with delayed union do not heal in the expected time period. Causes of delayed union include infection, inadequate blood supply to bone and soft tissues, excessive distraction or compression of the bone ends, excessive loss of bone, poor immobilization at the fracture site, excessive stress protection of the fracture, interposition of soft tissue at the fracture ends, too much weight-bearing by the patient, and systemic factors.[16,26,29]

The first step in treating delayed union is to identify the cause. Noninfected delayed union can sometimes be treated conservatively by adding a splint for greater stability or changing a patient's activity level. Sometimes, a highly comminuted fracture shows delayed union because of an extreme loss of blood supply, which resolves if given additional time. If gross malalignment, instability, loosening of implants, or infection has occurred, surgical intervention is usually necessary. Infected bone heals if kept rigidly stable, but this is extremely difficult in these species.[16,26,29]

Nonunion

In fracture nonunion, the fracture has not healed and, without surgical intervention, will not heal. The causes are the same as those of delayed union. Nonunion fractures have been classified by Weber and Cech as either viable (vascular) or nonviable (avascular).[39] Clinical characteristics of a nonunion are movement and pain at the fracture site. The patient is non-weight-bearing lame and usually has severe disuse atrophy of the muscles. On radiographs, either excessive callus (viable nonunion) or no callus (nonviable nonunion) may be seen. The clinician can visualize an increased gap between the bone ends, obliteration of the marrow cavity, osteopenia from disuse, or excessive callus with no bridging across the fracture. Regardless of the cause of the nonunion, additional surgery is needed. Rigid stability and a bone graft are necessary to stimulate bone production. If infection is still the inciting cause, aggressive wound management also is indicated.[16,26,29]

Malunion

Malunions are fractures that heal in an abnormal position. This can result in an abnormal or painful gait caused by limb shortening or angular or rotational deformity. Degenerative joint disease can develop from abnormal joint alignment or weight-bearing forces. The usual causes are improper alignment or loss of alignment at the time of fracture fixation; this underscores the need for close monitoring of the fracture after surgery.

Malunions may be nonclinical and may not need any intervention. If correction will improve the function of the limb, surgery is indicated. This may involve osteotomy of the bone in different fashions or the use of distraction osteogenesis if shortening of the limb is severe.[2,16] Remember that these species are small and that ring fixators are usually impractical. Because of their small size, light body weight, and locomotive stance, these animals seem to tolerate severe deformities with minimal clinical significance.

Posttraumatic Osteomyelitis

Posttraumatic osteomyelitis is another potential complication of fractures in rabbits, ferrets, and small mammals. This is a posttraumatic or postoperative infection of the bone caused by wound contamination, bone avascularity, and the presence of a suitable environment (e.g., hematoma). An infected wound needs more than 10^5 organisms per gram of tissue to induce posttraumatic osteomyelitis. Therefore good surgical debridement and copious lavage are very important in managing open fractures. Adhering to strict sterile surgical technique, careful wound handling, hemostasis, and anatomic closure helps prevent posttraumatic osteomyelitis.[5]

Posttraumatic osteomyelitis is fairly common in rabbits. Radiographically, rabbits with posttraumatic osteomyelitis show periosteal reactions, osteolysis, and sometimes an involucrum (Fig. 35-4).[42] In my experience, organisms most commonly found on culture are *Pseudomonas* species. Rabbits develop caseous, nondraining abscesses; thus typical drainage techniques are not useful. Treatment of osteomyelitis in rabbits must be aggressive. Collect samples for aerobic and anaerobic cultures,

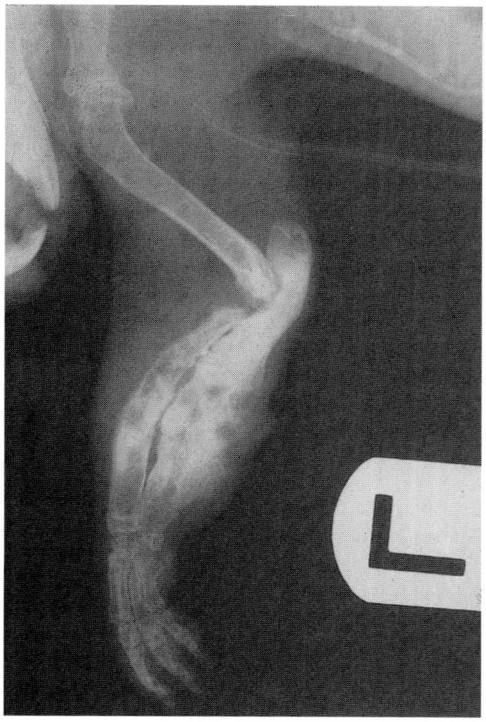

Figure 35-4 Severe posttraumatic osteomyelitis in the radius/ulna of a rabbit.

debride the wound, and administer an appropriate antibiotic. Additionally, antibiotic-impregnated beads are strongly recommended for use in rabbits. Local administration of antibiotics that are eluted over time may not be inactivated by the loss of blood supply to the infected, traumatized area.[12,21,22,37,40] Many in vitro studies show varied results depending on the antibiotic used, antibiotic form used (powder vs liquid), antibiotic concentration, carrier medium (polymethylmethacrylate or hydroxyapatite cement), and carrier medium surface area.[12,21,22,37,40] Many recent studies have shown efficacy with a variety of antibiotics (cephalosporins and aminoglycosides), with significant elution occurring within the first 48 hours and then continued elution from 2 weeks to months.[12,14,21,22,37,40]

Antibiotic-impregnated beads are being used clinically in rabbits for osteomyelitis with perceived success (see Chapter 34). Because antibiotic beads may continue to elute over extended periods of time, leaving them permanently at the infected site may be advantageous.[12,14] Also, many owners do not want a second surgery to remove the beads.

When using impregnated beads, use an appropriate antibiotic and dose. Higher doses elute more antibiotic[12,40]; however, some can reach toxic levels if too much antibiotic is placed locally. Beads can be made with special bead molds or injected into syringes and then cut to an appropriate size or placed on the suture. All uses must be performed under sterile conditions.

A similar type of abscess can develop in small rodents, but the incidence of posttraumatic osteomyelitis appears to be low. Ferrets with posttraumatic osteomyelitis have manifestations similar to those of dogs and cats. Therefore treatment and the use of drainage systems can be similar. In severe cases, antibiotic-impregnated beads can be used as well.

When treatment for posttraumatic osteomyelitis is unsuccessful, which is common in rabbits, amputation of the limb is the only option. This is a salvage procedure that is reserved for only those animals for which prognosis for successful treatment is very poor.

AMPUTATIONS

Amputation is indicated in small mammals when orthopedic trauma is so severe that it is unmanageable or when treatment of posttraumatic osteomyelitis is unsuccessful. It is also an option if the owner has severe financial constraints and cannot afford necessary follow-up bandage care and radiographs. Fortunately, these species are very adaptable to amputation of a single limb and ambulate well on three legs. Even large rabbits can adapt to the loss of a rear leg.

The level of amputation chosen depends on where the injury has occurred. In the foreleg, removing the scapula is easier and more cosmetic than amputating at the scapular-humeral joint. Some surgeons prefer to leave the scapula because it serves as a protective barrier to the chest wall. A hindleg amputation is more cosmetic if the amputation is midfemoral rather than at the coxofemoral joint. I disarticulate the limb at the coxofemoral joint only if the infection or injury is so close to the joint that a good resection is not possible.

Surgical approaches to amputation of the limbs are very similar to those for other small animals. The bones of rabbits have such thin cortices that they will shatter if cut with a bone cutter. Use either Gigli saw wire or a power saw to make a straight bone cut. Take care to leave enough soft tissue to cover the remaining bone at closure. Refer to anatomic texts for locations and variations of the soft tissues in these species.[1,20]

ELBOW LUXATIONS

Elbow luxations are another common condition seen in rabbits and ferrets (Fig. 35-5, *A*). These animals have non–weight-bearing lameness of the limb and a very painful, swollen elbow joint. Although this can result from trauma, there may be no known trauma history. Rabbits may have a predisposition for elbow luxations similar to that in certain breeds of dogs.

Treatment consists of reducing the elbow and then keeping it reduced in extension while the soft tissues scar down to keep it in place. The closed reduction is maintained by placing a splint made from Orthoplast, Vet-lite, or an aluminum rod (Fig. 35-5, *B*). Although immobilizing the shoulder joint is the proper technique for this type of injury in other mammals, immobilizing the shoulder joint in a rabbit is very difficult. A splint placed at the midhumerus can be successful, but such a splint must be monitored closely. Joints that reduce easily also reluxate easily.

Many elbow luxations need internal fixation to heal. For internal fixation, place a transarticular pin through the joint and then place a light Orthoplast or Vet-lite splint (Fig. 35-5, *C* and *D*). The transarticular pin keeps the joint reduced while the splint prevents full weight-bearing by the rabbit. The pin must be removed in approximately 3 weeks. The splint is usually needed for support for another 2 to 3 weeks after pin removal. Elbow luxation repair is usually successful with this

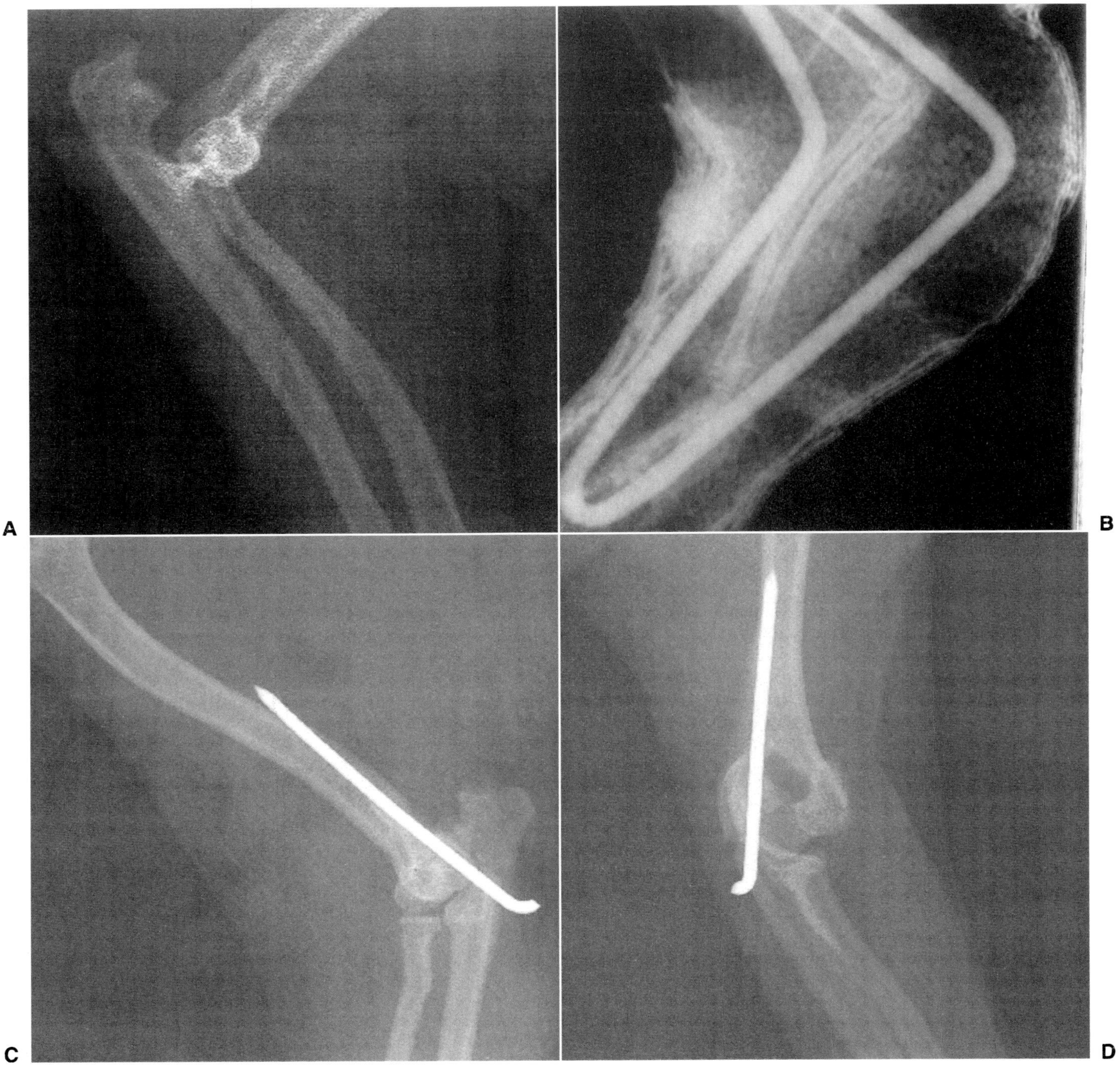

Figure 35-5 A, Radiograph of elbow luxation in a ferret. B, Radiograph of a reduced elbow luxation stabilized with a spica splint in a rabbit. C and D, Radiographs of a ferret elbow luxation reduced with a transarticular pin repair.

technique; if it is not, a transarticular external fixator can be placed.

REFERENCES

1. An NQ, Evans HE: Anatomy of the ferret. *In* Fox JG, ed. Biology and Diseases of the Ferret. Philadelphia, Lea & Febiger, 1988, pp 14-65.
2. Anson LW: Malunions. Vet Clin North Am Small Anim Pract 1991; 21:761-780.
3. Anson LW: Emergency management of fractures. *In* Slatter D, ed. Textbook of Small Animal Surgery, 2nd ed. Vol 2. Philadelphia, WB Saunders, 1993, pp 1603-1610.
4. Backstrom AS, Tulamo R-M, Raiha JE, et al: Intramedullary fixation of cortical bone osteotomies with absorbable self-reinforced fibrillated poly-96L/4D-lactide (SR-PLA96) rods in rabbits. Biomaterials 2001; 22:33-43.

5. Braden TD: Posttraumatic osteomyelitis. Vet Clin North Am Small Anim Pract 1991; 21:781-811.
6. Brinker WO, Hohm RB, Prieur WD: Manual of Internal Fixation in Small Animals. New York, Springer-Verlag, 1984.
7. Brinker WO, Piermattei DL, Flo GL: Handbook of Small Animal Orthopedics and Fracture Treatment, 2nd ed. Philadelphia, WB Saunders, 1990, p 5.
8. Brown SG, Kramers PC: Indirect (secondary) bone healing. *In* Bojrab MJ, ed. Disease Mechanisms in Small Animal Surgery, 2nd ed. Philadelphia, Lea & Febiger, 1993, pp 671-677.
9. DeCamp CE: External coaptation. *In* Slatter D, ed. Textbook of Small Animal Surgery, 2nd ed. Vol 2. Philadelphia, WB Saunders, 1993, pp 1661-1676.
10. DeYoung DJ, Probst CW: Methods of internal fracture fixation. *In* Slatter D, ed. Textbook of Small Animal Surgery, 2nd ed. Vol 2. Philadelphia, WB Saunders, 1993, pp 1610-1640.
11. Egger EL: External skeletal fixation. *In* Slatter D, ed. Textbook of Small Animal Surgery, 2nd ed. Vol 2. Philadelphia, WB Saunders, 1993, pp 1641-1661.
12. Ethell MT, Bennett RA, Brown MP, et al: In vitro elution of gentamicin, amikacin and ceftiofur from polymethylmethacrylate and hydroxyapatitie cement. Vet Surg 2000; 29:375-382.
13. Gordon LE, Thacher C, Kapatkin A: High-rise syndrome in dogs: 81 cases (1985-1991). J Am Vet Med Assoc 1993; 202:118-122.
14. Holcombe SJ, Schneider RK, Bramlage LR, et al: Use of antibiotic-impregnated polymethylmethacrylate in horses with open or infected fractures or joints: 19 cases (1987-1995). J Am Vet Med Assoc 1997; 211:889-893.
15. Kaderly RE: Primary bone healing. Semin Vet Med Surg (Small Anim) 1991; 6:21-25.
16. Kaderly RE: Delayed union, nonunion, and malunion. *In* Slatter D, ed. Textbook of Small Animal Surgery, 2nd ed. Vol 2. Philadelphia, WB Saunders, 1993, pp 1676-1685.
17. Kapatkin AS, Matthiesen DT: Feline high-rise syndrome. Compend Contin Educ Pract Vet 1991; 13:1389-1394.
18. Laftman P, Nilsson OS, Brosjo O, et al: Stress shielding by rigid fixation studied in osteotomized rabbit tibiae. Acta Orthop Scand 1989; 60:718-722.
19. Leighton RL: Principles of conservative fracture management: splints and casts. Semin Vet Med Surg (Small Anim) 1991; 6:39-51.
20. McLaughlin CA, Chiasson RB: Laboratory Anatomy of the Rabbit, 2nd ed. Dubuque, IA, William C. Brown, 1979, pp 7-31.
21. Miclau T, Dahners E, Lindsey RW: In vitro pharmacokinetics of antibiotic release from locally implantable materials. J Orthop Res 1993; 11:627-632.
22. Nijhof MW, Stallmann HP, Vogely C, et al: Prevention of infection with tobramycin-containing bone cement or systemic cefazolin in an animal model. J Biomed Mater Res 2000; 52: 709-715.
23. Paavolainen P, Karaharju E, Slatis P, et al: Radiographic evaluation of fracture healing after rigid plate fixation: experiments in the rabbit. Acta Radiol Diagn (Stockh) 1981; 22:697-702.
24. Papagelopoulos PJ, Giannarakos DG, Lyritis GP: Suitability of biodegradable polydioxanone materials for the internal fixation of fractures. Orthop Rev 1993; 22:585-593.
25. Perren SM: Primary bone healing. *In* Bojrab MJ, ed. Disease Mechanisms in Small Animal Surgery, 2nd ed. Philadelphia, Lea & Febiger, 1993, pp 663-670.
26. Robello GT, Aron DN: Delayed and nonunion fractures. Semin Vet Med Surg (Small Anim) 1992; 7:98-104.
27. Schelling SH: Secondary (classical) bone healing. Semin Vet Med Surg (Small Anim) 1991; 6:16-20.
28. Schrader SC: Complications associated with the use of Steinmann intramedullary pins and cerclage wires for fixation of long-bone fractures. Vet Clin North Am Small Anim Pract 1991; 21:687-703.
29. Summer-Smith G: Delayed unions and nonunions, diagnosis, pathophysiology, and treatment. Vet Clin North Am Small Anim Pract 1991; 21:745-760.
30. Terjesen T: Bone healing after metal plate fixation and external fixation of the osteotomized rabbit tibia. Acta Orthop Scand 1984; 55:69-77.
31. Terjesen T: Healing of rabbit tibial fractures using external fixation: effects of removal of the fixation device. Acta Orthop Scand 1984; 55:192-196.
32. Terjesen T: Plate fixation of tibial fractures in the rabbit: correlation of bone strength with duration of fixation. Acta Orthop Scand 1984; 55:454-456.
33. Terjesen T, Johnson E: Effect of fixation stiffness on fracture healing: external fixation of tibial osteotomy in the rabbit. Acta Orthop Scand 1986; 57:146-148.
34. Thaller SR, Huang V, Tesluk H: Use of biodegradable plates and screws in a rabbit model. J Craniofac Surg 1992; 2:168-173.
35. Tomlinson J: Complications of fractures repaired with casts and splints. Vet Clin North Am Small Anim Pract 1991; 21:735-744.
36. Toombs JP: Principles of external skeletal fixation using the Kirschner-Ehmer splint. Vet Clin North Am Small Anim Pract 1991; 6:68-74.
37. Trippel SB: Antibiotic-impregnated cement in total joint arthroplasty. J Bone Joint Surg 1986; 68A:1297-1302.
38. Wang GJ, Dunstan JC, Reger SI, et al: Experimental femoral fracture immobilized by rigid and flexible rods (a rabbit model). Clin Orthop 1981; 154:286-290.
39. Weber BG, Cech O: Pseudoarthrosis: Pathology, Biomechanics, Therapy, Results. Bern, Switzerland, Hans Huber, 1976.
40. Weisman DL, Olmstead ML, Kowalski JJ: In vitro evaluation of antibiotic elution from polymethylmethacrylate (PMMA) and mechanical assessment of antibiotic-PMMA composites. Vet Surg 2000; 29:245-251.
41. Whitney WO, Mehlhaff CJ: High-rise syndrome in cats. J Am Vet Med Assoc 1987; 191:1399-1403.
42. Worlock P, Slack R, Harvey L, et al: An experimental model of post-traumatic osteomyelitis in rabbits. Br J Exp Pathol 1988; 69:235-244.

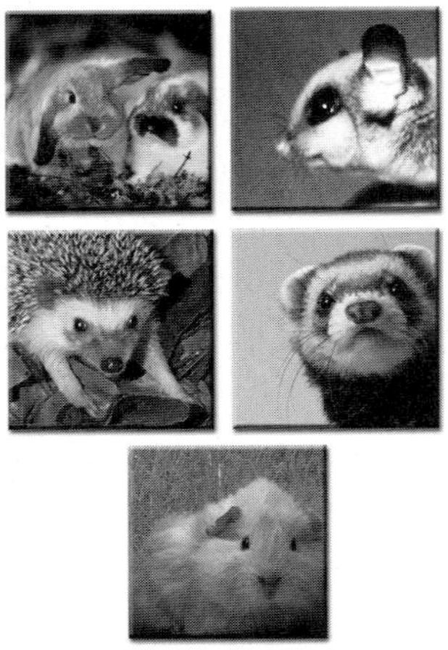

CHAPTER 36

Small Mammal Endoscopy

Stephen J. Hernandez-Divers, BVetMed, MRCVS, Diplomate Zoological Medicine, and Michael J. Murray, DVM

Endoscopy is the visual examination of internal structures with an endoscope. The endoscope can be used in any hollow or viscous organ (e.g., mouth, ear, trachea, or esophagus) or, by insufflation, in any potential space (e.g., peritoneal cavity or bladder). Endoscopy has proved to be a useful diagnostic tool in veterinary medicine, providing direct visualization and biopsy of internal organs.[3] In the field of zoological medicine, diagnostic endoscopy has shown great promise in a variety of species but has probably been most used by avian veterinarians.[4,5] Endoscopy of small mammals, specifically rabbits, is a novel use of this equipment but one that holds great promise for improved disease diagnosis and management.[1]

ENDOSCOPY EQUIPMENT

We prefer the use of the 2.7-mm rigid, rod-lens Hopkins telescope (Karl Storz Veterinary Endoscopy America Inc., Goleta, CA), 18 cm in length and with a 30-degree viewing angle, because of its versatility in exotic pet practice, the variety of available accessories, and the dedicated company support (Fig. 36-1). The telescope is housed inside a protective sheath and connected to a xenon light source by a light guide cable. Endoscopic instruments of particular interest include the biopsy forceps, grasping forceps, single-action scissors, fine aspiration and injection needle with Teflon guide, and wire retrieval basket. For laparoscopy, we prefer insufflating with a dedicated endoflator with medical-grade carbon dioxide gas and a Veress pneumoperitoneum needle. Sterile saline can be beneficial for irrigation and to improve visualization of internal structures, especially epithelial or mucosal surfaces. The modern endovision cameras greatly enhance the endoscopist's capabilities and are available in both European PAL and U.S. NTSC formats. Recording still images and video are also practical means of marketing endoscopic procedures to small herbivore owners and keepers. More complete reviews of endoscopic equipment are available.[3,5] To prevent postoperative infection, endoscopic instruments must be properly sterilized. The three practical options are gas sterilization with ethylene oxide gas, hydrogen peroxide vapor, and 2% glutaraldehyde solution.

ENDOSCOPIC PROCEDURES

For all procedures described, general anesthesia is recommended. Any contraindication for general anesthesia is often a contraindication for endoscopy. Participating in a course on endoscopic techniques and practicing on necropsy specimens are strongly recommended before working with client-owned animals.

Otoscopy

To examine the ear canal of a rabbit, position the animal in sternal recumbency with an assistant supporting the rabbit's head and holding the pinna erect. Gently insert the telescope down the external ear canal until the aural sulcus, a blind-ending diverticulum off the vertical canal, is seen. Continue advancing ventrally until the vertical canal deviates medially and becomes the horizontal canal before terminating at the oval tympanum. Epithelial lesions and exudate are often visible, and the integrity of the tympanum can be easily assessed (Plate 1). Tympanic perforation and otitis media, if present, will be evident. As needed, take a biopsy of any lesion and collect samples of exudate for cytologic, histopathologic, and microbiologic examination. Irrigate with sterile saline and clear debris as necessary. Use chemical cleansing agents only after samples for microbiologic culture are collected or if culture is not required.

Rhinoscopy

For rhinoscopy of a rabbit, position the intubated animal in sternal recumbency with the head held down. Flush both nares with sterile saline to clear mucus and debris from the nose. Depending on the size of the rabbit, an examination sheath may or may not be used with the telescope. However, use extreme care when working with the unprotected telescope to prevent

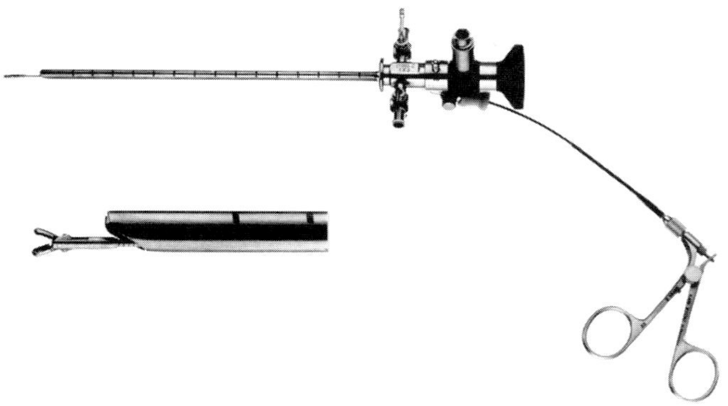

Figure 36-1 The 2.7-mm Hopkins telescope housed within the 14.5-Fr sheath with biopsy instrument in situ. The sheath offers two ports for insufflation and irrigation. *(Courtesy Karl Storz Veterinary Endoscopy America Inc.)*

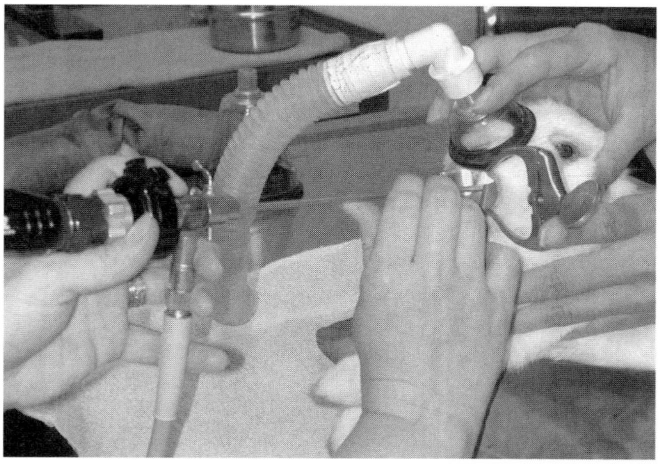

Figure 36-2 By using a nose cone for anesthetic delivery, a self-retaining oral speculum can be placed to permit endoscopic examination of the oral cavity. In this photograph, the upper arcade of a rabbit is being examined. A 180-degree rotation of the telescope permits examination of the lower arcade. *(Courtesy Stephen Hernandez-Divers, Ithaca, New York, and Michael Murray, Monterey, California.)*

damage to the instrument. With an assistant supporting the head, gently advance the endoscope into one nostril past the alar fold. The first area encountered is the nasal meatus, which is divided into dorsal, middle, and ventral areas (Plate 2). Advance the telescope further caudal to the dorsal and ventral nasal conchae (moving the telescope between the dorsal and ventral areas can be difficult in small rabbits). Finally, the cranial aspects of the ethmoid labyrinth are visible. Because the nasal membranes are highly vascular, take care to avoid trauma and subsequent hemorrhage. Irrigating with saline greatly aids visibility of these structures. Collect biopsy samples of lesions and exudate as necessary. Biopsy instruments may need to be inserted independently of the telescope if the small working space precludes the use of a sheath. Hemorrhage after biopsy is minor.

Oral Cavity

The very small oral commissure tends to preclude a thorough examination of the cheek teeth in rabbits and rodents. As a result, malocclusion tends to progress undetected until it becomes severe enough to elicit overt clinical signs. The rigid endoscope is ideally suited to examine the oral cavity in these small mammals and offers considerable advantages over a standard otoscope.[5] As an alternative to the Hopkins telescope, an 8.5-cm otoendoscope (Karl Storz Veterinary Endoscopy) can be used to examine the oral cavity and offers the advantage of not requiring a protective sheath.

Food material is often retained in the mouth after eating, especially in guinea pigs. Therefore fasting small mammals for 1 to 4 hours before examination may be helpful. With the patient appropriately sedated or anesthetized, hold the mouth open with a self-retaining mouth gag and a cheek retractor to enhance visibility of the dental arcades (Spectrum Surgical Supply, Stow, OH) (Fig. 36-2). Insert the telescope within its protective sheath into the oral cavity. Examine the upper arcades with the endoscope in its normal position (30-degree reflection up). Then, to examine the lower arcades, take advantage of the 30-degree offset by rotating the telescope 180 degrees. This allows a good view of the lower teeth (if a camera is used, it should *not* be rotated; rotate just the telescope).

Evaluate every tooth, including the lingual, buccal, and occlusal aspects (Plate 3). Use an appropriately sized and curved dental probe to palpate each tooth, attempting to detect movement or other evidence of disease. Additionally, pay particular attention to the gingiva. Chinchillas often have a subgingival point on the buccal aspect of the first upper premolar as the sole cause of "slobbers." Most commonly, malocclusion involves overgrowth of the lower arcade to the lingual aspect and of the upper arcade to the buccal aspect of the oral cavity. If left untreated, severe tongue injury and laceration can occur. In guinea pigs with severe malocclusion, the mandibular teeth can actually bridge and entrap the tongue.

Once identified, trim the maloccluded teeth with either a motorized dental handpiece or rongeurs (see Chapter 34). When using the latter, take exceptional care to avoid fracturing the tooth. Because of the possibility of fractures, the dental handpiece is preferred. To avoid damage to the telescope, remove it while trimming and reinsert it after the dental procedure is finished to verify all points have been trimmed.

Tracheal Intubation

In addition to limiting access to oral structures, the small oral commissure of small herbivores drastically limits access to the caudal oropharynx, including the glottis. As a result, tracheal intubation tends to be a "blind" procedure with varying degrees of success. This limited ability to routinely and consistently establish a patent airway may pose significant problems during the anesthetic management of these species. As a further complication of the problems associated with intubation, the laryngeal structures can be extensively traumatized during attempts to blindly pass an endotracheal tube.

Similar to other small herbivores commonly encountered in practice, the larynx of rabbits is situated caudal and slightly ventral to the angle of the jaw. Rabbits are obligate nasal breathers and the anatomy of their larynx is somewhat different than that of dogs or cats. The epiglottis is a relatively large structure with a butterfly-shaped distal aspect that is normally entrapped on the dorsal surface of the soft palate (Plate 4). This arrangement permits passage of air directly from the nasopharynx into the larynx and trachea without entering into the oral cavity.

The rigid endoscope is easily used as an aid to place an endotracheal tube. This can be performed by either slipping the endotracheal tube over the endoscope or passing the tube beside it (Plate 5). Remember, only tubes with an inside diameter greater than that of the telescope, in most cases 3.0 mm and greater, can be fit over the instrument. As the instrument is slowly advanced into the caudal oral cavity, apply gentle pressure on the dorsal soft palate to free the epiglottis and reveal the glottal opening. Slowly advance the endotracheal tube, the tip of which should be lubricated with a sterile xylocaine gel, between the arytenoid cartilages and into the trachea. Manipulate the beveled tip of the endotracheal tube to facilitate the movement of the tube between the vocal folds. After placing the tube, remove the endoscope and secure the tube to the rabbit in a normal fashion.

Vaginoscopy/Cystoscopy

Cystoscopy is a technique to diagnose and potentially treat diseases of the lower urinary tract.[2] In rabbits, transurethral cystoscopy is limited to females. Endoscopic evaluation of the lower urinary tract is possible in males; however, it usually requires some form of abdominal approach to the bladder. Similarly, vaginoscopy is used to diagnose diseases of the distal reproductive tract. The most common indication of vaginoscopy is as an adjunct to cystoscopy in the diagnostic workup of hematuria because bloody urine is often associated with uterine adenocarcinoma, endometrial hyperplasia, or uterine polyps (Plate 6).

With the animal appropriately anesthetized, place it in dorsal (preferred), ventral, or lateral recumbency. Create an optical cavity by infusing warmed sterile saline through the infusion port of the sheath system. An egress path must be established as well: as the bladder fills, open the egress path to protect against bladder rupture. Also, palpate the bladder frequently to ensure that overfilling does not occur. Examine all portions of the lower urinary tract; it is usually necessary to rotate the telescope 180 degrees for a complete evaluation. Collect diagnostic samples for histopathologic or microbiologic examination. Cystoscopic examination is particularly helpful in animals with urolithiasis. In some patients, the cystoscope can be used intraoperatively to aid in retrieving small uroliths from the neck of the bladder.

Vaginoscopy may be indicated in rabbits with suspected vaginal or cervical disease or as an adjunct to cystoscopy in rabbits with hematuria of suspected genital tract origin. In female rabbits that have bloody urine, a unilateral, blood-tinged discharge, which can result from uterine neoplasia or other endometrial disease, is often visible from one cervix. The technique for vaginoscopy is similar to that for cystoscopy; bear in mind that the reproductive tract is dorsal to the urinary tract. Again, egress for infused fluids must be facilitated. Slow infusion rates are typically adequate to distend the vagina in most small mammals.

Laparoscopy

Laparoscopy requires insufflating the abdomen and creating a pneumoperitoneum, which places increased pressure on the diaphragm. To perform this procedure in a rabbit, the anesthetized animal must be intubated and provided with some form of respiratory support. The Vetronics Ventilator (Bioanalytical Systems, Inc., West Lafayette, IN) has proved useful for intermittent positive-pressure ventilation in small mammals that undergo laparoscopy. For this procedure, position the rabbit according to the organs of interest; however, abdominal fat can mask certain structures such as the kidneys, uteri, and ovaries. We prefer a left flank approach to examine the liver, stomach, jejunum, spleen, cecum, sacculus rotundus, ampulla coli, ascending colon, and left kidney. A right flank approach is useful to examine the liver, duodenum, pancreas, cecum, and right kidney. Use a ventral midline approach to examine the liver, stomach, jejunum, and cecum.

The technique for laparoscopy in rabbits and other small mammals is the same as that in dogs.[3] Preinflate the abdomen to 8 to 12 mm Hg with carbon dioxide and a Veress pneumoperitoneum needle. Remove the Veress needle and perform a 1- to 2-cm cut-down procedure at the proposed entry site. To reduce gas leakage around the telescope, minimize the length of the incision in the muscles or linea alba. Once the telescope is in place, attach the insufflator to one of the ports on the sheath and adjust the pressure setting to maintain the desired pneumoperitoneum. Proceed with the examination of the organ(s) of interest and collect biopsy or microbiologic samples as needed (Plate 7). A biopsy of the liver, spleen, or pancreas can be performed easily; however, a biopsy of the kidneys requires incising the perirenal fat (Plate 8). Because of possible intestinal perforation and peritonitis, do not biopsy the intestinal wall unless grossly proliferative lesions are present.

The endoscope is no longer the extraordinary tool of the board-certified specialist but an essential instrument of any clinician who regularly treats exotic animals. The current indications for small herbivore endoscopy include examining and collecting diagnostic samples from the ear, mouth, nose, glottis, trachea, esophagus, vagina, bladder, and visceral organs.[1] Other indications for endoscopy will undoubtedly become apparent as the true potential of this technology in ferrets, rabbits, and rodents is realized.

ACKNOWLEDGMENTS

We thank Karl Storz Veterinary Endoscopy, The University of Georgia, and the Avian and Exotic Clinic of Monterey Peninsula for their continued support of exotic animal endoscopy.

REFERENCES

1. Divers SJ, Mitchell M: Endoscopic evaluation of lagomorphs. *In* Zwart P, ed. Proceedings of the European Association of Zoo and Wildlife Veterinarians. Paris, 1999, pp 221-226.
2. Rudd RG, Hendrickson DA: Minimally invasive surgery of the urinary system. *In* Freeman LJ, ed. Veterinary Endosurgery. St Louis, Mosby, 1999, pp 226-236.
3. Tams TR: Small Animal Endoscopy, 2nd ed. St Louis, Mosby, 1999.
4. Taylor M: Endoscopic examination and biopsy techniques. *In* Ritchie BW, Harrison GJ, Harrison LR, eds. Avian Medicine: Principles and Application. Lake Worth, FL, Wingers Publishing, 1994, pp 327-354.
5. Taylor M, Murray MJ: Endoscopic surgery. Semin Avian Exotic Pet Med 1999; 8:99-141.

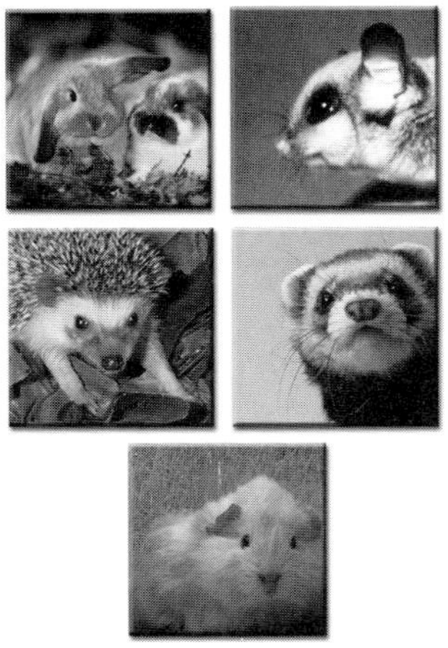

CHAPTER 37

Radiology and Ultrasound

Joseph D. Stefanacci, VMD, Diplomate ACVR, and
Heidi L. Hoefer, DVM, Diplomate ABVP

Radiography of exotic pets can be challenging. Small patient size and unique physiologic characteristics, such as rapid respiratory rate, can present technical dilemmas to the practitioner. However, with modern radiologic equipment and a better understanding of the use of anesthetics in these patients, the practitioner can take radiographs of most animals. Proper restraint and positioning are essential to ensure correct radiographic interpretation. The use of special x-ray cassettes in combination with the appropriate film provides the necessary radiographic detail and minimizes radiation exposure to personnel and patient.

Rigid restraint is paramount to produce diagnostic films. Several factors must be considered when you prepare an animal for radiography: the area to be radiographed, the temperament of the animal, and its general state of health. Most small mammals tolerate radiographic procedures well, but be careful with very stressed or debilitated patients. Treatment and clinical stability of the patient are the primary concerns, and radiography may often be postponed to minimize patient risk. Place dyspneic animals in an oxygen cage before taking radiographs; when taking radiographs of them, consider using injectable tranquilizers or gas anesthesia and an oxygen mask to minimize stress.

For ventrodorsal and lateral films of the body, manual restraint can sometimes be used. However, ferrets and small rodents can be difficult to restrain for any length of time, and they often need to be sedated for radiography. The choice of anesthetic agent varies with the individual practitioner and the area of radiographic interest. Isoflurane or sevoflurane delivered by face mask is convenient and safe in most animals. In excitable or fractious animals, induce anesthesia in an induction chamber and use a face mask for maintenance. To take radiographs of the head and neck, injectable agents such as ketamine and diazepam (ketamine 2.5-5.0 mg/kg plus diazepam 2.5-5.0 mg/kg in the same syringe given as an intravenous bolus) can be used to sedate an animal for short periods. For lengthy procedures such as a skull series, intubating the animal is preferable but can be difficult to impossible in small species.

Because motion artifact is a common problem, the use of x-ray–generating equipment capable of producing 300 mA in $^1/_{120}$ (0.008) second is a minimum requirement.[1] Larger, three-phase generators that can produce 1000 to 1200 mA are ideal because time stops are even shorter. Most radiographs can be exposed for $^1/_{120}$ (0.008) to $^1/_{60}$ (0.016) second with excellent results. Incremental adjustments of kilovoltage are necessary through a range of 40 to 70 kV (peak). A telescoping x-ray tube stand that can be moved along the x-ray table and adjusted in height is helpful. The ability to change the focal film distance (distance from the x-ray tube to the film) is useful to produce magnified views of anatomic areas of interest.[1] For a horizontally directed x-ray beam, a tube stand that can rotate 90 degrees is needed. With this tube stand, standing lateral radiographs of an animal can be obtained to evaluate gravity-dependent and non–gravity-dependent physiologic substances, including gas and fluid.

Fine or detail-intensifying screens or cassettes can be used for radiographs of most species (e.g., Curix Fine, Agfa, Orangeburg, NY; Quanta Detail, E.I. DuPont, Wilmington, DE; Lanex Fine, Eastman Kodak, Rochester, NY). These screens, combined with the proper x-ray film (Curix Detail RPIL, Agfa; Cronex 10, E.I. DuPont; TMG film, Eastman Kodak) maximize anatomic detail (bone, lung) while minimizing exposure time. For ultrafine detail in exotic pet radiography, the Min R mammography system (Eastman Kodak) can be used. We use Min R single-intensifying screen cassettes with Min R single-emulsion film for best results. One set of techniques that I (H. H.) use for tabletop mammography radiographs of small mammals requires 10 mA with a kilovoltage range of 62 to 68. With any film/screen combination, position animals less than 10 cm in thickness directly on the x-ray cassette. Animals thicker than 10 cm can be positioned on the x-ray table, with the film/cassette placed in the Bucky tray, under a grid.

The standard radiographic views are the lateral and the ventrodorsal (or dorsoventral) views. Because of the relatively small patient size, whole-body radiography can usually be done. This is often the easiest way to obtain a study and allows quick examination of the entire patient. Special radiographic projections, such as oblique and magnified views, can be attempted to evaluate certain body parts of interest, such as the skull. Thorough technical knowledge and familiarity with anatomy are necessary to successfully obtain and interpret these more difficult views.

Contrast radiography can be performed in small mammals. Although sometimes technically difficult to perform, contrast radiographs can provide important information that supports a clinical diagnosis. Gastrointestinal disease, such as mechanical obstruction from foreign body ingestion or hairball impaction in ferrets and rabbits, often can be delineated in an upper gastrointestinal contrast study. For a gastrointestinal contrast study, administer 10 to 15 mL/kg barium sulfate liquid (Novopaque 30% w/v, Picker Int., Highland Heights, OH) by mouth or stomach tube. If perforation is suspected, iohexol (Omnipaque, Winthrop Pharmaceuticals Inc, New York, NY) can be used in place of barium at the same dose or diluted 1 : 2 in water. Take sequential radiographs at 15- to 30-minute intervals until all the contrast media is in the large bowel. Take extra care with rabbits when gastric tubes are used; their small oropharynx and short neck make passing a gastric tube difficult. Esophageal structure and function can be evaluated with barium sulfate paste (Esophotrast Cream, Rhone-Poulenc Rorer Pharmaceuticals, Inc., Collegeville, PA). Megaesophagus in ferrets is easily assessed with this technique.

For urinary tract problems such as cystic or renal calculi in rabbits, ferrets, and guinea pigs, an intravenous iodinated contrast agent such as iothalamate sodium or meglumine (Conray, Mallinckrodt Medical, St. Louis, MO) (2 mL/kg) produces a good excretory urogram. Calculus location or renal function can be determined before surgery by this technique. If a urinary catheter can be placed, inject meglumine through it into the bladder for cystography. Expanding the urinary bladder to palpable turgidity allows detection of filling defects, diverticulae, or aberrant bladder location.

Interpreting radiographs of small mammals follows guidelines similar to those for all other animals. When evaluating radiographs, note changes in the radiographic signs of size, shape, number, location, margination, and opacity for each projection while considering the small body size and described anatomic variations of the animal.[2] Knowledge of normal anatomy is required; for example, the thorax of rodents is not clearly visualized because of its small size, and abdominal organs in guinea pigs can be obscured by gaseous cecal dilatation. Practice and patience ensure successful radiographic evaluation of these exotic pets.

REFERENCES

1. Silverman S: Diagnostic imaging of exotic pets. Vet Clin North Am Small Anim Pract 1993; 23:1287-1299.
2. Rübel GA, Isenbügel E, Wolvekamp P: Atlas of Diagnostic Radiology of Exotic Pets. Philadelphia, WB Saunders, 1991.

A

B

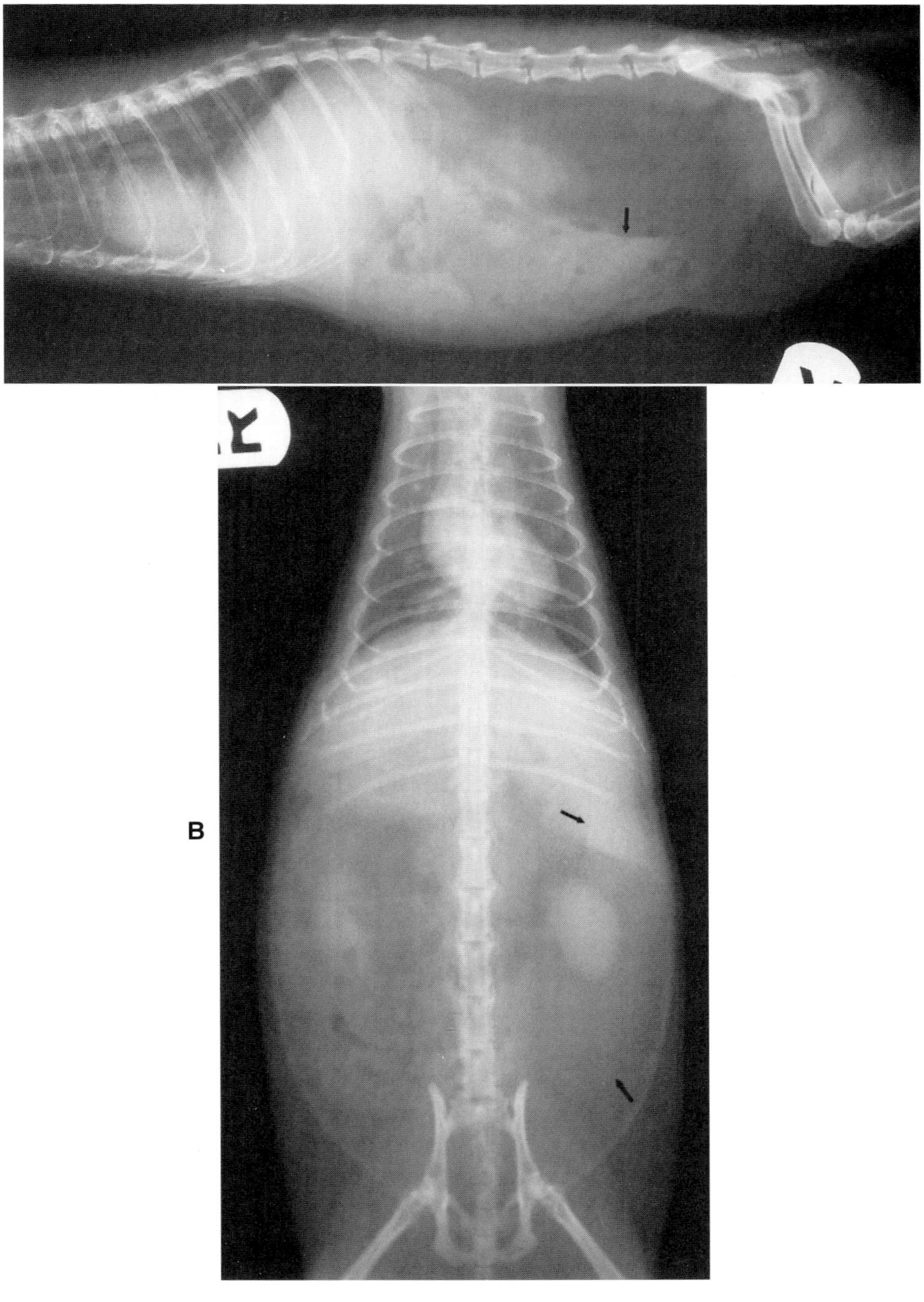

Figure 37-1
A and B. The normal ferret.

SIGNALMENT Four-year-old spayed female ferret.

RADIOGRAPHIC FINDINGS Splenomegaly is a common finding *(arrows)*. The large amount of intraperitoneal fat improves visualization of organs such as the spleen and kidneys. Normal ferrets may have a small amount of gas in the gastrointestinal tract.

A

B

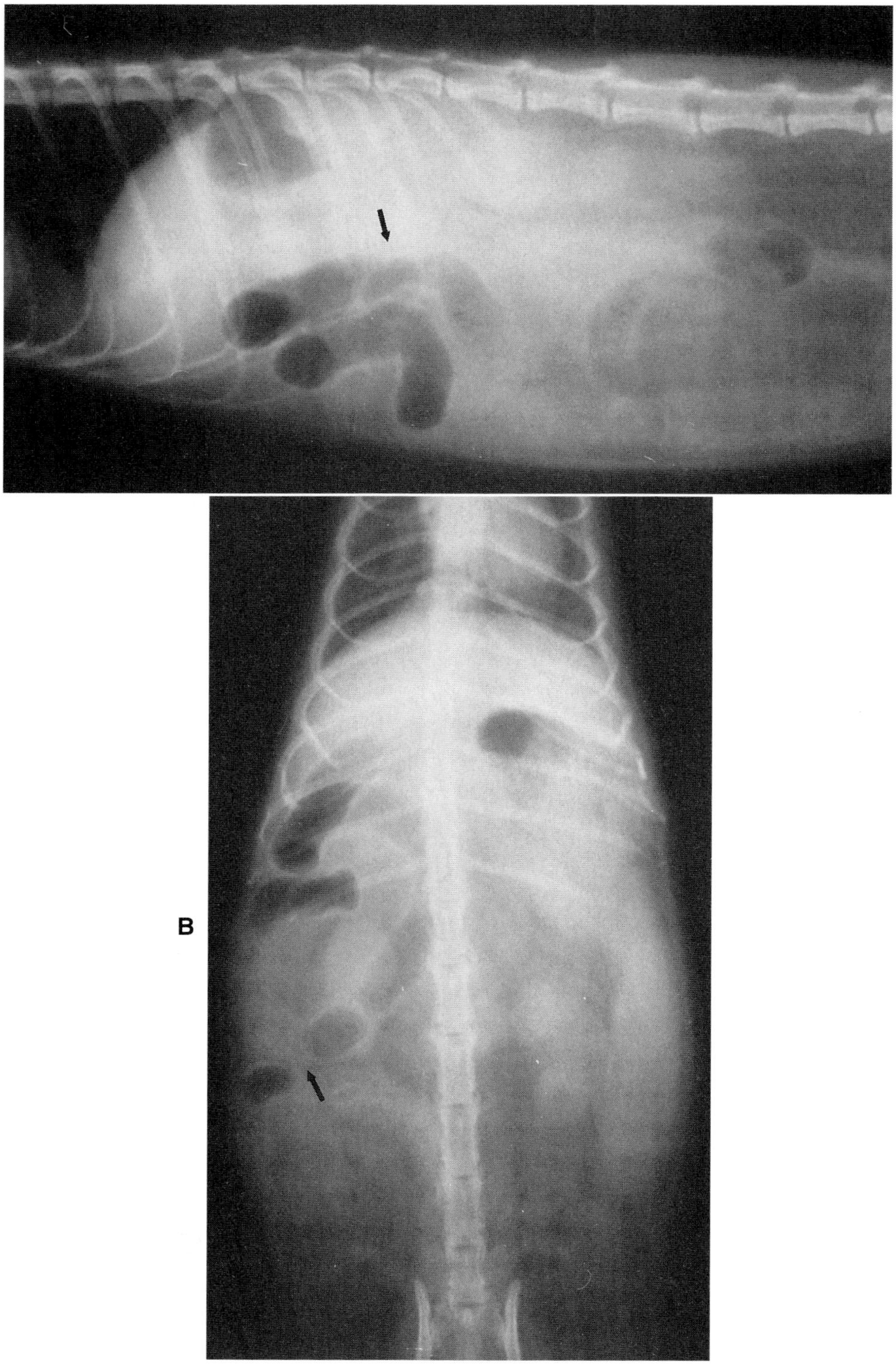

Figure 37-2
A and B.

SIGNALMENT — Spayed female ferret, 1.5 years old.

HISTORY — Anorexia, lethargy, and vomiting.

RADIOGRAPHIC FINDINGS — Several small bowel segments are abnormally dilated with gas and fluid (*arrows*). Note the "stacked" appearance of these loops in the lateral view.

FINAL DIAGNOSIS — Segmental small intestinal ileus caused by a foreign body (rubber eraser).

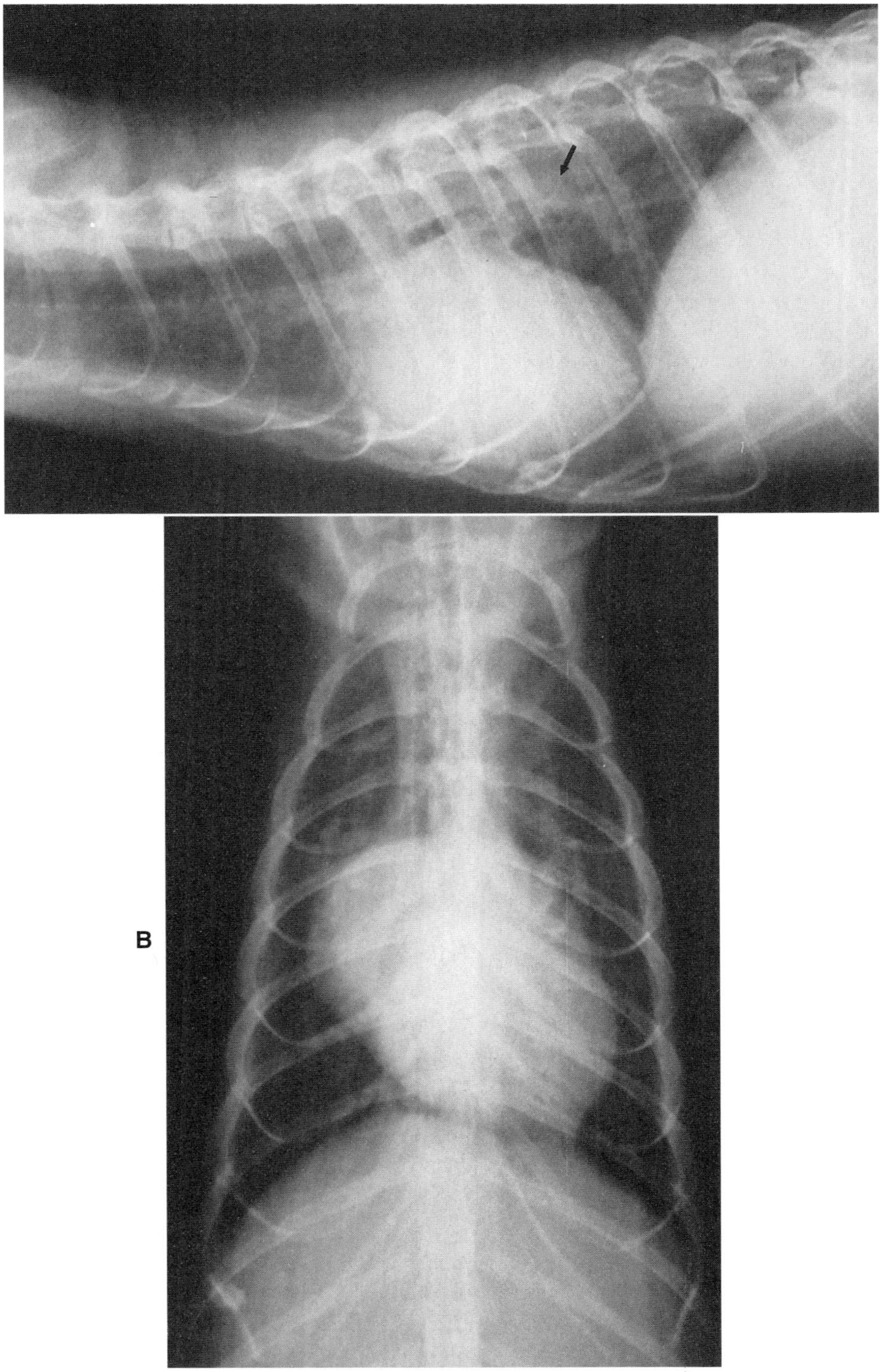

Figure 37-3
A and B.

SIGNALMENT	Five-year-old castrated male ferret.
HISTORY	Lethargy, tachypnea, and respiratory distress.
RADIOGRAPHIC FINDINGS	Generalized cardiomegaly is causing dorsal deviation of the trachea. An increase in pulmonary opacity is visible in the perihilar region (*arrow*). Pulmonary blood vessels are congested.
FINAL DIAGNOSIS	Dilated cardiomyopathy with mitral and tricuspid regurgitation.

A

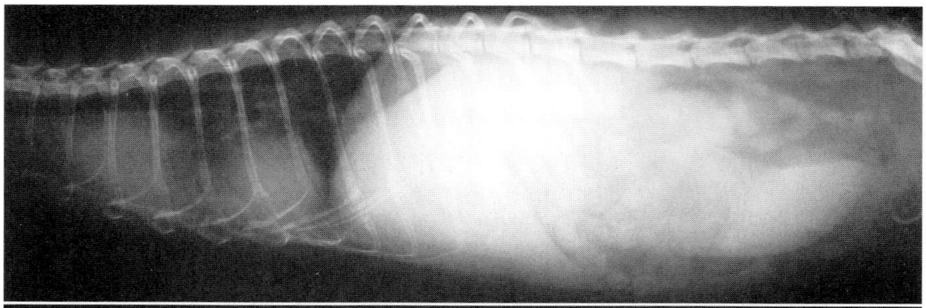

B

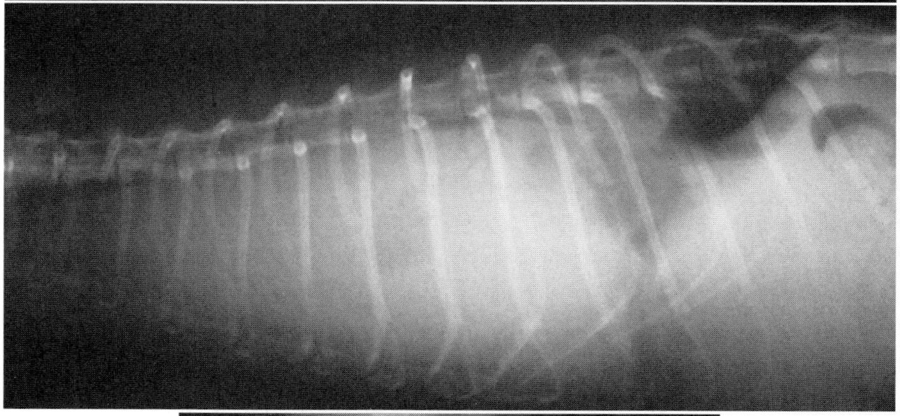

C

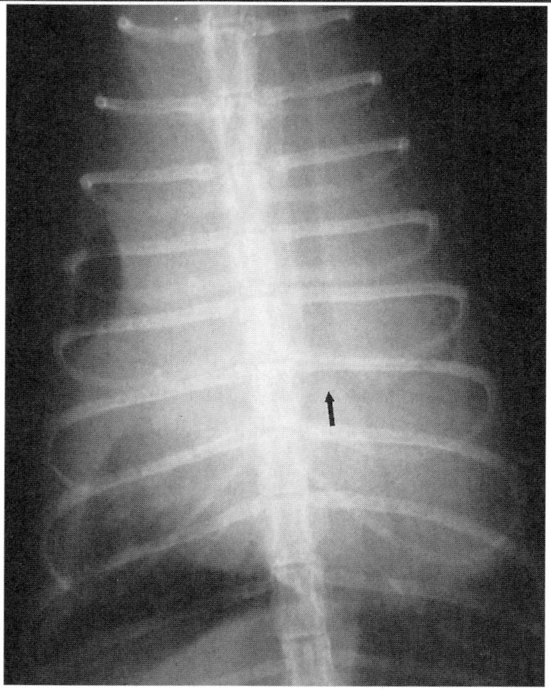

Figure 37-4, A

SIGNALMENT	Seven-month-old castrated male ferret.
HISTORY	Painful abdomen, diarrhea, and lethargy.
RADIOGRAPHIC FINDINGS	A large cranial mediastinal soft tissue mass is seen (lateral view only). Hepatomegaly and splenomegaly are present.
FINAL DIAGNOSIS	Lymphoma.

Figure 37-4, B and C

SIGNALMENT	One-year-old spayed female ferret.
HISTORY	Tachypnea, weight loss, and inappetence.
RADIOGRAPHIC FINDINGS	A general increased opacity is present within the thoracic cavity. The cardiac silhouette is obscured by radiographic silhouetting, but the tracheal bifurcation at the hilus is caudally displaced to the ninth intercostal space (*arrow*). Pleural effusion is present in the right side.
FINAL DIAGNOSIS	Cranial mediastinal mass consistent with lymphoma. Pleural effusion.

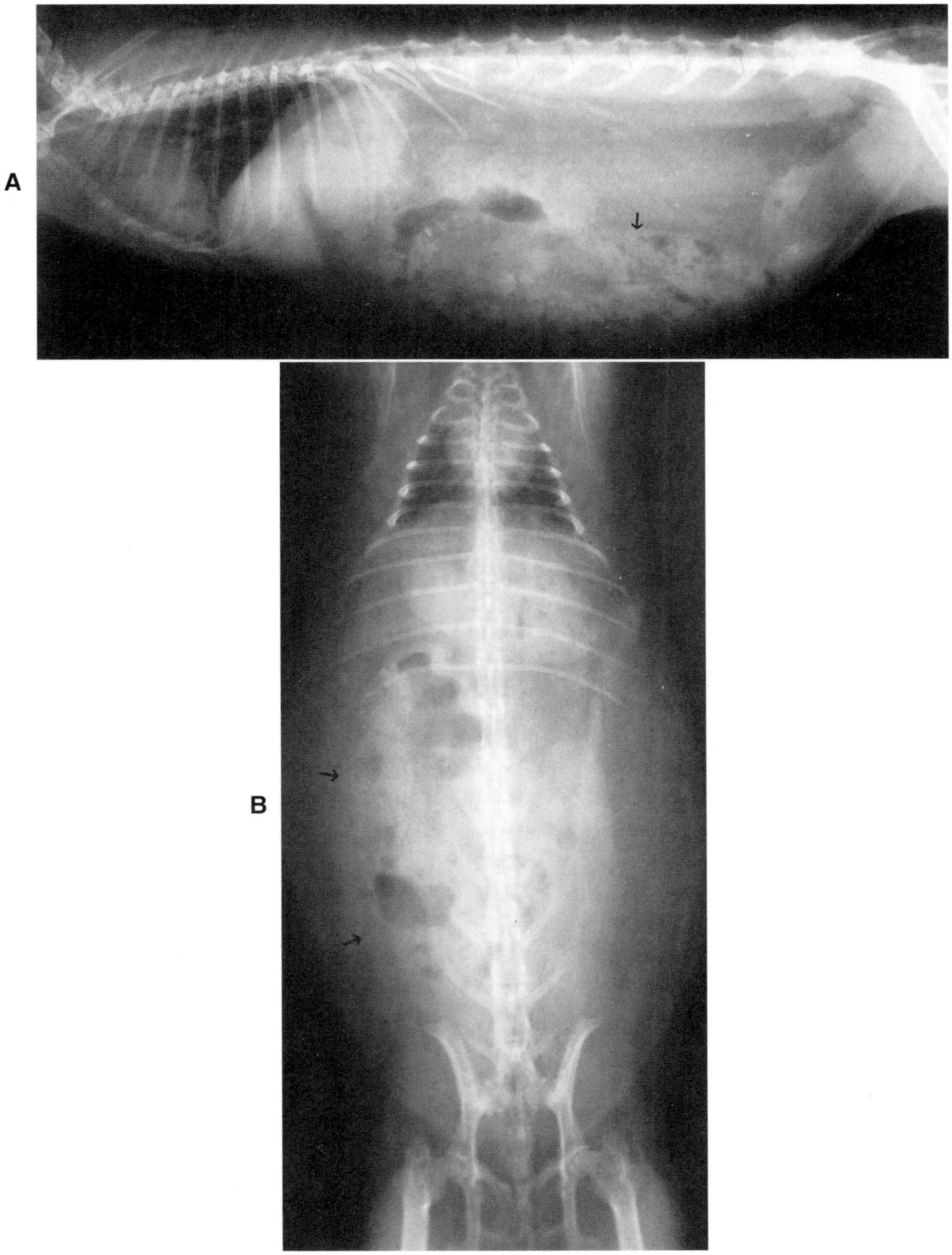

Figure 37-5
A and B, The normal rabbit.

SIGNALMENT Three-year-old intact female rabbit.

RADIOGRAPHIC FINDINGS Body cavity size disparity is again exemplified. The cranial lung lobes are small and poorly visualized. The caudal lung lobes are well aerated. The cecum *(arrows)* is usually seen in the right hemiabdomen and contains varying amounts of gas and ingesta. A large amount of retroperitoneal fat is displacing the kidneys ventrally (lateral view).

A

B

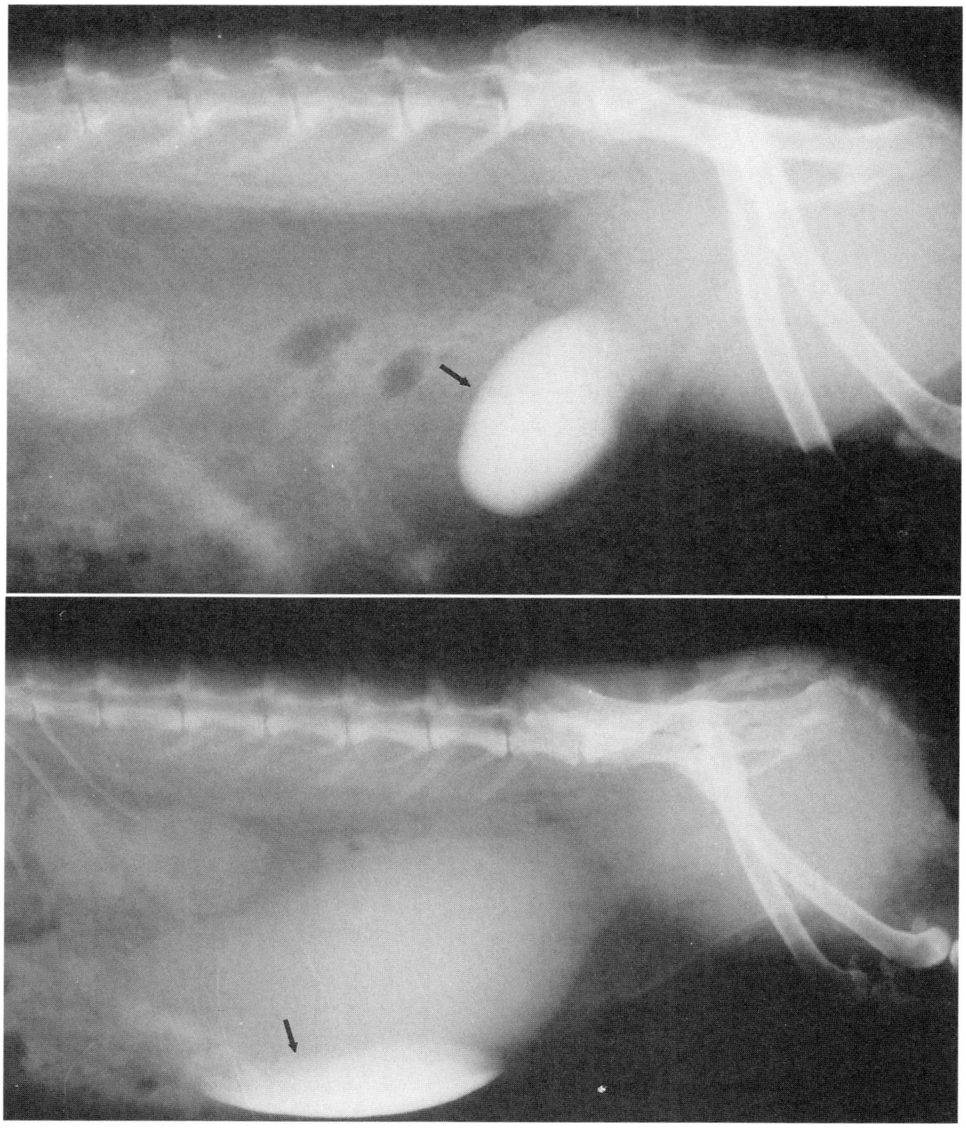

Figure 37-6, A

SIGNALMENT	Three-year-old castrated male rabbit.
HISTORY	White, chalky urine. Fed an alfalfa-rich diet.
RADIOGRAPHIC FINDINGS	The urinary bladder is moderately distended. A homogeneous mineral opacity is present in the bladder (*arrow*).
FINAL DIAGNOSIS	Calciuria caused by hypercalcemia from diet.

Figure 37-6, B

SIGNALMENT	Five-year-old castrated male rabbit.
HISTORY	Urine dribbling and perineal scalding.
RADIOGRAPHIC FINDINGS	The urinary bladder is severely distended and contains a mixture of fluid and mineral opacities. A hyperopaque mineral layer is seen in a nondependent location (*arrow*).
FINAL DIAGNOSIS	Hypotonic urinary bladder. Calciuria with thick, adherent sediment.

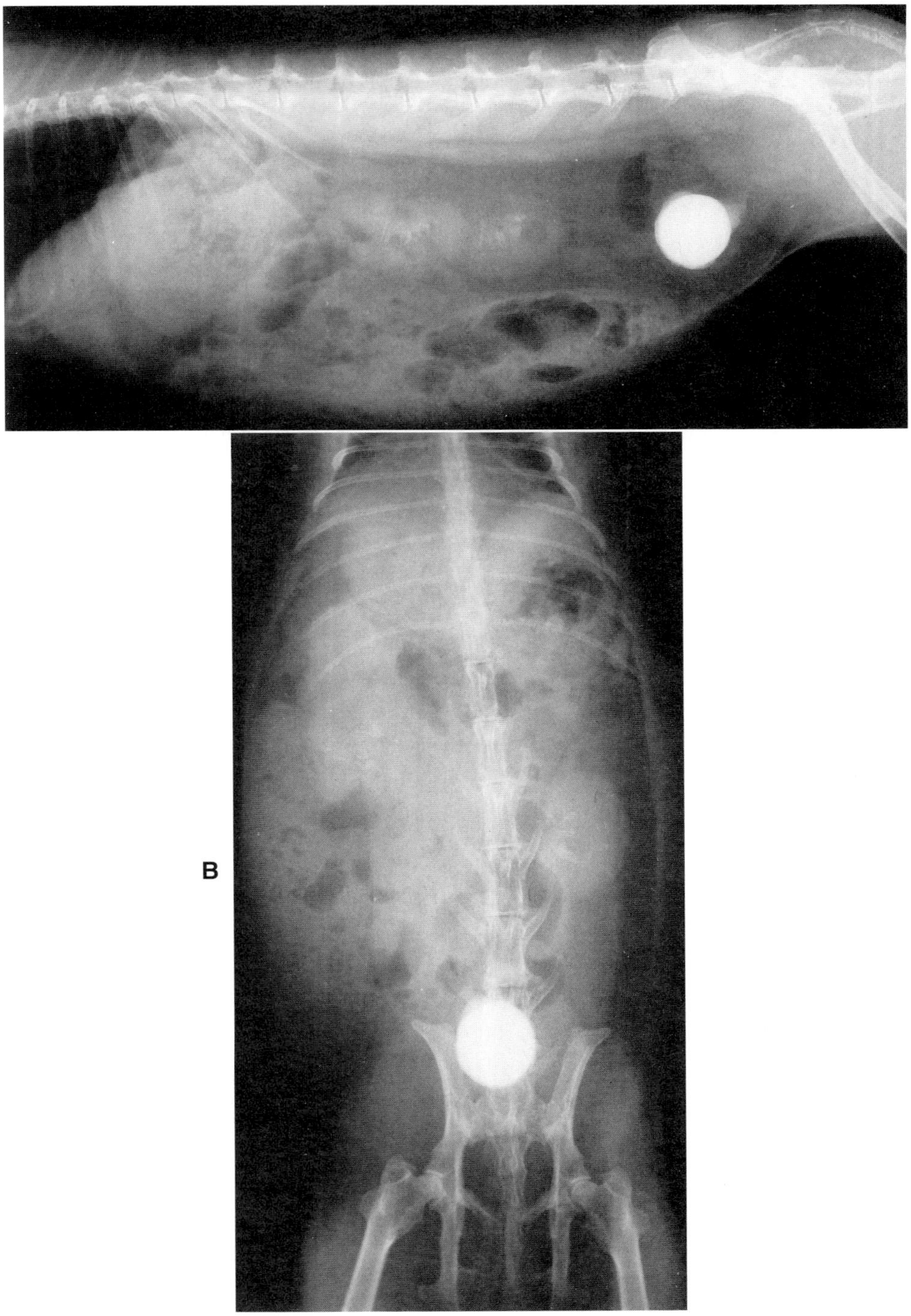

Figure 37-7
A and B.

SIGNALMENT Eight-year-old intact, male dwarf rabbit.

HISTORY Hematuria.

RADIOGRAPHIC FINDINGS A large, round mineral opacity is visible in the caudoventral abdomen, in the same radiographic plane as the urinary bladder. Bilateral renal linear mineral striations are present.

FINAL DIAGNOSIS Cystic calcium oxalate caculus. Bilateral renal diverticular mineralization. Calciuria.

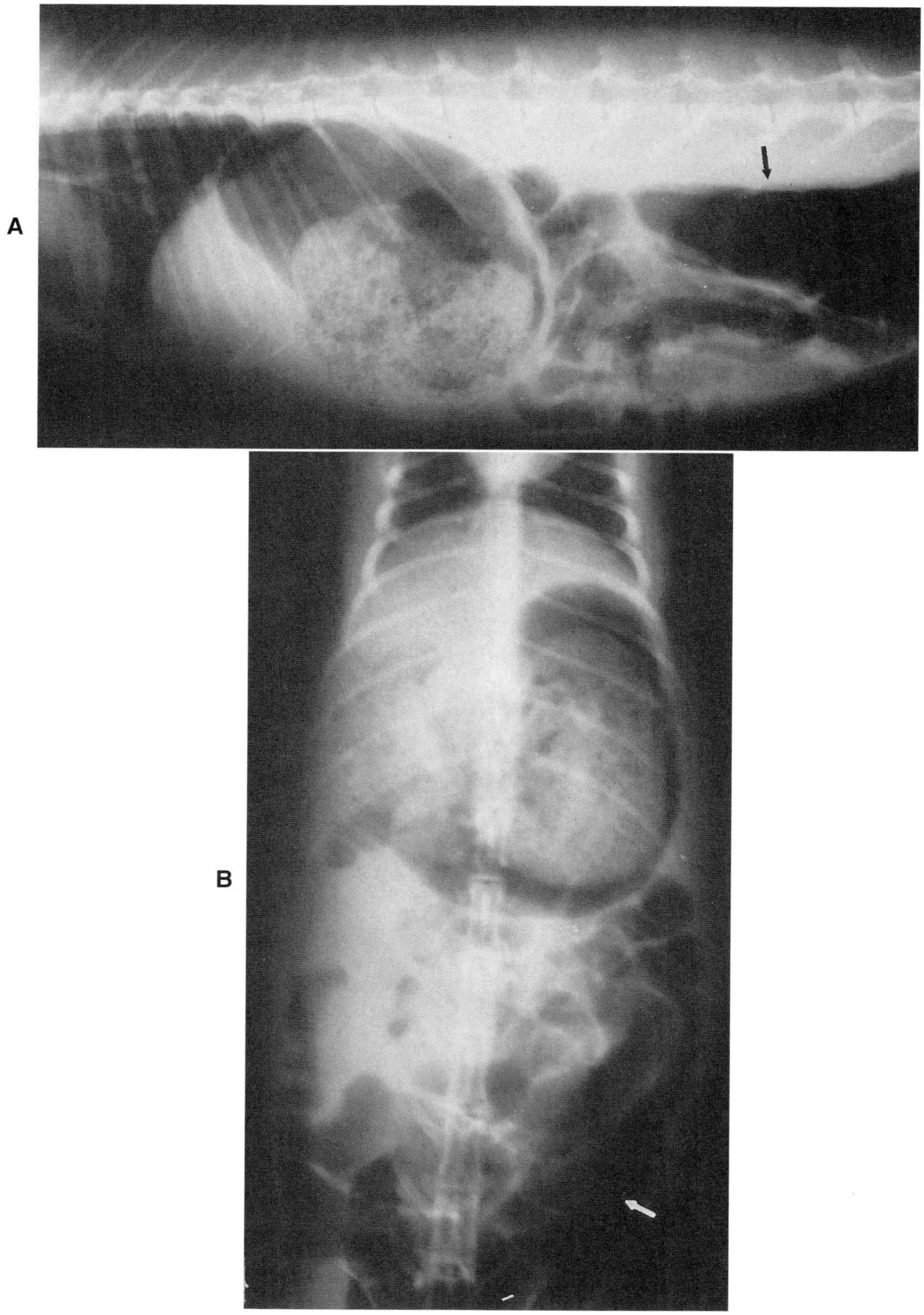

Figure 37-8
A and B.

SIGNALMENT	Three-year-old, intact female dwarf rabbit.
HISTORY	Anorexia, decreased stool excretion, lethargy, and dehydration.
RADIOGRAPHIC FINDINGS	A large intragastric mass is visible, associated with gastric distention and gas accumulation. Multiple intestinal loops are dilated and contain gas. The cecum (*arrow*) is large and gas filled.
FINAL DIAGNOSIS	Gastric stasis. Intestinal ileus. Suspected gastrointestinal hypomotility.

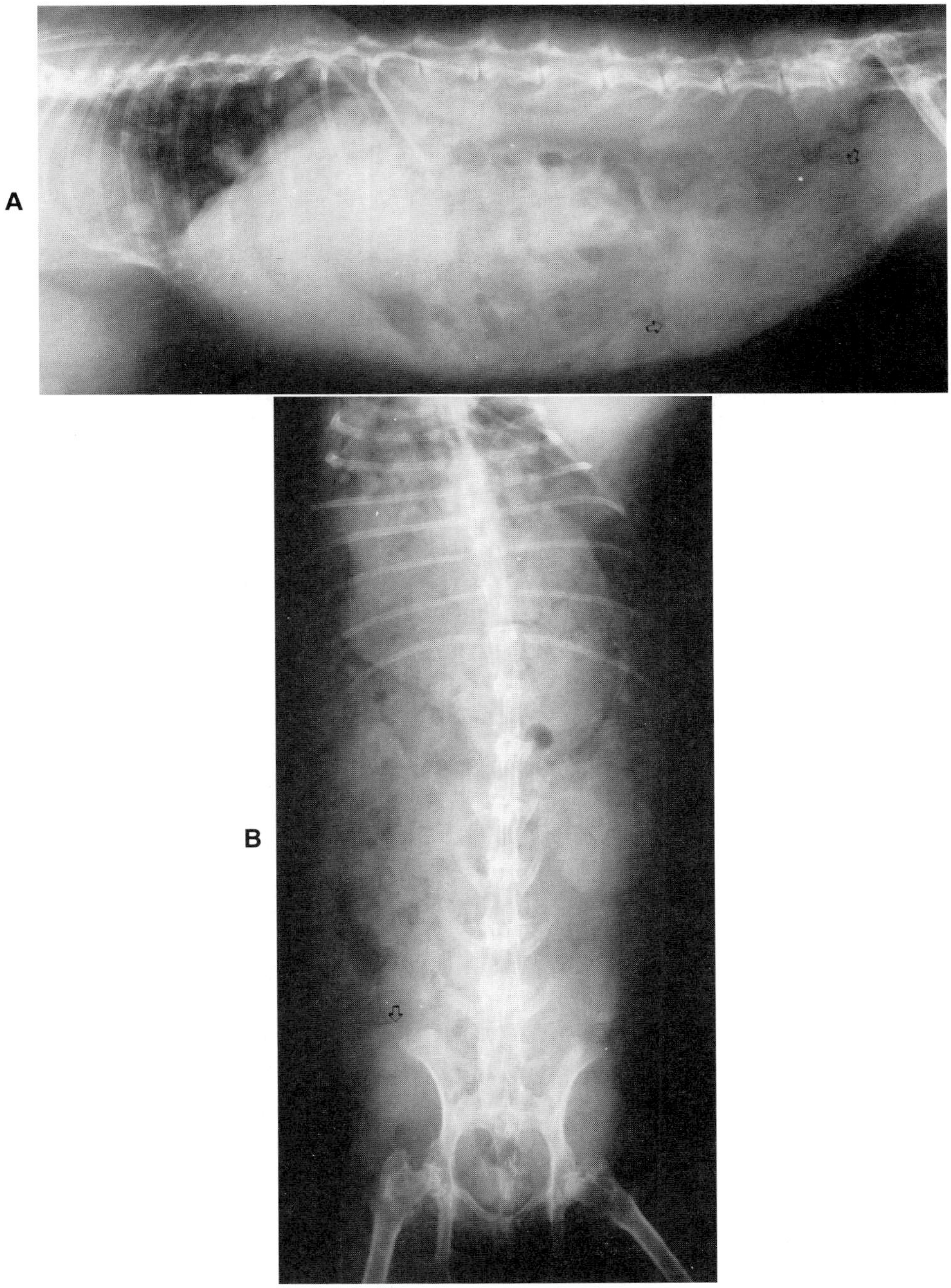

Figure 37-9
A and B.

SIGNALMENT	Five-year-old intact, female lop rabbit.
HISTORY	Large axillary mass.
RADIOGRAPHIC FINDINGS	A large soft tissue mass with mineralization is seen at the left thoracic body wall. A large, tubular soft tissue mass with mineralization is observed in the caudal abdomen (*arrows*). Pulmonary nodules are located throughout the lung lobes.
FINAL DIAGNOSIS	Uterine adenocarcinoma. Pulmonary metastasis.

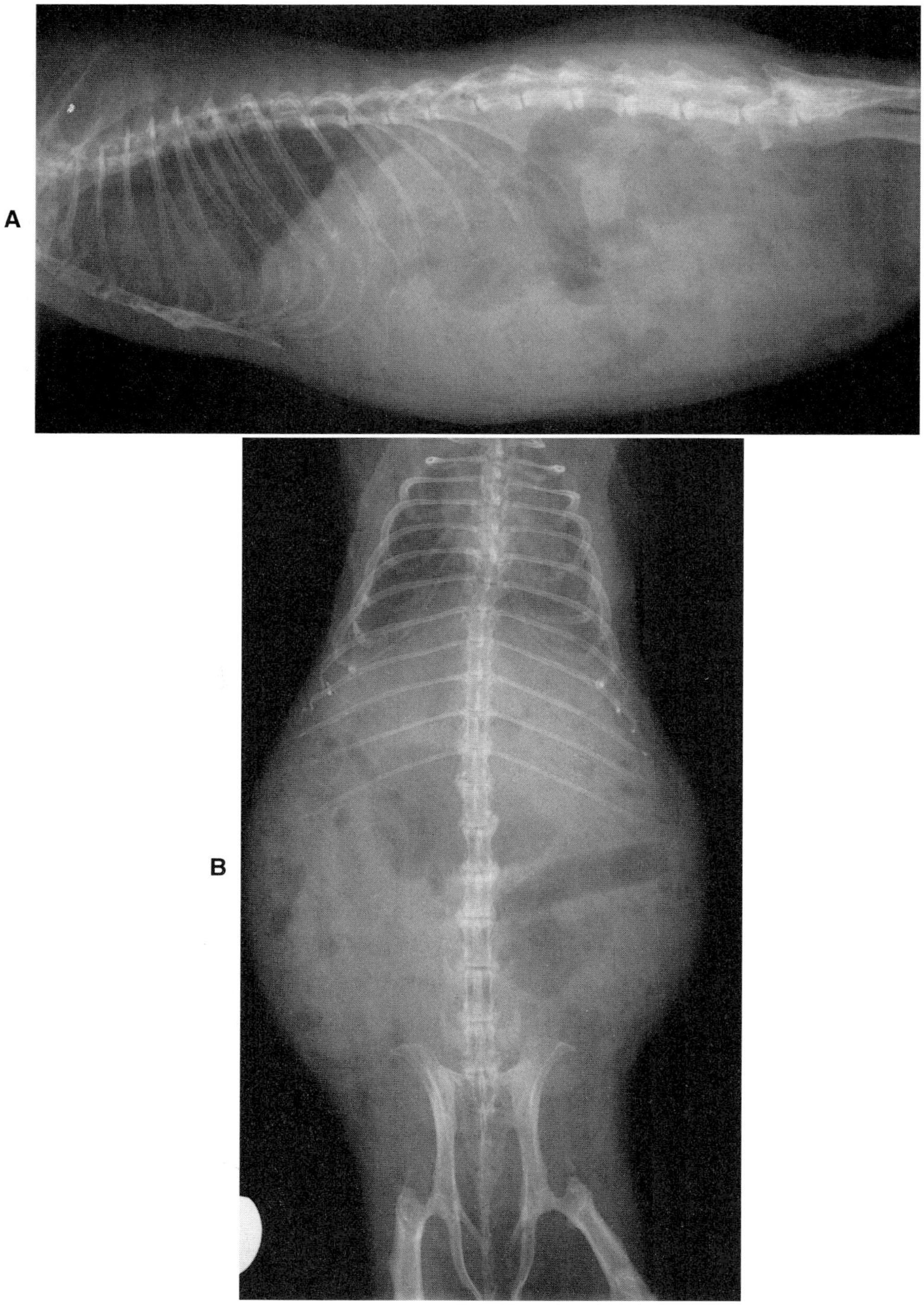

Figure 37-10
A and B, The normal guinea pig.

SIGNALMENT	Two-year-old intact, female guinea pig.
RADIOGRAPHIC FINDINGS	The abdominal cavity is relatively large. The gastrointestinal tract of this herbivore contains varying amounts of ingesta and gas. Because of this, visualization of abdominal viscera is usually poor. The cranial lung lobes are small and typically not well visualized; the caudal lung lobes are large and well aerated.

A

B

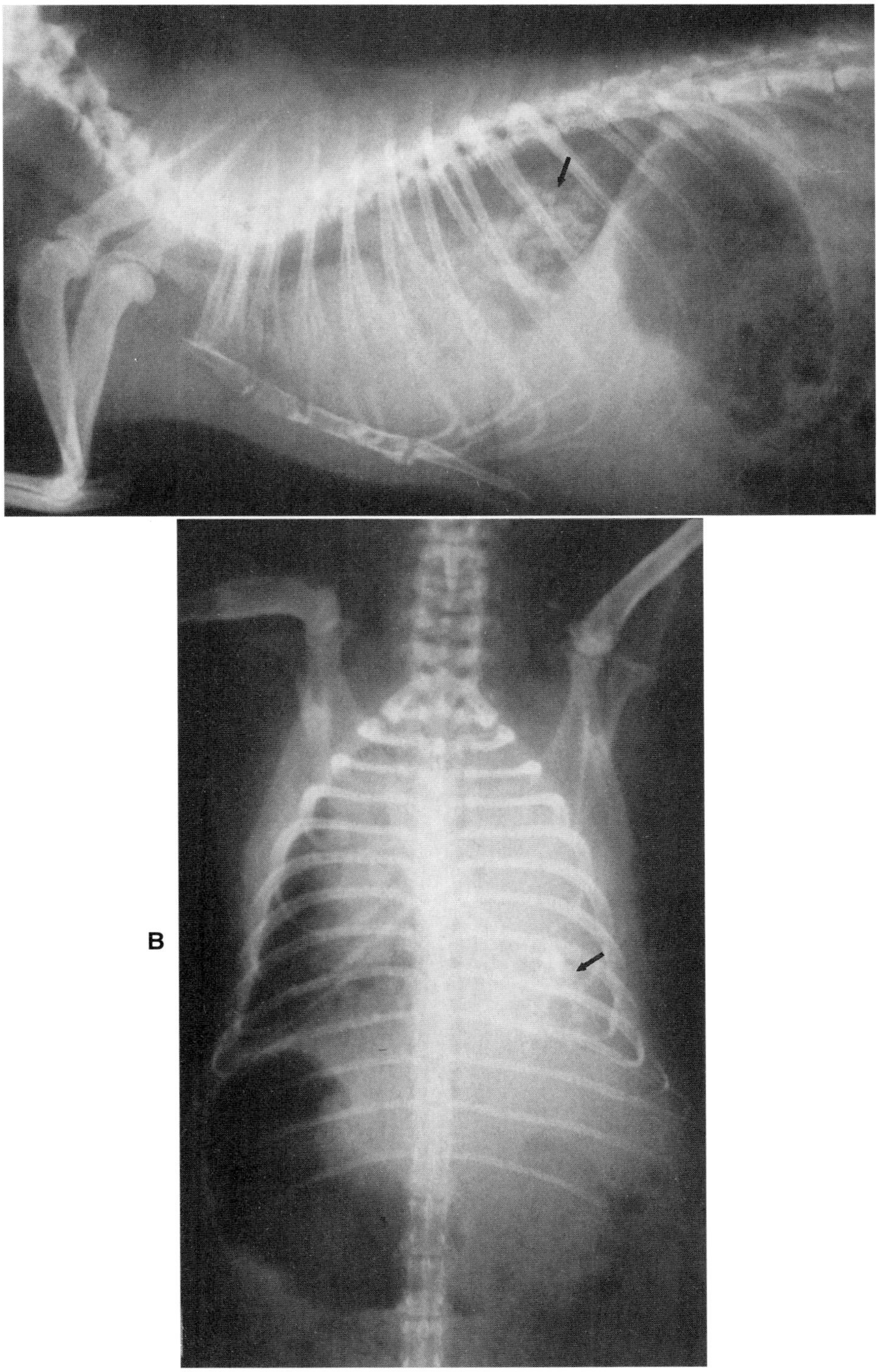

Figure 37-11
A and B.

SIGNALMENT	Two-year-old female guinea pig.
HISTORY	Dyspnea, inappetence, and weight loss.
RADIOGRAPHIC FINDINGS	The right hemithorax has a general increased opacity. Focal mineral opacities are in the right caudal lung lobe area (*arrow*). The cardiac silhouette is obscured on this side.
FINAL DIAGNOSIS	Chronic, calcified, pyogranulomatous pneumonia, right caudal lung lobe.

A
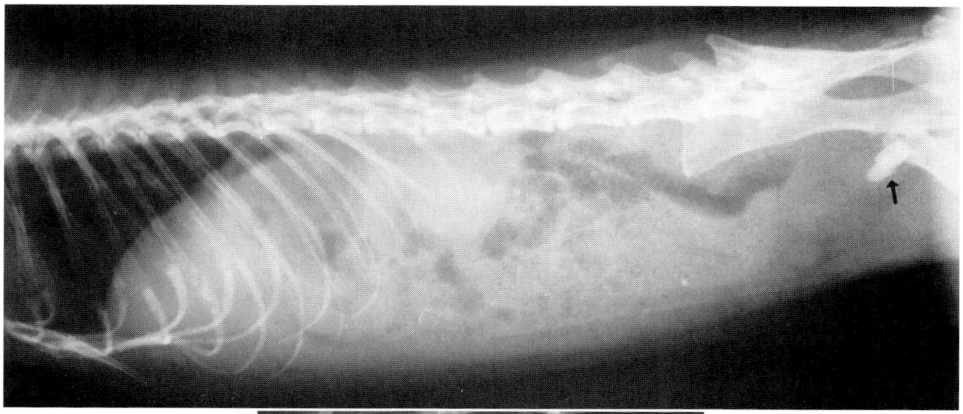

B
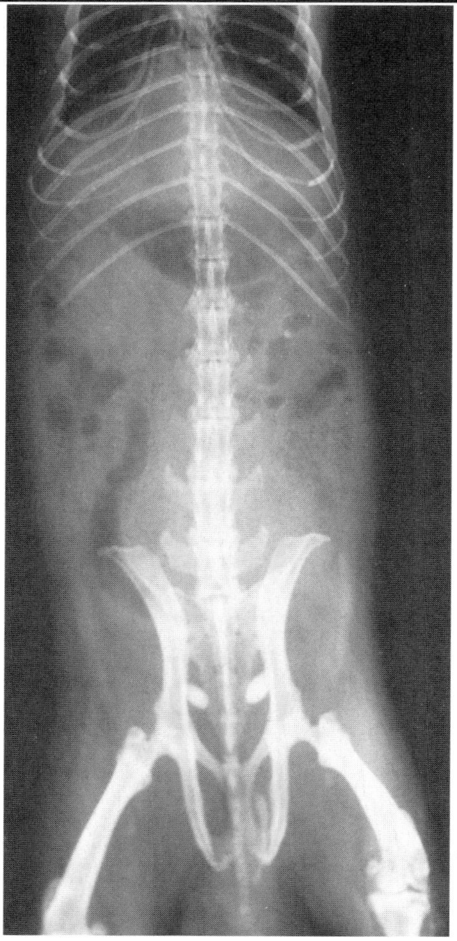

Figure 37-12
A and B.

SIGNALMENT	Five-year-old intact, male guinea pig.
HISTORY	Weight loss and abdominal discomfort.
RADIOGRAPHIC FINDINGS	Oval mineral opacities are present bilaterally in the caudal abdomen, adjacent to the urinary bladder (*arrow*).
FINAL DIAGNOSIS	Bilateral ureteral calcium oxalate calculi.

A

B

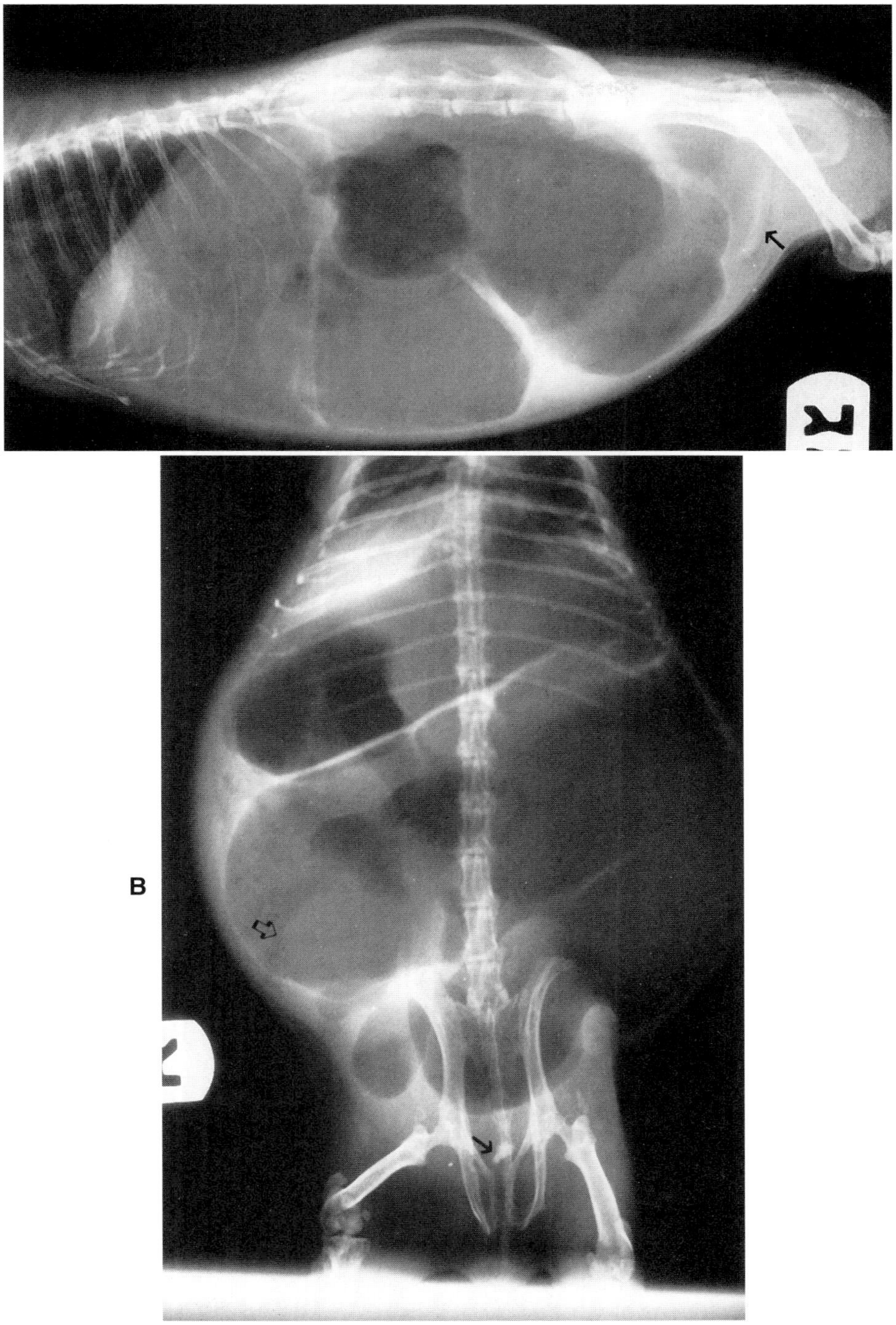

Figure 37-13
A and B.

SIGNALMENT Five-year-old intact, female guinea pig.

HISTORY Distended abdomen and inappetence.

RADIOGRAPHIC FINDINGS The cecum and stomach are severely dilated. In the ventrodorsal view, an oval-shaped soft tissue mass can be seen in the right caudal abdomen (*open arrow*). Mineral opacity is seen in the urinary bladder (*solid arrow*).

FINAL DIAGNOSIS Right cystic ovary. Gastrointestinal dilation of unknown cause. Calciuria.

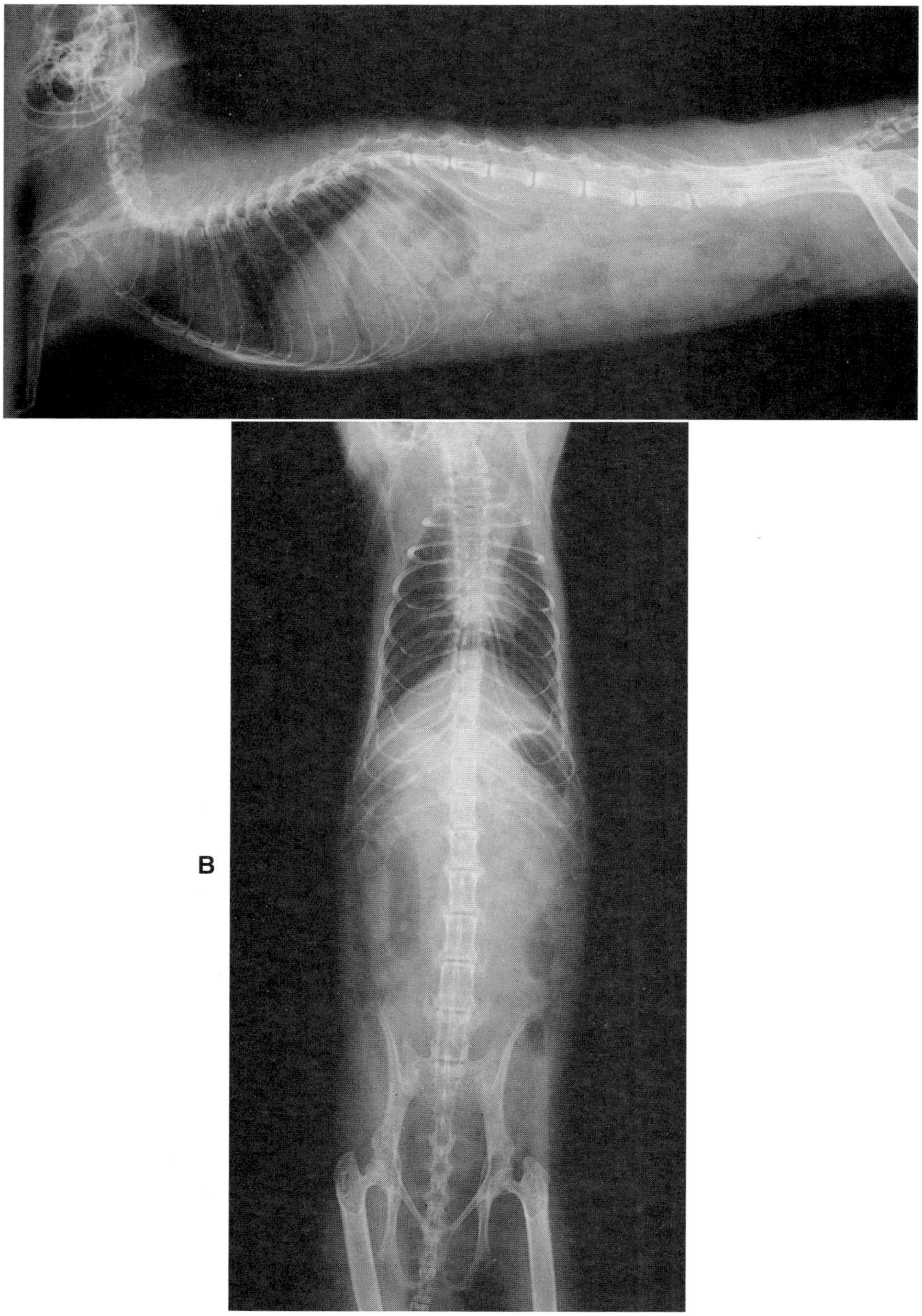

Figure 37-14
A and B, The normal chinchilla.

SIGNALMENT Three-year-old intact, female chinchilla.

RADIOGRAPHIC FINDINGS As in other hindgut fermenters, variable amounts of gastrointestinal gas and ingesta are present in the abdomen, and serosal detail is poor. The small body size allows full survey radiographs. Note the large, thin-walled auditory bullae in the lateral view.

A

B

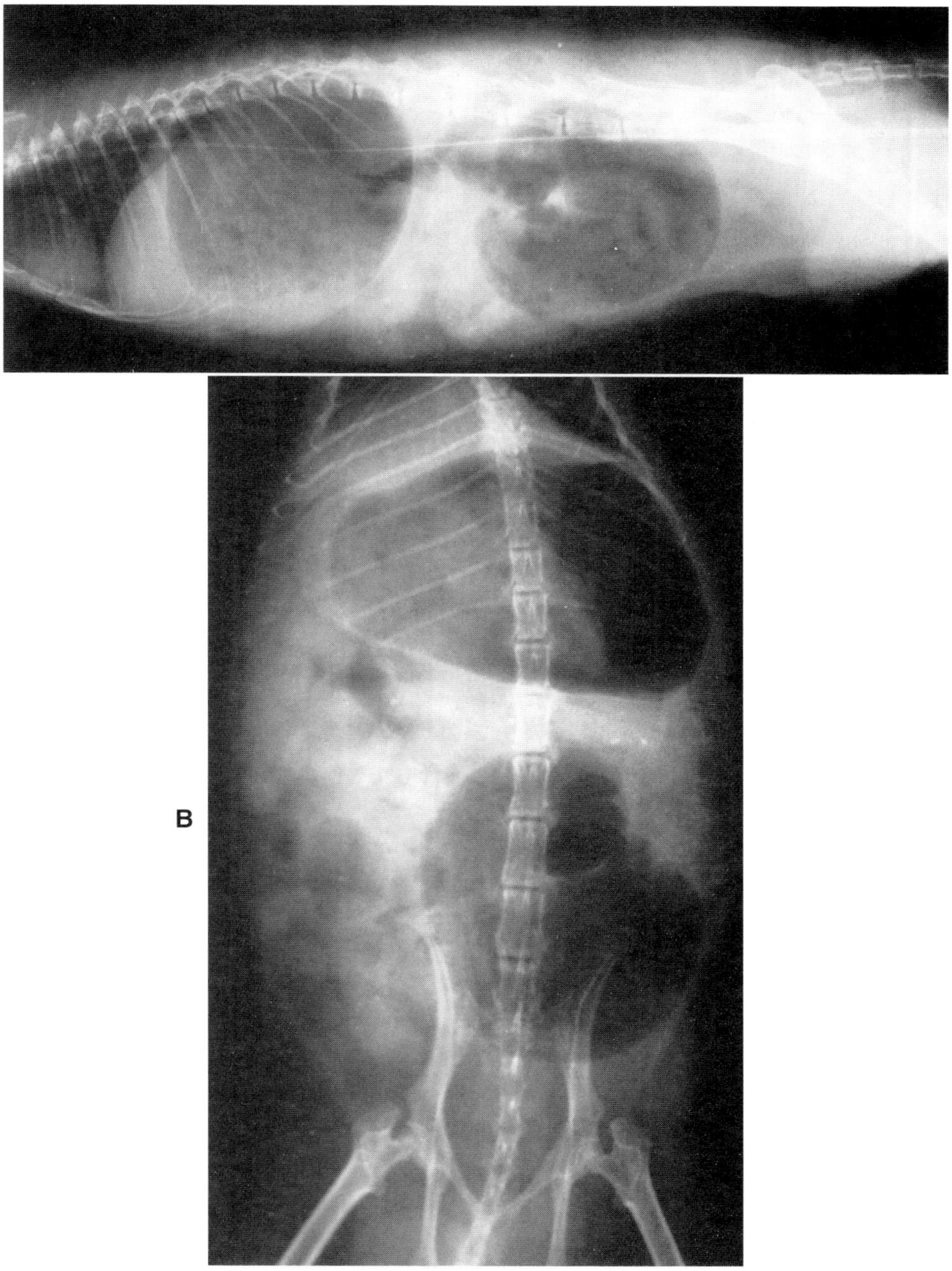

Figure 37-15
A and B.

SIGNALMENT: Four-year-old intact, male chinchilla.

HISTORY: Anorexia and lethargy.

RADIOGRAPHIC FINDINGS: The stomach and cecum are severely dilated. Ingesta is present in the stomach and in much of the small intestinal tract. The linear horizontal white line seen in the lateral view is an artifact.

FINAL DIAGNOSIS: Segmental mechanical ileus of the cecum caused by hairball impaction at the ileocecal junction.

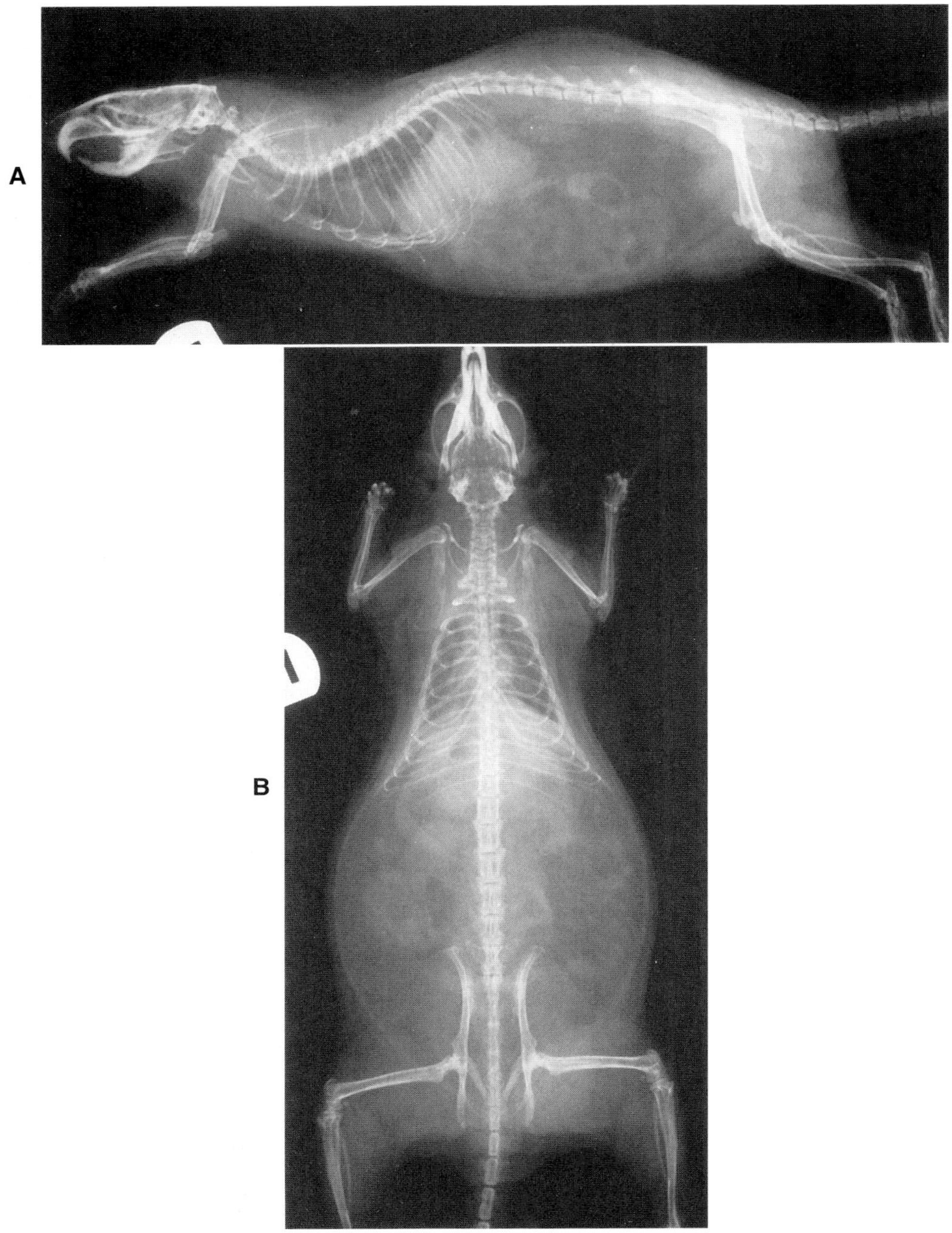

Figure 37-16
A and **B**, The normal rat.

SIGNALMENT Intact female rat, 1.5 years old.

RADIOGRAPHIC FINDINGS A major disparity in body cavity size is observed. The abdomen is much larger than the thorax, making visualization of thoracic structures difficult. The heart and caudal lung lobes are seen and can be evaluated. Feces and a small amount of gas are in the large intestine. Isoflurane anesthesia was used for restraint.

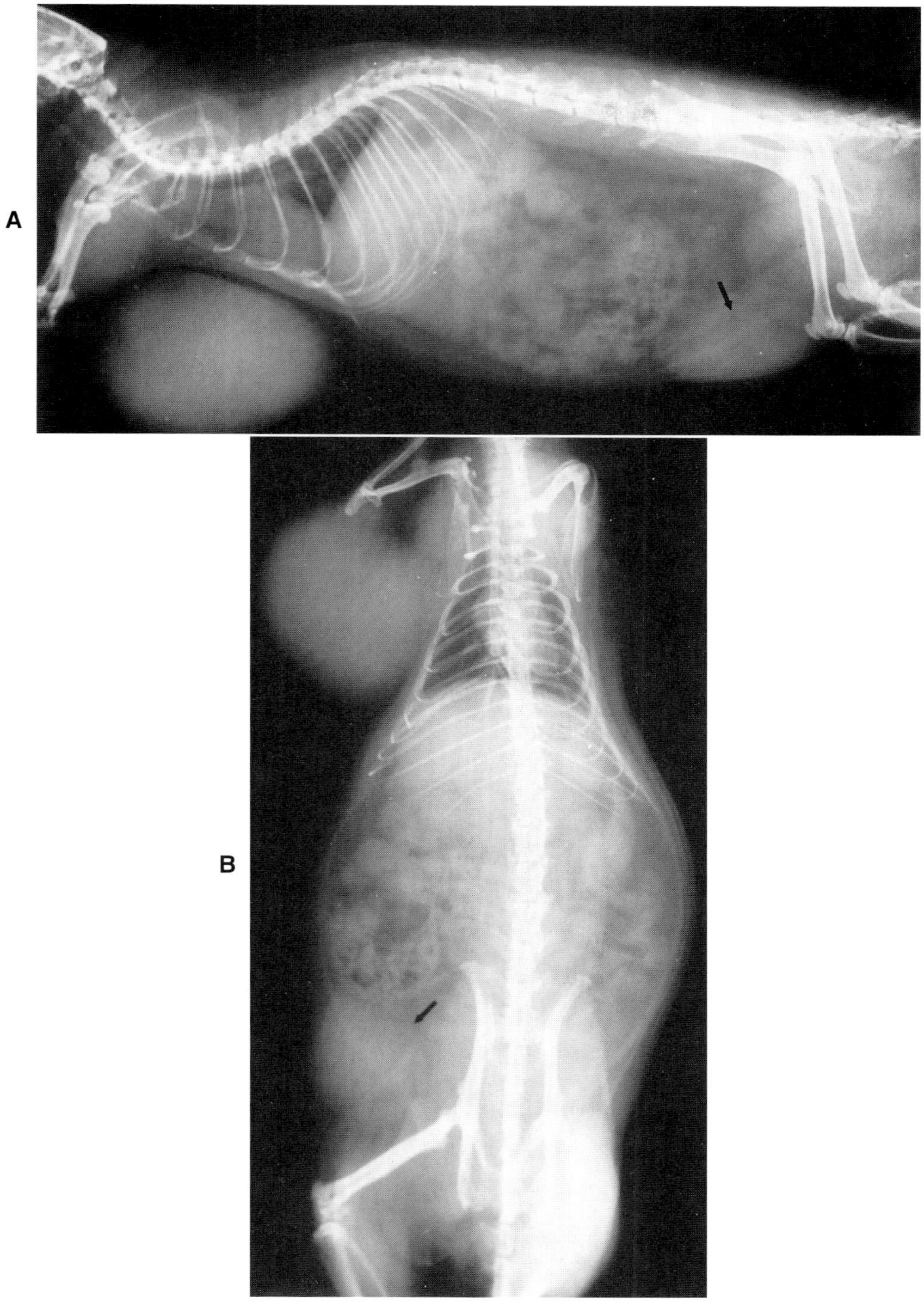

Figure 37-17
A and B.

SIGNALMENT Female rat, 1.5 years old.

HISTORY Rapidly enlarging axillary mass.

RADIOGRAPHIC FINDINGS A large, round soft tissue mass is seen in the right axillary region. A second, similar, smaller mass is present in the right caudoventral body wall (*arrow*).

FINAL DIAGNOSIS Mammary gland adenocarcinoma.

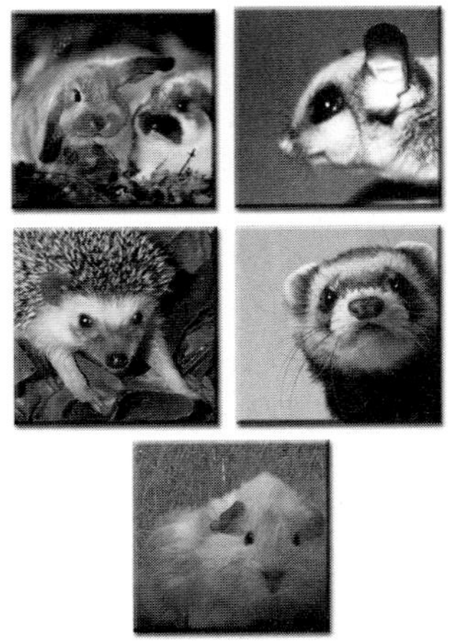

CHAPTER 38

Cytology and Hematology of Small Mammals

James Walberg, DVM, Diplomate ACVP, and
Andrew S. Loar, DVM, Diplomate ACVIM

This chapter provides photomicrographs and other information for practitioners and technicians on selected topics in cytology and hematology of small mammals. Most of the conditions described can be accurately diagnosed in-house without the delay and expense inherent with a commercial laboratory. Many pathologists are not comfortable with interpreting cytologic preparations from these animals, in part because they may not be familiar with many of their clinical diseases.

The same principles of cytology used in other animals can be applied to small mammals. A few references specifically address hematology and cytology in small mammals[6,8,13,14]; however, information in cytology texts that primarily pertain to dogs and cats is also easily applied to these species.[1,2,11] For example, an excellent reference on cutaneous lesions is found in a text concerning dog and cat dermatology.[12]

For some instances of infectious diseases in this chapter, material from other species was used. The organisms are the same, independent of the infected species. Wright's, Gram, and acid-fast stains are used in these photomicrographs. We do not use Diff-Quik or other forms of three-step quick stains for the following reasons: (1) Diff-Quick–type stains are expensive and labor intensive when especially large numbers of slides are being stained; (2) Diff-Quik stains can be easily contaminated with bacteria and fungal elements (e.g., thick smears or those that have not dried allow for contamination of the stain in the Copland jars); and (3) Diff-Quik staining is sometimes unpredictable, and these stains may produce a variable staining of mast cell granules.

Most photomicrographs were taken under immersion oil (100× lens) so that optimum details can be shown. The diagnosis can often be made on 40× magnification. For best optical resolution on 40× magnification (high dry), place immersion oil on the stained dried smear, then place a rectangular glass coverslip on the drop of oil. The slide can be evaluated on high dry (40× lens) without getting oil on the lens. If you wish to use the 100× lens, remove the coverslip or place a drop of oil on top of the coverslip.

REFERENCES

1. Baker R, Lumsden JH: Color Atlas of Cytology of the Dog and Cat. St Louis, Mosby, 2000.
2. Cowell RL, Tyler RD, Meinkoth JH: Diagnostic Cytology and Hematology of the Dog and Cat, 2nd ed. St Louis, Mosby, 1999.
3. Edwards DF: Actinomycosis and nocardiosis. *In* Green CE, ed. Infectious Diseases of the Dog and Cat, 2nd ed. Philadelphia, WB Saunders, 1998, pp 303-313.
4. Erdman SE, Li X, Fox JG: Hematopoietic diseases. *In* Fox JG, ed. Biology and Diseases of the Ferret, 2nd ed. Philadelphia, Williams & Wilkins, 1998, pp 231-246.
5. Fox JG: Bacterial and mycoplasmal diseases. *In* Fox JG, ed. Biology and Diseases of the Ferret, 2nd ed. Philadelphia, Williams & Wilkins, 1998, pp 321-354.
6. Fudge AM, ed: Laboratory Medicine: Avian and Exotic Pets. Philadelphia, WB Saunders, 2000.
7. Greene CE: *Clostridium perfringens* infection. *In* Greene CE, ed. Infectious Diseases of the Dog and Cat, 2nd ed. Philadelphia, WB Saunders, 1998, pp 243-248.
8. Hawkey CM, Dennett TB: Comparative Veterinary Hematology. Ames, Iowa State University Press, 1989.
9. Manning PJ, Wagner JE, Harkness JE: Biology and diseases of guinea pigs. *In* Fox JG, Cohen BJ, Loew FM, eds. Laboratory Animal Medicine. Orlando, Academic Press, 1984, pp 149-181.
10. Moore DM: Hematology of the guinea pig (*Cavia porcellus*). *In* Feldman BF, Zinkl JG, Jain NC, eds. Schalm's Veterinary Hematology, 5th ed. Philadelphia, Lippincott Williams & Wilkins, 2000, pp 1107-1110.
11. Raskin RE, Meyer DJ: Atlas of Canine and Feline Cytology. Philadelphia, WB Saunders, 2001.
12. Scott DW, Miller WH, Griffin CE: Dermatoses of pet rodents, rabbits, and ferrets. *In* Scott DW, Miller WT, Griffin CE, eds. Muller and Kirk's Small Animal Dermatology, 6th ed. Philadelphia, WB Saunders, 2001, pp 1415-1458.
13. Smith CA, Andrews CM, Collard JK, et al: Color Atlas of Comparative, Diagnostic, and Experimental Hematology. London, Wolfe Publishing, 1994.
14. Smith SA: Specific species appropriate hematology. *In* Feldman BF, Zinkl JG, Jain NC, eds. Schalm's Veterinary Hematology, 5th ed. Philadelphia, Lippincott Williams & Wilkins, 2000, pp 1096-1119.
15. Walton RM, Hendrick MJ: Feline Hodgkin's-like lymphoma: 20 cases (1992-1999). Vet Pathol 2001; 38:504-511.

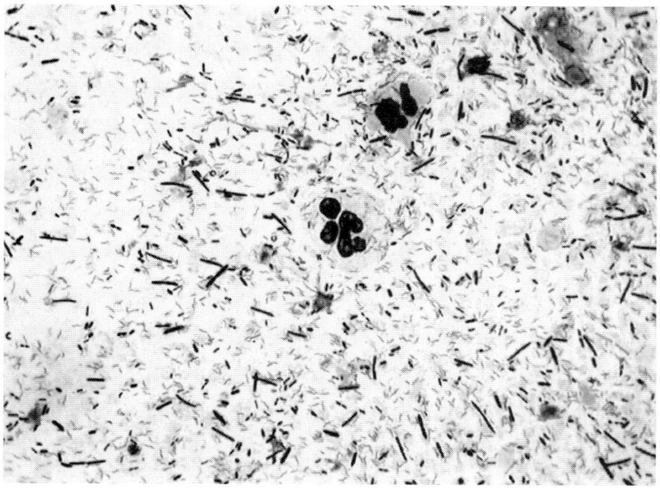

Figure 38-1 *Campylobacter* species: canine fecal smear (Wright's stain, ×100). This fecal smear shows numerous *Campylobacter* species organisms (lighter-staining smaller bacteria), a mixed population of bacterial rods, and two degenerating neutrophils. The characteristic "gull wing" formations (visible on the surface of the neutrophil) are chains of three to five of these slender, gram-negative, comma-shaped or curved motile rods. The organisms have the same morphologic characteristics in all species of animals. *Campylobacter* are often overlooked because of their small size. Animals can be carriers, in which case usually only very low numbers are seen. These organisms can be either the primary cause of diarrhea or act as secondary pathogens in conjunction with other enteric bacteria. *Campylobacter* species are difficult to culture. Neutrophils are not seen in normal stool and indicate an active infection. *Campylobacter jejuni-coli* is zoonotic.[5]

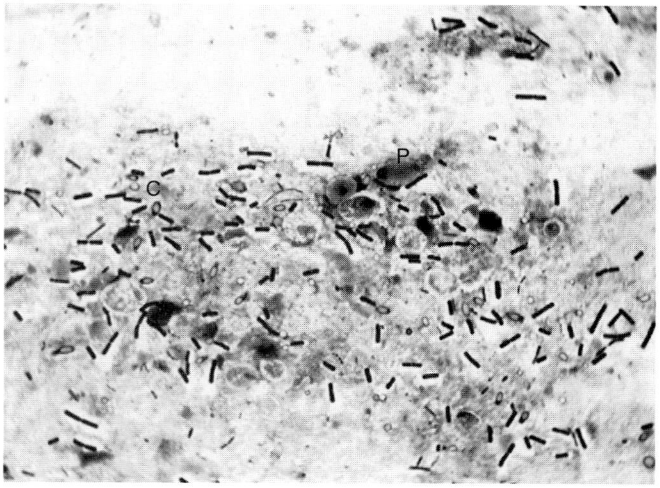

Figure 38-2 *Clostridium* species: ferret fecal smear (Gram stain, ×100). Numerous spore-forming clostridial organisms (likely *C. perfringens*) are seen. *Clostridium* species are gram-positive, anaerobic bacilli with clear, round to ovoid spores that bulge when they sporulate. Depending on where the spore is located, clostridial organisms have been described as having "safety pin" or "tennis racket" morphologic features. In its vegetative state, *C. perfringens* is a normal inhabitant of the gastrointestinal tract. However, when it undergoes endogenous sporulation, it releases enterotoxin that can result in watery to mucohemorrhagic diarrhea. Endogenous sporulation can occur after antimicrobial therapy or in conjunction with an alkaline environment, viral enteritis, alterations in diet, and immunosuppression. More than five spore-forming bacteria per oil immersion field are significant. Food can also be the source of enterotoxin, in which case the feces would not contain the sporulated bacteria (exogenous enterotoxication). Commercial tests are available that identify clostridial toxin (latex agglutination, enzyme-linked immunosorbent assay, and polymerase chain reaction).[7] *C*, Clostridial spore; *P*, unidentified protozoal cyst.

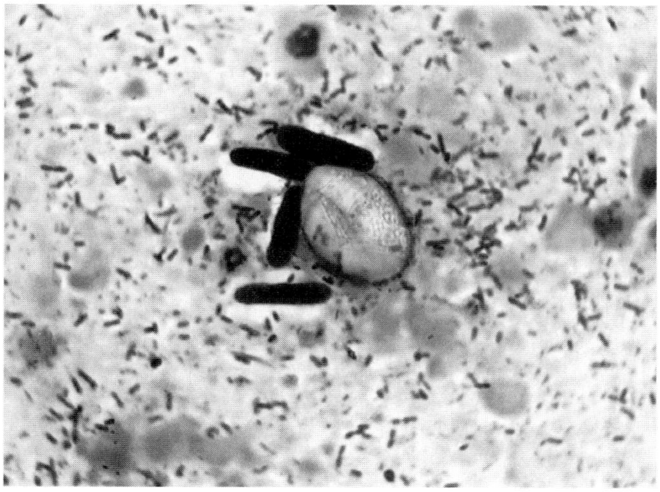

Figure 38-3 *Saccharomyces* species: rabbit fecal smear (Gram stain, ×100). This slide demonstrates four yeast organisms, *Cyniclomyces guttulatus* (more commonly referred to as *Saccharomyces* species), and one *Eimeria* protozoal cyst. *C. guttulatus* is a normal inhabitant of the cecum of rabbits and is a member of the Saccharomyces family. This gram-positive yeast can be seen in direct smears and fecal flotations and is sometimes mistaken for protozoa. Bacteria in this photo are in a different plane and appear out of focus.

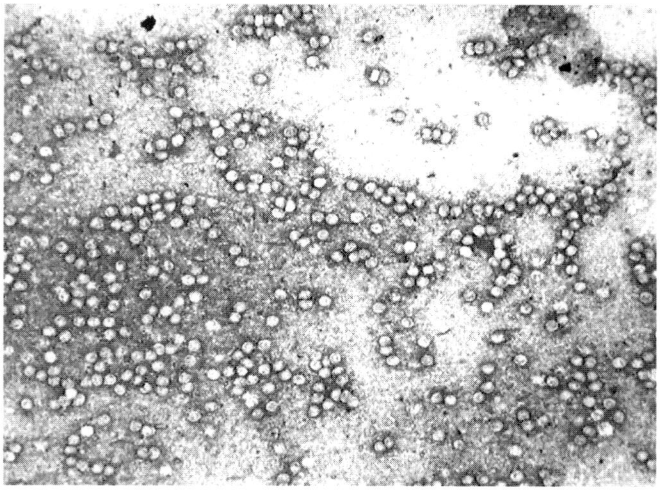

Figure 38-4 *Cryptosporidium* species: fecal smear (Wright's stain [also Plate 9, acid-fast stain], ×40). Numerous *Cryptosporidium* species oocysts are visible. When *Cryptosporidium* cause diarrhea, the organisms are numerous and easy to see. These protozoal cysts, 4 to 7 μm in diameter, are approximately the size of a red blood cell and are weakly acid-fast positive (Plate 9).

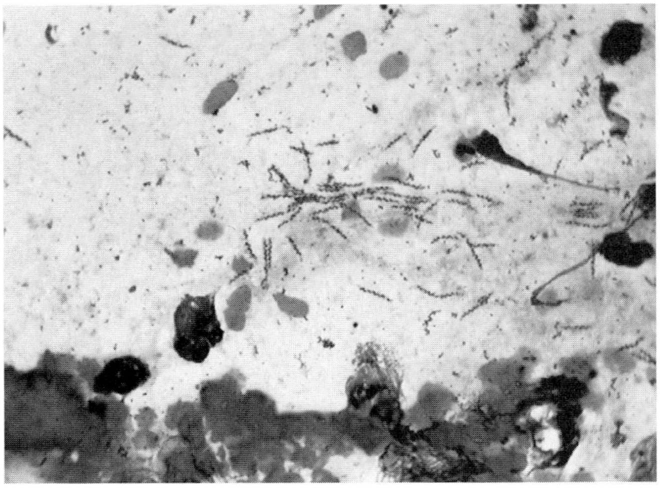

Figure 38-5 *Helicobacter* species: imprint from feline gastric mucus (Diff-Quik stain, ×100). These are typical *Helicobacter* bacteria. *Helicobacter* species are gram-negative, curved to spiral-shaped bacteria. There is more than one morphologic type. This figure shows the distinctive spiral-shaped form measuring 7 to 10 μm in length. *Helicobacter* species are easy to identify morphologically but extremely difficult to grow on culture media. Even with selective media, oral bacteria or reflux bacteria from the duodenum often overgrow these fastidious organisms. In our experience, the spiral form is easily discerned in cytologic preparations from dogs and cats but not from ferrets. Possibly, the long spiral form is not very common in ferrets (J. W. personal observation); thus methods other than cytologic examination should be used for diagnosis. A diagnosis of *Helicobacter* infection is made either by demonstrating the bacteria in cytologic preparations or by identifying the histologic lesion of follicular gastritis in endoscopic biopsy samples. An indirect diagnosis can be made by obtaining a positive result of a urea test on a fresh, unfixed biopsy specimen. *Helicobacter* species produce large amounts of urease, a feature of the organism used in commercial test kits for in-house testing. Commercially available urea slants are less expensive and can be substituted for the commercial kits (PML Microbiologicals, Wilsonville, OR). The slants are yellow/orange and change to pink/red, often within an hour after the organism has been added. The urea slant test detects any urease-producing bacteria, and a positive result is only presumptive for *Helicobacter* species. A biopsy sample of an affected stomach typically reveals chronic (lymphocytic) follicular gastritis.[5]

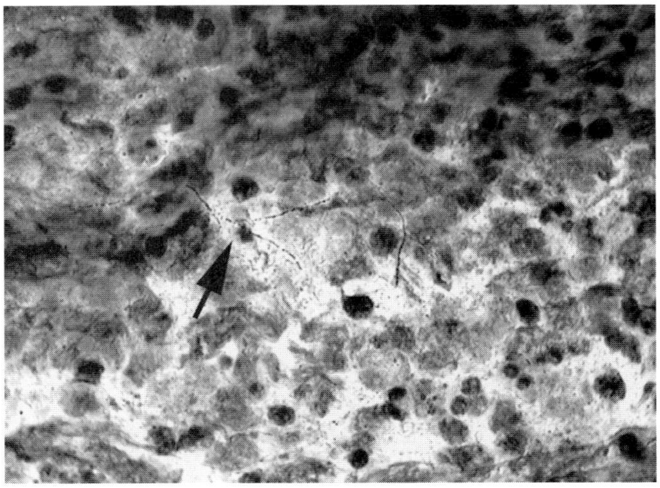

Figure 38-6 *Actinomyces* species: aspirate of a mandibular abscess from a rabbit (Wright's stain, ×100). Most of the cells are necrotic and cannot be identified (granules of heterophils are faintly visible). The bacterium here (*arrow*) is gram positive, branching, beaded, and filamentous, typical of *Actinomyces* species. These bacteria are anaerobic or microaerophilic and do not readily grow without special conditions (may take up to 2 weeks) and thus the incidence is likely underreported. Cytologic examination is especially useful in identifying this organism. *Actinomyces* species are generally seen in conjunction with other bacteria.[3]

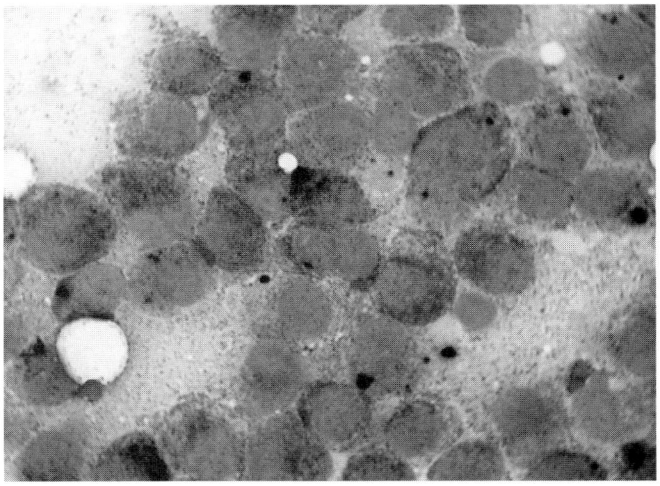

Figure 38-7 Melanoma: aspirate of a cutaneous neoplasm from a hamster (Wright's stain, ×100). This round cell tumor (also known as a *discrete cell* because the cell membrane is distinct) contains blackish granules in the cytoplasm and the background. The nuclei vary in size and have prominent nucleoli (nucleoli are not well seen in the black-and-white photos) and a stippled nuclear chromatin pattern. Melanomas occur in many species and can have variable amounts of melanin in the cytoplasm. Melanin must be demonstrated to make a definitive diagnosis. Sometimes so much pigment is present that it appears as if black ink has been aspirated. At the other extreme, amelanotic melanomas contain no or very little melanin. Melanomas are the most frequently reported cutaneous tumors in hamsters.[12]

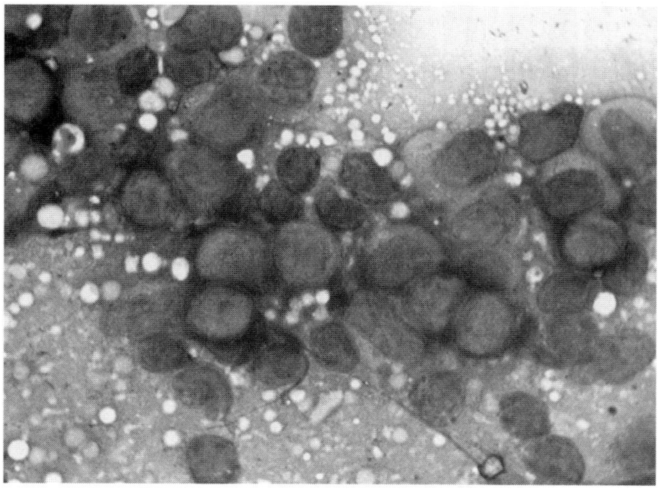

Figure 38-8 Cutaneous lymphoma: aspirate of a cutaneous neoplasm from a ferret (Wright's stain, ×100). This round cell tumor contains no granules in the cytoplasm. These cells show anisokaryosis and occasionally prominent nucleoli. The chromatin pattern varies from stippled to clumped. The clumping is uniform in one cell and may indicate reduplicated chromatin before mitosis or abnormal numbers of chromosomes (polyploidy). Note the pale basophilic background with lipid droplets suggestive of either lymph fluid or cytoplasm from lysed cells. This aspirate is from a ferret that had a previous diagnosis of visceral lymphosarcoma and suddenly developed numerous cutaneous nodules. Cutaneous lymphosarcoma, which involves the epidermis and ulcerates, is typically T-cell lymphoma (sometimes called mycosis fungoides or epitheliotropic lymphosarcoma), whereas cutaneous lymphoma that is subcutaneous (extranodal) can be either B- or T-cell lymphoma (J. W. personal observation). Samples from round cell tumors that are nondiagnostic on cytologic examination can be stained by immunoperoxidase methods to further characterize the tumor.

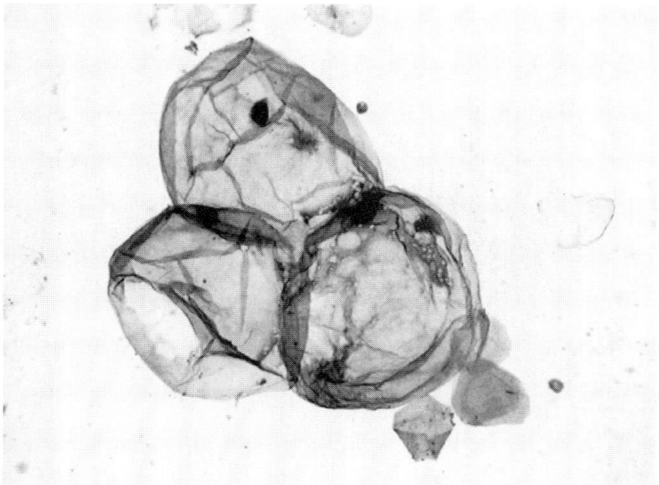

Figure 38-10 Lipoma: aspirate of a subcutaneous mass from a guinea pig (Wright's stain, ×40). Lipomas occur in most mammals. Because of the large size and thin cytoplasmic membrane, these cells often rupture, leaving only oily fat droplets. Lipocytes can be seen singly or in clumps. Notice the wrinkled cytoplasm, probably caused by the alcohol-based stain that dehydrates the cell. Fat accumulates around lymph nodes and may be all that is retrieved from a lymph node aspirate in small mammals.

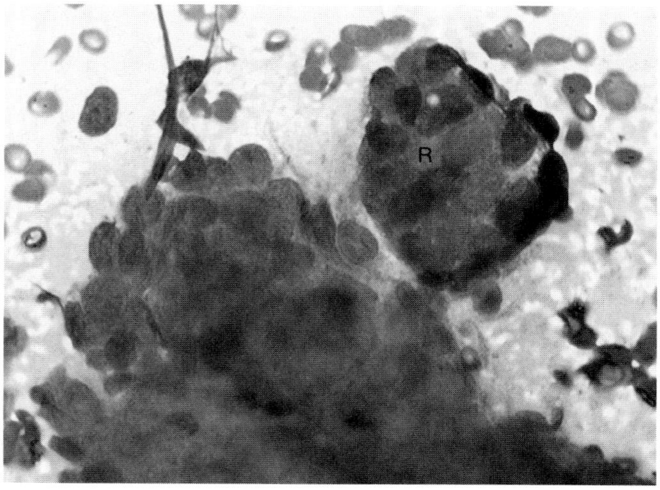

Figure 38-9 Carcinoma: aspirate of a cutaneous neoplasm from a hamster (Wright's stain, ×100). Carcinoma cells exfoliate in cohesive clusters and often stain darkly. In contrast to round cell tumors, individual cells may be difficult to identify. In the upper right of the photo, a rosette, or acinar structure, with nuclei arranged in a circle around a central lumen, is present. These structures suggest the tissue is of glandular epithelial origin.

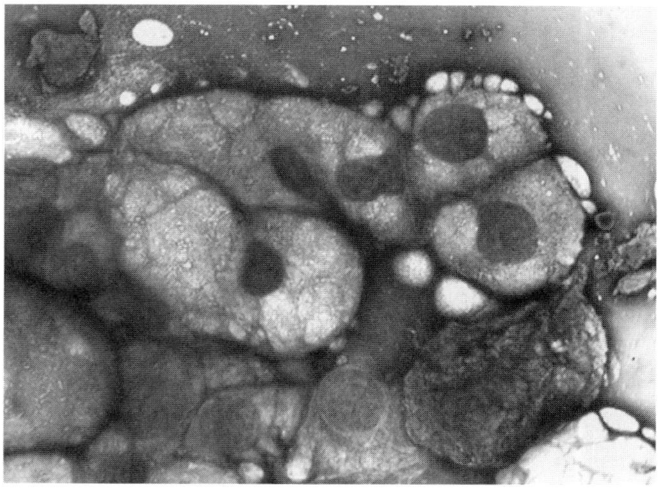

Figure 38-11 Chordoma: imprint from a lesion on the tail of a ferret (Wright's stain, ×100). The large foamy cells are referred to as *physaliferous cells* and are distinctive of chordoma. A characteristic amphophilic/cartilaginous matrix is also present. The incidence of chordomas is higher in ferrets than in other animals. Chordomas are also reported in rats, cats, and humans and are thought to originate from primitive notochord tissue, possibly within an intervertebral disc. Although chordomas most commonly involve the tail, they have been reported in the cervical spine of ferrets. They can be locally invasive. Metastases have only been reported in rats.

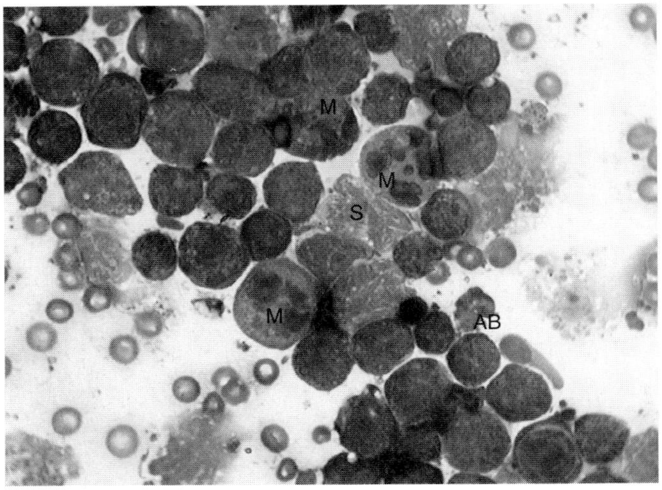

Figure 38-12 Lymphosarcoma: abdominal fluid from a ferret with multicentric lymphosarcoma (Wright's stain, ×100). When lymphosarcoma exfoliates into body cavities, the fluid is generally very highly cellular and contains a monotypic population of immature atypical lymphoid cells. This field has at least three mitotic figures. Notice the coarse stippling and irregular clumping of nuclear chromatin and the dark blue cytoplasm. Dark blue cytoplasm is typically a feature of lymphoblasts, whereas clumping of nuclear chromatin is generally associated with maturity (asynchrony of nucleus and cytoplasm). Smudge cells are also visible and can be associated with necrosis or damage of cells during sampling. An apoptotic body (fragment of a dying cell containing both nuclear material and cytoplasm) is present. *M,* Mitotic figure; *S,* smudge cell; *AB,* apoptotic body.

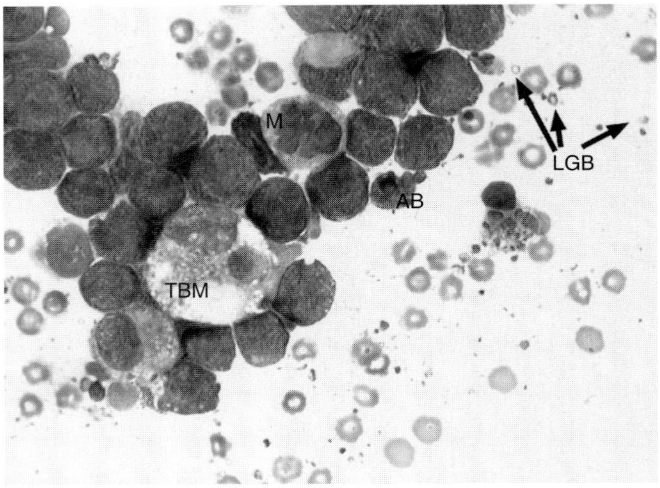

Figure 38-13 Lymphosarcoma: smear from the same abdominal fluid as Figure 38-12 (Wright's stain, ×100). This smear is similar to Figure 38-14 but also shows a tingible body macrophage and a few cytoplasmic fragments (also known as lymphoglandular bodies). These additional features are often seen in association with lymphosarcoma. Tingible body macrophages are activated macrophages cleaning up nuclear debris. Lymphoglandular bodies are seen whenever an increased production of lymphoid cells is present. These features by themselves, however, are not diagnostic of lymphosarcoma. *LGB,* Lymphoglandular bodies; *TBM,* tingible body macrophage; *AB,* apoptotic body; *M,* mitotic figure.

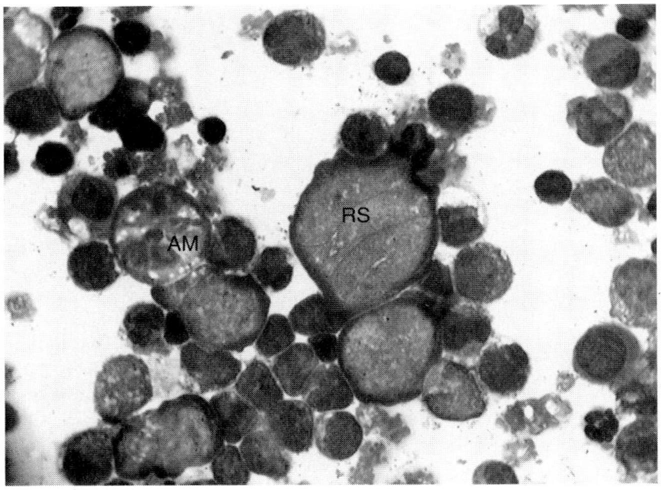

Figure 38-14 Lymphoma with Reed-Sternberg–like cell: cytospin preparation from a thoracic fluid sample in a ferret (Wright's stain, ×100). These Reed-Sternberg (*RS*)–like cells have been described in high-grade polymorphous lymphosarcomas in older ferrets.[4] These cells are distinctive giant cells that are binucleated or lobulated. The nuclei often appear as mirror images of one another and contain prominent nucleoli. In human beings, RS cells are seen in Hodgkin's disease; they are also described in feline lymphoma.[15] The ferret RS cell is not as distinctive as the human cell. Hodgkin's disease is not a recognized entity in the ferret. Also note the abnormal mitotic figure (*AM*). Because of the similarity in color of the nucleus and cytoplasm in this black-and-white photograph, one of the two nuclei is indistinct.

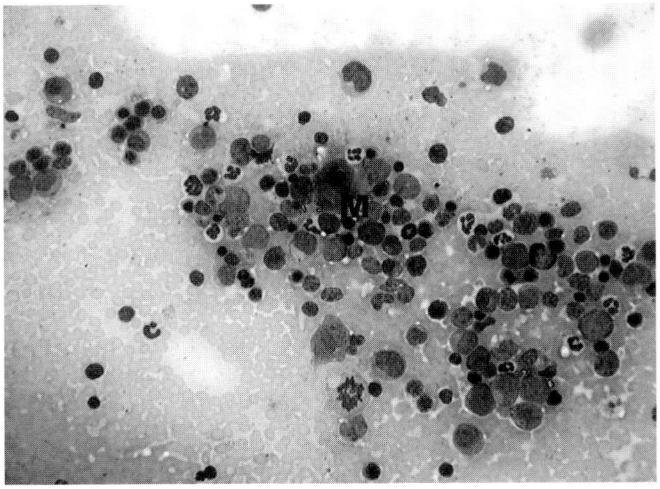

Figure 38-15 Splenic extramedullary hematopoiesis (EMH): aspirate from the spleen of a ferret (Wright's stain, ×40). In our experience, EMH is the most common diagnosis of splenic aspirate samples from ferrets. Notice the mixed population of hematopoietic cells, including a megakaryocyte. It is important to scan on a lower magnification to assess degree of cellularity. *M,* Megakaryocyte.

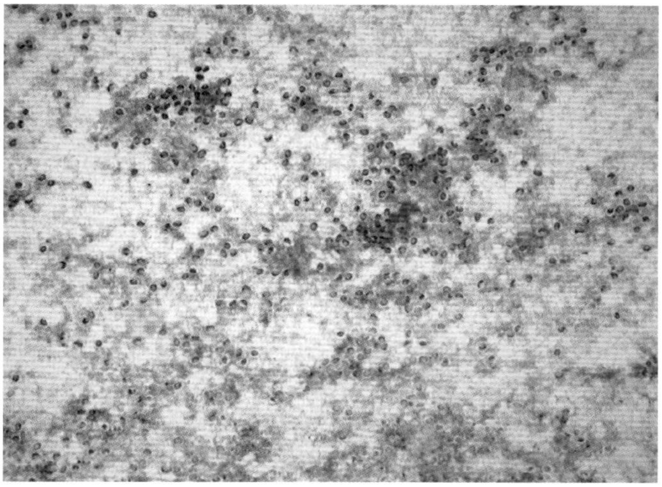

Plate 9 (see also Figure 38-4) Fecal smear (acid-fast stain, ×40). Numerous *Cryptosporidium* oocysts are present. When *Cryptosporidium* cause diarrhea, the organisms are numerous and easily identified. These protozoal cysts, 4 to 7 μm in diameter, are approximately the size of a red blood cell and are weakly acid-fast positive. The acid-fast stain used here (TB Quick Stain, Becton Dickinson Microbiology Systems, Sparks, MD) is a "cold" acid-fast stain and in our experience is easy to use and works well. An acid-fast stain specifically designed for *Cryptosporidium* species is not necessary (J. W., personal observation).

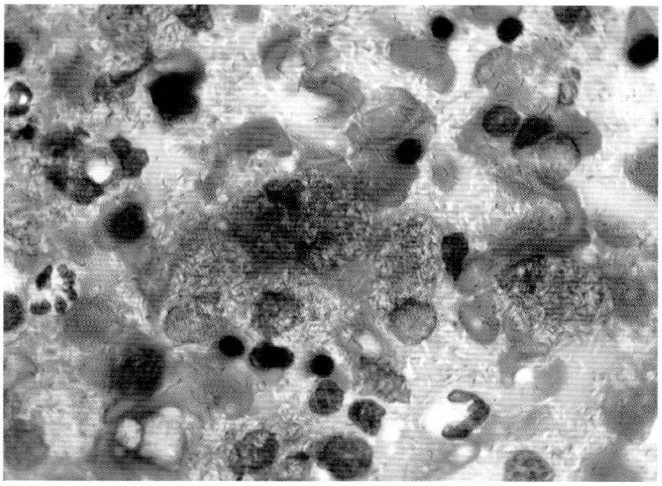

Plate 10 Mycobacteria: lymph node aspirate from a cat (Wright's stain counterstained with acid-fast stain, ×100). Numerous negative-staining bacilli are observed both within macrophages and free in the background. Counterstaining with a cold acid-fast stain (TB Quick Stain, Becton Dickinson Microbiology Systems) shows distinct, acid-fast–positive organisms. (Although not a recognized technique, counterstaining a Wright's-stained smear will stain some of the organisms and was used here because no unstained specimens were available for staining.) The morphologic features are similar in all species of animals. Mycobacteria are either weakly gram positive or are not readily stained by Gram stain because of waxy material in the cell wall. Typically, when acid-fast organisms are so numerous, they are often *Mycobacterium avium*.

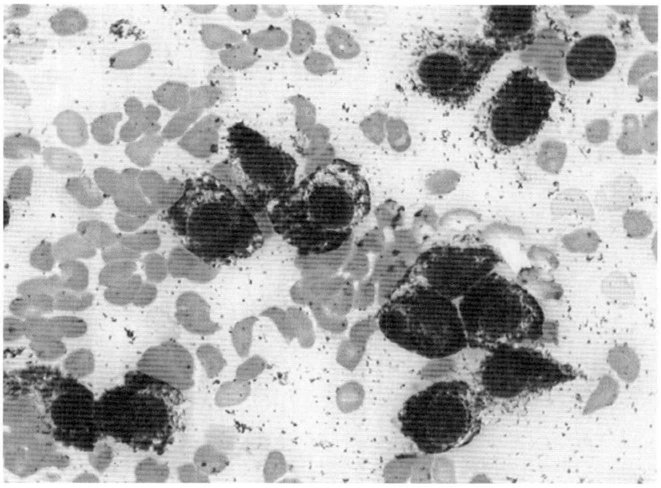

Plate 11 Aspirate of a cutaneous neoplasm in a ferret (Wright's stain, ×100). This round cell tumor contains characteristic purple or metachromatic granules in the cytoplasm characteristic of a mast cell tumor. The granules are purplish and not as distinct as those in other mammals. Mast cell tumors are described in the skin of ferrets and typically do not metastasize. The characteristic granules can be leached out in Diff-Quik stains. Without the granules, a diagnosis cannot be made with certainty. Granules from basophils can leach out as well; for this reason, we do not routinely use Diff-Quik stain.

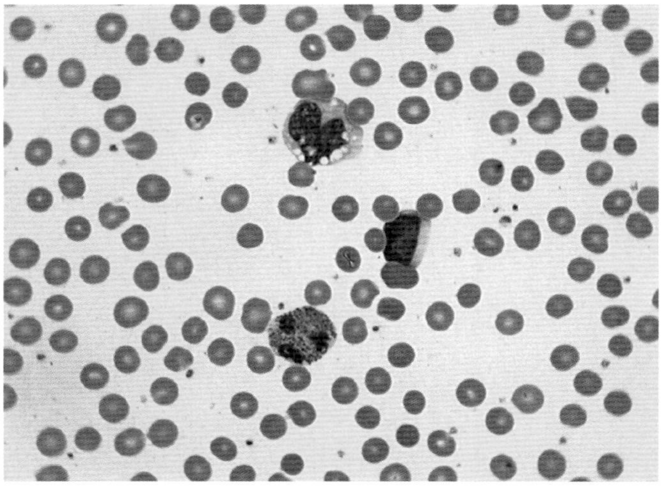

Plate 12 Rabbit peripheral blood (Wright's stain, ×100). This field shows the three common types of white blood cells in peripheral blood (monocyte, lymphocyte, and heterophil). The rabbit heterophil is analogous to the neutrophil in other species and is frequently mistaken for an eosinophil. Monocytes have a light blue cytoplasm and are occasionally vacuolated. Platelets in rabbits are small. Note a platelet adherent to a red blood cell adjacent to the monocyte.

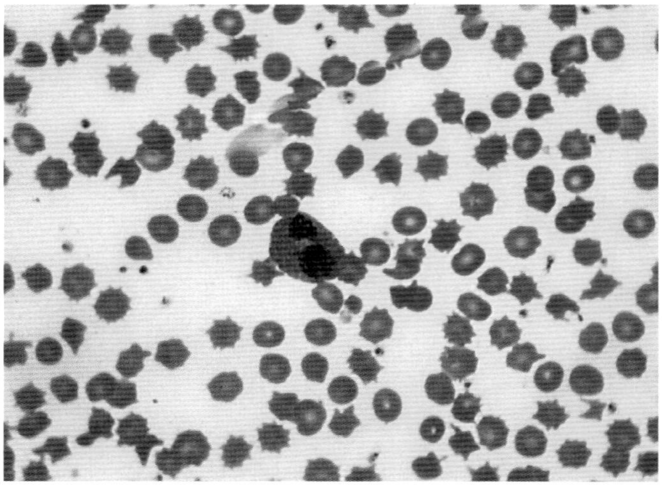

Plate 13 Rabbit peripheral blood (Wright's stain, ×100). This is a rabbit eosinophil. These cells are rare but distinct from heterophils in that they are larger, have larger granules that are more tightly packed, and have subtly different tinctorial properties. Note the crenation of most of the red blood cells. Crenated erythrocytes (echinocytes) have spicules that are evenly spaced and about the same size. Echinocytes are usually an artifact that can be associated with excess ethylenediamine tetraacetic acid (EDTA) anticoagulant or prolonged storage of blood, or they are a nonspecific finding in a variety of pathologic conditions.

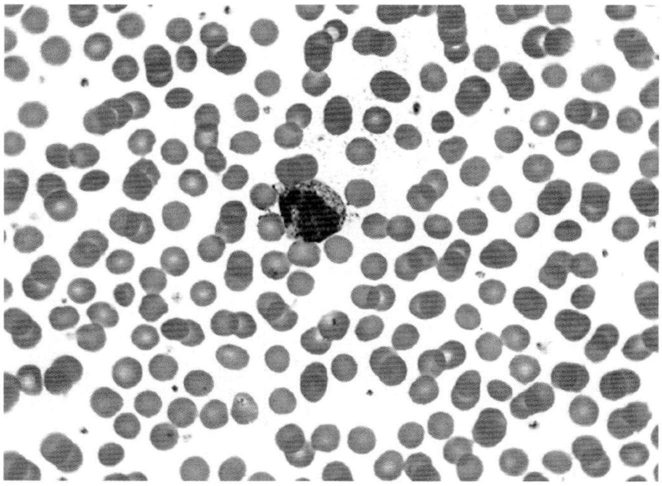

Plate 14 Rabbit peripheral blood (Wright's stain, ×100). This is a rabbit basophil. Basophils are distinctive cells with purplish granules stippling the cytoplasm. They are more frequently observed than eosinophils and occur with approximately the same frequency in rabbits as eosinophils do in other species (J.W., personal observation).

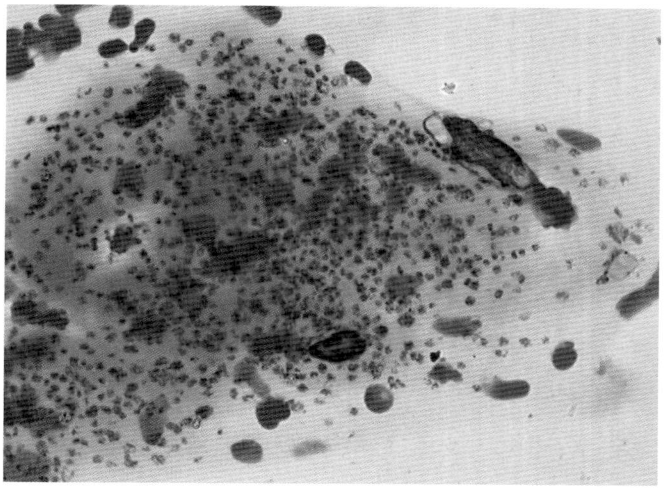

Plate 15 Rabbit peripheral blood (Wright's stain, ×100). This is a platelet and fibrin clot with two trapped white blood cells (monocyte and lymphocyte). Microscopic clots are more frequently observed at the trailing edge of a blood smear and are frequently seen in peripheral blood from rabbits (J.W., personal observation). This area should be scanned for clots and platelet clumps, which should be noted on the differential count. Platelets and white blood cells are not evenly dispersed in clotted blood, which compromises the accuracy of the automated or estimated counts.

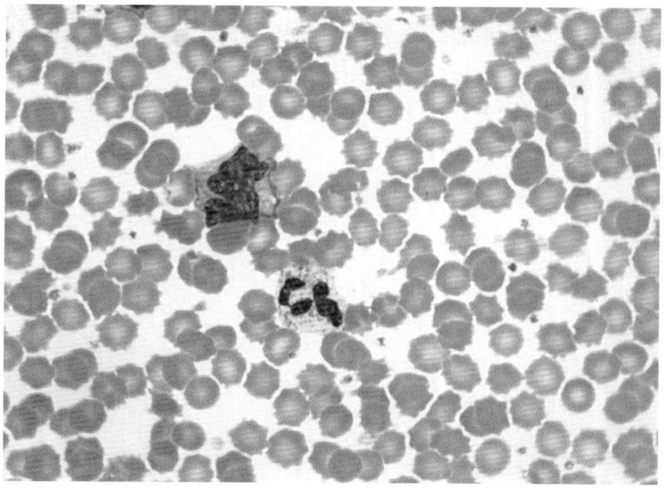

Plate 16 Guinea pig peripheral blood (Wright's stain, ×100). This field shows a monocyte and a neutrophil. Neutrophils are sometimes referred to *pseudoeosinophils* because of the distinct small eosinophilic granules.

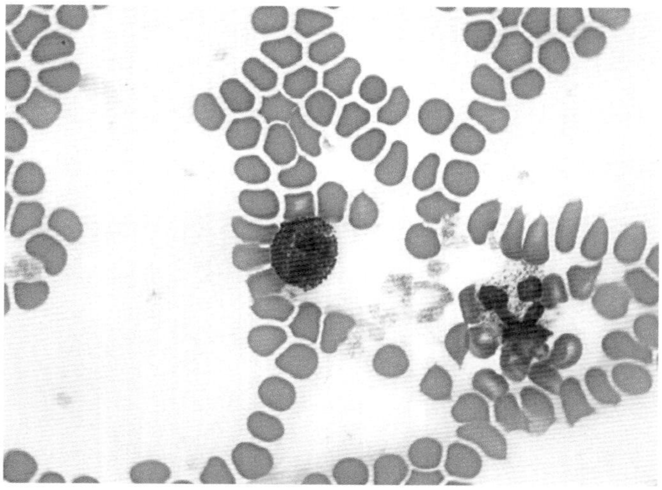

Plate 17 Guinea pig peripheral blood (Wright's stain, ×100). This is an eosinophil and is easily recognized by its distinctive large granules (compare with the granules in the nearby degenerating neutrophil).

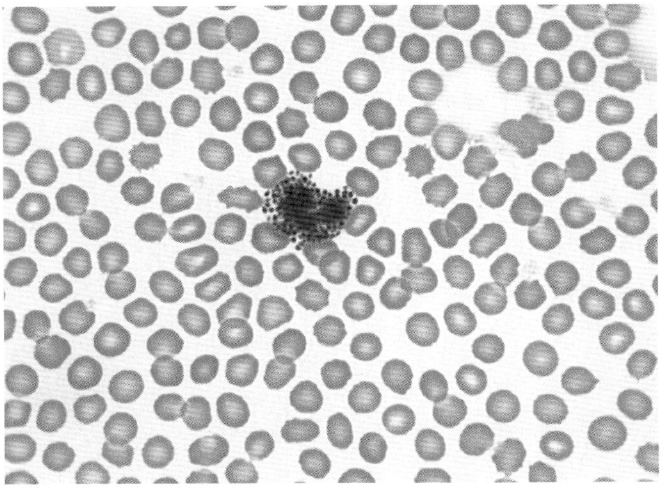

Plate 18 Guinea pig peripheral blood (Wright's stain, ×100). This is a basophil and is easily recognized, although granules may leach out with Diff-Quik stains.

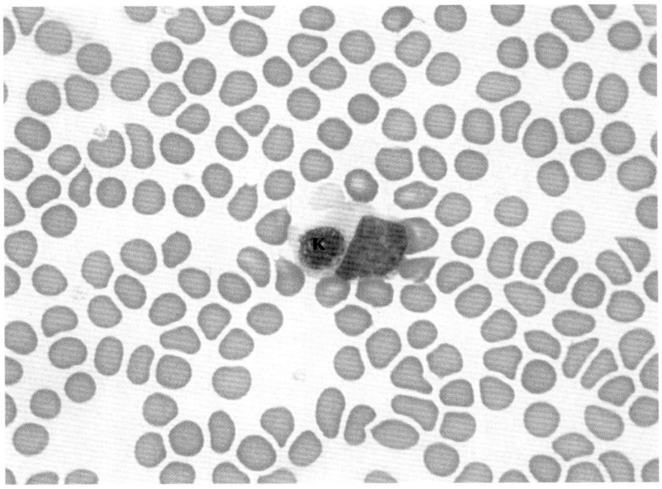

Plate 19 Lymphocytes are the predominant type of white blood cell in guinea pigs. This lymphocyte contains a Kurloff's body *(K)*, which is typically solitary, reddish in Wright's stain, and large (up to 8 μm in diameter). Sometimes it is difficult to distinguish the nucleus from a Kurloff's body. Lymphocytes containing Kurloff's bodies, also known as Foa-Kurloff cells, account for 3% to 4% of peripheral leukocytes. They are unique to the guinea pig, and are generally regarded as the equivalent of large granular lymphocytes (natural killer cells) in other mammals.[9,10]

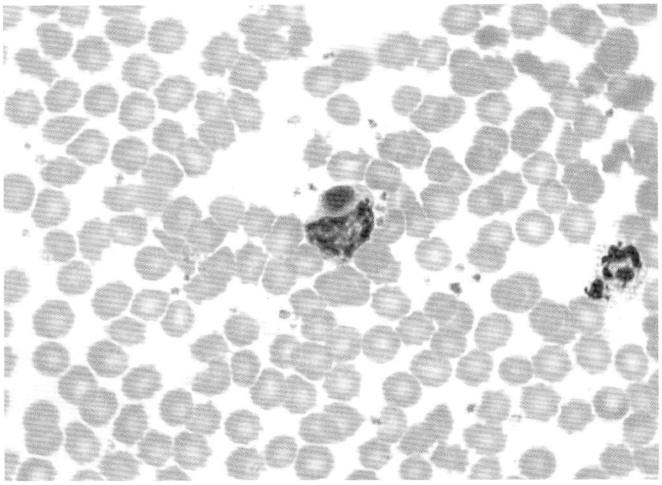

Plate 20 Guinea pig peripheral blood (Wright's stain, ×100). A rounded, large Kurloff's body is present within the lymphocyte.

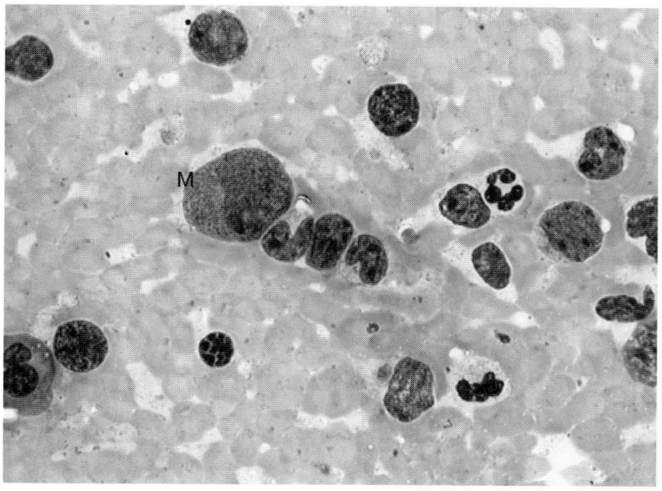

Figure 38-16 Splenic extramedullary hematopoiesis: aspirate from the spleen of a ferret (Wright's stain, ×100). Detail from Figure 38-15 showing, from left to right, a neutrophilic myelocyte with granules in the cytoplasm, a metamyelocyte, a rubricyte (crowded), and another metamyelocyte. *M,* Myelocyte.

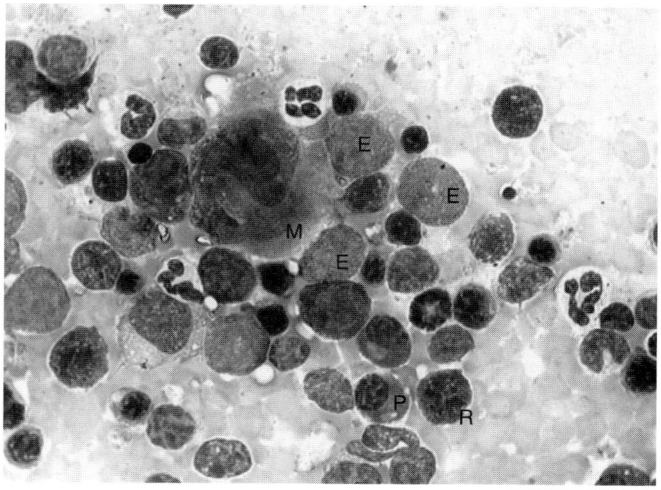

Figure 38-17 Spleen extramedullary hematopoiesis: aspirate from the spleen of a ferret (Wright's stain ×100). Detail from Figure 38-15 showing a megakaryocyte, eosinophilic myelocytes and metamyelocytes, prorubricyte, rubricyte, metarubricyte, and plasma cell. The rubricyte and plasma cell overlap in the morphology. Notice the plasma cell has a lower nucleus to cytoplasmic ratio, eccentric location of the nucleus, and perinuclear halo. *M,* Megakaryocyte; *E,* eosinophilic myelocyte; *R,* rubricyte; *P,* plasma cell.

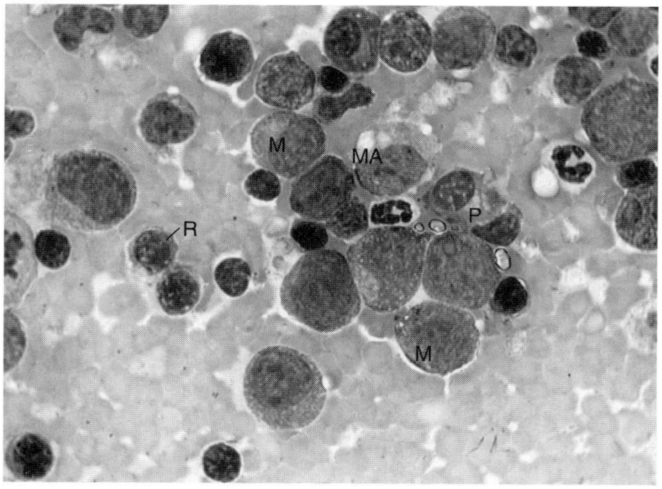

Figure 38-18 Spleen extramedullary hematopoiesis: aspirate from the spleen of a ferret showing mostly myelocytes (Wright's stain, ×100). These cells vary in size even though they are at the same stage of maturation (crowding or thick smears can prevent cells from spreading out, making them difficult to identify). Also present are plasma cells, rubricytes, and occasional macrophages. Most enlarged ferret spleens show EMH. Lymphosarcoma is a differential diagnosis for splenomegaly but should result in a monotypic population of generally immature lymphoid cells. *M,* Myelocyte; *P,* plasma cells; *R,* rubricytes; *MA,* macrophage.

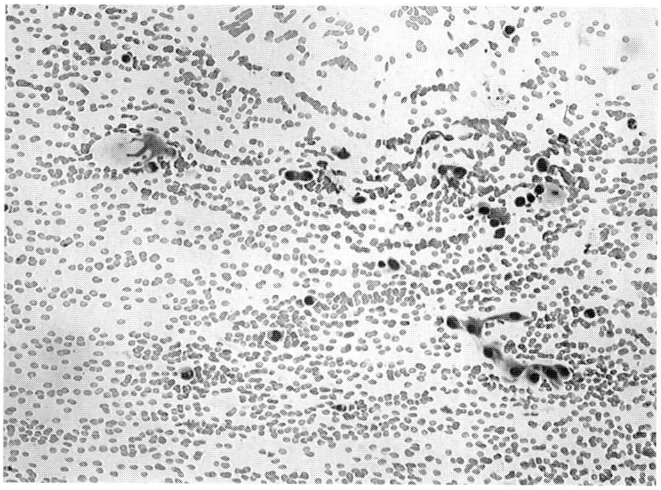

Figure 38-19 Synovial fluid from a guinea pig (Wright's stain, ×20). The findings are compatible with degenerative joint disease with normal viscosity and recent hemorrhage. Notice the "wind rowing" of cells. This feature, in which red blood cells or nucleated cells line up in parallel rows, is seen in material that is highly viscous such as synovial fluid. Any sample of a joint fluid aspirate should be cultured and smears prepared for cytologic examination and Gram stain, if appropriate. The most valuable test is the direct smear. From a direct smear, an estimated and differential cell count can be performed. Synovial fluid often becomes a gel at room temperature; this feature of the fluid (thixotropism) makes it difficult to perform cell counts.

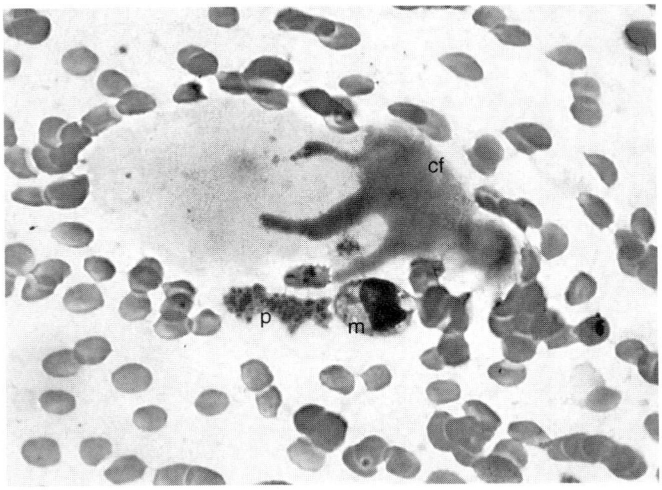

Figure 38-20 Synovial fluid from a guinea pig (Wright's stain, ×100). The presence of cartilage fragments indicates erosion of articular cartilage. Cartilage fragments vary in size and shape and have a characteristic metachromatic staining quality in Wright's stain. This fragment has a macrophage adjacent to it. A platelet clump is present, indicating that hemorrhage occurred during sampling. This cartilage fragment is an unusual shape and is recognized by its staining qualities. *cf*, Cartilage fragment; *p*, platelets; *m*, macrophage.

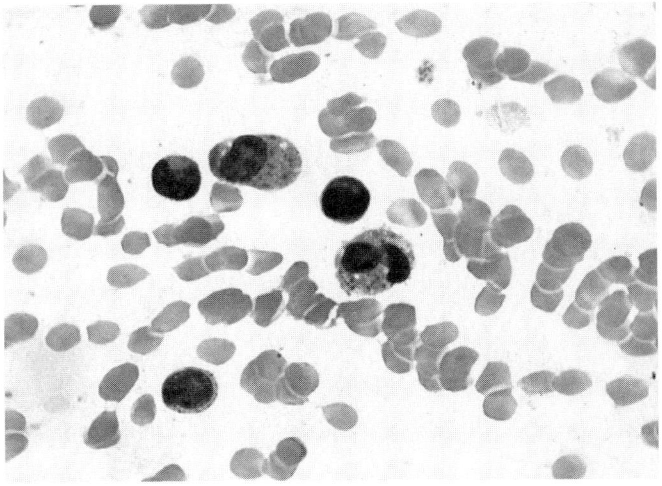

Figure 38-21 Synovial fluid from a guinea pig (Wright's stain, ×100). In degenerative joint disease, the types of cells observed are typically more than 90% mononuclear cells, that is, lymphocytes and monocytoid cells including macrophages. Note the azurophilic granules in the cytoplasm of the macrophages. These are likely lysosomes (membrane-bound packets of hydrolytic enzymes involved in intracellular digestion). Hemorrhage complicates interpretation of nucleated cells because some of the nucleated cells are inevitably leukocytes from the peripheral blood.

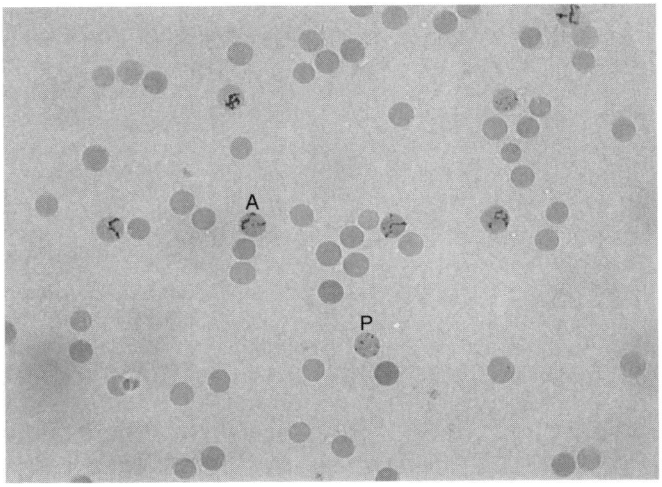

Figure 38-22 Reticulocyte: Ferret peripheral blood (reticulocyte stain, ×40). This slide was stained by the Unopette Test 5821 (Becton Dickinson, Franklin Lakes, NJ), which uses new methylene blue N in potassium oxalate to stain the cells. Two different types of reticulocytes (punctate and aggregate) that are similar to reticulocytes in cats are shown. Only the aggregate forms (denser and thicker particles) are typically counted in a reticulocyte count; if both are counted, they should be reported separately. Slides stained by this method can be counterstained with Wright's stain for ease of counting. *A*, Aggregate; *P*, punctate.

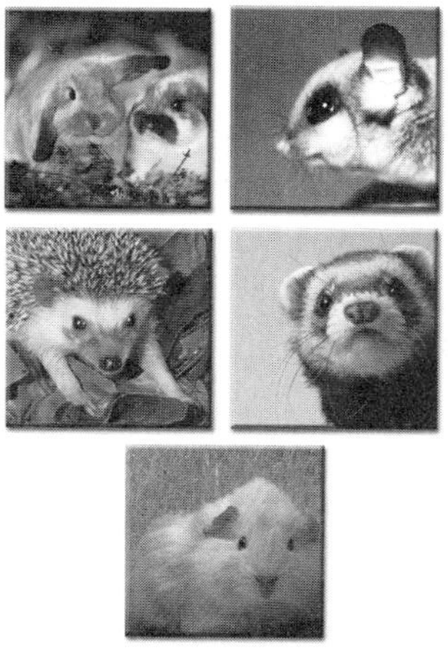

CHAPTER 39

Ophthalmologic Diseases in Small Pet Mammals

Alexandra van der Woerdt, DVM, MS, Diplomate ACVO, ECVO

RABBITS

Ophthalmic examination of rabbits can be performed easily.[43, 44] The eyes are laterally located and have a round pupil. Evaluation of a menace response is difficult, but most rabbits will react to bright light by squinting. The dorsal rectus muscle can usually be seen as a large striated band of tissue under the conjunctiva. Some rabbits do not respond to topical application of mydriatic agents because of the natural presence of atropinase. In these rabbits, the addition of 10% phenylephrine may help to obtain mydriasis. Rabbits have a merangiotic fundus. The well-myelinated optic nerve is present above the visual axis and has a deep optic cup. Retinal blood vessels are present in a linear streak medial and lateral to the optic nerve. An extensive venous plexus is present in the orbit. Tear production in rabbits can be measured by using Schirmer tear test strips. Average tear production is 5 mm/min (standard deviation, ±2.4 mm/min)[1]; however, very low values can be measured in some normal rabbits. Normal intraocular pressure measured by applanation tonometry is between 10 and 20 mm Hg.

The nasolacrimal system of rabbits has a single nasolacrimal punctum. The punctum is located in the ventral eyelid 3 mm from the eyelid margin, near the medial canthus and ventral to the lacrimal caruncle (Fig. 39-1).[5,24] The lacrimal sac is immediately rostral to the punctum and caudal to the nasolacrimal duct aperture. The nasolacrimal duct extends from the orbit to the nasal fossa and runs within the part of the maxilla that forms the lateral wall of the maxillary sinus.[24] Approximately 5 to 6 mm within the maxilla, the duct curves sharply and decreases in diameter.[5] At the level of the palatine bone, the nasolacrimal duct leaves the bony nasolacrimal canal and makes a sharp turn at the nasolacrimal duct flexure, which is located just caudal to the caudal limit of the incisor tooth roots. The nasolacrimal duct narrows at this flexure in normal rabbits. The duct then follows the ventral margin of the nasoturbinates and exits on the ventromedial aspect of the alar fold just caudal to the mucocutaneous junction of the nares.

Conjunctivitis and Epiphora

Conjunctivitis in rabbits is common. In normal rabbits with no ocular or respiratory disease, the most frequently isolated organisms from the conjunctival cul de sac include *Bacillus subtilis, Staphylococcus aureus, Bordetella* species, and *Pasteurella* species. However, *Pasteurella multocida* is a cause of conjunctivitis, epiphora, nasolacrimal duct obstruction, and dacryocystitis in rabbits.[24] Other infectious agents that have been associated with conjunctivitis in rabbits include *S. aureus, Pseudomonas* species, *Haemophilus* species, *Treponema paraluiscuniculi,* mycoplasma, chlamydiae, and myxoma virus. In a colony of rabbits with chronic conjunctivitis, *Streptococcus pyogenes,* nonhemolytic *Escherichia coli, Coynebacterium pyogenes, Haemophilus* species, *Neisseria* species, and *Lactobacillus* species were isolated from conjunctival samples. Mucopurulent conjunctivitis and blepharitis with corneal ulceration have been associated with *S. aureus* infection in a rabbit.[28] Treatment with topical gentamicin ophthalmic ointment and systemic gentamicin was curative. Other causes of conjunctivitis in rabbits include foreign bodies, entropion, distichia, trichiasis, and high ammonia or dust content in the environment. Dental disease, including root elongation and dental abscesses, is also associated with conjunctivitis.

Unilateral or bilateral epiphora can be present in rabbits without conjunctivitis. The discharge often has a white, gritty appearance and may be intermittent and resistant to treatment with topical antibiotics. Root elongation of the maxillary incisors is a common underlying cause.[16] The elongated roots can cause an obstruction of the nasolacrimal duct at its flexure just caudal to the roots of the incisors. Radiographs of the skull are needed to assess the incisors; excess curvature of the incisor roots is abnormal. In one report describing two affected rabbits, radiographs revealed a cystic dilation of the nasolacrimal duct immediately caudal to the duct flexure, and the incisors were more arched than in normal rabbits.[24] Irrigation of the

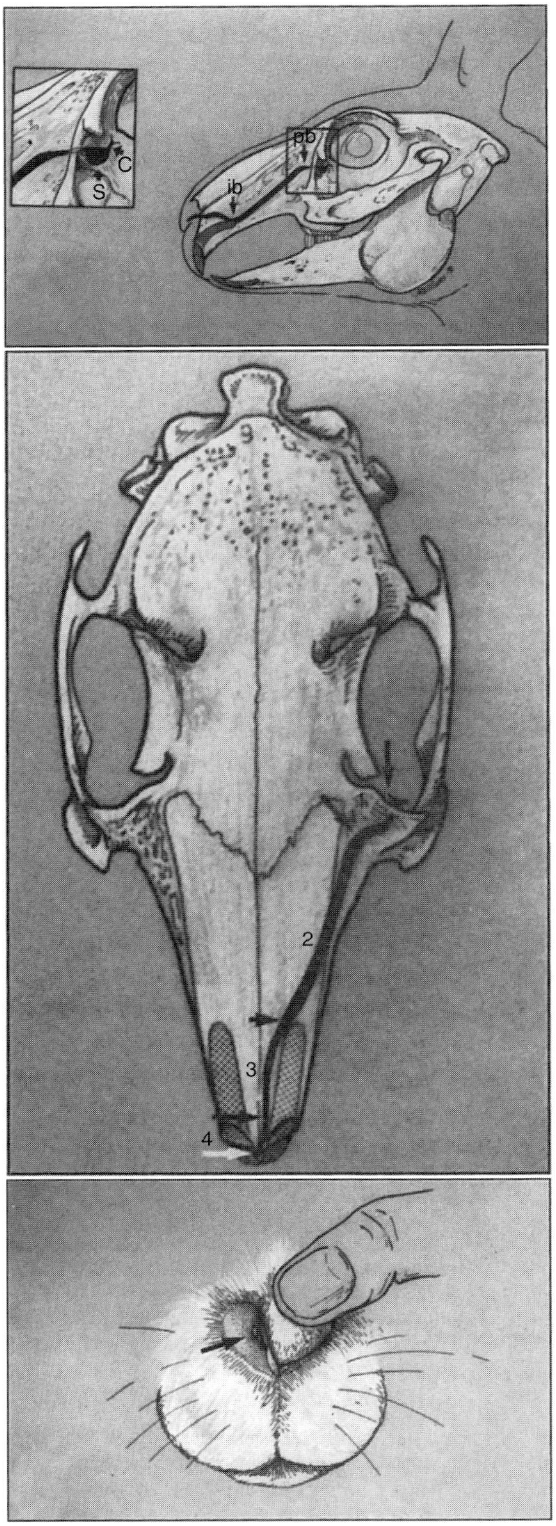

Figure 39-1 Diagram of the rabbit nasolacrimal duct. **A,** Lateral view with inset. The two sharp bends, the proximal maxillary bend (*pb*), and the bend at the incisor tooth (*ib*), are indicated. The inset shows the canaliculus (*C*) and the lacrimal sac (*S*). **B,** Dorsoventral view. *1,* Proximal portion of the duct extending from the punctum through the proximal maxillary curve; *2,* portion of the duct extending from the proximal maxillary curve to the base of the incisor tooth; *3,* portion of the duct extending from the base of the incisor tooth to the end of the lacrimal canal; *4,* distal portion of the duct extending from the end of the lacrimal canal to the nasal meatus. **C,** The nasal meatus of the nasolacrimal duct (*arrow*). The opening is enlarged for diagrammatic purposes. *(From Burling K, Murphy DJ, da Silva Curiel J, et al: Anatomy of the nasolacrimal duct and its clinical implications. Prog Vet Comp Ophthalmol 1991; 1:33-40.)*

nasolacrimal system in affected rabbits yielded opaque, white, gritty fluid. On cytologic examination, numerous macrophages, lipid-laden mesothelial cells, lipid droplets, and small numbers of bacteria and erythrocytes were present. The fluid cleared when ether was added, suggesting the presence of triglycerides or cholesterol. However, the role of lipid secretion in the pathogenesis of the obstruction was unknown. Bacteriologic culture of fluids used to irrigate the nasolacrimal ducts of both normal and affected rabbits yielded similar bacterial isolates; therefore, microorganisms apparently are not important in the pathogenesis of epiphora in rabbits. Bacterial isolates included *Staphylococcus, Pseudomonas, Moraxella,* and *Neisseria* species; *Oligella urethralis, Streptococcus viridans,* and *Bordetella bronchiseptica.* Inflammation was present in the nasolacrimal system of one rabbit.

In rabbits with epiphora, the diagnostic value of bacterial culture of the irrigation fluid is questionable. Skull radiographs are useful to detect underlying dental disease. Dacryocystorhinography using contrast material injected into the nasolacrimal system can help localize the site of obstruction, differentiate between a complete and partial obstruction, and identify any dilation.

Treatment of epiphora in rabbits can be frustrating. Irrigating the nasolacrimal duct is important to restore patency of the nasolacrimal system. After instilling a topical ophthalmic anesthetic, use a 23-gauge lacrimal cannula or a 24-gauge Teflon intravenous catheter to flush the duct (Fig. 39-2). Recurrence of the obstruction is common, and duct irrigation may need to be repeated every 2 to 3 days or weekly until a few consecutive clear irrigations are obtained. If topical antibiotic therapy is used, a broad-spectrum medication such as triple antibiotic solution is recommended. Topical nonsteroidal, anti-inflammatory ophthalmic medications, such as 0.03% flurbiprofen or 1% diclofenac, may help minimize irritation caused by the procedure. In rabbits with chronic or severe infections, concurrent topical ophthalmic and systemic antibiotic therapy may be needed. Suggested combinations include systemic enrofloxacin (Baytril, Bayer Corporation, Shawnee Mission, KS) and topical ciprofloxacin (Ciloxan, Alcon Laboratories, Inc., Fort Worth, TX) or gentamicin. In rabbits with evidence of underlying incisor root elongation, removal of the incisors can be considered in severe cases.

Cornea

Corneal dystrophy is the accumulation of cholesterol or lipid crystals in the cornea. This may develop spontaneously, as has been reported in American Dutch belted rabbits,[29] or from high dietary cholesterol. It also occurs in breeds that are predisposed to hypercholesterolemia, such as the Watanabe rabbit with heritable hyperlipidemia. In rabbits without systemic lipid

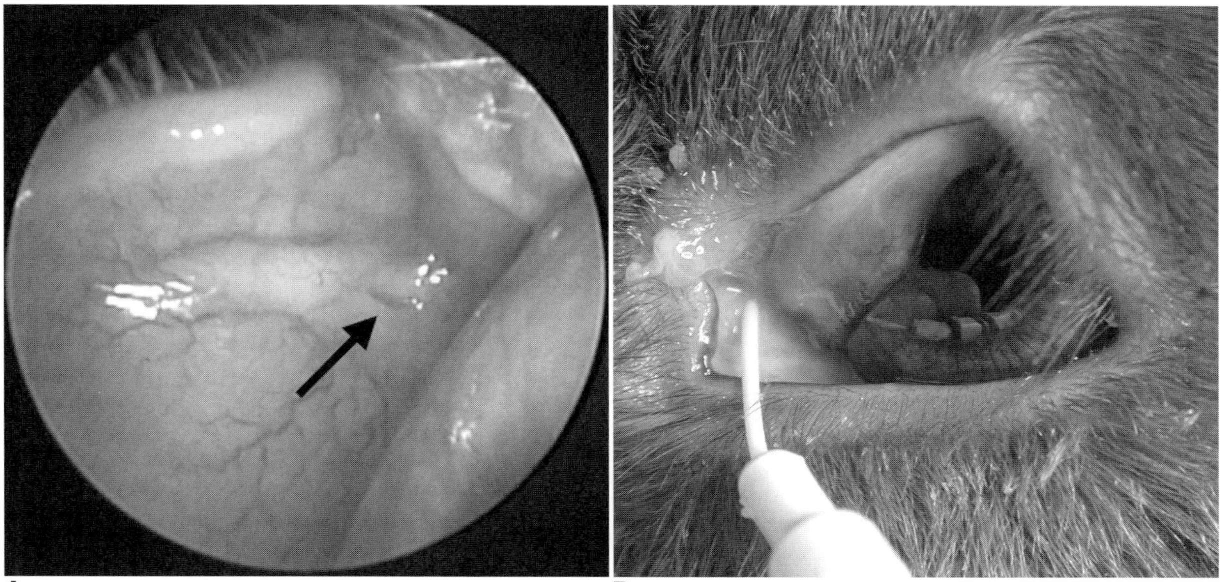

Figure 39-2 A, Rabbits have a single nasolacrimal punctum *(arrow)* in the ventral eyelid. B, Irrigation of the nasolacrimal duct in a rabbit with a 24-gauge Teflon intravenous catheter. *(A, Courtesy Susan Kelleher, DVM).*

abnormalities, spontaneous corneal dystrophy is usually bilateral and symmetrical and does not progress to visual impairment. In any rabbit with corneal dystrophy, carefully evaluate the fat content of the diet.

Progressive occlusion of the cornea with a conjunctival-like membrane is occasionally seen in rabbits.[12,35] Membranous corneal occlusion, or pseudopterygium, is a pain-free condition that may affect one or both eyes (Fig. 39-3). Ophthalmic examination reveals a circular membrane that originates at the limbus (the junction of the cornea and sclera) and gradually advances over the cornea. In severe cases, only a small central opening is present, allowing visibility of an otherwise normal globe. The membrane does not adhere to the cornea. The cause of this condition is unknown, although trauma has been suggested. Progressive membranous occlusion in rabbits has been compared with pterygium in humans. However, in humans the membrane is triangular and adherent to the cornea, whereas in rabbits it is nonadherent and circumferential from the limbus. Treatment with topical antibiotic or antibiotic-steroid medications has no effect. Surgically resecting the membrane and treating with topical antibiotics after surgery usually result in quick recurrence of the membrane. However, resecting the membrane a few millimeters beyond the limbus and treating with a topical antibiotic-steroid combination after surgery may prevent recurrence. Good results have also been obtained with surgical resection and the use of topical cyclosporine. Another described surgical technique is to incise the membrane into four quarters and suture each quadrant of the membrane to the inside of the eyelids.[35] With this technique, recurrence may be prevented for at least 1 year.

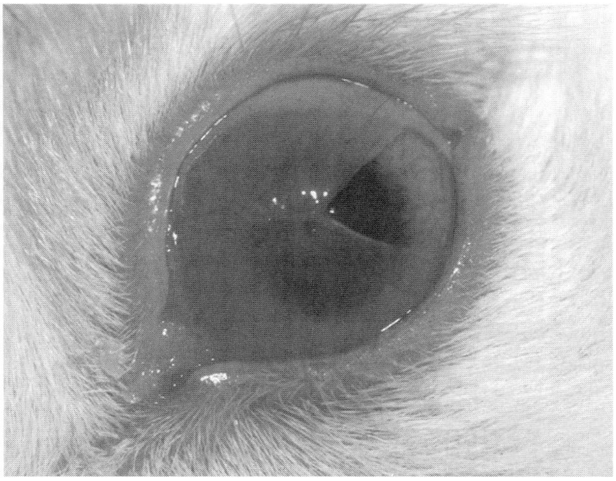

Figure 39-3 Progressive occlusion of the cornea with conjunctival-like tissue is present in this rabbit. The conjunctival-like tissue is not adhered to the cornea. The disease is not painful. *(Courtesy David Wilkie, DVM, MS.)*

Superficial, nonhealing corneal ulcers are occasionally seen in rabbits. Clinical signs are usually mild and include epiphora, conjunctival hyperemia, and blepharospasm. The ulcer is usually located in the paracentral cornea, is very superficial, and has redundant epithelial edges. The clinical appearance resembles an indolent ulcer, as seen in boxer dogs. Carefully examine the eyes of affected rabbits to eliminate potential causes such as abnormal hairs, lagophthalmos (inability to fully close the eyelid), facial nerve paralysis, or a foreign body. Treatment with a topical antibiotic solution or ointment usually fails to resolve the ulcer. Additional therapies such as corneal debridement, grid keratotomy, use of topical serum, application of corneal glue, tarsorrhaphy, or superficial keratectomy are usually necessary for the ulcer to heal.

Uveitis and Diseases of the Lens

Encephalitozoon cuniculi may cause granulomatous encephalitis and renal lesions in rabbits. Many rabbits infected with *E. cuniculi* are asymptomatic, but neurologic signs can include convulsions, tremors, torticollis, paresis, and coma. *Encephalitozoon cuniculi* infection has also been associated with phacoclastic uveitis. In one report, examination of phacofragmentation fluid from a rabbit revealed the presence of *E. cuniculi* DNA.[38] Most affected rabbits are young (less than 2 years), and dwarf rabbits appear predisposed to disease. Clinically, a white mass is often seen protruding into the anterior chamber (Fig. 39-4). Careful examination of the anterior segment of the eye with slit lamp biomicroscopy may reveal a break in the anterior lens capsule. The break is frequently hidden by inflammatory material and it may appear as if only the iris is involved in the inflammatory process. A focal cataract is often present in the area of the anterior lens capsule break. Signs of a severe pyogranulomatous anterior uveitis are usually present, such as conjunctival hyperemia, a swollen hyperemic iris, miosis, aqueous flare, and low intraocular pressure. The posterior segment of the eye is initially normal; however, if left untreated, severe uveitis and cataract formation can lead to blindness and possible phthisis bulbi or glaucoma. An abscess in the iris caused by *P. multocida* initially may resemble phacoclastic uveitis. Measuring serum antibody titers for *E. cuniculi* and *P. multocida* may aid in the differential diagnosis. Treatment of choice is surgical removal of the lens by phacofragmentation. Because of the rabbit's ability to regenerate a lens after this procedure, inserting an artificial lens after phacofragmentation is not recommended. Systemic treatment of *E. cuniculi* with albendazole (30 mg/kg PO q24h for 30 days, then 15 mg/kg PO q24h for an additional 30 days) has been reported.[38] More recently, fenbendazole (20 mg/kg q24h for 28 days) has proved effective in both preventing experimental *E. cuniculi* infection in rabbits and treating naturally infected, seropositive rabbits.[39] If the lens is not removed surgically, control of the uveitis with topical steroidal (such as 1% prednisolone acetate) and nonsteroidal anti-inflammatory medications as well as systemic fenbendazole or albendazole is necessary. Enucleation may be indicated if the uveitis cannot be controlled medically and a chronic painful eye is present.[46]

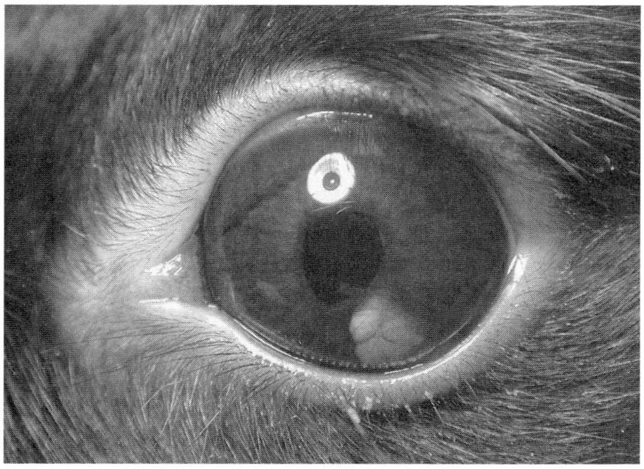

Figure 39-4 Rabbit infected with *Encephalitozoon cuniculi.* A white lesion is present in the iris, protruding into the anterior chamber. Lens involvement with cataract formation is present underneath the iridial lesion.

Glaucoma

Congenital glaucoma is inherited as an autosomal recessive trait in rabbits. In rabbits with glaucoma, the intraocular pressure is high as early as 3 months of age.[6] With increasing age, progressive buphthalmos with a markedly enlarged cornea, structural abnormalities of the iridocorneal angle, atrophy of the ciliary processes, and excavation of the optic nerve develop. Topical glaucoma medications used in dogs, such as 0.5% timolol maleate and 2% dorzolamide, may also be used in rabbits. Because response to therapy is unpredictable in rabbits, carefully monitor the intraocular pressure during treatment. Enucleation, inserting an intrascleral prosthesis, and laser cycloablation with a diode laser have also been used to manage glaucoma in pigmented pet rabbits. However, laser cycloablation cannot be used in albino rabbits. If left untreated in chronic cases, pressure-induced atrophy of the ciliary body may result in the intraocular pressure returning to normal.

Orbit

Retrobulbar disease processes are occasionally seen in rabbits. Clinical signs include progressive exophthalmos, protrusion of the third eyelid, and inability to retropulse the globe. Exposure keratitis may be present if the ability of the eyelids to close properly has been affected. Abscesses are a common cause of retrobulbar disease in rabbits, caused by infection with *P. multocida*[3] as well as other aerobic and anaerobic bacterial species. Dental disease with tooth root abscessation is often a predisposing factor, and a good dental examination and skull radiographs are indicated in any rabbit with a suspected retrobulbar mass (see Chapter 34). If available, a computed tomography scan is especially helpful in diagnosis (Fig. 39-5). Retrobulbar neoplasia is uncommon in rabbits.

An abscess in the retrobulbar space of a rabbit can be very difficult to treat. Because of the thick nature of the abscessed material, drainage of the abscess through the mouth, as performed in dogs and cats, may or may not be successful. If the abscess is caused by an abscessed tooth root, the tooth or teeth must be extracted to allow drainage and the rabbit must be treated with long-term systemic antibiotic therapy. In some cases, aggressive surgical debridement may be necessary. This may include exenteration of the orbit and sacrifice of a sighted eye. Even with aggressive surgical and medical management, the prognosis for recovery is always guarded. Anecdotal reports suggest some rabbits with retrobulbar abscesses respond to medical therapy with long-term (3 months) administration of benzathine/procaine penicillin G (for rabbits <2.5 kg, 75,000 U/rabbit SC q48h; for rabbits >2.5 kg, 150,000 U/rabbit SC q48h).[34]

Exophthalmos in obese rabbits may be caused by excessive fat deposition in the orbit. Periodic exophthalmos has been reported in rabbits with thymomas.[21,42] In one report, a localized myasthenia gravis associated with the thymoma was suggested as a cause.[42] More probably, the presence of a large intrathoracic mass obstructs blood flow in the right and left cranial vena cava, causing decreased vascular drainage from the head. Exophthalmos was also reported in a rabbit after chronic external jugular catheter placement[17] and has been seen clinically in a rabbit with

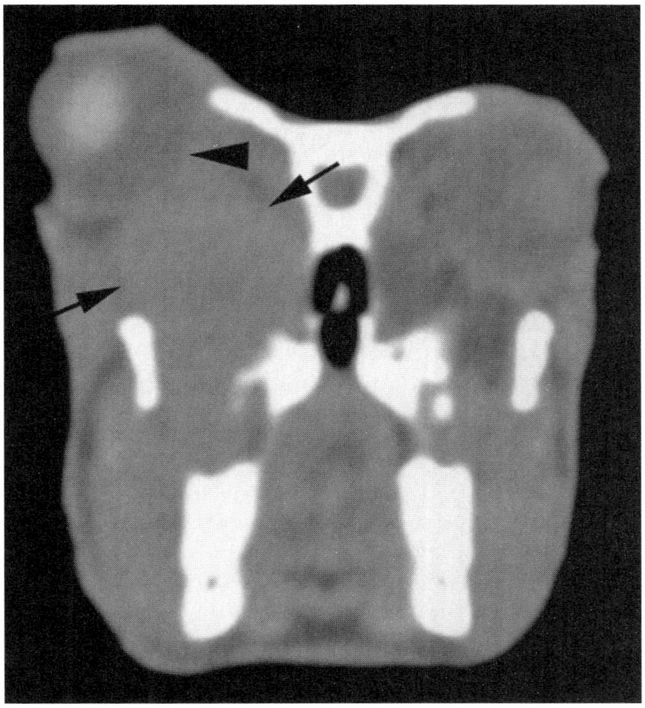

Figure 39-5 Computed tomographic scan of a rabbit with severe retrobulbar disease. A large mass (*arrows*) is present in the retrobulbar area, displacing the globe (*arrowhead*) dorsally and causing severe exophthalmos.

thrombosis of both external jugular veins after venipuncture and catheterization (K. Quesenberry, DVM, personal communication, 2002). Because the internal jugular veins of rabbits are relatively small, occlusion of the external jugular veins will compromise vascular drainage of the head. In the clinical case, the bilateral exophthalmos resolved spontaneously, presumably after the jugular veins became patent again (see Chapter 13).

Rabbits have several glands in the orbit. The lacrimal gland is located dorsolaterally, and the accessory lacrimal gland, divided into three lobes, is located along the caudal and ventral orbital margin. The superficial gland of the third eyelid is a small gland located near the cartilage of the third eyelid. The deep gland of the third eyelid, also known as the harderian gland, consists of two parts, a dorsal (white) and a ventral (pink) lobe. Prolapse of the deep gland of the third eyelid has been described in rabbits. Surgical correction with a pocket technique, as has been described in dogs, was successful in reducing the gland in one rabbit.[19]

FERRETS

Ferrets have prominent globes that are placed laterally in the skull, with very limited binocular vision. Their pupil is a horizontal slit and quickly responds to light. Topical 1% tropicamide may need to be applied to evaluate the fundus. Similar to dogs and cats, ferrets have a holangiotic retinal vascular pattern. The projection of retinal ganglion cells from the temporal area of the retina in albino ferrets differs from that of pigmented ferrets.[30] In pigmented ferrets, 6000 retinal ganglion cells project ipsilaterally to the brain, whereas in albino ferrets, only 1500 retinal ganglion cells project ipsilaterally. The significance of this difference has not been established.

Conjunctivitis in ferrets can be caused by viral or bacterial infection. Ocular signs of canine distemper virus, a fatal disease in ferrets, include mucopurulent oculonasal discharge, blepharitis, corneal ulcers, and keratoconjunctivitis sicca.[20] Conjunctival swelling and a proliferative lesion of the nictitans caused by infection with *Mycobacterium genavense* have been described in two ferrets. Other clinical signs in these ferrets included peripheral lymph node enlargement.[23]

Degeneration of corneal endothelial cells leading to progressive corneal edema and cloudiness of the cornea is seen in older mink (8-11 years).[15] Royal pastel females are predisposed. Unlike this disease in dogs, these mink do not develop corneal ulceration, pigmentation, or vascularization develop. There is no specific treatment for this condition, but symptomatic treatment with 5% sodium chloride solution or ointment 2 to 4 times a day may or may not improve corneal clarity.

A lymphoplasmacytic keratitis has been reported in a ferret with lymphoma.[33] An infiltrative lesion was present in the cornea that resembled corneal lesions reported in mink with Aleutian disease.

Cataracts are common in ferrets.[41] Progressive cataract formation has been reported in two genetically unrelated populations of ferrets.[26] In 1-year-old ferrets, cataracts were observed in 47% of animals examined. Severity ranged from clinically insignificant, small cataracts in the posterior cortex of the lens to blinding complete cataracts. By 18 months of age, cataracts were detected in virtually every animal, and in animals previously diagnosed, the cataracts had progressed. A genetically separate group had a combination of blinding cataract, microphthalmos, abnormal iris formation, and retinal detachment. In another ferret colony, microphthalmos, cataract, retinal dysplasia, and a persistent hyperplastic primary vitreous-type membrane were shown to be inherited as an autosomal dominant defect.[11] Dietary factors may play a role in the development of cataracts in ferrets. A diet high in fat or deficient in vitamin E or protein may promote cataract formation.[26]

Monitor the eyes of ferrets with cataracts regularly for the onset of secondary complications. Lens-induced uveitis can usually be controlled with topical 1% prednisolone acetate once or twice daily. Other complications caused by cataracts include lens subluxation or luxation and glaucoma. Ferrets that are blind because of cataracts usually adjust well in a home environment. However, cataract surgery can be performed successfully in ferrets. The lenses can be removed by phacofragmentation or by an extracapsular technique. Artificial lenses are not available in a size suitable for ferrets. Before cataract surgery, make sure the ferret becomes accustomed to frequent application of eye medications to facilitate easy treatment after surgery.

Retinal degeneration is seen in ferrets. Clinical signs are progressive loss of vision that may not be noticed until the disease is advanced. Ophthalmic examination reveals mydriasis with a very poor pupillary light reflex. Cataracts may or may not be present. Retinal vascular attenuation and tapetal hyperreflectivity are seen in the fundus. There is no treatment for retinal degeneration.

Lymphosarcoma is a common disease in ferrets. Although orbital involvement has only been reported in two ferrets,[25] it is occasionally seen clinically. Exophthalmos is often the presenting complaint. Ophthalmic examination reveals exophthalmos, decreased retropulsion of the globe, and protrusion of the third eyelid. Lagophthalmos may result in exposure keratitis with corneal ulceration and vascularization. In the two ferrets described, lymphosarcoma was also detected elsewhere in the body.[25] Peripheral lymph nodes were affected in one ferret, and involvement of the liver, spleen, intestines, kidneys, and adrenals was present in the other.

The diagnosis of retrobulbar lymphosarcoma can be confirmed by cytologic examination of a sample from the retrobulbar area obtained by fine-needle aspiration. However, this procedure may be difficult because of the limited size of the retrobulbar space. Instead, suspicion of orbital lymphosarcoma may be confirmed by obtaining samples for diagnostic tests elsewhere in the body, such as a fine-needle aspirate or wedge biopsy of an enlarged lymph node. Therapy of retrobulbar lymphosarcoma is directed at treating the disease systemically with prednisone or chemotherapeutic agents. If the corneal epithelium is intact, protect the eye with lubricating ophthalmic ointment applied 2 to 4 times daily. If an ulcer is present, treat with an antibiotic ophthalmic ointment, such as triple antibiotic or gentamicin ointment, applied 3 to 4 times daily. While treating the ferret for lymphosarcoma, temporary tarsorrhaphy may be necessary to protect the cornea if pronounced exophthalmos is present.

Zygomatic salivary gland mucocele is another reported cause of exophthalmos in ferrets.[27] Fine-needle aspiration of a soft fluctuant swelling dorsotemporal to the eye yields a tenacious, blood-tinged fluid. Surgical excision is usually curative (see Chapters 3 and 12).

GUINEA PIGS

Guinea pigs have a paurangiotic retina that appears avascular on examination. Their eyelids are open from birth, and they have a rudimentary third eyelid.

Conjunctivitis is common in guinea pigs (Fig. 39-6). One common cause is *Chlamydophila psittaci*,[20] which causes a self-limiting disease manifested by mild chemosis, ocular discharge, and follicle formation. Cytologic examination of a specimen from a conjunctival scraping may reveal intracytoplasmic inclusion bodies in epithelial cells. Treatment is generally considered unnecessary. Vitamin C deficiency in guinea pigs causes conjunctivitis with a flaky discharge. Treatment is directed at correcting the dietary deficiency.

A spontaneous outbreak of listerial keratoconjunctivitis has been reported in hairless guinea pigs.[9] Clinical signs ranged from serous lacrimation with hyperemic conjunctiva to purulent, ulcerative keratoconjunctivitis with corneal neovascularization. *Listeria monocytogenes* was cultured from the ocular discharge. Treatment was not attempted.

Blepharitis caused by dermatophyte infection may be seen in young guinea pigs.[3] Topical antifungal therapy is usually effective.

Lymphosarcoma is rare in guinea pigs but has been reported to infiltrate the cornea.[37] Lymphosarcoma should also be considered as a differential diagnosis of conjunctival masses in guinea pigs.[2] Another differential diagnosis for conjunctival nodules in guinea pigs is a syndrome known as "pea eye." These nodules are protrusions of portions of the lacrimal or zygomatic glands and appear pale or pink. Treatment is not necessary because animals are usually not bothered by their presence.

A corneal dermoid has been reported in a guinea pig from a commercial colony.[31] A circular mass with a hair protruding from the surface was present on the central cornea. If noticed in a clinical patient, treatment by superficial keratectomy is recommended.

Cataracts have been seen in clinical patients. Cataracts can be removed surgically, but the procedure is difficult because of the small size of the globe, the large size of the lens, and the difficulty of intubating a guinea pig for general anesthesia.

Osseous metaplasia of the mesectodermal trabecular meshwork occurs in guinea pigs (Fig. 39-7).[14] Clinically, an arc of white, opaque material is visible in the anterior chamber, covering the iridocorneal angle. Vessels may be present overlying the osseous choristoma. Hematopoietic active bone marrow is present. This is usually an incidental finding and no specific treatment is necessary.

As in rabbits and other rodents, exophthalmos in guinea pigs may be related to dental disease. A tooth root abscess of a molar

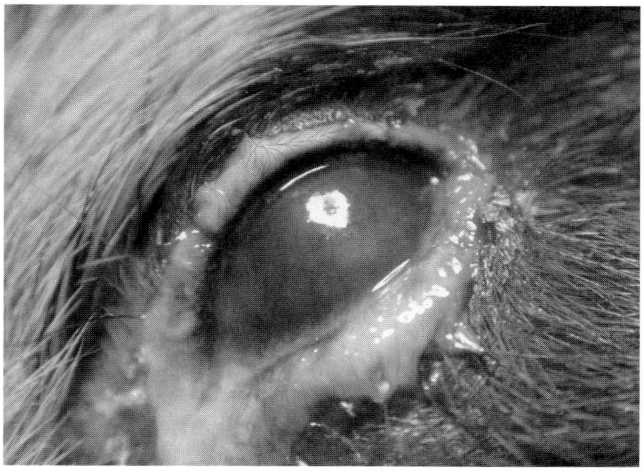

Figure 39-6 Conjunctivitis and keratitis in a guinea pig. Note the abundant mucopurulent discharge, corneal vascularization, and fibrosis.

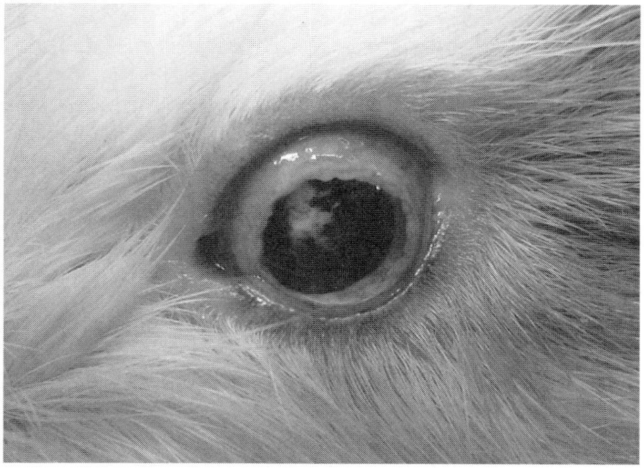

Figure 39-7 Osseous metaplasia of the mesectodermal trabecular meshwork in a guinea pig. White opaque material is present in the iridocorneal angle. *(From Brown C, Donnelly T: What's your diagnosis? Heterotopic bone in the eyes of a guinea pig. Lab Anim 2002; 31:23-25.)*

may result in maxillary sinusitis and orbital disease. Careful examination of the teeth is indicated in any guinea pig with exophthalmos.

CHINCHILLAS

Chinchillas have a vertical slit pupil and an anangiotic retina. Cataracts and asteroid hyalosis have been reported in older animals.[20]

The premolar, molar, and incisor teeth in chinchillas, as in guinea pigs, continue to grow and erupt throughout the animal's life. Insufficient wear can result in elongated roots of the premolar and molar teeth, resulting in progressive orbital disease including epiphora, decreased retropulsion of the globe, and proptosis (see Chapter 34). Computed tomography is more sensitive than radiographs in detecting early lesions.[10] The prognosis for advanced disease is poor.

RATS, MICE, AND HAMSTERS

The retina of rats, mice, and hamsters is holangiotic, with arteries and venules radiating from the optic nerve like spokes on a wheel. Rats have three lacrimal glands: intraorbital, extraorbital, and harderian.

Inbred strains of rats and mice are commonly used in commercial laboratories to study naturally occurring ophthalmologic diseases. Diseases involving all parts of the eye have been described. Common abnormalities include retinal degeneration, as in the RCS rat,[40] microphthalmos, and cataract. In addition to specific genetically determined ocular abnormalities in inbred strains, other spontaneous abnormalities occur. Ophthalmic examination of 6000 Sprague-Dawley rats revealed a focal linear retinopathy in 3% and a fundic coloboma in 0.5% of animals examined.[18] Spontaneous corneal degeneration has been described in Sprague-Dawley and Wistar rats,[4] and corneal dystrophy has been described in Fischer 344 rats.[22] Experimental infections also lead to ophthalmic abnormalities. Blepharitis with crust formation in the medial canthus and partial periocular alopecia were observed in mice experimentally infected with *Trypanosoma brucei*.[36]

Conjunctivitis in mice can be caused by numerous infectious agents, including *Pseudomonas aeruginosa*, *P. pneumotropica*, *Salmonella* species, *Streptobacillus moniliformis*, *Corynebacterium kutscheri*, Lancefield group C streptococci, *Mycoplasma pulmonis*, mousepox or ectromelia virus, Sendai virus, and lymphocytic choriomeningitis virus.[20] Bacteriologic culture and sensitivity testing may be indicated in individual rats and mice with persistent conjunctivitis. Epiphora in rats and mice can be caused by dental problems. Nasolacrimal duct obstruction can result from overgrowth or malocclusion of the incisors.

Chromodacryorrhea is red staining around the eyes seen in rats and mice. Inflammation of the harderian gland causes secretion of tears pigmented with porphyrin. Sialodacryoadenitis virus is a highly contagious coronavirus that replicates in the respiratory tract epithelium, causing rhinotracheitis, bronchitis, and alveolitis. The virus also causes sialoadenitis of the submandibular and parotid salivary glands and necrotizing dacryoadenitis of orbital and harderian lacrimal glands. Exophthalmos, epiphora, and keratoconjunctivitis may result. The infection usually resolves within 1 week in immunocompetent animals. In a study of athymic rats, infection persisted for more than 3 months, indicating that normal T-cell function is required for host defenses against the virus.[42] Infection with sialodacryoadenitis virus may also result in uveitis and multifocal retinal degeneration.[20] Complications from infection include corneal opacification, anterior and posterior synechiae, cataract, and glaucoma. Specific therapy is not available, and treatment is supportive only. Other causes for red tears include infection with parainfluenza virus type 3 or Sendai virus as well as pain or stress. Ammonia vapor from soiled bedding can act as an ocular irritant, predisposing animals to secondary infection. Keeping the housing areas well ventilated is important in preventing infection with sialodacryoadenitis virus.

Of clinical significance is the effect of xylazine on the lens in rats and mice. A reversible cataract has been observed after systemic use of xylazine. Transcorneal water loss and altered aqueous humor composition caused by corneal exposure have been suggested as a pathogenesis of cataract formation.[8]

In hamsters, keratoconjunctivitis can result from ammonia vapor from soiled bedding. Dental problems including tooth root infection may result in facial or retrobulbar abscesses, with hemifacial swelling, proptosis, and exposure keratitis as common sequelae. Treatment with systemic antibiotics is often unrewarding and such abscesses frequently result in death of the animal.[20]

Insidious globe enlargement with loss of vision has been reported in four hamsters.[13] Ophthalmic examination of these hamsters revealed an enlarged globe in both eyes, widely dilated pupils, lack of pupillary light reflex, a small optic nerve, and pale retinae. Histopathologic results suggested chronic open-angle glaucoma. Treatment of the suspected glaucoma was not attempted.

SUGAR GLIDERS

Sugar gliders have an avascular retina. Only a small residual tuft of fluorescein-impermeable vessels projects from the optic disc into the vitreous.[7]

Sugar gliders have prominent globes that are susceptible to trauma. Corneal ulcers may result from intraspecies fighting.[32] A retrobulbar abscess can result from a bite wound to the face or a molar root abscess. Corneal lipid infiltration may form in juvenile sugar gliders when the mother is fed a diet that is too high in fat. Although not reported, cataract formation is seen clinically.

REFERENCES

1. Abrams KL, Brooks DE, Funk RS, et al: Evaluation of the Schirmer tear test in clinically normal rabbits. Am J Vet Res 1990; 51:1912-1913.
2. Allgoewer I, Ewringmann A, Pfleghaar S: Lymphosarcoma with conjunctival manifestation in a guinea pig. Vet Ophthalmol 1999; 2:117-119.
3. Bauck L: Ophthalmic conditions in pet rabbits and rodents. Compend Contin Educ Pract Vet 1989; 11:258-266.
4. Bellhorn RW, Korte GE, Abrutyn D: Spontaneous corneal degeneration in the rat. Lab Anim Sci 1988; 38:42-50.
5. Burling K, Murphy CJ, da Silva Curiel J, et al: Anatomy of the rabbit nasolacrimal duct and its clinical implications. Progr Vet Comp Ophthalmol 1991; 1:33-40.

6. Burrows AM, Smith TD, Atkinston CS, et al: Development of ocular hypertension in congenitally buphthalmic rabbits. Lab Anim Sci 1995; 45:443-444.
7. Buttery RG, Haight JR, Bell K: Vascular and avascular retinae in mammals. A funduscopic and fluorescein angiographic study. Brain Behav Evol 1990; 35:156-175.
8. Calderone L, Grimes P, Shalev M: Acute reversible cataract induced by xylazine and by ketamine-xylazine anesthesia in rats and mice. Exp Eye Res 1986; 42:331-337.
9. Colgin LMA, Nielsen RE, Tucker FS, et al: Case report of listerial keratoconjunctivitis in hairless guinea pigs. Lab Anim Sci 1995; 45:435-436.
10. Crossley DA, Jackson A, Yates J, et al: Use of computed tomography to investigate cheek tooth abnormalities in chinchillas (*Chinchilla laniger*). J Sm Anim Pract 1998; 39:385-389.
11. Dubielzig RR, Miller PE: The morphology of autosomal dominant microphthalmia in ferrets. Proc Am Coll Vet Ophthalmol 1995; vol 2B:62.
12. Dupont C, Carrier M, Gauvin J: Bilateral precorneal membranous occlusion in a dwarf rabbit. J Sm Anim Exotic Anim Med 1995; 3:41-44.
13. Ekesten B, Dubielzig RR: Spontaneous buphthalmos in the Djungarian hamster (*Phodopus sungorus campbelli*). Vet Ophthalmol 1999; 2:251-254.
14. Griffith JW, Sassani JW, Bowman TA, et al: Osseous choristoma of the ciliary body in guinea pigs. Vet Pathol 1988; 25:100-102.
15. Hadlow WJ: Chronic corneal edema in aged ranch mink. Vet Pathol 1987; 24:323-329.
16. Harcourt-Brown F: Textbook of Rabbit Medicine. Oxford, Butterworth-Heinemann, 2002.
17. Hoyt RF Jr, Powell DA, Feldman SH: Exophthalmia in the rabbit after chronic external jugular catheter placement [abstract]. Proceedings American Association of Laboratory Animal Science Annual Meeting, 1994.
18. Hubert MF, Gillet JP, Durand-Cavagna G: Spontaneous retinal changes in Sprague Dawley rats. Lab Anim Sci 1994; 44:561-567.
19. Janssens G, Simoens P, Muylle S, et al: Bilateral prolapse of the deep gland of the third eyelid in a rabbit: diagnosis and treatment. Lab Anim Sci 1999; 49:105-109.
20. Kern TJ: Ocular disorders of rabbits, rodents, and ferrets. *In* Kirk RW, Bonagura JD eds.: Current Veterinary Therapy X. Philadelphia, WB Saunders, 1989, pp 681-685.
21. Kostolich M, Panciera RJ: Thymoma in a domestic rabbit. Cornell Vet 1992; 82:125-129.
22. Losco PE, Troup CM: Corneal dystrophy in Fischer 344 rats. Lab Anim Sci 1988; 38:702-710.
23. Lucas J, Lucas A, Furber H, et al: *Mycobacterium genavense* infection in two aged ferrets with conjunctival lesions. Aust Vet J 2000; 78:685-689.
24. Marini RP, Foltz CJ, Kersten D, et al: Microbiologic, radiographic, and anatomic study of the nasolacrimal duct apparatus in the rabbit (*Oryctolagus cuniculus*). Lab Anim Sci 1996; 46:656-662.
25. McCalla TL, Erdman SE, Kawasaki TA, et al: Lymphoma with orbital involvement in two ferrets. Vet Comp Ophthalmol 1997; 7:36-38.
26. Miller PE, Marlar AB, Dubielzig RR: Cataracts in a laboratory colony of ferrets. Lab Anim Sci 1993; 43:562-568.
27. Miller PE, Pickett JP: Zygomatic salivary gland mucocele in a ferret. J Am Vet Med Assoc 1989; 194:1437-1438.
28. Millichamp NJ, Collins BR: Blepharoconjunctivitis associated with *Staphylococcus aureus* in a rabbit. J Am Vet Med Assoc 1986; 189:1153-1154.
29. Moore CP, Dubielzig R, Glaza SM: Anterior corneal dystrophy of American Dutch belted rabbits: biomicroscopic and histopathologic findings. Vet Pathol 1987; 24:28-33.
30. Morgan JE, Henderson Z, Thompson ID: Retinal decussation patterns in pigmented and albino ferrets. Neuroscience 1987; 20:519-535.
31. Otto G, Lipman NS, Murphy JC: Corneal dermoid in a hairless guinea pig. Lab Anim Sci 1991; 41:171-172.
32. Pye GW, Carpenter JW: A guide to medicine and surgery in sugar gliders. Vet Med 1999; 94:891-905.
33. Ringle MJ, Lindley DM, Krohne SG: Lymphoplasmacytic keratitis in a ferret with lymphoma. J Am Vet Med Assoc 1993; 203:670-672.
34. Rosenfield ME: Successful eradication of severe abscesses in rabbits with long-term administration of penicillin G benzathine/penicillin G procaine. Available at: http://moorelab.sbs.umass.edu/~mrosenfield/bicillin/. Accessed May 17, 2002.
35. Schoofs S, Hanssen P: Epicorneal conjunctiva syndroom bij het konijn: een klinisch geval en chirurgische behandeling ervan. Vlaams Dierg Tijdschr 1998; 67:344-346.
36. Shapiro SZ, Thulin JD, Morton DG: Periocular and urogenital lesions in mice (*Mus musculus*) chronically infected with *Trypanosoma brucei*. Lab Anim Sci 1994; 44:76-78.
37. Steinberg H: Disseminated T-cell lymphoma in a guinea pig with bilateral ocular involvement. J Vet Diagn Invest 2000; 12:459-462.
38. Stiles J, Didier E, Ritchie B, et al: *Encephalitozoon cuniculi* in the lens of a rabbit with phacoclastic uveitis: confirmation and treatment. Vet Comp Ophthalmol 1997; 7:233-238.
39. Suter C, Müller-Doblies UU, Hatt J-M, et al: Prevention and treatment of *Encephalitozoon cuniculi* infection in rabbits with fenbendazole. Vet Rec 2001; 148:478-480.
40. Tso MOM, Zhang C, Abler AS, et al: Apoptosis leads to photoreceptor degeneration in inherited retinal dystrophy of RCS rats. Invest Ophthalmol Vis Sci 1994; 35:2693-2699.
41. Utroska B, Austin WL: Bilateral cataracts in a ferret. Vet Med/Sm Anim Clin 1979; 1176-1177.
42. Vernau KM, Grahn BH, Clarke-Scott HA, et al: Thymoma in a geriatric rabbit with hypercalcemia and periodic exophthalmos. J Am Vet Med Assoc 1995; 206:820-822.
43. Wagner F, Heider HJ, Gorig C, et al: Augenkrankheiten beim Zwergkaninchen. Teil 1: Anatomie, untersuchungsgang, erkrankungen der Augenlider, der Konjunktiva und des Tranennasengangs. Tierarztl Prax 1998; 26:205-210.
44. Wagner F, Heider HJ, Gorig C, et al: Augenkrankheiten beim Zwergkaninchen. Teil 2: Erkrankungen der kornea, intraokulare und retrobulbare erkrankungen sowie neoplasien. Tierartztl Prax 1998; 26:345-350.
45. Weir EC, Jacoby RO, Paturzo FX, et al: Persistence of sialodacryoadenitis virus in athymic rats. Lab Anim Sci 1990; 40:138-143.
46. Wolfer J, Grahn B, Wilcock B, et al: Phacoclastic uveitis in the rabbit. Progr Vet Comp Ophthalmol 1993; 3:92-97.

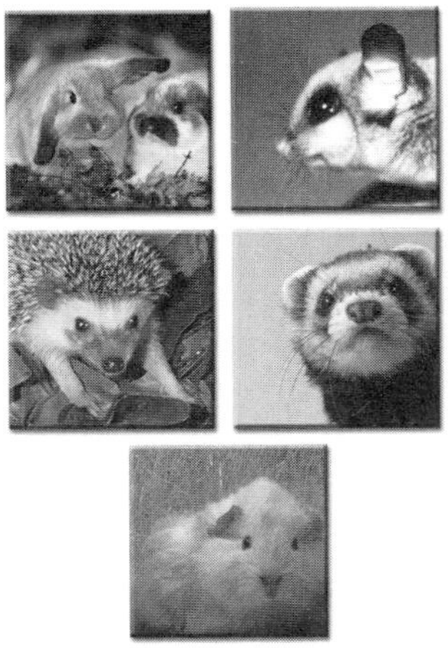

CHAPTER 40

Zoonotic Diseases

Mark A. Mitchell, DVM, MS, PhD, and
Thomas N. Tully, Jr., DVM, MS, Diplomate ABVP

BACTERIAL DISEASES
VIRAL DISEASES
PARASITIC DISEASES
MYCOTIC DISEASES
ALLERGIC REACTIONS

Nontraditional small mammals are growing in popularity as companion animals. The most common species treated by veterinarians include rabbits (*Oryctolagus cuniculus*), ferrets (*Mustela putorius*), mice (*Mus musculus*), rats (*Rattus norvegicus*), chinchillas (*Chinchilla lanigera*), golden hamsters (*Mesocricetus auratus*), Mongolian gerbils (*Meriones unguiculatus*), guinea pigs (*Cavia porcellus*), African pygmy hedgehogs (*Atelerix albiventris*), and sugar gliders (*Petaurus breviceps*). Small mammals are relatively inexpensive pets that often do not require the intensive care or attention that is required of dogs and cats. Because of these perceived advantages, ferrets, rabbits, and rodents are frequently purchased as first pets for children. Unfortunately, most pet owners are unaware of the zoonotic risks associated with owning these nontraditional pets. However, this also extends to medical and veterinary professionals, who are also often unfamiliar with the common zoonotic agents associated with these animals. Specific reports of zoonotic cases attributed to nontraditional species are rare. However, because of their increasing popularity and the amplified exposure to children and individuals with compromised immune systems (e.g., organ transplantation, immunosuppressive drug therapy, immunosuppressive diseases), there is a potential increase in the number of zoonotic cases correlated with small mammal ownership.

The majority of disease conditions associated with nontraditional mammalian pets are related to allergies, bites, and scratches. Dander from these nontraditional species can cause cutaneous and respiratory allergies in susceptible individuals. Many bite and scratch wounds inflicted by these pets can develop into bacterial or viral infections. Pet owners can avoid bite injuries if they understand the behavior of their pet. These animals should be primarily handled during peak activity hours. Certain rodents, such as the hamster, will assume a defense posture by rolling on their dorsum and will vocalize to ward off any perceived dangerous advances from humans. Most bite injuries are related to nocturnal/crepuscular species, such as the hamster, and can be avoided if owners are educated as to the most appropriate times to handle their pet.

This chapter focuses on the zoonotic potential of disease transmission to the typical companion animal owner. Individuals who work with large collections of ferrets, rabbits, and rodents found in laboratory animal settings or breeding facilities have a higher potential for exposure.

BACTERIAL DISEASES

Bordetella bronchiseptica is a gram-negative rod that has been attributed to high morbidity and mortality rates in guinea pigs.[2] Hamsters and mice do not appear to be as sensitive to this pathogen as other rodents.[24] *B. bronchiseptica* can be isolated from clinically normal rodents and lagomorphs. Clinical signs in affected rodents and lagomorphs are generally associated with the respiratory system and are characterized by nasal and ocular discharge, coughing, sneezing, and pneumonia. *B. bronchiseptica* has been associated with respiratory tract infections in humans. Although rodents and lagomorphs pose minimal risk in the dissemination of this bacterium to humans, at-risk individuals should take specific precautions to reduce exposure. Pet dogs are a greater risk to humans than nontraditional mammals for this organism through increased mouth-to-face contact.

Campylobacteriosis is a serious zoonotic disease responsible for the loss of millions of dollars annually in medical expenses. Contaminated food (e.g., poultry) is the primary cause of campylobacteriosis in the United States. Although nontraditional small mammals may harbor *Campylobacter jejuni* or *C. pylori*, they are low risk for transmission of this organism to their owners. Incubation of *Campylobacter* species is approximately 2 to 5 days, and the disease is generally self-limiting (10-14 days) in the immunocompetent host.[8] Ferrets that have recovered from campylobacteriosis may shed the bacteria for more than 140 days.[8] A 9-month bacteriologic survey of biomedical research ferrets suggests that ferrets may pose a special threat to individuals working with ferret colonies. In the study, *C. jejuni* and *C. coli* were isolated from 18% of the ferrets being tested.[8] Although no cases of ferret-associated campylobacteriosis have been reported, the prevalence of *Campylobacter* species in these ferrets suggests that they may serve as a source of infection.

Corynebacterium kutscheri is a gram-positive bacillus that is routinely isolated from the nasopharynx of rats. This microbe has also been isolated from clinically normal mice and hamsters. Most rodents that harbor this microbe are asymptomatic; however, acute clinical disease has been reported in susceptible animals. Affected rodents are generally in poor condition and may develop cutaneous abscesses, nasal and ocular discharge, and arthritis. Because this pathogen has been isolated from a human case of chorioamnionitis, rodents should be considered a potential reservoir for the disease.

Francisella tularensis is the causative agent of rabbit fever, or tularemia. This gram-negative coccobacillus is primarily a pathogen of wild rodents and lagomorphs. Captive rodents and lagomorphs generally are not considered important reservoirs for this microbe. The domestic cat is actually more likely to serve as a reservoir for this microbe than other domestic species because of its possible contact with infected wildlife. *F. tularensis* can be transmitted by aerosolization, direct contact, or ectoparasites (fleas and ticks). Affected individuals may develop cutaneous lesions, respiratory disease, or meningitis (Fig. 40-1).

Leptospira interrogans is frequently isolated from wild rodents. Individuals working with wild rodents or in areas where high densities of wild rodents are concentrated may be at risk of contracting leptospirosis. *L. interrogans, L. grippotyphosa,* and *L. icterohaemorrhagiae* have been isolated from ferrets. Individuals that have contact with ferrets used for hunting may also be predisposed to leptospirosis. Transmission may occur from direct contact or aerosolization of contaminated urine. Affected individuals may have chills, fever, and malaise or septicemia and generalized organ dysfunction. Although captive, nontraditional small mammals are not generally considered to be a source of *L. interrogans* for humans, these animals can serve as reservoirs for the spirochete and appropriate precautions should be taken to prevent exposure.

Listeria monocytogenes is a gram-positive, non–spore-forming rod. Ferrets may serve as a source of the *Listeria* organism because it has been isolated from the liver and lung tissue of infected animals. Listeriosis was also identified in ferrets that were experimentally infected with canine distemper virus. The common finding in many ferret listeriosis cases is that they were immunocompromised animals. Because adrenal gland disease is a common finding in geriatric ferrets, and *L. monocytogenes* is ubiquitous in the environment, caretakers should take appropriate precautions to minimize exposure of this pathogen to the ferret.

Ferrets are extremely sensitive to mycobacteriosis. *Mycobacterium avium, M. bovis,* and *M. tuberculosis* have all been isolated from ferrets. Most mycobacteriosis cases reported in ferrets are from Europe, where ferrets are still used for hunting and are often fed uncooked meat and meat by-products. *Mycobacterium* species can be transmitted to humans from ferrets through aerosolization of contaminated respiratory secretions or direct skin contact. Ferret owners should be instructed to only offer cooked meat to their animals, thereby reducing the likelihood of introducing pathogens to their colony.

Pasteurella multocida is a gram-negative rod that is an opportunistic pathogen of lagomorphs and rodents. In rabbits, *P. multocida* can cause multisystem disease and is difficult to eradicate. Because this organism is ubiquitous in the environment, inoculation of this organism into bite injuries or scratches received from lagomorphs or rodents can occur. In humans, *P. multocida* has been associated with multisystem disease. Susceptible individuals, including young children and immunocompromised adults, should practice strict hygiene after handling these animals. Bite or scratch injuries should be immediately disinfected and a physician contacted for additional information for wound management.

Rat-bite fever (RBF) is a rare but serious zoonosis caused by *Streptobacillus moniliformis* and *Spirillum minus* (Fig. 40-2). These microbes are considered indigenous flora in rats and may be isolated from the nasopharynx. Laboratory and pet rats are considered the primary reservoir for RBF, although wild rats and mice may also serve as competent reservoirs for these microbes. These bacteria are primarily transmitted from a bite. The incubation for streptobacillary RBF in humans is approximately 3 to 10 days, whereas spirillary RBF is 1 to 6 days. The clinical signs attributed to RBF are generally observed at approximately the same time

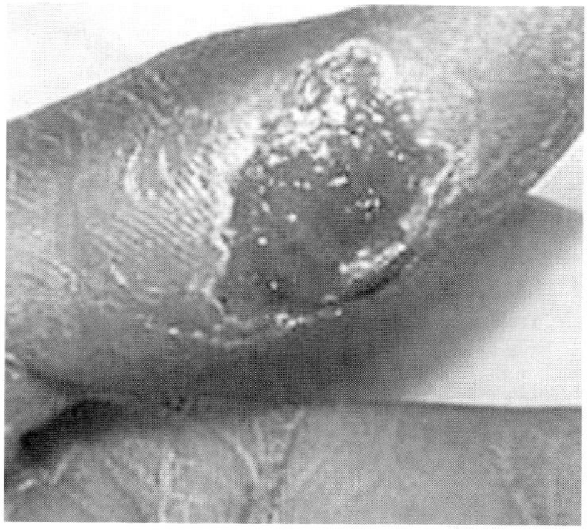

Figure 40-1 Finger of a human infected with *Francisella tularensis*.

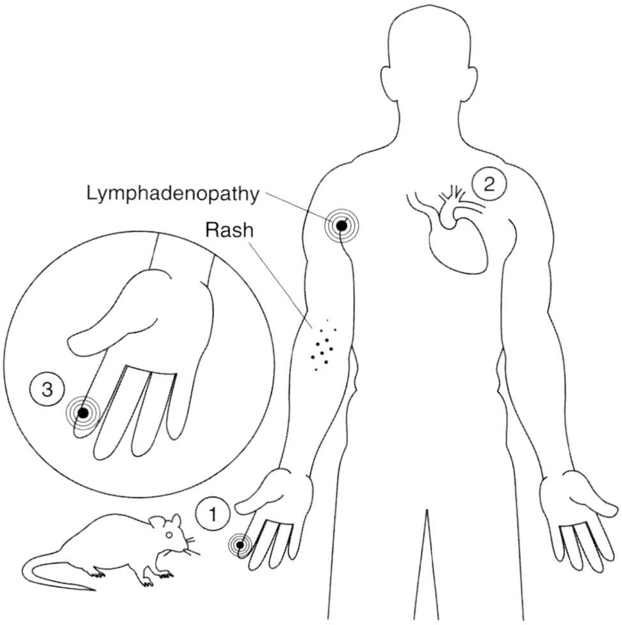

Figure 40-2 Rat-bite fever in humans is initiated with a bite that compromises the protective epithelial barrier. *1,* Entry wound (rat bite); *2,* spread of infection; *3,* disease ulceration at entry site.

the bite wound is healing and include relapsing fever, chills, vomiting, myalgia, and regional lymphadenopathy. Individuals infected with *S. moniliformis* frequently have a maculopapular rash on their extremities. The maculopapular rash does not occur with spirillary RBF. Rat-bite wounds should be immediately disinfected to reduce the likelihood of transmitting these bacterial pathogens.

Salmonella species are gram-negative facultative anaerobes that are ubiquitous in the environment. This microbe has been associated with both enzootic and epizootic outbreaks in captive rodent and lagomorph colonies.[6,11,18,22] Salmonella have also been isolated from other nontraditional small mammals, including sugar gliders, African hedgehogs, and ferrets.[25] All vertebrate species should be considered susceptible to salmonella infection. There are more than 2400 different *Salmonella* serotypes, and they should all be considered pathogenic. *S. enteritidis* and *S. typhimurium* are the two most common serotypes isolated from rodents and lagomorphs, whereas *S. tilene* appears to be the most common serotype isolated from sugar gliders and hedgehogs.[12,25] *S. typhimurium*, *S. hadar*, *S. kentucky*, and *S. enteritidis* have been isolated from ferrets.[12,25] Most rodents and ferrets appear to be asymptomatic reservoirs for this microbe. One exception is the guinea pig, which can develop life-threatening septicemia. Salmonella are primarily transmitted by the fecal-oral route or from contaminated fomites but can also can be transmitted by aerosol through the conjunctiva in some species.[16] Affected vertebrates may have anorexia, weight loss, enteritis, lymphadenopathy, or septicemia. Reproductive disorders, including abortions and premature birth, have also been associated with salmonella infections in rodents and lagomorphs. Humans who contract salmonellosis from these animals may have headaches, nausea, vomiting, abdominal pain, enteritis, or septicemia.[23] The incubation of salmonella in humans is approximately 6 to 48 hours. Humans can acquire salmonella from either direct or indirect exposure to mammal reservoirs. In 1994, a case of hedgehog-associated salmonellosis in a 10-month-old girl from Washington was attributed to indirect contact with the family's breeding colony of hedgehogs.[14] Because of the inherent zoonotic risks associated with the ownership of these and other pets, pet ownership should involve adult supervision. Strict hygiene, including hand washing with soap, should be practiced to reduce the risk of exposure. The recommendations for reducing the risk of reptile-associated salmonellosis formulated by the Association of Reptile and Amphibian Veterinarians and the Centers for Disease Control and Prevention would also be appropriate to distribute to owners of nontraditional small mammals.[3]

Streptococcus pneumoniae are gram-positive cocci. Although this pathogen has been isolated from several different mammalian species, the rat and guinea pig appear to be the most susceptible. There are a number of different serotypes that affect rats (II, III, VIII, XVI, and XIX) and guinea pigs (III, IV, and XIX). Several of these serotypes can also infect humans. Transmission of this pathogen is generally through aerosolization of contaminated respiratory secretions or by direct contact. Affected rodents may have pneumonia and torticollis. Humans infected with *S. pneumoniae* may have respiratory and meningeal disease.

There have been three major pandemics of plague during the history of civilization. *Yersinia pestis*, the causative agent of plague, is generally transmitted by flea-borne vectors, although it can also be spread by contaminated respiratory secretions with the pneumonic form (Figs. 40-3 and 40-4). The primary vector for *Y. pestis* is the rodent flea (*Xenopsylla cheopis*), although *Thrasis*, *Diamanus*, *Hoplopsyllus*, and *Dropsylla* species and *Orchopeas sexentatus* are also competent vectors. In the United States, *Y. pestis* is limited to the West and may be spread by domestic species. Because captive nontraditional pet mammals can also serve as competent hosts for many of the vectors reported for this pathogen, precautions should be taken to prevent the introduction of flea vectors into the home. Although there are no cases of plague associated with nontraditional pets in the United States, guinea pigs have been associated with plague in Andean countries, where they are raised for food.[20]

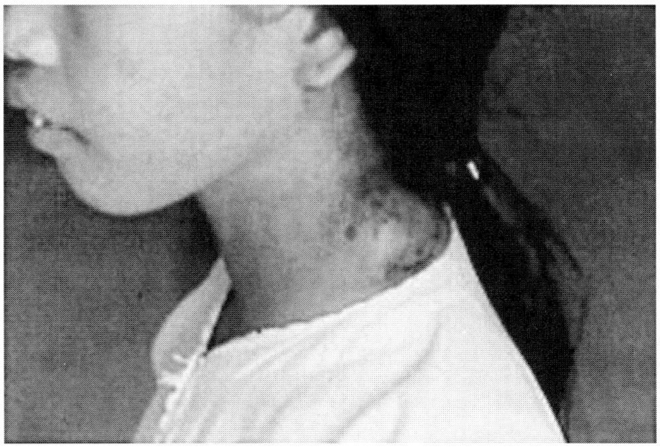

Figure 40-3 Enlarged lymph node (bubo) in a human infected with *Yersinia pestis*. (From www.insecta-inspecta.com.)

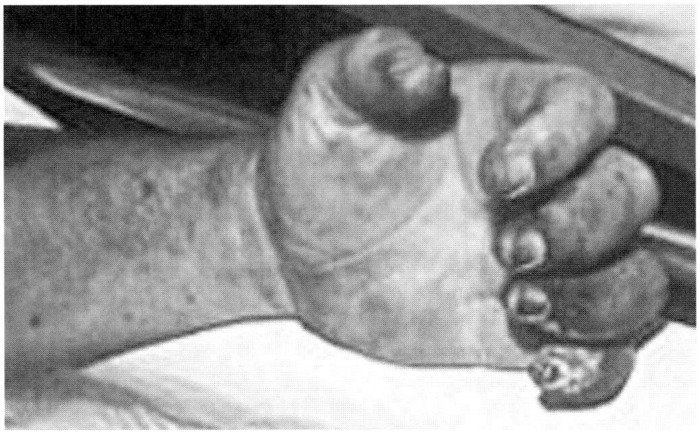

Figure 40-4 Vascular compromise associated with disseminated intravascular coagulation in a patient with the septicemic form of *Yersinia pestis*. (From www.insecta-inspecta.com.)

Yersinia pseudotuberculosis and *Y. enterocolitica* are opportunistic gram-negative coccobacilli that are routinely isolated from clinically normal rodents and lagomorphs. *Y. pseudotuberculosis* has been associated with epizootics in guinea pig colonies worldwide, rats from Japan, and hares from Europe.[1] Affected animals generally have weight loss and enteritis. Mortality rates can approach 75%. Wild rodents are considered to play an important role in the transmission of this pathogen. Although captive rodents have not been identified as an important source of infection for humans, they certainly could serve as competent reservoir of the bacteria in the human environment.

Y. enterocolitica has been associated with epizootics in chinchillas from Europe, Mexico, and the United States.[1] Septicemia was a common finding, and affected animals had enteritis and weight loss. Studies evaluating the prevalence of enterocolitic yersiniosis in wild rodent populations from Czechoslovakia, Scandinavia, and Chile suggest that the prevalence of this pathogen in wild rodents is low (4%-26%). Although pathologic lesions, including abscesses of the liver and intestinal lesions, have been reported in wild rodents, the majority of the wild rodents screened for this pathogen are normal. The biotypes characterized in rodents are not the same biotypes that infect humans. Although rodents are not considered an important source of enterocolitic yersiniosis in humans, veterinarians and animal caretakers should practice strict hygiene and take appropriate precautions when working with infected rodents and lagomorphs.

VIRAL DISEASES

Type A and B influenza viruses from the family Orthomyxoviridae are common pathogens of both ferrets and humans. These viruses can be transmitted between humans and ferrets by aerosolization. The disease is characterized in both humans and ferrets by a mucopurulent nasal and ocular discharge, sneezing, lethargy, fever, and inappetence. Pneumonia can develop in immunocompromised individuals. The influenza virus is apparently widespread in some ferret colonies. To reduce the likelihood of transmission of the virus between the two hosts, it is important to isolate infected ferrets from humans and vice versa.

Hantaan disease has been associated with epidemics in the United States, Japan, and Eurasia. This virus is transmitted through direct contact and aerosolization. Infected rodents are generally asymptomatic. Although this virus is generally associated with wild rodents, outbreaks have also been attributed to laboratory rodents in Europe and Japan. Affected individuals reported flu-like symptoms, fever, myalgia, and oliguria. Rodents should be screened for the virus before incorporating them into a colony.

Lymphocytic choriomeningitis (LCM) is caused by RNA arenavirus. The mouse is the primary reservoir for this virus, although the hamster and guinea pig are also competent reservoirs. This virus is transmitted by horizontal and vertical routes in rodents.[1] Affected rodents are generally asymptomatic, although clinical disease, including weight loss, photophobia, tremors, and convulsions, may occur.[12] Humans may become infected with LCM from exposure to contaminated feces or urine or from a bite. Affected humans frequently report clinical symptoms consistent with a flu, including malaise, headaches, fever, myalgia, and arthritis. Fatal aseptic meningitis or meningoencephalitis is rare. An epidemic of LCM occurred in 1973 to 1974 and was associated with hamsters being produced by a single facility in Birmingham, AL.[4] There were more than 181 human cases reported from 12 states. Humans working closely with large populations of rodents or wild rodents should practice strict hygiene and wear protective clothing to reduce the likelihood of exposure.

Rabies is caused by a negative-strand RNA lyssavirus. All mammals should be considered competent reservoirs for this virus; however, the majority (more than 90%) of reported cases are associated with wildlife.[17] Rabies has been isolated from ferrets, lagomorphs, and various rodent species, including rats, squirrels, and woodchucks. Although lagomorphs are not considered an important reservoir for rabies, a recent report of rabies in domestic rabbits suggests that pet owners and veterinarians should take appropriate precautions when animals have clinical signs associated with rabies infection. A rabies vaccination (Imrab 3, Merial, Athens, GA) has been approved for use in ferrets. Veterinarians should strongly recommend vaccinating ferrets against rabies. Although the risk of contracting rabies is extremely low, unvaccinated ferrets that bite a human must, by law, be euthanatized and submitted for rabies testing. Pet owners should take the appropriate precautions to limit contact between pets housed outdoors and wildlife.

Reoviruses are found in a number of different vertebrate hosts. Mouse reovirus type 3 has been associated with morbidity and mortality in suckling mice. Affected animals may be jaundiced, stunted, develop oily hair, and have diarrhea. This virus is spread through both horizontal and vertical routes. Reovirus type 3 has been associated with disease in humans, causing enteritis in susceptible, particularly immunocompromised, people who come into contact with infected mice. Immunocompromised individuals should therefore avoid contact with reovirus-infected mice.

In 2003, a rare zoonotic viral disease outbreak occurred in the United States. Monkeypox virus, a member of the orthopoxvirus group, was responsible for the outbreak. Monkeypox has similar clinical manifestations as smallpox and primarily occurs in the rainforest countries of central and west Africa.[9] This was the first report of the disease in the United States; and community-acquired monkeypox had never been reported outside of Africa.

Until the latest outbreak, most of the concerns for zoonotic infection have been in primate research and laboratory animal facilities, especially those housing Asian macaques.[7] Human-to-human contact has been reported, but rarely occurs.[7] In the 2003 U.S. outbreak, the majority of people who contracted clinical illness were exposed through close contact with sick captive prairie dogs (*Cynomys* species). It is believed that the prairie dogs became infected after they were exposed to a sick Gambian giant pouched rat (*Aterurus* species) or a shipment of similar animals. Animal species that are potential carriers of monkeypox and/or showing disease signs of a nonspecific nature should be quarantined, stabilized, and reported to state public health officials.

The clinical signs of monkeypox reported in animals during the 2003 U.S. outbreak included fever, cough, blepharoconjunctivitis, lymphadenopathy, and nodular rash. Traditionally, monkeypox has been associated with a high morbidity rate and a low to variable mortality rate in humans (1%-10% case fatality rate in African outbreaks). Humans can be exposed from direct contact with an infected animal's body fluids or bite wounds.[9] The smallpox vaccine, now available, will protect humans against monkeypox infection.[9] Morbidity and mortality rates for animals are variable.

If monkeypox is suspected in a case, the clinic should be contacted before arrival. The owners should protect themselves against potential exposure by quarantining the animal and wearing masks and gloves when the animal needs to be handled. Currently, all animals suspected of being infected with monkeypox or exhibiting clinical illness should be euthanatized and undergo necropsy. If the animal is not exhibiting clinical signs, then there is no recommendation by the Centers for Disease Control and Prevention for euthanasia, even with the knowledge of an animal's possible exposure to a confirmed case of monkeypox.

The 2003 monkeypox outbreak is an example of a rare emerging viral disease in the United States. Veterinarians should be aware that they are often the first line of defense when an unusual form of morbidity and mortality in animals is encountered. Communication with local, regional, state, and national public health officers is important when trying to identify a series of unusual animal disease presentations and conditions.

PARASITIC DISEASES

Cryptosporidiosis is a common zoonotic disease. *Cryptosporidium parvum* does not appear to be host specific and may infect a wide range of mammals. A 6-month study evaluating three serial fecal samples from a group of ferrets being received at a biologic research facility found that 66% of the animals had cryptosporidiosis.[19] Ferrets with cryptosporidiosis are generally asymptomatic, although postmortem examination has revealed mild pathologic changes in some clinically normal animals. Individuals with compromised immune systems, such as children and those with acquired immunodeficiency virus (AIDS), should limit their contact with *Cryptosporidium*-positive ferrets. Fatal intestinal cryptosporidiosis has also been reported in African hedgehogs, suggesting that these animals may also pose a zoonotic threat to human caretakers.[10]

Although there are no serious zoonotic diseases that can be spread from rabbits to healthy humans, immunocompromised (i.e., AIDS) patients may contract *Encephalitozoon cuniculi*. In one report, three patients with human immunodeficiency virus had *E. cuniculi*, with one of the patients having clinical manifestations of disease with the parasite (severe interstitial pneumonitis).[5] The symptoms abated and the parasite excretion ceased when these patients were treated with albendazole.

The two main *Giardia* species that infect rodents are *G. duodenalis* and *G. muris*. Clinical signs vary depending on the species of *giardia* and the species of animal infected. The clinical disease in man primarily affects the gastrointestinal tract but other body systems may be involved including the joints, specifically the synovial surfaces, and hypersensitivity reactions.[15] Transmission is direct through fecal-oral contamination of the trophozoite and cyst form of the organism. Diagnosis and treatment of the affected animals to prevent further shedding and proper hygiene after handling animals will prevent the spread and transmission of this protozoal parasite to humans.

Hymenolepis species is a cestode that infects rodents. *H. diminuta* has been identified in rats, hamsters, and mice, whereas *H. nana* is found mainly in mice and rats. Humans can become infected with this parasite by ingesting contaminated feces. Indirect infection can occur when insects ingest the tapeworm eggs, which then develop into cysticercoid larvae in the indirect host's body. Although most infected humans are asymptomatic, particularly with *H. diminuta*, clinical disease can occur with heavy infections because of the absorption of metabolic waste produced by a heavy worm burden and gastrointestinal irritation.[13] Children are more likely to be clinically affected than adults. Affected individuals may have abdominal cramping, nausea, vomiting, and diarrhea. The cestodes *Taenia taeniaeformis* of rats and mice and *T. serialis* found in rabbits can cause clinical illness in people when infected animals are consumed.

Sarcoptic mange, caused by *Sarcoptes scabiei*, affects many mammalian species. Affected animals often have severe, intense pruritus, scales, crusts, erythema, and generalized alopecia. Pododermatitis and self-mutilation are common findings in ferrets. Humans who become infected with sarcoptic mange may have wheals, vesicles, papules, and intense pruritus develop. Infected animals should be quarantined from other animals and only handled with gloves to reduce exposure. Lime sulfur shampoos, ivermectin, and selamectin may be used to treat affected animals.

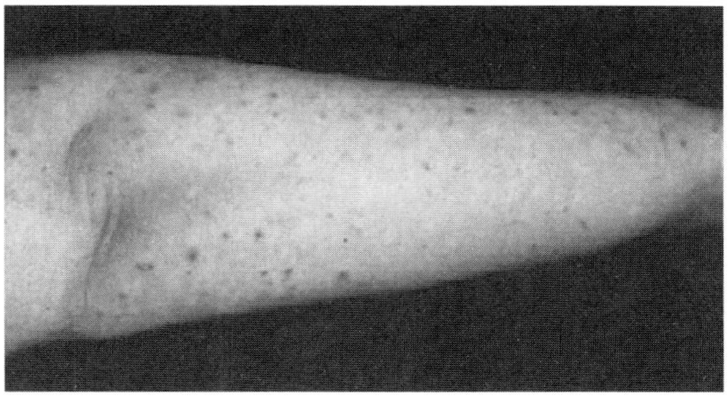

Figure 40-5 Dermatitis in a human caused by *Cheyletiella* species infestation.

Trixacarus caviae is an ectoparasite of guinea pigs. In general, guinea pigs infested with *T. caviae* are asymptomatic. However, animals that are maintained in poor conditions or are stressed may have generalized clinical signs, including alopecia, intense pruritis, scales, crusts, and hyperkeratosis. Pet owners, especially children, may become infected with *T. caviae* from direct contact with infected guinea pigs. Affected individuals generally have mild dermatitis. *T. caviae* is very difficult to eliminate in affected guinea pigs. Intensive environmental cleaning and management along with therapeutic treatment with ivermectin or selamectin have been effective.

Liponyssus bacoti, the tropical rat mite, will bite humans. Although this parasite mainly feeds on the rat host and lives within the animal's bedding, it is the transfer of other infectious diseases through the bite of the mite that is of medical concern. *L. bacoti* can transmit murine typhus, Q fever, and *Y. pestis*.[12] Treatment and prevention follow the same environmental and therapeutic protocols as described for other skin mite species.

Cheyletiella parasitovorax is an ectoparasite that infests domestic rabbits. This mite is generally found on the hair shaft and in the keratin layer of the skin. Infested rabbits may be asymptomatic or have alopecia and scaling. In severe cases, rabbits with cheyletiellosis appear to have "walking dandruff." The life cycle of this mite is 35 days, and the parasite generally does not survive for more than 10 days off of the rabbit host. Humans who become infested with this mite generally develop focal to multifocal dermatitis (Fig. 40-5). Papular and pruritic eruptions on the arms, thorax, waist, and legs have been described. The mite does not reproduce on the human host; therefore the infestation is generally self-limiting. Pet owners should be instructed to limit contact with infested rabbits during the treatment period, and gloves should be worn when contact is necessary.

MYCOTIC DISEASES

Trichophyton species (usually *T. mentagrophytes*) is an opportunistic fungal disease of mammals. "Ringworm" has been isolated from rodents, lagomorphs, ferrets, hedgehogs, and marsupials. Affected animals may be asymptomatic or have focal to multifocal alopecia. Depending on the degree of pruritus associated with the infection, crusts, scabs, and excoriations may also be present. Approximately 25% of the human ringworm cases reported annually are attributed to animal contact.[21] Affected humans may be asymptomatic or have alopecia and crusts, similar to the lesions identified in pet animals. To a lesser extent, *Microsporum canis* may affect rodents, with active lesions in humans most often found on the scalp. Topical application of antimycotics is the recommended treatment in infected humans.

ALLERGIC REACTIONS

It has been estimated that between 11% and 15% of people exposed to rodent and lagomorph species have allergic reactions develop.[10] Human allergic reactions to small mammal skin and fur antigens can present as respiratory, ocular, skin, or anaphylactic clinical signs. Many people are allergic to one animal's antigen, although multiple allergies involving small mammals may occur. The most common small animal antigens are, in descending order, rats, guinea pigs, rabbits, mice, hamsters, and gerbils. Respiratory reactions to aerosolized rat urine are particularly severe because of the life-threatening pulmonary effects of the tissue response to the antigenic components of the urinary compounds.[12] Antihistamine treatment is recommended for people with allergic reactions; reducing exposure to the antigenic compounds will decrease hypersensitivity reactions.

Although zoonotic diseases rarely result from our interactions with nontraditional small mammals maintained as companion animals, it is an area of importance to veterinarians. Understanding the zoonotic potential of small animal diseases is essential not only to protect the health of the veterinarians and their staff, but also to educate and inform their pet-owning clients.

REFERENCES

1. Acha F, Szyfres B: Zoonoses and Communicable Diseases Common to Man and Animals, 2nd ed. Washington, DC, Pan American Health Organization, 1987.
2. Anderson LC: Guinea pig medicine and husbandry. Vet Clin North Am Small Anim Pract 1987; 17:1045-1060.
3. Bradley T, Angulo F, Mitchell MA: Public health education on *Salmonella* spp. and reptiles. J Am Vet Med Assoc 2001; 219:754-755.
4. Deibel R, Woodall JP, Decher WJ, et al: Lymphocytic choriomeningitis virus in man: serologic evidence of association with pet hamsters. J Am Med Assoc 1975; 232:501-504.
5. Deplazes P, Mathis A, Baumgartner R, et al: Immunologic and molecular characteristics of *Encephalitozoon*-like microsporidia isolated from humans and rabbits indicate that *Encephalitozoon cuniculi* is a zoonotic parasite. Clin Infect Dis 1996; 22:557–559.
6. Duthie RC, Mitchell CA: *Salmonella enteritidis* infections in guinea pigs and rabbits. J Am Vet Med Assoc 1931; 78:27-41.
7. Fenner F: Poxviruses of laboratory animals. Lab Anim Sci 1990; 40:469-480.
8. Fox JG, Ackerman JL, Taylor NS: *Campylobacter jejuni* in the ferret: a model of human campylobacteriosis. Am J Vet Res 1987; 48:85-90.
9. Fox JG, Newcomer CE, Rozmiarek H: Selected zoonoses. *In* Fox JG, Anderson LC, Loew FM, et al, eds. Laboratory Animal Medicine, 2nd ed. San Diego, Academic Press, 2002, pp 1059-1105.
10. Graczyk TK, Cranfield MR, Dunning C, et al: Fatal cryptosporidiosis in a juvenile captive African hedgehog (*Atelerix albiventris*). J Parasitol 1998; 84:178-180.
11. Habermann RT, Williams FP: Salmonellosis in laboratory animals. J Natl Cancer Inst 1958; 20:933-947.
12. Harkness JE, Wagner JE: The Biology and Medicine of Rabbits and Rodents. Baltimore, Lea & Febiger, 1995, pp 103-284.
13. Jueco NL. *Hymenolepis nana* infection. *In* Steele JH, Jacobs L, Arambulo P, eds. Handbook Series in Zoonosis. Section C: Parasitic Zoonosis. Vol 1. Boca Raton, FL, CRC Press, 1982, pp 283-287.
14. Lipsky S, Tanino T: African pygmy hedgehog-associated salmonellosis—Washington. MMWR Morb Mortal Wkly Rep 1995; 44:462-463.
15. Meyer EA, Jarroll EL: Giardiasis. *In* Steele JH, Jacobs L, Arambulo P, eds. Handbook Series in Zoonosis. Section C: Parasitic Zoonosis. Vol 1. Boca Raton, FL, CRC Press, 1982, pp 25-40.
16. Moore B: Observations pointing to the conjunctiva as the portal of entry in *Salmonella* infection of guinea pigs. J Hyg (Lond) 1957; 55:414-433.
17. Morrison G: Zoonotic infections from pets. Understanding the risks and treatment. Postgrad Med 2001; 110:24-26, 29-30, 35-36.
18. Olson GA, Shields RP, Gaskin JM: Salmonellosis in a gerbil colony. J Am Vet Med Assoc 1977; 171:970-972.
19. Rehg JE, Gigliotti F, Stokes DC: Cryptosporidiosis in ferrets. Lab Anim Sci 1988; 38:155-158.
20. Ruiz A: Plague in the Americas. Emerg Infect Dis 2001; 7:539-540.
21. Ryan CP: Animals in schools and rehabilitation facilities. So Calif Vet Med Assoc 1998; 9:6,16.
22. Steffen EK, Wagner JE: *Salmonella enteritidis* serotype Amsterdam in a commercial rat colony. Lab Anim Sci 1983; 33:454-456.
23. Turnbull PCB: Food poisoning with special reference to *Salmonella*—its epidemiology, pathogenesis, and control. Clin Gastroenterol 1979; 8:663-713.
24. Winsser J: A study of *Bordetella bronchiseptica*. Proc Anim Care Panel 1960; 10:87-104.
25. Woodward DL, Khakhria R, Johnson WM: Human salmonellosis associated with exotic pets. J Clin Micro 1997; 35:2786-2790.

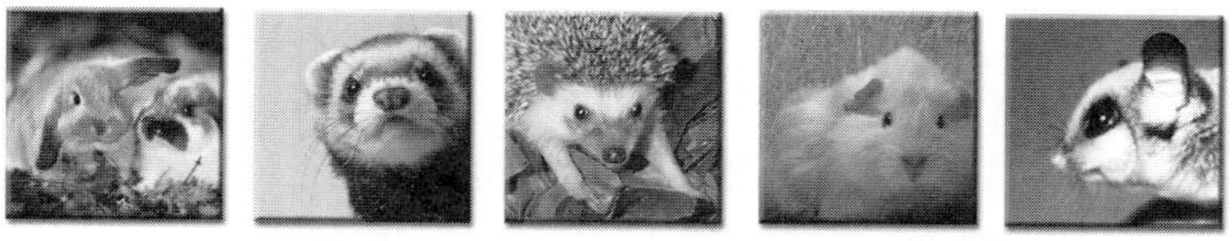

SECTION SEVEN

SPECIAL TOPICS

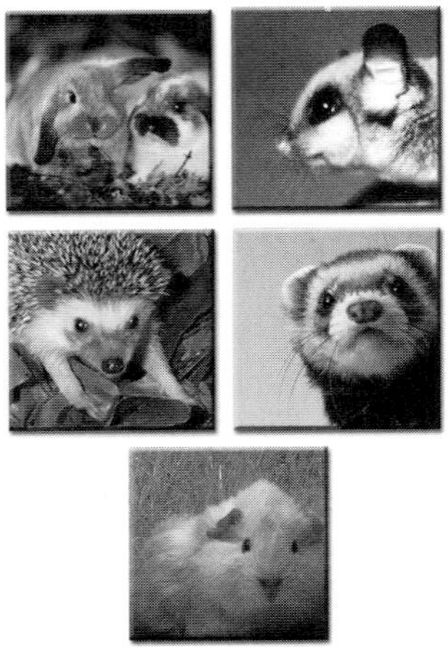

CHAPTER 41

Formulary

James K. Morrisey, DVM, Diplomate ABVP, and
James W. Carpenter, MS, DVM, Diplomate ACZM

This formulary presents the antimicrobial agents (Table 41-1); antifungal agents (Table 41-2); antiparasitic agents (Table 41-3); chemical restraint, anesthetic, and analgesic agents (Table 41-4); and miscellaneous agents (Table 41-5) most commonly used in ferrets, rabbits, guinea pigs, chinchillas, hamsters, rats, mice, prairie dogs, hedgehogs, and sugar gliders. There are many specific circumstances and drug types that cannot be included in this chapter. The reader is referred to other, more comprehensive formularies[1] and the literature for this information. Additionally, specific chapters in this book may have dosages that are different or not mentioned in this chapter.

It should be noted that most of these dosages are extralabel and based on empirical data, observation, and experience. To date, very few drugs are approved by the Food and Drug Administration for use in small mammals kept as nontraditional pets, such as the animals discussed in this book. The Animal Medicinal Drug Use Clarification Act enables veterinarians to use drugs approved for human and other animal use on animals other than those for which they are approved, if the reasoning is sound. This act requires that owners sign an informed consent form for extralabel drug use. Because most drugs are not approved by the Food and Drug Administration for use in these animals, it may be warranted for the owners to sign a consent form when registering their pet.

Because pharmacokinetic studies are lacking in these pet species, it is important to know some of the pharmacobiologic, physiologic, and anatomic characteristics of these animals. Drug uptake and use depend on many factors, including age, body fat, sex, physiology (gastrointestinal, hepatic, renal, etc), illness, diet, fasting state, and others. For example, it is well known that hindgut fermenters, such as rabbits and guinea pigs, do not tolerate some oral antibiotics, such as penicillins, because they can cause a fatal enterotoxemia. The complete list of this information is beyond the scope of this chapter and the reader is referred to the chapters on anatomy and physiology of each species elsewhere in this book. Because these dosages are often empirical, it is helpful to know the basic pharmacologic features and the side effects of the drugs being used for maximum safety and efficacy. It is important to inform the owner or technical staff of clinical signs that may indicate toxicity. This information is available in the drug inserts, the *Physician's Desk Reference*, and other formularies.[1,2] Allometric scaling may also be helpful in prescribing drugs in this formulary to other species.

Most of the drugs given to these nontraditional pet species are given parenterally or orally in the form of suspensions. There has been little research on the efficacy of various drug suspensions in these patients. It is essential for practitioners to have a good working relationship with a licensed compounding pharmacist. These pharmacists will ensure that the drug is placed in the appropriate media to remain viable in suspension and can warn of potential risks associated with this media.

It is important to obtain a definitive diagnosis whenever possible to avoid the problems associated with the empirical dosages and to improve efficacy in these species. Antibiotics should be selected based on culture and sensitivity results whenever possible. The use of more pathogen-specific antimicrobials will decrease the potential for resistant bacteria and often narrows the potential side effects.

We have attempted to verify and double-check all dosages presented in this formulary. However, despite these efforts, errors in the original sources or in the preparation of this chapter may have occurred. All users of this reference should therefore empirically evaluate all dosages to determine that they are reasonable before use. We assume no responsibility for and make no warranty regarding results obtained from the dosages listed.

REFERENCES

1. Carpenter JW, ed: Exotic Animal Formulary, 3rd ed. Philadelphia, WB Saunders, 2004.
2. Smith DA, Burgmann PM: Formulary. *In* Hillyer EV, Quesenberry KE, eds. Ferrets, Rabbits, and Rodents: Clinical Medicine and Surgery. Philadelphia, WB Saunders, 1997, pp 392-403.

TABLE 41-1
Antimicrobial Agents

Agent	Dosage								
	Ferrets	**Rabbits**	**Guinea Pigs**	**Chinchillas**	**Hamsters**	**Rats/Mice**	**Prairie Dogs**	**Hedgehogs**	**Sugar Gliders**
Amikacin	8-16 mg/kg SC, IM, IV divided q8-24h	5-10 mg/kg SC, IM, IV divided q8-24h	10-15 mg/kg SC, IM, IV divided q8-24h	10-15 mg/kg SC, IM, IV divided q8-24h	10 mg/kg SC, IM q12h	10 mg/kg SC, IM q12h	5 mg/kg SC, IM q12h	—	—
Amoxicillin	10-30 mg/kg PO q8-12h	Do not use	Do not use	Do not use	Do not use	—	15 mg/kg PO, SC q12h (use with caution)	15 mg/kg PO, IM q12h	30 mg/kg PO, IM divided q12-24h
Amoxicillin/ clavulanic acid	12.5-25 mg/kg PO q8-12h	Do not use	Do not use	Do not use	Do not use	—	—	12.5 mg/kg PO q12h	12.5 mg/kg PO, SC divided q12-24h
Ampicillin	5-30 mg/kg SC, IM, IV q8-12h	Do not use	Do not use	Do not use	Do not use	20-50 mg/kg PO, SC, IM q12h	—	10 mg/kg IM q12h	—
Cephalexin	15-30 mg/kg PO q8-12h	11-22 mg/kg PO q8h	50 mg/kg PO divided q12-24h	—	—	—	—	—	30 mg/kg PO, SC divided q12-24h
Chloramphenicol	25-50 mg/kg PO q12h	30-50 mg/kg PO q12h	50 mg/kg PO q8-12h	50 mg/kg PO q8-12h	30-50 mg/kg PO q8-12h	30-50 mg/kg PO q8-12h	50 mg/kg PO, SC, IM q12h	30-50 mg/kg PO q12h	—
Chlortetracycline	—	50 mg/kg PO q12h	—	50 mg/kg PO q12h	20 mg/kg PO, SC q12h	10 mg/kg PO, SC q12h (R); 25 mg/kg PO, SC q12h (M)	—	—	—
Ciprofloxacin	10-30 mg/kg PO q24h	10-20 mg/kg PO q12-24h	5-15 mg/kg PO q12-24h	5-15 mg/kg PO q12-24h	10 mg/kg PO q12h	10 mg/kg PO q12h	5-20 mg/kg PO q12h	5-20 mg/kg PO q12h	10 mg/kg PO q12h
Clindamycin	5-10 mg/kg PO q12h	Do not use	Do not use	Do not use	Do not use	—	—	5.5 mg/kg PO q12h	—
Doxycycline	—	2.5 mg/kg PO q12h	2.5 mg/kg PO q12h	2.5 mg/kg PO q12h	2.5 mg/kg PO q12h	5 mg/kg PO q12h; 100 mg/kg SC q7d (long-acting form)	2.5 mg/kg PO q12h	—	—
Enrofloxacin*	5-15 mg/kg PO, SC, IM q12h	5-15 mg/kg PO, SC, IM q12h	5-15 mg/kg PO, SC, IM q12h	5-15 mg/kg PO, SC, IM q12h	5-10 mg/kg PO, SC, IM q12h	5-10 mg/kg PO, SC, IM q12h	5-10 mg/kg PO, SC, IM q12h	2.5-10 mg/kg PO, SC, IM q12h	5 mg/kg PO, SC, IM q12h
Erythromycin	10 mg/kg PO q6h	Do not use	Do not use	Do not use	Do not use or use with caution	20 mg/kg PO q12h	—	10 mg/kg PO q12h	—
Gentamicin	5 mg/kg SC, IM q24h (use with caution or avoid use)	4 mg/kg SC, IM q24h (use with caution or avoid use)	5-8 mg/kg SC, IM divided q8-24h	5-8 mg/kg SC, IM divided q8-24h	5-8 mg/kg SC, IM divided q8-24h	5-10 mg/kg SC, IM divided q8-24h	—	—	2 mg/kg SC, IM divided q12-24h
Metronidazole	15-20 mg/kg PO q12h	20 mg/kg PO q12h	20 mg/kg PO q12h	10-20 mg/kg PO q12h (use with caution)	20 mg/kg PO q12h	10-40 mg/kg PO q24h (R)	20-40 mg/kg PO q12h	20 mg/kg PO q12h	25 mg/kg PO q12h

TABLE 41-1
Antimicrobial Agents—cont'd

Agent	Dosage								
	Ferrets	Rabbits	Guinea Pigs	Chinchillas	Hamsters	Rats/Mice	Prairie Dogs	Hedgehogs	Sugar Gliders
Neomycin	10 mg/kg PO q6-8h q12h	30 mg/kg PO q12h	15 mg/kg PO q12h	15 mg/kg PO q12h	30 mg/kg PO q12h	25 mg/kg PO q12h	25 mg/kg PO q12h	—	—
Penicillin G	40,000 IU/kg SC q24h	40-60,000 IU/kg SC q48h (use with caution)	Do not use	Do not use	—	22,000 IU/kg SC, IM q24h (R)	—	40,000 IU/kg SC, IM q24h	—
Tetracycline	20-25 mg/kg PO q8-12h	50 mg/kg PO q8-12h	10 mg/kg PO q8-12h (use with caution)	10-20 mg/kg PO q8-12h	10-20 mg/kg PO q8-12h	10-20 mg/kg PO q8-12h	10-20 mg/kg PO q8-12h	—	—
Trimethoprim-sulfa	15-30 mg/kg PO, SC q12h	30 mg/kg PO, SC q12h	15-30 mg/kg PO, SC q12h	15-30 mg/kg PO, SC q12h	15-30 mg/kg PO, SC q12h	15-30 mg/kg PO, SC q12h	15-30 mg/kg PO, SC q12h	30 mg/kg PO q12h	15 mg/kg PO q12h
Tylosin	10 mg/kg PO, SC q8-12h	10 mg/kg PO, SC q12h	10 mg/kg PO, SC q12h (use with caution)	10 mg/kg PO, SC q12h	2-8 mg/kg PO, SC q12h (use with caution)	10 mg/kg PO, SC q12h	—	10 mg/kg PO, SC q12h	—

*The oral route of administration is preferable; limit subcutaneous and intramuscular routes of administration because of potential tissue necrosis at injection site.

TABLE 41-2
Antifungal Agents

Agent	Dosage								
	Ferrets	Rabbits	Guinea Pigs	Chinchillas	Hamsters	Rats/Mice	Prairie Dogs	Hedgehogs	Sugar Gliders
Griseofulvin	25 mg/kg PO q12h	12.5 mg/kg PO q12h	15-25 mg/kg PO q24h	25 mg/kg PO q24h	25 mg/kg PO q24h	25 mg/kg PO q24h	25 mg/kg PO q24h	50 mg/kg PO q24h	—
Ketoconazole	10-30 mg/kg PO q12-24h	10-40 mg/kg PO q24h	—	—	10 mg/kg PO q24h	20 mg/kg PO q24h	—	10 mg/kg PO q24h	—
Lime sulfur dip (2.5%)	Dip q7d	Dip q7d × 4 treatments	Dip q7d	Dip q7d × 4 treatments	Apply topically q7d	Apply topically q7d	—	—	NA

NA, Not applicable.

TABLE 41-3
Antiparasitic Agents

	Dosage								
Agent	**Ferrets**	**Rabbits**	**Guinea Pigs**	**Chinchillas**	**Hamsters**	**Rats/mice**	**Prairie Dogs**	**Hedgehogs**	**Sugar Gliders**
Amitraz	0.3% solution topically q7d	—	0.3% solution topically q7d	—	1.4 mL/L topically q7d	1.4 mL/L topically q7d	—	0.3% solution topically q7d	—
Carbaryl 5% powder	Apply topically q7d	Apply topically q7d	Apply topically q7d	Apply topically q7d	Apply topically q7d	Apply topically q7d	Apply topically q7d	—	Apply topically sparingly
Fenbendazole	20 mg/kg PO q24h × 5 days	10-20 mg/kg PO, repeat in 14 days	20 mg/kg PO q24h × 5 days	20 mg/kg PO q24h × 5 days	20 mg/kg PO q24h × 5 days	20 mg/kg PO q24h × 5 days	25 mg/kg PO q24h × 5 days or q14d	—	20 mg/kg PO q24h × 3 days
Fipronil	1 pump of spray or 1/5 of cat tube q30-60d	Toxic; do not use	—	—	7.5 mg/kg topically q30-60d	7.5 mg/kg topically q30-60d	1/2 kitten dose topically	—	—
Imidacloprid	1 cat dose topically q30d	1 cat dose topically q30d	—	—	—	—	1/2 kitten dose topically	—	—
Ivermectin	0.2-0.4 mg/kg PO, SC, repeat in 14 days; 0.05 mg/kg PO, SC q30d (heartworm prevention or microfilaricide)	0.2-0.4 mg/kg SC q10-14d	0.2-0.4 mg/kg SC q10-14d	0.2-0.4 mg/kg SC q10-14d	0.2-0.4 mg/kg SC q10-14d	0.2-0.4 mg/kg SC q10-14d; 2 mg/kg topically on back (M)	0.2-0.4 mg/kg SC q10-14d	0.2-0.4 mg/kg SC q10-14d	0.2 mg/kg SC q10-14d
Lime sulfur dip (2.5%)	Dip q7d	Dip q7d	Dip q7d	Dip q7d	Dip q7d	Dip q7d	Dip q7d	—	—
Lufenuron	30-45 mg/kg PO q30d	30 mg/kg PO q30d	—	—	—	—	—	—	—
Metronidazole	20 mg/kg PO q12h	20 mg/kg PO q12h	25 mg/kg PO q12h	50 mg/kg PO q12h (use with caution)	70 mg/kg PO q8h	10-40 mg/rat PO q24h	40 mg/kg PO q24h	25 mg/kg PO q12h	25 mg/kg PO q12h
Milbemycin oxime	1.15-2.33 mg/kg PO q30d	—	—	—	—	—	—	—	—

TABLE 41-3
Antiparasitic Agents—cont'd

	Dosage								
Agent	Ferrets	Rabbits	Guinea Pigs	Chinchillas	Hamsters	Rats/Mice	Prairie Dogs	Hedgehogs	Sugar Gliders
Piperazine adipate	—	500 mg/kg PO q24h × 2 days	4-7 mg/mL drinking water × 3-10 days	500 mg/kg PO q24h	3-5 mg/mL drinking water × 7 days, off 7 days, repeat	4-7 mg/mL drinking water × 3-10 days	—	—	—
Piperazine citrate	50-100 mg/kg PO, repeat in 14 days	200 mg/kg PO, repeat in 14 days	10 mg/mL drinking × 7 days, off 7 days, repeat	100 mg/kg PO q24h × 2 days	10 mg/mL drinking water × 7 days, off 7 days, repeat	4-5 mg/mL drinking water × 7 days, off 7 days, repeat	4-5 mg/mL drinking water × 7 days, off 7 days, repeat	—	—
Praziquantel	5-10 mg/kg PO, SC, IM, repeat in 10 days	5-10 mg/kg PO, SC, IM, repeat in 10 days	5-10 mg/kg PO, SC, IM, repeat in 10 days	5-10 mg/kg PO, SC, IM, repeat in 10 days	6-10 mg/kg PO, SC, repeat in 10 days	6-10 mg/kg PO, SC, repeat in 10 days	6-10 mg/kg PO, SC, IM, repeat in 10-14 days	7 mg/kg PO, SC, repeat in 14 days	—
Pyrantel pamoate	4.4 mg/kg PO, repeat in 14 days	5-10 mg/kg PO, repeat in 14 days	—	—	—	—	5 mg/kg PO q7d × 3 treatments	—	—
Pyrethrin products	Topically as directed q7d	Topically as directed q7d	Topically as directed q7d	Topically as directed q7d	Topical powder 3×/wk, shampoo q7d	Topical powder 3×/wk, shampoo q7d	Topically as directed q7d	—	Topically as directed q7d
Sulfadimethoxine	50 mg/kg PO once, then 25 mg/kg q24h × 9 days	50 mg/kg PO once, then 25 mg/kg q24h × 10-20 days	25-50 mg/kg PO q24h × 10 days	25-50 mg/kg PO q24h × 10 days	25-50 mg/kg PO q24h × 10-14 days	10-15 mg/kg PO q12h	25 mg/kg PO q24h × 7-10 days	2-20 mg/kg q24h PO, SC, IM × 2-5 days, off 5 days, repeat once	—
Selamectin	6 mg/kg topically	6 mg/kg topically	6 mg/kg topically	—	—	—	—	6 mg/kg topically	—
Sulfamerazine	—	100 mg/kg PO	1-5 mg/mL drinking water	1-5 mg/mL drinking water	1 mg/mL drinking water	1 mg/mL drinking water	—	—	—
Sulfaquinoxaline	—	1 mg/mL in drinking water	1 mg/mL drinking water	—	1 mg/mL drinking water	1 mg/mL drinking water	—	—	—
Thiabendazole	—	50-100 mg/kg PO q24h × 5 days	100 mg/kg PO q24h × 5 days	50-100 mg/kg PO q24h × 5 days	100 mg/kg PO q24h × 5 days	100 mg/kg PO q24h × 5 days	—	—	—

TABLE 41-4
Chemical Restraint, Anesthetic, and Analgesic Agents

	Dosage								
Agent	**Ferrets**	**Rabbits**	**Guinea Pigs**	**Chinchillas**	**Hamsters**	**Rats/Mice**	**Prairie Dogs**	**Hedgehogs**	**Sugar Gliders**
Acepromazine	0.1-0.5 mg/kg SC, IM	0.5-1.0 mg/kg IM	0.5-1.0 mg/kg IM	0.5-1.0 mg/kg IM	0.5-1.0 mg/kg IM	0.5-1.0 mg/kg IM	0.5-1.0 mg/kg IM	—	—
Acetylsalicylic acid	0.5-22 mg/kg PO q8-24h	10-100 mg/kg PO q8-24h	50-100 mg/kg PO q4h	—	240 mg/kg PO q24h	100-120 mg/kg PO q4h	—	—	—
Atipamazole	1 mg/kg SC, IM, IV	Give same volume SC, IP, IV as medetomidine	1 mg/kg SC	—	—	1.0-2.5 mg/kg IP (M)	—	0.3-0.5 mg/kg IM	—
Atropine	0.04 mg/kg SC, IM, IV	0.1-0.5 mg/kg SC, IM*	0.1-0.2 mg/kg SC, IM	0.1-0.2 mg/kg SC, IM	0.1-0.4 mg/kg SC, IM	0.1-0.4 mg/kg SC, IM	0.04-0.1 mg/kg SC, IM	0.01-0.04 mg/kg SC, IM	0.01-0.02 mg/kg SC, IM
Buprenorphine	0.01-0.03 mg/kg SC, IM, IV q8-12h	0.01-0.05 mg/kg SC, IM, IV q6-12h	0.05 mg/kg SC q8-12h	0.05 mg/kg SC q8-12h	0.1-0.5 mg/kg SC q8h	0.02-0.5 mg/kg SC, IP, IM q6-12h (R); 0.05-2.5 mg/kg SC, IP, IM q6-12h (M)	0.03-0.06 mg/kg SC, IM q8-12h	0.01 mg/kg SC, IM q6-8h	—
Butorphanol	0.05-0.5 mg/kg SC, IM q8-12h	0.1-1.0 mg/kg SC, IM, IV q4-6h (higher doses may be given)	0.4-2.0 mg/kg SC q4h	0.2-2.0 mg/kg IM q4h	.1-5 mg/kg SC q4h	1-2 mg/kg SC q4h (R); 1-5 mg/kg SC q4h (M)	0.1-0.5 mg/kg SC, IM q8h	0.05-0.40 mg/kg SC q6-8h	0.5 mg/kg IM q8h
Carprofen	1 mg/kg PO q12-24h	1-2.2 mg/kg PO q12h	1-2 mg/kg PO q12-24h	4 mg/kg PO q24h	—	5-10 mg/kg PO (R)	1 mg/kg PO q12-24h	—	—
Diazepam	1-2 mg/kg IM	1-3 mg/kg IM, IV	0.5-3.0 mg/kg IM	—	3-5 mg/kg IM	3-5 mg/kg IM	0.4-0.6 mg/kg IM	0.5-2.0 mg/kg IM	0.5-1.0 mg/kg IM
Enflurane	2% maintenance	To effect; MAC = 2.9%	To effect; MAC = 2.17%	To effect	To effect	To effect	To effect	To effect	To effect
Flunixin meglumine	0.3-2.0 mg/kg SC q12-24h	1.1 mg/kg SC, IM q12h	2.5-5.0 mg/kg SC q12-24h	1-3 mg/kg SC q12h	2.5 mg/kg SC q12-24h	2.5 mg/kg SC q12-24h	—	—	0.1 mg/kg IM
Glycopyrrolate	0.01 mg/kg IM	0.01-0.02 mg/kg SC	0.01-0.02 mg/kg SC	0.01-0.02 mg/kg SC	0.01-0.02 mg/kg SC	0.01-0.02 mg/kg SC	0.01-0.02 mg/kg SC	—	—
Ibuprofen	1 mg/kg PO q12-24h	2-7.5 mg/kg PO q12-24h	10 mg/kg PO q4h	—	—	10-30 mg/kg PO q4h (R); 7-15 mg/kg PO q4h (M)	—	—	—
Isoflurane	2%-3% maintenance	1.50%-1.75% maintenance; MAC = 2.05%	0.25%-4.0% maintenance	0.25%-4.0% maintenance	0.25%-4.0% maintenance	0.25%-4.0% maintenance	1.75%-2.5% maintenance	0.25%-4.0% maintenance	0.25-4.0% (generally 1%-3%) maintenance
Ketamine	10-50 mg/kg IM	20-50 mg/kg IM; 15 mg/kg IV	22-44 mg/kg IM	20-40 mg/kg IM	20-40 mg/kg IM	22-44 mg/kg IM	20-40 mg/kg IM	5-20 mg/kg IM	20 mg/kg IM
Ketamine/ acepromazine	20-35 mg/kg (K)/ 0.20-0.35 mg/kg (A) SC, IM	40 mg/kg (K)/ 0.5-1.0 mg/kg (A) IM	—	40 mg/kg (K)/ 0.5 mg/kg (A) IM	—	—	40-50 mg/kg (K)/ 0.4-0.5 mg/kg (A) IM	—	10 mg/kg (K)/ 1 mg/kg (A) SC

TABLE 41-4
Chemical Restraint, Anesthetic, and Analgesic Agents—cont'd

	Dosage								
Agent	**Ferrets**	**Rabbits**	**Guinea Pigs**	**Chinchillas**	**Hamsters**	**Rats/Mice**	**Prairie Dogs**	**Hedgehogs**	**Sugar Gliders**
Ketamine/ diazepam	10-20 mg/kg (K)/ 1-2 mg/kg (D) IM	10-15 mg/kg (K)/ 0.3-0.5 mg/kg (D) IM, IV	20-30 mg/kg (K)/ 1-2 mg/kg (D) IM	20-40 mg/ kg (K)/1-2 mg/kg (D) IM	—	—	20-30 mg/kg (K)/ 0.4-0.6 mg/kg (D) IM	—	—
Ketamine/ medetomidine	5-8 mg/kg (K)/ 0.08-0.1 mg/kg (M) IM	0.35 mg/kg (M) IM/5-20 mg/kg (K) IV 15 min later	40 mg/kg (K)/ 0.5 mg/kg (M) IM, IP	—	75 mg/kg (K)/ 1 mg/kg (M) IM, IP	50-75 mg/kg (K)/1 mg/kg (M) IP (mice)	10-20 mg/kg (K)/ 0.5 mg/kg (M)	5 mg/kg (K)/0.1 mg/kg (M) IM	—
Ketamine/ midazolam	5-10 mg/kg (K)/ 0.25-0.5 mg/kg (M) IV	25 mg/kg (K)/ ≤2 mg/kg (M) IM	5-10 mg/kg (K)/ 0.5-1.0 mg/kg (M) IM	5-10 mg/kg (K)/ 0.5-1.0 mg/kg (M) IM	—	—	5-10 mg/kg (K)/ 0.5-1.0 mg/kg (M) IM	—	—
Ketoprofen	1 mg/kg PO, SC, IM q24h	1 mg/kg IM q12-24h	1 mg/kg SC, IM q12-24h	1 mg/kg SC, IM q12-24h	—	—	1-3 mg/kg SC, IM q12-24h (doses of 3-5 mg/kg have been used)	—	—
Medetomidine	0.1 mg/kg SC, IM	0.25 mg/kg IM	0.3 mg/kg SC, IM	—	0.1 mg/kg SC, IM	0.1 mg/kg SC	0.5 mg/kg IM	0.1 mg/kg IM	—
Meperidine	5-10 mg/kg SC, IM, IV q2-4h	5-10 mg/kg SC, IM q2-3h	20 mg/kg SC, IM q2-3h	10-20 mg/kg SC, IM q6h	20 mg/kg SC, IM q2-3h	20 mg/kg SC, IM q2-3h	—	—	—
Midazolam	0.3-1.0 mg/kg SC, IM	≤2 mg/kg IM, IV	1-2 mg/kg IM	1-2 mg/kg IM	1-2 mg/kg IM	1-2 mg/kg IM	1-2 mg/kg IM	—	—
Morphine	0.5-5.0 mg/kg SC, IM q2-6h	2-5 mg/kg SC, IM q2-4h	2-5 mg/kg IM q4h	—	2-5 mg/kg SC q2-4h	2-5 mg/kg SC q2-4h	—	—	—
Oxymorphone	0.05-0.20 mg/kg SC, IM, IV q8-12h	0.05-0.20 mg/kg SC, IM q8-12h	0.2-0.5 mg/kg SC, IM q6-12h	—	0.2-0.5 mg/kg SC, IM q6-12h	0.2-0.5 mg/kg SC, IM q6-12h	—	—	—
Pentobarbital	1-2 mg/kg PO q12h†	20-45 mg/kg IV, IP	30-45 mg/kg IP	35-40 mg/kg IP	50-90 mg/kg IP	30-45 mg/kg IP (R); 50-90 mg/kg IP (M)	—	—	—
Propofol	2-5 mg/kg IV	2-15 mg/kg IV	—	—	—	—	3-5 mg/kg IV	—	—
Sevoflurane	To effect	To effect; MAC = 3.7%	To effect	To effect	To effect	To effect	To effect	To effect	To effect
Tiletamine/ zolazepam	12-22 mg/kg IM (seldom indicated)	3 mg/kg IM (not recommended)	—	20-40 mg/kg IM	—	20-40 mg/kg IM (R)	4-40 mg/kg IM	1-5 mg/kg IM	—
Xylazine	1 mg/kg SC, IM	1-5 mg/kg SC, IM	—	—	—	—	—	0.5-1.0 mg/kg IM	—
Yohimbine	0.5 mg/kg IM	0.2-1.0 mg/kg IM, IV	—	—	—	—	—	0.5-1.0 mg/kg IM	—

*Some doses have been as high as 3 mg/kg SC because many rabbits possess serum atropinase.
†Use oral elixir for seizure control.
MAC, Minimum alveolar concentration.

TABLE 41-5
Miscellaneous Agents

Agent	Dosage								
	Ferrets	Rabbits	Guinea Pigs	Chinchillas	Hamsters	Rats/Mice	Prairie Dogs	Hedgehogs	Sugar Gliders
Calcium EDTA	20-30 mg/kg SC q12h	27 mg/kg SC q6-12h	30 mg/kg SC q12h	30 mg/kg SC q12h	—	—	25 mg/kg SC q6-12h	—	—
Cimetidine	10 mg/kg PO, SC, IM, IV q8h	5-10 mg/kg PO, SC, IM, IV q8-12h	5-10 mg/kg PO, SC, IM, IV q6-12h	5-10 mg/kg PO, SC, IM, IV q6-12h	5-10 mg/kg PO, SC, IM, IV q6-12h	5-10 mg/kg PO, SC, IM, IV q6-12h	5-10 mg/kg PO, SC, IM, IV q6-12h	—	—
Cisapride	0.5 mg/kg PO q8-12h	0.5 mg/kg PO q8-12h	0.5 mg/kg PO q8-12h	0.5 mg/kg PO q8-12h	0.1-0.5 mg/kg PO q12h	0.1-0.5 mg/kg PO q12h	5-10 mg/kg PO, SC, IM, IV q8-12h	—	—
Diazoxide	10-20 mg/kg PO q12h	—	—	—	—	—	—	—	—
Dexamethasone	0.5-2.0 mg/kg SC, IM, IV	0.5-2.0 mg/kg PO, SC q12h	0.5-2.0 mg/kg IM, SC, IV	0.5-2.0 mg/kg SC, IM, IV	0.5-2.0 mg/kg SC, IM, IV	0.5-2.0 mg/kg SC, IM, IV	0.5-4.0 mg/kg SC, IM, IV	0.1-1.5 mg/kg IM	0.1-0.6 mg/kg SC, IM, IV
Digoxin	0.005-0.01 mg/kg PO q12-24h	0.005-0.01 mg/kg PO q24-48h	—	—	0.05-0.1 mg/kg PO q12-24h	—	0.01-0.05 mg/kg PO q12-24h	—	—
Diphenhydramine	0.5-2.0 mg/kg PO, SC, IM q8-12h	2 mg/kg PO, SC q8-12h	5 mg/kg SC PRN	1-2 mg/kg PO, SC q12h	1-2 mg/kg PO, SC q12h	1-2 mg/kg PO, SC q12h	1-2 mg/kg PO, SC q12h	—	—
Enalapril	0.25-0.5 mg/kg PO q24-48h	—	—	—	—	—	0.25-0.5 mg/kg PO q12h	—	—
Epinephrine	0.02 mg/kg SC, IM, IV, IT	0.2 mg/kg IV (cardiac arrest)	0.003 mg/kg IV	—	—	—	—	—	—
Furosemide	2 mg/kg PO, SC, IM, IV q8-12h	2-5 mg/kg PO, SC, IM, IV q12h	2-5 mg/kg PO, SC q12h	2-5 mg/kg PO, SC q12h	2-10 mg/kg PO, SC q12h	2-10 mg/kg PO, SC q12h	1-4 mg/kg PO, SC q12h	2.5-5.0 mg/kg , PO, SC, IM q8h	—
Human chorionic gonadotropin	100 IU/animal IM, repeat in 14 days	20-25 IU/animal IV	1000 IU/animal IM, repeat q7-10d	—	—	—	—	—	—
Hydroxyzine	2 mg/kg PO q8h	2 mg/kg PO q8-12h	—	—	—	—	—	—	—

TABLE 41-5
Miscellaneous Agents—cont'd

Agent	Dosage								
	Ferrets	Rabbits	Guinea Pigs	Chinchillas	Hamsters	Rats/Mice	Prairie Dogs	Hedgehogs	Sugar Gliders
Iron dextran	10 mg/kg IM once	4-6 mg/kg IM once	—	—	—	—	—	25 mg/kg IM	—
Metoclopramide	0.2-1.0 mg/kg PO, SC, IM q6-8h	0.5 mg/kg PO, SC q8-24h	0.2-1.0 mg/kg PO, SC, IM q12h	0.2-1.0 mg/kg PO, SC, IM q12h	0.2-1.0 mg/kg PO, SC, IM q12h	0.2-1.0 mg/kg PO, SC, IM q12h	0.2-1.0 mg/kg PO, SC, IM q12h	—	—
Oxytocin	0.2-3.0 IU/kg SC, IM	0.1-3.0 IU/kg SC, IM	0.2-3.0 IU/kg SC, IM, IV	0.2-3.0 IU/kg SC, IM, IV	0.2-3.0 IU/kg SC, IM, IV	0.2-3.0 IU/kg SC, IM, IV	0.2-3.0 IU/kg SC, IM, IV	—	—
Potassium citrate	—	33 mg/kg PO q8h	10-30 mg/kg PO q12h	—	—	—	—	—	—
Prednisone	0.5-2.0 mg/kg PO q12-24h	0.5-2.0 mg/kg PO q12h	0.5-2.2 mg/kg PO, SC, IM	0.5-2.2 mg/kg PO, SC, IM	0.5-2.2 mg/kg PO, SC, IM	0.5-2.2 mg/kg PO, SC, IM	0.5-2.2 mg/kg PO, SC, IM	2.5 mg/kg PO, SC, IM q12h	—
Sucralfate	25 mg/kg PO q8h	25 mg/kg PO q8-12h	25-50 mg/kg PO	25-50 mg/kg PO	25-50 mg/kg PO	25-50 mg/kg PO	25-50 mg/kg PO	10 mg/kg PO q8-12h	—
Theophylline	4.25 mg/kg PO q8-12h	—	—	—	—	—	10 mg/kg PO q8-12h	—	—
Vitamin A	—	—	500-5000 IU/kg IM	—	500-5000 IU/kg IM	—	—	400 IU/kg IM q24h × 10 days	500-5000 IU/kg IM
Vitamin B complex*	1-2 mg (thiamine)/kg SC, IM	—	0.02-0.2 mL/kg SC, IM	0.02-0.2 mL/kg SC, IM	0.02-0.2 mL/kg SC, IM	0.02-0.2 mL/kg SC, IM	0.02-0.2 mL/kg SC, IM	1 mL/kg SC, IM	0.02-0.2 mL/kg SC, IM
Vitamin C	—	—	50-100 mg/animal PO, SC q24h (for deficiency)	—	—	—	—	50-200 mg/kg PO, SC q24h	—
Vitamin K	Use feline dose	1-10 mg/kg IM prn	1-10 mg/kg IM prn	1-10 mg/kg IM prn	1-10 mg/kg IM prn	1-10 mg/kg IM prn	1-10 mg/kg IM prn	—	—

*Use concentration formulated for small animals.

INDEX

Page numbers followed by "f" indicate figures; page numbers followed by "t" indicate tables.

P